Magnetic Resonance
in
Epilepsy

Neuroimaging Techniques

Second Edition

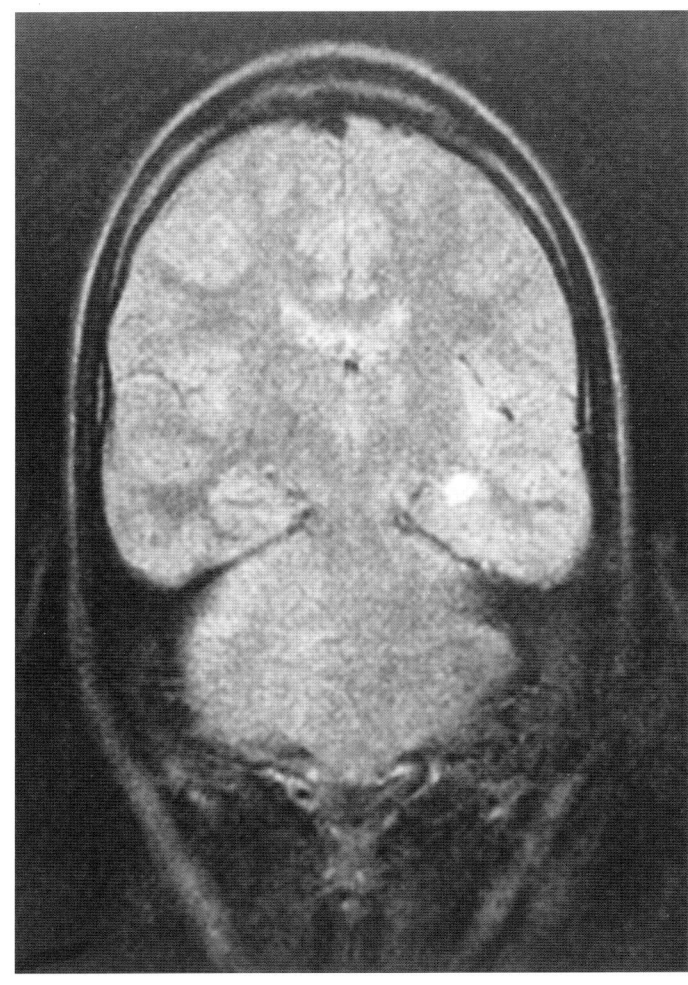

Frontispiece One of the earliest images of hippocampal sclerosis detected by magnetic resonance imaging. Coronal T2-weighted image showing increased signal abnormalities from the hippocampus. Pathologic analysis confirmed the diagnosis. Magnetic resonance image obtained at the Montreal Neurologic Institute on a Philips Gyroscan 0.5 T unit in 1986.

Magnetic Resonance in Epilepsy

Neuroimaging Techniques

Second Edition

Ruben I. Kuzniecky, M.D., F.A.A.N.

Graeme D. Jackson, B.SC.(HONS), MB.BS., M.D., F.R.A.C.P.

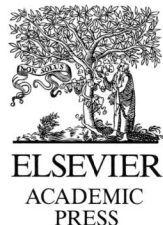

ELSEVIER

ACADEMIC
PRESS

AMSTERDAM • BOSTON • HEIDELBERG • LONDON
NEW YORK • OXFORD • PARIS • SAN DIEGO
SAN FRANCISCO • SINGAPORE • SYDNEY • TOKYO

Elsevier Academic Press
30 Corporate Drive, Burlington, MA 01803, USA
525 B Street, Suite 1900, San Diego, California 92101-4495, USA
84 Theobald's Road, London WC1X 8RR, UK

∞ This book is printed on acid-free paper

Library of Congress Cataloging-in-Publication Data
Application submitted

British Library Cataloguing in Publication Data
A catalogue record for this book is available from the British Library

ISBN: 0-12-431152-0

For all information on all Academic Press publications
visit our Web site at www.books.elsevier.com

Printed in China
05 06 07 08 09 9 8 7 6 5 4 3 2 1

Dedication

To my father whose eternal spirit lives in us.

Ruben Kuzniecky

To Ruth, Daniel, Hannah and Joseph for providing the meaning.

Graeme Jackson

Contents

List of contributors ix
Editors xi
Foreword xiii
Fred Andermann
Preface to the Second Edition xv
Acknowledgments xvii

1. Introduction to epilepsy 1
Graeme D. Jackson, Ruben I. Kuzniecky and Samuel F. Berkovic

2. Principles of magnetic resonance imaging 17
Graeme D. Jackson, Ruben I. Kuzniecky and Gaby S. Pell

3. Brain anatomy 29
Henri Duvernoy

4. Temporal lobe epilepsy 99
Graeme D. Jackson, Regula S. Briellmann and Ruben I. Kuzniecky

5. Extra-temporal lobe epilepsy 177
Ruben I. Kuzniecky and Graeme D. Jackson

6. MRI in special conditions associated with epilepsy 197
Ruben I. Kuzniecky and Graeme D. Jackson

7. Malformations of cortical development 221
A. James Barkovich

8. Structural analysis applied to epilepsy 249
Andrea Bernasconi

9. Imaging and neuropsychology 271
Michael M. Saling

10. Functional MRI in epilepsy 281
Jeffrey R. Binder and John A. Detre

11. Magnetic resonance neurophysiology: simultaneous EEG and fMRI 299
Anthony B. Waites, David F. Abbott, Steven W. Fleming and Graeme D. Jackson

12. MR diffusion and perfusion imaging in epilepsy 315
Alan Connelly

13. Magnetic resonance spectroscopy 333
    Magnetic resonance spectroscopy: principles and techniques
    Biochemistry for magnetic resonance spectroscopy
    Clinical applications of magnetic resonance spectroscopy in epilepsy
Hoby Hetherington, Ognen Petroff, Graeme D. Jackson, Ruben I. Kuzniecky,
Regula S. Briellmann and R. Mark Wellard

14. Single-photon-emission computed tomography in epilepsy 385
Christopher C. Rowe

15. Positron-emission tomography in epilepsy 395
Csaba Juhàsz, Diane C. Chugani, Otto Muzik and Harry T. Chugani

16. Magnetoencephalography in epilepsy 413
Robert C. Knowlton and William W. Sutherling

Index 433

List of Contributors

David F. Abbott, Ph.D.   *Brain Research Institute, Melbourne, Victoria, Australia*

A. James Barkovich, M.D.   *Department of Radiology, Neuroradiology Section, University of California San Francisco, San Francisco, CA, USA*

Samuel F. Berkovic, M.D.   *Epilepsy Research Collaborative Centre, University of Melbourne, Melbourne, Victoria, Australia*

Andrea Bernasconi, M.D.   *Montreal Neurological Institute, McGill University, Montreal, Québec, Canada*

Jeffrey R. Binder, M.D.   *Department of Neurology, Medical College of Wisconsin, Milwaukee, WI, USA*

Regula S. Briellmann, M.D.   *Brain Research Institute and University of Melbourne, Melbourne, Victoria, Australia*

Diane C. Chugani, Ph.D.   *PET Center, Children's Hospital of Michigan, Wayne State University School of Medicine, Detroit, MI, USA*

Harry T. Chugani, M.D.   *PET Center, Children's Hospital of Michigan, Wayne State University School of Medicine, Detroit, MI, USA*

Alan Connelly, Ph.D.   *Radiology and Physics Unit, Institute of Child Health, University College London, London, UK*

John A. Detre, M.D.   *Departments of Neurology and Radiology, University of Pennsylvania, Philadelphia, PA, USA*

Henri Duvernoy, M.D.   *Laboratoire d'Anatomie, Université de Franche-Comté, Besançon, France*

Hoby Hetherington, Ph.D.   *Gruss Magnetic resonance Research Center, Albert Einstein College of Medicine, Yeshiva University, New York, NY, USA*

Steven W. Fleming, B.Eng. (Elec.)   *Brain Research Institute, Melbourne, Victoria, Australia*

Csaba Juhász, M.D., Ph.D.   *PET Center, Children's Hospital of Michigan, Wayne State University, Detroit, MI, USA*

Robert C. Knowlton   *University of Alabama at Birmingham, School Of Medicine, UAB Epilepsy Center, UAB-HSF MEG Laboratory, Birmingham, AL, USA*

Otto Muzik, Ph.D.   *PET Center, Children's Hospital of Michigan, Wayne State University School of Medicine, Detroit, MI, USA*

Gaby S. Pell, Ph.D.   *Brain Research Institute, Melbourne, Victoria, Australia*

Ognen Petroff, M.D.   *Department of Neurology, Yale School of Medicine, New Haven, CT, USA*

Christopher Rowe, M.D.   *Department of Nuclear Medicine, Austin Hospital, University of Melbourne, Melbourne, Australia*

Michael M. Saling, Ph.D.   *Department of Psychology, Austin Hospital, University of Melbourne, Melbourne, Australia*

William W. Sutherling, M.D.   *Neuromagnetism Laboratory, Epilepsy and Brain Mapping Program, Huntington Hospital and Epilepsy Monitoring Unit, Pasadena, CA, USA*

Anthony B. Waites, Ph.D.   *Brain Research Institute, Melbourne, Victoria, Australia*

R. Mark Wellard, Ph.D.   *Brain Research Institute, Melbourne, Victoria, Australia*

Editors

Ruben I. Kuzniecky, M.D., F.A.A.N.
Professor, Neurology
Co-Director, NYU Epilepsy Center
New York University Medical School
New York, USA

Graeme D. Jackson B.Sc. (Hons), MB.BS., M.D., F.R.A.C.P.
Professor of Medicine and Radiology
University of Melbourne
Director, Brain Research Institute
Melbourne, Australia

Foreword

It is at times difficult to predict from the outset how our understanding of neurologic disease and of brain function may be enhanced by the development and application of a new technology. Roentgen's discovery of X-rays, for instance, allowed an initially unforeseen extension of our senses and opened a new era of modern medicine.

Despite the extraordinary insight of early neurologists like Jackson and Gowers, the mechanisms of epilepsy remained the subject of intuitive analysis and, even in the 1920s, there was still some question whether pyknolepsy was epileptic or not. All this changed with the discovery of the electroencephalogram by Hans Berger. It opened a window on the physiology of epilepsy that in turn fueled research and undreamed progress in our understanding of the working of the brain. The EEG complemented clinical localization, and the electroclinical correlation became the gold standard for our understanding and formulation of the different forms of epilepsy.

The advent of computed tomography revolutionized neurologic diagnosis and lightened the burden of neurologic dysfunction by removing the torture of pneumoencephalography. Then came magnetic resonance imaging! Previously, few neurologists were aware of it, and then only as an interesting exercise in physics. The early reports about its usefulness in epilepsy were disappointing. Excitement, however, was soon kindled when epileptologists, such as Sam Berkovic in our group and others as well, first realized that one could now actually see the amygdala and the hippocampus during life.

Ruben Kuzniecky was part of this early wave of enthusiasm and chose magnetic resonance imaging pathologic correlations in temporal lobe epilepsy as the subject of his debut in clinical research. On the other side of the globe, Graeme Jackson, working with Bladin and Berkovic, became similarly enthralled by the spell of modern imaging of epileptic disorders. Information mushroomed and our understanding of the mechanisms of epilepsy was greatly enhanced.

Since the first edition of this book there have been new technical developments such as diffusion and perfusion MRI. These, I hope, will be subjected to further clinical validation in the field of epilepsy and permit new approaches in patients with status epilepticus and should clarify also the spread of epileptic discharge. Spike-dependent FMRI permits the marriage of electrophysiology and imaging. Quite surprising results are emerging, which should lead to new insights on the mechanisms not only of focal, but also of generalized epilepsy.

The investigation of patients with epilepsy is in a continuous process of evolution. In particular, one can say without exaggeration that magnetic resonance imaging and now magnetic resonance spectroscopy have and continue to revolutionize our concepts of epilepsy. Recently, the indications and methods of presurgical evaluation have been completely altered by the utilization of magnetic resonance techniques, with reduction in morbidity, improved accessibility, and reduced costs.

Medical administrators and economists are still not always aware of the need for congruent information from the different imaging and other sources in the localization of the epileptic process. This should include, in addition to high-quality MRI, magnetoencephalography and positron emission tomography, highlighting the need for congruence of these different techniques in order to obtain the best possible localization. Important challenges remain: for instance, the demonstration of imaging changes in mild cortical dysplasia, a test of the ingenuity of the physicists working in this rapidly expanding field.

It seemed appropriate to bring together in one volume current concepts of epilepsy, the insights derived from the new technology, emerging approaches to investigation of patients, and the prospect of future technological advances and their clinical application. This timely volume will focus attention of imagers, physicists, and neuroradiologists on the problems of epilepsy and provide epileptologists, neurologists, and neurosurgeons with the information required to optimally use this technology for the benefit of epileptic patients.

Fred Andermann, M.D.
Montreal, Canada

Preface to the Second Edition

When we wrote the first edition of this book it was a time when the role of magnetic resonance in epilepsy was still being defined. One major issue in the field was what role MR imaging had in the diagnosis of hippocampal sclerosis (the most common cause of intractable epilepsy). Amazingly, it was widely felt that MR imaging without crude volumetric analysis was unable to routinely detect hippocampal sclerosis. Functional MRI was only just being described. The first edition attempted to pull together the knowledge required to effectively use MR in answering clinical and research questions in epilepsy. In effect, we were just entering the imaging era of epilepsy. This field continues to grow and this has motivated us to undertake this second edition so that those beginning in the field and those who would like to review the wide range of techniques that can help with their clinical and research question can access a source for this. We have enlisted the help of more co-authors who can give deep insights into the relevant parts of these growing fields of MR as they are relevant to epilepsy.

Now it is abundantly clear what the development of high-resolution brain imaging techniques, particularly MR imaging, has meant to the study and treatment of epilepsy. The multiplanar capability and high-resolution MR imaging of brain structures remains unmatched by any other current imaging technique. Similarly, the sensitivity of MR for the detection of small brain lesions is unsurpassed. MR offers high-resolution anatomic imaging and also has the ability to provide dynamic information about brain regions activated during various physiologic tasks. In addition, metabolic imaging using MR spectroscopy has now emerged as a technology with wide applications in the study of brain function and disease states. The prospect for these technologies is great with the advent of routinely available high-field imaging systems. These MR technologies continue to evolve rapidly and will continue to modify the way we study the central nervous system, its functions, and its common disorders. As well as rapid changes in the available technology, the way we interpret and apply the findings obtained using this technology requires ever-increasing sophistication on the part of the interpreting specialist, and the analysis methods teams that are increasingly important in dealing with this wealth of data. It is important to understand that a 'routine study' may no longer be adequate for many problems, and that optimizing the MR investigation is necessary. Increasingly, patients will have many MR sessions, starting with a screening examination, returning for a focused study based on clear ideas of probable disease areas and epileptological hypotheses, and finally returning for advanced investigations that cannot be performed in all cases. This requires very close communication between the physician, the physicist, and the imaging specialist and the analysis team.

The aim of this second edition of *Magnetic Resonance in Epilepsy* is to update readers about this rapidly changing field and its application to human epilepsy. We have retained in part the organization of the first edition with the first three chapters devoted to an introduction to principles that we feel are needed to more fully understand the context of neuroimaging findings. The first chapter is an introduction to epilepsy, written largely for those not familiar with the field. Chapter 2 similarly deals with the principles of MR in a way that is intended to provide an overview of major issues that allow the non-physicist an understanding of how MR works. We hope this will help in understanding the specific findings of later chapters. We felt that Chapter 3 by Henry Duvernoy was a masterpiece in the first edition. There it dealt primarily with the anatomy of the hippocampus and temporal lobe. As the focus of MR has increasing expanded to deal with issues of abnormalities beyond the temporal lobe, so this chapter has been expanded to include anatomic and MRI details of the entire brain. We strongly believe that the detection of what is abnormal is based on a detailed and deep understanding of normal brain anatomy as demonstrated by classical sectional anatomy (almost equivalent to high-resolution MRI).

Chapters 4–7 discuss epilepsy first from the viewpoint of the site of seizure origin (Chapters 4 – temporal – and 5 – extratemporal). This reflects our clinical interest relevant to the investigation of patients with epilepsy. Chapters 6 and 7 approach the MR findings from an etiologic viewpoint. The common acquired causes for epilepsies (Chapter 6) are followed by a discussion of malformations of cortical development (Chapter 7). Chapter 8 is devoted to advances in structural analysis of MRI, which increasingly allows the detection of subtle cortical abnormalities that are often the basis of epilepsy .

Chaper 9 provides a discussion of language and memory from the viewpoint of the epilepsy neuropsychologist. While we could have placed this in the initial part of the book as essential principles, the advent of fMRI of language and memory (Chapter 10) needs to be understood along with this perspective.

The linkage of the spatial resolution and sensitivity of fMRI with the temporal resolution of electroencephalography (Chapter 11) promises to be revolutionary for our understanding of epilepsy process in the intact whole brain. This promises to have clinical applicability in many situations as well.

Techniques such as perfusion and diffusion imaging, DWI (Chapter 12) and MRS (Chapter 13), are important research tools in epilepsy that are rapidly developing and being applied to problems in clinical practice. Chapters 14–16 discuss the role of other imaging techniques in epilepsy such as PET, SPECT, and magnetoencephalography. It is with wonder that we see how these new techniques have advanced the field.

We do not discuss computed tomography imaging in this book. CT technology continues to develop and, although we do not recommend CT studies for the investigation of epilepsy, it will be interesting to see how this technology develops in the next decade.

We hope that the reader will find in this book a valuable source of information on MR and the role of neuroimaging in epilepsy. The success of this book will only be measured by how helpful it is to those who use it for research, education, and clinical care. As we wrote in 1995 in the preamble to our first edition, 'MR technology is rapidly changing but we trust that the guiding principles of MR as described in this book may apply to technology and applications of this technology yet to come'. In retrospect, we think we were correct. We are confidently courageous to repeat the same message again. Ultimately, our hope is that the knowledge obtained from this book will be usefully applied to the investigation and treatment of those most afflicted: patients with epilepsy.

Welcome to the neuroimaging era of epilepsy!

Ruben I. Kuzniecky, New York, USA
Graeme D. Jackson, Melbourne, Australia
July 2004

Acknowledgments

We are indebted to the many teachers who inspired and encouraged us to undertake our paths in clinical research that led to the original project and the second edition of this book. We specially thank the individuals who have contributed their efforts to chapters in this second edition. We recognize them as authors and great authorities in their field.

We thank Richard Morawetz and James Hugg who provided assistance, advice and material for this book and the late Dr. John Whitaker, Chair of Neurology at UAB, who supported our initial MRI efforts.

We thank the directors of the Brain Research Institute; Chris Blake, Tom Buchan, Margaret Jackson, Anne Ward and Mark Jones, who have done much to encourage advanced MR research in Australia. Jennifer Williams supported the fledgling institute. John Balla and Peter Bladin were great early career teachers and mentors. Sam Berkovic, John Duncan and David Gadian have always given support and encouragement in research. Jewell Gardner and Lucy Holloway helped with many details of this second edition.

We also thank the MRI technical, clinical and research staff at UAB, the Brain Research Institute, and Austin Health for their many contributions to our work and aspects of this book.

Many thanks to Faye Clark and Perry Smith for graciously providing us with a most wonderful venue to retreat at Lake Martin, Alabama, to finish this book. Special thanks to Dr. Noelle Gracy from Academic Press who undertook the initiation of this project and completed it with us, Anne Russum who patiently finished the project and Claire Jennings who graciously organized and worked on many aspects of this book.

To our partners, Yvonne and Ruth, who supported without protest the many hours we spent away from home and our children. We love you dearly.

Finally, our thanks and thoughts go out to our patients and their families. We believe that what we have learned over the past decade has had an important impact on the life of many patients. Hopefully, their issues will further serve as inspiration to all of us to advance our understanding to the benefit of those affected by epilepsy.

CHAPTER 1

Introduction to Epilepsy

Graeme D. Jackson, Ruben I. Kuzniecky and Samuel F. Berkovic

"Today, epilepsy has more secrets to confide to the neurologist or neurosurgeon who can understand the 'tongue' she speaks."

Wilder Penfield, 1974 (age 83).

The origin of the modern view of epilepsy is generally considered to have been the studies and work of John Hughlings Jackson (Fig. 1.1). He was appointed assistant physician to the National Hospital for the Relief and Cure of the Paralysed and Epileptic (now the National Hospital for Neurology and Neurosurgery), Queen Square, London in 1862 at the age of 27. Jackson's wife developed focal motor seizures following a cerebral thrombosis, and it is this form of epilepsy, with its typical march of symptoms, that became known as jacksonian epilepsy. This work was in the context of a developing view of neurology that was beginning to relate cortical functions to specific locations within the brain (1). In 1873 Jackson presented his classic definition of epileptic seizures, which was 'occasional sudden excessive, rapid and local discharges of gray matter (2, 3).' This view established partial seizures as being truly epileptic in origin. At that time William Gowers, J. Hughlings Jackson, Victor Horsley, and David Ferrier were developing concepts of cortical localization and of epilepsy, which were to have far reaching consequences. The combination of basic scientific research and clinical findings enabled Jackson's ideas to be confirmed by Ferrier in experiments in primates using techniques of cortical stimulation (4). As a consequence, brain functions were able to be localized and the view developed that localization of the site of origin of seizures was possible based on their clinical symptoms – in particular the symptoms at the start of the clinical seizure.

ORIGINS OF SEIZURE SURGERY

Using this concept of brain localization and using clinical symptoms as a guide to the site of the seizure focus (jacksonian seizures), a neurosurgeon in Glasgow, William Macewen, correctly localized a frontal meningioma and operated in 1879 (5). Following tumor removal the patient both survived and became seizure-free. At the National Hospital

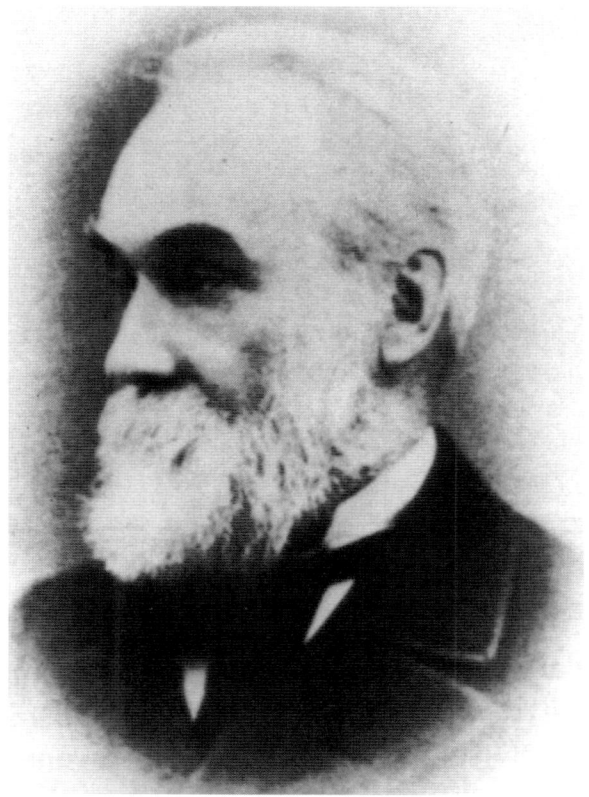

FIG. 1.1. John Hughlings Jackson, London (1835–1911).

in London, Victor Horsley operated on three patients with epileptogenic lesions in 1886 (6). The first of these was a patient of Jackson's, and present in the operating theater were Horsley, Jackson, and Ferrier. This represents the origin of epilepsy surgery for the treatment of epilepsy. Although these early cases were successful, establishing the principle of seizure control by surgical removal of the 'seizure focus,' the overall success of surgery for epilepsy was poor and eventually operative treatment fell into disuse until the 'modern era' represented by Penfield and colleagues at the Montreal Neurologic Institute. What now seem like simple measures, such as anesthesia, antisepsis, and antibiotics, made a large impact on the feasibility and safety of neurosurgery for epilepsy, as they did in many other areas of medicine.

Despite major developments in the understanding of the process of epilepsy and the propagation and spread of seizures, the central issues and principles on which this surgery was based have, at their core, remained largely unchanged to the present day. That is, if the seizure focus can be accurately localized, then surgical removal of that focus will alleviate the occurrence of seizures. What has changed to a remarkable extent is the technological environment in which this work can be carried out. Major milestones have been the advent of the electroencephalogram (EEG) and more recently neuroimaging techniques, represented in their most dramatic form by magnetic resonance imaging (MRI). The data and criteria by which the diagnosis of seizure localization is made continues to develop and this book examines the role of MR in this evaluation process: this development has changed the face of epilepsy diagnosis, management and treatment. In addition to its initial revolutionary role in surgical treatment of epilepsy, MRI has altered the understanding of, and clinical approach to, many forms of focal and generalized epilepsy.

THE MODERN ERA

During the 20th century, Wilder Penfield (Fig. 1.2), who founded the Montreal Neurologic Institute in 1934, became the leading figure in the further development of both the surgical treatment of epilepsy and the structural localization of brain functions. In common with Jackson, his extensive writings, coupled with a clear, detailed, and objective skill in observation, provided a wealth of information, which is of relevance to this day. From his observations, Penfield recognized the dramatic vascular changes that occur during seizures (7). Despite the subsequent emphasis, as a consequence of the development of the powerful EEG technology, on the electrical events that occur during seizures, Penfield retained his interest in these vascular changes throughout his life (8). With the advent of ictal imaging technologies, such as SPECT (9) and functional MRI, the legacy of his observations remain relevant to the interpretation of blood flow changes during ictal events. Although he died in 1976 at the age of 85, before the development of medical nuclear magnetic

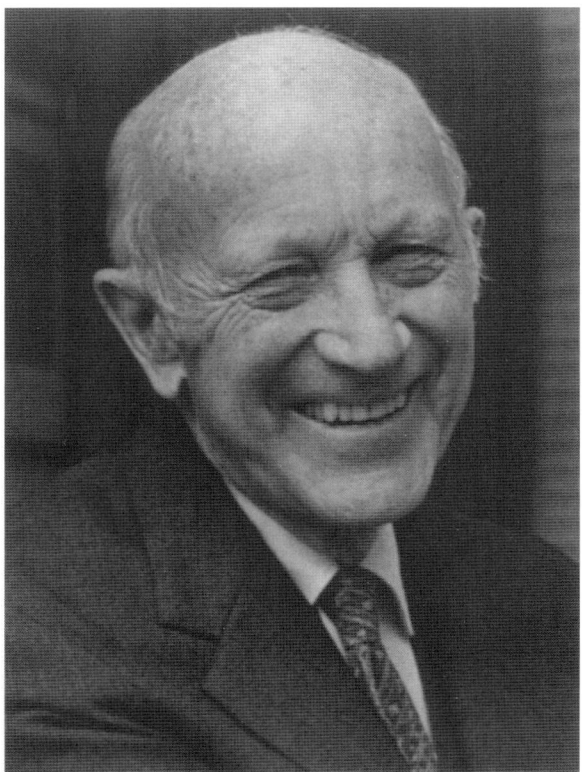

FIG. 1.2. Wilder Penfield, Montreal (1891–1976).

resonance technology, he clearly foresaw that new technology would reveal many new aspects of epilepsy and brain functions.

ELECTROENCEPHALOGRAM DEVELOPMENT

In 1929, Berger published the technique of EEG (10), which, in his study, was based on a single-electrode contact. This important technology was subsequently developed by many researchers to provide a means whereby seizures could be localized without characteristic and localizing ictal clinical symptoms. This was a very exciting development in neurology as it enabled the totally noninvasive investigation of brain function with an objective technique that provided information independent of the clinical examination. This eventually shifted the emphasis from epilepsy originating in eloquent areas of cortex such as the motor strip (because of the ability to localize these events) and enabled temporal lobe seizures to be localized on the basis of the electroencephalographic localization of the electrical activity associated with the seizure.

The EEG technology developed to the point that in 1951 Bailey (neurosurgeon) and Gibbs (electroencephalographer) published a series of 25 patients who underwent temporal lobe resection based only on EEG criteria (11) without supporting clinical localization. The results were encouraging and helped establish the EEG as the prime method of seizure localization, to the extent that epileptic syndromes often became referred to as electro-clinical diagnoses (showing how important this investigation modality had become in the practice of epilepsy). Over the next 30 years the study of epilepsy was dominated by the technical development of, and understanding of the information obtained from, the EEG (12, 13). During this period, surgery, as a treatment of epilepsy, also gained considerable ground.

MAGNETIC RESONANCE IMAGING

Magnetic resonance techniques were first applied to human studies in the late 1970s (12) and the routine clinical availability of MRI began in the mid 1980s. MRI enables a detailed view of the fine structure of the living brain, which had previously only been possible after death (by post-mortem examination). It soon became apparent that MRI could add another powerful dimension to the problem of localizing where seizures originate by demonstrating the location and nature of structural brain abnormalities. Small tumors, many which had been undetected by CT scanning, were commonly found in these patients (13–17).

Less apparent, but especially important, lesions such as hippocampal sclerosis were initially thought to be largely undetectable using MR (14, 16, 18). The development of MR techniques for the detection of hippocampal sclerosis figured prominently in the first edition of this book and remains central to epilepsy practice. Even in the case of tumors, however, a new issue arose. There is an apparent dissociation in some cases between the site of the EEG abnormality and the imaging abnormality. The issue then becomes: which is most important; to resect the structural lesion or to resect the area of EEG abnormality? The answer to this could only have been addressed in the MR era of epilepsy surgery. Most studies suggest that removal of the structural abnormality, when it can be detected, is critical for good post-surgical outcome (19, 20).

Magnetic resonance also opened Pandora's box on malformations of cortical development, which are a major cause of hitherto unexplained epilepsies (21). While classical neuropathology on autopsy specimens had led to the recognition of severe developmental abnormalities, it was only with the advent of MR that more subtle varieties were properly appreciated. Understanding and interest in this area has exploded in the last few years, largely due to the impetus of MRI (Box 1.1).

Improvements in instrumentation, sequence development and interpretative skills have enabled ever more subtle lesions to be detected. MR is now an obligatory part of the investigation of all patients with epilepsy, although the yield may be low for certain clearly defined idiopathic syndromes.

STRUCTURAL VERSUS FUNCTIONAL ABNORMALITY

The distinction between the structural lesion that may underlie the epileptic process, the area that produces

---

BOX 1.1 Classification Scheme: Malformations of Cortical Development

I. Malformations Due to Abnormal Neuronal and Glial Proliferation or Apoptosis
  A. Decreased proliferation/increased apoptosis: microcephalies
    1. Microcephaly with normal to thin cortex
    2. Microlissencephaly (extreme microcephaly with thick cortex)
    3. Microcephaly with polymicrogyria/cortical dysplasia
  B. Increased proliferation/decreased apoptosis (normal cell types): megalencephalies
  C. Abnormal proliferation (abnormal cell types)
    1. Non-neoplastic
      a. Cortical hamartomas of tuberous sclerosis
      b. Cortical dysplasia with balloon cells
      c. Hemimegalencephaly (HMEG)
    2. Neoplastic (associated with disordered cortex)
      a. Dysembryoplastic neuroepithelial tumor (DNET)
      b. Ganglioglioma
      c. Gangliocytoma
II. Malformations Due to Abnormal Neuronal Migration
  A. Lissencephaly/subcortical band heterotopia spectrum
  B. Cobblestone complex
    1. Congenital muscular dystrophy syndromes
    2. Syndromes with no involvement of muscle
  C. Heterotopia
    1. Subependymal (periventricular)
    2. Subcortical (other than band heterotopia)
    3. Marginal glioneuronal
III. Malformations Due to Abnormal Cortical Organization (Including Late Neuronal Migration)
  A. Polymicrogyria and schizencephaly
    1. Bilateral polymicrogyria syndromes
    2. Schizencephaly (polymicrogyria with clefts)
    3. Polymicrogyria with other brain malformations or abnormalities
    4. Polymicrogyria or schizencephaly as part of multiple congenital anomaly/mental retardation syndromes
  B. Cortical dysplasia without balloon cells
  C. Microdysgenesis
IV. Malformations of Cortical Development, Not Otherwise Classified
  A. Malformations secondary to inborn errors of metabolism
    1. Mitochondrial and pyruvate metabolic disorders
    2. Peroxisomal disorders
  B. Other unclassified malformations
    1. Sublobar dysplasia
    2. Others

Modified from reference 22.

---

symptoms, and the epileptogenic zone has been clearly made (see Engel 1993 (1) and references therein). In addition to remarkable advances in structural imaging, MR spectroscopy (MRS), functional MRI (fMRI) of brain function and very recently, fMRI of epileptic activity have changed our understanding and clinical practice in epileptology. No one could have predicted the remarkable ability that MR techniques have for investigating noninvasively brain structure, function biochemistry, and metabolism.

In 1967, Penfield, aged 76, published a paper with the title of 'Epilepsy, the great teacher: the progress of one pupil (23).' The sentiment of this paper is no less true today than ever, and MR technology may provide many new insights and lessons if we can learn to use and apply it well.

DEFINITIONS, TERMINOLOGY AND CLASSIFICATION

Epilepsy terminology can sometimes seem very difficult to understand. It is a field that has much confusing and residual outdated terminology. The terminology, and indeed the knowledge this terminology relates to, has changed rapidly over a relatively short time. It is therefore important to have at least a few clear concepts and to understand something about the current definition and significance of terms relating to epilepsy, in order to make any sense of the field.

An additional problem is the residue of many terms and concepts that no longer relate to current classifications and views of epilepsy. For example, the terms petit mal (meaning small seizure) and grand mal (meaning large seizure) date from the early concepts of epilepsy proposed by the French school of epileptology (which established an outstanding epilepsy tradition) and these terms are still often used. Many new meanings have been attached to these old concepts (often used in different ways even when referring to the same patient) and, as these concepts no longer fit our view of seizures, the use of these terms adds confusion rather than clarification. Terms such as 'grand mal' no longer have any part in a modern classification of seizures yet are a constant source of confusion to those who deal with epilepsy. (Generally 'tonic–clonic seizure,' a description of the seizure type, is what is meant by 'grand mal seizure;' see below.)

While this book does not take on fully the task of dealing with general concepts of epilepsy, a few essential definitions and the concepts on which they are based must be established in order to understand the context into which we place MR findings.

Important Concepts of Epilepsy

Epileptic seizures can be defined as the clinical manifestations of abnormal excessive neuronal activity in the gray matter of the cerebral cortex. Although abnormal electrical activity usually manifests itself through predictable clinical features, it may be silent (pure electrographic events) or it may exhibit clinical features (therefore a seizure), which may either relate to the site of this seizure or correspond to regions indirectly activated by a discharge beginning at some distant site. *Epilepsy* is a chronic disorder that has as its major symptom events (epileptic seizures) that are only manifested periodically. If we define epilepsy in this way it must be defined in terms not of fixed underlying damage to the cerebral cortex but of these transient functional events. This may not be the only possible definition of epilepsy; however, it is largely these episodic events that most trouble the patient and that treatment is designed to prevent.

While the first task of the practicing epileptologist is often to determine whether a transient event is an epileptic event or not (for example a pseudoseizure), we will not deal with this issue here. We now consider only those events that are epileptic in nature.

In general, epileptic conditions can be thought of in three broad categories. In the first place seizures can occur in a normal brain, precipitated by specific factors (such as hypoxia or hypoglycemia). This type of seizure may be experienced by anyone, depending on the circumstances. Second, seizures can occur in an apparently structurally normal brain, but with a known tendency to seizures, whether genetic, biochemical, or otherwise. Finally, seizures can occur in a brain that has a definite structural abnormality, either focally or diffusely (24). While this may seem an obvious distinction, it is essential to determine which category any given patient fits into, and it is not always immediately obvious which situation applies. In order to make this distinction the clinical history (the context) and investigations such as EEG (function) and MRI (brain structure) may be essential. To begin the process of analysis (and subsequently to be able to communicate our findings) the following definitions may be usefully applied:

Epilepsy is a general term that cannot be considered a diagnosis. To say that a person has epilepsy is not in any way specific, and should not be considered to be a complete diagnosis. While it may give a general indication of the nature of a problem, it is so nonspecific as to be almost meaningless in many contexts. 'Epilepsy' encompasses a large number of conditions that can manifest as a variety of seizure types.

Epileptic Seizures

Epileptic seizures are transient events consisting of abnormal brain function. Hughlings Jackson (2) proposed in 1870 that they were "occasional excessive and disorderly discharges of nervous tissue." With the advent of the EEG, this definition, in terms of electrical events in the brain, has become widely accepted, and many might consider a seizure to be an electroclinical event. It is clear, however, that an epileptic seizure consists of transient, complex alterations in blood flow, metabolism, and biochemistry, and changes in neurotransmitters as well as electrical events. With powerful new methods of noninvasive investigation of brain structure and function, our concepts of what an epileptic seizure is are starting to change as this information becomes increasingly available. The essential feature of an epileptic seizure is that it is a transient event, and it is the symptom of 'epilepsy' that troubles the patient. Regardless of what the underlying abnormality of the brain is, epileptic seizures are transient episodes that disturb the normal function of the brain.

BOX 1.2 Abridged Version of the International Classification of Seizures

1. Partial (focal, local) seizures
   A. Simple partial seizures
   B. Complex partial seizures
   C. Partial seizures evolving to secondary generalized seizures
2. Generalized seizures (convulsive or nonconvulsive)
   A. Absence seizures
   B. Myoclonic seizures
   C. Clonic seizures
   D. Tonic seizures
   E. Tonic–clonic seizures
   F. Atonic seizures
3. Unclassified epileptic seizures

From reference 26.

The international league against epilepsy (ILAE) classification of epileptic seizures proposed by the Commission on Classification and Terminology (1981) (25) divides seizures into those that are generalized from the beginning, and those that are partial or focal at the beginning. The partial seizures are divided, according to whether or not consciousness is disturbed, into simple partial and complex partial seizures (Box 1.2). This box gives a summary of the full classification.

The current classification system emphasizes features of the clinical seizure that can be used to make some assumptions or preliminary hypotheses about the underlying mechanism of the seizure disorder. Specifically, the presence of partial seizures implies that the seizures begin in a specific, possibly localized, site. The presence of generalized seizures provides no evidence to suggest a focal structural lesion (although it in no way excludes this) and it is more likely that either a widespread abnormality, or no detectable abnormality is present. Although the seizure type may suggest the likelihood of an underlying abnormality it must be considered as only a starting point. The type of seizure is not a diagnosis but a symptom and therefore the concept of an epilepsy syndrome is a useful one.

As noted above, epileptic seizures are transient episodes manifested as abnormal clinical behavior. As well as the clinical context of epilepsy, one can also define epilepsy in terms of functional events that occur at specific times. These events can be studied through EEG or estimating blood flow changes with positron-emission tomography (PET) or single-photon-emission computed tomographic (SPECT) techniques (or, more recently, fMRI). One can also view the process of epilepsy in terms of the underlying abnormality of the cerebral cortex that gives rise to these transient events. Using the simple concept of partial or generalized epilepsy (see below), one can presume that, in the first situation, a small area of dysfunction, either anatomical or biochemical, will be present. Conversely in generalized epilepsy, one may postulate that large brain areas are abnormal or that there are generalized underlying abnormalities that form the basis of these seizures.

While it may not always be possible to precisely define all these events, it can be proposed that a complete description of any epilepsy or epileptic disorder will require definition of the clinical episodes (demonstrated by the clinical semiology, video monitoring to demonstrate the seizure events), transient functional events (partly illustrated by the ictal EEG, ictal SPECT, and functional MRI), and the fixed underlying structural and biochemical abnormality of the brain (as shown in part by MRI, PET, SPECT, MRS, and the neuropsychological deficit).

Epilepsy Syndromes

The first 'modern' classification of epileptic seizures, as presented above (25), has proved to be very useful for the description of a patient's symptoms, but in the MR era the problem often is that is often only the first step in the diagnostic process. When the clinical and electrographic features are associated with a recognizable grouping of features such as age of onset, genetics, and course, they may constitute an epilepsy syndrome (27). Clear examples include juvenile myoclonic epilepsy, a form of idiopathic generalized epilepsy, and benign rolandic epilepsy, classified within the idiopathic partial epilepsies. In these conditions, a genetic defect may determine the clinical and EEG features. In the new approach to classification discussed below only certain defined, specified, and agreed syndromes are included. This is a work in progress but we believe that it is a very sensible development and one that we fully endorse. In the MR context we note that the syndrome of mesial temporal epilepsy (29) has been proposed as a good example of lesional epilepsy, although this is not fully accepted as an agreed syndrome by the ILAE commission.

Conceptually, the epilepsies are the diseases that cause recurrent epileptic seizures. Often these diseases are not known, or cannot be defined in terms of underlying pathophysiology and etiology. Therefore empirically defined clusters of the clinical and investigation features of these patients are collected into categories of classification known as epilepsy syndromes.

Epilepsy syndromes are symptom complexes that include information from the main investigation modalities such as EEG and now MRI. The International Classification of the Epilepsies and Epileptic Syndromes (30, 31) groups the epilepsies according to whether they are localization-related (partial) or generalized, and whether they are idiopathic or symptomatic (Box 1.3). As more detailed information becomes widely available from MRI and molecular genetics, the classification needs to change in recognition of knowledge of underlying basis of the epilepsy. As noted above, the defined list of epilepsy syndromes no longer tries to be inclusive but to list defined entities as these become more fully understood. The ILAE 1989 system needed to be fully

BOX 1.3   Abridged Version of the International
Classification of Epilepsies

1. Localization-related epilepsies
   Idiopathic, e.g. benign childhood epilepsy with centrotemporal
      spikes
   Symptomatic, e.g. frontal, temporal, occipital, and parietal lobe
      epilepsies (partial epilepsies)
2. Generalized epilepsies
   Idiopathic, e.g. absence epilepsy (childhood or juvenile)
   Juvenile myoclonic epilepsy (JME)
   Symptomatic, e.g. Lennox–Gastaut syndrome
3. Epilepsies undetermined whether focal or generalized,
      e.g. Landau–Kleffner syndrome
4. Special syndromes, e.g. febrile convulsions

From reference 28.

inclusive of all cases of epilepsy. The benefit of the new proposal is that it can list as syndromes only those entities that are more clearly defined. One example of this would be temporal lobe epilepsy with hippocampal sclerosis.

With both approaches, an epilepsy syndrome is empirically defined and therefore is different from a specific disease or a pathologically defined disorder such as tuberous sclerosis or Aicardi 'syndrome' (25) where the seizures are a major symptom of a defined disease. Epileptic syndromes do not necessarily imply a common etiology. There are no ideal classifications; however the most widely used classification scheme in current use (abbreviated in Box 1.3) is that of the International League Against Epilepsy (1985) (30, 31). Many of these syndromes are electroclinical syndromes, reflecting the era when this classification arose. MRI and other investigations have been difficult to incorporate into this conceptual framework, leading to the concept of 'axis' so that new information can be incorporated while retaining the benefits of the very successful electroclinical syndrome concept with which we are all so familiar.

The recent approach to classification has been led by the ILAE. Engle (22) clearly articulates the benefits of using a number of axes that may give conceptually different information about the epilepsy syndrome. This scheme remains under development but provides important concepts for the classification of epilepsy. We support this scheme as the current most sensible way of bringing genetic and imaging information into a successful framework of previously existing electroclinical syndromes. It allows us to move forward in times of technological change while being 'backward compatible' with prior art. These developments are central to how we will all view our patients in the near future. As written by Engel (32), with our editing:

it is anticipated that seizures and syndromes will not be organized into fixed dichotomous classifications, but rather categorized in various ways for various purposes.

Axis 1 consists of a description of the ictal semiology, using a standardized Glossary of Descriptive Terminology. The description of the ictal event, without reference to etiology, anatomy, or mechanisms, can be very brief or extremely detailed, as required for clinical or research purposes. ... Communication among clinicians, and among researchers, will be greatly enhanced by the establishment of standardized terminology for describing ictal semiology.

Axis 2 is the epileptic seizure type, or types, experienced by the patient, derived from a list of accepted seizure types, which represent diagnostic entities with etiologic, therapeutic, and/or prognostic implications. Localization within the brain should be specified when this is appropriate, and in the case of reflex seizures, the specific stimulus will also be specified here. The Task Force has constructed a list of accepted epileptic seizure types, including forms of status epilepticus, and precipitating factors for reflex seizures. Seizure types have been divided into self-limited seizures and continuous seizures, and further divided into generalized seizures and focal seizures, but it is anticipated that other approaches to organization, categorization, and classification of seizure types will be devised for specific purposes.

Axis 3 is the syndromic diagnosis derived from a list of accepted epilepsy syndromes, although it is understood that a syndromic diagnosis may not always be possible. The recommended list distinguishes between epilepsy syndromes and conditions with epileptic seizures that do not require a diagnosis of epilepsy, and also identifies which syndromes are still in development. It is important to stress that the list ... contains syndromes that are still under discussion, such as the new concept of Idiopathic generalized epilepsies with variable phenotypes, and the Reflex epilepsies, and that the Task Force will continue to revise this list based on the results of further deliberations, input from the membership, and new information. As with epileptic seizures, it is anticipated that different approaches to organization, categorization, and classification of epilepsy syndromes will be created for specific purposes. ...

Axis 4 will specify etiology when this is known. The etiology could consist of a specific disease derived from a classification of diseases frequently associated with epileptic seizures or syndromes, a genetic defect, or a specific pathological substrate. ...

Axis 5 is an optional designation of the degree of impairment caused by the epileptic condition.

Most of the cases of epilepsy dealt with in the first edition of this book focused on the symptomatic (or secondary) partial group of epilepsies. This was because the major contribution of MR was to imaging of various structural abnormalities. When the first edition was written 10 years ago, it was debated whether hippocampal sclerosis could be reliably seen with MR techniques (33). Now any center where the MR diagnosis is not virtually as good as the pathologic diagnosis should not be involved in epilepsy surgery. As can be seen by the organization of later chapters, MR has moved into advanced diagnosis of structural abnormalities that are very subtle. Issues arise as to whether we only see abnormalities that cause epilepsy or whether the increased sensitivity shows us the consequences of epileptic seizures. MR also shows us structural and metabolic abnormalities of the brain that will soon move into the routine clinical assessment of epilepsy surgery programs.

Things have changed, but in many ways they have remained the same – detecting the structural basis of epilepsy is the main issue. Weighting the findings in an appropriate way for ongoing management is the skill needed.

Advanced MR techniques need to be known about, used, and understood by epilepsy clinicians. Functional MRI and EEG in the magnet is giving insights into generalized epilepsy circuits that may have important clinical implications in the near future. Placing these advances in a diagnostic framework will be increasingly important. The basis of understanding all this new information is good clinical epileptology.

EPIDEMIOLOGY OF EPILEPSY

How Common is Epilepsy?

The prevalence of epilepsy has been estimated as 5–8/1000 (27, 30, 31) with similar rates in China, Europe, and the Unites States despite methodological differences. Higher rates have been reported in some countries but it is unclear whether exceptionally higher prevalences are truly representative or are related to unusual circumstances. Prevalence rates are age-specific (30) with increased prevalence from childhood to adolescence with an increase after age 70.

The incidence of epileptic seizures (the number of new cases in a population over time) is approximately 30–50/100 000 person-years (34). Incidence is high during the first year of life, declines thereafter until middle age, and then rises sharply after age 60 (27). In any population, epilepsy manifested by partial onset seizures is the most frequently occurring single seizure type. The incidence of partial seizures remains constant through life, with an incidence of 20/100 000 until age 65, when the incidence rises to 80/100 000. Prevalence studies suggest that epilepsy with partial seizures comprises 40–60% of all newly diagnosed cases (30, 34–41).

The natural history of this group of patients is difficult to determine because of methodological problems in studies of this subject; however, it would seem that between 50% and 60% of patients with newly diagnosed complex partial seizures can be expected to achieve complete control of their seizures, and the majority of these will eventually be able to be managed without antiepileptic medications. About 30–40% will have no improvement in seizure control, or will worsen. Young onset (under 2 years), a large number of seizures, the presence of secondarily generalized seizures, and a history of status epilepticus or febrile seizures are factors associated with a bad outcome (31, 34, 42–44).

Consequences of Intractable Epilepsy

Intractable epilepsy is a very disabling condition. The incidence of early death in this group is high. In some studies up to 1% of patients with intractable epilepsy die per year (31, 45). The risk of sudden unexpected death (SUDEP) appears to be twice as high than in the general population. Sudden unexpected death in epilepsy appears to be more likely if seizures are not controlled (40–42). A higher number

suffer significant injury. In addition to this clear medical injury, the social consequences of intractable seizures can be disabling. Psychosocial patterns and independence are not established normally through the developing and adolescent years. A patient with intractable seizures cannot hold a driving license, and is so precluded from many social interactions and vocational opportunities. The public loss of body control that occurs during major seizures can be psychologically and socially disabling both personally and in the work place (46). This social impairment can have major consequences even after successful epilepsy surgery that renders the patient seizure-free (47–49).

MECHANISMS OF EPILEPSY

In 1885, Gowers posed one of the most fundamental questions about epilepsy. Is epilepsy a disease process that occurs before the first seizure or is it an ongoing process starting after the first seizure? In his monograph on *Epilepsy and other chronic convulsive disorders* (50), Gowers wrote:

The effect of a convulsion on the nerve centers is such as to render the occurrence of another seizure more easy, to intensify the predisposition which already exists. Thus every fit may be said to be, in part, the result of those which have preceded it, and the cause of those which follow it. The search for the causes of epilepsy must thus be chiefly an investigation into the conditions which precede the occurrence of the first fit.

The question of whether the process of epilepsy can be prevented or reversed at its onset is still debated (51). This most basic question of the mechanism of intractability is still not satisfactorily answered.

Attempts to understand the basic mechanisms of epilepsy have depended greatly on the investigation of animal models of epilepsy. The choice of model depends on the question being asked of the experiments. Several models have provided insights into possible mechanisms. A detailed discussion of these models is beyond the scope of this introduction, but each model, such as the amygdala kindled rat (52, 53) has provided important insights, and testable hypotheses, about possible mechanisms that may apply to human epileptic processes (54). It is only with the advent of the techniques of investigation that have become possible with MR technology that some of these hypotheses can be tested, in vivo, in human epilepsy.

Mechanisms of Epileptogenesis

The question of what epilepsy is and what underlies the epileptic seizure is one that has been at the heart of the study of epilepsy from ancient times. One is always amazed when reading through the old, and not so very old, literature about some of the concepts that have been held about epilepsy until recent times. Even well into this century, it was common, particularly in the UK, for epilepsy to be managed in mental asylums. Some of this stigma of 'madness' associated with the presence of epilepsy still persists. Until the time of J. Hughlings Jackson in the late 19th century (2, 3) the disorder we now know as complex partial epilepsy (manifested as complex partial and partial seizures) was not considered to be true epilepsy. Partial seizures were considered only to be 'epileptiform.' It was through the studies of Jackson that the epileptic nature of the partial epilepsies was accepted.

In the earliest of writings, epilepsy, known as 'the sacred disease' was thought to be caused by possession by evil spirits or gods. Treatment therefore involved the use of religious, occult, and magical powers. The term 'epilepsy', first coined in the writings of Hippocrates, is derived from the Greek word that means 'a taking hold of or seizing'. Even at the end of the 19th century it was possible for a medical practitioner specializing in the treatment of epilepsy (who most appropriately should remain anonymous) to advocate in a lecture in New York that various forms of mutilation were appropriate for the treatment of epilepsy, including castration, as convulsions were known to originate in the testes and masturbation was known to exacerbate epileptic seizures. Even Gowers (at a much earlier time) considered castration to be an appropriate surgical treatment for epilepsy in some cases (50).

A More Modern View of Epileptogenesis

In the context of the modern discipline of neuroscience, this question of the mechanism of epilepsy has taken on a new impetus. In the most general terms it may be considered that neurons, in their normal functions, are characterized by the ability to be excited and to discharge. It is this very quality, when the discharges occur abnormally, that is part of the basic process of epileptogenesis. Both normal and abnormal brain may generate seizures. What has become clear is that no single mechanism underlies all epileptiform activity (55). It is more likely that there are a number of mechanisms underlying the epilepsies.

A further difficulty in this research is to differentiate between factors that cause the epilepsy in the first place and factors that are the consequence of the epilepsy. By the time the diagnosis of epilepsy is made, many events may have occurred that are secondary to the fact of the epilepsy itself (50). It is clear that epileptogenesis is a process that is based on normal brain tissue characteristics. These may have been modified, exaggerated, or released from normal physiological controls. It is probable that epileptiform activity is the consequence of normal, indeed necessary, aspects of normal brain tissue behavior. The most important normal features are excitability of neurons and plasticity of the cellular machinery that underlies the processes of learning, development, and recovery from brain damage.

Basic Mechanisms of Epilepsy

The basic mechanisms of epilepsy can be considered at many levels. These include:

- molecular defects in inherited epilepsies
- cell biology changes inside the neuron or at the cell membrane (especially ion channels)
- alterations in neuronal architecture or populations
- abnormalities in connections between proximate neurons
- alterations in neuronal networks within the cortex or between cortex and subcortical structures.

Fundamentally, as originally posited by Hughlings Jackson, seizures are generated from cortical gray matter. The only 'modern' qualification to this is that the cortical neurons may sometimes be misplaced as heterotopic gray matter. Thus, in various malformations of cortical development, seizures may be generated from anatomically subcortical structures. Second, from a physiological viewpoint epilepsy has been viewed as abnormal excitability of single cells ('the epileptic neuron') or as abnormalities of synchronization in neuronal networks. It is likely that there are elements of both general processes in all epilepsies.

We are in an exciting state of development in the understanding of epilepsies driven by recent technological and scientific advances. The revolution in molecular genetics has enabled discovery of genes underlying certain epilepsies, which will allow understanding of these epilepsies 'from the bottom up'. Rapid advances in developmental neurobiology have led to new insights into brain development that are crucial to understanding childhood epilepsies. The discovery that the adult brain can generate new neurons, especially in the temporal lobe, has fundamentally altered thinking about brain plasticity and epileptogenesis.

It is not the purpose of this book to explore in detail the research in all of the area of epileptogenesis but rather to give some idea of the range and scope of this area of research. Some brief notes therefore are in order.

Molecular Genetics

All human epilepsies have a genetic component, but in most the inheritance is complex, with a mixture of genetic and acquired factors. An enlarging number of syndromes have been described with major gene effects (usually autosomal dominant) and in some of those syndromes the fundamental molecular lesions are known. At the time of writing, all but one of the major genes discovered for human epilepsies code for ion channel subunits. Ion channels are multi-subunit complexes in cell membranes that regulate the flow of ions in and out of cells, or between intracellular compartments. They are fundamental to the mechanism of action potentials and hence to normal neuronal excitability. These are broadly divided into ligand-gated and voltage-gated channels – the former alter ion specific fluxes in response to the binding of neurotransmitter ligands, the latter in response to changes in membrane voltage (56–62).

Ligand-gated channel genes include nicotinic receptor subunit genes that cause autosomal dominant nocturnal frontal lobe epilepsy and gamma-amino butyric acid (GABA)$_A$ receptor subunits associated with various forms of generalized epilepsy. Voltage-gated channel genes include: potassium channel genes causing benign familial neonatal convulsions; sodium channel genes causing generalized epilepsy with febrile seizures plus severe myoclonic epilepsy in infancy and benign familial neonatal–infantile seizures; and chloride channel genes associated with generalized epilepsy. The only nonchannel gene definitively associated with human epilepsy to date is *LGI1*, mutated in autosomal partial epilepsy with auditory features. This gene, of unknown function, is possibly related to genes responsible for brain development.

Surprising insights from these discoveries include the observation that genetic abnormalities, presumably expressed in all cells, can cause focal epilepsies – this remains unexplained. Second, mutations in the same gene can be associated with both benign self-limiting epilepsies and severe progressive epileptic encephalopathies.

Transmitter Systems

Several transmitter systems have been intensively studied in regard to the problem of epileptogenesis. Prominent in these investigations is the hypothesis that epileptiform activity is generated by a loss of GABA-ergic inhibition. GABA is the primary inhibiting neurotransmitter in cortical structures (63). GABA inhibition is important in chronic models of epilepsy and in clinical epileptic conditions and has recently been shown to be involved in some genetic epilepsies (see above) (64). Molecular changes in GABA subunit composition underlie some genetic epilepsies but alterations in subunit stoichiometry and receptor density may underlie epileptogenesis in certain circumstances. This has been the basis of much research and has led to the development of several new antiepileptic drugs based on their ability to enhance the actions of GABA.

There are, however, a large number of different GABA-ergic subsystems. There are at least two major forms of GABA receptor: the GABA$_A$ and the GABA$_B$ receptor, each with multiple subtypes. Binding of GABA to the GABA$_A$ receptor leads to opening of the chloride channel. Many antiepileptic drugs appear to act on this receptor. For example, benzodiazepines bind to the GABA receptor complex and increase the binding efficacy of the receptor for GABA itself (65). It has been hypothesized that repetitive or intense activity in the postsynaptic target cell may decrease GABA$_A$ receptor efficacy. This may reduce the inhibitory influence

of these circuits, leading to hyperexcitability. The GABA$_B$ receptor is linked to a potassium channel (66), and activation induces hyperpolarization in many cells (67). This is an important mechanism as virtually all neurons in the hippocampus use GABA as a transmitter (68–70). It is suggested that even a minor decrease in GABA inhibition may lead to spontaneous epileptiform activity (71).

Glutamate has long been recognized as important in fast excitatory synaptic transmission in the cortex and hippocampus. It is clear that this is also a very complex system. The primary receptors appear to be divided into two groups according to whether they prefer *N*-methyl D-aspartate (NMDA)-type receptors or non-NMDA receptors (which are more sensitive to other excitatory amino acids such as kainate and quisqualate). NMDA function is potentially important, as NMDA channel antagonists can block the burst discharges in some models of epileptogenesis (72). In fact, some NMDA receptor antagonists are being studied in clinical trials. The mechanisms by which these antiepileptic activities are achieved is uncertain (73, 74).

Neuronal Circuits

As well as these questions of basic neurotransmitters and receptors, it has become clear that the circuitry of the neurons may also be abnormal in patients with epilepsy (75–87). There is a form of reorganization, characterized by sprouting of axonal branches and terminals, that occurs as a result of seizures in human hippocampal tissue as well as in animal models (88, 89). Most of these studies show concurrent loss of cells associated with this axonal sprouting. It has been suggested that the sprouting axons replace the neurons at the synaptic sites where cell death has removed the presynaptic elements. This process appears to provide cells with additional recurrent excitatory feedback that can increase the excitability of the circuits. The discovery that neurogenesis can occur in the human brain has led to the idea that cellular proliferation (in addition to cell loss) may be part of the plastic process underlying epileptogenesis.

Cell loss is common in the epileptic brain (90) and sclerosis is seen as a potential trigger for significant reorganization in neuronal circuits. One likely theory is that calcium influx to the cell, which is mediated by excitation of NMDA receptors, may lead to cellular destruction (91). It has been postulated that there is a relationship between NMDA receptor density and the regions that are susceptible to excitotoxic damage.

Despite these exciting developments in the understanding of cellular processes, it is clear that epilepsy itself is a function of large populations of synchronously active neurons. Generally, epilepsy is associated with abnormal discharges in gray matter structures such as the cortex and hippocampus. It is also clear that systems such as the hippocampus, entorhinal cortex, and piriform cortex are capable of marked hyperexcitable discharge without the presence of clear initiating factors such as tumors or areas of dysplasia, which are commonly found as the basis of focal seizures in the cerebral cortex itself (92–95).

The most basic question of where epileptiform activity begins and how it spreads remains difficult to answer at this theoretical level. The onset of epileptiform activity presupposes that an epileptic focus must exist where the seizure originates. Even at this level of analysis, however, this concept can be challenged. It can be suggested that some regions (in experimental animals) that are particularly sensitive to stimulation, such as the area tempesta, may not constitute epileptic foci but rather may serve only as triggers. The focus itself may be another discrete group of neurons such as the CA1 pyramidal cell neurons in the hippocampus. Similarly, whatever is needed to initiate a seizure (the focus itself) may be widely distributed over quite a large brain region, including the hippocampus and entorhinal cortex. The epileptic focus is a concept that can be considered in several ways. By this, we mean that the focus may not be the same as the site where the EEG first appears, and even this may not correlate with the pathological findings. Similarly, the 'pacemaker' or 'generator' region of the seizure focus may not be synonymous with these other regions. (See Fig. 1.3 below.)

Mechanisms of Seizure Spread

If we put aside this question of how to define a seizure focus for a moment, then the way in which the epileptic activity spreads from the focus to the other regions of the brain is also of importance. The dominant mechanism of seizure spread could be assumed to be release of excitatory transmitter at the terminals, which depolarizes the postsynaptic terminals. Similarly, accumulation of extracellular potassium or other substances may be responsible for increasing the regional excitation. It has even been suggested that the spread of seizures may depend on some gating mechanism. In this regard the activity of the dentate gyrus has been suggested to be critical for the spread of seizures to other parts of the brain (82, 96).

There are many methodological problems in investigating the fundamental mechanisms of epilepsy. There are many types of epilepsy models, which may contribute to our understanding of basic mechanisms in different ways. The mechanisms may, of course, not be the same in each of these models, and it is not necessarily the aim of these studies to come up with a 'unified' model of epilepsy.

In general terms, there are acute models of epilepsy and chronic models of epilepsy. The acute models usually involve systemic administration or topical application of convulsant substances or a sudden insult such as electrical stimulation or metabolic derangement. Chronic models, on the other hand, can be induced by permanent structural lesions and by repetitive electrical stimulation of the brain (kindling) or they can occur spontaneously in genetically epileptic animals. These models have been widely used for the assessment of new drugs in the treatment of epilepsy.

Some of these concepts and mechanisms of epilepsy do not necessarily relate to the clinical distinction between partial and generalized epilepsy. In the case of the clinical problem of epilepsy surgery, one can reduce the argument to the simple question of whether there is a discrete epilepsy focus to be removed or whether the aim of surgery is simply to interrupt some critical circuitry that is required to generate the hyperexcitability associated with seizures. A classic example of this latter approach would be the use of corpus callosotomy.

The Issue of Secondary Epileptogenesis

In animal models, secondary epileptogenesis can be demonstrated in the kindling model, where repeated subconvulsive electrical stimulation of the amygdala for just a few seconds once or twice a day can lead to the development of partial epilepsy in these animals (52–54, 97). There can even be the development of spontaneous seizures arising from the contralateral (nonstimulated) side. These spontaneous seizures may persist after stimulation is discontinued, thus mimicking chronic epilepsy. The evidence for this process occurring in humans is controversial (24). It can also be demonstrated in the phenomenon of the mirror focus (97), where a toxic or other lesion is applied focally to the cortex. The site of injury may give rise to a primary epileptic focus. If, however, the animal is observed for a prolonged period (days, weeks, or months) spontaneous epileptiform potentials are observed in the hemisphere contralateral to the primary focus.

How these observations in animal models relate to the origins of human epilepsy and to the secondary effects of seizures seen in the human brain remains controversial. Morrell used the criteria of unequivocal evidence of independent interictal or ictal epileptiform discharges in the hemisphere contralateral to a well defined tumor to demonstrate the phenomenon of the mirror focus in humans. He showed an incidence of up to 36% of what he called 'secondary epileptogenesis,' with 15% of patients having clinical attacks arising from this focus. While the demonstration of secondary epileptogenesis in humans is indirect, many epileptologists would accept the possibility of secondary epileptogenesis in their patients. It is possible that this phenomenon is the basis of the well-described 'dual pathology' of hippocampal sclerosis in patients with a tumor or other lesion elsewhere. The alternative view is that damage occurs bilaterally at the time of the original epileptogenic insult and that these bilateral findings simply reflect the distribution of this pathology.

Seizure-induced Brain Damage

Perhaps of equal interest is the secondary damage to the brain that has been postulated to occur secondary to the occurrence of seizures themselves (98–125). This is an enormously difficult area and has been the subject of a recent book in itself, so the most superficial treatment of this issue is the following. (See also Chapter 4.)

It seems clear that progressive neurological deterioration in some patients with epilepsy occurs. This deterioration may relate to the occurrence of seizures or clusters of seizures rather than to the underlying condition in some individuals. Prolonged status epilepticus can give rise to brain damage. On the other hand, many patients who have many seizures continue to function at a high level all their lives and do not seen to show secondary damage to the brain. This argument is also confounded by the fact that it is difficult to exclude the possibility that seizures may reflect the presence of an underlying process that may be the primary cause (rather than the seizures themselves) of this demonstrated neurological deterioration.

Therefore we can only conclude with some speculations (and opinions) – that sometimes seizures damage the brain but do not always do so. Furthermore, hippocampal sclerosis may occur as a primary lesion that is the consequence of unknown insults, but hippocampal sclerosis can also arise as a secondary lesion (like kindling) as a consequence of seizures originating elsewhere. In this latter instance, even if the initial seizures arise elsewhere, the hippocampus may become the primary seizure focus later in life. It is our opinion that the noninvasive techniques of MR investigation of the human brain that are described in this book provide the means whereby these issues can be more fully addressed.

AN IMAGING VIEW

We think the following concepts are of value in conceptualizing the type of information provided by the various methods of investigation.

- epileptogenic region.
- epileptogenic lesion.
- pacemaker zone.

Epileptogenic Region

The epileptogenic region is based on the assumption that an area of brain parenchyma is abnormal and epileptogenic. This region is conceptually and practically the most difficult to define with certainty. Methodological questions remain an issue in defining this region. Is the epileptogenic region defined by EEG, PET, semiology, or pathology? It is clear, however, that this region always includes the pacemaker zone and, in the vast majority of cases, also contains the epileptogenic lesion (Fig. 1.3). However, in some circumstances the epileptogenic region may not include the totality of a lesion or may border the margins of the epileptogenic lesion (Fig. 1.3B, C).

Epileptogenic Lesion

The epileptogenic lesion is defined as the structural abnormality that is presumed to be the basis of the seizures. Most commonly the lesion is a marker for the underlying epilepsy and may vary from gross to subtle and from strictly circumscribed to more diffuse. In most cases, the lesion is intimately associated with the pacemaker zone and is included in the epileptogenic region (Fig. 1.3). Nonetheless, in rare cases a lesion may be present and may not have any epileptogenic significance; furthermore, more than one lesion may be present although only one of them is associated with the epileptogenic focus.

Pacemaker Zone

Finally, the pacemaker zone can be defined as the locus of the seizures. It is difficult to define what constitutes the pacemaker zone. A good example is a patient with temporal lobe epilepsy of mesial temporal origin (Fig. 1.3D). The pacemaker zone is localized to the mesial temporal structures, which are atrophic and on pathology demonstrate neuronal loss and astrocytosis. EEG abnormalities extend beyond the pacemaker and epileptogenic lesion. Another example is when the pacemaker zone and the epileptogenic lesion are intimately associated but the epileptogenic region involves the entire temporal lobe (Fig. 1.3E).

When other features are added to a particular problem such as the one described above, other questions may surface. For example, in some patients with mesial temporal seizures the aura consists of viscerosensory manifestations. Hippocampal atrophy may be present on MRI and confirmation of the seizure focus in the mesial temporal region is achieved with EEG. Removal of the mesial structures renders the patient free of partial complex events but s/he continues to have the same aura. Has the pacemaker zone been removed or have we only disconnected some temporal lobe structures needed for seizure generation and propagation? In most cases of lesional neocortical epilepsy, we presume that the pacemaker zone is localized within or in close intimacy to the lesion and that removal of the lesion results in obliteration of both elements (Fig. 1.3A).

Problems of Epilepsy that Magnetic Resonance Techniques Must Address

Epilepsy constitutes an important clinical problem and also provides an important challenge to our understanding of subtle forms of brain damage. It is a condition in which seizures are a symptom of focal or generalized brain abnormality and it is a disorder primarily of gray matter. In many cases a focal structural or EEG abnormality can be defined. In intractable cases the clinical problem requires precise definition of normal and abnormal brain structure and function

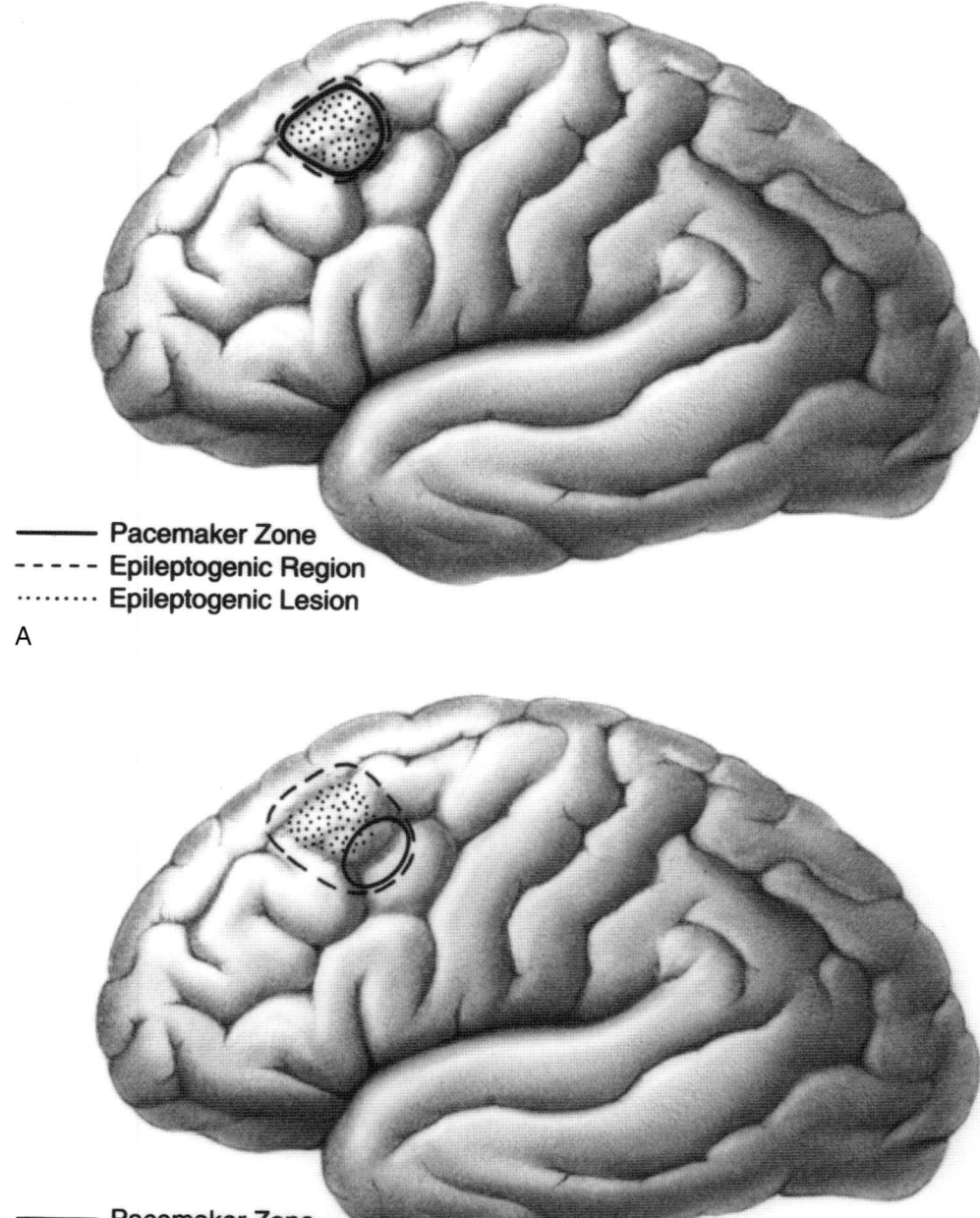

Pacemaker Zone
----- Epileptogenic Region
········· Epileptogenic Lesion

A

Pacemaker Zone
----- Epileptogenic Region
········· Epileptogenic Lesion

B

FIG. 1.3. A. A patient with focal seizures arising from the left middle frontal gyrus. The epileptogenic region is intimately associated with the epileptogenic lesion and the pacemaker zone. In this case there is complete concordance among these three areas. **B.** There is an epileptogenic lesion localized to the left middle frontal gyrus. EEG abnormalities were recorded over a larger region of the cerebral contex that surrounds the epileptogenic lesion. The pacemaker zone appears to partially involve the epileptogenic region, which in turn is fully contained in the epileptogenic region. In this cases there is not complete concordance between the regions.

Continued

if surgical treatment of the disorder is to be considered. In many cases the underlying cause of the damaged or abnormal area of the brain is not known. Understanding of the basic neurobiology of the functional event of the seizure and the relationship of seizure generating neural circuits to the underlying brain structure is a main goal of the clinical and research effort.

The problem of epilepsy necessitates understanding of brain structure, function, and biochemistry in normal and pathological states. The central problems in the understanding and management of epilepsy continue to be:

• To determine whether the epilepsy syndrome is generalized (no defined site of seizure onset, i.e. onset

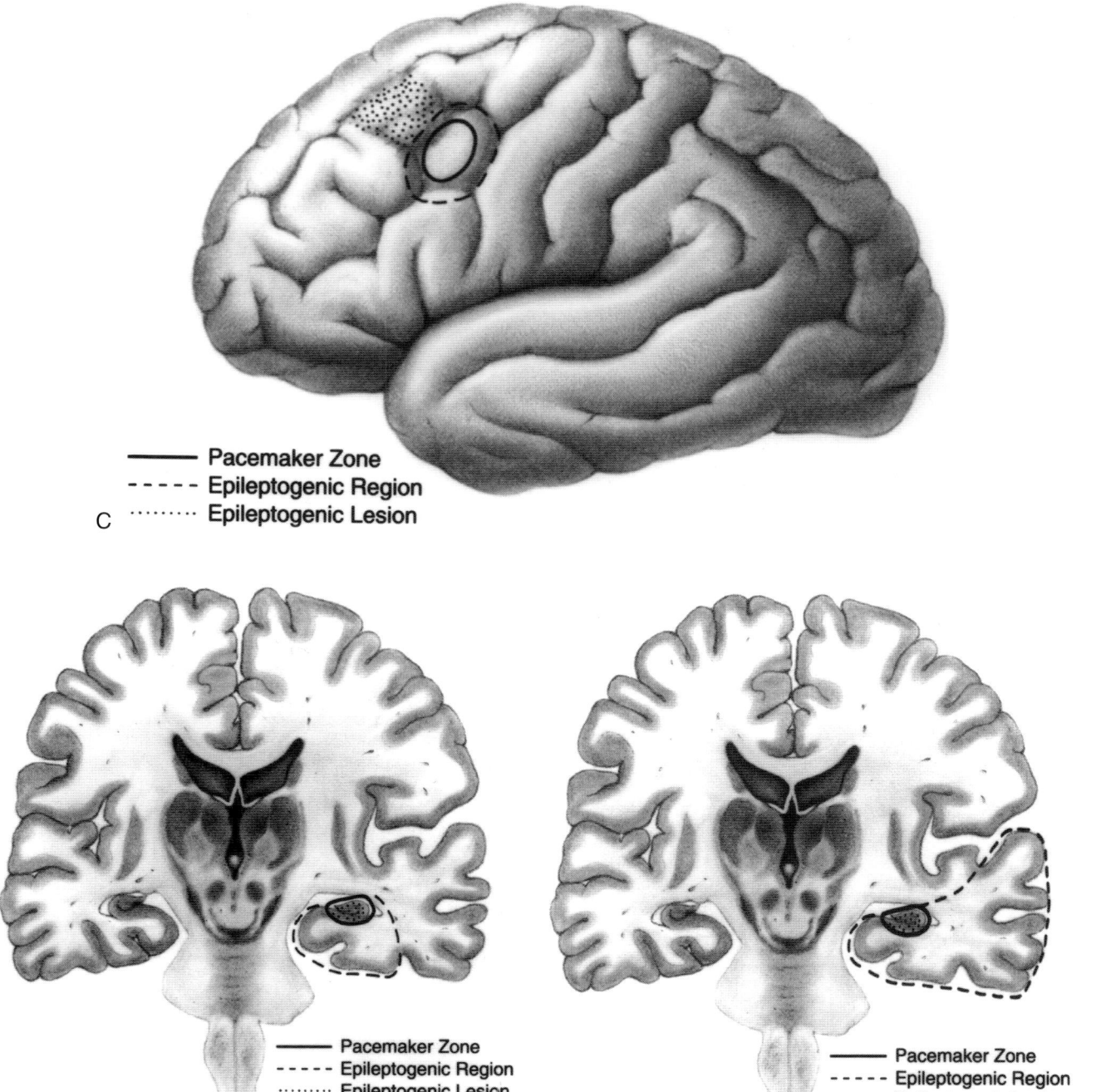

FIG. 1.3. *Cont'd.* **C.** With a similar lesion, the electrophysiological data do not include the epileptogenic lesion, and the epileptogenic region is only at the margin of the lesion. **D.** The idealized case of mesial temporal epilepsy where there is left hippocampal sclerosis and good concordance between the pacemaker zone and the lesion and the epileptogenic region is well localized to this area. **E.** In another patient with left temporal lobe seizures, the epileptogenic region extends well beyond the pacemaker zone and the epileptogenic lesion of hippocampal sclerosis.

almost simultaneous in all or many parts of the brain) or partial (focal or localized seizure onset, with or without subsequent generalized spread).

To understand the neurobiological basis of this distinction.

• To define whether a structural abnormality of the brain exists that may give rise to the epilepsy disorder and to distinguish this from the secondary effects of seizures.

• If partial, to define the location and extent of the region (or regions) responsible for the generation of the seizures, and how functional events relate to the underlying structural abnormality. It is clinically important to understand if seizures begin in a specific location, or are part of a more widespread epileptogenic circuit. Increasingly fMRI/EEG techniques seem to show epileptic circuits that may be important in understanding seizure generation.

- To understand which lesions are epileptogenic and what abnormalities of structure and function define such areas. What defines the tissue that, in itself, is epileptogenic, as opposed to that which is merely abnormal (possibly as a result of seizure effects)?
- To determine the effects of seizures on the brain. Under what circumstances do seizures cause damage (e.g. cellular damage, neuronal loss, hippocampal sclerosis) and how much is it the disease or condition that gives rise to the epilepsy disorder that causes the observed damage/abnormality of the brain?
- To identify important functional areas of cortex (motor, sensory, language, memory) that must be preserved if a neurosurgical procedure is to be performed for treatment of intractable seizures. To more broadly define what predicts a good outcome in terms of seizures, function, and psychosocial functioning.

Noninvasive investigations contribute to the solution of these problems by identifying gray matter lesions such as hippocampal sclerosis, replacing the use of invasive methods used to localize the site of seizure origin, defining the nature and extent of the structural, functional and metabolic abnormalities of the seizure focus, and determining preoperatively factors that influence the likely seizure and functional outcome from surgical treatment. Increasingly, many aspect of the physiology of the epilepsy condition can be studied with MR techniques. These dramatic new frontiers in MR technology have been added to this volume on MR in epilepsy.

This book attempts to either answer these questions, or to point toward techniques, interpretation, and potential studies that will allow us to do so using MR technology. MR has both enormous achievements and enormous potential yet to be harnessed for the understanding and definition of brain abnormalities in diseases of the brain such as epilepsy. It has generated an excitement that must, in days past, have been associated with the discovery of X-rays and the advent of EEG technology.

REFERENCES

1. Engel JJ. *Surgical treatment of the epilepsies*, 2nd ed. New York: Raven Press, 1993.
2. Jackson JH. A study of convulsions. *Trans St Andrews Med Grad Assoc* 1870;3:162–207.
3. Jackson JH. Observations on the anatomical, physiological, pathological investigations of epilepsies. *West Riding Lunatic Asylum Rep* 1873;3:315.
4. Ferrier D. On the localisation of the functions of the brain. *Br Med J* 1874;2:766–767.
5. Macewen W. Tumor of the dura matter removed during life in a person affected with epilepsy. *Glasgow Med J* 1879;12:210.
6. Horsley V. Brain surgery. *Br Med J* 1886;2:670–675.
7. Penfield W. The evidence for a cerebral vascular mechanism in epilepsy. *Ann Intern Med* 1933;7:303–310.
8. Penfield W. Remarks on incomplete hypothesis for the control of cerebral circulation. *J Neurosurg* 1971;35:124–127.
9. Berkovic SF, Newton MR, Chiron C, Dulac O. Single photon emission tomography. In: Engel JJ, ed. *Surgical treatment of the epilepsies*, 2nd ed. New York: Raven Press, 1993:233–243.
10. Berger H. Uber das Elektrenkephalogram des Menschen. *Arch Psychiatr Nervenkr* 1929;87:527–570.
11. Bailey P, Gibbs FA. The surgical treatment of psychomotor epilepsy. *JAMA* 1951;145:365–370.
12. Gadian DG. *Nuclear magnetic resonance and its applications to living systems*. New York: Oxford University Press, 1982.
13. Aaron J, New PFJ, Strand R, et al. NMR imaging in temporal lobe epilepsy due to gliomas. *J Comput Assist Tomogr* 1984;8:608–613.
14. Sperling MR, Wilson C, Engel JJ, et al. Magnetic resonance imaging in intractable partial epilepsy: correlative studies. *Ann Neurol* 1986;20: 57–62.
15. Duncan R, Patterson J, Hadley DM, et al. CT, MR and SPECT imaging in temporal lobe epilepsy. *J Neurol Neurosurg Psychiatry* 1990;53: 11–15.
16. Ormson MJ, Kispert DB, Sharbrough FW, et al. Cryptic structural lesions in refractory partial epilepsy: MR imaging and CT studies. *Radiology* 1986;160:215–219.
17. Bergen D, Bleck T, Ramsey R, et al. Magnetic resonance imaging as a sensitive and specific predictor of neoplasms removed for intractable epilepsy. *Epilepsia* 1989;30:318–321.
18. Heinz ER, Heinz TR, Radtke R, et al. Efficacy of MRI vs CT in epilepsy. *Am J Neuroradiol* 1988;9:1123–1128.
19. Fish D, Andermann F, Olivier A. Complex partial seizures and small temporal or extratemporal structural lesions: surgical management. *Neurology* 1991;41:1781–1784.
20. Cascino G, Kelly PJ, Sharbrough FW, et al. Long-term follow-up of stereotacticl Lesionectomy in partial epilepsy: predictive factors and electroencephalographic results. *Epilepsia* 1992;33:639–644.
21. Barkovich AJ, Kuzniecky RI, Dobyns WB, et al. A classification scheme for malformations of cortical development. *Neuropediatrics* 1996;27:59–63.
22. Barkovich AJ, Kuzniecky RI, Jackson GD, et al. Classification system for malformations of cortical development: update 2001. *Neurology* 2001;57:2168–2178.
23. Penfield W. Epilepsy, the great teacher: the progress of one pupil. *Acta Neurol Scand* 1967;43:1–10.
24. Engel JJ. *Seizures and epilepsy*. Philadelphia: Davis, 1989.
25. Aicardi J. *Diseases of the nervous system in childhood*. London: MacKeith Press, 1992.
26. Commission on Classification and Terminology of the International League Against Epilepsy. Proposal for revised clinical and electroencephalographic classification of epileptic seizures. *Epilepsia* 1981;22:489–501.
27. Annegers JF, Hauser WA, Elveback LR. Remission of seizures and relapse in patients with epilepsy. *Epilepsia* 1979;20:729–737.
28. Commission on classification and terminology of the international league against epilepsy: A revised proposal for the classification of epilepsy and epileptic syndromes. *Epilepsia* 1989;30:268–278.
29. Weiser HG, Engel JJ, Williamson PD, et al. Surgically remedial temporal lobe syndromes. In: Engel JJ, ed. *Surgical treatment of the epilepsies*, 2nd ed. New York: Raven Press, 1993.
30. Hauser WA, Annegers JF, Kurland LT. Prevalence of epilepsy in Rochester, Minnesota 1940–1980. *Epilepsia* 1990;32:429–445.
31. Hauser WA. The natural history of temporal lobe epilepsy. In: Luders HA, ed. *Epilepsy surgery*. New York: Raven Press, 1992:133–141.
32. ILAE Task Force on Classification and Terminology. A proposed diagnostic scheme for people with epileptic seizures and with epilepsy: report of the ilae task force on classification and terminology. Brussels: ILAE, 2003. Available on line at www.epilepsy.org/ctf/over_frame.html.
33. Jackson GD, Berkovic SF, Tress BM, et al. Hippocampal sclerosis can be reliably detected by magnetic resonance imaging. *Neurology* 1990;40:1869–1875.

34. Sander JW. The epidemiology of epilepsy revisited. *Curr Opin Neurol* 2003;16:165–170.

35. Granieri E, Rosati G, Tola R, et al. A descriptive study of epilepsy in the district of Coppara, Italy: 1964–1978. *Epilepsia* 1983;24:502–514.

36. Crombie DL, Cross KW, Fry RJ, et al. A survey of the epilepsies in general practice: a report of the research committee of the Royal College of General Practitioners. *Br Med J* 1960;2:416–422.

37. Sander JW, Shorvon SD. Incidence and prevalence studies in epilepsy and their methodological problems. *J Neurol Neurosurg Psychiatry* 1987;50:829–939.

38. Shinnar S, Pellock JM. Update on the epidemiology and prognosis of pediatric epilepsy. *J Child Neurol* 2002;17(Suppl 1):S4–S17.

39. Frey LC. Epidemiology of posttraumatic epilepsy: a critical review. *Epilepsia* 2003;44(Suppl 10):11–17.

40. Cowan LD. The epidemiology of the epilepsies in children. *Ment Retard Dev Disabil Res Rev* 2002;8:171–181.

41. Van Cott AC. Epilepsy and EEG in the elderly. *Epilepsia* 2002; 43(Suppl 3):94–102.

42. Tomson T. Mortality in epilepsy. *J Neurol* 2000;247:15–21.

43. Sillanpaa M. Long-term outcome of epilepsy. *Epileptic Disord* 2000;2:79–88.

44. Ficker DM. Sudden unexplained death and injury in epilepsy. *Epilepsia* 2000;41(Suppl 2):S7–S12.

45. Klennerman P, Sander JW, Shorvon SD. Mortality in patients with epilepsy. *J Neurol Neurosurg Psychiatry* 1993;56:149–152.

46. Taylor DC. Epilepsy as a chronic sickness: remediating its impact. In: Engel J Jr, ed. *Surgical treatment of the epilepsies*, 2nd ed. New York: Raven Press, 1993:11–22.

47. Wilson SJ, Saling MM, Lawrence J, Bladin PF. Outcome of temporal lobectomy: expectations and the prediction of perceived success. *Epilepsy Res* 1999;36:1–14.

48. Wilson SJ, Bladin PF, Saling MM, et al. The longitudinal course of adjustment after seizure surgery. *Seizure* 2001;10:165–172.

49. Wilson S, Bladin P, Saling M. The 'burden of normality': concepts of adjustment after surgery for seizures. *J Neurol Neurosurg Psychiatry* 2001;70:649–656.

50. Gowers WR. *Epilepsy and other chronic convulsive disorders*. New York: William Wood, 1885.

51. Reynolds EH, Elwes RDC, Shorvon SD. Why does epilepsy become intractable? *Lancet* 1983;2:952–954.

52. Adamec RE. Does kindling model anything clinically relevant? *Biol Psychiatry* 1990;27:249–279.

53. Cain DP. Transfer of kindling: clinical relevance and a hypothesis of its mechanism. *Prog Neuropsychopharmacol Biol Psychiatry* 1985; 9:467–472.

54. Delgado EA, Ward AJ, Woodbury DM, Porter RJ. New wave of research in the epilepsies. *Adv Neurol* 1986;44:3–55.

55. Wyllie E, Chee M, Granstrom ML, et al. Temporal lobe epilepsy in early childhood. *Epilepsia* 1993;34:859–868.

56. Scheffer IE, Berkovic SF. The genetics of human epilepsy. *Trends Pharmacol Sci* 2003;24:428–433.

57. Noebels JL. The biology of epilepsy genes. *Annu Rev Neurosci* 2003; 26:599–625.

58. Willmore LJ, Ueda Y. Genetics of epilepsy. *J Child Neurol* 2002; 17(Suppl 1):S18–S27.

59. Kaneko S, Okada M, Iwasa H, et al. Genetics of epilepsy: current status and perspectives. *Neurosci Res* 2002;44:11–30.

60. Berkovic SF, Mulley JC. The first gene for an idiopathic epilepsy: a fruitful collaboration of Australian clinical research and molecular genetics. *Aust NZ J Med* 1996;26:154–156.

61. Serratosa JM. Genetics of the partial epilepsy. *Neurologia* 1996;11 (Suppl 4):53–57.

62. Berkovic SF. Epilepsy genes and the genetics of epilepsy syndromes: the promise of new therapies based on genetic knowledge. *Epilepsia* 1997;38(Suppl 9):S32–S36.

63. Kohling R. Neuroscience. GABA becomes exciting. *Science* 2002;298:1350–1351.

64. Franck JE, Kunkel DD, Baskin DG, Schwartzkroin PA. Inhibition in kainate-lesioned epileptogenic hippocampi: physiologic, autoradiographic and immunocytochemical observations. *J Neurosci* 1988;8: 1991–2002.

65. Olsen RW. The GABA postsynaptic membrane receptor ionophore complex. *Mol Cell Biochem* 1981;39:261–279.

66. Dutar P, Nicoll RA. Pre- and postsynaptic GABA receptors in the hippocampus have different pharmacological properties. *Neuron* 1988;1:585–591.

67. Newberry NR, Nicoll RA. A bicuculline-resistant inhibitory post-synaptic potential in rat hippocampal pryamidal cells in vitro. *J Physiol (Lond)* 1984;348:239–254.

68. Swartz BE, Halgren E, Delgado-Escueta AV, et al. Neuroimaging in patients with seizures of probable frontal lobe origin. *Epilepsia* 1989;30:547–558.

69. Swartz BE, Halgren E, Delgado EA, et al. Multidisciplinary analysis of patients with extratemporal complex partial seizures. I. Intertest agreement. *Epilepsy Res* 1990;5:61–73.

70. Swartz BE, Tomiyasu U, Delgado-Escueta AV, et al. Neuroimaging in temporal lobe epilepsy: test sensitivity and relationships to pathology and postoperative outcome. *Epilepsia* 1992;33:624–634.

71. Chagnac-Amitai Y, Connors BW. Horizontal spread of synchronized activity in neocortex and its control by GABA-mediated inhibition. *J Neurophysiol* 1989;61:747–758.

72. Herron CE, Williamson R, Collingridge GL. A selective *N*-methyl-D-aspartate antagonist depresses epileptiform activity in rat hippocampal slices. *Neurosci Lett* 1985;61:255–260.

73. Anderson WW, Swartzwelder HS, Wilson WA. The NMDA receptor antagonist 2-amino-5-phosphono-valerate blocks stimulus train-induced epileptogenesis but not epileptiform bursting in the rat hippocampal slice. *J Neurophysiol* 1987;57:1–21.

74. McNamara JO. Development of new pharmacological agents for epilepsy: lessons from the kindling model. *Epilepsia* 1989;30 (Suppl 1):513–518.

75. Bartolomei F, Wendling F, Bellanger JJ, et al. Neural networks involving the medial temporal structures in temporal lobe epilepsy. *Clin Neurophysiol* 2001;112:1746–1760.

76. Blumenfeld H, Taylor J. Why do seizures cause loss of consciousness? *Neuroscientist* 2003;9:301–310.

77. Blumenfeld H, Westerveld M, Ostroff RB, et al. Selective frontal, parietal, and temporal networks in generalized seizures. *Neuroimage* 2003;19:1556–1566.

78. Blumenfeld H. From molecules to networks: cortical/subcortical interactions in the pathophysiology of idiopathic generalized epilepsy. *Epilepsia* 2003;44(Suppl 2):7–15.

79. Jefferys JG. Experimental neurobiology of epilepsies. *Curr Opin Neurol* 1994;7:113–22.

80. Jefferys JG. Models and mechanisms of experimental epilepsies. *Epilepsia* 2003;44(Suppl 12):44–50.

81. Kubova H, Moshe SL. Experimental models of epilepsy in young animals. *J Child Neurol* 1994;9(Suppl 1):S3–S11.

82. Lopes da Silva F, Blanes W, Kalitzin SN, et al. Epilepsies as dynamical diseases of brain systems: basic models of the transition between normal and epileptic activity. *Epilepsia* 2003;44(Suppl 12):72–83.

83. Lopes da Silva FH, Blanes W, Kalitzin SN, et al. Dynamical diseases of brain systems: different routes to epileptic seizures. *IEEE Trans Biomed Eng* 2003;50:540–548.

84. McCormick DA, Contreras D. On the cellular and network bases of epileptic seizures. *Annu Rev Physiol* 2001;63:815–846.

85. Moshe SL, Brown LL, Kubova H, et al. Maturation and segregation of brain networks that modify seizures. *Brain Res* 1994;665: 141–146.

86. Steinlein OK, Noebels JL. Ion channels and epilepsy in man and mouse. *Curr Opin Genet Dev* 2000;10:286–291.

87. Swann JW, Smith KL, Lee CL. Neuronal activity and the establishment of normal and epileptic circuits during brain development. *Int Rev Neurobiol* 2001;45:89–118.

88. Davenport CJ, Brown WJ, Babb TL. Sprouting of GABAergic and mossy fiber axons in dentate gyrus following intrahippocampal kainate in the rat. *Exp Neurol* 1990;109:180–190.

89. Sutula T, Cascino G, Cavazos J, et al. Mossy fiber synaptic reorganization in the epileptic human temporal lobe. *Ann Neurol* 1989;26:321–330.

90. Meldrum BS, Corsellis JAN. *Epilepsy*. New York: John Wiley, 1984.

91. Choi DW, Rothman SM. The role of glutamate neurotoxicity in hypoxic ischemic neuronal death. *Ann Rev Neurosci* 1990;13:171–182.

92. Babb TL, Lieb JP, Brown WJ, et al. Distribution of pyramidal cell density and hyperexcitability in the epileptic human hippocampal formation. *Epilepsia* 1984;25:721–728.

93. Babb TL, Brown WJ, Pretorius J, Lieb JP. Temporal lobe volumetric cell densities in temporal lobe epilepsy. *Epilepsia* 1984;25:729–740.

94. Babb TL, Brown WJ. Pathological findings in epilepsy. In: Engel J Jr, ed. *Surgical treatment of the epilepsies*. New York: Raven Press, 1987:511–540.

95. Babb TL, Pretorius JK. Pathological substrates of epilepsy. In: Wylie E, ed. *The treatment of epilepsy: principles and practice*. Philadelphia: Lea & Febiger, 1993:55–70.

96. Dzhala VI, Staley KJ. Transition from interictal to ictal activity in limbic networks in vitro. *J Neurosci* 2003;23:7873–7880.

97. Wada JA, Mizoguchi T, Komai S. Kindling epileptogenesis in orbital and mesial frontal cortical areas of subhuman primates. *Epilepsia* 1985;26:472–479.

98. Holmes GL. Seizure-induced neuronal injury: animal data. *Neurology* 2002;59(Suppl 5):S3–S6.

99. Aiyathurai EJ, Boon WH. The probable mechanisms of brain damage and epilepsy in febrile convulsions, Singapore syndrome and Reye's syndrome. *Acta Paediatr Jpn* 1989;31:245–258.

100. Bengzon J, Kokala Z, Elmer E, et al. Apoptosis and proliferation of dentate gyrus neurons after single and intermittent limbic seizures. *Proc Natl Acad Sci* 1997;94:10432–10437.

101. Bengzon J, Mohapel P, Ekdahl CT, Lindvall O. Neuronal apoptosis after brief and prolonged seizures. *Prog Brain Res* 2002;135:111–119.

102. Blennow G, Brierley JB, Meldrum BS, Siesjo BK. Epileptic brain damage: the role of systemic factors that modify cerebral energy metabolism. *Brain* 1978;101:687–700.

103. Borges K, Gearing M, McDermott DL, et al. Neuronal and glial pathological changes during epileptogenesis in the mouse pilocarpine model. *Exp Neurol* 2003;182:21–34.

104. Bouilleret V, Nehlig A, Marescaux C, Namer IJ. Magnetic resonance imaging follow-up of progressive hippocampal changes in a mouse model of mesial temporal lobe epilepsy. *Epilepsia* 2000;41:642–650.

105. Briellmann RS, Jackson GD, Kalnins R, Berkovic SF. Hemicranial volume deficits in patients with temporal lobe epilepsy with and without hippocampal sclerosis. *Epilepsia* 1998;39:1174–1181.

106. Briellmann RS, Newton MR, Wellard RM, Jackson GD. Hippocampal sclerosis following brief generalized seizures. *Neurology* 2001;57:315–317.

107. Briellmann RS, Berkovic SF, Syngeniotis A, et al. Seizure-associated hippocampal volume loss: a longitudinal MR-study of temporal lobe epilepsy. *Ann Neurol* 2002;51:641–644.

108. Chang LB, Lirng JF, Teng MM, et al. Sequential MRI studies of a patient with complex partial status – a case report. *Kaohsiung J Med Sci* 2001;17:633–637.

109. Corsellis JA, Bruton CJ. Neuropathology of status epilepticus in humans. *Adv Neurol* 1983;34:129–139.

110. Duncan JS. Seizure-induced neuronal injury: human data. *Neurology* 2002;59:S15–S20.

111. Fujikawa DG, Itabashi HH, Wu A, Shinmei SS. Status epilepticus-induced neuronal loss in humans without systemic complications or epilepsy. *Epilepsia* 2000;41:981–991.

112. Heinemann U, Buchheim K, Gabriel S, et al. Cell death and metabolic activity during epileptiform discharges and status epilepticus in the hippocampus. *Prog Brain Res* 2002;135:197–210.

113. Jackson GD, Chambers BR, Berkovic SF. Hippocampal sclerosis: development in adult life. *Dev Neurosci* 1999;21:207–214.

114. Kälviäinen R, Salmenperä T, Partanen K, et al. Recurrent seizures may cause hippocampal damage in temporal lobe epilepsy. *Neurology* 1998;50:1377–1382.

115. Meldrum BS. Cell damage in epilepsy and the role of calcium in cytotoxicity. *Adv Neurol* 1986;44:849–855.

116. Najm IM, Wang Y, Shedid D, et al. MRS metabolic markers of seizures and seizure-induced neuronal damage. *Epilepsia* 1998;39:244–250.

117. Nohira V, Lee N, Tien RD, et al. Magnetic resonance imaging evidence of hippocampal sclerosis in progression: a case report. *Epilepsia* 1994;35:1332–1336.

118. Perez ER, Maeder P, Villemure KM, et al. Acquired hippocampal damage after temporal lobe seizures in 2 infants. *Ann Neurol* 2000;48:384–387.

119. Sasahira M, Simon RP, Greenberg DA. Neuronal injury in experimental status epilepticus in the rat: role of hypoxia. *Neurosci Lett* 1997;222:207–209.

120. Scott RC, Gadian DG, King MD, et al. Magnetic resonance imaging findings within 5 days of status epilepticus in childhood. *Brain* 2002;125:1951–1959.

121. Scott RC, King MD, Gadian DG, et al. Hippocampal abnormalities after prolonged febrile convulsion: a longitudinal MRI study. *Brain* 2003;126:2551–2557.

122. Sloviter RS. Permanently altered hippocampal structure, excitability, and inhibition after experimental status epilepticus in the rat: the 'dormant basket cell' hypothesis and its possible relevance to temporal lobe epilepsy. *Hippocampus* 1991;1:41–66.

123. Sloviter RS. Status epilepticus-induced neuronal injury and network reorganization. *Epilepsia* 1999;40(Suppl 1):S34–S39; discussion S40–S41.

124. Tasch E, Cendes F, Li LM, et al. Neuroimaging evidence of progressive neuronal loss and dysfunction in temporal lobe epilepsy. *Ann Neurol* 1999;45:568–576.

125. VanLandingham KE, Heinz ER, Cavazos JE, Lewis DV. Magnetic resonance imaging evidence of hippocampal injury after prolonged focal febrile convulsions. *Ann Neurol* 1998;43:413–426.

CHAPTER 2

Principles of Magnetic Resonance Imaging

Graeme D. Jackson, Ruben I. Kuzniecky and Gaby S. Pell

INTRODUCTION

The aim of this chapter is to provide a basic discussion of concepts in magnetic resonance imaging (MRI), written from the perspective of the nonphysicist. It does not attempt to describe in detail the basic phenomena of the MR experiment. There are many excellent accounts of the physics of MR and for this purpose we recommend several excellent texts listed at the end of this chapter. We have not made it our task to provide another version of these descriptions. Rather, what we have attempted to do is to discuss in simple terms what we see as essential concepts of MR. We hope that this will be an easily read chapter that will introduce the reader to important concepts in MR and will both provide a context for further reading and stimulate the desire to read these more basic texts.

Here, we will introduce and discuss concepts that we feel are essential knowledge for those dealing with MR investigations in clinical practice. These concepts are important for those ordering an MR study, for those involved in carrying out and interpreting such studies, and for the clinician who eventually has to make a clinical decision based on this information. While not everyone on the team needs to be an expert, all need some basic knowledge in order for this powerful technology to be used appropriately, and for communication between the different members of the team to occur with better understanding. The power and diversity of MR techniques means that the clinical issues, the MR technology, and the particular MR investigation must be integrated in order to optimize the information obtained from these studies. Unless the neuroimaging specialist, the physicist and the clinician all have a mutual basis for the discussion of both clinical and MR issues, and are capable of operating as a team, then optimal clinical examinations

cannot be expected. Ultimately it will be the patient who will suffer the consequences of the failure to fully utilize this resource.

Therefore, we raise issues and concepts that we feel are important to the understanding of the MR study from a clinical perspective. The aim of this chapter is to provide a basic knowledge for the clinical user. We trust the omissions and simplifications are not too great, and the perspective understandable.

The Many Types of Magnetic Resonance Examination

Magnetic resonance, unlike computed tomography (CT) or other imaging modalities, is a collection of techniques that enable many aspects of the structure, biochemistry, and function of the brain to be identified completely noninvasively. The scanner is still the standard 'workhorse' for the acquisition of anatomic images. Even for this standard procedure, there are a number of choices that have to be made by the operator in order to acquire the most informative information. It is, therefore, important when considering a specific pathology that the technique is 'optimized' in order to identify the pathologic substrate that is the subject of the investigation. There are many choices of imaging sequence, orientation, slice thickness, and imaging time, all of which can contribute to optimization of the imaging. This often needs to be defined for each pathologic entity that is to be investigated, and it cannot be assumed that simple or 'routine' imaging is adequate for the acquisition of images that will allow the identification of all important abnormalities.

Magnetic resonance techniques can also do more than noninvasively acquire pictures of slices through the brain. Three-dimensional data sets can be acquired, which allows reformatting of the two-dimensional image in any plane and with any slice thickness. This is akin to the ability to reformat (or remontage) the electroencephalogram (EEG) data after it is acquired if it is acquired digitally. This is important for dealing with partial volume effects and for volume measurement techniques. Techniques are also available that can help to quantify tissue characteristics such as the T2 or T1 relaxation times. This requires different sequences and provides different information from that obtained with standard anatomic imaging techniques. MR can also identify biochemical aspects of a selected region of the brain by MR spectroscopy (MRS) and can provide low-resolution images of these metabolites using chemical shift imaging (CSI). These techniques can be used to identify specific metabolites and their relative concentrations in specific areas of the brain (Chapter 13).

Functional MRI (fMRI) takes MR technology into the field of imaging brain function as well as structure. The noninvasive nature of MR techniques and the high spatial resolution of MR hold great promise for the investigation of many aspects of brain function, both in normal states and in pathologic conditions. fMRI is now available on most clinical scanners in conjunction with the rapid imaging technique of echo-planar imaging. Although there is much yet to learn about this technique and its implications, it extends the importance of MR into many new areas. This provides a practical means of achieving the dream of being able to link brain structure and function by noninvasive investigations in the same subject during the same integrated examination.

These are the techniques that give rise to the clinical information that is the subject of this book. Before considering these techniques and their clinical applications specifically, it is important to discuss some general principles that apply to all these techniques. As we have already emphasized, the aim of this is to introduce concepts that we believe should be familiar to all who spend time using imaging techniques in the care of patients with epilepsy. It is not intended to provide a detailed explanation of basic principles or to be a substitute for a text in this area.

Terminology

The importance of nuclear magnetic resonance (NMR) in the field of neurology, and in particular in the field of epilepsy, can be compared to the impact on medicine that has followed from such major discoveries and developments as the X-ray and the EEG. The basic principle upon which all NMR experiments have been based was described by Block and Purcell in the mid 1940s. That is, *if certain nuclei are placed in a magnetic field, they are able to 'absorb' energy in a specific radio frequency range, and signal can be recorded as a result of this energy exchange as these nuclei return to their original state.* This phenomenon is the basic principle of NMR. In recent years, the word 'nuclear' has been dropped because of its association with the concept

of radiation. MR techniques do not rely on ionizing radiation and are not associated with exposure to any radioactivity at all.

Some Basic Principles of Magnetic Resonance Physics

Magnetic Properties of Atomic Nuclei

The technique of MRI is based on the intrinsic properties of atomic nuclei of charge, spin, and magnetism. The magnetic property is especially enhanced in certain naturally occurring nuclei such as ^{1}H (protons), ^{31}P (phosphorus), and ^{23}Na (sodium) and these are the nuclear species that are commonly investigated with NMR. The nuclei can be considered as tiny bar magnets and, when positioned in an external magnetic field, will align themselves along the direction of the field in the same way that a compass needle aligns itself with magnetic north. But the nucleus differs from this simple model in that it possesses another intrinsic property, nuclear spin (or spin angular momentum), and can be considered as spinning continuously around the nuclear axis. The combination of nuclear magnetism and spin confers properties on the nuclei that have an analogy with a spinning top that has tipped from the vertical direction. In the same way that the top rotates around both its own axis and the vertical direction of the gravitational field, the nucleus rotates around both the direction of an external magnetic field and its own axis (Fig. 2.1). This frequency of the *precession* around the magnetic field is characteristic of the particular nucleus and the direct linear relationship between frequency and the strength of the magnetic field is fundamental to NMR. For example, the improvement of signal-to-noise ratio (SNR) in MR images acquired in a 3 T scanner is improved with respect to images acquired in a standard 1.5 T scanner by a direct result of the doubling of the fundamental precession frequency that this relationship predicts.

In fact, two discrete possibilities exist for the direction of the precession: one for the nucleus aligned along the direction of the external magnetic field (represented in Fig. 2.1) and another one in the opposite direction (anti-aligned).

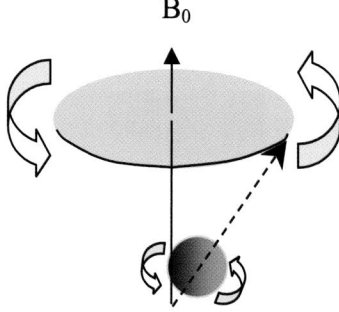

FIG. 2.1. A nucleus in the presence of an external magnetic field, B_0. As a consequence of the intrinsic properties of spin and magnetism, it will also rotate around not only its own axis but also the axis of the external magnetic field. This is known as precession.

As expected, the former state of alignment is preferred and the majority of nuclei in a large 'ensemble' or collection of nuclei will assume this state (low energy). However, a certain proportion of the nuclei will be anti-aligned (high energy) and it is this population difference that underlies the phenomenon of NMR. In the presence of a pulse of electromagnetic waves whose energy corresponds to the difference between these two states, the energy from these waves will be absorbed by the system – a process of resonance (hence nuclear magnetic 'resonance') – and the populations of spins in the two states will be equalized. The frequency region of the electromagnetic spectrum (in the order of tens of megahertz) that is suitable for this purpose is known as radiofrequency (RF).

This perturbed state is temporary and, once the application of the electromagnetic waves is terminated, the nuclei will return to the initial state. The energy previously absorbed by the system will hence be returned in the form of a signal that can be detected by a suitably placed receiver coil. By imposing conditions on the system using magnetic field gradients (see later), this signal will reflect not only the nuclear species from which it originated but also its spatial location. A spatially encoded map of these signals – an MR image – can thereby be formed. The nucleus of the hydrogen atom (^1H) – the proton – is especially suitable for this technique and since water (H_2O) forms more than 80% of the human body, imaging with 'proton MRI' has revolutionized the clinical imaging of soft tissue.

For a more detailed discussion of the principles of physics that give rise to the MR signal, and how this is then manipulated to create an image, refer to one of the texts listed at the end of this chapter.

The Energy Used in Magnetic Resonance and Its Biological Effects

The energy which is used in the process by which the MR image is acquired is not known to cause any harmful biologic effects. As compared to both X-rays (as in CT) and radioisotopes (as in positron-emission tomography, PET, and single-photon-emission CT, SPECT), the energy used in MR imaging is nine orders of magnitude (1,000,000,000 times) less than the energy of X-rays and radioisotopes. It is known to be largely the high energy of the radiation (in X-rays) that causes biologic damage to cells (particularly their DNA), and therefore, even from first principles, the extremely low energy of the radiofrequency electromagnetic radiation employed in MR studies (when compared to X-rays) is far less likely to cause significant biologic damage.

X-Rays Compared to Magnetic Resonance

It is worth keeping in mind that the basic principle of X-rays and NMR signals are fundamentally different.

X-ray images stem from the interaction between the X-rays themselves and the electron cloud of the atoms. This is a 'diffraction technique' and the resolution that can be obtained is therefore related to the wavelength of the radiation (X-rays are high-frequency electromagnetic radiation with high energy). If MR were to use this principle, then the wavelength is so long (low-frequency and low-energy electromagnetic radiation) that the smallest object that could be seen using radiofrequency diffraction (at these energy levels) would be of the order of meters in size. In contrast to this, the NMR is a 'resonance technique' and stems from intrinsic properties of the nucleus described in the previous section.

Magnetic Resonance Signal and Spectroscopy

It should be understood that the standard MR image derives from the relatively strong signal that comes from hydrogen protons (^1H). This is simply because this signal is so strong that we can generate good SNR, and good spatial resolution as a result of this. MR signal can also arise from other nuclei; in particular ^{13}C, ^{19}F, ^{23}Na, and ^{31}P, which are currently used principally in research studies. These nuclei produce smaller signals as the result of a combination of the naturally occurring proportions of these nuclei in the body and the lower intrinsic NMR sensitivity of these species. While these so-called multinuclear studies suffer from relatively low levels of SNR and resolution, they can provide important information about biochemical and metabolic processes.

The technique classification of MRS describes the monitoring of these nuclei with NMR. It represents a simplified form of imaging without spatial encoding in which the intensity of the NMR signal is examined as a function of spectral frequency (see paragraphs below). It has become increasingly common to combine spectroscopy with methods of spatial localization in order to generate spatially encoded metabolite information and even low-resolution images. Common techniques for spatial localization are known as chemical shift imaging (CSI), point-resolved spectroscopy (PRESS), and image selected in vivo spectroscopy (ISIS).

The frequency of the energy that is absorbed by the 'visible' atomic nuclei (those with magnetic properties) when they are placed in a magnetic field depends on many factors such as the exact type of nucleus, the field strength of the external magnetic field, and the physical and chemical environment that the nucleus finds itself in. It is this latter property – the fact that the physical–chemical environment of the nucleus affects the frequency of the MR signal – that is so important for MR spectroscopy studies.

Chemical Shift

The effects of the local environment of the molecule acts to alter the effect of the applied magnetic field at the nucleus of interest. Specifically, the applied magnetic field acts to induce currents in the electron clouds about the nucleus, which in turn causes an opposing magnetic field. The magnetic field felt at the nucleus is then the difference of the applied magnetic field and the field generated by the electrons. For example, the hydrogen nucleus absorbs and transmits energy at different frequencies depending on the environment in which the nucleus finds itself. This phenomenon is known as 'chemical shift'. The resonant frequency of protons in water is, therefore, slightly different from the frequency of hydrogen nuclei in a different chemical environment. For example, a molecule of ethanol (at low resolution) displays a ^{1}H spectrum consisting of three resonances rising from the each of the three types of ^{1}H nucleus (Fig. 2.2). The relative positions of these resonances are invariant with field strength, such that resonances are reported in terms of their chemical shift in units of units of 10^{-6} (ppm, parts per million) of the applied field strength.

The chemical shift of the nucleus of interest, therefore, provides biochemical information about its environment. A typical proton spectrum is shown in Fig. 2.3A. A chemical shift is seen in hydrogen nuclei from protons in fat, in metabolites such as choline, creatine, *N*-acetyl-aspartate (NAA), and also from those in glutamate, lactate, and other substances. This provides the basis for the identification of these substances in living tissue. In a similar manner, a phosphorus spectrum provides information about important phosphorus-containing metabolites such as adenosine triphosphate (ATP) and phosphoesters (Fig. 2.3B). Clinically relevant information is mostly obtained from this region of the proton spectrum.

Signal Strength of Brain Metabolites

In proton MRS, the maximum strength of the signal we can detect depends on the concentration of the chemical in which the hydrogen nucleus is located. The signals from metabolites such as NAA (arising from the ^{1}H nucleus but with a different frequency from the water signal because of

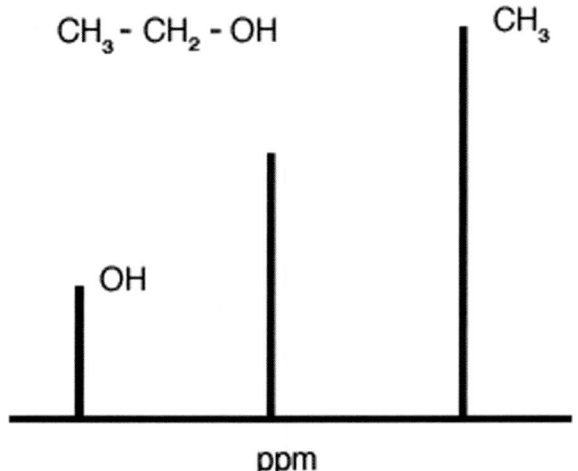

FIG. 2.2. Schematic of the spectrum of ethanol at low resolution.

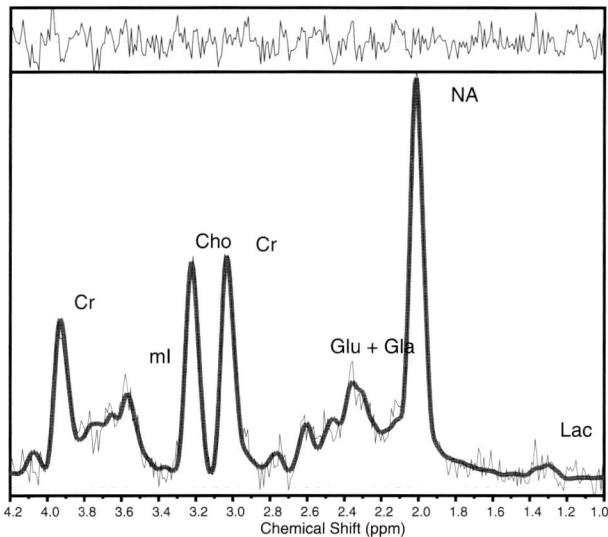

A

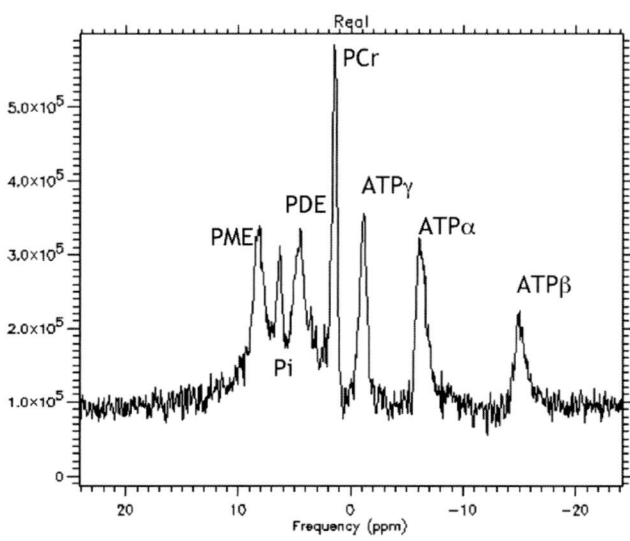

B

FIG. 2.3. A. Proton spectrum of the human frontal lobe at 3 T, showing multiple peaks from Cr (creatine and phosphocreatine) and peaks from NAA (*N*-acetyl aspartate), Cho (choline and choline-containing compounds), and myoinositol (ml). The dark line is the fitted spectrum using a basis set acquired on the system and applied by LC Model. The residual of the fit is listed in the upper panel. **B.** Phosphorus spectrum from the human brain at 3 T showing three peaks from ATP (adenosine triphosphate), PCr (phosphocreatine), PDE (phosphodiesters), Pi (inorganic phosphate), and PME (phosphomonoesters).

its different chemical environment) are about 1/10 000 the intensity of the water signal in the proton spectra. The presence of a large water signal is essential for imaging brain anatomy but is a major problem for proton spectroscopy as the water signal tends to 'drown out' these smaller signals. Therefore, to see these signals one needs to reduce the intensity of the water signal by special techniques ('water suppression') in order to be able to concentrate on this region of the spectrum, which is composed of signals of such low intensity. Similarly, the signal from the relatively concentrated extracranial fat component is usually unwanted and can interfere with the spatial localization imposed by more complicated MRS techniques such as CSI ('chemical shift artifact'). Various methods of 'spectral editing' can be used to eliminate this extracranial lipid component.

The Three Magnetic Fields Used in MR Studies

There are three separate magnetic fields generated by different equipment in an MR system, all of which are important for the generation and interpretation of signals that are used in clinical studies. Inside the main magnetic field (generated by the superconducting magnet) are contained two distinct electromagnet systems, which supply additional magnetic fields. The magnetic field gradient set that is used in the standard method of spatial localization with standard MR imaging is located between the main magnet and the bore of the magnet (covered by the plastic finish that is seen when looking into the bore). Another system (the RF coil) is physically located within the main magnet bore and is usually in close association with the part of the body that is to be imaged. This is the component that we can see attached to the patient during an imaging study.

The Main Magnetic Field

The strongest magnetic field, denoted B_0, therefore usually referred to in magnetic resonance as the main magnetic field or simply as 'the magnet', is measured in teslas (standard units of magnetic field strength). There are several designs of magnet, but at higher field strengths ($>0.5\,T$) the main magnetic field is usually created by superconducting electromagnets which require cooling with liquid helium. Therefore, $1.5\,T$ refers to a system in which the main magnet generates a homogeneous magnetic field of this strength within the bore of the magnet. It is essential that this main magnetic field is as homogeneous as possible within the area in which MR studies are performed, as small variations in the magnetic field (by the field gradients and the RF coil) are used to encode information such as spatial position. For this reason inhomogeneities caused by, for example, metal will distort the homogeneous field and will grossly interfere with image quality. In fact, the degree of field inhomogeneity is required to be better than $100\,ppm$ within the region of interest for imaging and considerably better for useful spectroscopic investigations. In order to improve the field characteristics, magnet systems are delivered with shim coils, which act as a direct means to improve the degree of homogeneity.

The Magnetic Field Gradients

Magnetic field gradients modify the main magnetic field so that the magnetic field varies with spatial position in a linear manner within the magnet bore. They are commonly denoted G_x, G_y, and G_z to describe physical gradients in the three principal directions. These extra magnetic fields are generated by a set of three gradient coils that are placed within the magnet bore. As a consequence of these gradients, the same nuclei at different positions along the gradient direction will experience a slightly different total magnetic field, and therefore precess with a slightly different frequency. Since this distribution of precessional frequencies is imposed on the system and is therefore known, it can be used to allocate spatial information to the signal generated with the result that an image can be reconstructed.

The Radiofrequency Pulse

As previously described, signal formation in NMR is a consequence of the transmission of a short-lasting RF pulse to the spin system at a frequency close to the energy difference between the two energy states that the nuclei can exhibit (this process is known as excitation). It can be shown that this corresponds to a pulse of oscillating magnetic field that is itself precessing at the fundamental precessional frequency of the nucleus in question. This magnetic field, denoted the B_1 field, is generated by yet another system within the bore of the magnet that is generally known as the RF coil. The direction of this RF pulse needs to be perpendicular to the main magnetic field for the energy to be efficiently absorbed. It is this oscillating field that excites the nuclei and results in the generation of a signal. The same coil is usually used to detect the resulting NMR signal after the excitation stage has been terminated. The coil is then known a combined 'transmitter-receiver' coil.

Pulse Sequences

The main magnetic field is static and does not change. The other two magnetic fields can be switched on or off. A pulse sequence is a combination, or sequence, of radiofrequency and gradient pulses that are used to affect the tissue magnetization in specific ways in order to generate a signal that can then be analyzed to create an image (or a spectrum). Specific pulse sequences have particular properties that can be used to generate different contrast (for example T1 and T2 weighting). Some typical sequences will be discussed shortly.

Many pulse sequences use so-called 90° or 180° RF pulses or combinations of these, and it is helpful to understand what these are. As previously described, when a sample is placed in an external magnetic field, the nuclei in the sample are either aligned or anti-aligned with the main field, with an excess of nuclei in the former state. This creates a net magnetic 'vector' – also known as net 'magnetization' – which is effectively the sum effect of the large group of nuclei (or 'spins') in the sample. The vector is aligned with the direction of the main field (conventionally called the longitudinal or z-direction). The RF pulse is applied in a direction that is perpendicular to this direction (the *xy*-plane, known also as the 'transverse plane') and induces a rotation of this net magnetic vector around the direction of the RF magnetic field. The degree of rotation induced by this pulse can be shown to be proportional to the duration and the amplitude of the RF pulse. A 90° pulse therefore describes an RF pulse that rotates the net magnetization vector by this amount. The vector is thereby rotated into the transverse, *xy*-plane where a signal can be detected by the receiver coil. It should be noted that signals cannot be detected in the longitudinal plane. A 180° pulse will be twice as strong and can be used to either invert the magnetization in the *z*-direction or to reverse the direction of the magnetization when it is already in the *xy*-plane (see spin echo imaging). These manipulations are crucial to obtaining MR signals. The strength of the RF pulses have to be calibrated at the beginning of each study. Manipulation of the magnetic field in this way is essential for all aspects of imaging and for generating tissue contrast.

THE MAGNETIC RESONANCE IMAGE

There are a large number of techniques that can be used to generate an MR image and for the optimization of contrast, which will allow pathologic areas of the brain to be identified. The general principle is that *if the lesion is not seen on a particular MR study it does not mean that it cannot be seen using other MR techniques.*

There are a large number of operator-dependent choices that will determine the sensitivity of the MR technique, and as a consequence the clinical MR examination has to be planned according to what information is most important to identify. What is seen in the MR image depends on factors such as the SNR, the contrast between different tissues, the amount of partial voluming within the sample, the slice thickness, and the spatial resolution of the image. As these things often are related in such a way that improving one of them worsens another, it is important to understand something of these relationships in order to be able to 'optimize' the MR examination.

The Ideal Imaging Sequence

For maximum image quality, we would like to have good SNR, high resolution, good contrast between the different tissues we want to visualize, no artifacts such as partial volume or motion, and we would also like the time to acquire the images to be as short as possible. We have listed some of these properties in Box 2.1.

The Concept of 'Optimization'

In the following section we will deal briefly with each of these issues. It should be emphasized here that our aim in

---

> **BOX 2.1** The Ideal MR Sequence Should Have
>
> - High signal-to-noise ratio
> - High spatial resolution
> - Thin slices or three-dimensional data sets
> - High contrast between normal tissues
> - High contrast between pathologic and normal tissue
> - No artifacts (e.g. motion, partial volume)
> - Short acquisition time
> - Quiet pulse sequences

considering these problems is to provide the minimum practical guidance as to what factors may be important (and we think need to be known by all who have an interest in MR imaging) in the acquisition of useful MR images. Again this section is intended to provide an overview of important issues rather than being a substitute for a basic text on MR imaging.

It will quickly become clear that, as in life, we cannot have everything all the time and that compromises must be made. This introduces the concept of *optimizing* the images that are acquired in order to solve the clinical problem that we are faced with. It is of no use to have a technically impressive method of image acquisition, or a short imaging time, if the information these images provide do not allow the appropriate clinical diagnosis.

What optimization means may differ among the different specialists dealing with imaging. To the neurologist, optimization may mean making the diagnosis with the greatest sensitivity and specificity possible *regardless of imaging time* while, to the busy neuroimaging service, optimization may mean producing images that allow the diagnosis with the greatest sensitivity and specificity *within a specified examination time*. Similarly, the production of beautiful-appearing images may be of no value if there is no contrast between the pathologic region and normal tissue. For this reason, among many others, it has become essential for neurologists, neuroradiologists, and physicists to work together, all with a basic understanding of the types of compromise that are being made in the imaging so that the optimized diagnostic studies are performed. This is essential both in clinical practice and in clinical research.

Signal-to-Noise-Ratio

The SNR reflects the amount of meaningful signal (which will make up the image) that is detected compared to the amount of random signal (or noise) that is also detected (which does not reflect meaningful information). If the magnitude of the random signal is too high with respect to the magnitude of the meaningful signal then it may be impossible to construct an image of sufficient diagnostic quality.

In MRI, for a given pulse sequence and for given pulse parameters, the SNR is directly proportional to two main factors – the voxel size and the square root of the number of data acquisitions. The voxel is the element of three-dimensional space whose volume is given by the product of the slice thickness and the in-plane resolution. The in-plane resolution is, in turn, determined by the field-of-view (FOV) and the matrix size in the x- and y-directions of 'frequency encoding' and 'phase encoding' respectively. A single acquisition is the acquisition of one complete data set (all phase encode steps) and takes a fixed amount of time depending on the acquisition parameters specified. If, for example, we acquire this information four times, the signal will be four times as great but, as the noise does not add coherently, it will be only twice as big (noise increases by the square root of n (SYMBOL)) resulting in a SNR which is twice as great.

$$SNR \propto slice\ thickness \bullet \sqrt{\frac{(NEX) \bullet (FOV)^2}{(N_x \bullet N_y)}}$$

where NEX = the number of times the slice is acquired (all phase steps repeated), FOV = the field of view, N_y = the number of phase encoding steps, and N_x = the number of frequency encoding steps.

It should be noted that this acquisition does not take into account the imaging time, and other texts should be consulted for a more detailed explanation of the complex interactions of pulse parameters on the SNR.

It can be seen from the equation that certain tradeoffs between certain desired aspects of the scanning procedure have to be made. For example, thinner slices improve the signal resolution in the through-slice direction but will have a lower SNR and in routine imaging a compromise is made between slice thickness and the number of acquisitions. Similarly, improvements in the in-plane resolution are at the expense of a decreased SNR. Note also that there is a proportionally increased effect of slice thickness that cannot be easily regained by increasing the number of times the image is acquired. For example, to acquire an image with the same SNR and with half the slice thickness, the number of acquisitions of the slice would have to be increased by a factor of four (effectively quadrupling the acquisition time).

In this way, SNR competes with in-plane spatial resolution, slice thickness, and acquisition time. As an alternative way of viewing this interaction, a high level of SNR in a voxel can be viewed as money in the bank. We can decide how to spend it; we can choose to buy increased spatial resolution, thinner slices, or shorter imaging time. Each of these has a different value. Unfortunately, as in the real world, the money eventually runs out and we have to make some choices as to what we really want. The choice is made even harder because NEX and FOV do not seem to play fair; we have to spend a lot of SNR to gain a little improvement in resolution (meaning that they are expensive), and we do not really gain as much extra SNR as we would expect by increasing the time taken for the image acquisition. In this way we have to optimize the imaging parameters to acquire the information we need. Obtaining the clinical information

that is required depends on the particular optimization for the things that are wanted. Is it in-plane spatial resolution, slice thickness, contrast, SNR, or imaging time? These decisions must be made by consultation between all members of the team.

In-plane Spatial Resolution

The in-plane spatial resolution is determined by the matrix size and the size of the FOV; that is how many voxels we divide the area we are imaging into. A typical matrix in clinical practice is 256 × 256, which means that the whole image is divided, in two dimensions, into an array of this many compartments or picture elements (pixels). The actual size of the pixels will depend on the FOV. If we know the third dimension of the slice thickness as well we can determine the voxel volume, i.e. the volume of tissue from which the signal in each element arises. As discussed in the previous paragraphs, improved resolution is at the expense of SNR. The voxel size is therefore determined by the tradeoff.

Zero Filling

An alternative matrix, such as a 256 × 128 matrix, gives pixels that are not square. In this case, there are 256 samples of the echo in the x-direction (frequency encoding) and 128 steps in the y-direction (phase encoding). As will be discussed shortly, for standard imaging the total acquisition time is directly proportional to the number of the phase-encoding steps (and not the frequency-encoding steps) and the time taken to acquire each one of them (the repetition time, TR).

With the acquisition of these rectangular pixels, the resolution in the phase encoding direction is halved with respect to the 256 × 256 acquisition but the acquisition time is also halved. In fact, the image reconstruction of such a matrix can be manipulated to produce a square 256 × 256 matrix by use of the process known as zero-filling. Nevertheless, the 'true' resolution in the phase-encoding direction is unchanged by this process. The consequence of this acquisition scheme is an improvement of the SNR by a factor of 2 × √2, with contributions from the differing resolution (×2) and acquisition time (√2).

Asymmetric Field of View

Another alternative for scan time reduction is the acquisition of an asymmetric field of view. The same size of pixel is acquired but over a zoomed FOV in the y-direction. The spatial resolution is unchanged relative to the square 256 × 256 scan and the acquisition time is reduced. Care must be taken, however, that the FOV in the y-direction is sufficient to contain the extent of the sample in that direction so that image artifacts do not arise.

Slice Thickness

The slice thickness determines the through-plane resolution. The relationship of slice thickness and SNR has already been discussed. Another important issue when deciding on the optimal in-plane and though-plane resolution is that of partial voluming. This is the 'mixing' of signals from different tissue types within the same voxel, which leads to a blurring of the signal intensities. The smaller the voxel size, the better will be the suppression of partial volume effects. However, this will be at the cost of acquisition time.

Problems of Movement

Motion is a major problem in standard MRI pulse sequences such as the spin echo, in which the image is acquired one phase-encoding step at a time rather than in a single shot. This can be considered to be analogous to acquiring a photographic image at low light intensity. If the shutter of the camera is left open for several minutes, the effects of motion can be considerable (we have all taken that photograph in dim light that was ruined by motion effects). The effect is significant in the MR image not just because of gross head movements but also because of pulsations from blood vessels, eye movement, and respiration, which is intrinsic to the biologic system being imaged. This causes image ghosting, but in MRI this blurring due to motion effects occurs *only* in the phase-encode direction (because of the way the image is acquired).

Imaging Time

We will discuss the factors that give contrast in normal scans (e.g. T1-weighted, and T2-weighted contrast) shortly. Here we will consider how repetition time affects the time taken to acquire the scan as well as the issues of SNR ratio and spatial resolution.

For standard acquisition methods such as spin echo, the time taken to acquire an image is proportional to the number of phase-encode steps multiplied by the time taken to acquire each of these phase-encode steps. This duration between one phase-encode step and the next is known as the repetition time, or TR. It would seem that short TR sequences would give shorter imaging time without losing SNR or spatial resolution. But the TR can be critical for the generation of tissue contrast. It is usually of no use to acquire an image that does not have any contrast between gray and white matter, even if there is strong signal from both of them. Some sequences can use short TR methods to generate contrast, and in some it is essential for the generation of contrast that the tissue magnetization 'relaxes' between excitations (see below). Therefore shortening the TR of a sequence to reduce imaging time needs to be considered carefully.

Contrast

The aim of clinical imaging is to distinguish the structures of the object with such sharpness and accuracy that there is no doubt as to the visualization of the object in the image. A high degree of contrast is therefore a necessity for efficacious imaging. The contrast in MRI is a direct consequence of the relative signal intensities from different tissue types. The aim will always still be to obtain the optimal SNR and therefore, for example, moving to a higher field strength should improve the contrast. The magnetic field strength is an example of an 'extrinsic' contrast parameter and other such parameters determined by the pulse sequence parameters have been discussed in previous sections. The relative levels of signal intensity also depend on several 'intrinsic' factors. The common, and possibly the most important, ones from a medical imaging viewpoint are proton density contrast and contrast as a result of the NMR relaxation time, T2 and T1. The other intrinsic components of the signal that can generate contrast include T2* contrast, diffusion contrast, chemical shift, perfusion contrast, temperature, and bulk flow.

Proton Density Contrast

There is a simple principle that the amount of signal in a given voxel will be dependent on the number of protons in that voxel that can give signals. Therefore if the tissues have differing proton densities, there will be contrast generated between them. In the brain, the principal tissue types have similar proton density – gray matter/white matter contrast in proton-density-weighted images is poor.

Relaxation Times

The equilibrium state of the spin system corresponds to an initial magnetization vector that is aligned along the z-direction. As previously described, subsequent to say, a 90° RF pulse, the net magnetization arising from the spins would precess indefinitely in the transverse plane. This is not a practical reality and the relaxation times describe the return of the spin system to the equilibrium state.

T1 Relaxation Time

The T1 relaxation time is also known as the spin lattice relaxation time or the longitudinal relaxation time. T1 describes the recovery of the magnetization vector to the z-direction. It is governed by exchanges of energy at a particular range of frequencies between the relaxing spin and the surrounding 'lattice.' In fact, the T1 time is given by the time required for the system to recover to 63% of its equilibrium value. For any given nucleus, the T1 depends on the following parameters:

- the type of the nucleus
- the resonant frequency (i.e. related to the field strength)
- the temperature
- the microviscosity, or the mobility of the observed spin
- the presence of large molecules in the immediate vicinity
- the presence of paramagnetic ions and molecules in the vicinity.

In practical purposes, the length of T1 governs the rate at which the sample can be excited. A longer T1 requires that excitation of the sample be at a slower rate so as to allow sufficient magnetization to recover along the longitudinal axis prior to each RF pulse. Differences in T1s of the water resonances from various tissues forms the basis of many imaging sequences to discriminate cerebrospinal fluid water (long T1) from gray matter (shorter T1) and white matter (shortest T1).

T2 Relaxation Time

The T2 relaxation time is also known as the spin–spin relaxation time or the transverse relaxation. This relaxation time describes the loss of 'phase' in the transverse plane. When the spins are first placed in the transverse plane by an RF pulse, they will all be rotating around the z-direction in phase with each other. However, this state does not persist, as a result of intrinsic effects (T2) and magnetic field inhomogeneities (T2′) such that the nuclei in different locations and states begin to precess at a slightly faster or slower rate. This leads to a loss of phase (or 'coherence') that is described by the T2 relaxation times. It should be noted that this process occurs independently of T1 relaxation. T2* describes the combined effects of T2 and T2′ sources of transverse signal dephasing. A spin echo is commonly used to provide T2 contrast while a gradient echo image displays T2* contrast.

The T2 relaxation time is dependent on the following parameters:

- the observation frequency (field strength, although this is much less crucial than for T1)
- the temperature
- the mobility of the observed spin (microviscosity)
- the presence of large molecules, paramagnetic ions and molecules.

PULSE SEQUENCES

Types of Sequence

The main pulse sequence types can be divided into two classifications – spin echo and gradient echo. The main sequence types are therefore:

- spin echo, e.g. SE, FSE
- inversion recovery
- gradient echo, e.g. FLASH, GRASS
- other sequences, e.g. EPI, SENSE, SMASH.

There are many acronyms for specific pulse sequences which can usually be better understood if they can be related to one of these main types.

Spin-echo Sequence

A spin echo is produced by a combination of a 90° and a 180° pulse. These pulses are known as the excitation and refocusing pulses respectively. After the initial application of the 90° pulse, the net magnetization is placed in the transverse plane. T1 relaxation subsequently induces the return of the magnetization to the main field direction. Similarly, T2 and T2* induce a loss of coherence (dephasing) in the transverse plane. The magnetization vector therefore appears to fan out in the xy-plane. In order to rephase these spins and thereby produce a secondary signal, a 180° pulse is applied at a time TE/2 after the 90°, where TE is known as the echo time. This pulse refocuses the transverse magnetization, producing a 'rephased' signal, known as a 'spin echo', centered on a time TE after the 90° pulse. Field inhomogeneities are rephased by the refocusing pulse and the echo signal is a reflection of T2 relaxation from the initial excitation (as described above, T2* is a combination of T2 and T2′ effects). The pulse sequence repeats after a time TR time, during which time the magnetization can recover by T1 relaxation.

By manipulating the echo time (or TE) by altering the timing of the 180° pulse with respect to the 90° pulse, differences in tissue signal as a result of T2 contrast are obtained (this is T2-weighting). Lengthened TE times provides increasingly improved T2-weighting but this is at the cost of decreased signal which is decaying according to T2. The TR time is also important in the contrast provided by the spin-echo sequence. For full recovery of the magnetization to the equilibrium z-direction, the TR has to be long (approximately five times the T1 of the tissue). With repeated 90° pulses, the initial signal size we see in the xy-plane will be dependent on the amount of magnetization that has recovered back to the z-direction during the previous TR period (dependent on the T1 relaxation time). This introduces T1 contrast into short TR spin-echo sequences, which can provide useful contrast. Since T1- and T2-weighting provide opposite contrast in spin-echo imaging, the T2-weighting is usually minimized in this case with use of a short TE.

A rapid implementation of the standard spin-echo sequence is known alternatively as fast spin echo (FSE), turbo spin echo (TSE), or rapid acquisition with relaxation enhancement (RARE). The sequence makes use of multiple 180° pulses (i.e. 90°–180°–180°– ...) to refocus the magnetization on more than one occasion in each pass. The principle of this sequence is that a multiple-echo sequence can contribute more than one phase-encode line to an image during each TR period. The acquisition time is reduced by a factor corresponding to the number of refocusing pulses. Disadvantages are increased RF absorption (specific absorption rate, SAR) and modified T2-contrast effects.

Inversion Recovery

An early method of acquiring T1-weighted images was using an inversion recovery sequence (IR). This is essentially a spin-echo technique with a preceding 180° pulse which can be thought of inverting the magnetization from initial alignment with the z-direction (+z) to anti-alignment (−z). The subsequent recovery of the magnetization to the +z direction is governed by T1 relaxation so the image will have a very flexible degree of T1-weighting.

Image acquisition was commonly achieved with a spin-echo module; however, the sequence was long, and multiple slice acquisition was complicated. Inversion recovery is now usually implemented with rapid imaging techniques such as echo planar imaging.

Gradient-echo Sequences

As an alternative method of spin rephasing after an initial 90° pulse to the spin echo, the gradient-echo sequence employs a changing gradient rather than an additional RF pulse. A dephasing gradient pulse −G is instead applied along the frequency (x) direction, which is followed by a rephasing gradient +G of the opposite polarity. Reversing the sign of the gradient reverses the direction of the precession of the spins in the xy-plane. Therefore, the spins begin to rephase and an echo known as a gradient echo forms at a time TE after the 90° pulse. The gradient echo forms when the phase of all the spins in the excited slice becomes zero. By way of contrast with spin echoes, gradient echoes do not refocus the effects of static field inhomogeneities (T2′) and the signal is therefore T2*-weighted. The advantage of the gradient-echo method is the possibility of manipulating the amount of signal that recovers to the z-direction before each repeated phase-encoding step by a combination of reduced TR and RF flip angles (<90°). Imaging times can thereby be substantially reduced. Many variants of the rapid gradient-echo sequence have been developed with names such as FLASH, GRASS, and FSIP. Differing degrees of contrast can be obtained with modified treatment of remaining transverse magnetization between steps and also by including a preparation period with, for example, a prior inversion pulse, to generate enhanced T1-weighting.

Echo Planar Imaging Sequence

Echo planar imaging (EPI) is the fastest imaging sequence currently available and has the potential to revolutionize many aspects of MR technology. It is a rapid MRI technique that is capable of producing tomographic images at video rates. It is a single-shot method and imaging times are in the order of 100 ms for a 128 × 128 matrix. An initial 90° (gradient-echo EPI) or 90°–180° (spin-echo EPI) combination of pulses tips the magnetization into the transverse plane. A rapid switching of a strong gradient then form a series of gradient echoes, each with a different degree of phase encoding. This means that an entire image can be acquired in a single excitation rather than one, or only a few, during each excitation of the slice.

The echo planar technique depends on specialized equipment, including strong gradient fields that are capable of rapid switching. This creates technical demands but the equipment is now fairly standard on clinical MR scanners. With the increasing use of fMRI in clinical studies in which the speed of acquisition is crucial, this technique has become increasingly used in the clinical domain. The rate of change of the magnetic field during gradient changes is such that induced current can be caused in biologic material (therefore stimulation). Although this was considered to be a potential danger in the initial stages of using this technique, it does not seem to have been a major problem as it is below the threshold for causing biologic damage. The sequence suffers from an increased sensitivity to signal loss from sources of susceptibility differences in the sample.

Functional Magnetic Resonance Imaging

The most important application appears to be in the area of fMRI of the brain. During brain activity there is a rapid momentary increase in the blood flow to the specific areas in the brain. The increase in circulation effectively provides an increase in oxygen, which is paramagnetic and which affects relaxation times of the local brain tissues. The difference in these relaxation times relative to surrounding tissues causes a contrast between the tissues. More specifically, deoxyhemoglobin and oxyhemoglobin are chemically different. Deoxyhemoglobin has an unpaired electron and is therefore paramagnetic while oxyhemoglobin is not. Paramagnetic substances cause a disturbance in the local magnetic field and cause loss of signal due to an increased rate of dephasing. This is predominantly a T2* effect since it include the contribution of static field inhomogeneities (see section on T2 relaxation times above). An activated area therefore exhibits a temporary increase in signal on T2*-weighted images as a result of the decreased concentration of deoxyhemoglobin during the activation.

Gradient-echo images are especially suitable for fMRI because of to their intrinsic T2*-weighting. Spin-echo imaging can also be used since T2 contrast is produced by spins moving through the static fields in the vicinity of the blood vessels. Because this effect is small compared to the overall signal (approximately 2% at 1.5 T for gradient-echo imaging with visual activation), it is best seen as the difference between images acquired during activation and those acquired in the baseline or resting state. As images need to be acquired with an optimal time resolution to sample the rapidly changing tissue oxygenation state, gradient echo EPI has become the sequence of choice for fMRI. For further details see Chapter 10.

Diffusion Contrast

Diffusion images are sensitive to the translational, microscopic motion of water protons in tissue. For the diffusion of water molecules within tissue, this displacement will be affected by phenomena such as restricted diffusion, in which molecules are confined within borders, and the permeability of the cell membranes through which the water molecules diffuse. For this reason, the measured tissue diffusion coefficient, known as an apparent diffusion coefficient (ADC), is closely related to the biophysical environment of the tissue water and can be used to describe cell function and structure. It is termed an apparent measure since the motion of water molecules in tissue is modulated by a number of factors other than brownian motion, including chemical exchange, cell membrane permeability, and structural restriction.

In order to sensitize a pulse sequence to diffusion, pairs of gradient pulses are used. For static spins, perfect rephasing occurs. However, if the spin has moved during or between the application of these gradients, the phase shift accumulated during the first gradient is not reversed by the phase dispersion caused by the second gradient pulse, since the spin's position and, therefore, the phase has altered. A net attenuation of the signal results due to incomplete rephasing of diffusing spins occurs and this signal loss can be directly related to the ADC. Diffusion sensitivity can be affected by changes in ionic homeostasis due to impairments in blood flow.

Diffusion gradients can be incorporated into a large variety of MRI pulse sequences, including EPI. The early sensitivity of diffusion imaging to the tissue damage induced by a stroke has motivated the most important clinical use of diffusion imaging in the evaluation of cerebral ischemia.

Diffusion Tensor Imaging

Diffusion is a three-dimensional process and water mobility may be facilitated along one axis of a structure. The measured ADC along this orientation will be larger than in other directions. The directional dependence of diffusion is known as diffusion anisotropy and is especially apparent in brain white matter, in which diffusion mobility is greater along the nerve axon fibers. Along other directions, diffusion is considered as being restricted. The diffusion coefficient is therefore better represented within brain tissue by a rank-3, two-dimensional tensor that takes into account molecular displacements in the x, y and z directions (diagonal terms) and also their possible coupling terms (nondiagonal terms).

The measurement of the full diffusion tensor can be achieved with multiple measurements using different combinations of gradient pulses in the three gradient axes. This technique is known as diffusion tensor imaging (DTI) and offers the capability to assess white matter fiber organization in healthy and diseased states. Furthermore, three-dimensional visualization of the white matter structures is currently being attempted in various laboratories. Various combinations of tensor parameters can be used to summarize the tensor in a more meaningful manner, such as fractional anisotropy (FA).

Perfusion Imaging

The level of cerebral perfusion is an important indicator of tissue viability and function, and perfusion imaging attempts to directly quantify regional blood flow in the brain. At the capillary level, blood flow can be thought of as irrigating or perfusing a volume of tissue. Since flow at the level of the microcirculation is not a vector quantity, the scalar unit of cerebral blood flow (CBF) is described in terms of the volume of blood perfusing a unit volume of tissue per unit time. The most common units are ml/100 g/min. The CBF of brain gray matter in man is approximately 60 ml/100 g/min.

Cerebral blood volume can be measured with contrast-agent-based perfusion techniques that sample the washout of a gadolinium-based tracer during a single pass. The past 10 years have seen the development of an alternative, non-invasive MRI technique for quantitative measurements of cerebral perfusion that uses tissue water as an endogenous, freely diffusable tracer. The techniques are based on the differentiation of flowing arterial water spins and static tissue spins by the magnetic labeling of one compartment with respect to the other. The blood water spins are delivered to the brain voxel where they are extracted from the capillary bed and join the larger pool of tissue water. The exchange between the magnetically labeled water in blood and tissue leads to a change in tissue magnetization that can be detected by MRI.

The goal of these so-called arterial spin-labeling (ASL) methods is to extract and analyze the flow-related magnetization change. The tagged images are alternated with control images in which the flow label is not applied. The signal difference between these two images directly reflects local quantitative perfusion, since the static tissue signal is eliminated. Variants of this technique include FAIR, QUIPSS, and CASL. These techniques have been used to study a wide variety of pathologies such as stroke and epilepsy.

Parallel Imaging

Rapid imaging has taken a big leap forward with the development of parallel imaging techniques such as SENSE and SMASH, in which multiple receiver coils are used to boost the imaging time. The improvement in scan time is related to the number of receiver coils but the relationship is not linear. For a fixed scan time, the techniques can be used to boost spatial and temporal resolution or to improve patient coverage. Fast cardiac studies of a single heartbeat are now feasible and the liver can be imaged in a single breath-hold. The benefits of the parallel imaging techniques are enhanced at high-field with scan time increases of up to six or eight times possible at 3 T. Commercial 1.5 T and 3 T systems are now available from the major manufacturers with parallel imaging provided as standard.

FURTHER READING

Abragam A. Principles of nuclear magnetism. Oxford: Clarendon Press, 1961.

Bloch F, Hansen WW, Packard ME. Nuclear induction. *Phys Rev* 1946;69:127.

Buxton RB. *An introduction to functional magnetic resonance imaging: principles and techniques.* Cambridge: Cambridge University Press, 2001.

Calamante F, Thomas DL, Pell GS, et al. Measuring cerebral blood flow using magnetic resonance imaging techniques. *J Cereb Blood Flow Metab* 1999;19:701–735.

DeGraaf R. *In vivo NMR spectroscopy: principles and techniques.* New York: John Wiley, 1999.

Detre JA, Leigh JS, Williams DS, Koretsky AP. Perfusion imaging. *Magn Reson Med* 1992;23:37–45.

Farrar TC, Becker ED. Pulse and Fourier transform NMR. *Introduction to theory and methods.* New York: Academic Press, 1971.

Fukushima E, Roeder SBW. *Experimental pulse NMR: a nuts and bolts approach.* New York: Addison Wesley, 1981.

Gadian DG. *NMR and its applications to living systems*, 2nd ed. Oxford: Oxford University Press, 1996.

Haacke EM, Brown RW, Thompson MR, Venkatesan R. *Magnetic resonance imaging: physical principles and sequence design.* New York: John Wiley, 1999.

Jezzard P, Matthews PM, Smith SM, eds. *Functional magnetic resonance imaging: an introduction to methods.* Oxford: Oxford University Press, 2001.

Jones DK, Williams SC, Gasston D, et al. Isotropic resolution diffusion tensor imaging with whole brain acquisition in a clinically acceptable time. *Hum Brain Mapping* 2002;15:216–230.

Knowles PF, Marsh D, Rattle HWE. *Magnetic resonance of biomolecules.* London, Wiley 1976.

Morris PG, Morris SC. *Nuclear magnetic resonance imaging in medicine and biology.* Oxford: Clarendon Press, 1988.

Moseley ME, Kucharczyk J, Mintorovitch J, et al. Diffusion-weighted MR imaging of acute stroke: correlation with T2-weighted and magnetic susceptibility-enhanced MR imaging in cats. *Am J Neuroradiol* 1990;11:423–429.

Pruessmann KP, Weiger M, Scheidegger MB, Boesiger P. SENSE: sensitivity encoding for fast MRI. *Magn Reson Med* 1999;42:952–962.

Purcell EM, Torrey HC, Pound RV. Resonance absorption by nuclear magnetic moments in a solid. *Phys Rev* 1946;69:37–38.

Rinck P. *Magnetic resonance in medicine*, 4th ed. Malden, MA: Blackwell Science, 2001.

Sodickson DK, Manning WJ. Simultaneous acquisition of spatial harmonics (SMASH): ultra-fast imaging with radiofrequency coil arrays. *Magn Reson Med* 1997;38:592–603.

Stark DD, Bradley WG, Bradley WG. *Magnetic resonance imaging*, 3rd ed. St Louis, MO: Mosby, 1999.

Wehrli FW, Shaw D, Kneeland BJ, eds. *Biomedical magnetic resonance imaging: principles methodology and applications.* Weinberg: VCH Publishing, 1988.

Wehrli FW. *Fast scan magnetic resonance: principles and applications.* New York: Raven Press, 1991.

Westbrook C, Kaut C. *MRI in practice*, 2nd ed. Malden, MA: Blackwell Science, 1998.

CHAPTER 3

Brain Anatomy

Henri Duvernoy

INTRODUCTION

An overview of the general organization of the human cerebral surface will allow the position of hippocampus to be appreciated before moving on to study its anatomy. (For more information about the surface cortical anatomy see reference 1.)

The hemispheres are divided into frontal, temporal, parietal, and occipital lobes by fissures and sulci (central sulcus, lateral, parieto-occipital, and temporo-occipital fissures). The lateral surface of the *frontal lobe* is divided into precentral, superior (F1), middle (F2), and inferior (F3) gyri by three sulci: superior frontal, inferior frontal, and precentral. The middle frontal gyrus is often subdivided into superior and inferior parts by the middle frontal sulcus (Figs 3.1, 3.2). The inferior surface of the frontal lobe, often called the orbital lobe, is composed of the lateral, medial, anterior, and posterior orbital gyri and by the gyrus rectus (Figs 3.5, 3.6).

The *temporal lobe* is situated on the lateral, inferior, and medial aspects of the hemisphere. Four sulci – the superior temporal (or parallel), inferior temporal, lateral occipitotemporal and medial occipitotemporal (or collateral) – divide the temporal lobe in five gyri: superior temporal (T1), middle temporal (T2), inferior temporal (T3), fusiform (T4), and parahippocampal (T5).

The *occipital lobe,* like the temporal lobe, is visible on the lateral, inferior, and medial aspects of the hemisphere. Its anatomy is intricate. Sulci and gyri are difficult to identify. Nevertheless, the occipital lobe can be divided into six gyri: superior (01), middle (02), and inferior (03), occipital gyri, fourth occipital gyrus (04), lingual gyrus (05), and cuneus (06).

On the lateral surface of the hemisphere, the superior, middle, and inferior gyri are separated from each other by the superior and inferior occipital sulci. The large middle occipital gyrus is often subdivided into superior and inferior parts by the lateral occipital sulcus (Figs 3.1, 3.9). On the inferior and medial surfaces, the lateral temporo-occipital, collateral, and calcarine sulci delimit the inferior occipital, fourth occipital, and lingual gyri and the cuneus. The lateral surface of the *parietal lobe* is divided by the intraparietal sulcus into three gyri: the postcentral, superior (P1), and inferior (P2) parietal gyri. The inferior parietal gyrus is itself subdivided into supramarginal and angular gyri. The superior parietal gyrus lies on the superior margin of the hemisphere and overlaps its medial surface, where it is called precuneus (Figs 3.1, 3.3, 3.9, 3.10).

A supernumerary lobe, the *limbic lobe,* is often described on the medial and inferior aspects of the hemisphere (Figs 3.3, 3.19). The limbic lobe is delimited by the limbic fissure, which is mainly composed of the cingulate and collateral sulci. The limbic lobe may be divided into a large limbic and slender intralimbic gyri. The *limbic gyrus* is successively made up of the subcallosal gyrus, the cingulate gyrus, and the isthmus, which together belong, from an anatomical point of view, to the frontal and parietal lobes, and the parahippocampal gyrus (T5), which is part of the temporal lobe (see above).

The uncus or anterior part of the parahippocampal gyrus curves posteriorly and overlaps the parahippocampal gyrus; only the anterior segment of the uncus belongs to the parahippocampal gyrus and so to the limbic gyrus, whereas its posterior segment is a part of the intralimbic gyrus.

The *intralimbic gyrus* is mainly formed by the *hippocampus,* the hippocampus bordering the parahippocampal gyrus (Fig. 3.19) belongs to the temporal lobe from an anatomical point of view (Fig. 3.17) and to the limbic lobe functionally. It is a cortical fold, which bulges into the floor of the temporal horn of the lateral ventricle. After opening the temporal horn and removing the choroid plexuses (Fig. 3.18), the hippocampus appears as an arc, medially concave, which may look like a sea horse. This arc is composed of three segments: a head or anterior part, transversally oriented, a body or middle part, which is sagittally oriented, and a tail or posterior part, again transversally oriented and situated beneath the splenium.

STRUCTURE OF THE HIPPOCAMPUS

For more information about the hippocampal structures and functions see references 2–56.

The hippocampus is formed by two cortical laminae embedded in each other, the cornu ammonis and the gyrus dentatus (Fig. 3.20). The cornu ammonis is linked to the parahippocampal gyrus by the subiculum, a transitional cortex. According to the different aspects of the pyramidal neurons, the *cornu ammonis* can be divided into four fields: CA1, which is linked to the subiculum; CA2; CA3, in contact with the ventricular cavity; and CA4, in close contact with the gyrus dentatus. The endoventricular aspect of the cornu ammonis is covered by a thin lamina of white matter, the alveus, which joins the fimbria. The fimbria extends backwards into the crus of the fornix.

The *gyrus dentatus* is a narrow dorsally concave lamina mainly composed of small rounded cells, the granular neurons. The gyrus dentatus, by its concavity, encloses the CA4 field of the cornu ammonis. These two structures form together the area dentata. The superficial part of the gyrus dentatus, visible on the medial aspect of the temporal lobe, is called margo denticulatus or dentes of the gyrus dentatus and is separated from the subiculum by a narrow hippocampal sulcus. The cornu ammonis, gyrus dentatus and subiculum are joined together to constitute a functional unit, the hippocampal formation, belonging to the limbic system. A large amount of information, originating from wide association areas, projects to the entorhinal area and then to the subiculum. From the subiculum, fibers successively reach the gyrus dentatus, CA3, CA1, and then return to the subiculum. Thus, the subiculum seems to be the center of this chain. It sends the definite responses, which return to the associative areas by way of the fimbria, fornix, and thalamus or directly through the entorhinal cortex.

Through these wide cortical connections, the *hippocampal formation* is mainly involved in the creation of memory, in association with the amygdala. Lesions of the hippocampal formation mainly located in CA1, which shows a selective vulnerability to hypoxia (CA1 is known as 'the vulnerable sector' of the cornu ammonis), produce anterograde amnesia characterized by defects in remembering events that occur after the appearance of the lesion.

HIPPOCAMPAL ANATOMY

The aspects of the hippocampal body, head, and tail will be studied in succession.

Hippocampal Body

The hippocampal body (Figs 3.18, 3.20, 3.24, 3.25, 3.27, 3.34) presents the most typical aspect of the hippocampal anatomy and is made up of the cornu ammonis and the gyrus dentatus, which form two U-shaped interlocking laminae. The cornu ammonis is a strongly convex protrusion in the floor of the temporal horn covered with alveus and limited medially by the fimbria and laterally by the collateral eminence.

The gyrus dentatus is a deep structure whose narrow superficial segment, the margo denticulatus, is partly hidden by the fimbria. The margo denticulatus is composed of rounded protrusions, which form the dentes of the gyrus dentatus, and is separated from the subjacent subiculum by an often ill-defined hippocampal sulcus.

Hippocampal Head

The hippocampal head (Figs 3.18, 3.23–3.25, 3.33, 3.40) is the voluminous anterior part of the arc of the hippocampus. It includes an intraventricular part and an extraventricular part. The intraventricular part is composed of several protrusions, the digitationes hippocampi, which are folds of cornu ammonis.

The extraventricular part, belonging to the posterior segment of the uncus, is divided into the apex (often wrongly called the intralimbic gyrus), the band of Giacomini, which prolongs the margo denticulatus in the uncus, and the gyrus uncinatus.

Hippocampal Tail

The hippocampal tail (Figs 3.18, 3.20, 3.29–3.32, 3.39, 3.41) is the slender posterior part of the hippocampal arc. Each of the constituents of the hippocampus can be found in the tail but with different names: thus the cornu ammonis becomes superficially the gyrus fasciolaris, which continues under the splenium as the subsplenial gyrus and further as the indusium griseum on the dorsal surface of the corpus callosum (Fig. 3.20). The superficial part of the gyrus dentatus forms the fasciola cinerea, which disappeared under the splenium. Folds of cornu ammonis sometimes lift the surface of the parahippocampal gyrus, producing the gyri of Andreas Retzius (Fig. 3.20).

RELATIONS OF THE HIPPOCAMPUS WITH THE SURROUNDING NERVOUS STRUCTURES

The hippocampus has important relationships with:

- the temporal horn
- the temporal lobe
- the mesencephalon.

The hippocampus bulges into the *temporal horn* of the lateral ventricle (Figs 3.17, 3.18) and is covered by voluminous choroid plexuses, with the exception of the digitationes hippocampi, which are free of them. The hippocampus is bordered laterally by the protrusion of the collateral eminence, which prolongs caudally by the collateral trigone, forming the floor of the ventricular atrium. Through the atrium, the temporal horn communicates with the occipital horn (Figs 3.19, 3.22, 3.23).

The hippocampus is situated on the medial aspect of the temporal lobe (Fig. 3.20). Through the temporal horn of the ventricle, the hippocampal head is covered by the amygdala (Figs 3.24, 3.25, 3.39–3.41) and the hippocampal body by the tail of the caudate nucleus and the stria terminalis (Figs 3.21, 3.27). The temporal stem, a narrow lamina of white matter, separates the temporal horn and the hippocampus from the superior and middle temporal gyri and the deep parallel (superior temporal) sulcus (Figs 3.24–3.28).

The arched right and left hippocampi surround the *mesencephalon* (Figs 3.22, 3.23) and the vessels which encircle it, especially the posterior cerebral and anterior choroid arteries and the basal veins. These vessels run into the subarachnoid cisterns lining the mesencephalon (Fig. 3.22), which are the interpeduncular cistern (Figs 3.35, 3.36) on the anterior aspect of the mesencephalon, the crural and ambient cisterns (Figs 3.26–3.31, 3.34–3.36) on its lateral aspect, and the quadrigeminal cistern on its posterior aspect (Figs 3.30, 3.33–3.37). The wing of the ambient cistern prolongs the ambient cistern in the lateral part of the transverse fissure, which is closed laterally by the choroid fissure in contact with the temporal horn (Figs 3.21, 3.30, 3.35, 3.36). Finally, the right and left hippocampi are in close contact with the free edge of the tentorial opening, especially at the uncal level (Fig. 3.23). In herniation of the temporal lobe, the uncus slips between the tentorial edge and the crus cerebri and may compress the mesencephalon and the posterior cerebral artery.

This brief anatomical study, which is a summary of a previous work, will make it easier to understand the coronal, axial, and sagittal sections on Figures 3.24–3.43 (see also hippocampal sections).

ACKNOWLEDGMENT

Figures 3.7, 3.8, 3.9, 3.10, 3.11 and 3.19 have been reproduced with permission from Springer Verlag (The Human Brain, Duvernoy, H., 1995, © Springer-Verlag).

REFERENCES

1. Duvernoy HM. The Human Brain. Surface, Blood Supply and Three-dimensional Sectional Anatomy, 2nd edn, New York: Springer Verlag Wien, 1991.
2. Amaral DG, Campbell MJ. Transmitter systems in the primate dentate gyrus. *Hum Neurobiol* 1986;5:169–180.
3. Amaral DG, Witter MP. The three-dimensional organization of the hippocampal formation: a review of anatomical data. *Neuroscience* 1989;3:571–591.
4. Angevine JB. Development of the hippocampal region. In: Isaacson RL, Pribram KH, eds. The hippocampus. I: Structure and development. New York: Plenum Press, 1975:61–94.
5. Babb TL, Brown WJ. Neuronal, dendritic, and vascular profiles of human temporal lobe epilepsy correlated with cellular physiology in vivo. In: Delgado-Escuela AV, Ward AA, Woodbury DM, Porter RJ, eds. Basis mechanisms of the epilepsies. Advances in Neurology. New York: Raven Press, 1986:949–966.
6. Babb TL, Brown WJ, Pretorius J, et al. Temporal lobe volumetric cell densities in temporal lobe epilepsy. *Epilepsia* 1984;6:729–740.
7. Benveniste H, Jorgensen MB, Sandberg M, et al. Ischemic damage in hippocampal CA1 is dependent on glutamate release and intact innervation from CA3. *J Cerebral Blood Flow Metab* 1989;9:629–639.
8. Blackstad TW. Commissural connections of the hippocampal region in the rat, with special reference to their mode of termination. *J Comp Neurol* 1956;105:417–538.
9. Blackstad TW. On the termination of some afferents to the hippocampus and fascia dentata. *Acta Anat* 1958;35:202–214.
10. Braak H. On the structure of the human archicortex. I – The cornu Ammonis. A Golgi and pigmentarchitectonic study. *Cell Tissue Res* 1974;152:349–383.
11. Chronister RB, White LE. Fiber architecture of the hippocampal formation: anatomy, projections and structural significance. In: Isaacson RL, Pribram KH. The hippocampus. I: Structure and development. New York: Plenum Press, 1975:9–39.
12. Crunelli V, Forda S, Kelly JS. Excitatory amino acids in the hippocampus: synaptic physiology and pharmacology. TINS 1985:26–30.
13. Duvernoy HM. The Human Hippocampus. Functional Anatomy, Vascularization and Serial Sections with MRI, 2nd edn, Springer Verlag Berlin Heidelberg, 1998.
14. Earle KM, Baldwin M, Penfield W. Incisural sclerosis and temporal lobe seizures produced by hippocampal herniation at birth. *Arch Neurol Gen Psychiatry* 1953;27:42.
15. Gastaut H, Lammers HJ. Anatomie du rhinencephale. Paris: Masson, 1961.
16. Green RC, Mesulam MM. Acetylcholinesterase fiber staining in the human hippocampus and parahippocampal gyrus. *J Comp Neurol* 1988;273:488–499.
17. Haigler HJ, Cahill L, Crager M, Charles E. Acetylcholine, aging and anatomy: differential effects in the hippocampus. *Brain Res* 1985;362:157–160.
18. Isaacson RL. The limbic system. New York: Plenum Press, 1974.
19. Johansen FF, Jorgensen MB, Ekström von Lubits DKJ, Diemer N. Selective dendrite damage in hippocampal CA1 stratum radiatum with unchanged axon ultrastructure and glutamate uptake after transient cerebral ischaemia in the rat. *Brain Res* 1984;291:373–377.
20. Liliequist B. The subarachnoid cisterns. An anatomic and roentgenologic study. *Acta Radiol* 1959;Suppl 185:61–71.

21. Lopes da Silva FH, Arnolds DEAT. Physiology of the hippocampus and related structures. *Ann Rev Physiol* 1978;40:185–216.

22. Lorente de No R. Studies on the structure of the cerebral cortex. II: Continuation of the study of the Ammonic system. *J Psychol Neurol* 1934;46:113–177.

23. Lynch G, Baudry M. The biochemistry of memory: a new and specific hypothesis. *Science* 1984;224:1057–1063.

24. Mani RB, Lohr JB, Jeste DV. Hippocampal pyramidal cells and aging in the human: a quantitative study of neuronal loss in sectors CA1 to CA4. *Exp Neurol* 1986;94:29–40.

25. Margerison JH, Corsellis JAN. Epilepsy and the temporal lobes. *Brain* 1966;89:499–536.

26. Milner PM. A cell assembly theory of hippocampal amnesia. *Neuropsychologia* 1989,27:23–30.

27. Morris RGM, Hagan JJ. Allocentric spatial learning by hippocampectomised rats: a further test of the 'spatial mapping' and 'working memory' theories of hippocampal function. *Q J Exp Psychol* 1986;38B:365–395.

28. Naidich TP, Daniels DL, Haughton VM, et al. Hippocampal formation and related structures of the limbic lobe: anatomic-MR correlation. Part I: Surface features and coronal sections. *Radiology* 1987;162: 747–754.

29. Nieuwenhuys R. Chemoarchitecture of the brain. Berlin: Springer, 1985.

30. Nieuwenhuys R, Voogd J, Van Huijzen CH. The human central nervous system. A synopsis and atlas. Berlin: Springer, 1978.

31. O'Keefe J, Nadel L. The hippocampus as a cognitive map. Oxford: Oxford University Press, 1978.

32. Olton DS, Wible CG, Shapiro ML. Mnemonic theories of hippocampal function. *Behav Neurosci* 1986;100:852–855.

33. Onodera H, Sato G, Kogure K. Lesions to Schaffer collaterals prevent ischemic death of CA1 pyramidal cells. *Neurosci Lett* 1986;68:169–174.

34. Press GA, Amaral DG, Squire LR. Hippocampal abnormalities in amnesic patients revealed by high-resolution magnetic resonance imaging. *Nature* 1989;341:54–57.

35. Rosene DL, VAN Hoesen GW. The hippocampal formation of the primate brain. A review of some comparative aspects of cyto-architecture and connections. In: Jones EG, Peters A, eds. Cerebral cortex, vol. 6. Further aspects of cortical function, including hippocampus. New York: Plenum Press, 1987:345–456.

36. Saunders RC, Rosene DL. A comparison of the efferents of the amygdala and the hippocampal formation in the rhesus monkey: I. Convergence in the entorhinal, prorhinal, and perirhinal cortices. *J Comp Neurol* 1988;271:153–184.

37. Scharrer E. Vascularization and vulnerability of the cornu Ammonis in the opossum. *Arch Neurol Psychiatry* 1940;44:483–506.

38. Schwerdtfeger WK. Structure and fiber connections of the hippocampus. A comparative study. In: Advances in anatomy, embryology and cell biology 83. Berlin: Springer 1984:74.

39. Schwerdtfeger WK. Light and electron microscopic data on field CA1 of the hippocampus of the squirrel monkey, *Saimiri sciureus*. *J Hirnforsch* 1986;27:521–532.

40. Shefer VFF. Hippocampal pathology as a possible factor in the pathogenesis of senile dementias. *Neurosci Behav Physiol* 1977;8,: 236–239.

41. Squire LR. Mechanisms of memory. Science 1986;232:1612–1619.

42. Squire LR, Zola-Morgan S. The medial temporal lobe memory system. *Science* 1991;253:1380–1386.

43. Sutherland RJ. The navigating hippocampus: an individual medley of movement, space, and memory. In: Buzsaki G, Vanderwolf CH. Electrical activity of the archicortex. Budapest: Akadémiai Kiado, 1985:255–279.

44. Sutula TH, Cascino G, Cavazos J, Parada I, Ramirez L. Mossy fiber synaptic reorganization in the epileptic human temporal lobe. *Ann Neurol* 1989;26:321–330.

45. Swanson LW. The hippocampus. New anatomical insights. TINS 1979: 9–12.

46. Teyler TJ, Discenna P. The topological anatomy of the hippocampus: a clue to its function. *Brain Res Bull* 1984;9:711–719.

47. Teyler TJ, Discenna P. The role of hippocampus in memory: a hypothesis. *Neurosci Biobehav Res* 1985;12:377–389.

48. Tryhubczak A. Myeloarchitectonics of the hippocampal formation in the dog. *Fol Biol* 1975;23:177–188.

49. Vanderwolf CH, Leung LWS, Stewart DJ. Two afferent pathways mediating hippocampal rhythmical slow activity. In: Buzsaki G, Vanderwolf CH. Electrical activity of the archicortex. Budapest: Akadémiai Kiado, 1985:47–66.

50. Van Hoesen GW. Neural systems of the non-human primate forebrain implicated in memory. OLTON DS. Memory dysfunctions: an integration of animal and human research from preclinical and clinical perspectives. *Ann NY Acad Sci* 1985;444:97–112.

51. Vogt C, Vogt O. Sitz und Wesen der Krankheiten im Lichte der topistischen Hirnforschung und des Variierens der Tiere, 1er Teil. Leipzig: Barth, 1937.

52. Walaas I. The hippocampus: In: Emson PC. Chemical neuroanatomy. New York: Raven Press, 1983:337–358.

53. West MJ, Gundersen HJG. Unbiased stereological estimation of the number of neurons in the human hippocampus. *J Comp Neurol* 1990; 296:1–22.

54. Yasargil MG. Microneurosurgery. vol. I: Microsurgical anatomy of the basal cisterns and vessels of the brain, diagnostic studies, general operative techniques and pathological considerations of the intra-cranial aneurysms. Stuttgart: Thieme, 1984.

55. Zola-Morgan S, Squire LR, Amaral DG. Human amnesia and the medial temporal region: enduring memory impairment following a bilateral lesion limited to field CA1 of the hippocampus. *J Neurosci* 1986;6:2950–2967.

56. Zola-Morgan S, Squire LR, Amaral DG. Lesions of the hippocampal formation but not lesions of the fornix or the mammillary nuclei produce long-lasting memory impairment in monkeys. *J Neurosci* 1989;9:898–913.

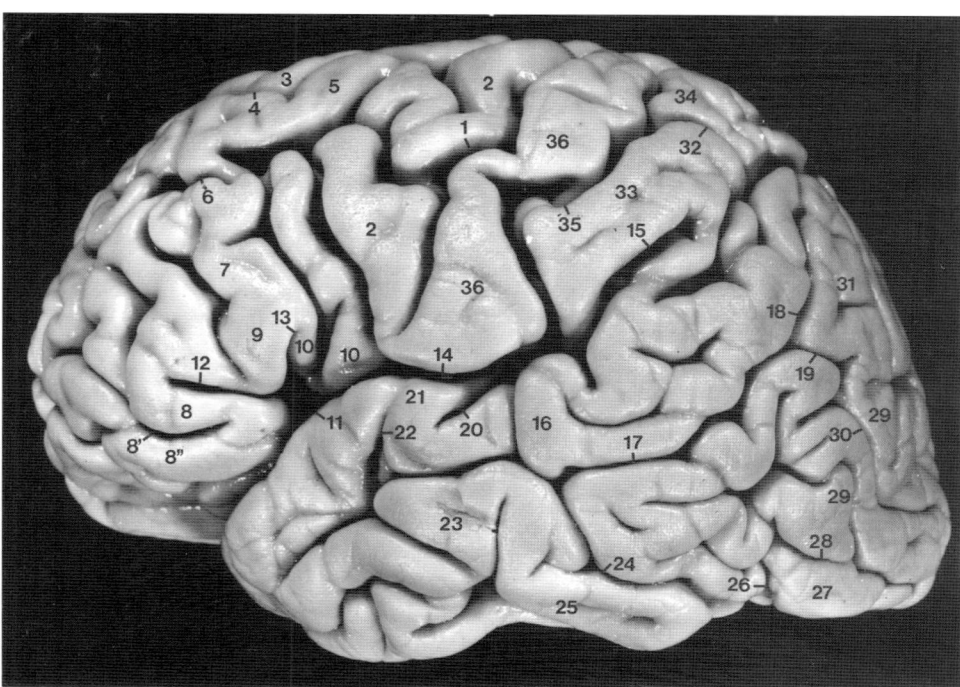

FIG. 3.1. Lateral aspect of the left hemisphere.

1 Central sulcus
2 Precentral gyrus
3 Superior frontal gyrus (F1)
4 Superior frontal sulcus
5 Middle frontal gyrus (F2)
6 Inferior frontal sulcus
7 Inferior frontal gyrus (F3)
8 Pars orbitalis
8′ Lateral orbital sulcus
8″ Lateral orbital gyrus
9 Pars triangularis
10 Pars opercularis
11 Lateral fissure, anterior segment
12 Horizontal ramus of lateral fissure
13 Vertical ramus of lateral fissure
14 Lateral fissure, middle segment
15 Lateral fissure, posterior segment
16 Superior temporal gyrus (T1)
17 Anterior segment of superior temporal sulcus

18 Ascending posterior segment of superior sulcus
19 Horizontal posterior segment of temporal sulcus
20 Transverse temporal sulcus
21 Transverse temporal gyrus
22 Sulcus acousticus
23 Middle temporal gyrus (T2)
24 Inferior temporal sulcus
25 Inferior temporal gyrus (T3)
26 Temporo-occipital incisure
27 Inferior occipital gyrus (O3)
28 Inferior occipital sulcus
29 Middle occipital gyrus (O2)
30 Lateral occipital sulcus
31 Angular gyrus
32 Intraparietal sulcus
33 Supramarginal gyrus
34 Superior parietal gyrus (P1)
35 Inferior postcentral sulcus
36 Postcentral gyrus

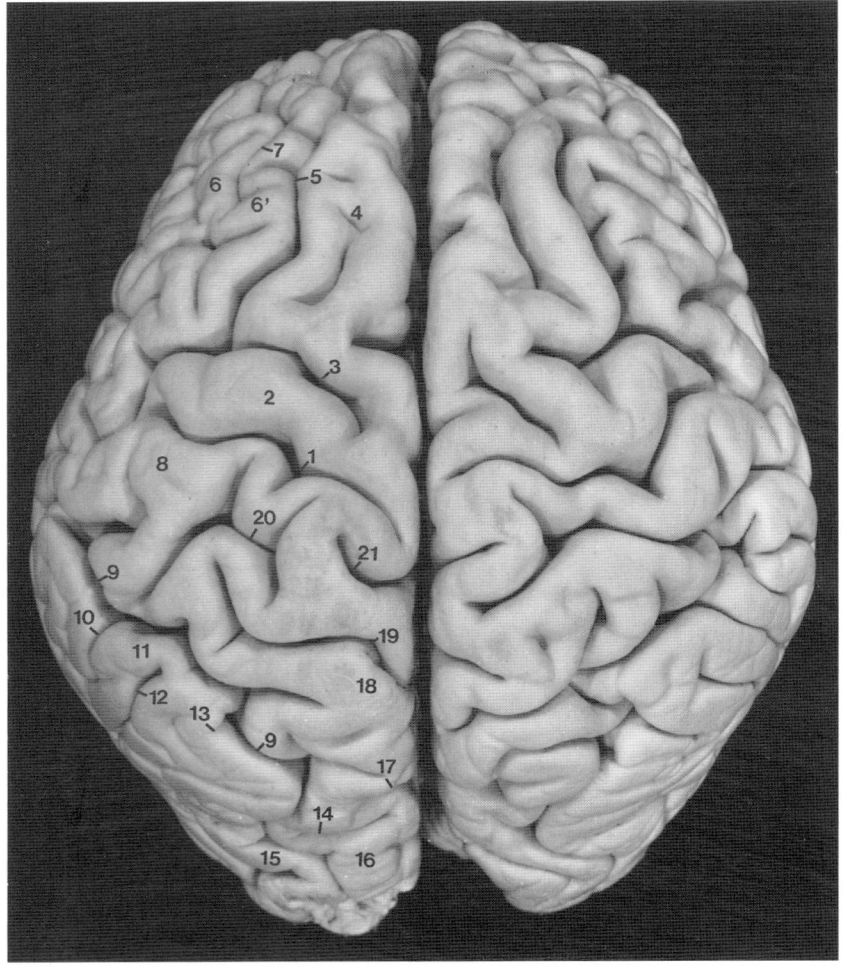

FIG. 3.2. Superior aspect of the left and right hemispheres.

1 Central sulcus
2 Precentral gyrus
3 Superior precentral sulcus
4 Superior frontal gyrus (F1)
5 Superior frontal sulcus
6,6″ Middle frontal gyrus
7 Middle frontal sulcus
8 Postcentral gyrus
9 Intraparietal sulcus
10 Sulcus intermedius primus (Jensen)
11 Angular gyrus
12 Superior temporal sulcus

13 Sulcus intermedius secundus
14 Transverse occipital gyrus
15 Middle occipital gyrus (O2)
16 Superior occipital gyrus (O1)
17 Parieto-occipital fissure
18 Superior parietal gyrus (P1)
19 Transverse parietal sulcus
20 Superior postcentral sulcus
21 Cingulate sulcus, marginal segment

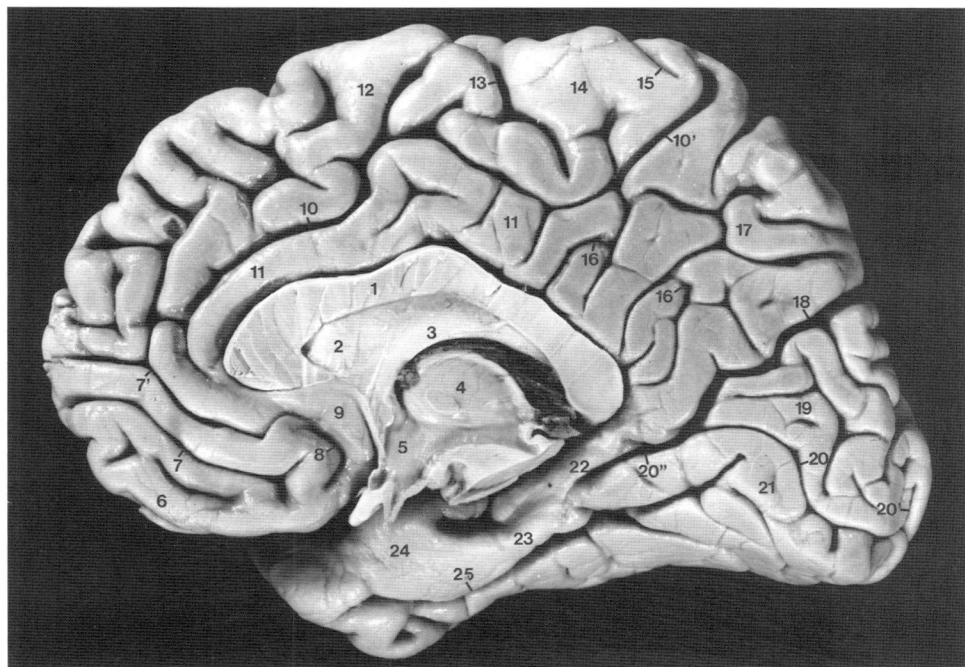

FIG. 3.3. Medial aspect of the right cerebral hemisphere.

1 Corpus callosum
2 Septum pellucidum
3 Fornix
4 Thalamus
5 Hypothalamus
6 Gyrus rectus
7,7' Suborbital sulci
8 Anterior paraolfactory sulcus
9 Subcallosal gyrus
10 Cingulate sulcus
10' Marginal segment of cingulate gyrus
11 Cingulate gyrus
12 Medial aspect of superior frontal gyrus (F1)
13 Paracentral sulcus
14 Paracentral lobule

15 Central sulcus
16 Subparietal sulcus
17 Precuneus
18 Parieto-occipital fissure
19 Cuneus
20 Calcarine sulcus
20' Retrocalcarine sulcus
20" Anterior calcarine sulcus
21 Lingulal gyrus
22 Isthmus
23 Parahippocampal gyrus
24 Uncus
25 Collateral sulcus

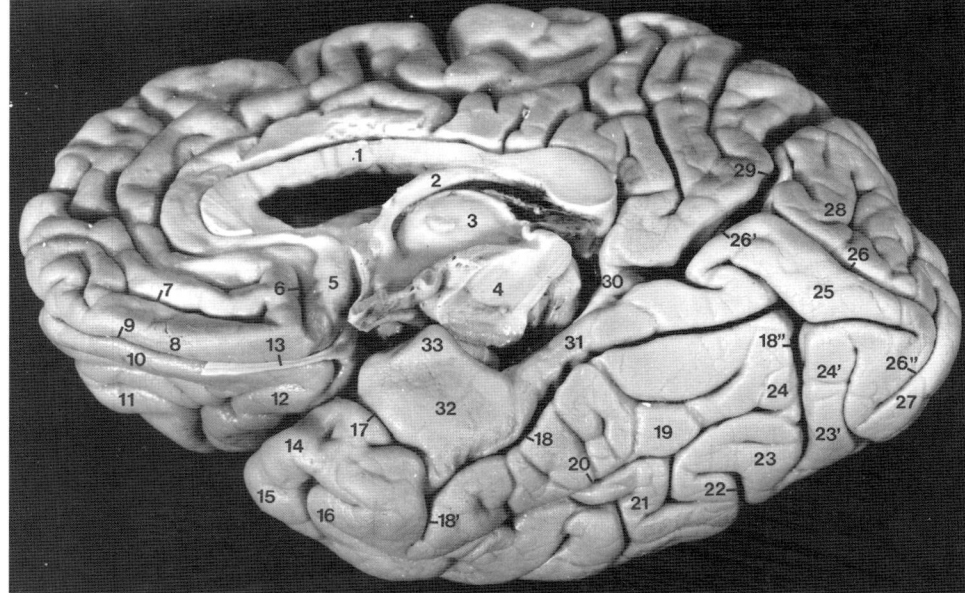

FIG. 3.4. Inferomedial aspect of the right cerebral hemisphere.

1 Corpus callosum
2 Fornix
3 Third ventricle
4 Cut surface of mesencephalon
5 Subcallosal gyrus
6 Anterior paraolfactory sulcus
7 Suborbital sulcus
8 Gyrus rectus
9 Medial orbital sulcus
10 Medial orbital gyrus
11 Anterior orbital gyrus
12 Posterior orbital gyrus
13 Olfactory tract
14 Temporal pole, superior temporal gyrus (T1)
15 Temporal pole, middle temporal gyrus (T2)
16 Temporal pole, inferior temporal gyrus (T3)
17 Rhinal sulcus
18 Collateral sulcus
18′ Anterior transverse collateral sulcus

18″ Posterior transverse collateral sulcus
19 Fusiform gyrus (T4)
20 Lateral occipitotemporal sulcus
21 Inferior temporal gyrus (T3)
22 Temporo-occipital incisure
23, 23′ Inferior occipital gyrus (O3)
24, 24′ fourth occipital gyrus
25 Lingual gyrus (O5)
26′ Calcarine sulcus
26″ Anterior calcarine sulcus
26 Retrocalcarine sulcus
27 Gyrus descendens
28 Cuneus (O6)
29 Parieto-occipital fissure
30 Isthmus
31 Parahippocampal gyrus (T5)
32 Piriform lobe (entorhinal area)
33 Gyrus ambiens

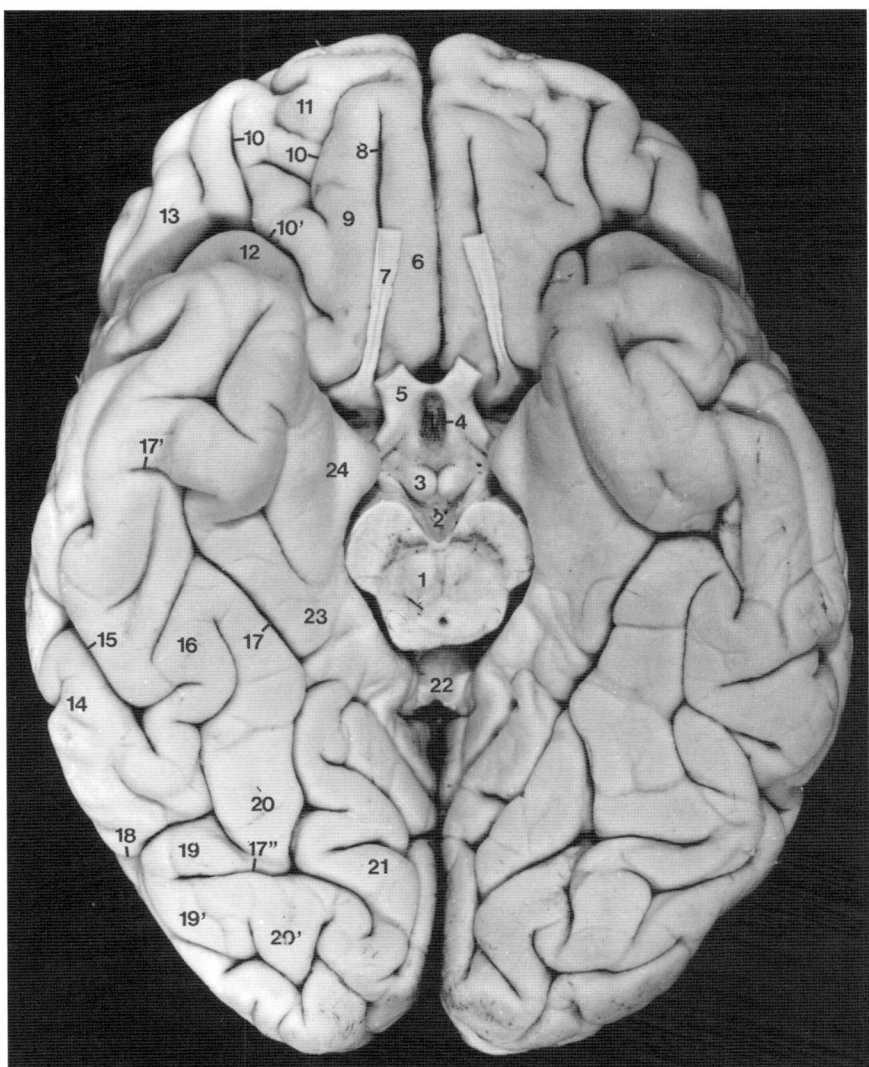

FIG. 3.5. Inferior aspect of the brain with cerebellum and brainstem removed.

1 Cut surface of mesencephalon
2 Interpeduncular fossa
3 Mamillary body
4 Hypophyseal stalk and median eminence
5 Optic chiasma
6 Gyrus rectus
7 Olfactory tract
8 Medial orbital sulcus
9 Medial orbital gyrus
10 H-shaped orbital sulcus
10′ Arcuate orbital sulcus
11 Anterior orbital gyrus
12 Posterior orbital gyrus
13 Lateral orbital gyrus
14 Inferior temporal gyrus (T3)

15 Lateral occipitotemporal sulcus
16 Fusiform gyrus (T4)
17 Collateral sulcus
17′ Anterior transverse collateral sulcus
18 Temporo occipital incisure
19 Inferior occipital gyrus (O3)
19′ Inferior occipital gyrus (O3)
20 Fourth occipital gyrus (O4)
20′ Fourth occipital gyrus
21 Lingual gyrus (O5)
22 Splenium
23 Parahippocampal gyrus
24 Uncus

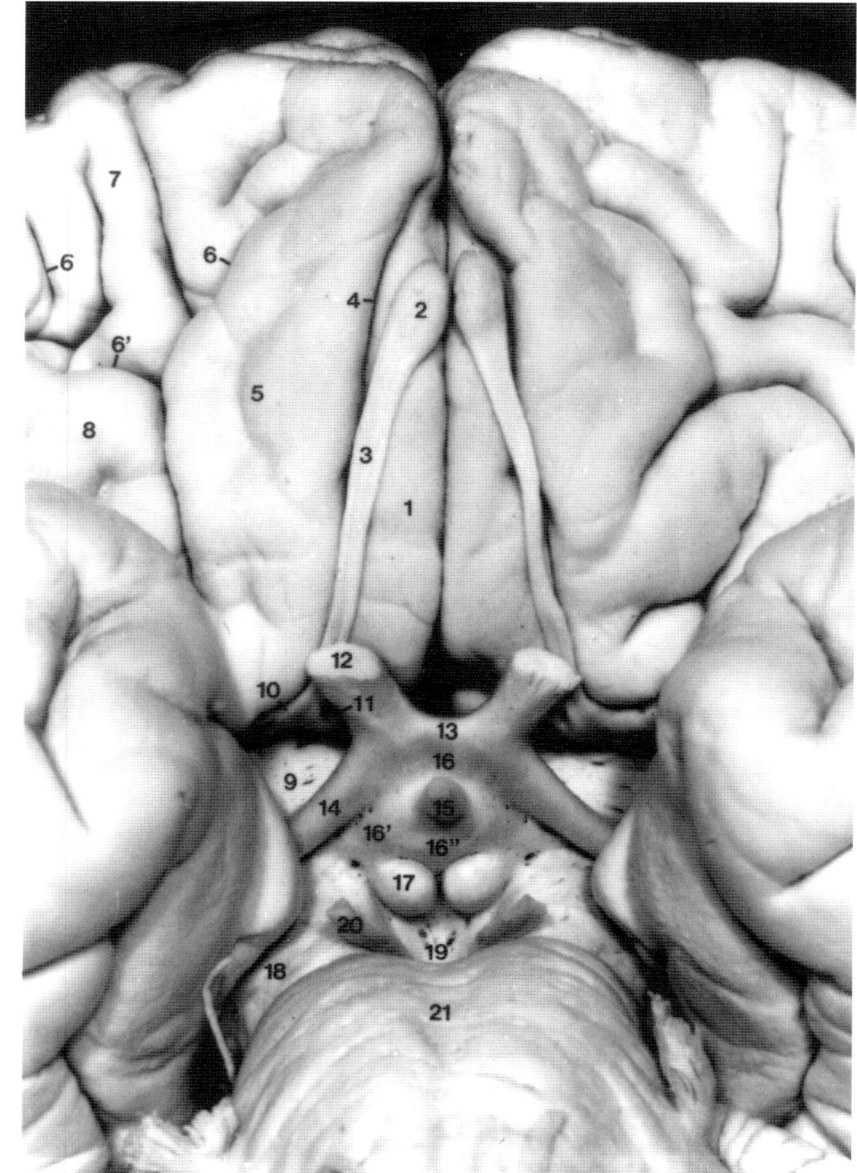

FIG. 3.6. Basal surface of the brain – orbital lobe.

1 Gyrus rectus
2 Olfactory bulb
3 Olfactory tract
4 Medial orbital sulcus
5 Medial orbital gyrus
6 H-shaped orbital sulcus
6' Arcuate orbital sulcus
7 Anterior orbital gyrus
8 Posterior orbital gyrus
9 Anterior perforated substance
10 Lateral olfactory stria
11 Medial olfactory stria
12 Optic nerve

13 Optic chiasma
14 Optic tract
15 Hypophysial stalk
16 Anterior tuber
16' Lateral tuber
16" Posterior tuber
17 Mamillary body
18 Crus cerebri
19 Interpeduncular fossa
20 Oculomotor nerve
21 Pons

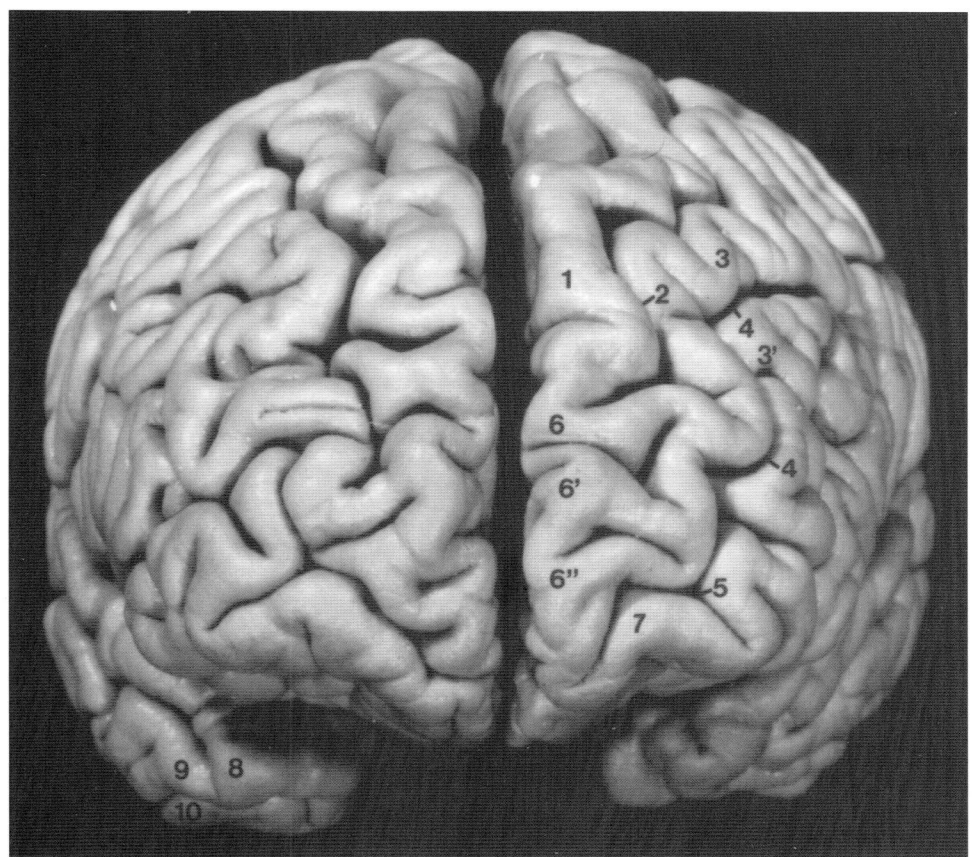

FIG. 3.7. Frontal pole, anterior aspect.

1 Superior frontal gyrus
2 Superior frontal sulcus
3,3′ Middle frontal gyrus (F2), superior and inferior parts
4 Middle frontal sulcus reaching 5

5 Frontomarginal sulcus
6,6′,6″ Superior, middle, and inferior transverse frontopolar gyri
7 Frontomarginal gyrus

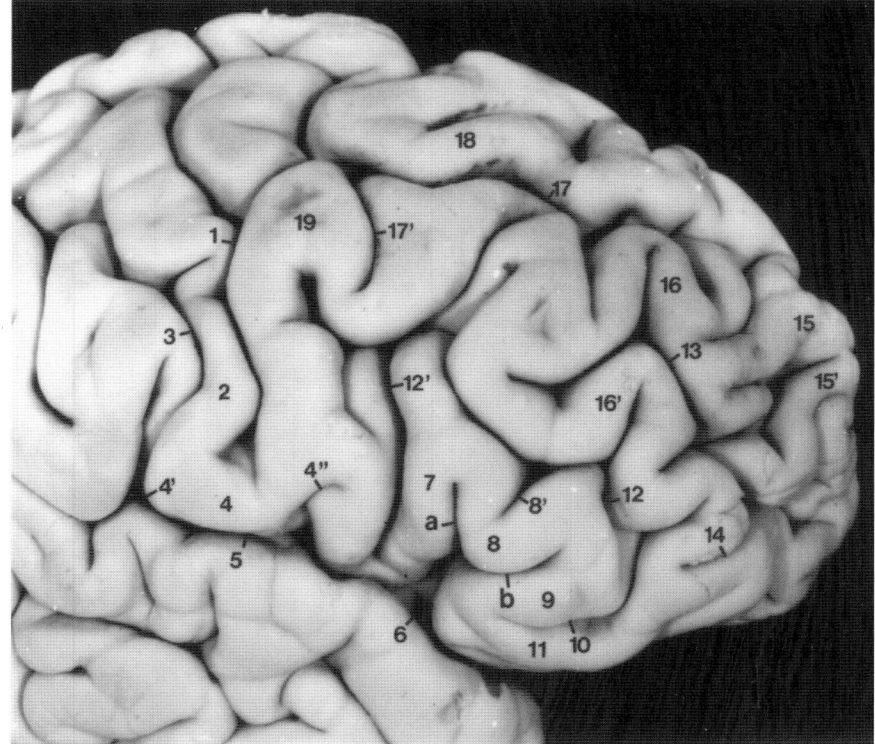

FIG. 3.8. Lateral aspect of the right frontal lobe.

1 Central sulcus
2 Postcentral gyrus
3 Inferior postcentral sulcus (ascending portion)
4 Subcentral gyrus
4′ Posterior subcentral sulcus
4″ Anterior subcentral sulcus
5 Lateral fissure, middle segment
6 Lateral fissure, anterior segment; a vertical and b horizontal ramus
7 Inferior frontal gyrus (F3), pars opercularis
8 Inferior frontal gyrus (F3), pars triangularis
8′ Sulcus triangularis
9 Inferior frontal gyrus (F3), pars orbitalis

10 Lateral orbital sulcus
11 Lateral frontal sulcus
12 Inferior frontal sulcus
12′ Inferior precentral sulcus
13 Middle frontal sulcus reaching 14
14 Frontomarginal sulcus
15 Superior frontopolar gyrus
15′ Inferior frontopolar gyrus
16,16′ Middle frontal gyrus (F2) superior and inferior parts
17 Superior frontal sulcus
17′ Superior precentral sulcus
18 Superior frontal gyrus
19 Precentral gyrus

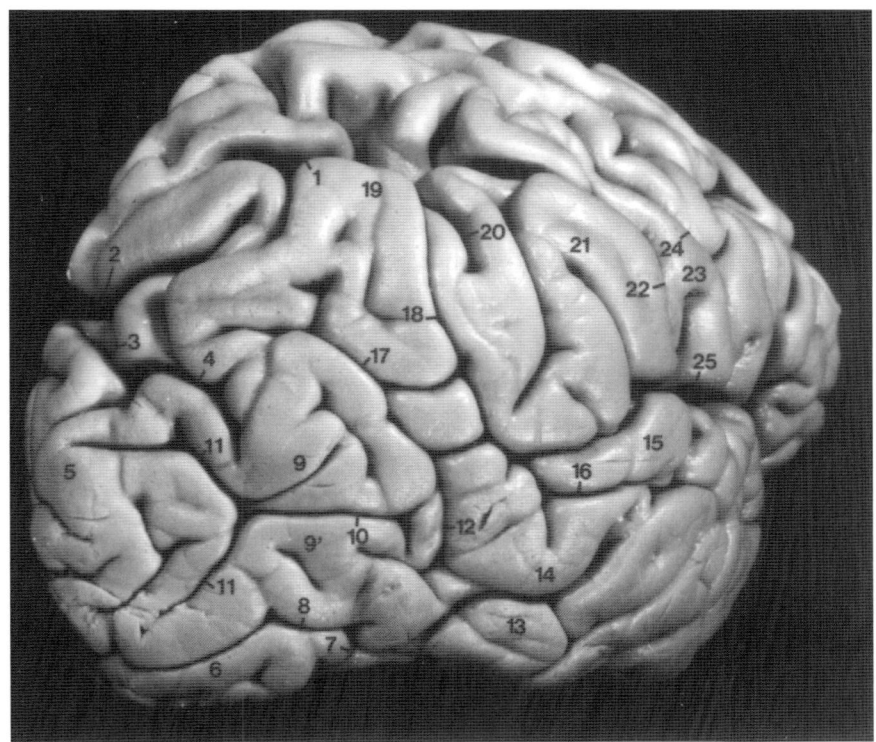

FIG. 3.9. Occipital pole, right hemisphere, lateral aspect.

1 Intraparietal sulcus
2 Parieto-occipital fissure
3 Intra-occipital sulcus
4 Transverse occipital sulcus
5 Superior occipital gyrus (O1)
6 Inferior occipital gyrus (O3)
7 Temporo-occipital incisure
8 Inferior occipital sulcus
9,9′ Middle occipital gyrus (O2)
10 Lateral occipital sulcus
11 Sulcus lunatus
12 Anterior occipital sulcus
13 Inferior temporal gyrus (T3)
14 Middle temporal gyrus (T2)
15 Superior temporal gyrus (T1)
16 Superior temporal sulcus
17 Superior temporal sulcus, horizontal posterior segment
18 Superior temporal sulcus, ascending posterior segment
19 Angular gyrus
20 Sulcus intermedius primus
21 Supramarginal gyrus
22 Inferior postcentral sulcus
23 Postcentral gyrus
24 Central sulcus
25 Lateral sulcus

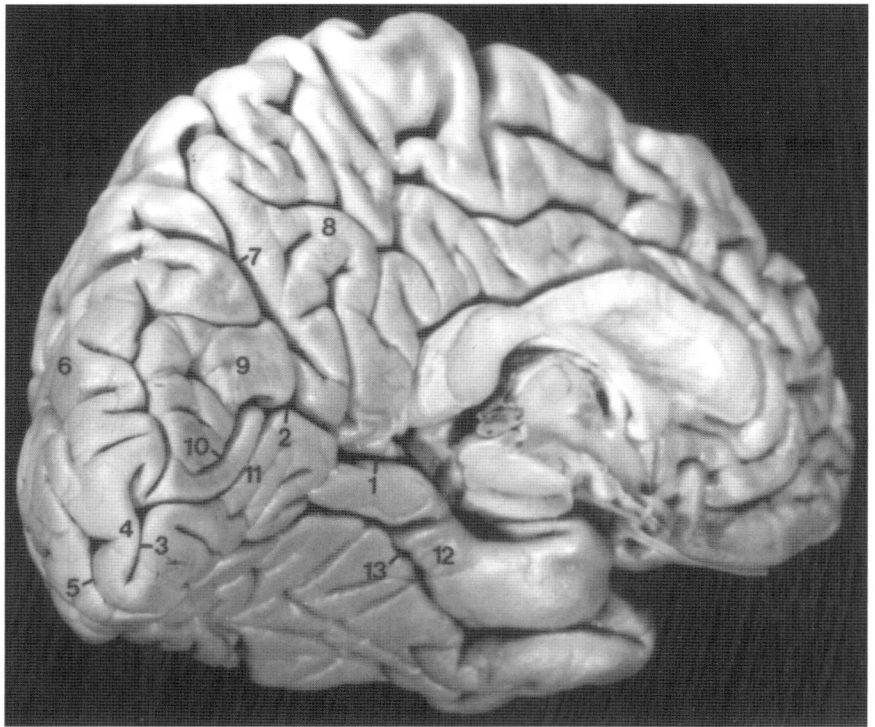

FIG. 3.10. Occipital pole, left hemisphere.

1 Anterior calcarine sulcus
2 Calcarine sulcus
3 Retrocalcarine sulcus
4 Gyrus descendens of Ecker
5 Occipitopolar sulcus
6 Superior occipital gyrus (O1)
7 Parieto-occipital fissure

8 Precuneus
9 Cuneus (O6)
10 Paracalcarine sulcus
11 Lingual gyrus (O5)
12 Parahippocampal gyrus (T5)
13 Collateral sulcus

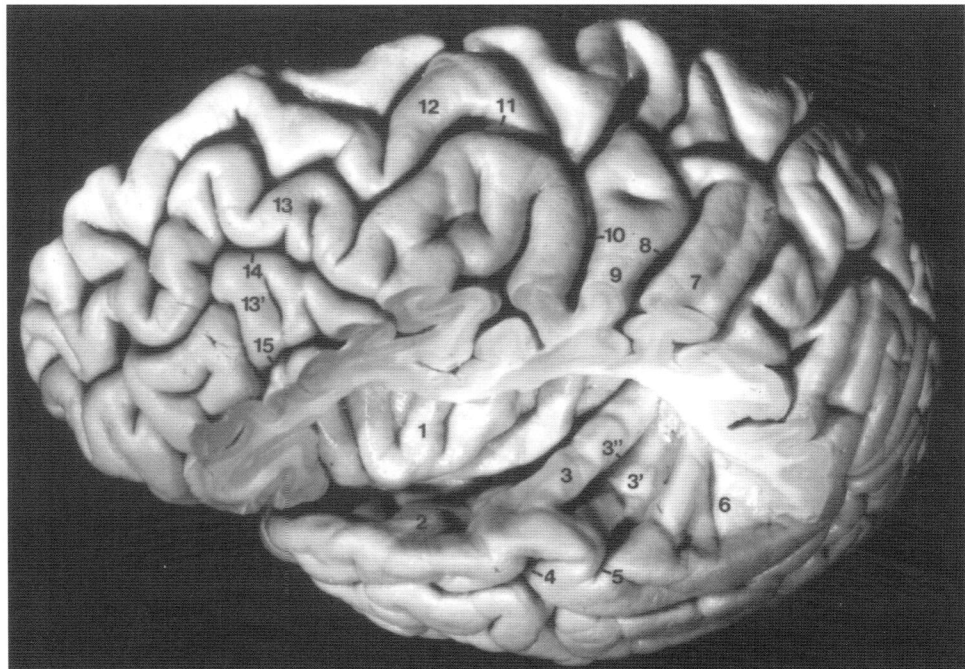

FIG. 3.11. Superior aspect of left superior temporal gyrus after ablation of the lower part of the frontal and parietal lobes.

1 Insula
2 Planum polare
3,3′ Anterior and posterior transverse temporal gyri (Heschel)
3″ Intermediate transverse temporal sulcus
4 Sulcus acousticus
5 Transverse temporal sulcus
6 Planum temporale
7 Postcentral gyrus
8 Central sulcus

9 Precentral gyrus
10 Superior central sulcus
11 Superior frontal sulcus
12 Superior frontal gyrus (F1)
13,13′ Middle frontal gyrus (F2), superior and inferior parts
14 Middle frontal sulcus
15 Inferior frontal sulcus

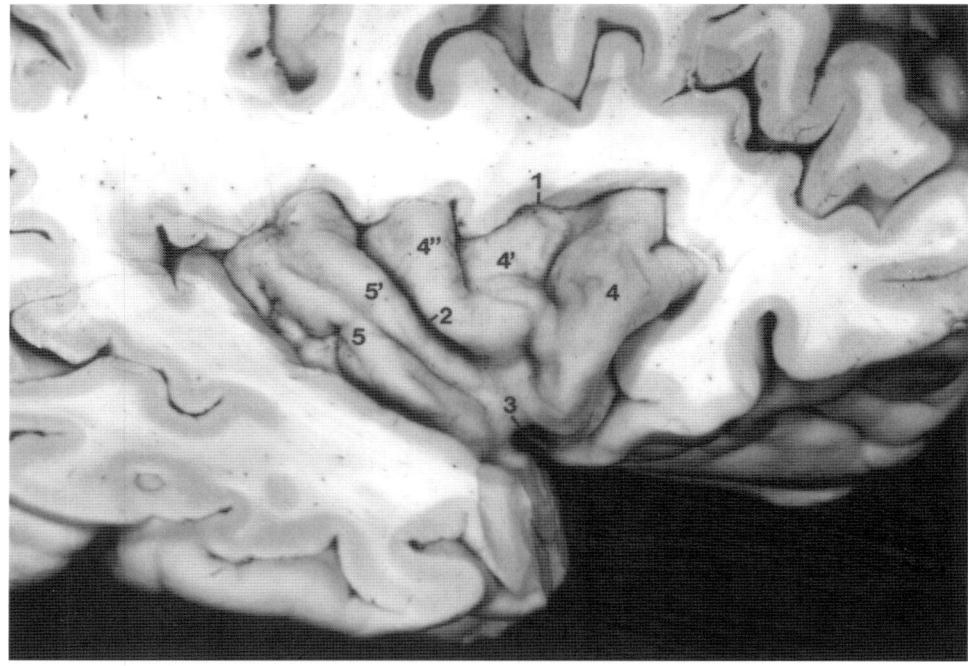

FIG. 3.12. Lateral aspect of the right insula after ablation of frontal, parietal, and temporal opercula.

1 Circular insular sulcus
2 Central insular sulcus
3 Falciform fold

4,4′,4″ Short insular gyri
5,5′ Long insular gyri

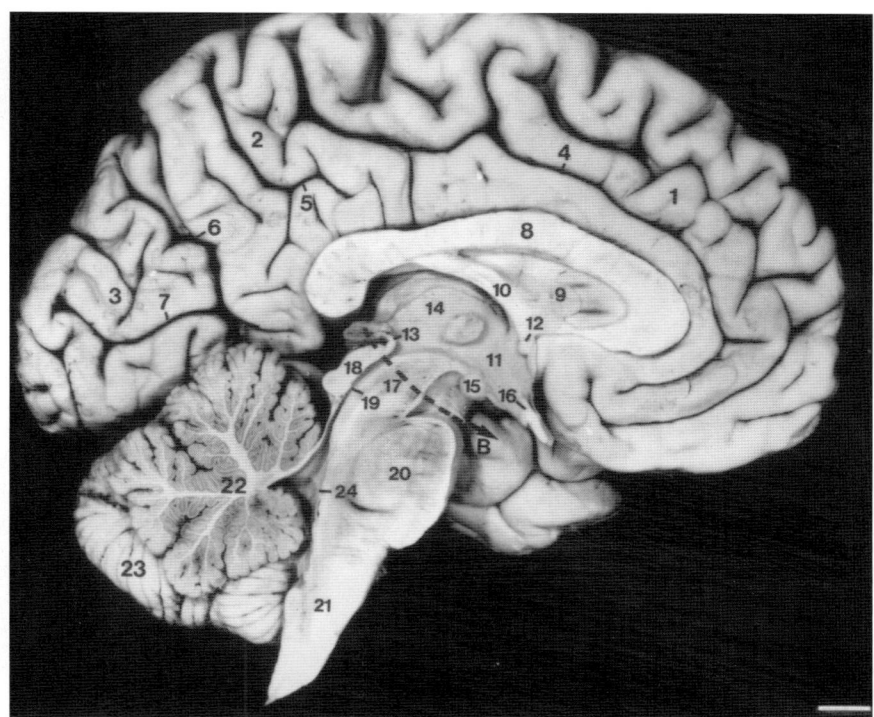

FIG. 3.13. Medial aspect of the left hemisphere observed after sagittal section of commissures and third ventricle. The inferior aspects of temporal and occipital lobes are hidden by brain stem and cerebellum.

1 Medial aspect of frontal lobe
2 Medial aspect of parietal lobe
3 Medial aspect of occipital lobe
4 Cingulate gyrus
5 Subparietal sulcus
6 Parieto-occipital fissure
7 Calcarine sulcus
8 Corpus callosum
9 Septum pellucidum
10 Fornix
11 Third ventricle
12 Anterior commissure
13 Posterior commissure

14 Thalamus
15 Mamillary body
16 Optic chiasma
17 Mesencephalon
18 Quadrigeminal plate
19 Cerebral aqueduct
20 Pons
21 Medulla
22 Cerebellum
23 Inferior cerebellum
24 Fourth ventricle

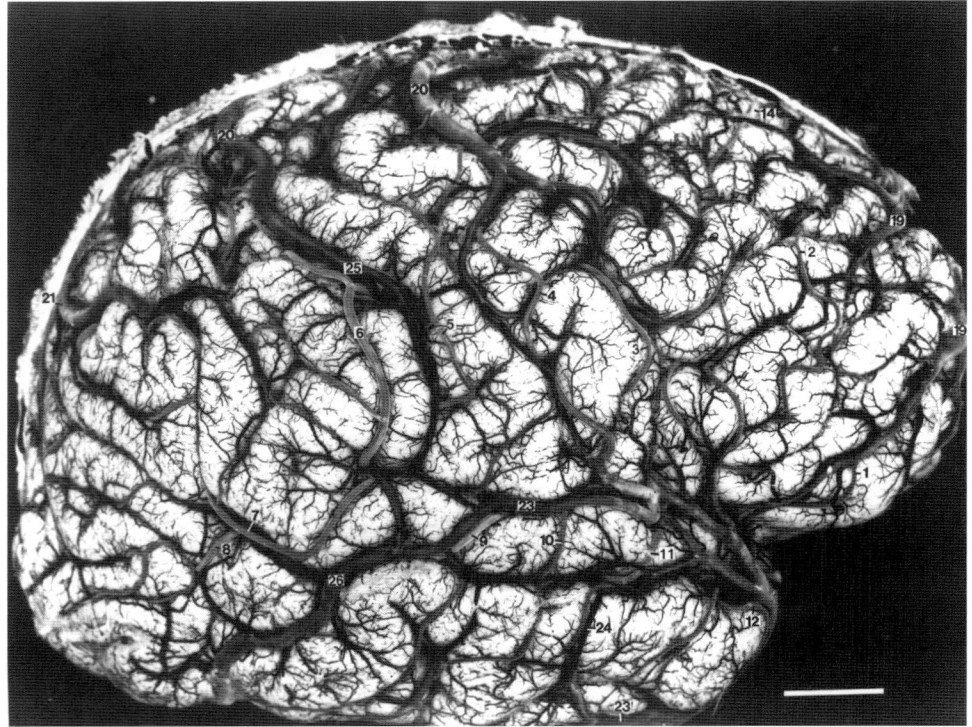

FIG. 3.14. Lateral view of a right cerebral hemisphere: leptomeningeal vessels.

1 Lateral orbitofrontal artery
2 Prefrontal artery
3 Precentral artery
4 Central artery
5 Anterior parietal artery
6 Posterior parietal artery
7 Angular artery
8 Temporo-occipital artery
9 Posterior temporal artery
10 Middle temporal artery
11 Anterior temporal artery
12 Temporopolar artery
13 Frontopolar arteries
14 Anterior internal frontal artery

15 Middle internal frontal artery
16 Posterior internal frontal artery
17 Paracentral artery
18 Internal parietal artery
19 Frontopolar cortical vein
20 Frontoparietal cortical veins
21 Parietal cortical veins
22 Superior occipital cortical vein
23 Sylvian cerebral vein
24 Lateral inferior temporal vein
25 Superior cortical anastomotic vein (Trolard)
26 Superior cortical anastomotic vein (Labbe)

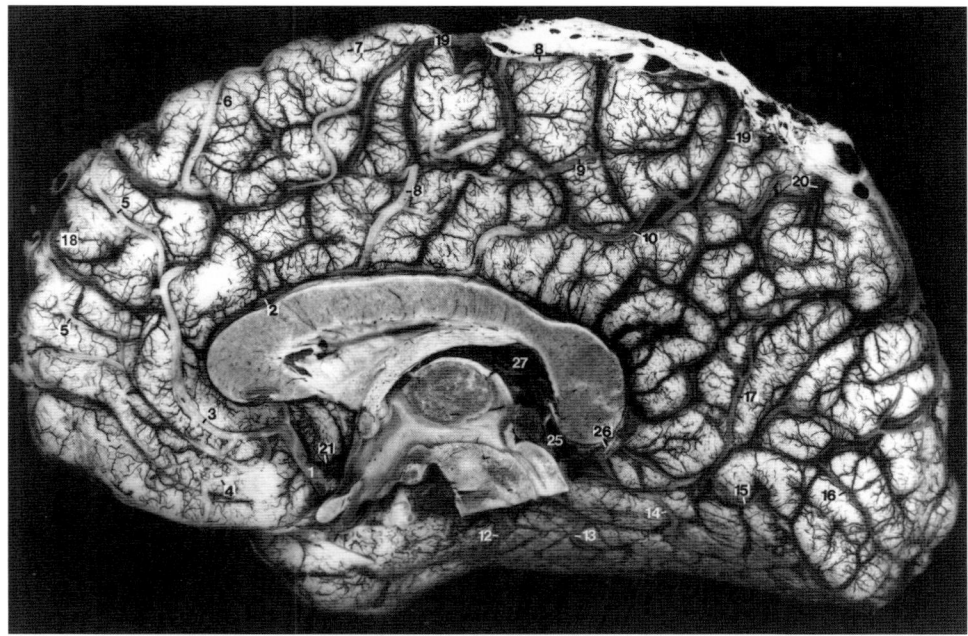

FIG. 3.15. Medial view of a right cerebral hemisphere: leptomeningeal vessels.

 1 Trunk of the anterior cerebral artery
 2 Pericallosal artery
 3 Callosomarginal or cingular artery
4,4′ Medial orbitofrontal arteries
 5 Frontopolar arteries
 6 Anterior internal frontal artery
 7 Middle internal frontal artery
 8 Posterior internal frontal artery
 9 Paracentral artery
10 Internal parietal arteries
11 Posterior cerebral artery
12 Anterior inferior temporal artery
13 Middle inferior temporal artery
14 Posterior inferior temporal artery

15 Occipitotemporal artery
16 Calcarine artery
17 Parieto-occipital artery
18 Frontopolar cortical vein
19 Frontoparietal cortical vein
20 Parietal cortical vein
21 Anterior cerebral vein
22 Venous drainage towards 23
23 Basal vein
24 Pericallosal vein
25 Great cerebral vein
26 Straight sinus
27 Internal cerebral vein

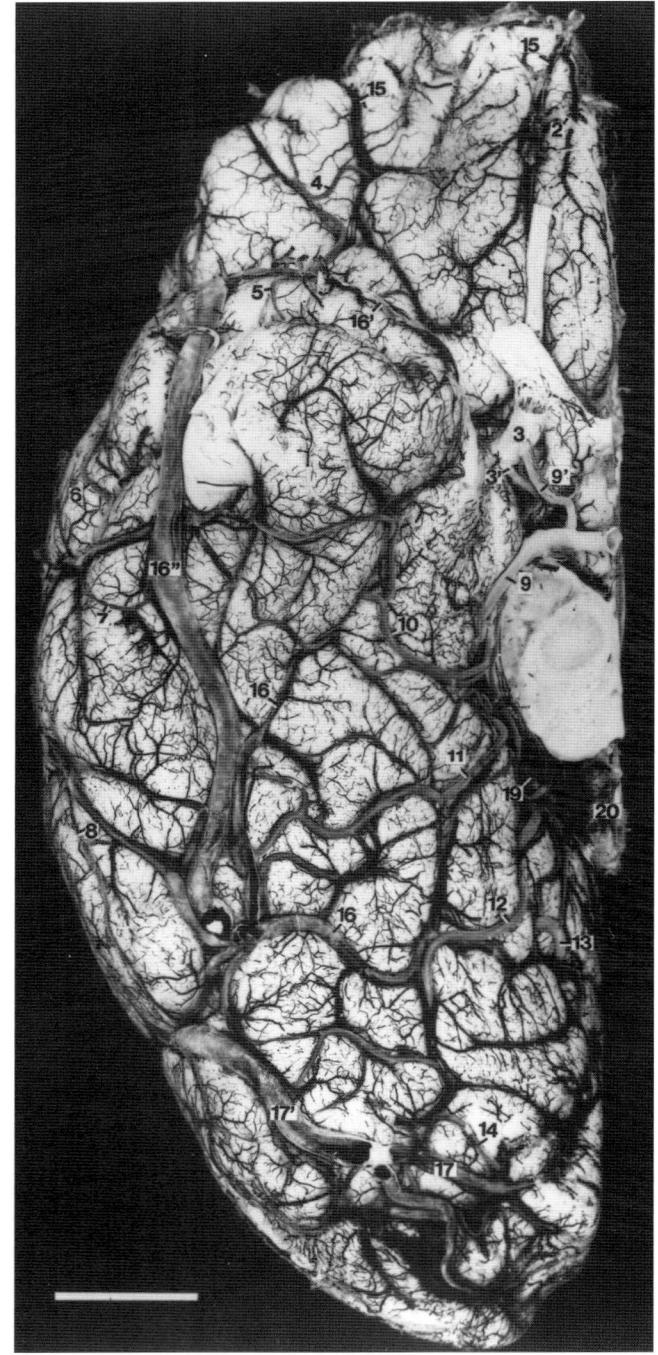

FIG. 3.16. Inferior view of a right cerebral hemisphere: leptomeningeal vessels.

1 Anterior cerebral artery
2 Medial orbitofrontal arteries
3 Middle cerebral artery
3′ Anterior choroidal artery
4 Lateral orbitofrontal artery
5 Temporopolar arteries
6 Anterior temporal artery
7 Middle temporal artery
8 Posterior temporal artery
9 Posterior cerebral artery
9′ Posterior communicating artery
10 Anterior inferior temporal artery

11 Middle inferior temporal artery
12 Posterior inferior temporal artery
13 Calcarine artery
14 Occipitotemporal artery
15,15′ Veins of the orbital lobe
16 Medial inferior temporal veins
16′,16″ Temporopolar veins
17 Inferior occipital veins
17′ Inferior anastomotic vein (Labbe)
19 Basal vein
20 Great cerebral vein

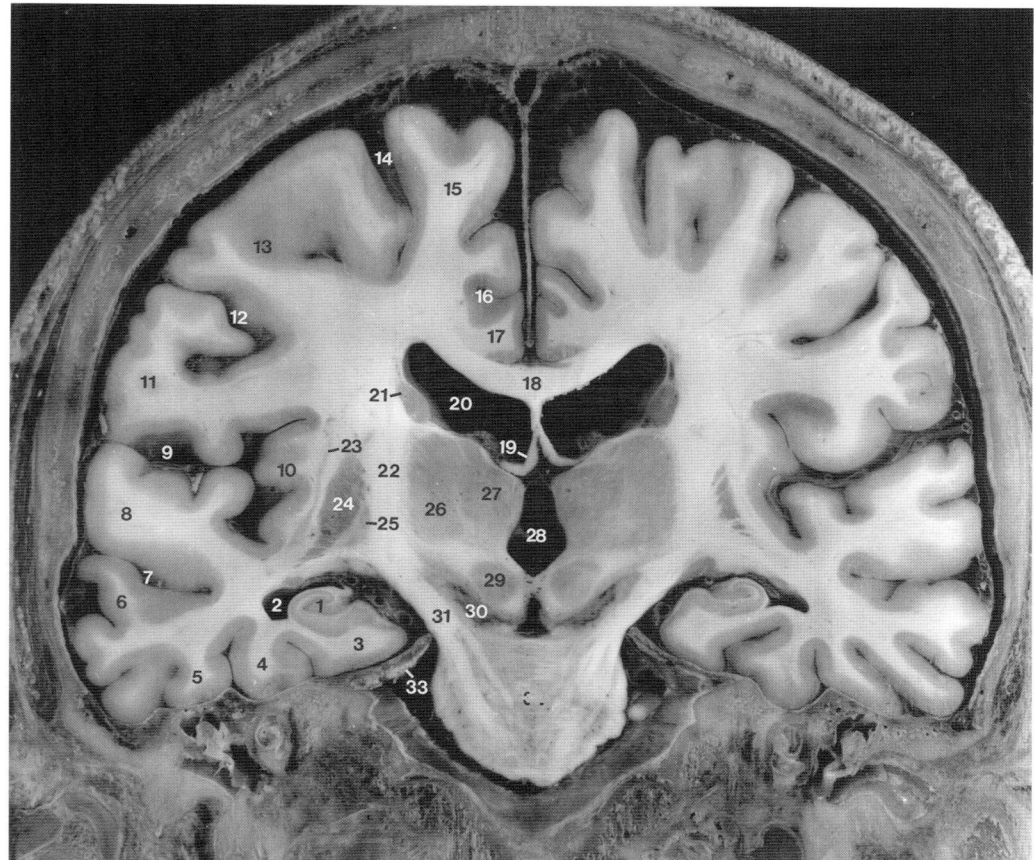

FIG. 3.17. Coronal section of the brain showing the general relations of the hippocampus with adjacent nervous structures.

1 Section of the hippocampus
2 Temporal horn of the lateral ventricle
3 Parahippocampal gyrus
4 Fusiform gyrus
5 Inferior temporal gyrus
6 Middle temporal gyrus
7 Superior temporal sulcus
8 Superior temporal gyrus
9 Lateral fissure
10 Insula
11 Postcentral gyrus
12 Central sulcus
13 Precentral gyrus
14 Precentral sulcus
15 Superior frontal gyrus
16 Cingulate sulcus
17 Cingulate gyrus

18 Corpus callosum
19 Fornix
20 Lateral ventricle
21 Caudate nucleus
22 Internal capsule, posterior limb
23 Claustrum
24 Putamen
25 Lateral pallidum
26 Ventral lateral thalamic nucleus
27 Dorsomedial thalamic nucleus
28 Third ventricle
29 Red nucleus
30 Substantia nigra
31 Crus cerebri
32 Pons
33 Tentorium cerebelli

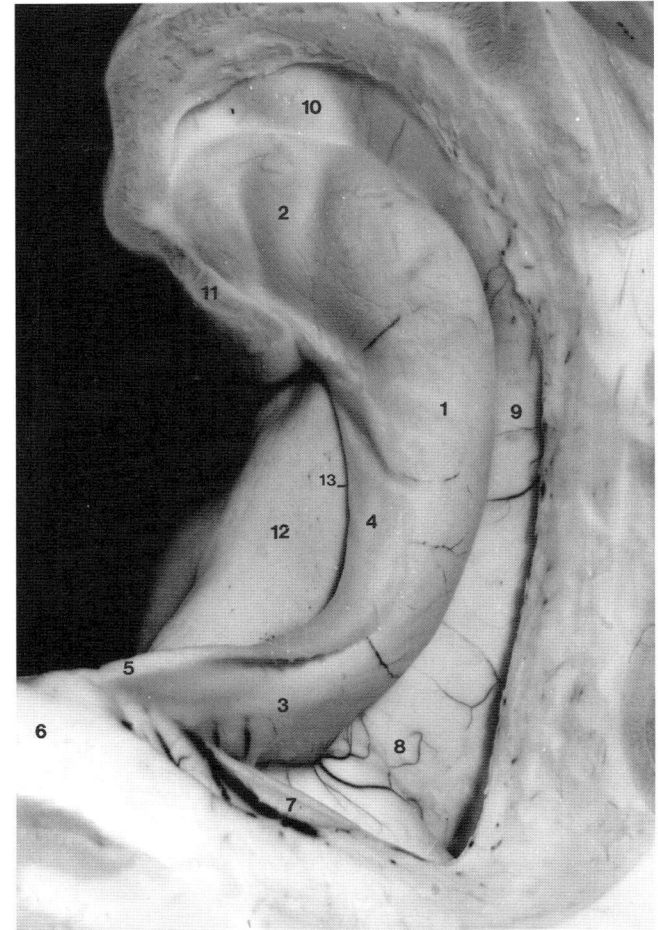

FIG. 3.18. Intraventricular aspect of the right hippocampus. The temporal horn of the lateral ventricle has been opened and the choroid plexuses have been removed.

1 Hippocampal body
2 Hippocampal head: digitationes hippocampi
3 Hippocampal tail
4 Fimbria
5 Crus of the fornix
6 Splenium of the corpus callosum
7 Calcar avis in the occipital horn
8 Collateral trigone

9 Collateral eminence
10 Uncal recess of the temporal horn (the amygdala overlying the hippocampal head has been removed)
11 Uncal part of the hippocampus
12 Parahippocampal gyrus (subiculum)
13 Hippocampal sulcus

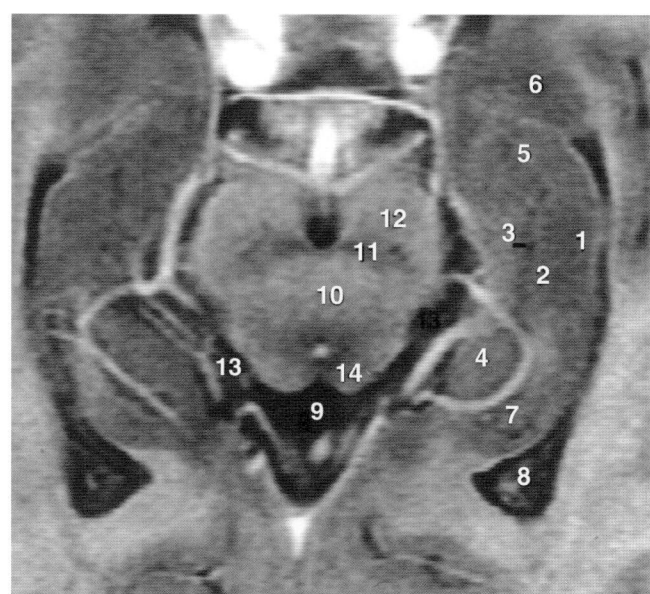

FIG. 3.19. MRI view of a section passing through the hippocampal axis (inverted T2-weighted image).

1 Hippocampal body, cornu ammonis
2 Hippocampal body, gyrus dentatus
3 Hippocampal sulcus
4 Subiculum
5 Hippocampal head
6 Amygdala
7 Hippocampal tail

8 Atrium of the lateral ventricle
9 Quadrigeminal cistern
10 Brachium conjunctivum
11 Substantia nigra
12 Crus cerebri
13 Ambient cistern
14 Colliculus

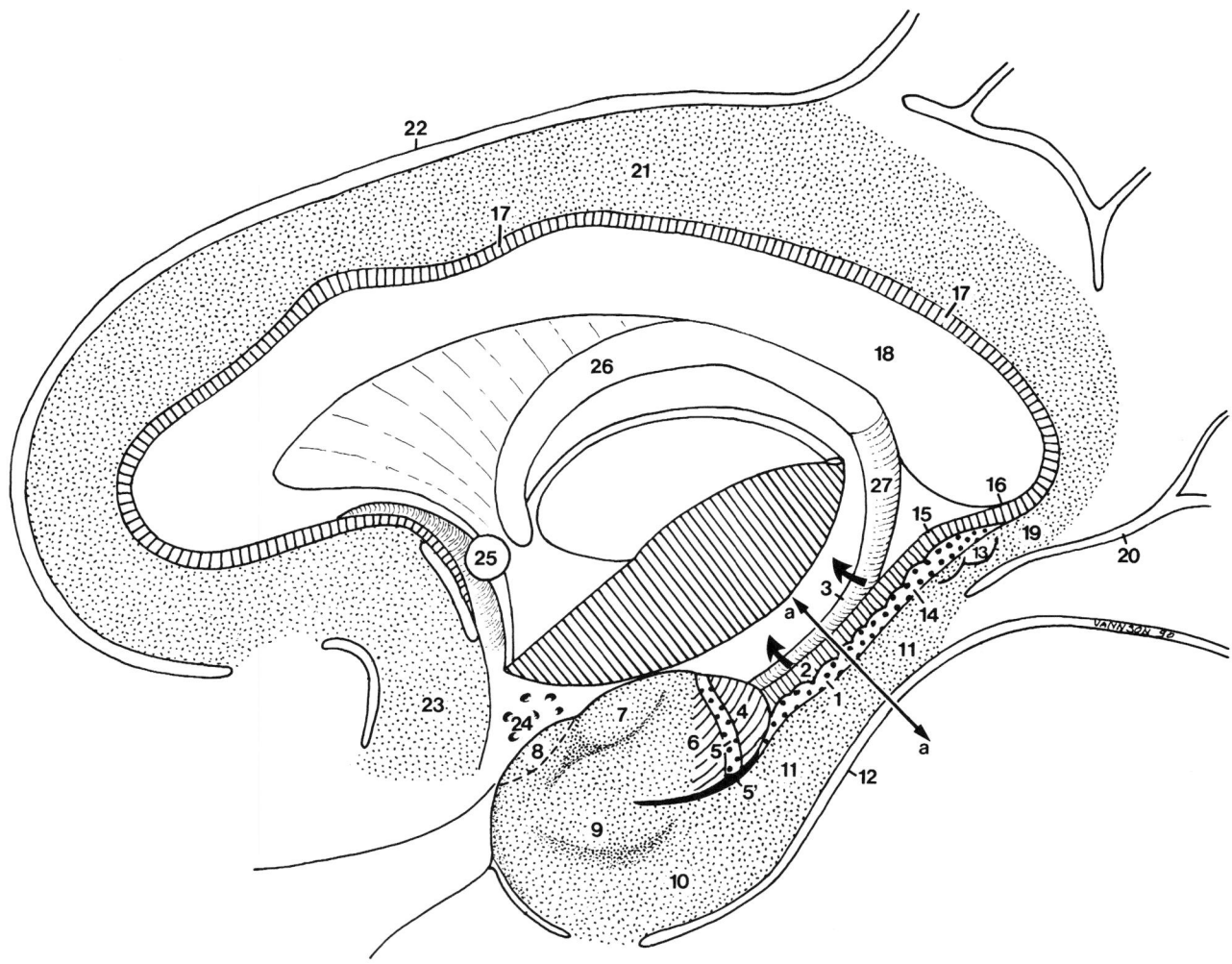

FIG. 3.20. Medial aspect of the hippocampus.

Hippocampal body:
1 Superficial part of the gyrus dentatus (margo denticulatus)
2 Cornu ammonis
3 Fimbria displaced upwards (arrows) to show the cornu ammonis

Hippocampal head (uncal part):
4 Apex of the uncus
5 Band of Giacomini (the uncal extension of the margo denticulatus (1))
5′ Uncal sulcus
6 Gyrus uncinatus

The anterior part of the uncus, which belongs to the parahippocampal gyrus (and is often called piriform lobe), is composed of :
7 Semilunar gyrus
8 Prepiriform cortex
9 Gyrus ambiens
10 Entorhinal area
11 Parahippocampal gyrus
12 Collateral sulcus

Hippocampal tail
13 Gyri of Andreas Retzius
14 Fasciola cinerea prolonging the gyrus dentatus
15 Gyrus fasciolaris which is the extension of the cornu ammonis in the tail
16 The gyrus subsplenialis prolongs the gyrus fasciolaris and is itself continued by the indusium griseum (17) on the dorsum of the corpus callosum (18)
19 Isthmus
20 Anterior calcarine sulcus
21 Cingulate gyrus
22 Cingulate sulcus
23 Subcallosal area
24 Anterior perforated substance
25 Anterior commissure
26 Fornix
27 Crus of the fornix

The dotted area indicates the limbic lobe. The a–a line indicates the plane of the section of Figure 3.21.

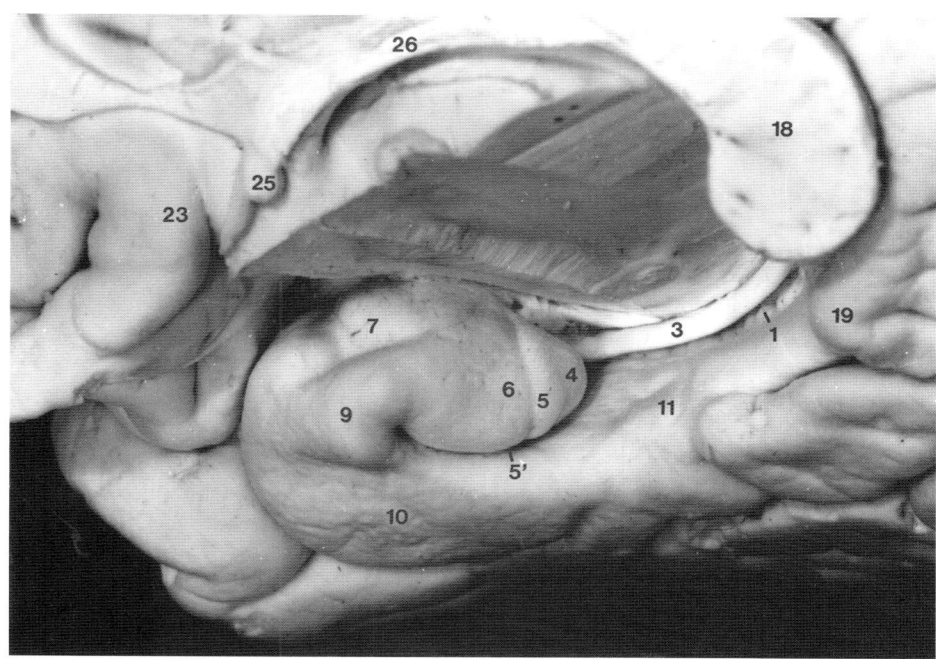

FIG. 3.20. *Cont'd.*

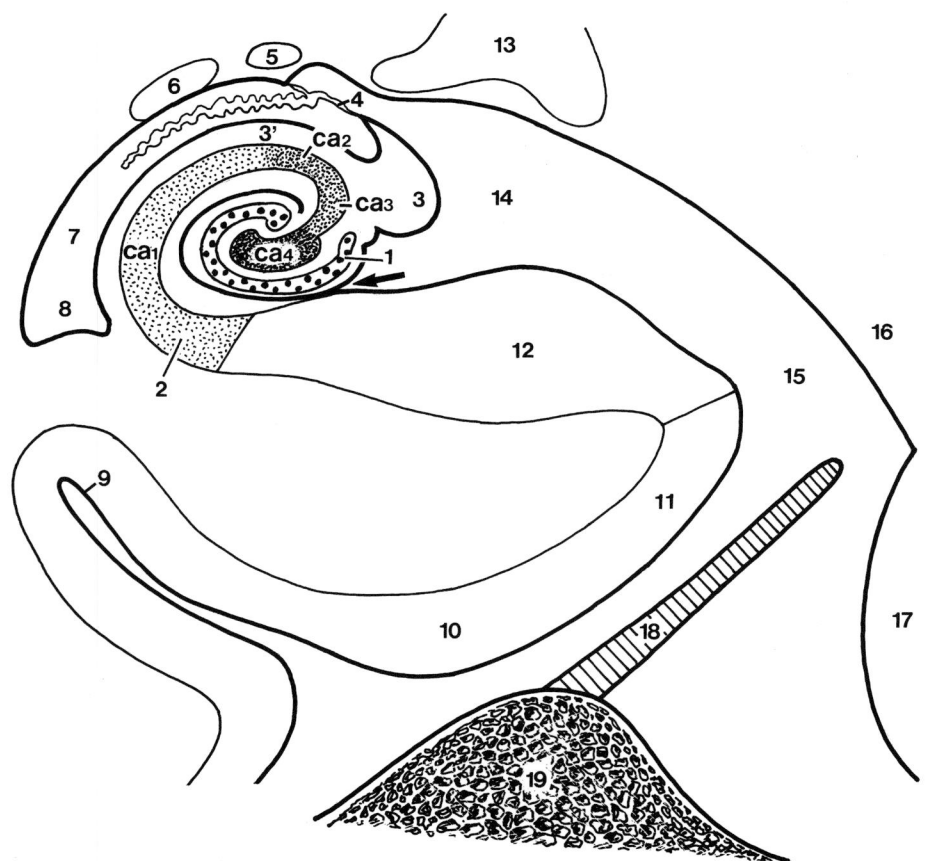

FIG. 3.21. Diagram of a transverse section of the hippocampus. The hippocampus is composed of two cortical layers, the gyrus dentatus (1) and the cornu ammonis (2), superficially separated by the hippocampal sulcus (arrow) and covered with fimbria (3) and alveus (3').

CA1, CA2, CA3, CA4 Fields of cornu ammonis
 4 Tela choroidea of the temporal horn (fissura choroidea)
 5 Stria terminalis
 6 Tail of caudate nucleus
 7 Temporal horn of the lateral ventricle
 8 Collateral eminence
 9 Collateral sulcus
10 Parahippocampal gyrus
11 Entorhinal area

12 Subiculum
13 Lateral geniculate body
14 Lateral part of the transverse fissure (wing of the ambient cistern)
15 Ambient cistern
16 Crus cerebri
17 Pons
18 Tentorium cerebelli
19 Temporal, petrous part

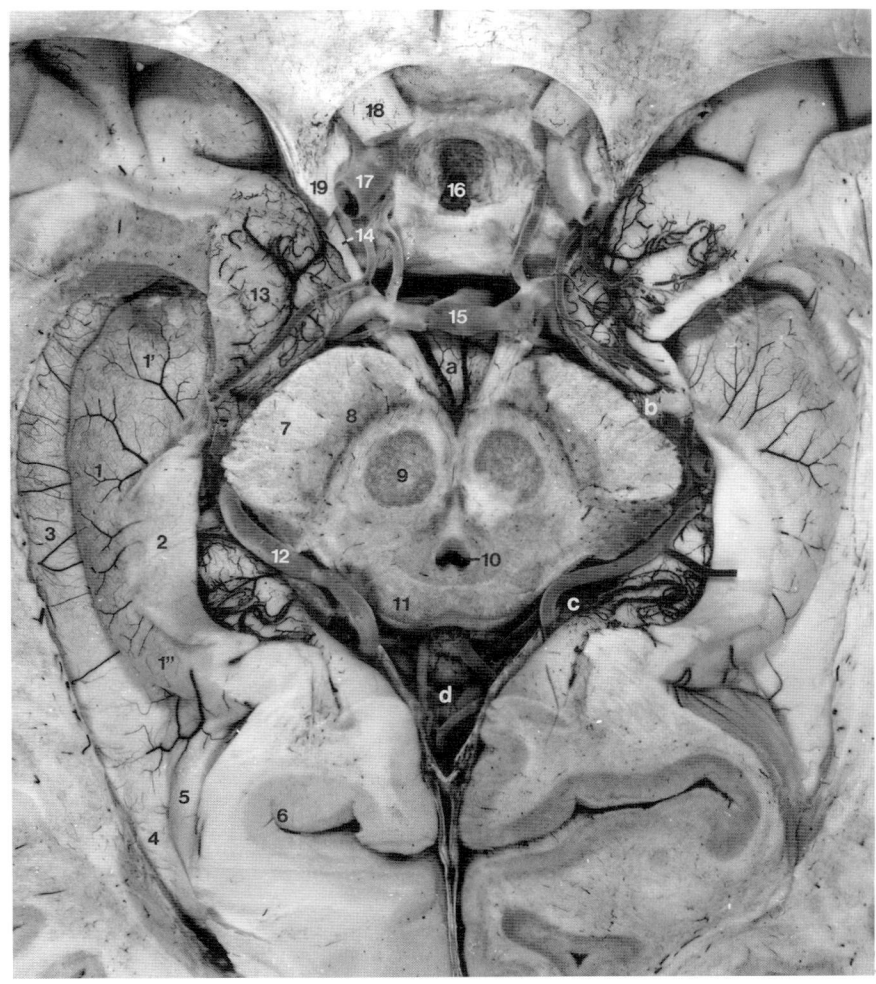

FIG. 3.22. Horizontal section of the upper mesencephalon. The temporal horns of the lateral ventricles have been opened and the choroid plexuses removed to show the right and left hippocampi.

1 Endoventricular view of the hippocampal body
1′ Endoventricular view of the hippocampal head (digitationes hippocampi)
1″ Endoventricular view of the hippocampal tail
2 Fimbria
3 Collateral eminence
4 Occipital horn of the lateral ventricle
5 Calcar avis
6 Anterior calcarine sulcus

The two hippocampi encircle the mesencephalon:
7 Crus cerebri
8 Substantia nigra
9 Red nucleus
10 Cerebral aqueduct

11 Superior colliculus
12 Posterior cerebral artery
13 Uncus
14 Oculomotor nerve
15 Basilar artery
16 Hypophysial stalk
17 Middle cerebral artery
18 Optic nerve
19 Anterior clinoid process.

Subarachnoid cisterns:
 a interpeduncular cistern
 b crural cistern
 c ambient cistern
 d quadrigeminal cistern

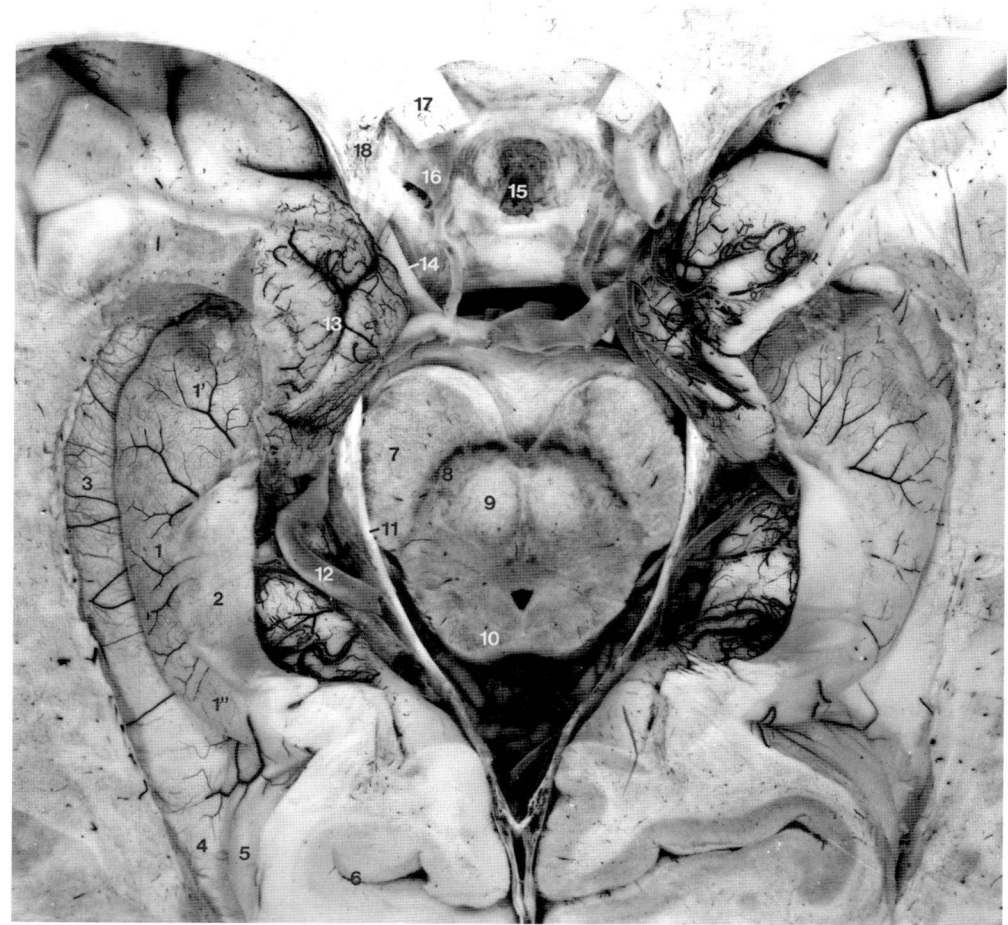

FIG. 3.23. Horizontal section of the lower mesencephalon. The temporal horns of the lateral ventricles have been opened and the choroid plexuses removed to show the right and left hippocampi.

1 Endoventricular view of the hippocampal body
1′ Endoventricular view of the hippocampal head (digitationes hippocampi)
1″ Endoventricular view of the tail
2 Fimbria
3 Collateral eminence
4 Occipital horn of the lateral ventricle
5 Calcar avis
6 Anterior calcarine sulcus
7 Crus cerebri
8 Substantia nigra
9 Superior cerebellar peduncle

10 Inferior colliculus
11 Free edge of the tentorium cerebelli, which delimits the tentorial opening, encircles the mesencephalon and is in close contact with the two hippocampi
12 Posterior cerebral artery
13 Uncus
14 Oculomotor nerve
15 Hypophysial stalk
16 Middle cerebral artery
17 Optic nerve
18 Anterior clinoid process

SECTIONAL ANATOMY OF THE HIPPOCAMPUS

Coronal, axial and sagittal sections of the hippocampus will be successively presented.

The bicommissural plane acted as a reference plane for axial sections parallel to this plane and for coronal sections perpendicular to it. Sagittal section are parallel to the median plane.

Some sections are parallel to a plane passing through the anterior commissure and the mamillary body (AC–MB plane), which is perpendicular to the hippocampal axis (Figs 3.25B, 3.27B and 3.29B) and one section is perpendicular to the AC–MB plane and parallel to the hippocampal axis (Fig. 3.19).

The illustrations for each section consist of a three-dimensional drawing that is then compared with the corresponding anatomical section and MRI.

The MRI views are courtesy of:

- the Department of Neuroradiology of the Quinze-Vingts Hospital, Paris (Professors E.A. Cabanis and M.T. Iba-Zizen)
- the Department of Neurology of the NYU School of Medicine, New York, NY (Dr R.I. Kuzniecky)
- the Department of Neuroradiology of the J. Minjoz Hospital, Besançon (Professor J.F. Bonneville and Dr. F. Cattin).

CORONAL SECTIONS OF THE HIPPOCAMPUS

The coronal views show eight sections moving progressively from anterior to posterior levels.

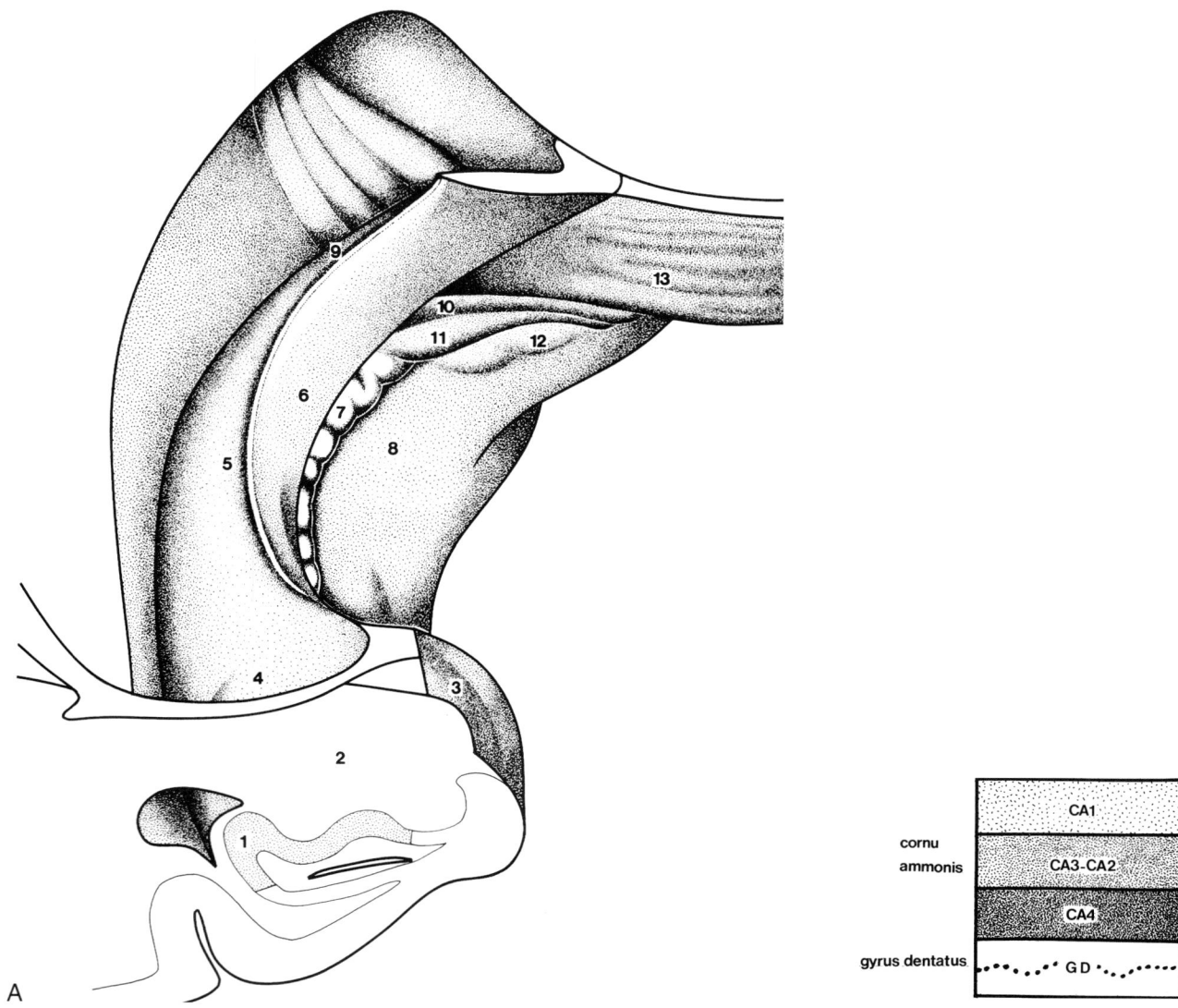

FIG. 3.24. Coronal section of the hippocampal head. **A.** Three-dimensional drawing. **B.** T1-weighted MR image. **C.** Anatomic section (posterior view).

1 Anterior apex of the hippocampal head (cornu ammonis)	16 Parahippocampal gyrus (entorhinal area)
2 Amygdala	17 Collateral sulcus
2′ Amygdala, lateral nucleus	18 Fusiform gyrus
2″ Amygdala, basal nucleus	19 Inferior temporal gyrus
2‴ Amygdala, cortical nucleus	20 Middle temporal gyrus
3 Uncus	21 Superior temporal gyrus
4 Hippocampal head	22 Lateral fissure
5 Hippocampal body	23 Precentral gyrus
6 Fimbria	24 Insula
7 Margo denticulatus	25 Claustrum
8 Parahippocampal gyrus (subiculum)	26 Caudate nucleus
9 Hippocampal tail	27 Internal capsule (genu)
10 Gyrus fasciolaris	28 Putamen
11 Fasciola cinerea	29 Lateral pallidum
12 Gyri of Andreas Retzius	30 Medial pallidum
13 Splenium	31 Column of fornix
14 Temporal stem	32 Optic tract
15 Temporal horn of the lateral ventricle	33 Third ventricle

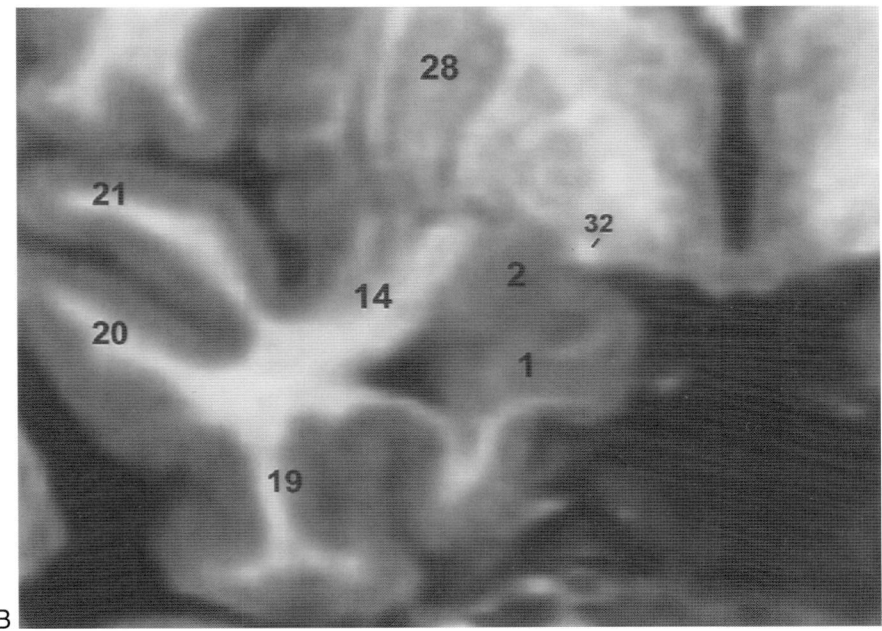

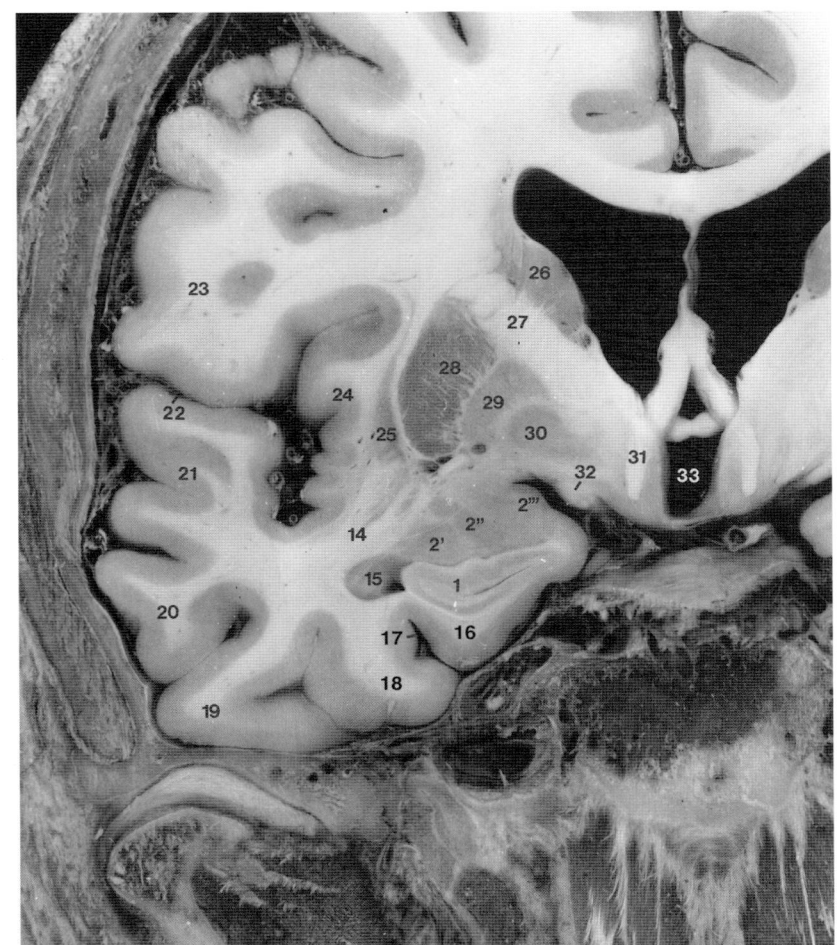

FIG. 3.24. *Cont'd.*

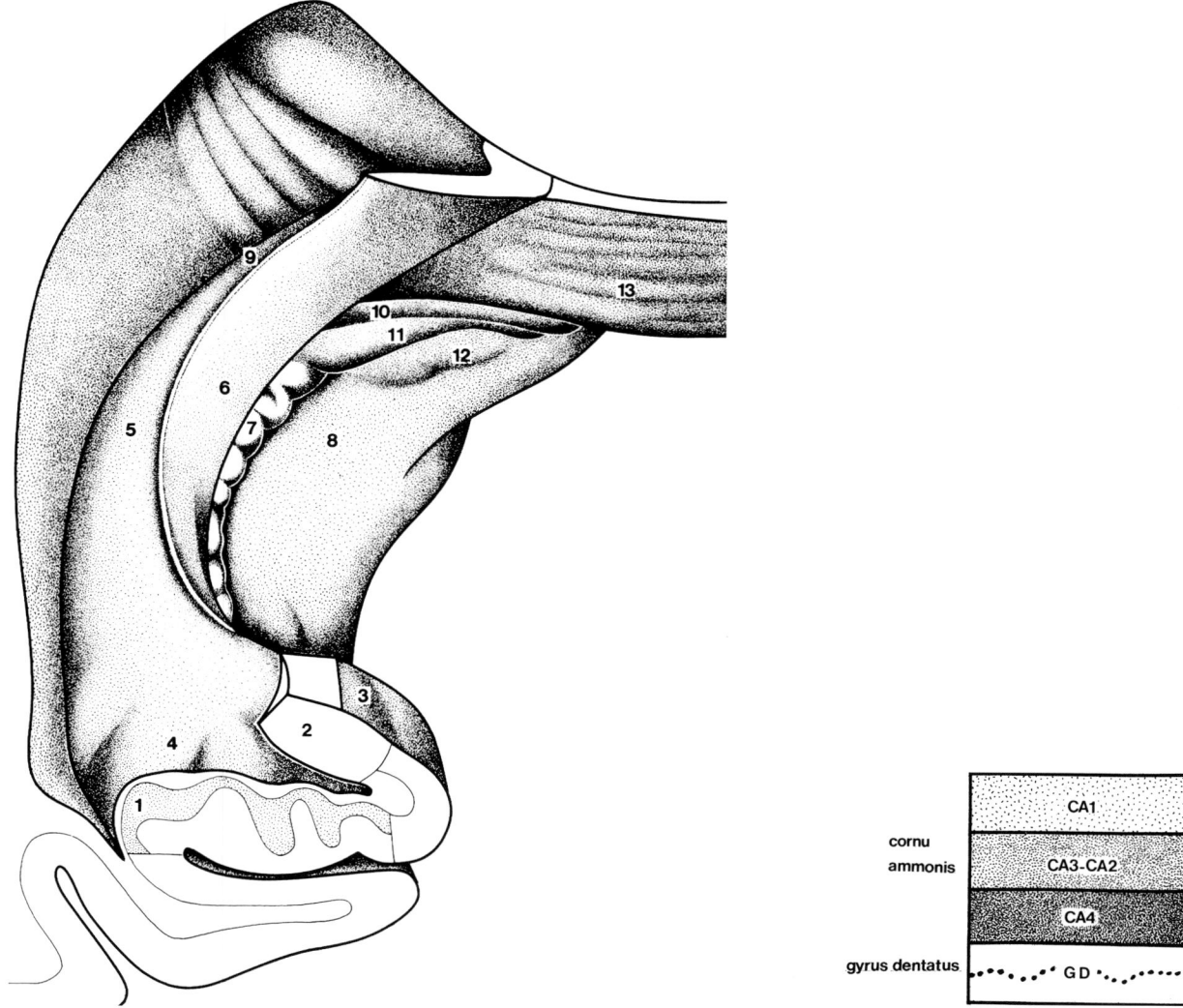

FIG. 3.25. Coronal section of the hippocampal head. **A.** Three-dimensional drawing. **B.** T1-weighted MR image. **C.** Inverted T2-weighted MR image. **D.** Anatomic section (posterior view).

1 Hippocampal head, digitationes hippocampi (cornu ammonis, cut surface)
2 Amygdala (cortical nucleus)
3 Uncus
4 Hippocampal head
5 Hippocampal body
6 Fimbria
7 Margo denticulatus
8 Parahippocampal gyrus (subiculum)
9 Hippocampal tail
10 Gyrus fasciolaris
11 Fasciola cinerea
12 Gyri of Andreas Retzius
13 Splenium
14 Temporal stem
15 Temporal horn of the lateral ventricle
16 Uncal sulcus
17 Subiculum
18 Parahippocampal gyrus
19 Collateral sulcus

20 Fusiform gyrus
21 Inferior temporal gyrus
22 Middle temporal gyrus
23 Parallel sulcus
24 Superior temporal gyrus
25 Lateral fissure
26 Precentral gyrus
27 Caudate nucleus
28 Internal capsule (genu)
29 Claustrum
30 Insula
31 Putamen
32 Lateral pallidum
33 Medial pallidum
34 Optic tract
35 Ventral anterior thalamic nucleus
36 Third ventricle
37 Mamillary body
38 Lateral ventricle
39 Corpus callosum

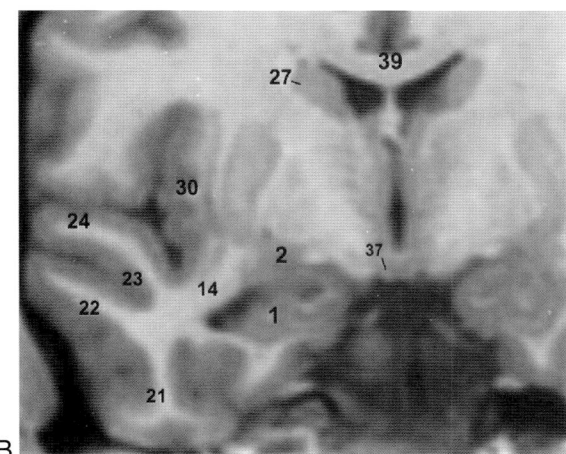

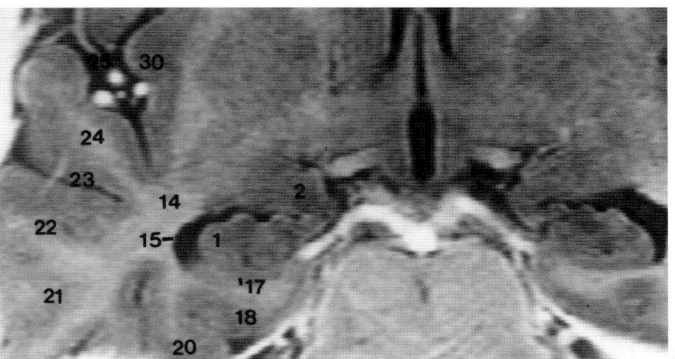

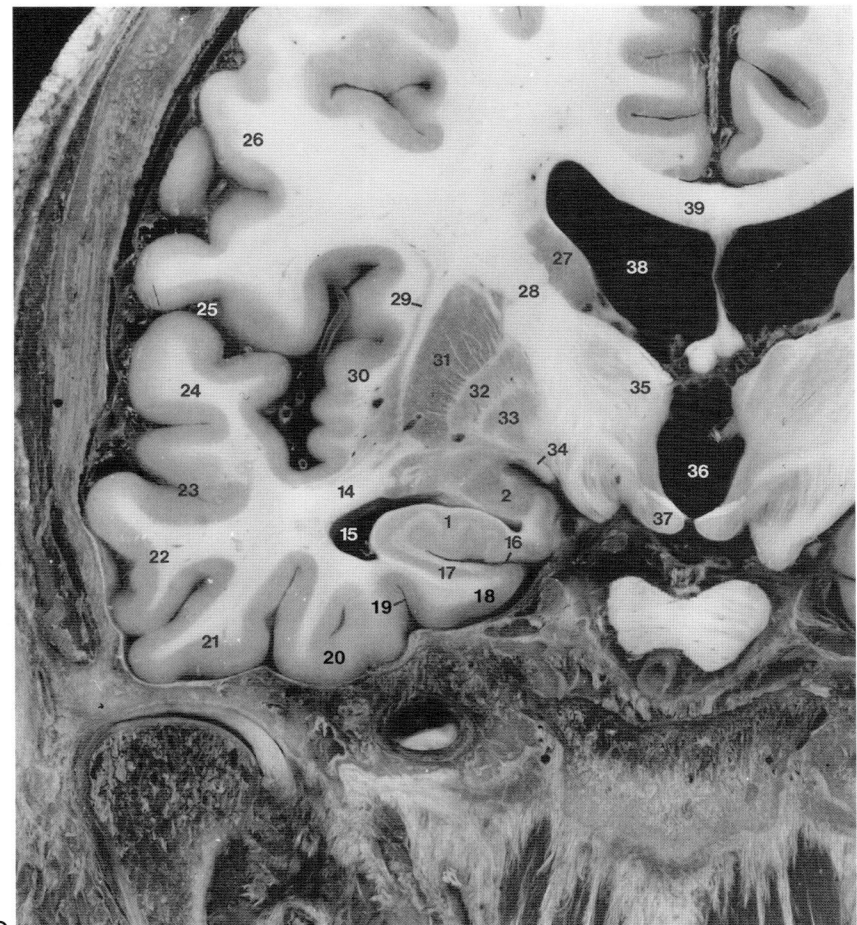

FIG. 3.25. *Cont'd.*

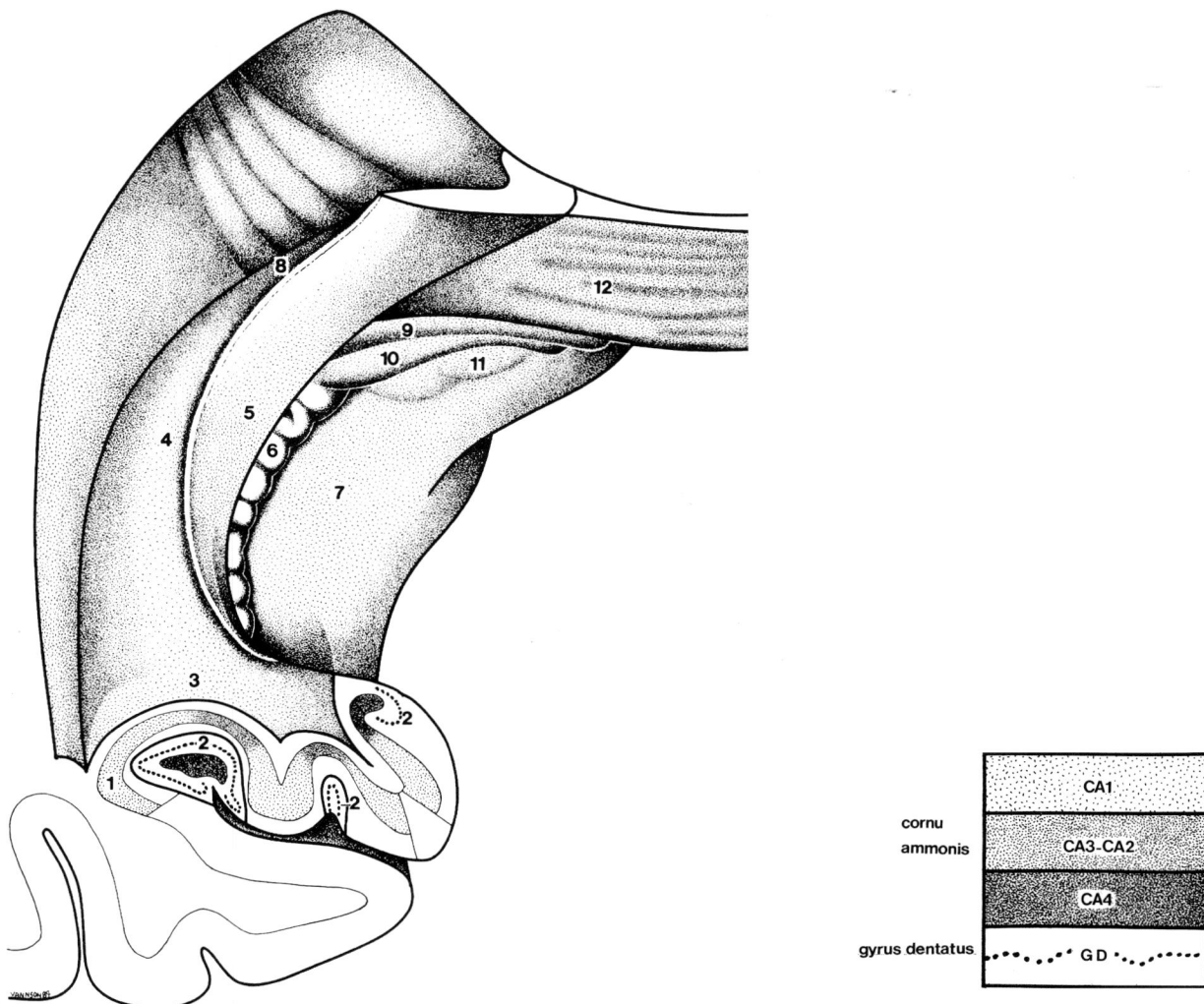

FIG. 3.26. Coronal section of the hippocampal head. **A.** Three-dimensional drawing. **B.** T1-weighted MR image. **C.** Anatomic section (posterior view).

1 Hippocampal head (cornu ammonis)
2 Hippocampal head (gyrus dentatus)
3 Hippocampal head (endoventricular aspect)
4 Hippocampal body
5 Fimbria
6 Margo denticulatus
7 Parahippocampal gyrus (subiculum)
8 Hippocampal tail
9 Gyrus fasciolaris
10 Fasciola cinerea
11 Gyri of Andreas Retzius
12 Splenium
13 Temporal stem
14 Temporal horn of the lateral ventricle
15 Uncal sulcus
16 Subiculum
17 Parahippocampal gyrus (entorhinal area)
18 Collateral sulcus
19 Fusiform gyrus
20 Inferior temporal gyrus
21 Middle temporal gyrus
22 Parallel sulcus
23 Superior temporal gyrus
24 Lateral fissure
25 Postcentral gyrus

26 Central sulcus
27 Precentral gyrus
28 Corpus callosum
29 Lateral ventricle
30 Caudate nucleus
31 Internal capsule, posterior limb
32 Insula
33 Claustrum
34 Putamen
35 Lateral pallidum
36 Medial pallidum
37 Optic tract
38 Anterior thalamic nucleus
39 Ventral lateral thalamic nucleus
40 Dorsomedial thalamic nucleus
41 Zona incerta
42 Subthalamic nucleus
43 Substantia nigra
44 Third ventricle
45 Interpeduncular fossa
46 Crus cerebri
47 Crural cistern
48 Posterior cerebral artery
49 Tentorium cerebelli
50 Pons

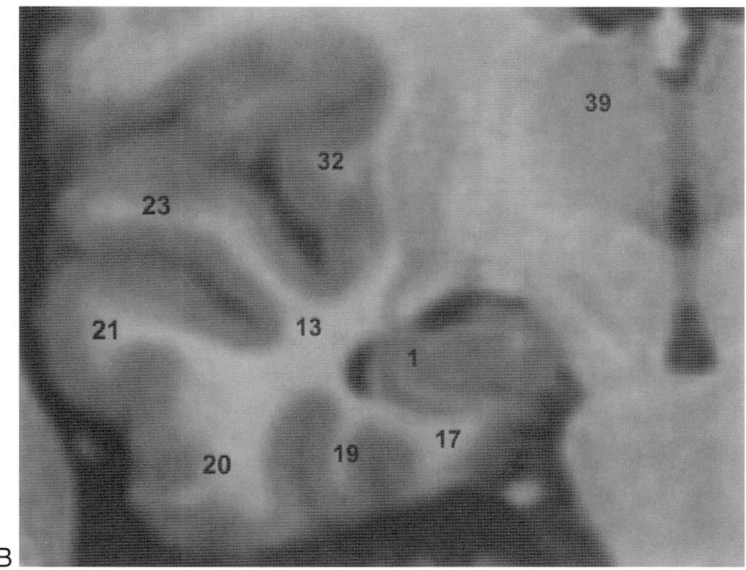

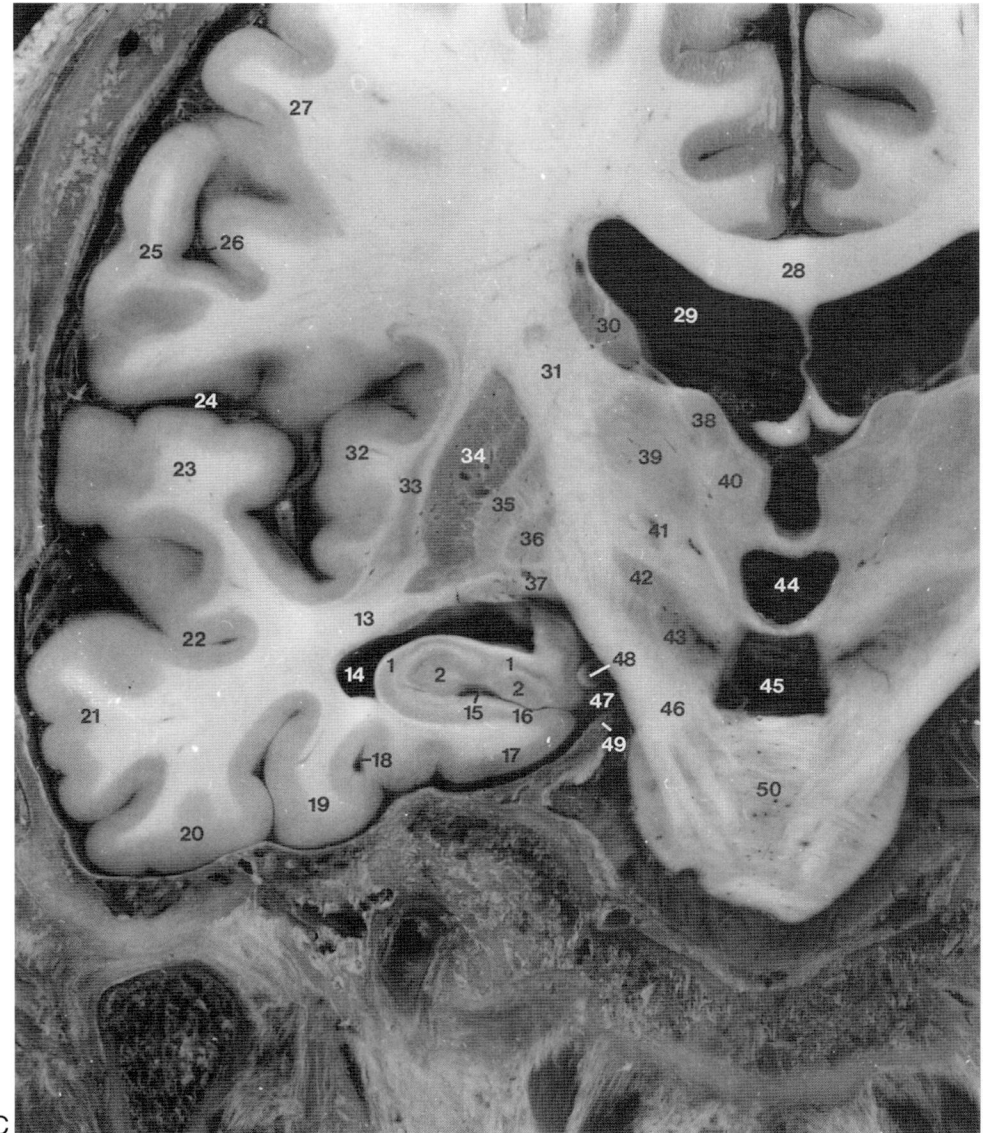

FIG. 3.26. Cont'd.

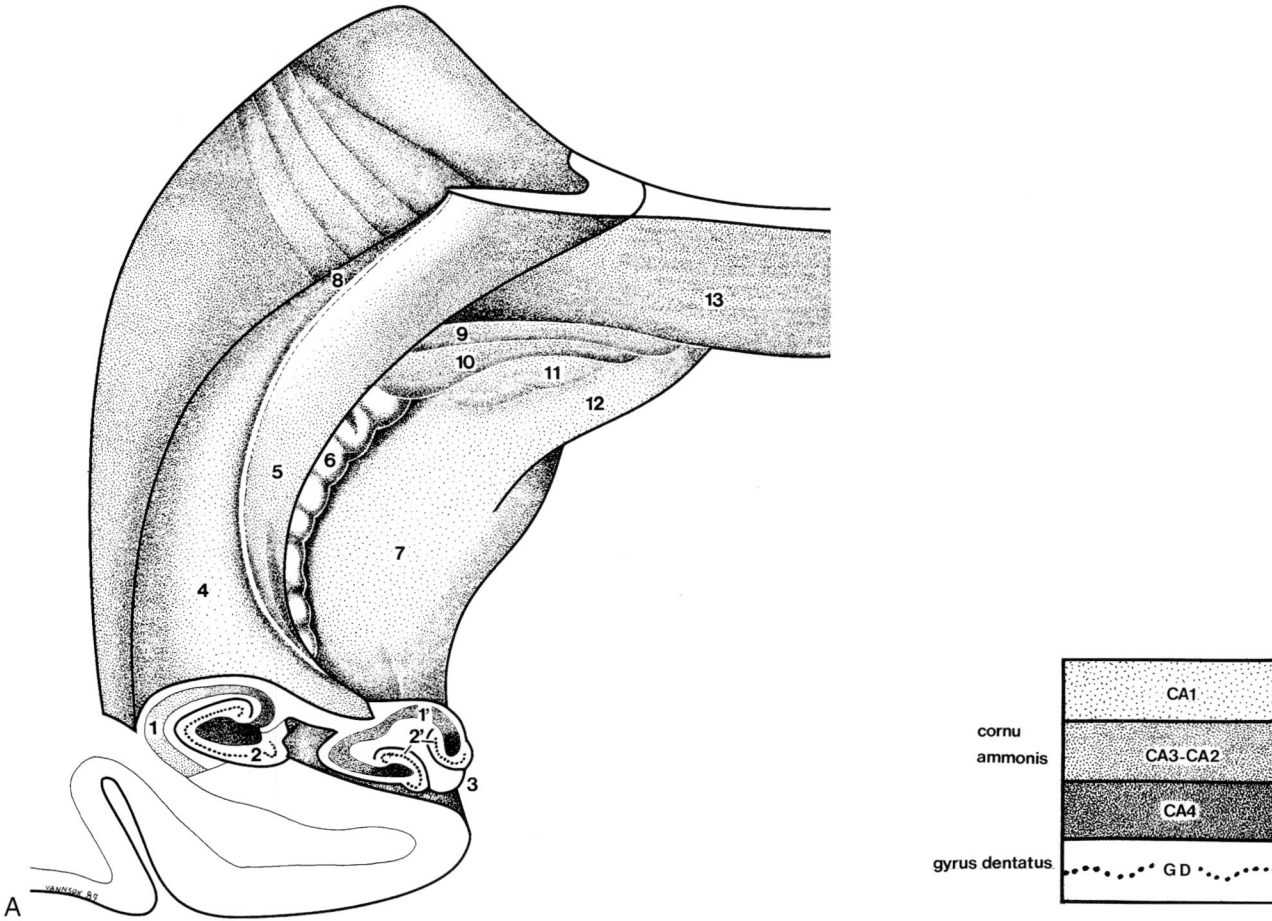

FIG. 3.27. Coronal section of the hippocampus. **A.** Three-dimensional drawing. **B.** Inverted T2-weighted MR image. **C.** T1-weighted MR image. **D.** Anatomic section (anterior view).

 1 Hippocampal body (cornu ammonis)
 1' Hippocampal head, uncal part, (cornu ammonis)
 1" Fimbria
 2 Hippocampal body (gyrus dentatus)
 2' Hippocampal head, uncal part (gyrus dentatus)
 3 Apex of the uncus
 4 Hippocampal body
 5 Fimbria
 6 Margo denticulatus
 7 Parahippocampal gyrus (subiculum)
 8 Hippocampal tail
 9 Gyrus fasciolaris
10 Fasciola cinerea
11 Gyri of Andreas Retzius
12 Isthmus
13 Splenium
14 Temporal stem
15 Temporal horn of the lateral ventricle
16 Tail of caudate nucleus
17 Subiculum
18 Parahippocampal gyrus (entorhinal area)
19 Fusiform gyrus
20 Inferior temporal gyrus
21 Middle temporal gyrus
22 Parallel sulcus
23 Superior temporal gyrus

24 Lateral fissure
25 Postcentral gyrus
26 Central sulcus
27 Precentral gyrus
28 Corpus callosum
29 Lateral ventricle
30 Fornix
31 Caudate nucleus
32 Internal capsule, posterior limb
33 Insula
34 Putamen
35 Lateral pallidum
36 Medial pallidum
37 Optic tract
38 Anterior thalamic nucleus
39 Dorsomedial thalamic nucleus
40 Ventral lateral thalamic nucleus
41 Third ventricle
42 Subthalamic nucleus
43 Substantia nigra
44 Red nucleus, anterior pole
45 Crus cerebri
46 Crural cistern and posterior cerebral artery
47 Tentorium cerebelli
48 Pons

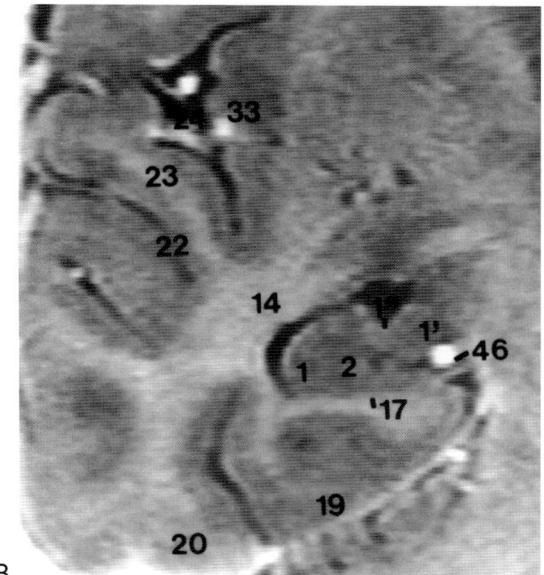

B

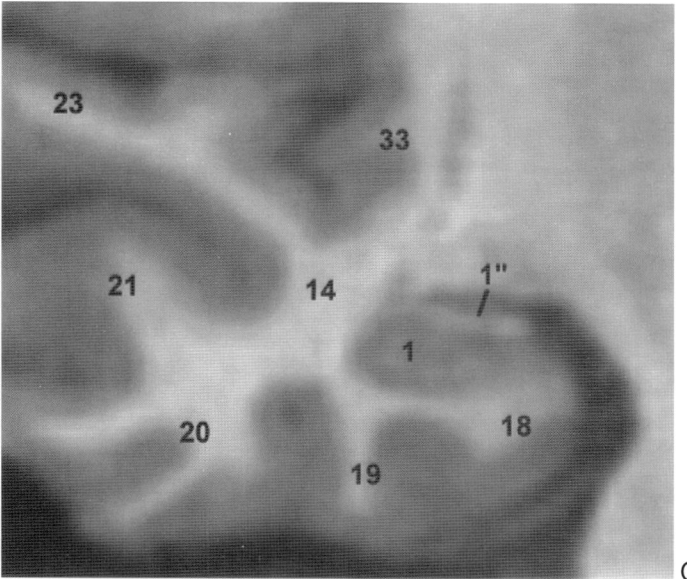

C

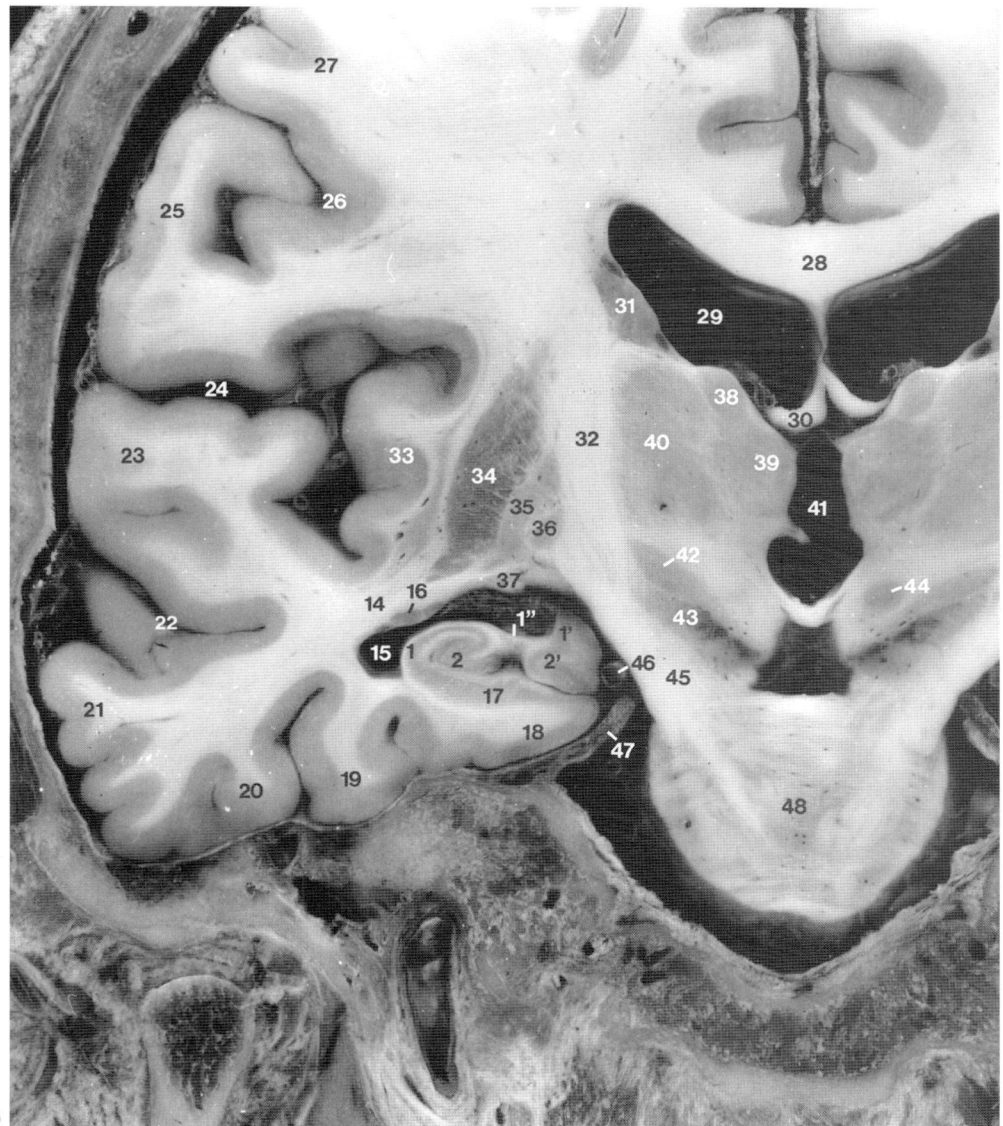

D

FIG. 3.27. *Cont'd.*

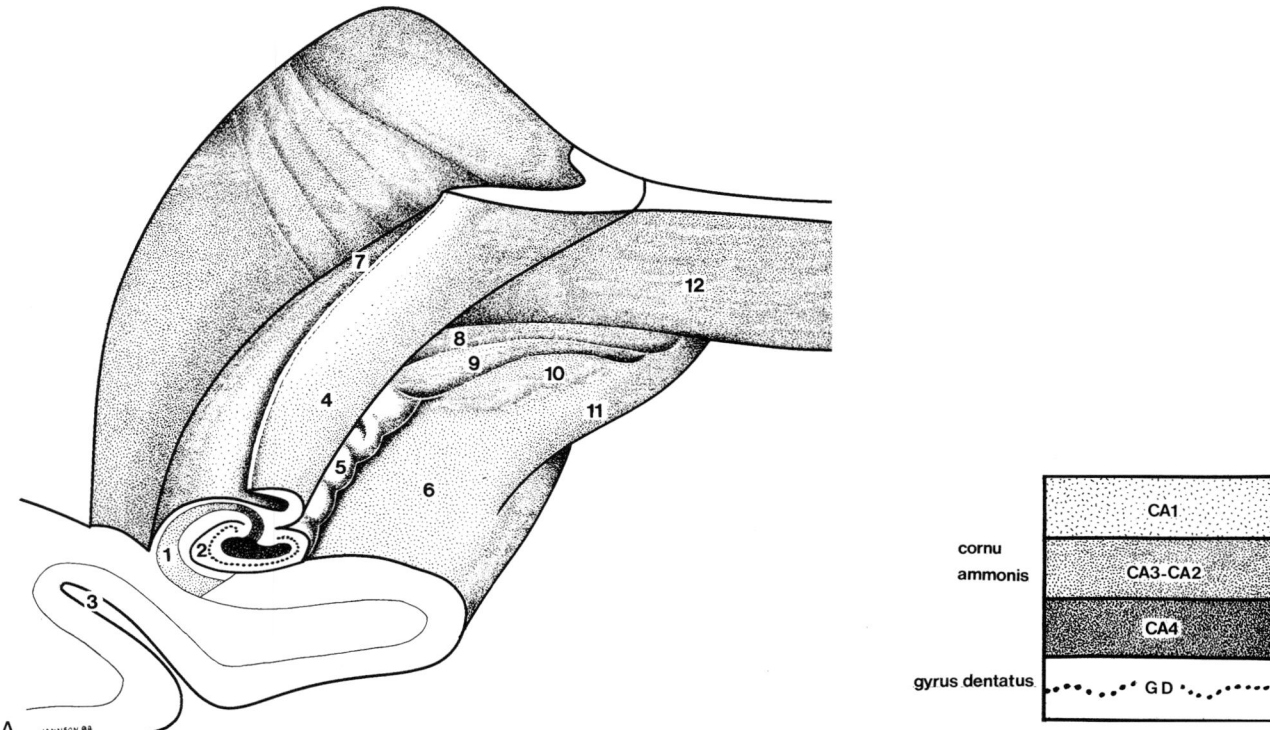

FIG. 3.28. Coronal section of the hippocampal body. **A.** Three-dimensional drawing. **B.** T1-weighted MR image. **C.** Inverted T2-weighted MR image. **D.** Anatomic section (posterior view).

1 Hippocampal body, cornu ammonis
2 Hippocampal body, gyrus dentatus
3 Collateral sulcus
3' Collateral eminence
4 Fimbria
5 Margo denticulatus
6 Parahippocampal gyrus (subiculum)
7 Hippocampal tail
8 Gyrus fasciolaris
9 Fasciola cinerea
10 Gyri of Andreas Retzius
11 Isthmus
12 Splenium
13 Temporal stem
14 Temporal horn of the lateral ventricle
15 Tail of caudate nucleus
16 Subiculum
17 Parahippocampal gyrus
18 Fusiform gyrus
19 Inferior temporal gyrus
20 Middle temporal gyrus
21 Parallel sulcus
22 Superior temporal gyrus
23 Lateral fissure

24 Transverse temporal (Heschl) gyrus
25 Postcentral gyrus
26 Central sulcus
27 Precentral gyrus
28 Corpus callosum
29 Lateral ventricle
30 Fornix
31 Caudate nucleus
32 Internal capsule, posterior limb
33 Insula
34 Putamen
35 Lateral pallidum
36 Optic tract
37 Ventral lateral thalamic nucleus
38 Dorsomedial thalamic nucleus
39 Ventral posterolateral thalamic nucleus
40 Red nucleus
41 Substantia nigra
42 Crus cerebri
43 Ambient cistern
44 Tentorium cerebelli
45 Pons
46 Internal ear

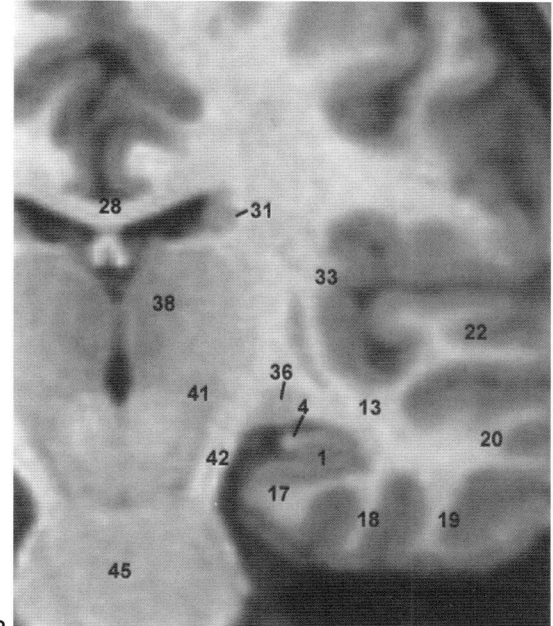

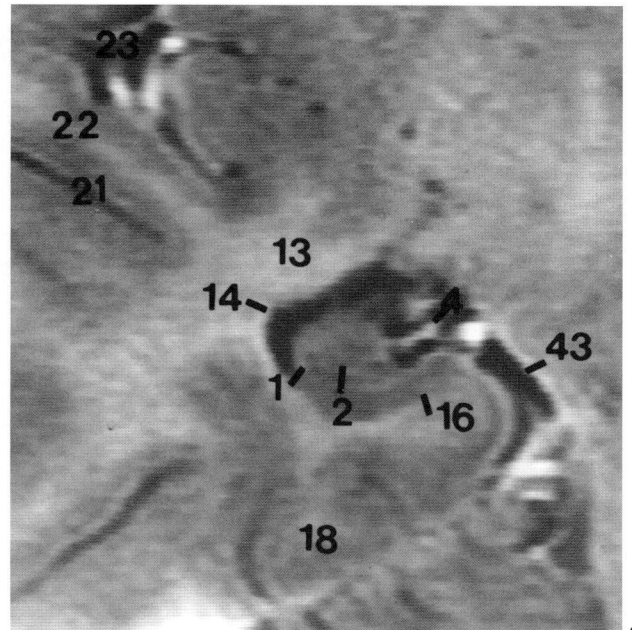

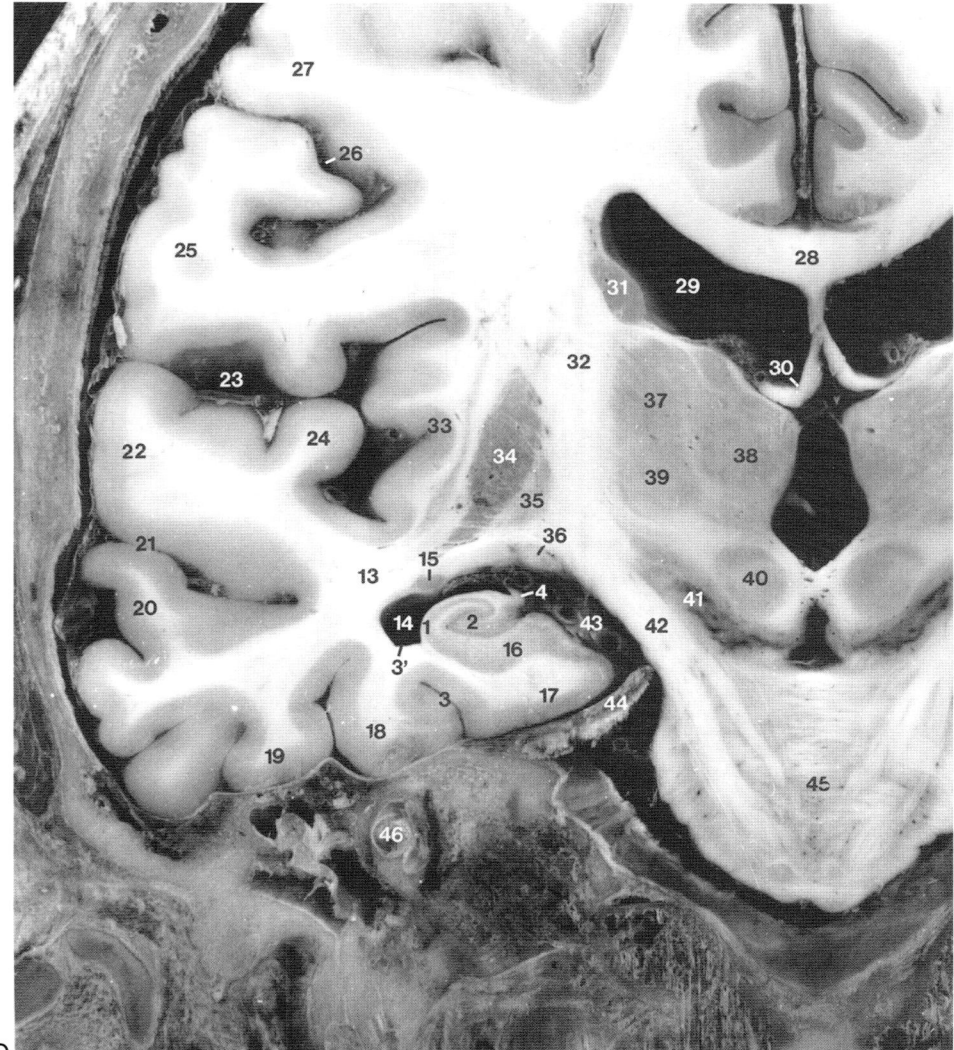

FIG. 3.28. *Cont'd.*

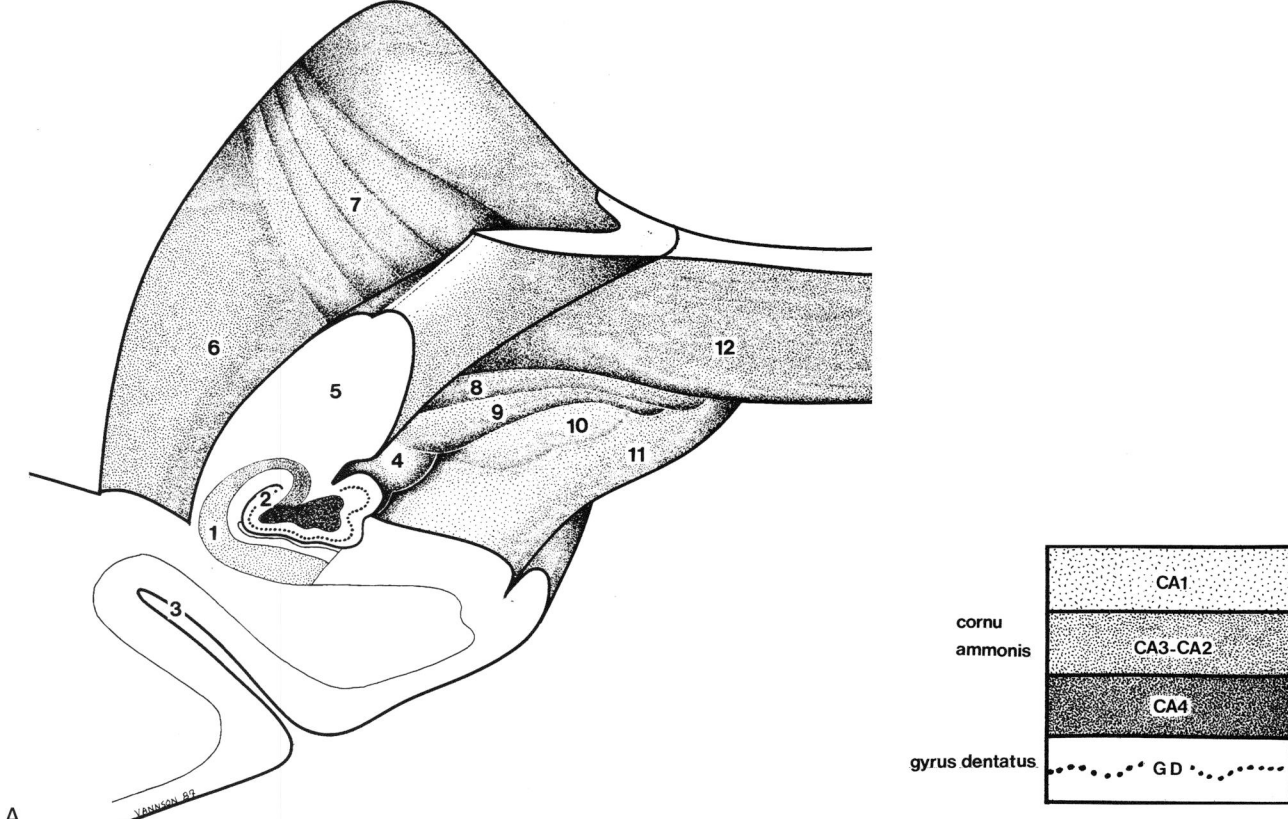

FIG. 3.29. Coronal section of the hippocampal tail. **A.** Three-dimensional drawing. **B.** T1-weighted MR image. **C.** Anatomic section (posterior view).

1 Hippocampal tail, cornu ammonis	19 Parallel sulcus
2 Hippocampal tail, gyrus dentatus	20 Superior temporal gyrus
3 Collateral sulcus	21 Lateral fissure
3′ Collateral eminence	22 Supramarginal gyrus
4 Margo denticulatus	23 Corpus callosum (splenium)
5 Crus of the fornix	24 Crus of the fornix
6 Collateral trigone	25 Lateral ventricle
7 Calcar avis	26 Caudate nucleus
8 Gyrus fasciolaris	27 Internal capsule, retrolentiform part
9 Fasciola cinerea	28 Pulvinar
10 Gyri of Andreas Retzius	29 Ambient cistern
11 Isthmus	30 Wing of the ambient cistern
12 Splenium	31 Quadrigeminal cistern
13 Temporal horn of the lateral ventricle	32 Superior colliculus
14 Tail of caudate nucleus	33 Tentorium cerebelli
15 Parahippocampal gyrus	34 Cerebellar hemisphere
15′ Subiculum	35 Superior cerebellar peduncle
16 Fusiform gyrus	36 Middle cerebellar peduncle
17 Inferior temporal gyrus	37 Pons
18 Middle temporal gyrus	38 Flocculus

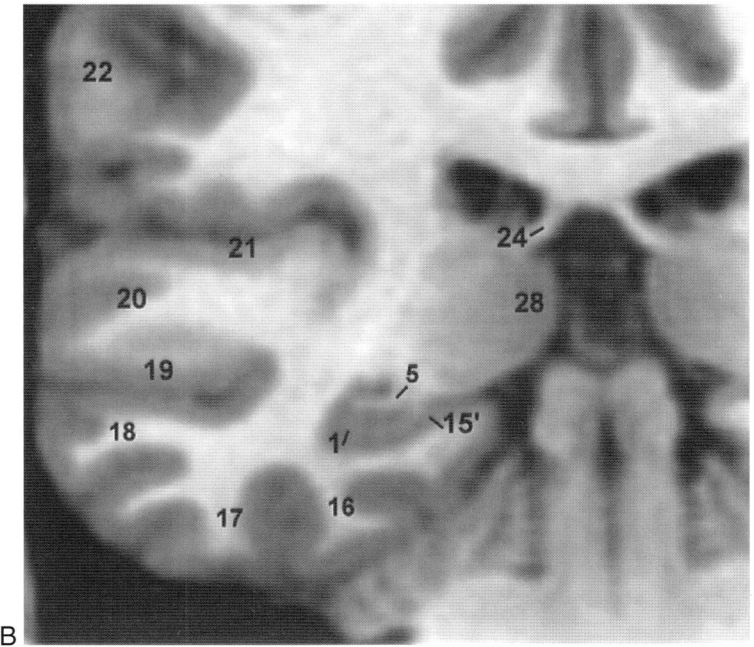

B

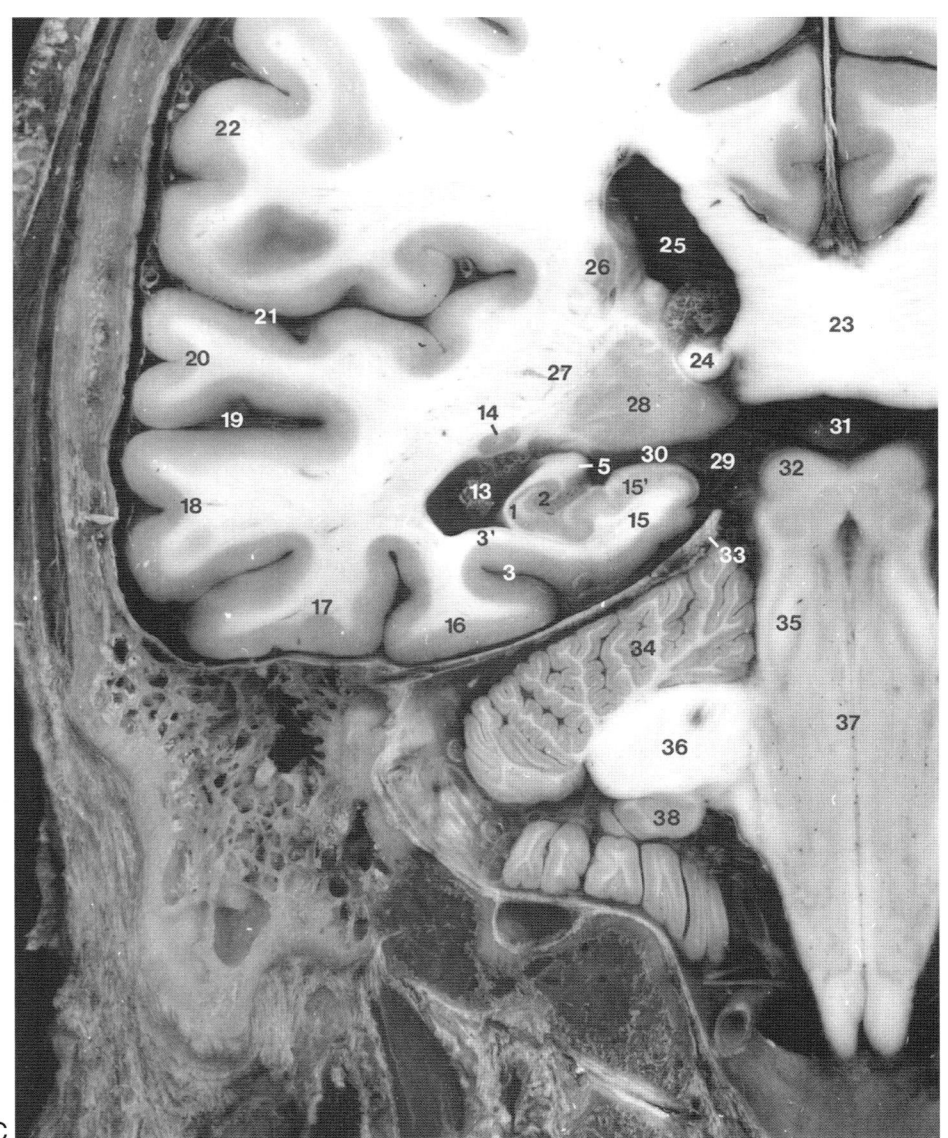

C

FIG. 3.29. *Cont'd.*

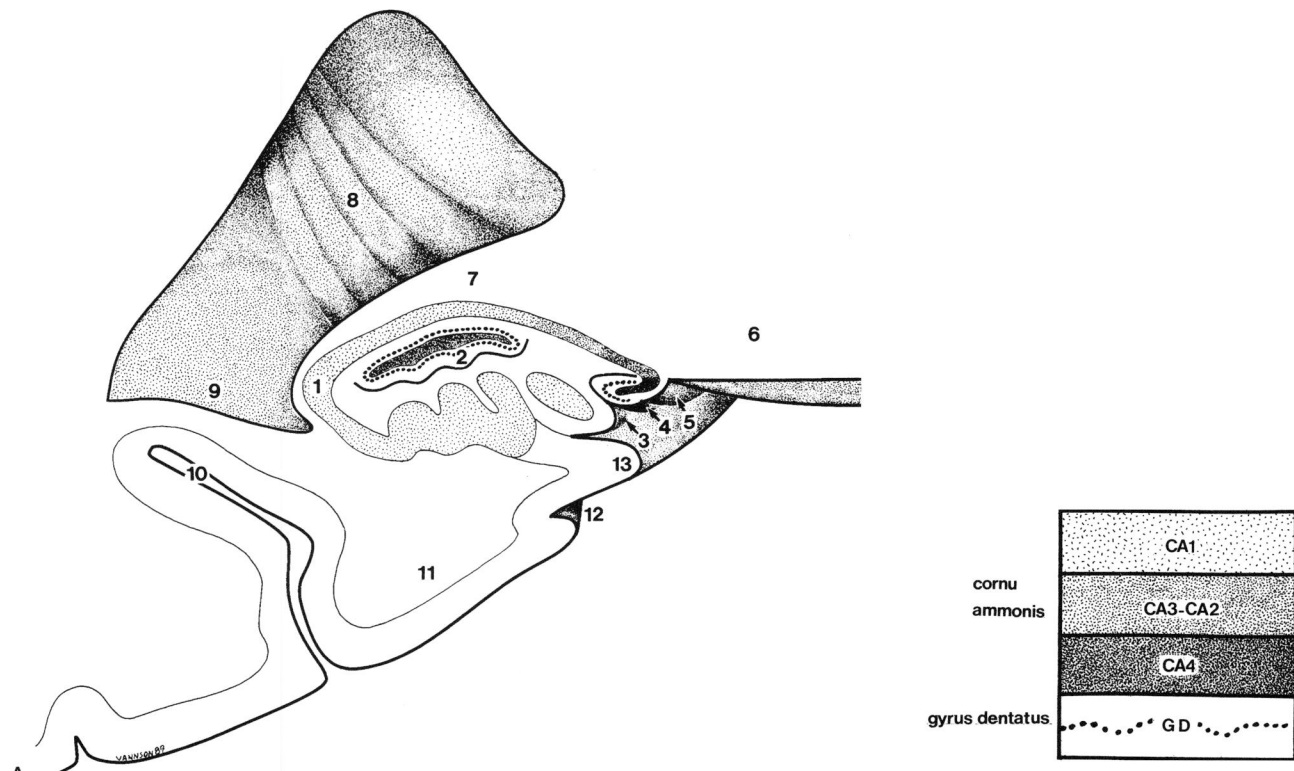

FIG. 3.30. Coronal section of the hippocampal tail. **A.** Three-dimensional drawing. **B.** T1-weighted MR image. **C.** Anatomic section (posterior view).

 1 Hippocampal tail, cornu ammonis
 2 Hippocampal tail, gyrus dentatus
 3 Gyrus of Andreas Retzius
 4 Fasciola cinerea
 5 Gyrus fasciolaris
 6 Corpus callosum, splenium
 7 Crus of the fornix
 8 Calcar avis
 9 Collateral trigone
10 Collateral sulcus
11 Parahippocampal gyrus
12 Anterior calcarine sulcus
13 Isthmus
14 Fusiform gyrus
15 Inferior temporal gyrus

16 Middle temporal gyrus
17 Parallel sulcus
18 Superior temporal gyrus
19 Lateral fissure
20 Supramarginal gyrus
21 Atrium of lateral ventricle
22 Quadrigeminal cistern
23 Ambient cistern
24 Superior colliculus
25 Tentorium cerebelli
26 Cerebellar hemisphere
27 Superior cerebellar peduncle
28 Middle cerebellar peduncle
29 Flocculus
30 Pons

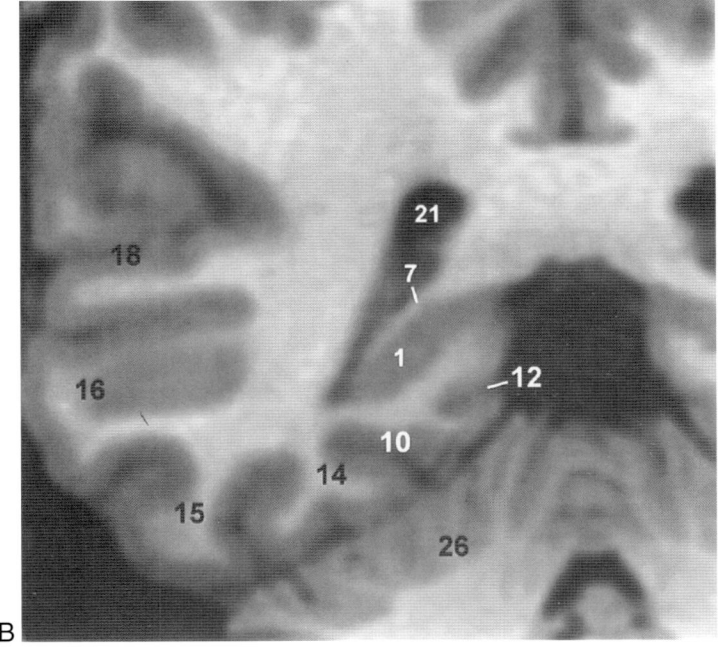

B

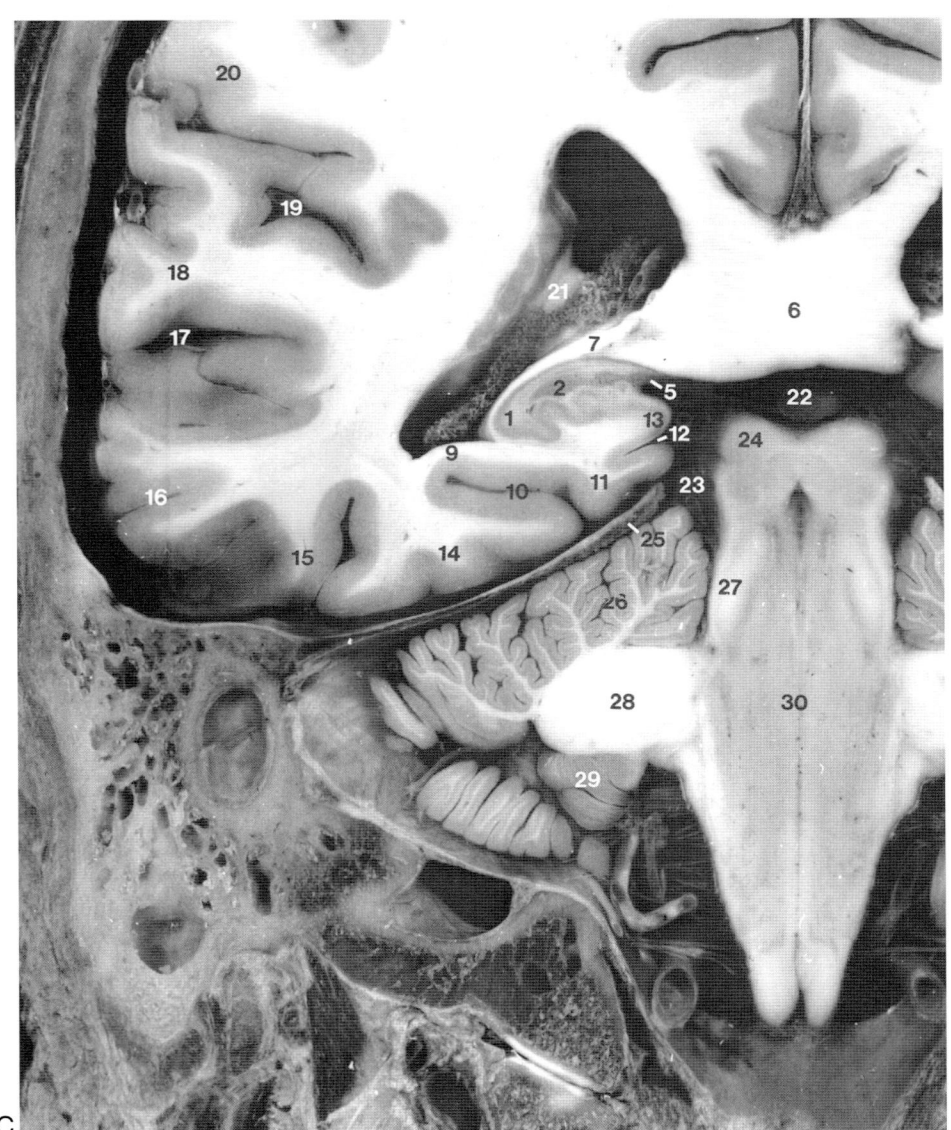

C

FIG. 3.30. *Cont'd.*

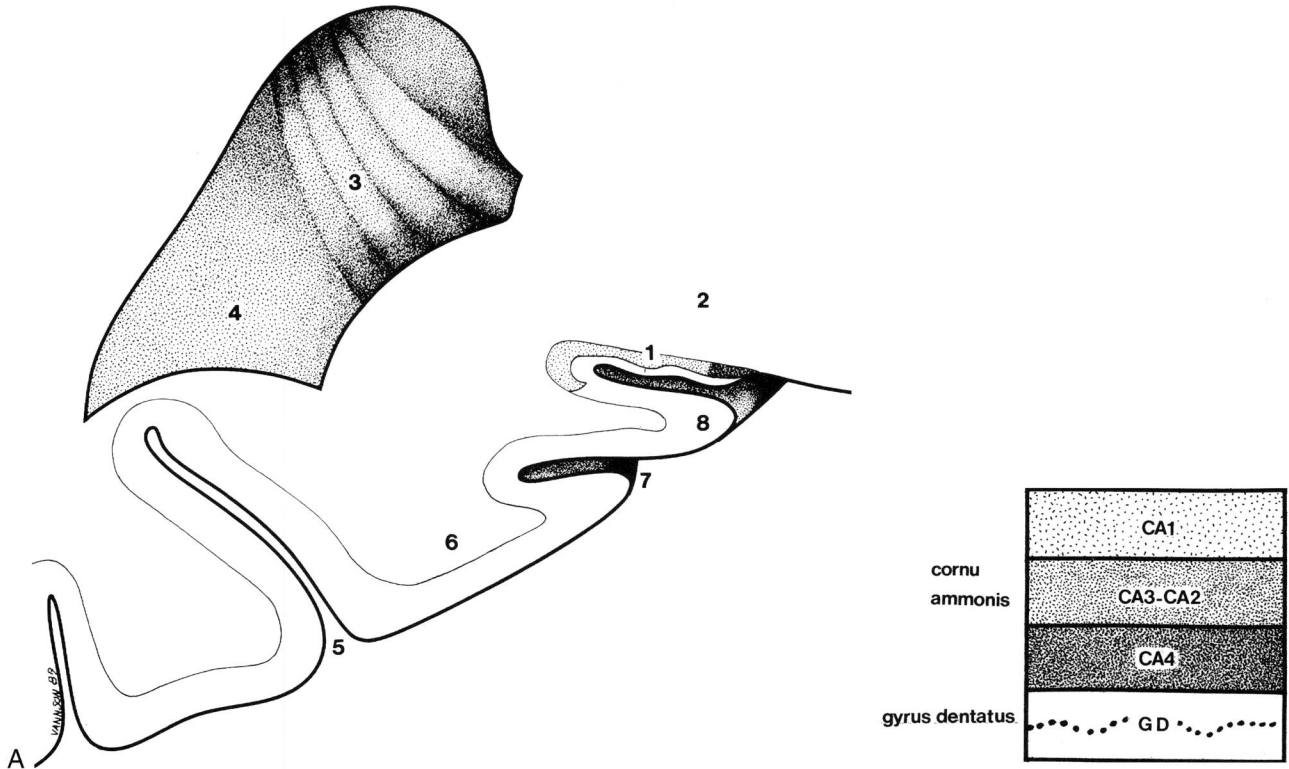

FIG. 3.31. Coronal section of the hippocampal tail. **A.** Three-dimensional drawing. **B.** T1-weighted MR image. **C.** Anatomic section (anterior view).

1 Hippocampal tail, subsplenial gyrus
2 Corpus callosum, splenium
3 Calcar avis
4 Collateral trigone
5 Collateral sulcus
6 Parahippocampal gyrus
7 Anterior calcarine sulcus
8 Isthmus
9 Fusiform gyrus

10 Inferior temporal gyrus
11 Middle temporal gyrus
12 Parallel sulcus
13 Superior temporal gyrus
14 Supramarginal gyrus
15 Atrium of the lateral ventricle
16 Tentorium cerebelli
17 Cerebellum
18 Fourth ventricle

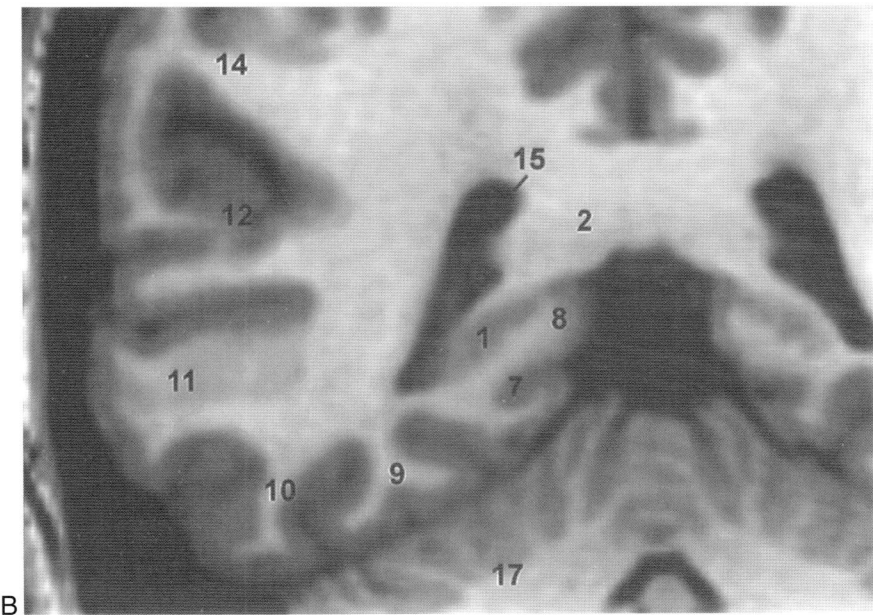

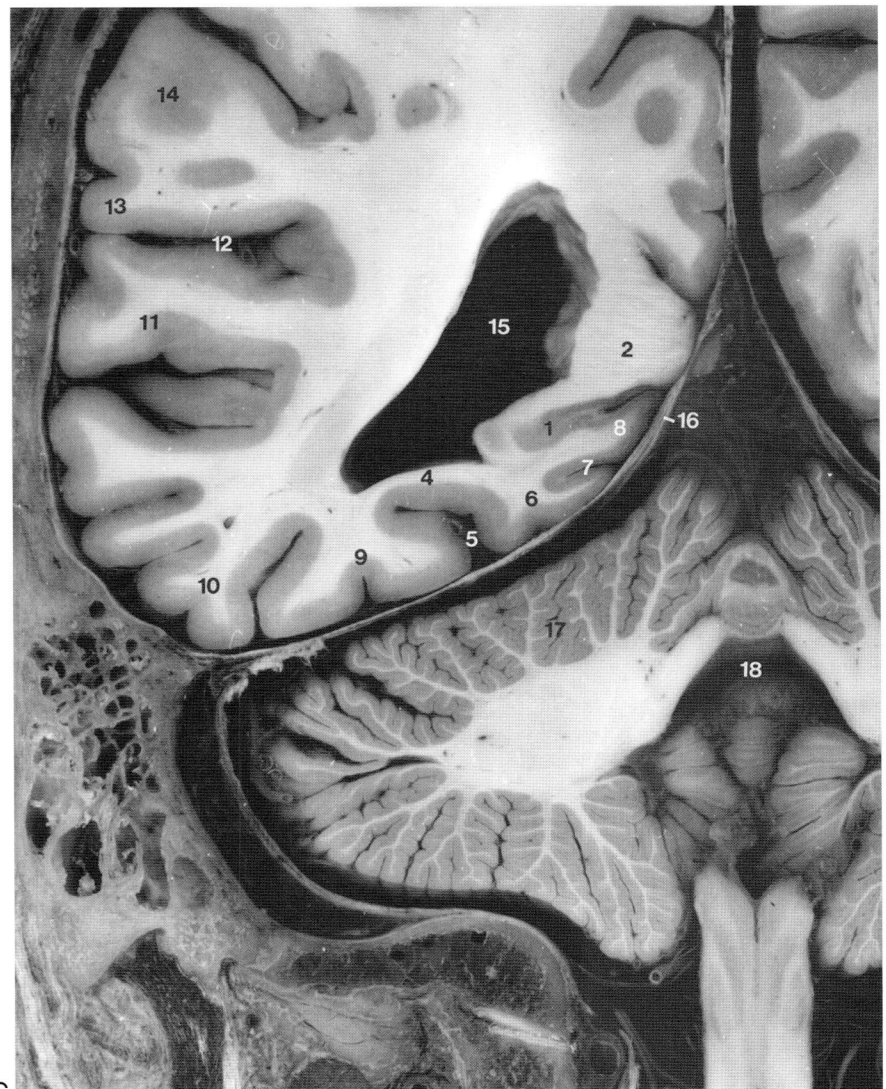

FIG. 3.31. *Cont'd.*

AXIAL SECTIONS OF THE HIPPOCAMPUS

The axial views show six sections progressing from upper to lower levels.

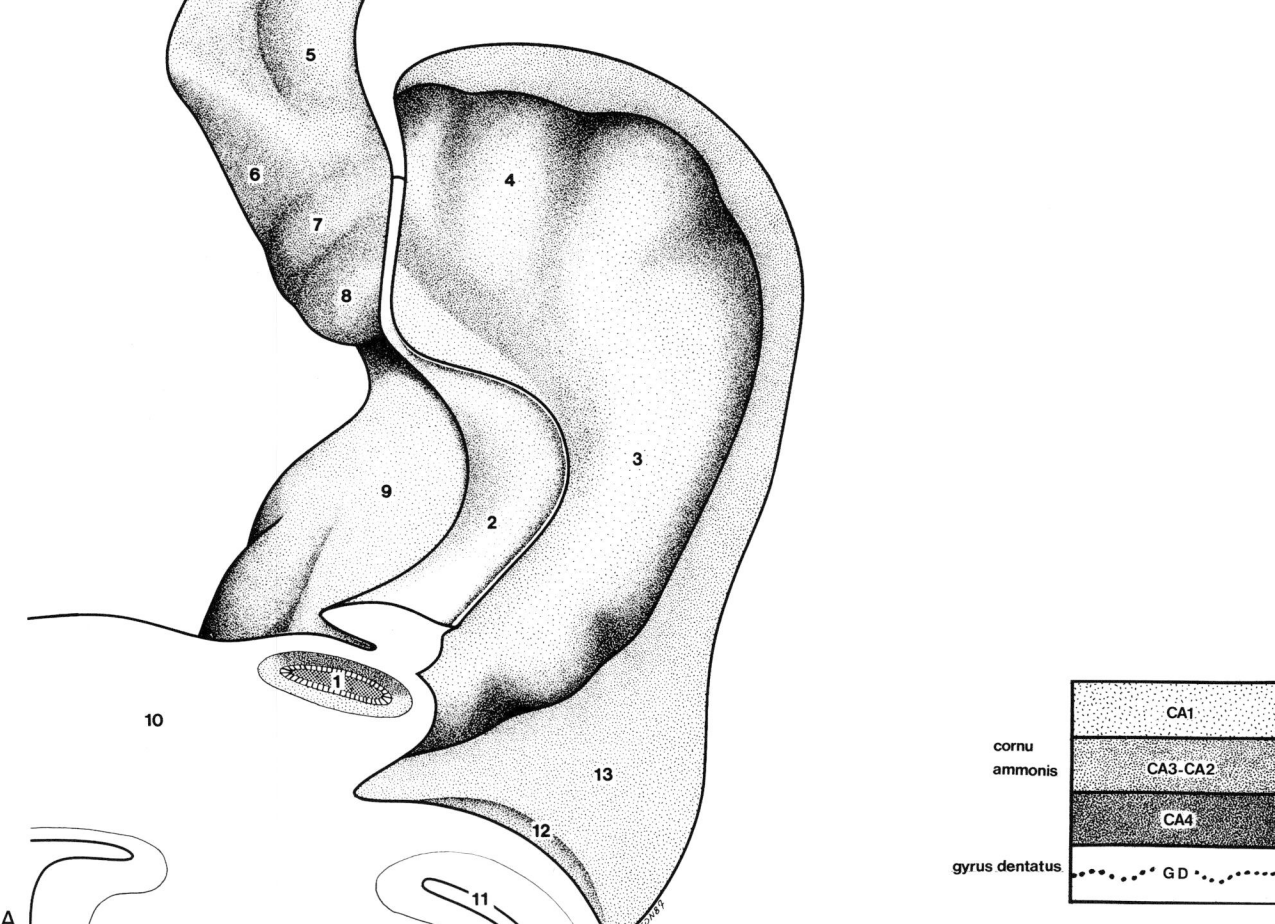

FIG. 3.32. Axial section of the hippocampus. **A.** Three-dimensional drawing. **B.** Anatomic section (inferior view).

 1 Hippocampal tail (cornu ammonis)
 2 Crus of the fornix
 3 Hippocampal body
 4 Hippocampal head (digitationes hippocampi)
 5 Semilunar gyrus
 6 Gyrus uncinatus
 7 Band of Giacomini
 8 Apex of the uncus
 9 Parahippocampal gyrus (subiculum)
10 Corpus callosum, splenium
11 Anterior calcarine sulcus
12 Calcar avis
13 Collateral trigone
14 Atrium of the lateral ventricle
15 Cingulate gyrus
16 Parieto-occipital fissure
17 Calcarine sulcus
18 Middle temporal gyrus
19 Parallel sulcus
20 Superior temporal gyrus
21 Lateral fissure
22 Lateral ventricle
23 Fornix
24 Caudate nucleus
25 Insula
26 Putamen
27 Internal capsule, anterior limb
28 Internal capsule, genu
29 Internal capsule, posterior limb
30 Anterior thalamic nucleus
31 Ventral lateral thalamic nucleus
32 Dorsomedial thalamic nucleus
33 Stria medullaris
34 Pulvinar
35 Tail of caudate nucleus
36 Third ventricle

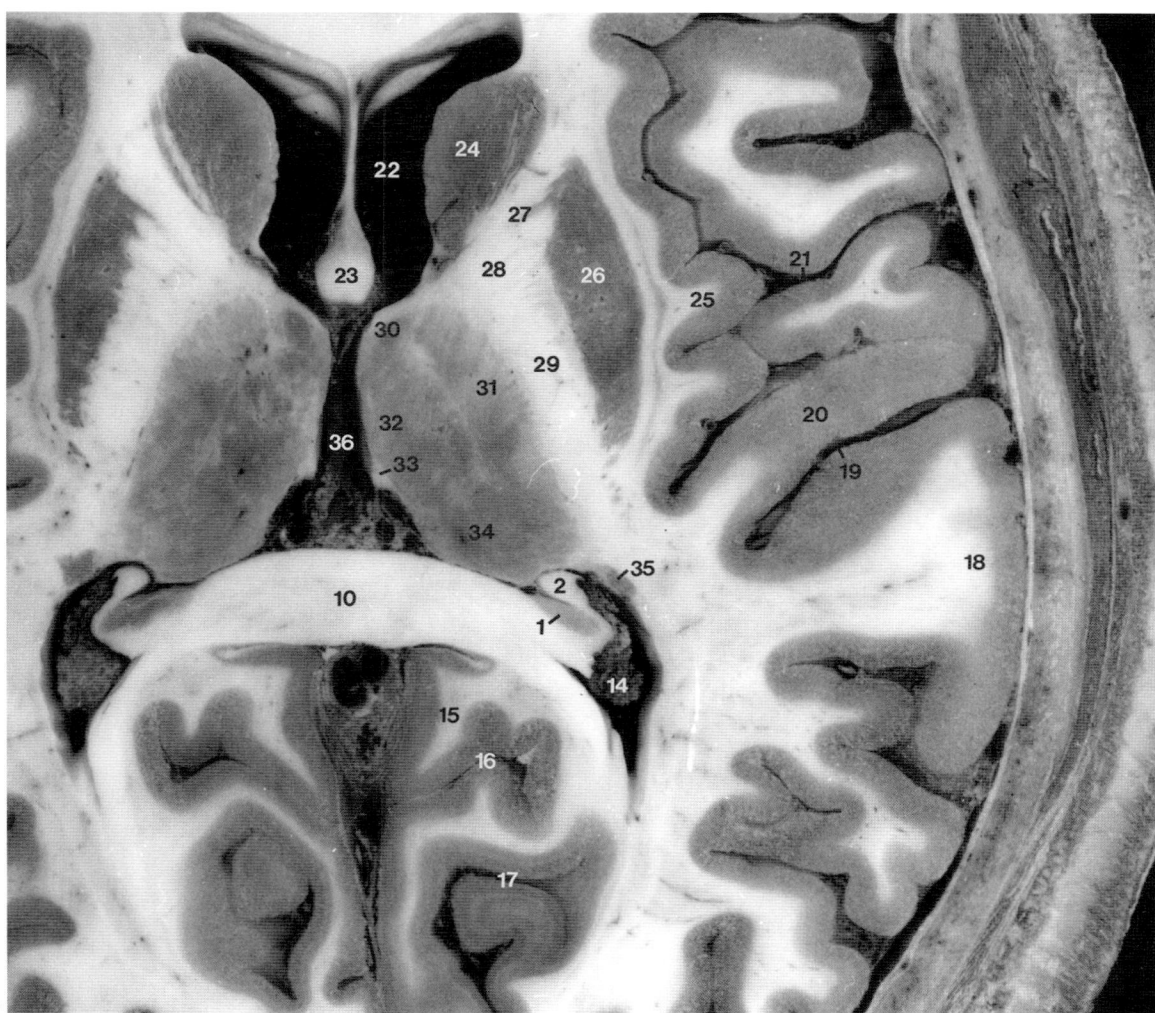

FIG. 3.32. *Cont'd.*

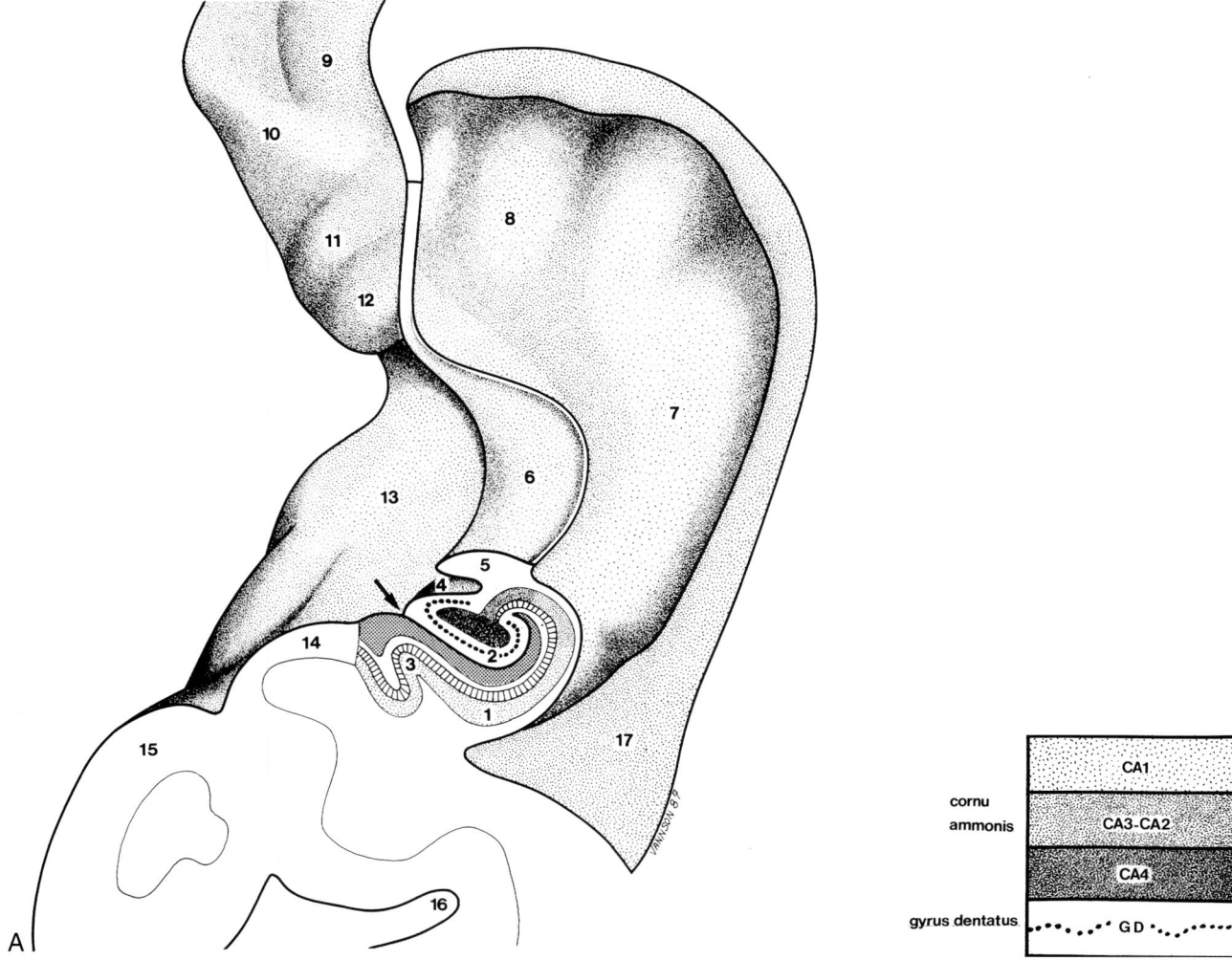

FIG. 3.33. Axial section of the hippocampus. **A.** Three-dimensional drawing. **B.** T1-weighted MR image. **C.** Anatomic section (inferior view).

1 Hippocampal tail, cornu ammonis
2 Hippocampal tail, gyrus dentatus
3 Gyrus of Andreas Retzius (folds of cornu ammonis)
4 Margo denticulatus
5 Cut surface of the fimbria
6 Fimbria
7 Hippocampal body
8 Hippocampal head (digitationes hippocampi)
9 Semilunar gyrus
10 Gyrus uncinatus
11 Band of Giacomini
12 Apex of the uncus
13 Parahippocampal gyrus (subiculum)
14 Subiculum (cut surface)
15 Isthmus
16 Anterior calcarine sulcus
17 Collateral eminence
18 Lingual gyrus
19 Calcarine sulcus
20 Middle temporal gyrus
21 Parallel sulcus

22 Superior temporal gyrus
23 Lateral fissure
24 Insula
25 Caudate nucleus
26 Fornix
27 Claustrum
28 Putamen
29 Lateral pallidum
30 Medial pallidum
31 Internal capsule, anterior limb
32 Internal capsule, genu
33 Internal capsule, posterior limb
34 Interthalamic adhesion
34′ Thalamus
35 Third ventricle
36 Pineal gland
37 Superior colliculus
38 Pulvinar
39 Quadrigeminal cistern
40 Occipital horn of the lateral ventricle

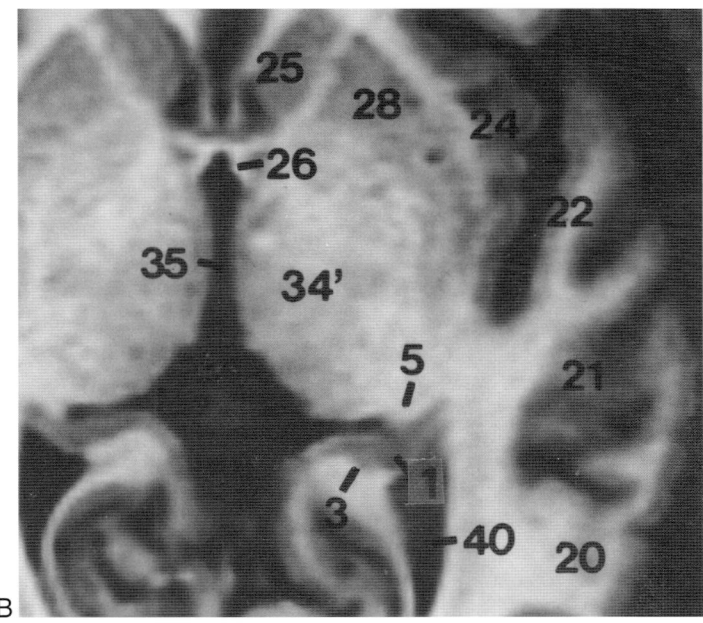

B

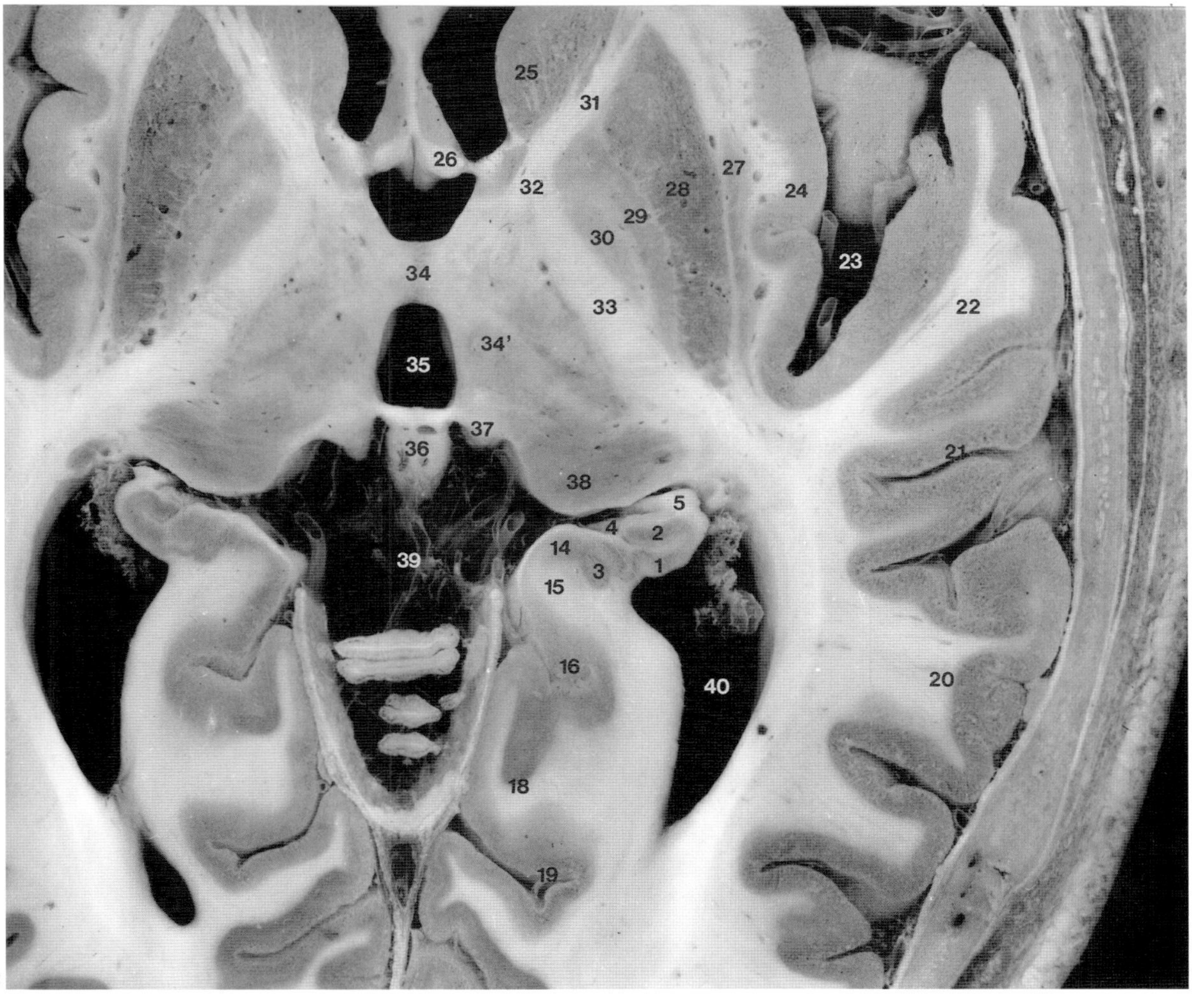

C

FIG. 3.33. *Cont'd.*

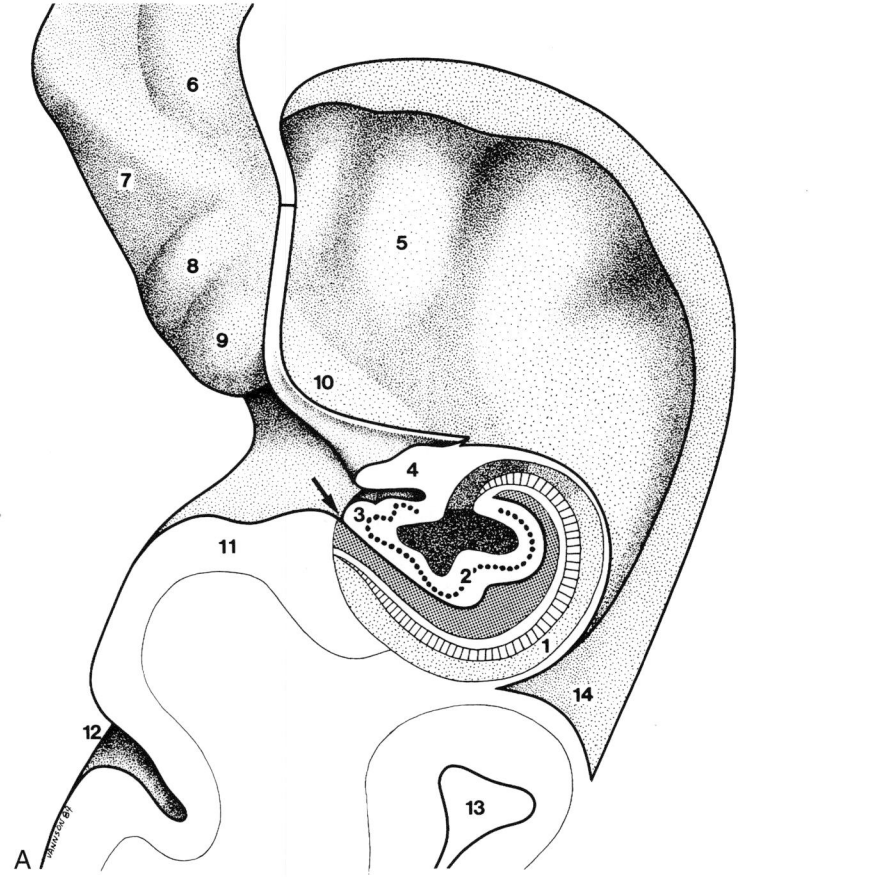

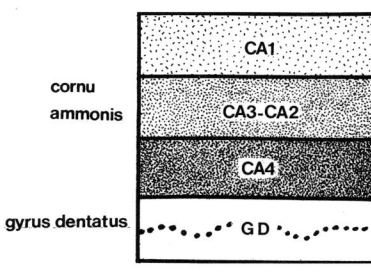

FIG. 3.34. Axial section of the hippocampus. **A.** Three-dimensional drawing. **B.** T2-weighted MR image. **C.** Anatomic section (inferior view).

1 Hippocampal body, cornu ammonis
2 Hippocampal body, gyrus dentatus
3 Margo denticulatus
4 Cut surface of the fimbria
5 Hippocampal head (digitationes hippocampi)
6 Semilunar gyrus
7 Gyrus uncinatus
8 Band of Giacomini
9 Apex of the uncus
10 Fimbria
11 Subiculum
12 Anterior calcarine sulcus
13 Collateral sulcus
14 Collateral eminence
15 Lingual gyrus
16 Middle temporal gyrus
17 Parallel sulcus
18 Superior temporal gyrus
19 Lateral fissure
20 Insula

21 Claustrum
22 Caudate nucleus
23 Anterior commissure
24 Putamen
25 Lateral pallidum
26 Medial pallidum
27 Anterior column of the fornix
28 Hypothalamus
29 Third ventricle
30 Mamillothalamic tract
31 Crus cerebri
32 Subthalamic nucleus
33 Red nucleus
34 Superior colliculus
35 Medial geniculate body
36 Lateral geniculate body
37 Cerebellum
38 Quadrigeminal cistern
39 Ambient cistern
40 Wing of ambient cistern (lateral part of the transverse fissure)

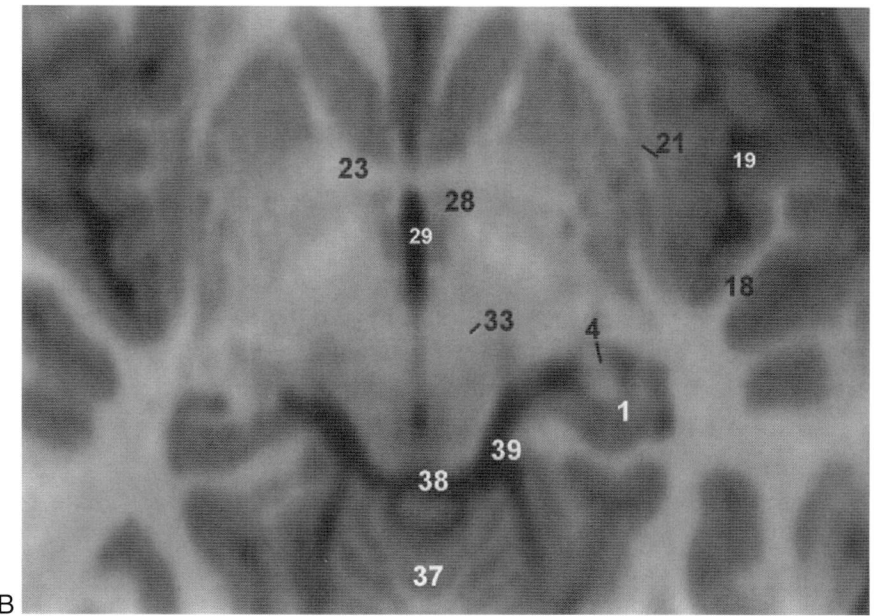

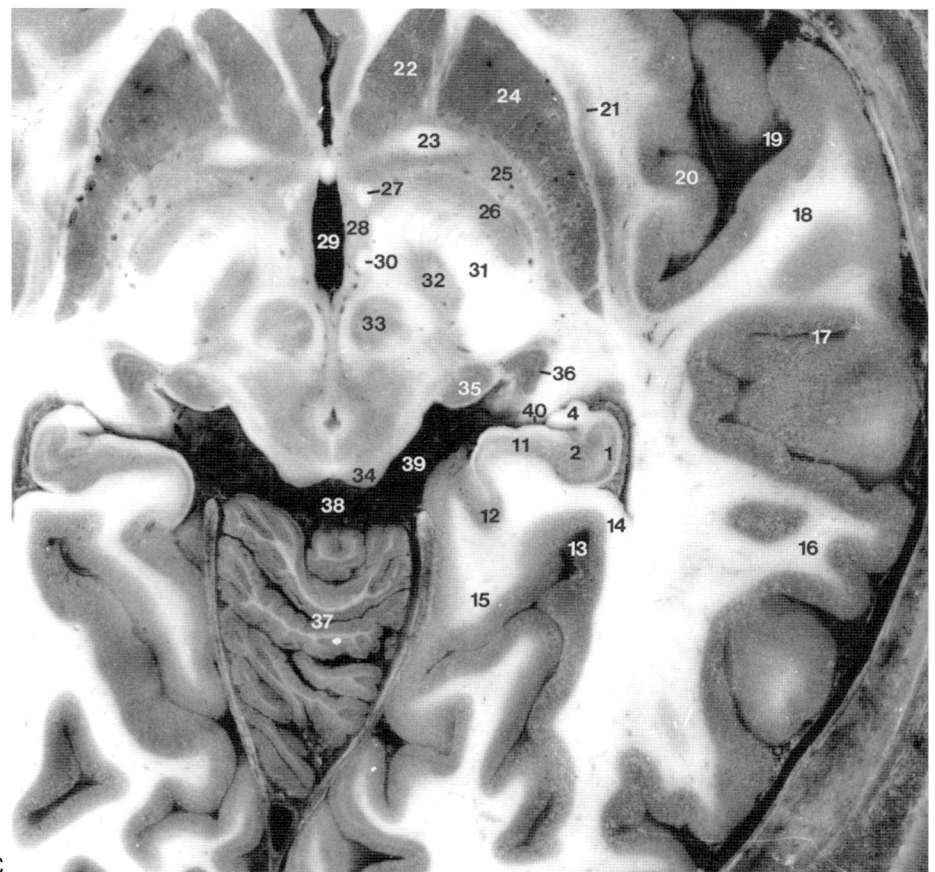

FIG. 3.34. *Cont'd.*

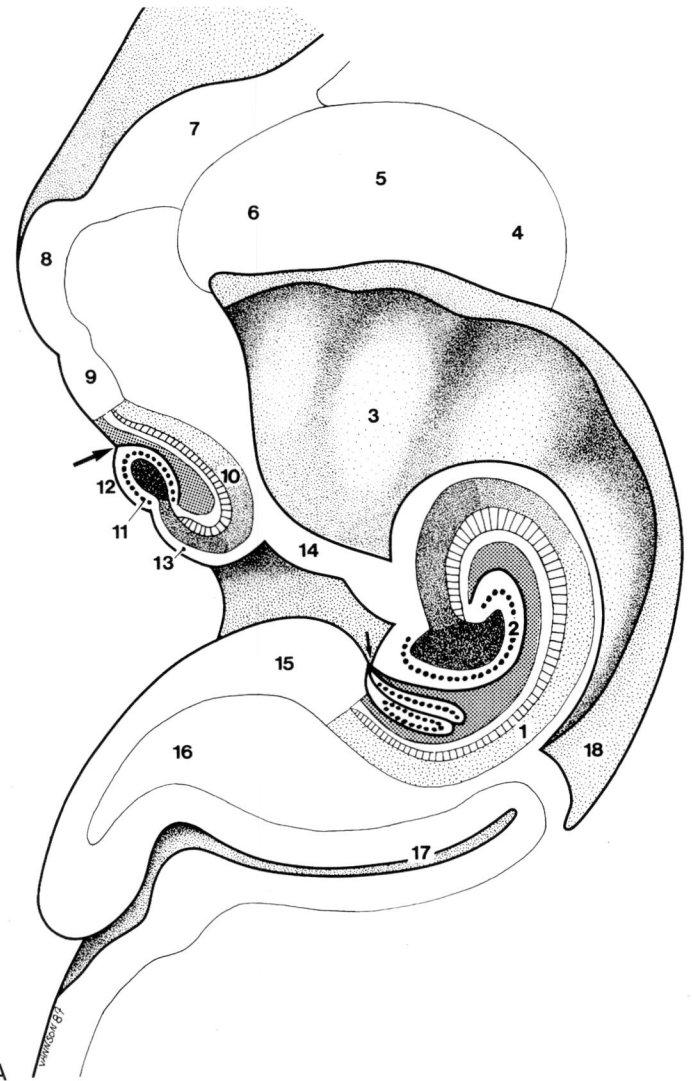

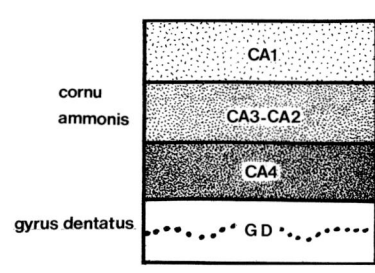

FIG. 3.35. Axial section of the hippocampus. **A.** Three-dimensional drawing. **B.** Inverted T2-weighted MR image. **C.** Anatomic section (superior view).

1 Hippocampal body, cornu ammonis
2 Hippocampal body, gyrus dentatus (an arrow indicates the hippocampal sulcus)
3 Hippocampal head, digitationes hippocampi
4 Amygdala, lateral nucleus
5 Amygdala, basal nucleus
6 Amygdala, accessory basal nucleus
7 amygdala, cortical nucleus
8 Gyrus uncinatus
9 Subiculum in the uncus
10 Hippocampal head, uncal part (cornu ammonis)
11 Hippocampal head, uncal part (gyrus dentatus)
12 Band of Giacomini (an arrow indicates the hippocampal sulcus)
13 Apex of the uncus
14 Fimbria
15 Subiculum
16 Parahippocampal gyrus
17 Collateral sulcus
18 Collateral eminence
19 Middle temporal gyrus

20 Parallel sulcus
21 Superior temporal gyrus
22 Lateral fissure
23 Insula
24 Nucleus accumbens
25 Anterior perforated substance
26 Optic tract
27 Third ventricle
28 Mamillary body
29 Red nucleus
30 Substantia nigra
31 Crus cerebri
32 Interpeduncular cistern
33 Crural cistern
34 Ambient cistern
35 Wing of the ambient cistern
36 Quadrigeminal cistern
37 Cerebellum
38 Tentorium cerebelli
39 Temporal horn of the lateral ventricle

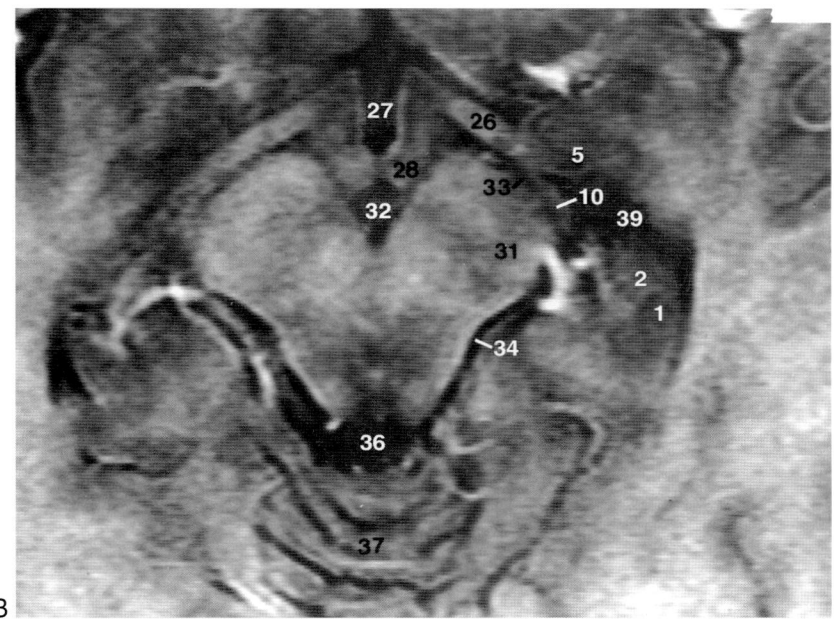

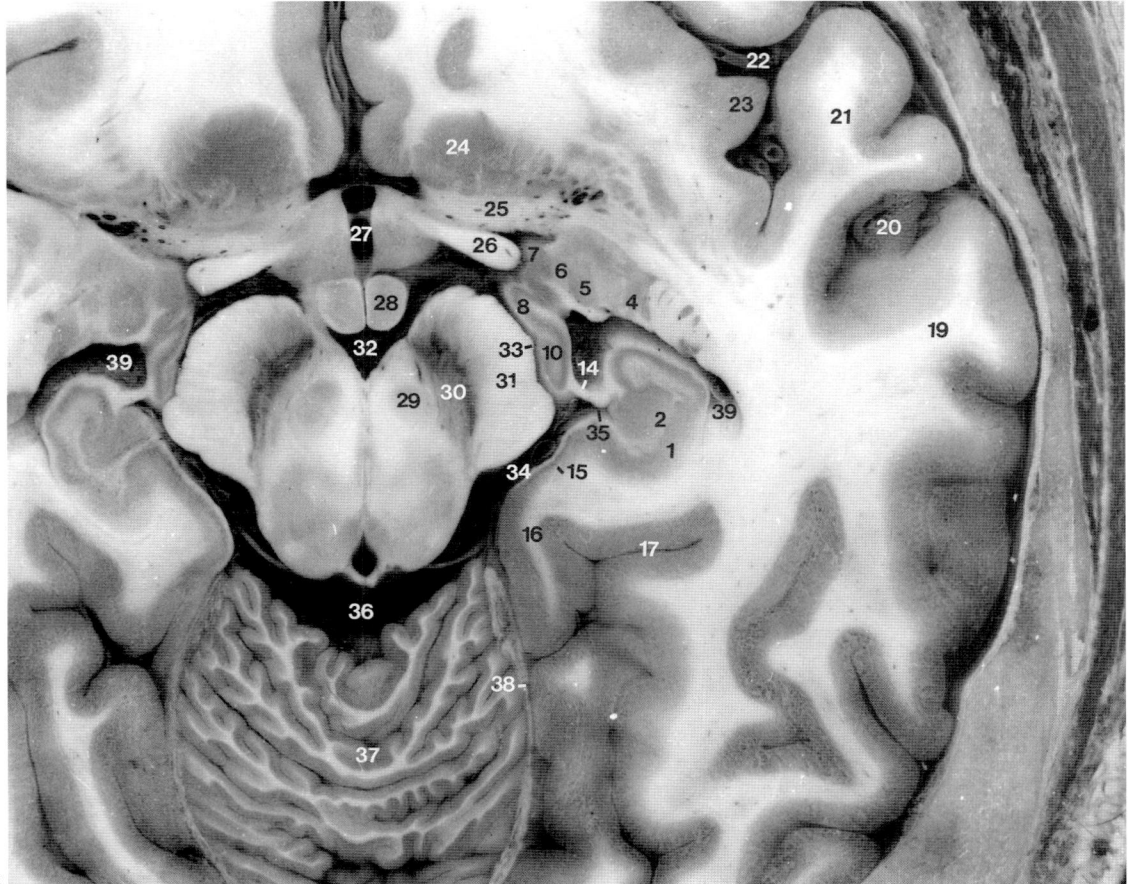

FIG. 3.35. *Cont'd.*

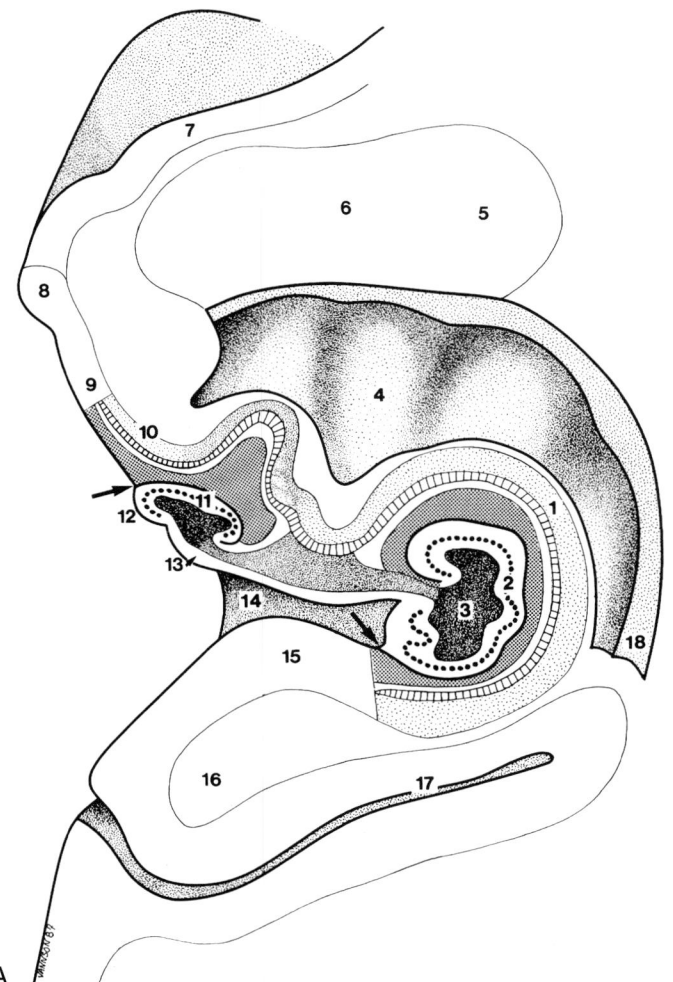

A

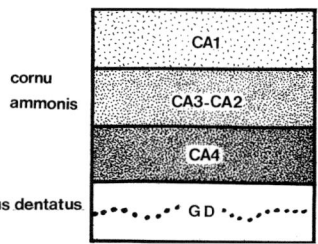

FIG. 3.36. Axial section of the hippocampus. **A.** Three-dimensional drawing. **B.** Inverted T2-weighted MR image. **C.** Anatomic section (superior view).

 1 Hippocampal head, cornu ammonis
 2 Hippocampal head, gyrus dentatus
 3 Hippocampal head, cornu ammonis
 4 Digitationes hippocampi
 5 Amygdala, lateral nucleus
 6 Amygdala, basal nucleus
 7 Gyrus ambiens
 8 Gyrus uncinatus
 9 Subiculum in the uncus
10 Cornu ammonis in the uncus
11 Gyrus dentatus in the uncus
12 Band of Giacomini (superficial part of the gyrus dentatus in the uncus)
13 Apex of the uncus
14 Uncal sulcus (arrows show the hippocampal sulcus)
15 Subiculum
16 Parahippocampal gyrus
17 Collateral sulcus
18 Collateral eminence

19 Middle temporal gyrus
20 Parallel sulcus
21 Superior temporal gyrus
22 Lateral fissure
23 Nucleus accumbens
24 Optic tract
25 Tuber
26 Third ventricle
27 Mamillary body
28 Superior cerebellar peduncle
29 Substantia nigra
30 Crus cerebri
31 Interpeduncular cistern
32 Crural cistern
33 Ambient cistern
34 Quadrigeminal cistern
35 Cerebellum
36 Tentorium cerebelli

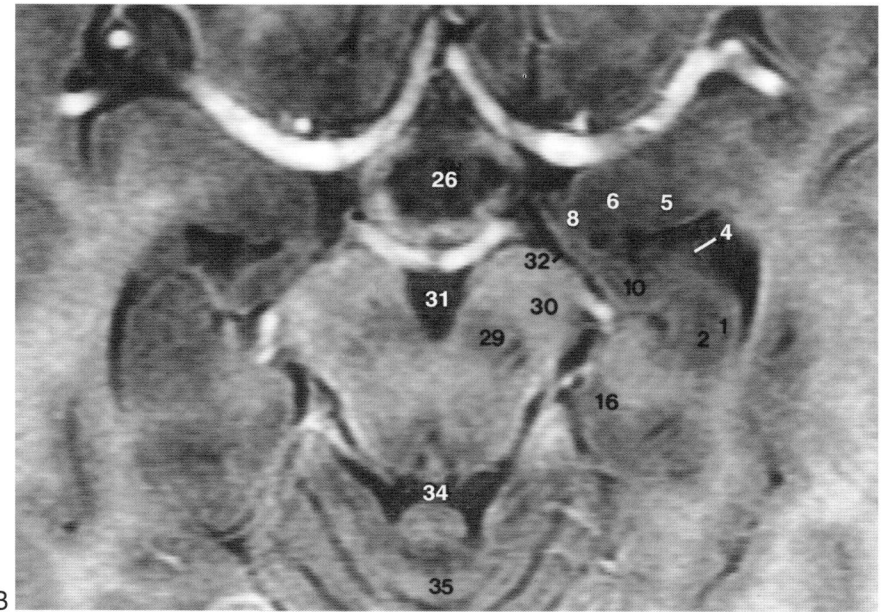

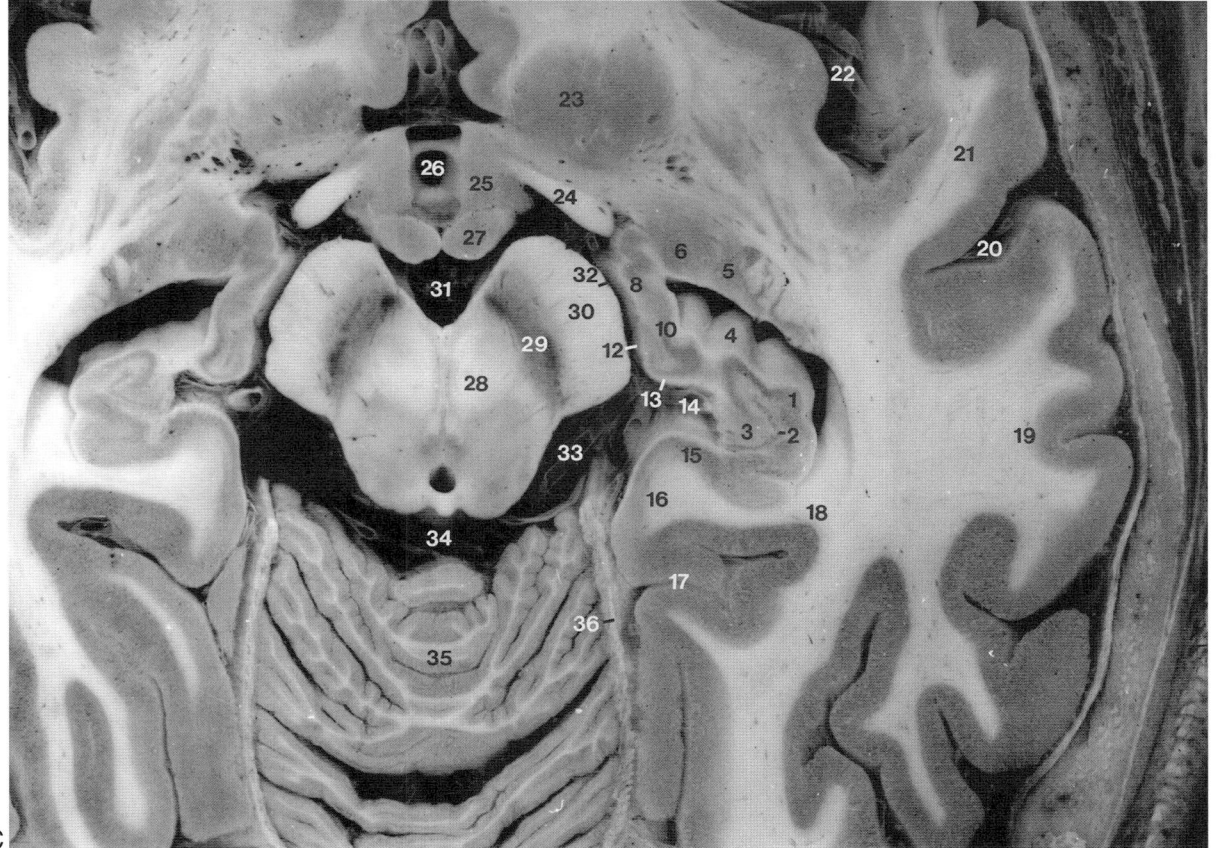

FIG. 3.36. *Cont'd.*

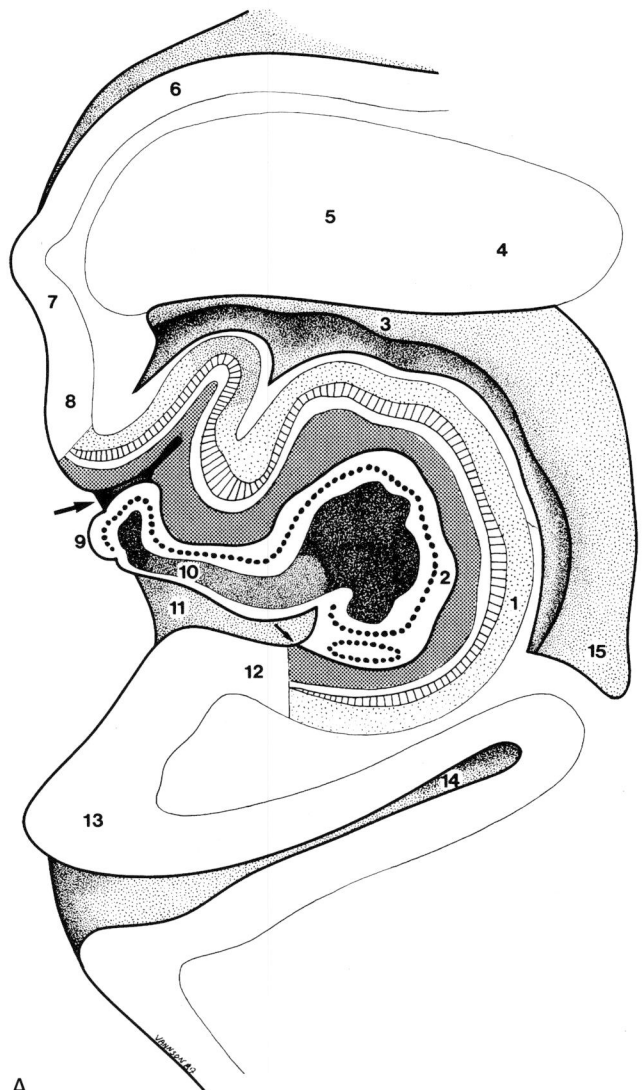

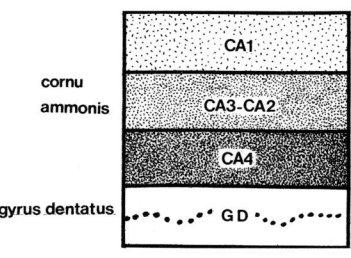

FIG. 3.37. Axial section of the hippocampus. **A.** Three-dimensional drawing. **B.** Inverted T2-weighted MR image. **C.** Anatomic section (inferior view).

1 Hippocampal head, cornu ammonis
2 Hippocampal head, gyrus dentatus
3 Temporal horn of the lateral ventricle
4 Amygdala, lateral nucleus
5 Amygdala, basal nucleus
6 Gyrus ambiens
7 Gyrus uncinatus
8 Subiculum in the uncus
9 Band of Giacomini (arrows indicate the hippocampal sulcus)
10 Apex of the uncus
11 Uncal sulcus
12 Subiculum
13 Parahippocampal gyrus
14 Collateral sulcus
15 Collateral eminence

16 Inferior temporal gyrus
17 Middle temporal gyrus
18 Superior temporal gyrus
19 Lateral fissure, basal part
20 Middle cerebral artery
21 Medial orbital gyrus
22 Gyrus rectus
23 Optic chiasma
24 Chiasmatic cistern
25 Oculomotor nerve
26 Basilar artery
27 Upper part of pons
28 Cerebellum
29 Tentorium cerebelli

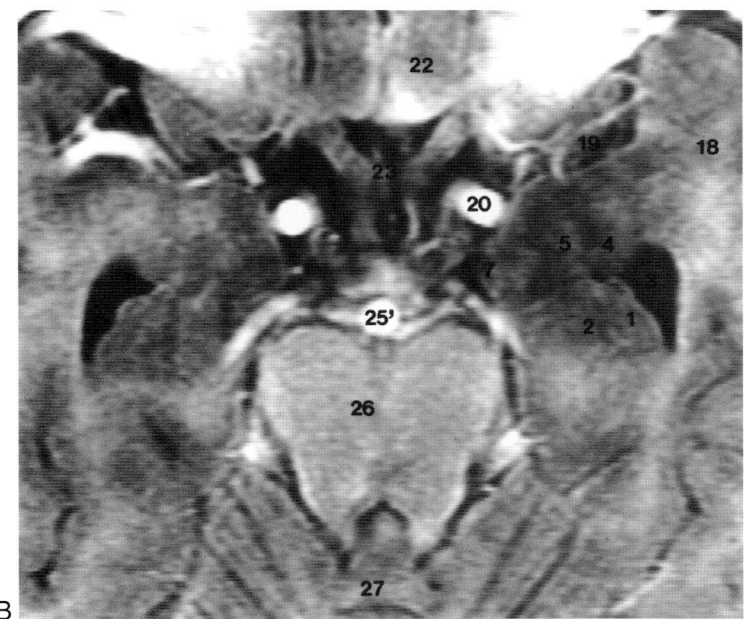

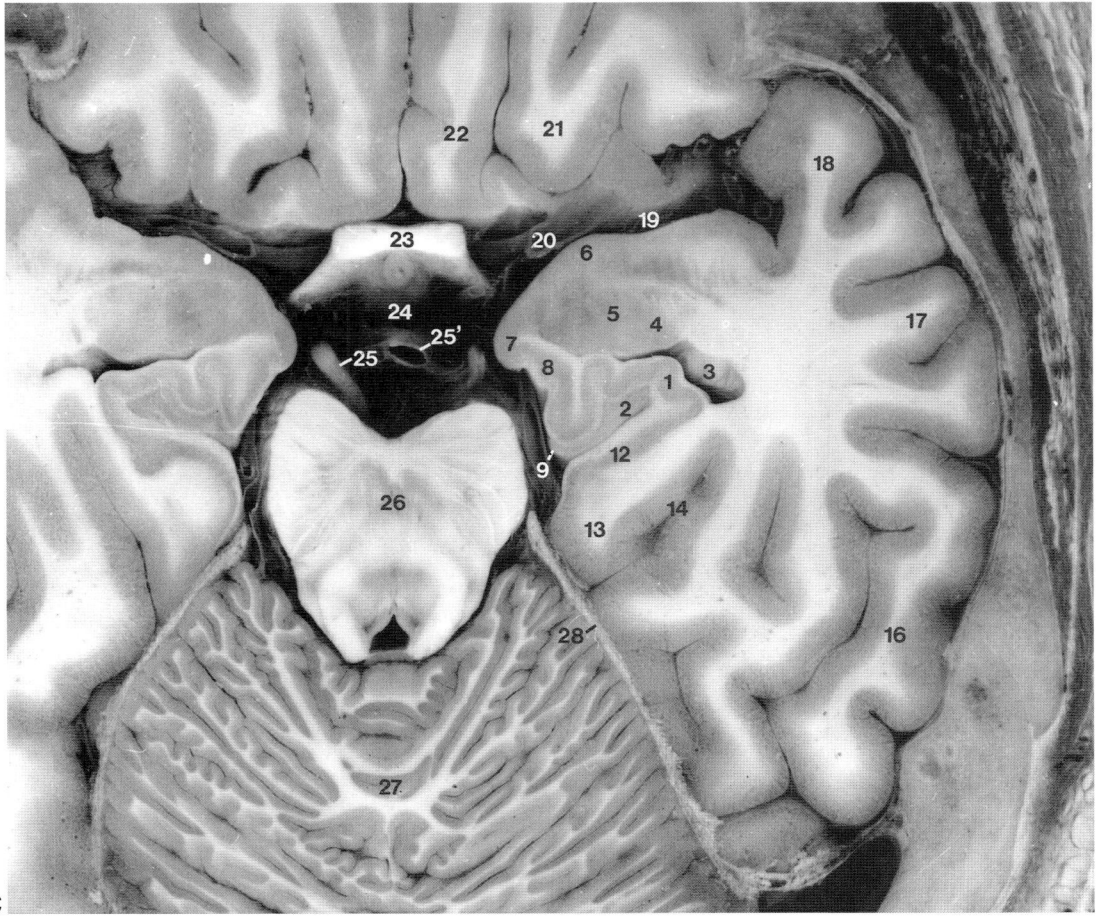

FIG. 3.37. *Cont'd.*

SAGITTAL SECTIONS OF THE HIPPOCAMPUS

The sagittal views show six sections progressing from medial to lateral levels.

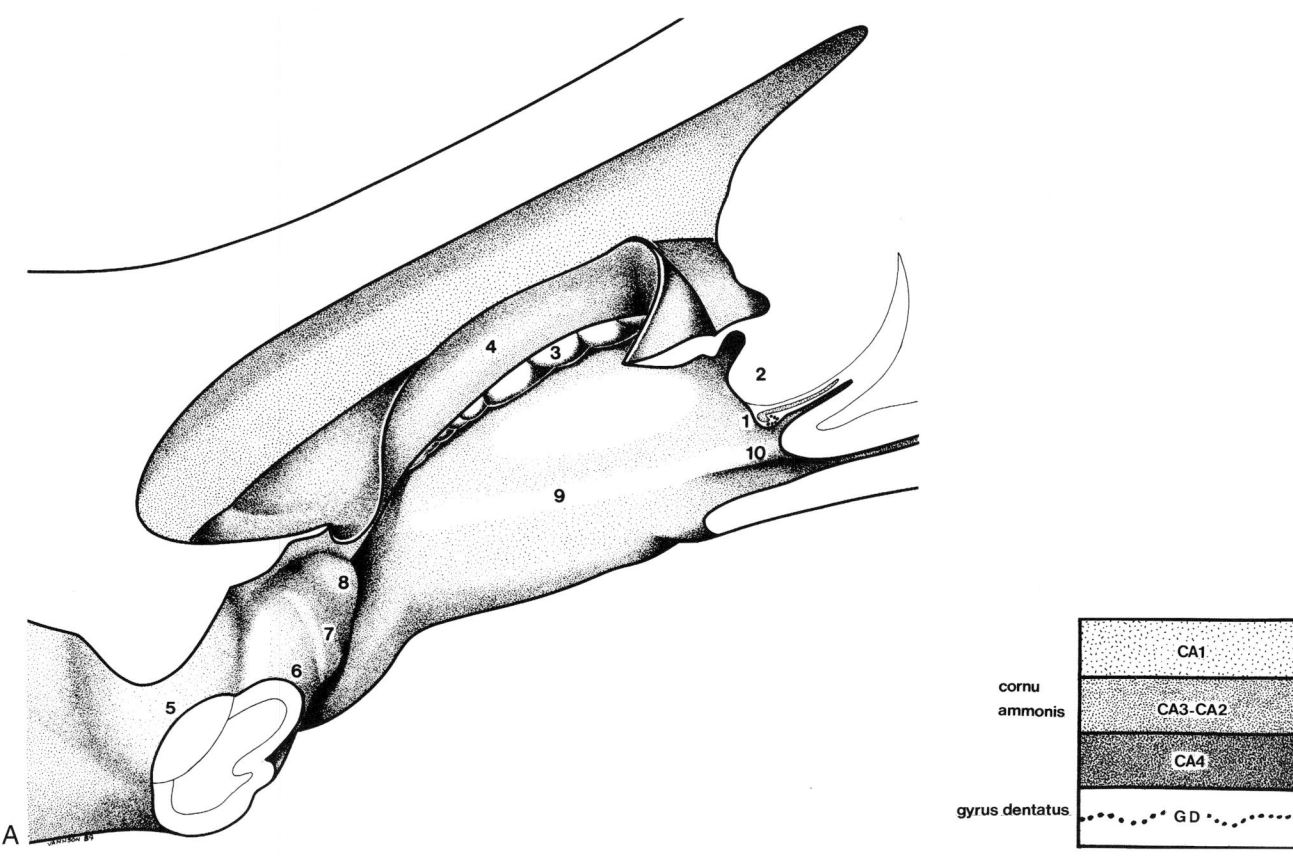

FIG. 3.38. Sagittal section of the hippocampus. **A.** Three-dimensional drawing. **B.** T1-weighted MR image. **C.** Anatomic section.

 1 Hippocampal head
 2 Splenium
 3 Margo denticulatus
 4 Fimbria
 5 Semilunar gyrus
 6 Gyrus uncinatus
 7 Band of Giacomini
 8 Apex of the uncus
 9 Parahippocampal gyrus
10 Isthmus
11 Occipital lobe
12 Parieto-occipital fissure

13 Crus of fornix
14 Lateral ventricle
15 Caudate nucleus
16 Putamen
17 Lateral pallidum
18 Medial pallium
19 Crus cerebri
20 Pulvinar
21 Medial geniculate body
22 Tentorium
23 Middle cerebral artery
24 Cerebellum

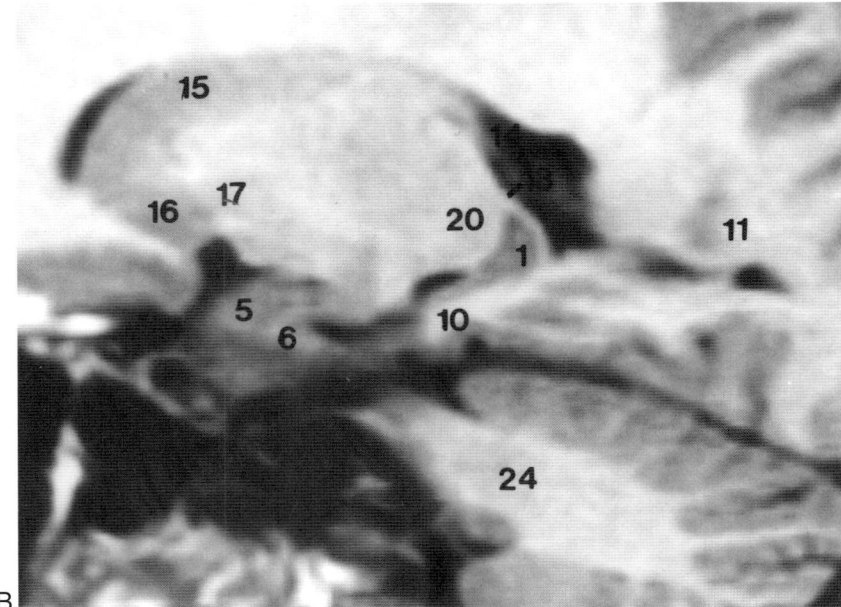

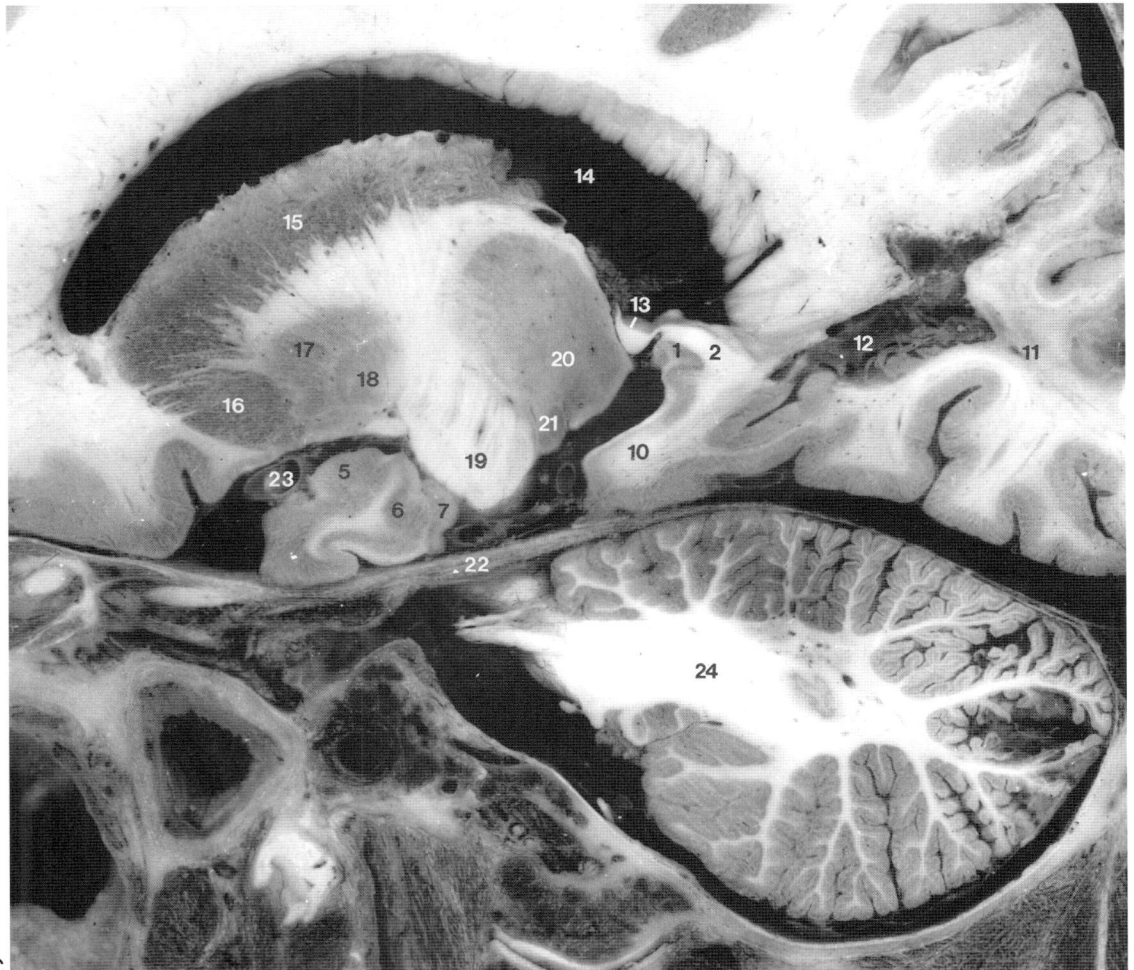

FIG. 3.38. *Cont'd.*

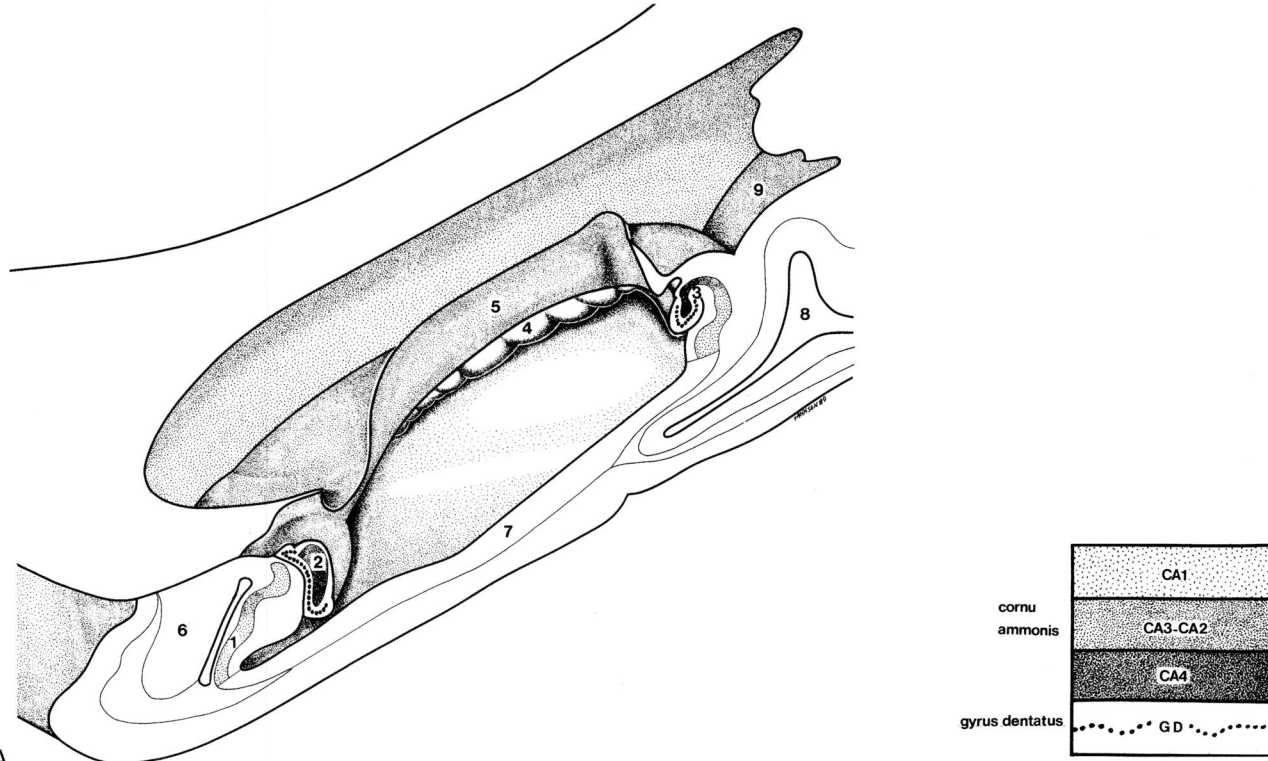

FIG. 3.39. Sagittal section of the hippocampus. **A.** Three-dimensional drawing. **B.** T1-weighted MR image. **C.** Anatomic section.

1 Hippocampal head, cornu ammonis
2 Hippocampal head, apex of the uncus
3 Hippocampal tail
4 Margo denticulatus
5 Fimbria
6 Amygdala
7 Temporal horn
8 Parahippocampal gyrus
9 Anterior calcarine fissure
10 Calcar avis
11 Occipital lobe
12 Lateral ventricle
13 Crus of the fornix
14 Pulvinar
15 Caudate nucleus
16 Putamen
17 Lateral pallidum
18 Medial pallidum
19 Middle cerebral artery
20 Tentorium cerebelli
21 Trigeminal cave
22 Trigeminal nerve
23 Cerebellum

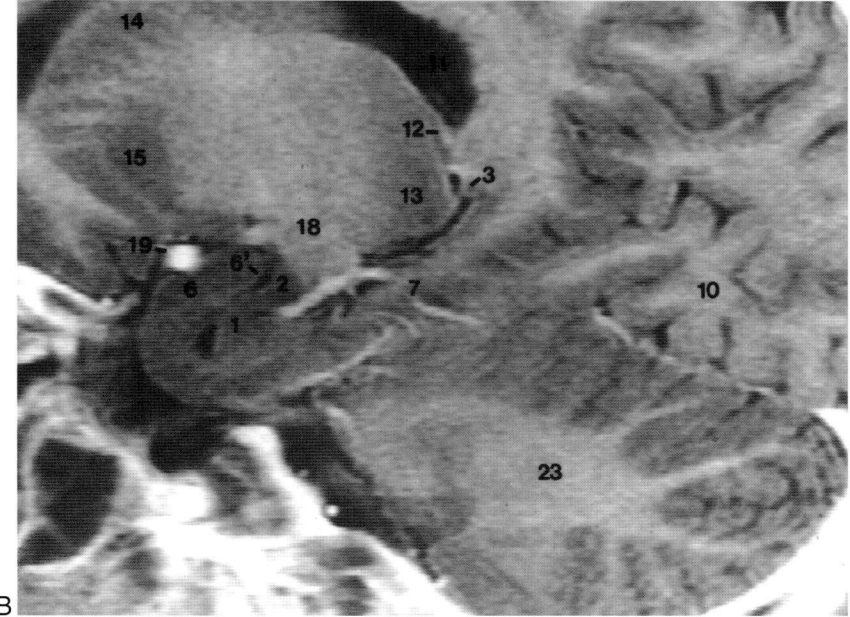

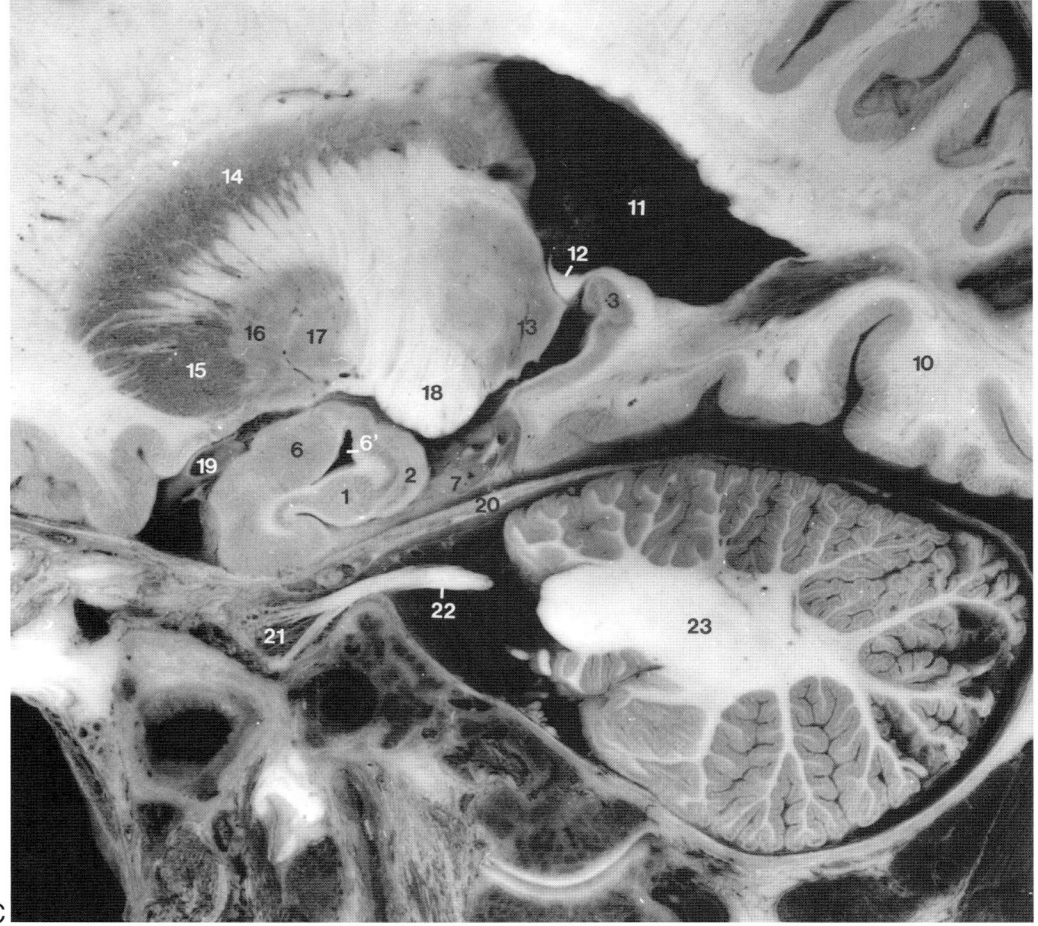

FIG. 3.39. *Cont'd.*

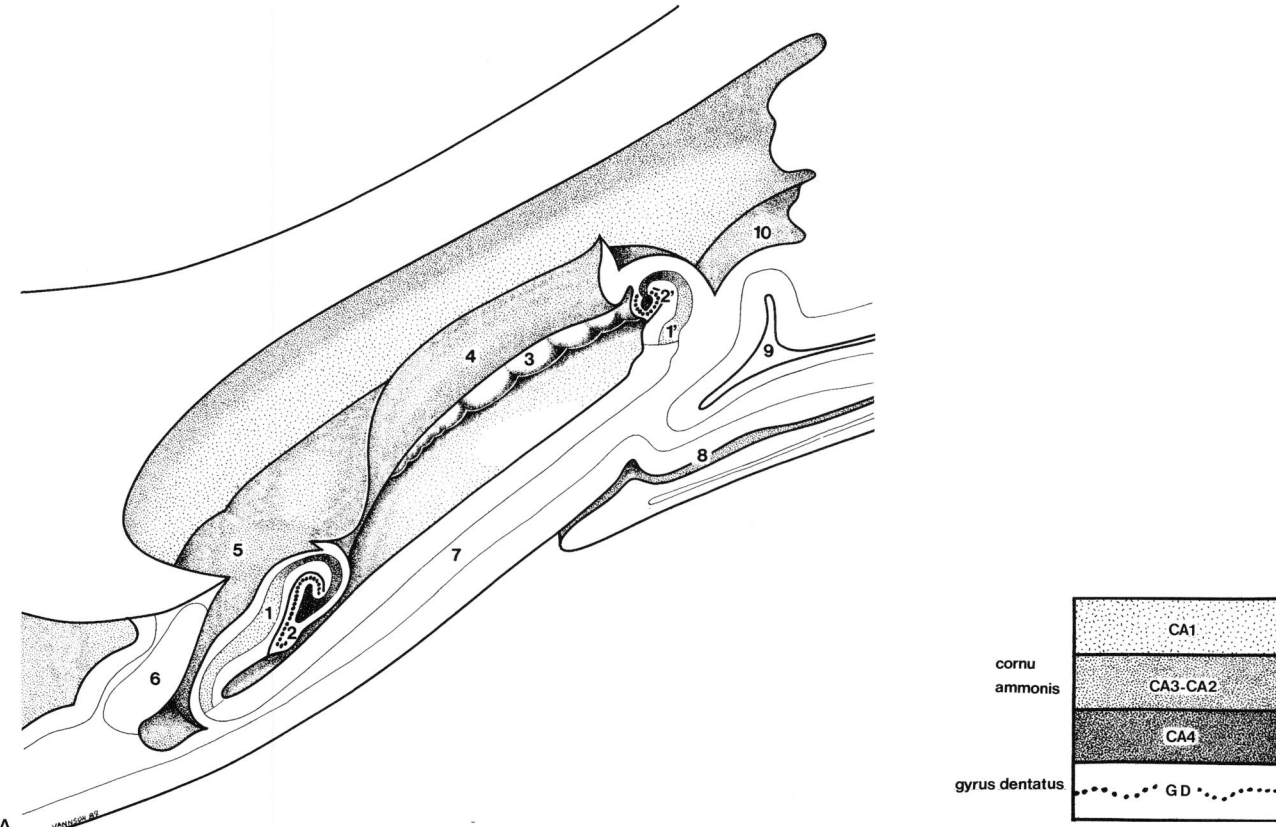

FIG. 3.40. Sagittal section of the hippocampus. **A.** Three-dimensional drawing. **B.** T1-weighted MR image. **C.** Anatomic section.

1 Hippocampal head, cornu ammonis
2 Hippocampal head, gyrus dentatus
1′ Hippocampal tail, cornu ammonis
2′ Hippocampal tail, gyrus dentatus
3 Margo denticulatus
4 Fimbria
5 Digitationes hippocampi
6 Amygdala
7 Parahippocampal gyrus
8 Collateral sulcus
9 Anterior calcarine sulcus
10 Calcar avis
11 Occipital lobe

12 Lateral ventricle
13 Caudate nucleus
14 Pulvinar
15 Internal capsule, posterior limb
16 Putamen
17 Lateral pallidum
18 Medial pallidum
19 Middle cerebral artery
20 Temporal horn lateral ventricle
21 Tentorium cerebelli
22 Cerebellum
23 Trigeminal nerve

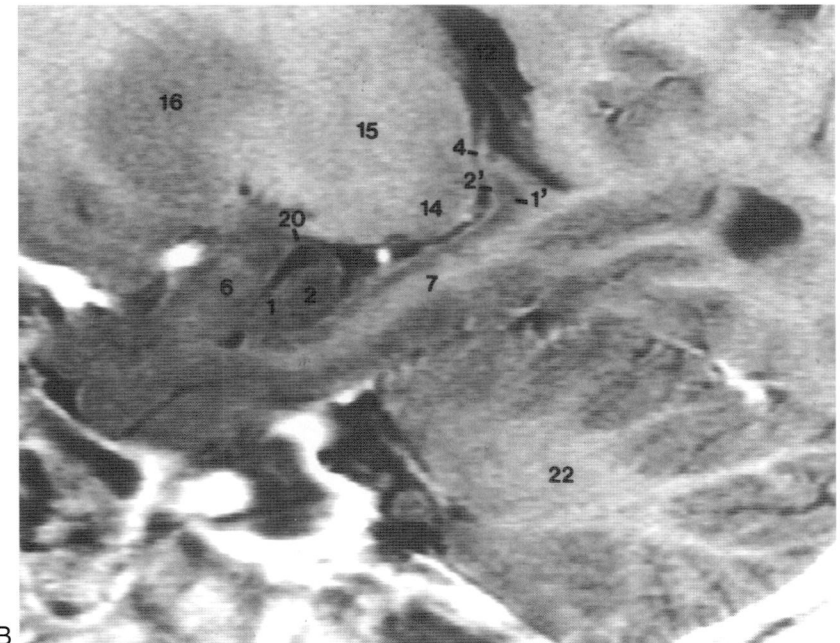

B

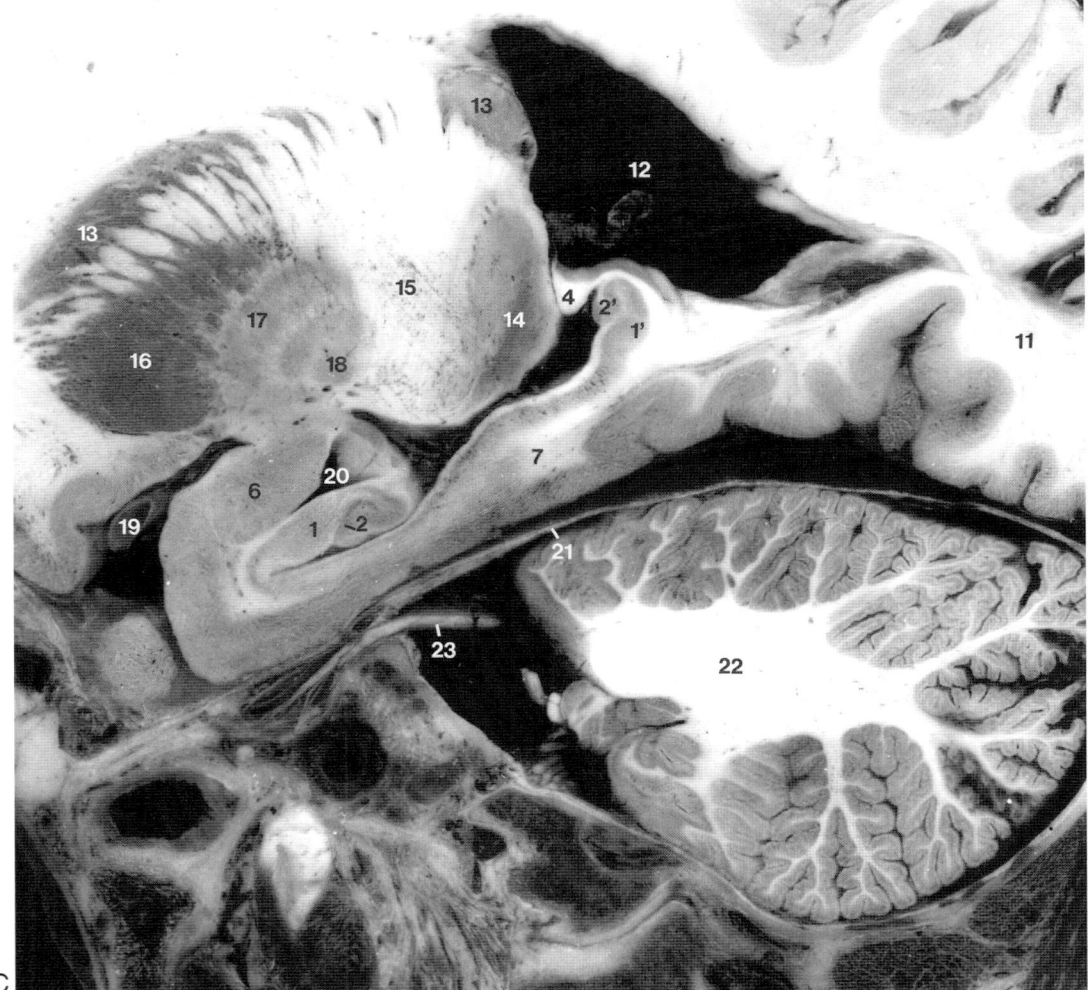

C

FIG. 3.40. *Cont'd.*

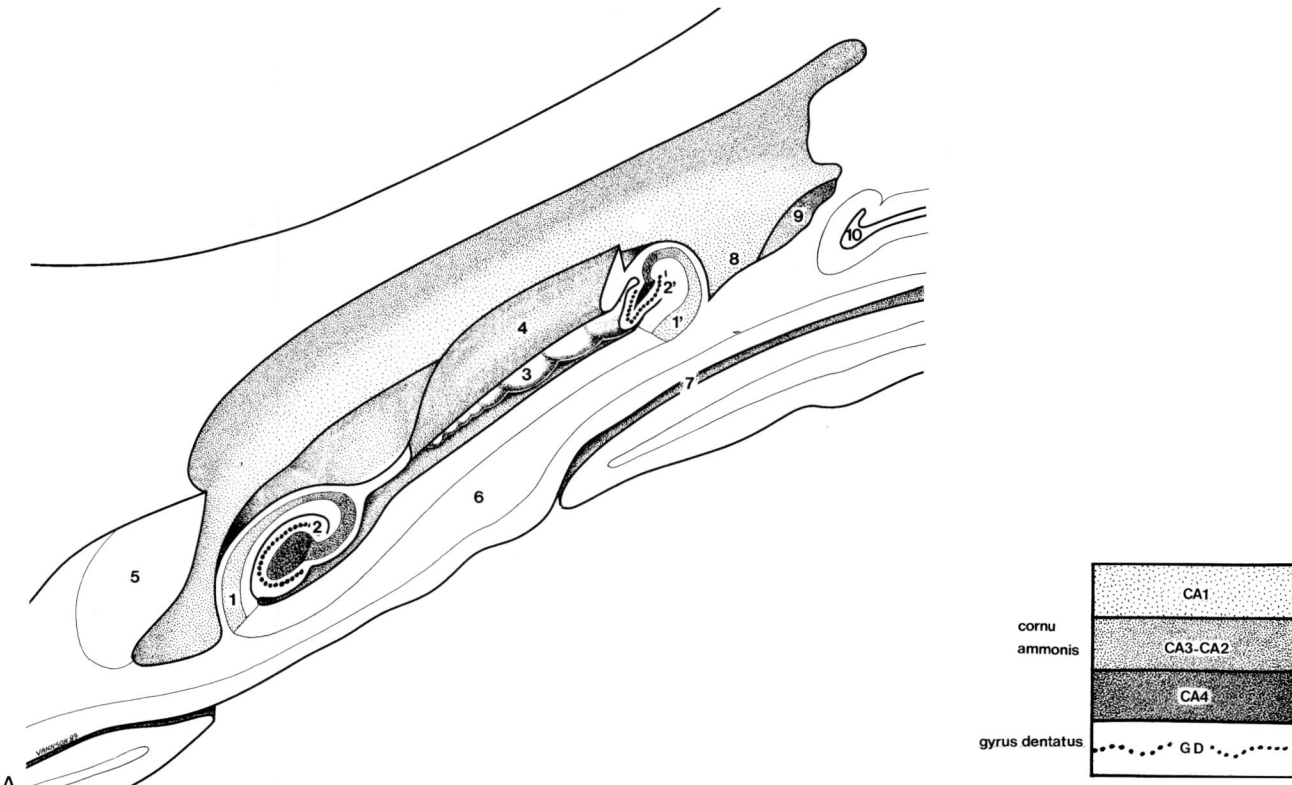

FIG. 3.41. Sagittal section of the hippocampus. **A.** Three-dimensional drawing. **B.** T2-weighted MR image. **C.** Anatomic section.

 1 Hippocampal head, cornu ammonis
 2 Hippocampal head, gyrus dentatus
 1′ Hippocampal tail, cornu ammonis
 2′ Hippocampal tail, gyrus dentatus
 3 Margo denticulatus
 4 Fimbria
 5 Amygdala
 6 Parahippocampal gyrus
 7 Collateral sulcus
 8 Collateral trigone
 9 Calcar avis
10 Calcarine sulcus

11 Occipital lobe
12 Lateral ventricle
13 Caudate nucleus
14 Internal capsule
15 Putamen
16 Lateral pallidum
17 Temporal horn, lateral ventricle
18 Middle cerebral artery
19 Tentorium cerebelli
20 Cerebellum
21 Internal carotid artery

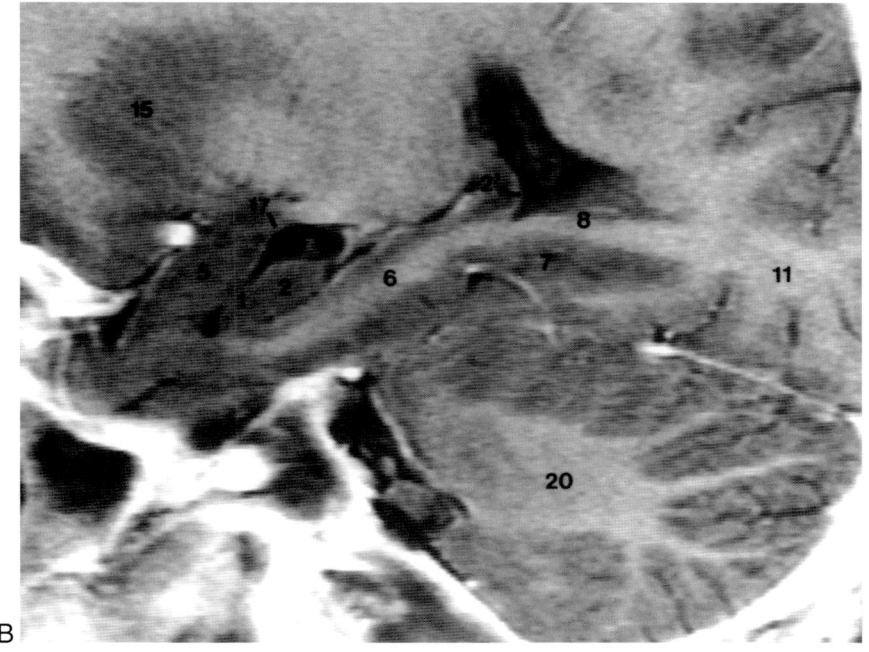

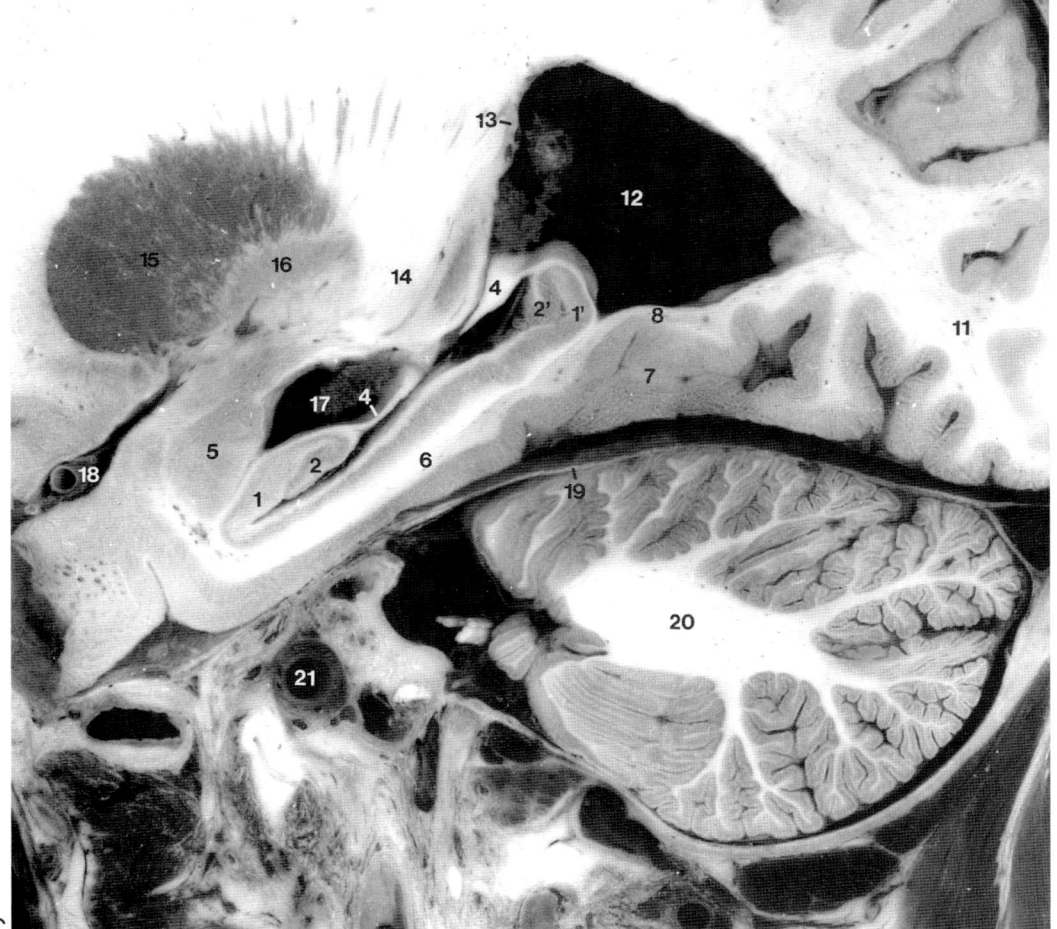

FIG. 3.41. *Cont'd.*

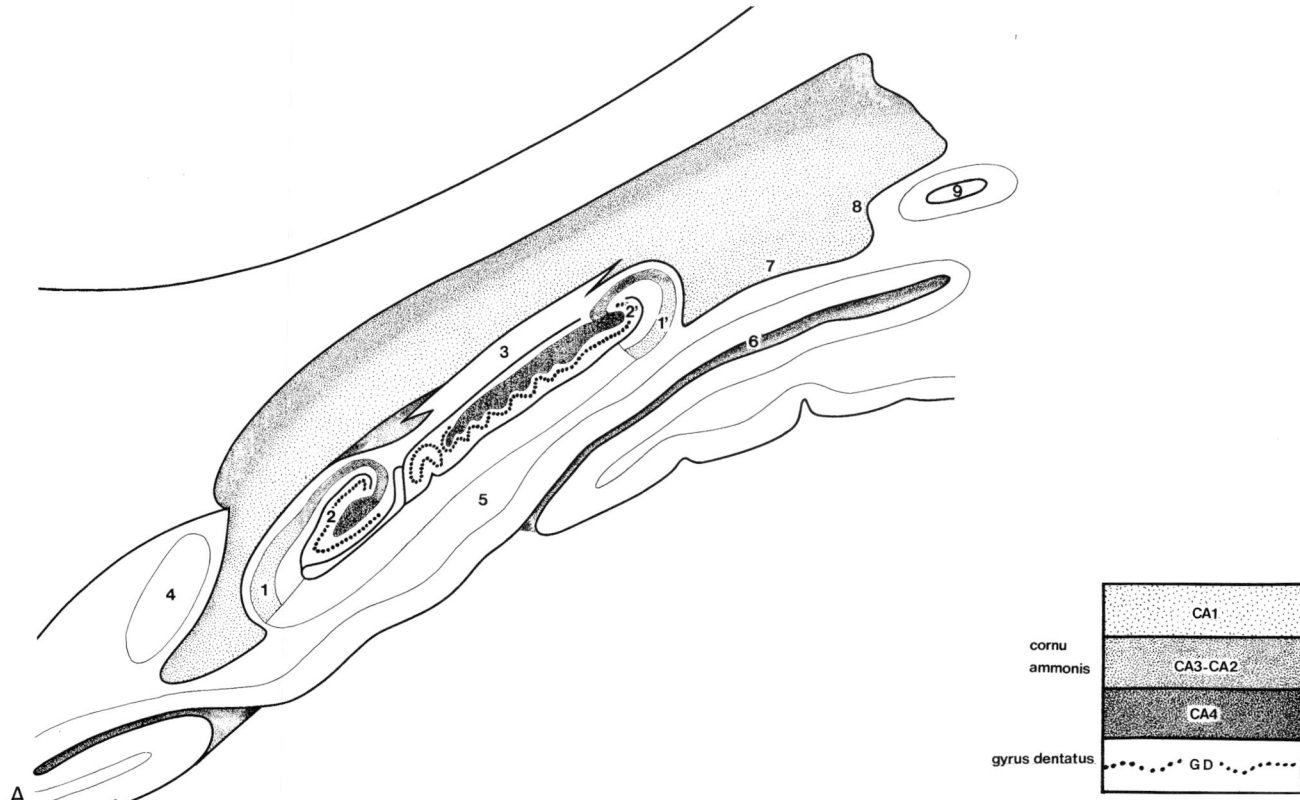

FIG. 3.42. Sagittal section of the hippocampus. **A.** Three-dimensional drawing. **B.** T2-weighted MR image. **C.** Anatomic section.

1 Hippocampal head, cornu ammonis
2 Hippocampal head, gyrus dentatus
1' Hippocampal tail, cornu ammonis
2' Hippocampal tail, gyrus dentatus
3 Fimbria
4 Amygdala
5 Parahippocampal gyrus
6 Collateral sulcus
7 Collateral trigone
8 Calcar avis

9 Calcarine sulcus
10 Occipital lobe
11 Atrium of the lateral ventricle
12 Temporal horn of the lateral ventricle
13 Putamen
14 Lateral pallidum
15 Tentorium cerebelli
16 Cerebellum
17 Internal carotid artery

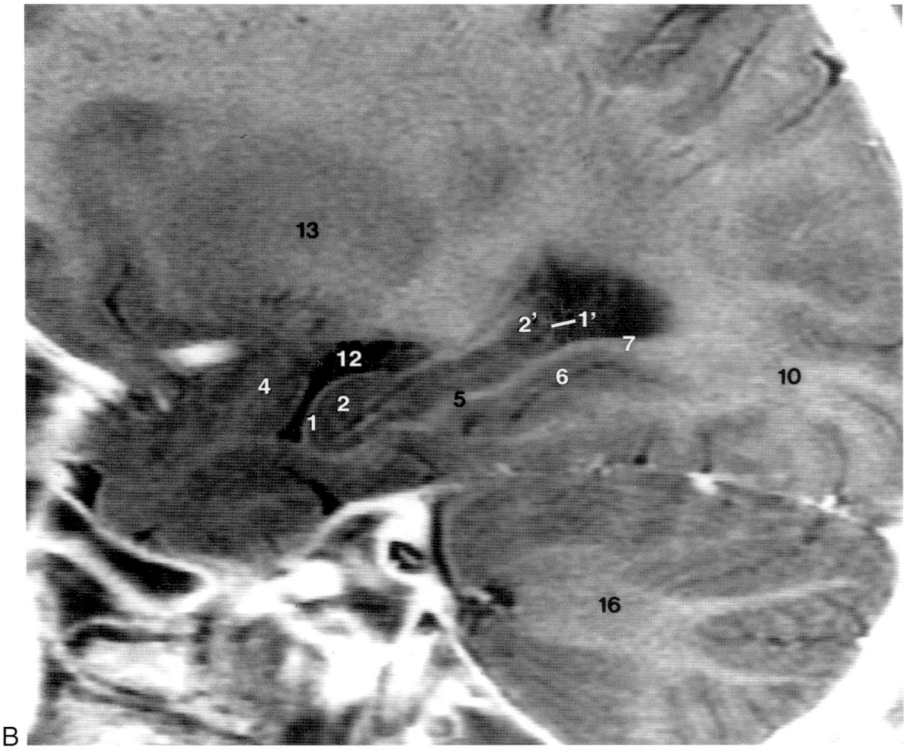

B

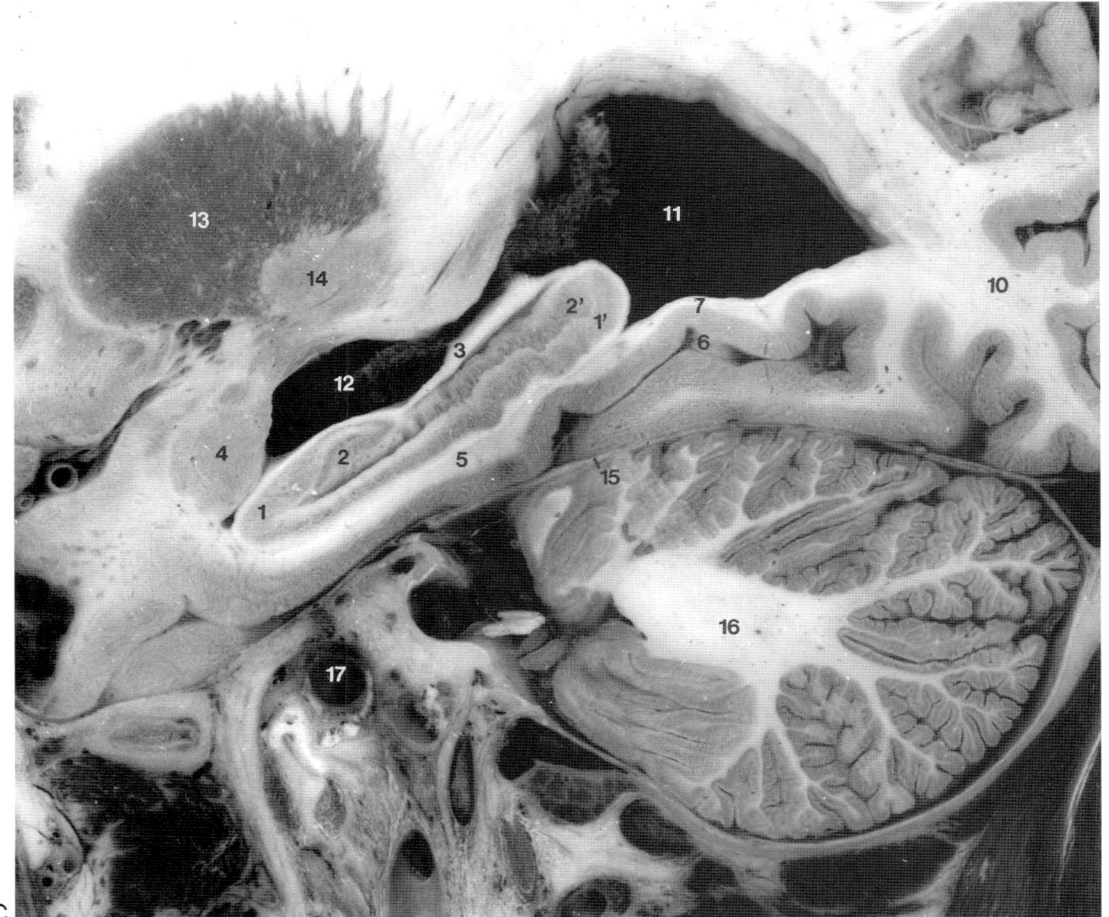

C

FIG. 3.42. *Cont'd.*

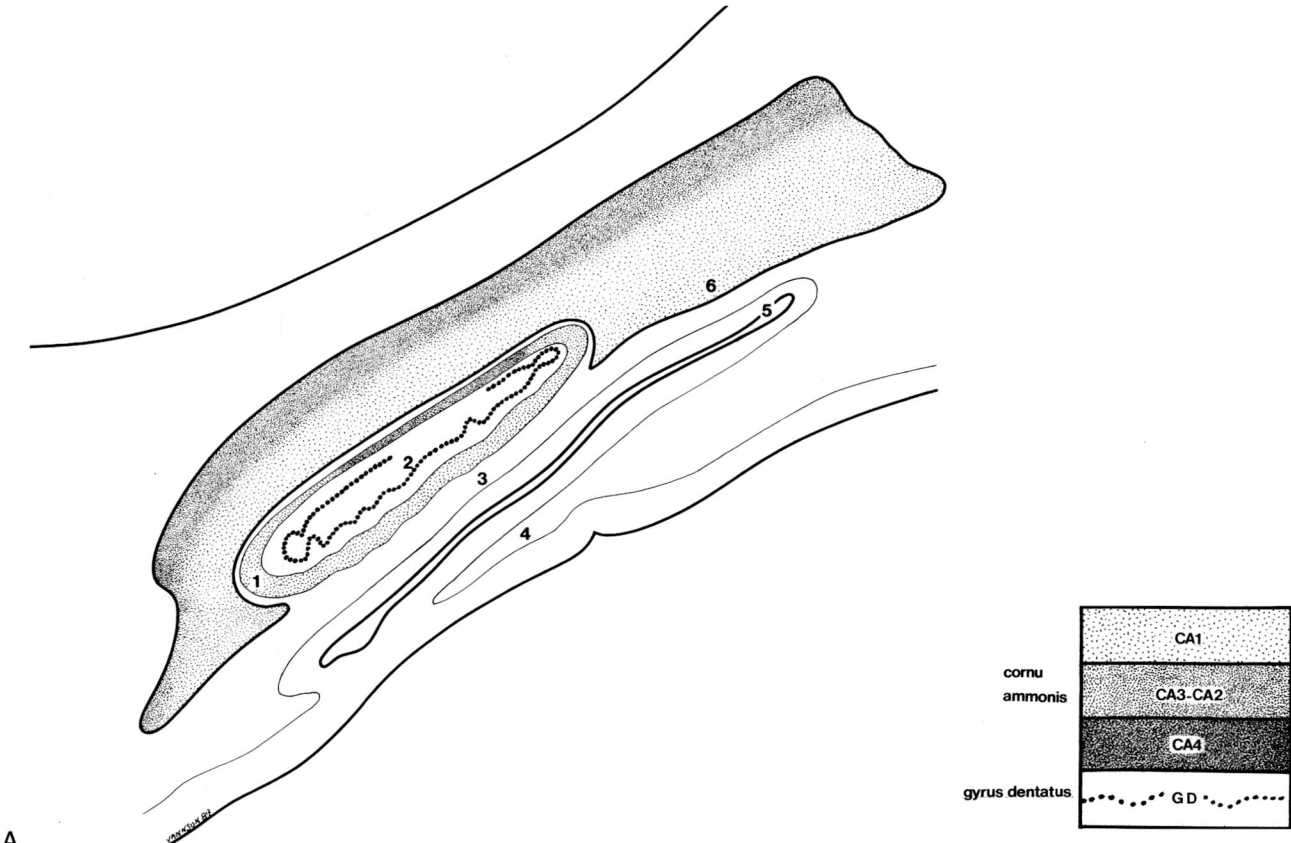

Fig. 3.43. Sagittal section of the hippocampus. **A.** Three-dimensional drawing. **B.** T2-weighted MR image. **C.** Anatomic section.

1 Hippocampal body, cornu ammonis
2 Hippocampal body, gyrus dentatus
3 Parahippocampal gyrus
4 Fusiform gyrus
5 Collateral sulcus
6 Collateral trigone
7 Occipital lobe
8 Atrium of the lateral ventricle
9 Alveus of the hippocampus

10 Temporal horn of the lateral ventricle
11 Putamen
12 Amygdala
13 Tentorium cerebelli
14 Cerebellum
15 Internal carotid artery
16 Internal jugular vein
17 Temporal, petrous part

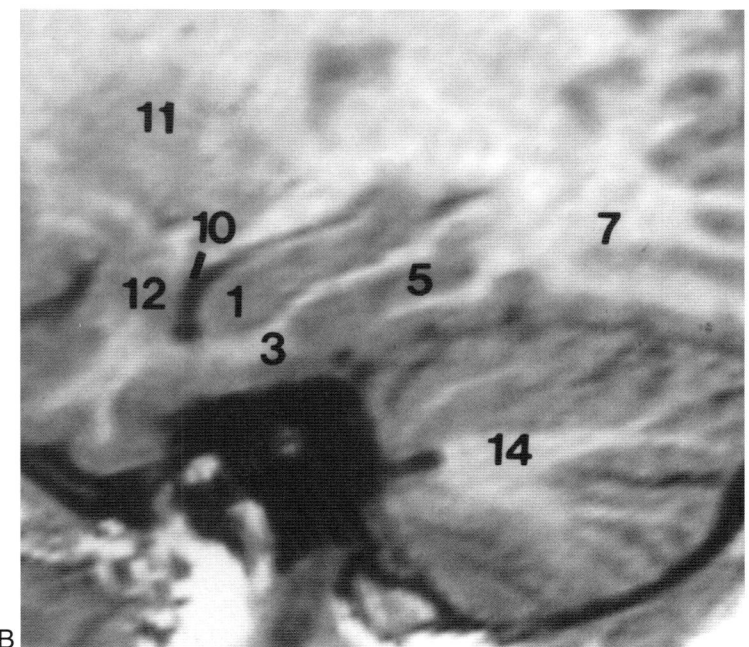

B

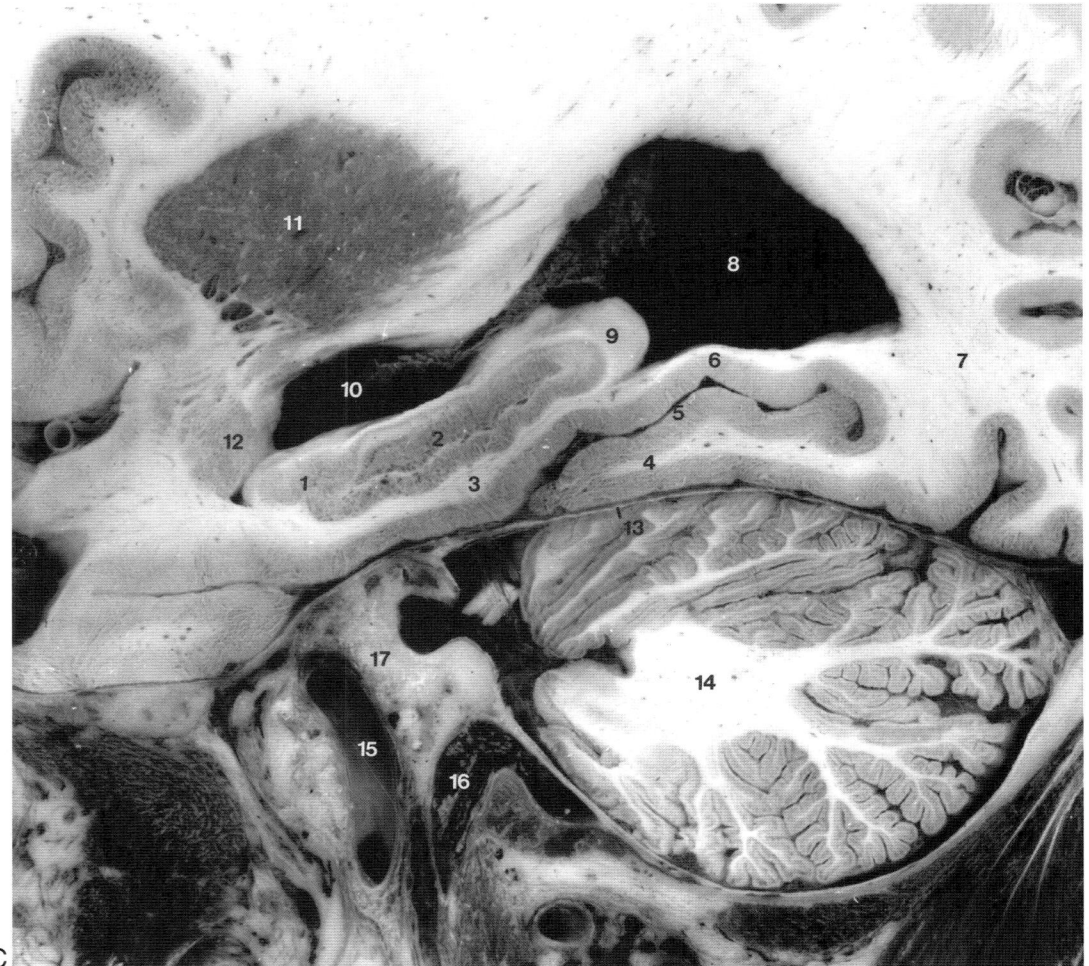

C

Fig. 3.43. *Cont'd.*

Temporal Lobe Epilepsy

Graeme D. Jackson, Regula S. Briellmann and Ruben I. Kuzniecky

"To be human is to have the experience of selfhood, a feeling of personal identity.

Memory is obviously necessary to ensure that the thread that binds our present existence to every one of its earlier stages remains unbroken.

[T]o what extent can [the study of temporal lobe epilepsy] … further our understanding of human temporal lobe function?"

Pierre Gloor, The temporal lobe and limbic system, 1997

INTRODUCTION

The aim of this chapter is to describe temporal lobe epilepsy (TLE) as we see it in the MRI era and to highlight information that we feel is essential for a proper understanding of the information available from MRI and for interpretation of this data.

The last 10 years have seen neuroimaging take on an increasingly important role in the management of epilepsy and to become essential in the surgical management of epilepsy. When one thinks about TLE, the issue of intractability and the possibility of surgery for cure of the epilepsy must come to mind. This process often starts with an anatomic assessment of the brain and, in epilepsy, this means an MRI study specifically optimized for the examination of the temporal structures.

New techniques, imaging sequences and analysis methods have appeared that give ever-greater sensitivity for detecting abnormalities of brain structure. Neuroimaging has also become a powerful and important physiologic probe of functions that were previously considered entirely the domain of electrophysiology. These startling advances are probably only the beginning, and future developments appear to offer as much excitement as have these past advances, and are specifically discussed in later chapters of this book.

The ever-expanding range of imaging options has also brought with it the question of cost-effectiveness of investigation and treatment. It used to be common practice to acquire all investigations in all patients. Increasingly patients are being streamlined into phases of investigation, with surgery being offered early on in certain well-defined categories. Do all patients need interictal and ictal SPECT, MRI, fMRI, MRS and PET?

Increasingly imaging studies are graded, and extra studies are based on algorithms that are weighted by what is found on MR and other investigations. Like the electroencephalogram (EEG), MR is not a single investigation. When one performs an EEG study, there are screening studies, special montages, activation studies (sleep deprivation, hyperventilation, and photic stimuli), and then long-term monitoring with video EEG. In MR also, multiple sessions addressing different issues may be needed in order to acquire all of the relevant imaging information.

Finding a lesion can be easy – being certain that there is no causative lesion in the brain can be much more difficult and may involve special studies and analytic methods.

CLINICAL FEATURES OF TEMPORAL LOBE EPILEPSY

The Temporal Lobe: Development and Functions

The temporal lobe is one of the last areas of the cortex to mature (Table 4.1). 50% of temporal lobes are myelinated at

Table 4.1. Brain Development

Primary neuralation	3–4 weeks
Secondary neuralation	4–7 weeks
Prosencephalon	2–3 months
Proliferation	3–4 months
Migration	3–5 months
Organization	5 months–years
Myelination	Birth–years

80 weeks (1). The temporal lobes are important for memory, hearing, and language, among other things. As Gloor has said, "To be human is to have the experience of selfhood, a feeling of personal identity." The temporal lobes may be essential for this and therefore essential for the human experience. Phylogenetically, the hippocampi subserved the purpose of smell and memory for smell may have been important for survival; hippocampal memory structures in humans may have evolved from this aspect of the olfactory system. We are all aware that smell can evoke vivid memories still. To study this subject further we refer to the masterly work of Gloor, completed and published posthumously (2).

How Do We Classify Temporal Lobe Epilepsy?

The International Classification of Epilepsies, Epileptic Syndromes, and Related Seizure Disorders recognizes several partial or focal epilepsies. TLE is classified as a symptomatic localization related epilepsy (3) (see chapter 1). Temporal lobe epilepsy is characterized by seizures originating in or primarily involving temporal lobe structures. Most clinicians distinguish mesial temporal epilepsy (4) from neocortical or lateral temporal lobe epilepsy (5–8). The medial structures that are important for the generation of seizures include the hippocampus, amygdala, and parahippocampal gyrus, although hippocampal sclerosis (HS) is by far the most common cause of intractable TLE. We discuss these in more detail below.

Seizures, 'Substrates' and 'Axes': A Changing Concept in the Imaging Era

The classification of the epilepsies (3) is based on the events associated with the seizure. Hence it is known as an electroclinical classification system and focuses mainly on the nature of the seizure events. The importance of considering substrates of the epilepsies is that the lesions that give rise to seizures are virtually not taken into account by this classification system. These substrates are present in the brain at all times, including in the interictal period. Hence, temporal lobe epilepsy, whether caused by a malignant or a benign tumour, HS, or focal dysplasia, would be syndromically identical. Clearly the disease is different in these cases and this has differing consequences for patients and their

management. There are now attempts to include these data by considering the data available along a number of major axes. This is discussed in detail in Chapter 1.

Temporal Lobe Epilepsy: The Clinical Problem

Definitions

In clinical practice, one divides intractable epilepsy into generalized and partial epilepsy (as described in Chapter 1). When the seizures affect consciousness (complex partial seizures) the most common site of seizure onset is the temporal lobe (9–13). Complex partial seizures are defined by the part of the brain from which the seizures arise. Therefore TLE is defined as epileptic seizures originating in, or *primarily involving*, temporal lobe structures (3,14–23). This is an important distinction when considering the mechanism and further management of these patients, in particular the possibility of surgical treatment of the epilepsy. Two major types of TLE are usually recognized: mesial TLE (MTLE), where the onset of seizures is from the hippocampus, amygdala, or other medial structures in the temporal lobe, and lateral (neocortical) TLE (less than 10% of TLE cases), where seizures arise from the temporal neocortex.

Complex partial seizures may also be caused by seizures that arise from extra-temporal-lobe structures (16, 24–30), often with seizure spread through the temporal lobe. While temporal lobe seizures may have isolated neocortical temporal or limbic onset without involvement of the other structures, in the majority of patients, seizure spread to adjacent areas occurs (9, 31–36).

Seizure Semiology

Seizures originating in temporal lobe structures are simple partial seizures (SPS), characterized by retention of consciousness and therefore often termed an 'aura', complex partial seizures (CPS) characterized by an impairment of awareness, and secondarily generalized tonic-clonic seizures.

'Auras' or simple partial seizures are common in mesial temporal epilepsy, particularly when the underlying cause is HS. In patients with HS, the most common aura is the 'abdominal aura' or rising epigastric sensation often described as nausea, an uncomfortable epigastric sensation, or 'butterflies in the stomach.' This sensation is described as 'rising' into the chest and neck. An unprovoked feeling of fear is common and may be present simultaneously with the epigastric aura (37). Other auras include déjà vu, jamais vu, tachycardia and palpitations, olfactory and gustatory hallucinations, and feelings of depersonalization. Auras or simple partial seizures have been reported to occur as part of the seizure semiology in 20–90% of patients (9, 10, 13, 38). Quesney (31) reported auras in 67% of patients with temporal lobe epilepsy. The reported variations stem from study methodology and from patient selection. Some patients may report auras during a specific time in their life. Not uncommonly, patients may report variations in auras depending on the type of drug treatment and some patients may lose their auras with specific drug regimens.

Among the auras or simple partial seizures, viscerosensory (epigastric, abdominal, nausea) and experiential (fear, déjà vu, etc.) phenomena are the most frequent, occurring in almost 50% of patients with temporal lobe epilepsy (10, 11, 39–41).

A commonly quoted aura is olfactory hallucinations (42–44); however, in our experience fewer than 5% of patients with temporal lobe seizures report this aura. Other auras reported in these patients include complex auditory, vestibular, and formed visual hallucinations. Motionless stare has been reported in many patients during temporal lobe attacks. Although previous studies suggested that this distinctive behavior is typical of temporal lobe epilepsy (18), other studies have not been able to confirm this finding. In fact, Quesney (31) found motionless stare in only 24% of cases in his series.

The second type of seizure is the 'complex partial seizure.' The phenomenology of the complex partial temporal lobe seizures includes a disruption of normal awareness, intrusion in the ability to respond to the environment, automatic behavior, and, commonly, amnesia. Seizure may typically begin with arrest of motor activity and a blank stare with impaired awareness and responsiveness. Then semipurposeful, involuntary, automatic motor behaviors (automatisms) develop. Ictal automatisms characteristically consist of prominent oroalimentary signs that include lip smacking, chewing, salivation, and swallowing. Speech disturbances (speech arrest, vocalization, humming, among others), are also common. Gestural changes and mimetic behavior such as grimacing, smiling, or laughing may be observed. Finally, many patients will develop hand (fumbling, pulling, picking type behavior) or ambulatory automatisms (17, 18, 45–50).

Motor phenomena – in particular, contralateral dystonic posturing of the upper limb – are reliable lateralizing findings of temporal lobe epilepsy onset (51, 52). Often, the patient may manifest automatisms of the contralateral hand during the ictal phase. Late and complex head turning is usually not a reliable sign of lateralization in temporal lobe because it probably reflects secondary spread (31). Following the ictal phase, confusion and abnormal behavior with amnesia may follow in what is considered the postictal period. Contralateral upper extremity hypokinesia is common and short-lasting.

Secondary generalization may occur in some patients and may take different forms (28, 38, 53–55). Secondary generalization is not typical in TLE. Nose-wipe at end of seizure is usually with the hand ipsilateral to the side of the seizure and occurs at the ictal-to-postictal transition (56–60). Postictal aphasia reliably lateralizes seizure onset to the dominant temporal lobe. Postictal anterograde or retrograde amnesia also occurs but is not reliably lateralizing.

Electroencephalographic Findings in Temporal Lobe Epilepsy

Interictal EEG studies in patients with temporal lobe epilepsy usually demonstrate anterior temporal or unifocal temporal lobe sharp activity (31, 61–67, 68). The occurrence of bitemporal independent epileptiform discharges in patients with temporal lobe seizures has been reported with varying frequencies ranging from 20% to 50% (31, 32, 34, 61, 69, 70). It is unclear, however, whether this frequency reflects a selection bias towards patients investigated for possible surgery, who are obviously the most severely affected. In the majority of patients, EEG findings may suggest lateralization, although not necessarily localization of the seizure focus. Anterior temporal and sphenoidal electrodes may provide a higher yield of positive EEGs and are useful for this purpose (9, 71), although the invasive nature of sphenoidal electrodes has led to decreased use in the era of neuroimaging. Ictal surface EEGs are usually abnormal during complex partial seizures of temporal lobe onset. Different patterns of ictal EEG abnormality have been described, the most characteristic being the presence of attenuation of background activity followed by rhythmic sharp activity recorded from the affected temporal lobe (Fig. 4.1). This may be followed by contralateral spread of the seizure discharges (24, 31, 61, 72–79, 4,68, 80).

An attempt has been made to subclassify temporal lobe epilepsy according to the region of ictal onset (24). This classification is based on depth EEG studies and is limited by the inherent characteristics of the sampling problem of depth electrodes, since only a few electrodes are used for recording a seizure originating at a distance but rapid spread may be misinterpreted as originating at the nearest depth electrode. This subclassification of seizures has not been widely accepted but the clinical features that were described for seizure onset in different parts of the temporal lobe is instructive. *Hippocampal–amygdalar* seizures are the most common (24, 31, 32, 81). Auras occur in 80–90% of patients and include déjà vu, epigastric sensations, fear, and other affective sensations. Consciousness is preserved initially but is lost with contralateral seizure spread. Oroalimentary automatisms and complex gestural features occur with seizure spread. The *temporal polar* seizures are very similar to hippocampal–amygdalar seizures. However, prominent early autonomic changes and oroalimentary automatisms are more common in this latter type. Auditory hallucinations are rare and may be more frequent in seizures arising from the lateral posterior neocortical region. Posterior *lateral temporal neocortical* seizures (neocortical TLE) are also characterized by vestibular and complex visual hallucinations. *Opercular–insular* onset seizures (also neocortical TLE) often manifest with auditory and visceral auras and prominent visceromotor phenomena. Finally, seizures with *frontobasal–cingulate* origin (again sometimes neocortical TLE, depending of the site of seizure origin) typically have prominent motor automatisms and loss of awareness.

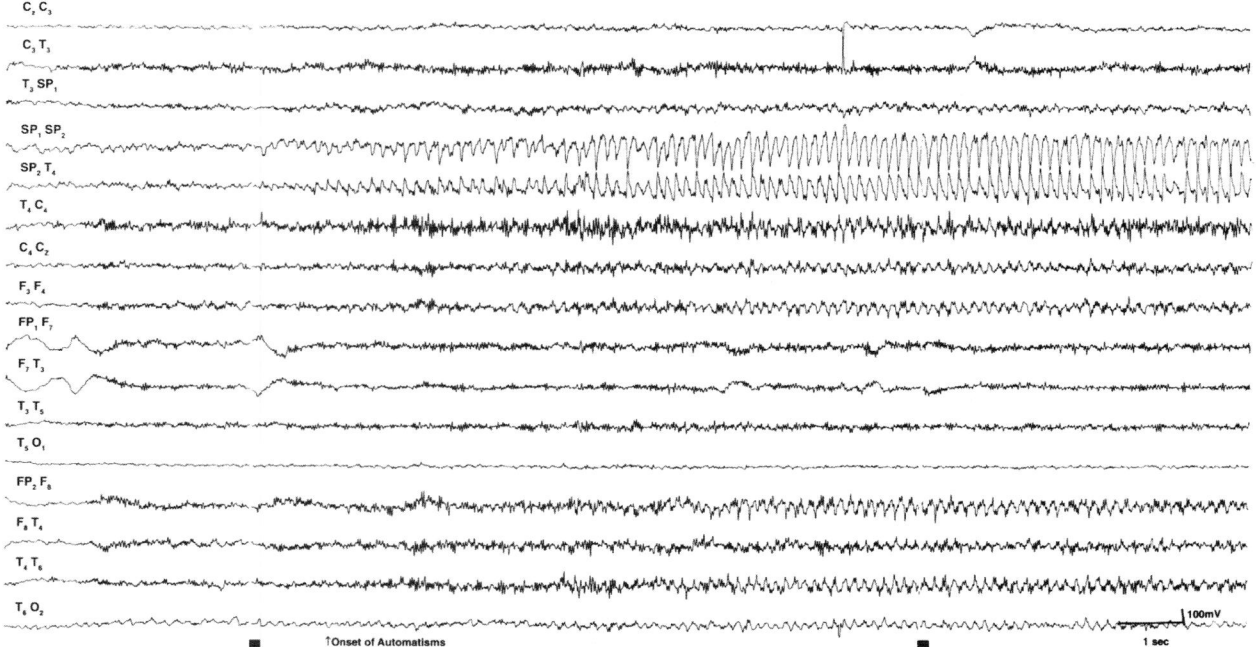

FIG. 4.1. Scalp ictal EEG recording with sphenoidal electrodes of a complex partial seizure characterized by automatisms and confusion. The EEG demonstrates rhythmic activity over the right temporal region involving the right sphenoidal electrode (SP_2).

Seizures with these characteristics often arise from the frontal lobe and spread posteriorly to involve mesial structures, and should not be classified under the temporal group.

Temporal Origin or Spread to Temporal Structures (Temporal Involvement)

It is clear that these clinical features of seizures, which reflect involvement of temporal lobe areas, fall into two major groups. One is primary temporal lobe onset seizures while the second group consists of seizures arising outside of the temporal lobe structures but rapidly and predominantly spreading to the temporal lobes. The temporal onset seizures then need to be divided into medial temporal onset (amygdala, hippocampus, entorhinal cortex and parahippocampal gyrus) and temporal neocortical, as discussed above.

Because of the impact of MRI, depth EEG studies are now infrequently performed in cases of TLE with structural abnormality such as HS. Historical data give insights into the areas of onset of temporal seizures. Depth EEG studies indicate that almost 50% of temporal lobe seizures arise from the hippocampus (32, 33, 72, 82–86). Amygdaloid-onset seizures are less frequent and may account for approximately 10% of temporal lobe epilepsy (9, 24, 31, 87–89). Neocortical seizures are even less frequent (1–10%). Conversely, regional onset (hippocampus, amygdala, and temporal neocortex) is common in temporal lobe seizures (32). Although they may provide a view of the relative frequency of onset of seizures in each region, these figures should be interpreted with care since they were derived from depth electrode studies, and were carried out with different methodologies.

Another important issue is whether most limbic seizures have focal or regional onsets involving single or multiple adjacent structures; again the data is variable but up to two-thirds of patients may have regional onset depending on the methodology and patient population (32). Nonetheless, these data support the long-held view that the mesial structures are important for the generation or propagation of ictal activity in temporal lobe seizures (9, 24).

The mesial initiation of most ictal patterns in temporal lobe epilepsy corresponds to the existence in pathologic material of a particular pattern of cell loss and astrocytic changes in specific areas of the hippocampus and amygdala. These changes are usually defined by the pathologist as representing *mesial temporal sclerosis* or *hippocampal sclerosis* (19, 22, 90–103) (Figs 4.2, 4.3). When only the hippocampus can be examined, the diagnosis of HS is made, although more widespread pathology may exist. The importance of detecting and diagnosing this entity, preoperatively, using MRI, in any patient and in particular in potential epilepsy surgical candidates, cannot be overemphasized. Based on the number of patients referred to specialized epilepsy centers, it is clear that complex partial seizures of temporal onset constitute the major seizure type. This is important because, among the approximately 8000 operative procedures for epilepsy carried out worldwide between 1986 and 1990, almost 60% were temporal lobe resections (35). While extratemporal epilepsy based on MRI lesions may be more common, these figures are likely to still be true. It should be noted here that there are often many psychosocial

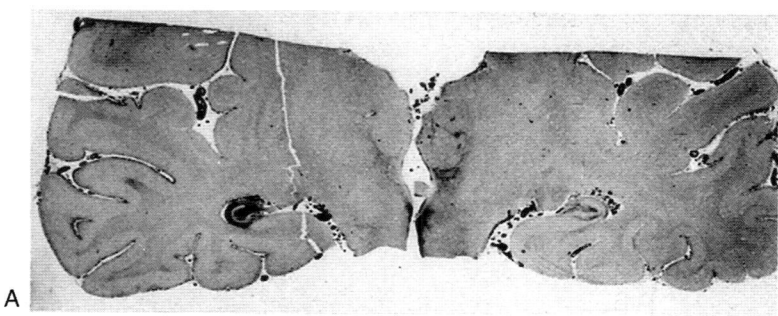

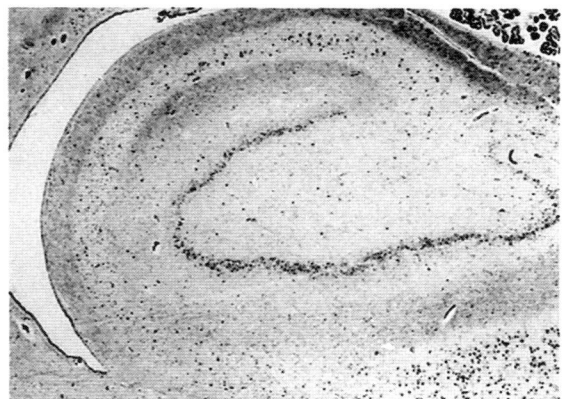

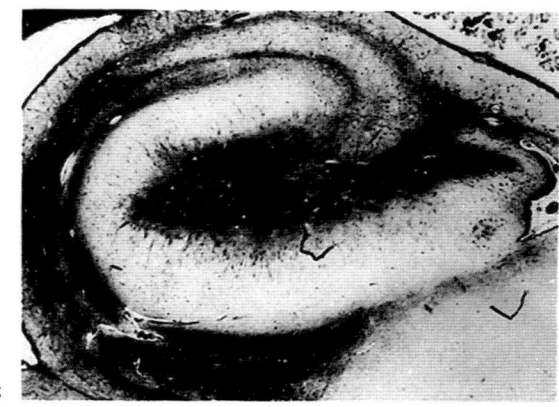

FIG. 4.2. A. Pathologic specimen demonstrating bilateral hippocampal atrophy with predominant asymmetrical gliosis in one hippocampus. **B, C.** Hippocampal sclerosis. Histologic specimens with Nissl stain (**B**) and Kanzler stain (**C**) show the presence of cell loss and astrogliosis in most hippocampal subfields, except for CA2 to CA3. (With permission from Meencke and Veith 1991 (97).)

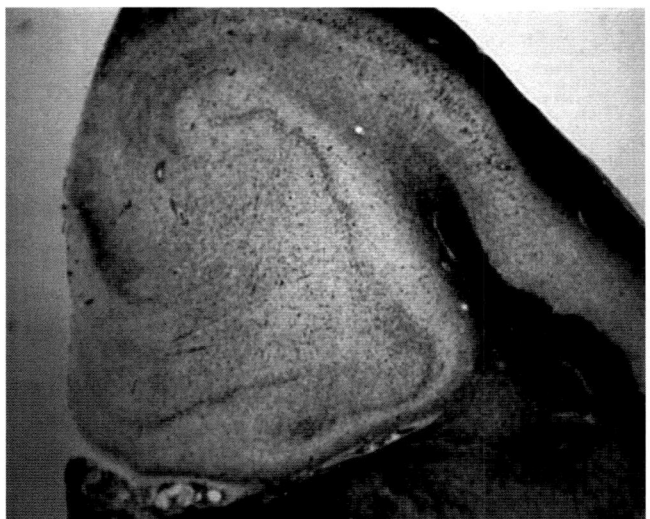

FIG. 4.3. Histopathologic features of hippocampal sclerosis on hematoxylin and eosin stain. There is loss of neurons in the CA1, CA3, and end folium (CA4) with relative sparing of the CA2 neurons. Diffuse gliosis and dispersion of dentate neurons is also seen.

and adjustment issues for the patient after surgical treatment. Management of the patient with intractable epilepsy needs to involve more than simply a focus on seizures (104–108) and references therein.

PATHOLOGIC FINDINGS IN TEMPORAL LOBE EPILEPSY

Mesial Temporal Sclerosis (Hippocampal Sclerosis)

Temporal lobe epilepsy is one of the most common medically intractable seizure disorders. Although often the most intractable, the outcome following surgery is best in this group. In such cases 70–80% of patients can expect to have a good seizure outcome (seizure free or only occasional seizures) (19, 21, 35, 54, 94, 109–124). Mesial temporal sclerosis is the most common abnormality found in the temporal lobes of these patients (11, 22, 96–100, 125–129). Mesial temporal or hippocampal sclerosis is generally considered to be a highly epileptogenic lesion. It is associated with mesial temporal seizures onset. It is usually presumed to be associated with the seizure disorder when it is present in the clinical context of intractable epilepsy, although it may be present with other identifiable pathology on the ipsilateral side in about 30% of cases. The reliable identification of HS using noninvasive MRI is of vital interest in the context of epilepsy surgery, and the use of an optimized MR technique for the noninvasive diagnosis of this lesion should be a mandatory part of the diagnostic workup of patients with intractable temporal lobe epilepsy.

The presence of amygdala sclerosis and gliosis and neuronal damage to the uncus and parahippocampal gyrus needs to be routinely assessed by MR epilepsy protocol studies. Despite major research advances (see later chapters) the unique anatomy of the hippocampus has meant that routine radiologic assessment of TLE cases continues to be focused primarily on the hippocampus. Regional abnormalities can be detected using a variety of MR techniques. As MR detection of brain abnormalities becomes ever more sensitive, the issue of which abnormalities are primary and which secondary and nonepileptogenic becomes an ever-increasing problem.

The terms 'hippocampal sclerosis' and 'mesial temporal sclerosis' are often used virtually interchangeably. We prefer to use the term 'hippocampal sclerosis' when only the hippocampus is being referred to, and 'mesial temporal sclerosis' to mean abnormalities of the hippocampus as well as other structures such as the amygdala, entorhinal cortex, and parahippocampal region.

It was not until the imaging era that it was possible to assess the degree of bilateral hippocampal damage in life. Similarly, the ability to assess whether there are other abnormalities in addition to HS is not possible by examination of the resection specimen, because only a limited amount of brain tissue is available for examination. To summarize our experience with imaging over the last decade or so, in the case of damage to the hippocampus we see areas in addition to the hippocampus that are abnormal by atrophy or by signal change. We also see cases where the abnormalities seem to be bilateral, and some in which the emphasis of abnormality is clearly lateralized. The MR cases we see are summarized in Figure 4.4. In addition, we see HS on its own, and with other definite lesions in the brain (Table 4.2).

This gives rise to the concept of three different types of HS (130). The first is when it is classical, as we have conceived of it since the time of Sommer (131). The second is where there are abnormalities in addition to the HS but these might be thought of as of a similar type to the HS (atrophy and signal changes in tissues beyond the hippocampus). This we have called HS+, the 'plus' meaning areas involved additional to the hippocampus. The third type of HS occurs in the presence of a distinct 'other' pathology such as a focal tumor. These we have called +HS, meaning that there is a consequent HS, possibly from the effects of seizures on the hippocampus, which originated in the 'other' lesion. We imply that the HS is secondary, which may or may not turn out to be the case. Nonetheless, this is a distinct MR-diagnosable type of HS, and one that is recognized with increasing frequency.

We have prefaced the presentation of the findings on the MR scans in these patients with these concepts so that the importance of the observations has a context.

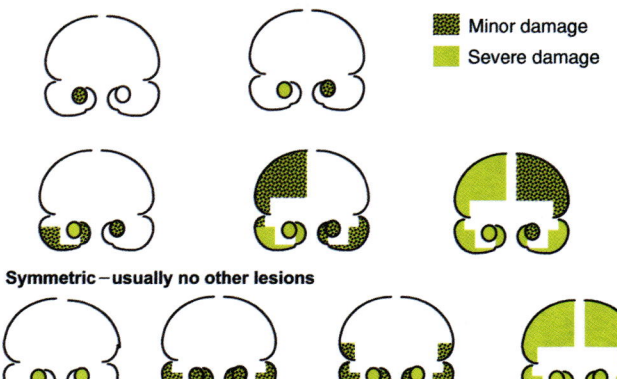

FIG. 4.4. The types of hippocampal sclerosis seen on MR studies. There are various degrees of asymmetric damage. As the ipsilateral damage becomes more severe, the more likely it is to find regional and contralateral damage of lesser degrees. In the case of the symmetric hippocampal sclerosis, the degree of damage equally involves regional structures on both sides. This suggests that there might be two fundamentally different mechanisms that cause hippocampal damage, and that the severity of the insult or the vulnerability of the subject might determine the final outcome. These patterns can be conceived of as being caused by seizure or other damage that is either lateralized (upper panels) or generalized (lower row).

Mesial Temporal Sclerosis: The Most Important Cause of Temporal Lobe Epilepsy

Terminology

The terms Ammon's horn sclerosis, mesial temporal sclerosis and hippocampal sclerosis are used almost interchangeably. However, these terms are, strictly, not synonymous since the distribution of pathologic changes is different between these entities (90, 95, 96, 126, 127). While, pathologically, mesial temporal sclerosis encompasses changes in the amygdala, hippocampus and the adjacent entorhinal cortex, the term *hippocampal sclerosis* refers to abnormalities in the CA1–CA4 areas and in the dentate gyrus and subiculum. In *Ammon's horn sclerosis*, the abnormalities are restricted to areas CA1 to CA4 exclusively. When interpreting pathologic material or MR studies, often only the hippocampal tissue or the hippocampal structure is examined and regional changes may only be implied.

Table 4.2. Hippocampal Sclerosis Variants: The Magnetic Resonance Era

Pure HS	+HS	HS+
Classical	Lesion plus HS	HS plus other abnormality
Rarely seen	Always ipsilateral	Contralateral
Only with	At least 30%	Hemisphere
'tunnel vision'	of HS	Cerebellum
techniques		

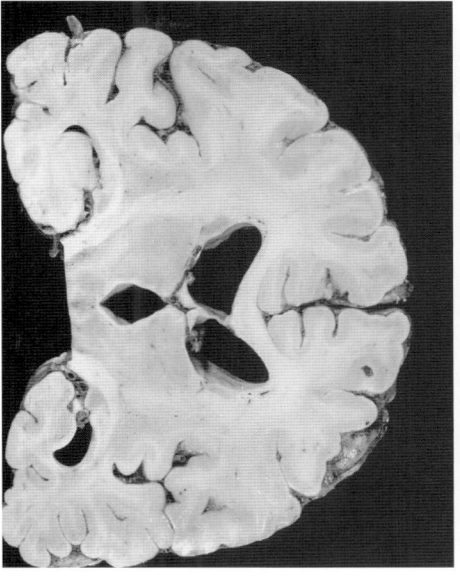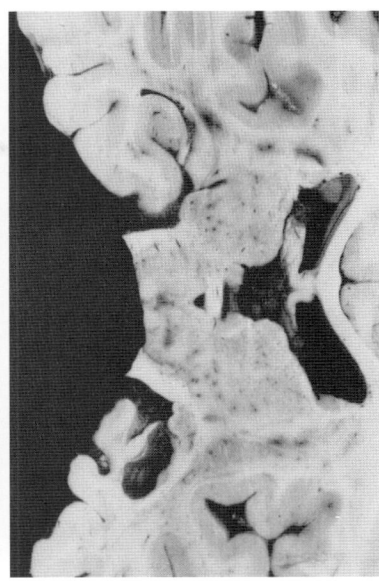

A   B

FIG. 4.6. Macroscopic specimens in two patients with complex partial seizures of temporal lobe origin caused by mesial sclerosis. Note severe unilateral hippocampal atrophy with temporal horn enlargement.

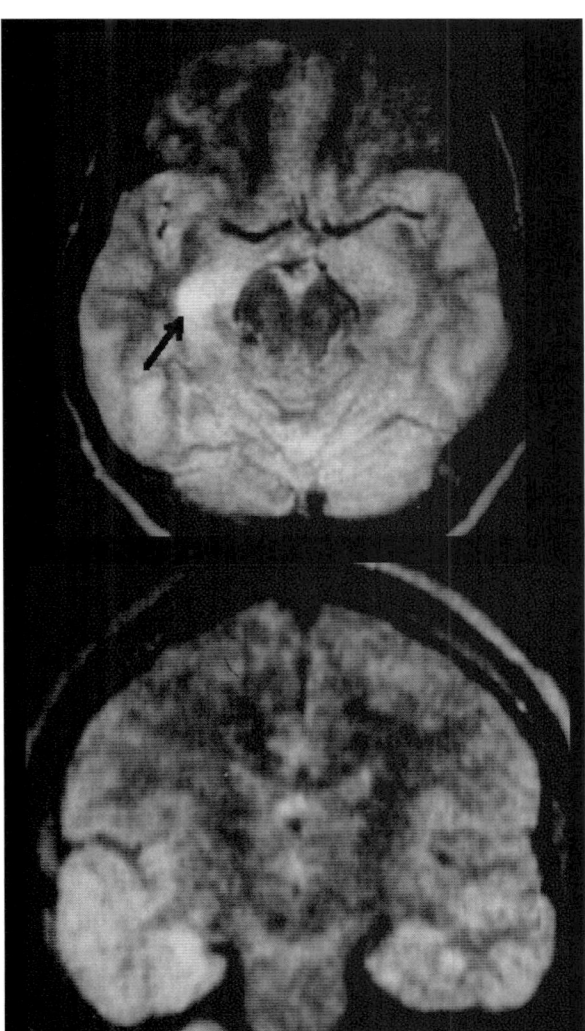

FIG. 4.5. This is an early study showing increased T2 weighted signal in the hippocampal region. Clearly there is some abnormality, but to specify hippocampal sclerosis on such images was not possible or reliable. Regional abnormality is seen in the right temporal lobe (on the left side of the image).

Since these terms were originally derived from pathologic findings, we should be careful when using MR as a method of implying these pathologies; one should not make a pathologic diagnosis of mesial temporal sclerosis unless abnormalities are demonstrated beyond the confines of the hippocampus. Conversely, because MR imaging (and sometimes pathologic assessment) often only looks at the hippocampus with high sensitivity, it is probable that many cases do have more regional abnormalities than is detected, as shown in diagrammatic form in Figure 4.4. Often areas such as the rest of the temporal lobe or the ipsilateral hemisphere are affected. Sometimes the changes are general and bilateral. In many cases HS is seen with more regional abnormality. It is likely that there is a range of causes of this damage that looks like an injury.

The alternative way of using the term 'mesial temporal sclerosis' is as a general term that covers any lesion that has gliosis as a feature in this region. The MR correlate of this can be seen in an early study of TLE (Fig. 4.5), and pathologic specimens (Fig. 4.6) where HS as well as regional signal change in the hippocampus is seen.

The diagnosis of mesial temporal sclerosis is typically made in the presence of neuronal loss greater than 30–50% cell loss in CA1 of the pyramidal cell layer of the hippocampus (usually a typical pattern of the cell loss is specified) (90, 91). This diagnosis is often based only on hippocampal evaluation, and often gliosis is not considered essential for this diagnosis. Implicit in this diagnosis is the assumption that HS is a continuum with severe neuronal loss and gliosis at one end and a small degree of cell loss at the other. Other findings are necessarily ignored. The same clinical consequences are assumed in terms of epileptogenicity.

Subtypes of Hippocampal Sclerosis

Since the macroscopic description of mesial sclerosis by Bouchet and Cazauvieilh in 1825 (132) and the first histologic

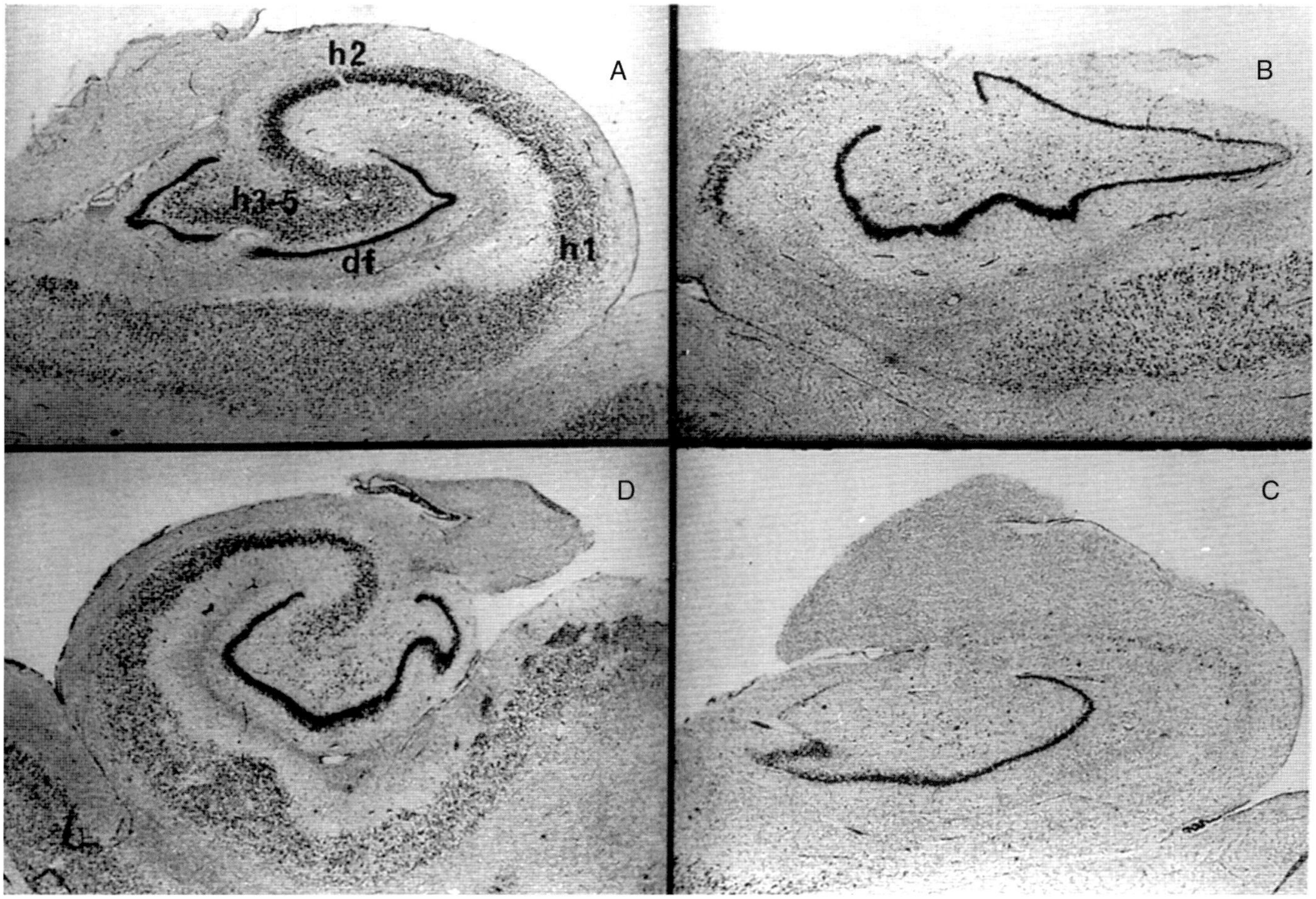

FIG. 4.7. Pathologic specimens demonstrating normal hippocampus and subtypes of hippocampal sclerosis. **A.** Normal hippocampal layers. **B.** Classical Ammon's horn sclerosis with prominent cell loss in CA1, CA4 and CA3. **C.** Total Ammon's horn sclerosis with massive cell loss in all subfields. **D.** End-folium sclerosis with isolated cell loss in the end-folium (With permission from Bruton 1988 (127).)

description of this entity in 1880 by Sommer (131), the morphologic changes of mesial sclerosis in temporal lobe seizures have been central to the understanding of epilepsy. Macroscopically, HS is characterized by an atrophic, small, firm hippocampus (Fig. 4.6).

This abnormality can be bilateral symmetrical or asymmetrical or unilaterally localized (Fig. 4.3) (97, 100, 126, 133, 134). Histologically, HS is characterized by the presence of neuronal cell loss and astrocytic proliferation in the fascia dentata, Ammon's horn, presubiculum and subiculum (Figs 4.7, 4.8). Pathologists have studied this condition, both qualitatively and, more recently, using quantitative techniques with cell counts. Using qualitative methods, Margerison and Corsellis in their classic study (126) divided HS into different subgroups. The most frequent form observed in their series was *classical Ammon's horn sclerosis* with primary nerve cell loss in the CA1 and CA 4 sections of the hippocampus with least damage to the CA2 regions. Less commonly, there is widespread cell loss through the entire hippocampus labeled *total Ammon's horn sclerosis* (Fig. 4.7). The third type is termed *end-folium sclerosis*, where cell loss is restricted to that region (Fig. 4.9).

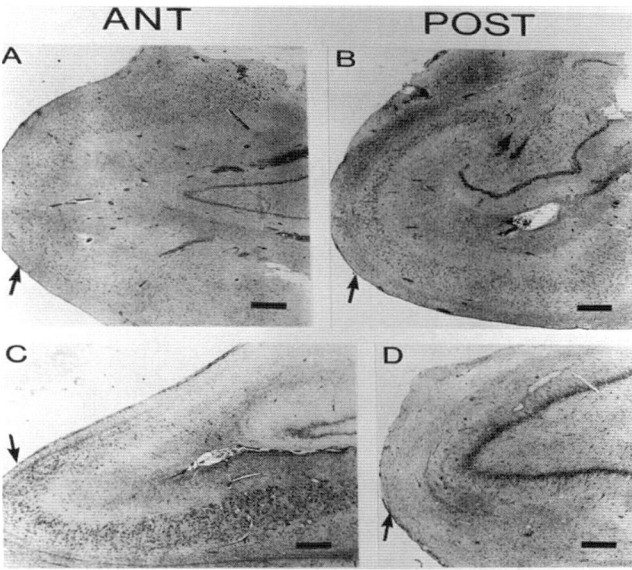

FIG. 4.8. Anterior versus posterior hippocampal cell loss. **A, B.** Cell loss is restricted to the anterior hippocampus with sparing of the posterior region (**B**). **C, D.** In contrast, **C** and **D** demonstrate minimal cell loss in the anterior hippocampus (**C**) with severe loss in the posterior section. (With permission from Babb et al. 1997.)

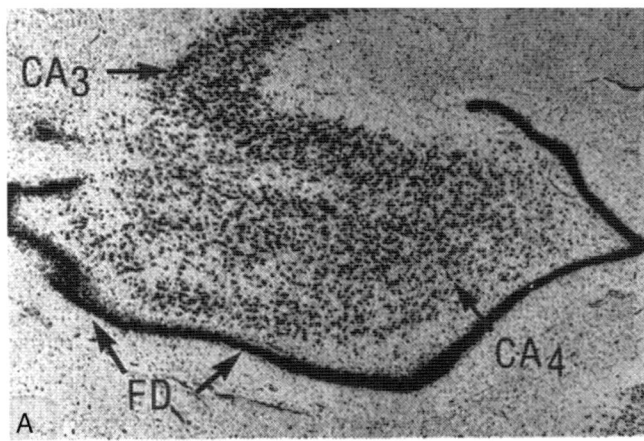

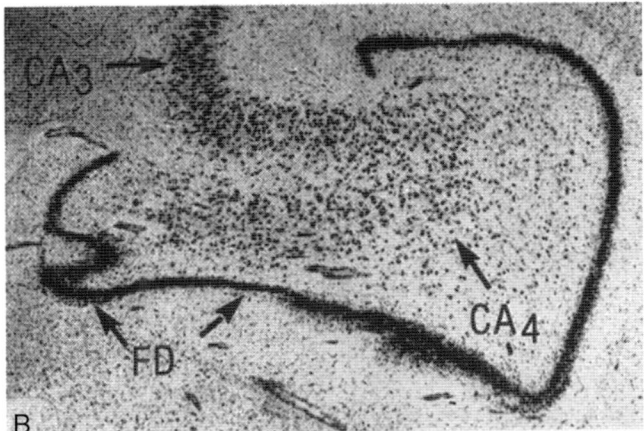

FIG. 4.9. End-folium sclerosis with minimal cell loss in CA3. Normal hippocampus (**A**) and TLE (**B**) showing primary cell loss in the CA4 region of the hippocampus. (With permission from Margerison and Corsellis, 1966 (126).)

In his classic review of the pathology of temporal lobe epilepsy, Bruton (127) reported that 43% of cases demonstrated mesial sclerosis without other pathology. Among those patients, 57% of the specimens had *classical sclerosis* while 39% had *total sclerosis*, and only 4% had *end-folium sclerosis*. In addition, he reported (127) that 27% of these patients demonstrated damage in the adjacent fusiform gyrus and that 76% of specimens revealed amygdaloid cell loss and gliosis. This is consistent with the findings from other studies (88, 98).

The degree of neuronal cell loss is variable but is typically defined as being more than 50% in the presence of gliosis (88, 92, 97, 98). However, a 25% cell loss in the hippocampus with associated gliosis has been described (92) and may also represent significant hippocampal damage. It is unlikely that the hippocampus is damaged in such a way that either 50% of neurons are lost (a common definition of HS) or no damage has occurred.

Hippocampal damage may either be a continuum, HS being a level of damage that can unequivocally be detected visually by a histopathology, or there may be different types of damage that cause different degrees of change in the hippocampus, and these have different clinical meanings.

This issue is a difficult one and as techniques become more sensitive the significance of subtle changes is important. For example, studies have shown subtle changes in the hippocampus on the contralateral side to classical HS, and in the ipsilateral hippocampus when the seizures originate in areas other than the mesial temporal lobe (135, 136). This damage may reflect secondary, possibly less epileptogenic effects of seizure spread. We need at present to keep an open mind about whether minor degrees of abnormality mean the same thing as classical changes.

Our MR experience leads us to believe that the pathologic entity of HS really comprises a range of abnormalities that have different features and different meanings in terms of seizure generation or secondary seizure effects depending on the context in which they are found (e.g. atrophy without signal change seems to suggest secondary effects in the hippocampus and may or may not be the primary epileptogenic lesion, while atrophy with signal change almost always appears to be highly epileptogenic). The different MR features of HS could facilitate a new way to evaluate and classify different types of hippocampal damage complementary to the pathologic evaluation of a resected specimen.

Quantitative Cell Counts

The reported incidence of pathologically verified HS in resected temporal lobe specimens is variable but ranges between 49% and 70% (90, 91, 127). Although methodologic differences and patient selection could considerably affect these numbers, the percentage of patients with this pathology has been remarkably consistent in all studies, even given different population bias, surgical versus nonsurgical groups, and using MR techniques of diagnosis compared to pathologic diagnosis. The incidence of HS in children had been considered to be different from that in the adult population but some studies suggest that this may not be the case (137–140). Therefore, it is likely that the quoted frequency is an accurate reflection of the biology of this disorder.

The best correlation can be found in the frequency of HS among autopsy studies of patients with temporal lobe epilepsy. Sano et al. (100) found HS in 58% of cases with temporal lobe seizures and Margerison et al. reported HS in 65% of autopsied cases (126). It is important to mention, however, that the diagnostic criteria of temporal lobe epilepsy used in some of these studies are not comparable to the one presently in use. It is likely that some patients with extra-temporal-lobe epilepsy were included in those earlier studies. Nonetheless, most studies are consistent in indicating this high frequency of HS in temporal lobe epilepsy.

Hippocampal Sclerosis in the Normal Population

Hippocampal sclerosis, even as defined by pure pathologic criteria, is not exclusively associated with temporal lobe epilepsy. Some authors have quoted frequencies of HS in autopsy series of patients with different forms of seizures as ranging from 20% to 80% (134). HS has not usually been found in MR series of normal controls, although there may be an incidence of typical HS in controls without epilepsy (141). This finding needs to be replicated in other centers but asymptomatic HS may exist. HS without epilepsy has also been described in relatives of temporal lobe epilepsy patients (142).

The problem with these figures is that both the pathologic and MR criteria for defining the entity and the patient populations need to be strict. Certainly, there are patients with HS who seem to have mild, easily controlled epilepsy and may never have been diagnosed as having epilepsy. We have personal experience of following several of these individuals over many years. While all we know of have had seizures without medication, at least one had mild complex partial seizures and managed to deny this while living an active employed life into his thirties. Medication abolished all events.

Meencke (97) and Peiffer (133, 134) have consistently found the frequency of HS in the general epileptic population at autopsy to be approximately 30% and insist there is an incidence of this entity in the normal population. Other autopsy studies indicate that up to 10% of controls (individuals without epilepsy) may have at least a subtle degree of HS (133, 134).

Hippocampal Sclerosis and the Epileptic Focus – What Makes it Epileptogenic?

Is HS itself an epileptogenic lesion? The answer to this is unequivocally yes. Are all degrees and types of hippocampal injury equally epileptogenic? As we have discussed above, there is evidence that not all damaged hippocampi have the same degree of epileptogenesis.

The patterns of cell loss in other conditions that produce hippocampal damage are different: in anoxic or other injuries, the entire CA fields may be damaged, including the presubiculum. The mechanisms underlying hippocampal damage in both epilepsy and ischemia may be related to the presence of high concentrations of glutamate receptors in CA1, CA3, and the dentate gyrus (143–149), which suggests that neuroexcitotoxic damage, and hence selective cell loss, may be an important part of the etiology of epileptogenic HS.

A number of other factors also seem to be important in the genesis of epilepsy in HS. Among these factors, the age at the time of initial precipitating injury and the type of insult may play an important role, although the mechanism for this is still unclear. Numerous studies indicate that prolonged febrile convulsions and status epilepticus occurring between ages 3 months and 7 years are crucial; below or above these ages, the subsequent course may be different (12, 13, 20, 23, 29, 49, 54, 94, 128, 150–153). It is therefore likely that injury occurring during a crucial window at an early age produces intrinsic reorganization of the hippocampus with the possibility of disruption of the normal balance between excitatory and inhibitory mechanisms (154–156).

Findings in human HS also suggest the presence of anomalous reorganization of mossy fibers in CA1, CA2, and subiculum. In fact, excessive GABA-ergic input may remain in human HS, facilitating initiation and propagation of seizure discharges (154, 157–159). It appears unlikely that HS exists in isolation, and other structures may therefore be as important for the generation and propagation of seizures in temporal lobe epilepsy. The failure of selective hippocampal lesions or even hippocampal removal to ablate seizures and the common persistence of auras after selective or radical temporal lobe resections is strong evidence for the role of other structures in temporal lobe epilepsy.

Amygdala Sclerosis

Gloor (9) has pointed out that the amygdala (and the entorhinal cortex) may play an important role in mesial sclerosis. Several lines of evidence support this contention. First, pathologic data (despite the difficulties of assessment due to the architecture of the amygdala) have repeatedly demonstrated neuronal loss and gliosis in the amygdala in the temporal lobes of patients with intractable epilepsy resected at surgery (12, 19, 94, 127), ranging from 50% to 75% (12, 88, 127). Second, surgical studies carried out at the Montreal neurologic institute indicate that removal of parts of the amygdala may be as important as resection of the hippocampus (9, 115, 160). Finally, imaging data derived with MRI have demonstrated the presence of signal changes and volume reductions both in association with HS and independently when the hippocampus has been assessed as normal (161–164). The quantification of this volume loss and signal changes may be as important for the amygdala as it has been for the hippocampus (165–172). This suggests that the amygdala can be both involved in the seizures of mesial temporal lobe epilepsy and an independent source for seizure generation.

Bilateral Hippocampal Sclerosis

Another important issue concerns the presence of unilateral and bilateral HS. As discussed above, autopsy studies have shown a variable incidence. Meencke (97) found bilateral lesions in 56%, while Sano et al. (100) found that 86% of brains of patients who died with epilepsy had bilateral HS. In contrast, Margerison and Corsellis (126) found bilateral lesions in only 47% of patients in their series. In some of these studies, the changes were restricted to the hippocampus in one-third of the specimens, underscoring the fact that HS was detected in the context of widespread injury. In fact, when predominantly unilateral HS was encountered, it was more restricted than in the bilateral cases. These studies have also suggested that bilateral lesions are more common with early perinatal disturbances (173), whereas, with late injuries, unilateral lesions were more common. In the group of patients with postnatal and early childhood lesions, 56% demonstrated bilateral lesions while 44% had unilateral pathology. In summary, pathologic data suggest that HS may be unilateral but often may occur bilaterally or asymmetrically, depending on the type and time of injury.

These pathologic data are supported by the findings using MR methods (162, 174–177, 130). To detect bilateral disease of the hippocampus, a technique of quantification is important (166, 178–180), as visual assessment relies heavily on a comparison between the ipsilateral and contralateral sides. T2 relaxometry demonstrates bilateral, usually asymmetrical changes in a similar proportion to that predicted by pathologic studies (135, 136).

It is clear that the majority of patients with intractable temporal lobe epilepsy referred for surgical intervention have mesial temporal sclerosis. The classic form appears to be strongly associated with an antecedent history of atypical febrile convulsions during childhood. These patients usually follow a rather characteristic clinical course, have often unilateral EEG findings, and outcome following surgery is excellent. Although the hippocampus itself has been the focus of our attention, other structures including the amygdala and parahippocampal gyrus probably play an important role in this condition. The present and future role of MRI in the anatomicopathologic dissection of these pathologies is therefore substantial. As the sensitivity of MR increases the populations that are studied may also change. Many of these issues were well known, although the knowledge about these conditions was largely derived from anatomicopathologic correlations. The major advance with imaging is that this knowledge can be applied to the living patient with MR studies that can detect these pathologically defined abnormalities. Beyond this, MR studies allow us to extend these historical observations as we can examine whole populations noninvasively.

MAGNETIC RESONANCE IMAGING OF TEMPORAL LOBE EPILEPSY

Commissions of the International League Against Epilepsy: Recommendations

Who Should Have an MRI?

The Commission on Neuroimaging of the International League against Epilepsy (ILAE) (181, 182) recommends that "[i]n the non-acute situation, the ideal practice is to obtain structural neuroimaging with MRI in all patients with epilepsy, except in patients with a definite electroclinical diagnosis of idiopathic generalized epilepsy (benign myoclonic epilepsy of infancy, childhood absence epilepsy, juvenile absence epilepsy, juvenile myoclonic epilepsy), or benign epilepsy of childhood with centrotemporal spikes." Even these excluded syndromes may offer a surprise, and numerous cases where structural abnormalities are found in these electroclinical syndromes have now been reported.

What Sequences Should be Done?

The Commission on Neuroimaging of the ILAE states that "MRI is essential for presurgical evaluation. ... Epilepsy surgery should never be contemplated without an MRI examination, apart from exceptional circumstances such as a specific contraindication (e.g. cardiac pacemaker)." They recommend that a minimum of both T1- and T2-weighted images be obtained and a three-dimensional volume acquisition with images be obtained or examined in coronal and axial orientations. It is clear that epilepsy is a specialist study in MRI and a 'routine' MRI study is not adequate for the problem of epilepsy surgery. The exact protocols will change with advances in technology as discussed in this volume (183).

Defining the Seizure Focus

The seizure focus in partial epilepsy has long been conceived of as having a brain abnormality, 'the epileptogenic lesion'; a pacemaker zone necessary for seizure generation, 'the ictal onset zone'; and a region of the brain that gives rise to the expression of the seizures, 'the symptomatogenic zone'. (These concepts are discussed in more detail in Chapter 1).

Clinical seizures, virtually by definition, demonstrate the symptomatogenic region of seizure involvement. This is the area of the brain that gives rise to clinical symptoms and is often a pointer to the area of the brain involved in seizures.

Prior to imaging techniques, EEG was the main way to tell what part of the brain was generating the seizures (Fig. 4.1). The EEG from the scalp reflects both the site of onset of seizures and its electrical spread. Although it has excellent resolution for the timing of events, EEG has poor sensitivity and poor spatial resolution. By the time electrical discharges are seen on the scalp recording, they may be a distance away from the 'seizure focus'.

Intracranial EEG is used to increase sensitivity, specificity and spatial resolution and hence is important in seizure surgery programs. It involves a major operation, and attendant risks, and still has a number of important drawbacks. It is primarily limited by the relatively small area that can be sampled. In imaging terms it has a very narrow field of view and it effectively ignores what is occurring away from the sampled area. For such a highly invasive diagnostic test it often does not provide definitive information (184). In the imaging era, intracranial studies are usually reserved for increasingly complex epilepsy.

The advent of MRI, ictal single-positron-emission computed tomography (SPECT) and positron-emission tomography (PET), and optimized imaging strategies has added direct noninvasively acquired knowledge about the lesions that are present in the brain of patients with epilepsy. These methods can also deliver information about focal brain activity as well, as is discussed in Chapter 11.

The purpose of defining the seizure focus is to remove it surgically and 'cure' the epilepsy. Increasingly, good outcome from seizures is seen to depend on complete resection of epileptogenic lesions over and above the ictal pacemaker zone, when this can be identified. The selection of surgical candidates increasingly depends on the presence of a structural abnormality and then confirmation of the epileptogenic nature of these abnormalities with functional methods such as ictal EEG and SPECT studies (185). Still, many cases of partial epilepsy appear to have no identifiable focal abnormality even in the best imaging and image interpretation centers. Part of this may result from the insensitivity of our methods, and part from the fact that the biology of seizure generation is not conveniently focal. MR methods are giving us a way to tackle these issues.

Mesial Temporal Sclerosis: Diagnosis with Magnetic Resonance Imaging

Generations of epileptologists have been fascinated with the issues that surround HS, including its origins and its causal relationship with epilepsy. Like many areas of science, the strongest opinions exist when the data is weakest. MRI has given us new insights into many of the questions that surround HS because it has given us new and compelling data. In some well studied cases, HS can be observed in relation to the onset and development of both the seizure process and the hippocampal damage. These privileged observations, in life, of patients with HS, including those not operated on, provide us with new insights into disease pathogenesis that are not possible with postsurgical or postmortem data. We therefore now reflect on a decade of observations in the MR era and bring together some of these findings into our current understanding of HS.

As we have discussed when reviewing the pathology of TLE with HS above, HS must be thought of as damage to the formed hippocampus (156). Pathologically it consists of loss of normal tissue (neuron loss and macroscopic atrophy) and gliosis and reorganization. In other words, it is a scar that appears to have occurred after the hippocampus was formed. Whether the event that caused this damage occurred in utero (making HS a 'developmental lesion') or after birth (an 'acquired lesion') is largely a semantic rather than an etiologic argument. A similar pattern of 'damage' can be induced in a range of animal models and human disease from a variety of stimuli that can be considered to be neurotoxic.

If we accept that HS is damage to the hippocampus, longstanding questions remain: What is or are the origins of HS? What is the mechanism of damage? When does the damage occur? What is the role of other lesions? Why is it often unilateral? We believe that answers to many of these questions are taking shape.

Imaging of the Normal Hippocampus

The hippocampus is in many ways an ideal structure for MR to examine. It is well defined, it has a convenient longitudinal orientation so that cross-sectional imaging gives an excellent view of its structure even with relatively thick slices, and MRI–pathologic correlations are possible because

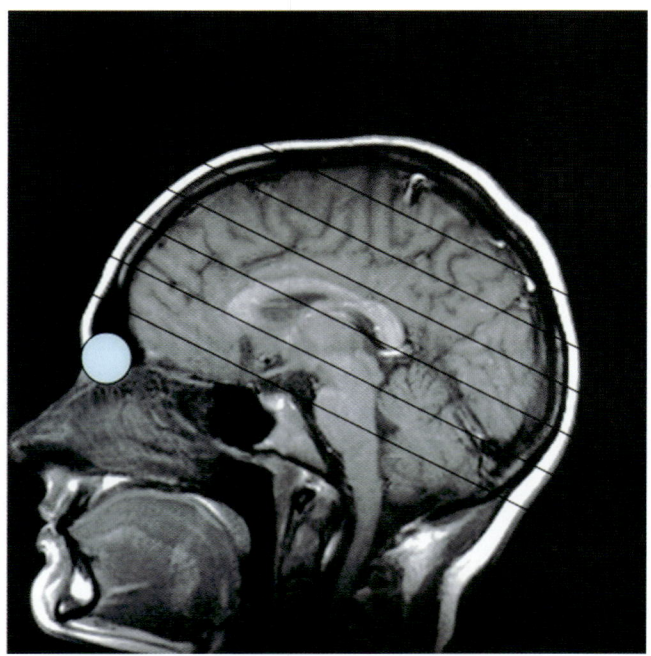
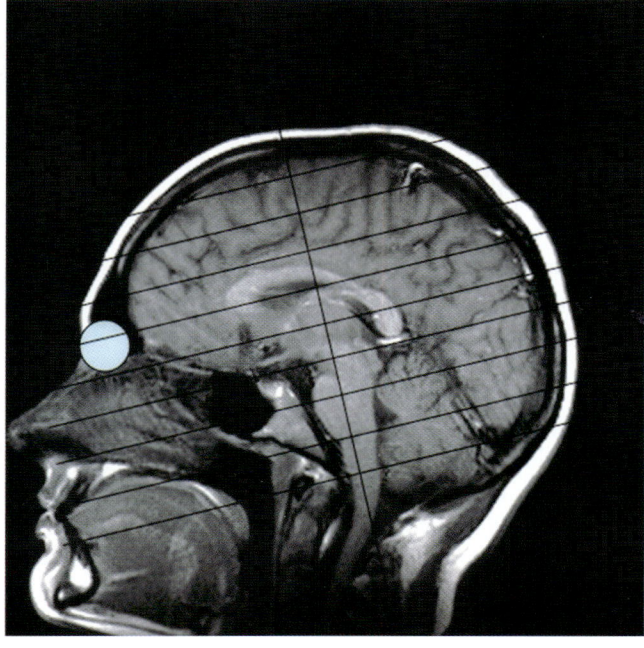

A   B

FIG. 4.10. A. The imaging axis typical for CT scanning is shown in this image. The location of the eye more laterally is approximated by the circle. This axis covers the brain in the minimum number of slices and does not directly expose the eye to radiation. This minimizes radiation exposure, particularly to the eye when compared to other axes. **B.** Parasagittal image showing the hippocampal axis. This is approximately perpendicular to and along the long axis of the brain stem.

Continued

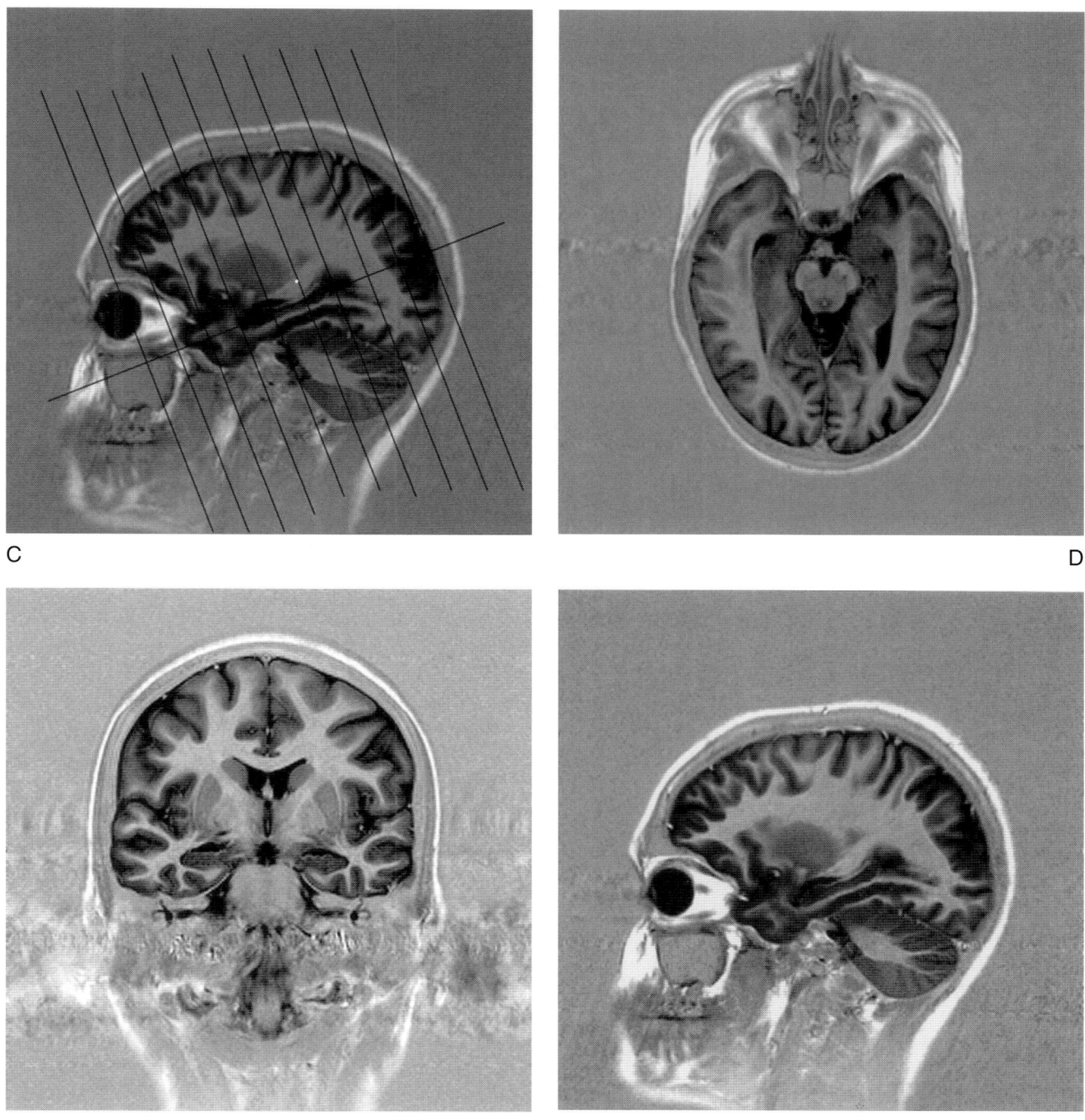

FIG. 4.10. *Cont.* **C.** If more lateral landmarks are used, the hippocampal axis is along the long axis of the hippocampus and perpendicular to this. Note that the orientation is similar to that shown in **B.** The eye is seen in this parasagittal image. **D.** If an image is taken in the plane shown in **C,** both hippocampi can be seen in the medial part of the temporal lobe. **E.** In this axis the coronal images cut through the hippocampus at right angles, giving the clearest possible assessment of size and internal structure. **F.** Parasagittal image through the hippocampus.

surgical removal is undertaken for the treatment of epilepsy. All this leads to great sensitivity and specificity in the MR assessment of the hippocampus, if the radiography of image acquisition and experience in interpretation are available.

The orientation of the hippocampus within the brain is shown in Figure 4.10. The traditional orientation of images is shown in Figure 4.10A. This axis was established in the CT era and allows coverage of the whole brain in the minimum

number of slices and avoiding the radiation-sensitive lens of the eye. This orientation is familiar to most radiologists. The orientation of the 'hippocampal axis' is shown in Figure 4.10B for comparison, and roughly corresponds to the long axis of the brain stem. It is best to orient coronal images perpendicular to the long axis of the hippocampus (Fig. 4.10C) and the axial images, or reconstructions, are done perpendicular to the coronal images. The normal hippocampus in representative

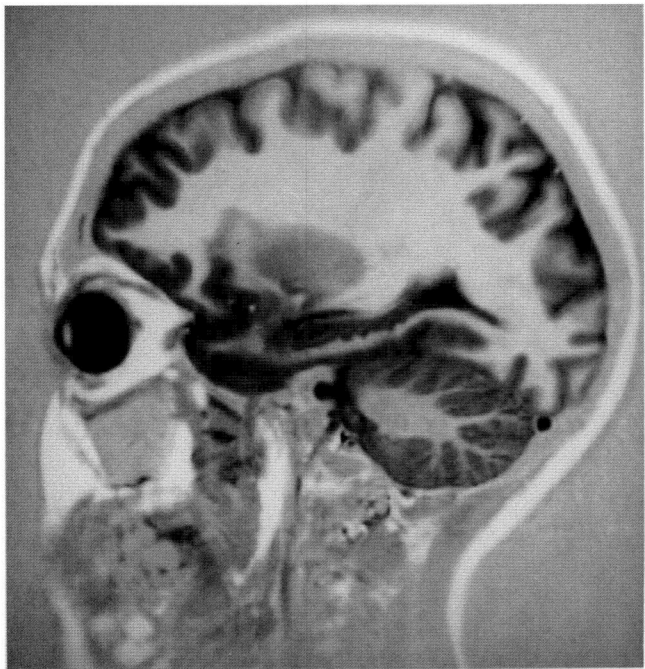

FIG. 4.11. Parasagittal image showing the indentations of the dentate at the inferior border of the hippocampus. In very thin slices this can give apparent asymmetry.

axial (Fig. 4.10D), coronal (Fig. 4.10E) and parasagittal (Fig. 4.10F) orientation are shown. Note that the whole length of the hippocampus can be seen in a single axial slice. In some circumstances these can be very important images.

The hippocampal axis is excellent for imaging most of the subcortical and temporal lobe structures (186). The parasagittal images (Fig. 4.11) show an important feature of the hippocampus – the indentations of the dentate on its inferior border. If thin images are taken, apparent asymmetry of the hippocampus in some slices can be attributable to the fact that the section passes through a different part of these indentations. Most images in this chapter are acquired in this orientation.

Methods of Detecting Pathology Using Magnetic Resonance: Principles

As described in previous chapters, conceptually, the detection of pathology by MRI in general, and of mesial sclerosis in particular, may be performed in three ways:

• The visual detection of abnormal tissue quality by contrast between normal and abnormal tissue. Signal is used to reflect the fact that the tissue composition is in some way abnormal. To do this, we can emphasize T1 or T2 relaxation times, MR spectroscopy, diffusion-weighted imaging, diffusion tensor imaging, or any other method of interrogating the makeup of brain tissue
• The visual detection of morphologic changes of a structure, which can demonstrate changes in size or appearance that reflect the underlying pathology

---

BOX 4.1. The MRI Features of Hippocampal Sclerosis

MORPHOLOGIC
   ▪ Atrophy
   ▪ Altered internal structure

SIGNAL
   ▪ Increased T2-weighted signal intensity
   ▪ Decreased T1-weighted signal intensity

• Advanced image analysis methods (dealt with in detail in Chapter 8).

We will discuss the details of the major MRI techniques, which have enabled the reliable noninvasive diagnosis of mesial temporal sclerosis and in particular of HS (187, 1881, 62).

Magnetic Resonance Features of Hippocampal Sclerosis that Allow a Visual Diagnosis

In line with our principles, stated above, the features of HS will include studies that demonstrate abnormality of the tissue composition, and abnormalities of morphology (Box 4.1).

Changes in Tissue Signal

Abnormal Hippocampal T2-Weighted Signal

Visual analysis of T2-weighted changes was the first method that demonstrated a correlation between hippocampal pathology and MR-detectable signal abnormality (Fig. 4.5) (162, 189–193).

In images that were not coronal in the hippocampal axis, regional signal change was more likely to be from gliosis or a foreign tissue lesion than HS. With optimized images it is clear that the signal can be seen to arise in the hippocampus itself (Figs. 4.12, 4.13). High signal in the mesial temporal region can occur from lesions in the parahippocampal gyrus, foreign tissue lesions, and hippocampal dysplasia (see below). Typical concern in interpreting hippocampal T2 signal is partial volume from the surrounding cerebrospinal fluid (CSF). This is largely dealt with by using fluid-attenuated inversion recovery (FLAIR) images (Fig. 4.14) where the CSF signal is nulled (dark). These images make the signal change more obvious, but it can usually be identified in the T2-weighted images. Another concern in the medial temporal region is high signal from flow artefact from flow in the carotid arterial system (Fig. 4.15), which can usually be easily recognized as such, and a number of focal high-signal areas such as fluid in the hippocampal fissure, which is a normal finding (Fig. 4.16).

Problems in interpretation often stem from a failure to appreciate the anatomy of the hippocampus. Correlation with

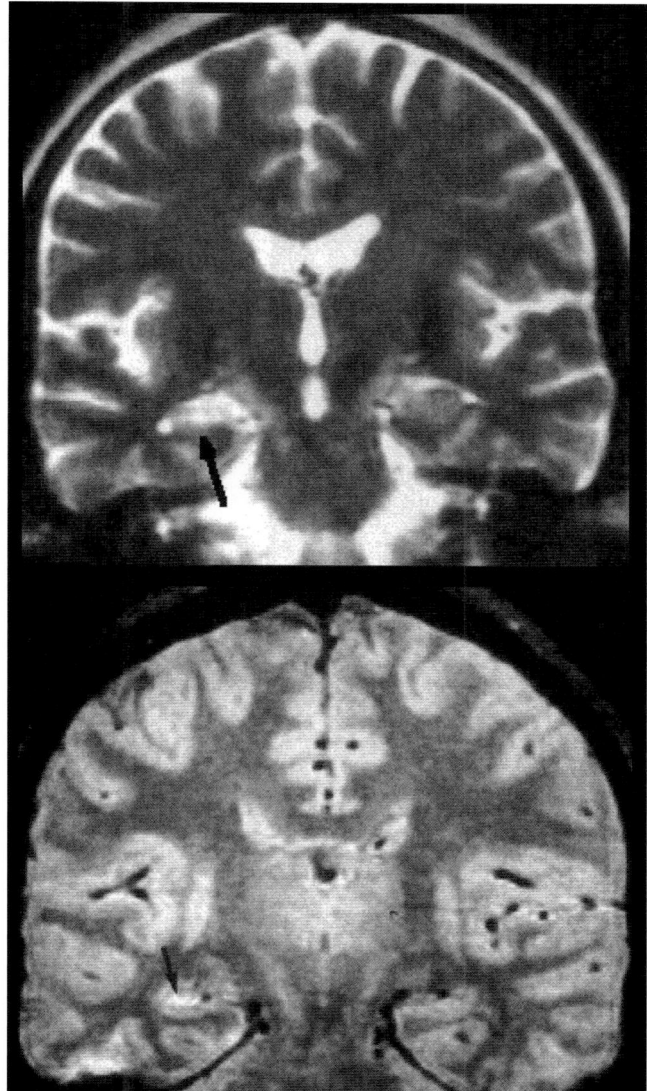

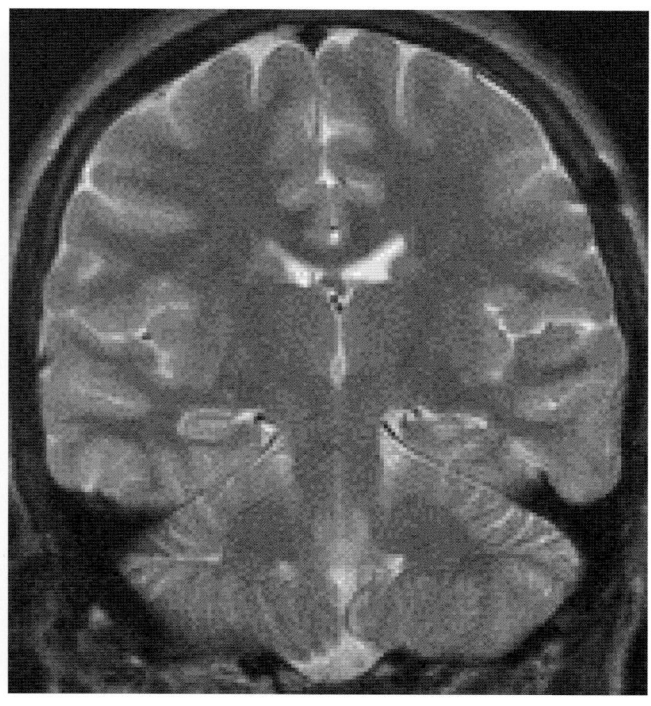

FIG. 4.12. Increased signal is seen in the heavily T2-weighted image (**A**) and the proton-density image (**B**). The MR shows typical hippocampal sclerosis on the left in a patient with TLE. This girl has the clinical history that is consistent with the idea of a syndrome of mesial temporal sclerosis. She had a prolonged febrile convulsion at 12 months of age, a silent period, and then her first seizure at 7 years of age. Her development was normal, VIQ 79, PIQ 94. Quantitative T2 and MRS were abnormal on the left.

the anatomical images can usually clarify where the signal abnormality arises. Orientation of the imaging slice perpendicular to the long axis of the hippocampus avoids significant partial volume effects in most cases. Once it is appreciated that one can have confidence in abnormal signal if it is anatomically localized to the hippocampal gray matter, the abnormal signal as a feature of HS is generally easily appreciated.

Although the abnormal T2 signal is a reliable finding for HS, one needs to be aware of a number of common problems. A problem may arise from the presence of normal dilatation of the hippocampal fissure. Although this may be incorrectly diagnosed as a high signal from the hippocampus, it is rare for it to be mistaken for HS in experienced hands. Lastly, bilateral hippocampal T2 signal abnormalities may be present which may create difficulties because of the lack of a contrast or control for comparison. These and other problems are usually resolved by using clearly defined

criteria for the diagnosis of HS in optimized images or by using more advanced methods of analysis or quantification when doubt exists.

Using optimized T2-weighted sequences (orientation and sequence) including CSF-nulled sequences such as the FLAIR sequence (194–201), one can easily detect the presence of increased signal from the hippocampal body. The high signal is localized to the hippocampal gray matter and usually can be seen in the middle of the structure if one uses the corresponding T1-weighted image for definition of anatomical detail (162, 175, 188, 202–204).

High signal on T2-weighted (including FLAIR images) has proved to be very reliable and sensitive, in experienced hands, for the detection of HS (174, 175, 202, 204). The quantification of T2 relaxation times has also confirmed that T2 signal abnormality is almost invariably present with HS even when this cannot be seen by visual analysis.

T2 MAP   T2w (TE=84ms)   T2 MAP   T2w (TE=84ms)

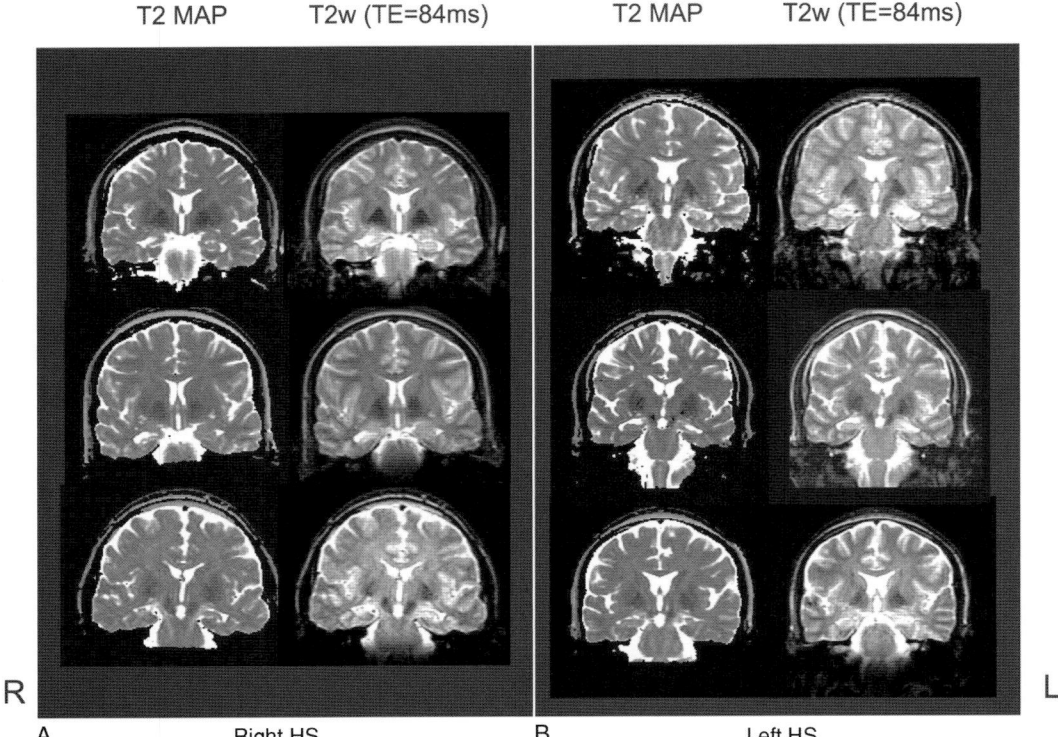

R   L
A   Right HS   B   Left HS

FIG. 4.13. Three examples of right hippocampal sclerosis are shown in **A** and three examples of left HS in **B**. The T2 map is shown on the left and the T2-weighted image on the right. Only one image from each set of coronal images is shown. Note the signal characteristics in the ipsilateral hippocampi.

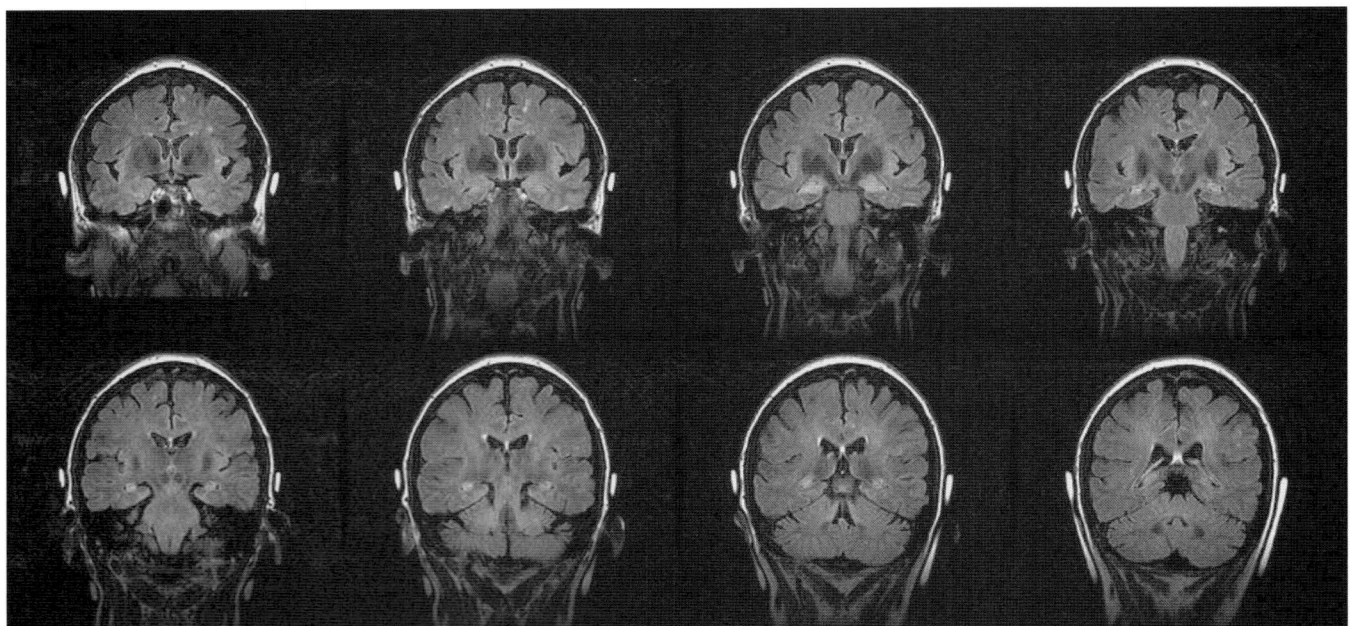

FIG. 4.14. Coronal FLAIR imaging through the length of the hippocampi in a patient with temporal lobe epilepsy. There is bilaterally increased FLAIR signal in both hippocampi, worse on the right. There was unilateral right hippocampal changes on T2-weighted imaging. The patient was operated successfully on the most abnormal (right) side. He is seizure-free after surgery.

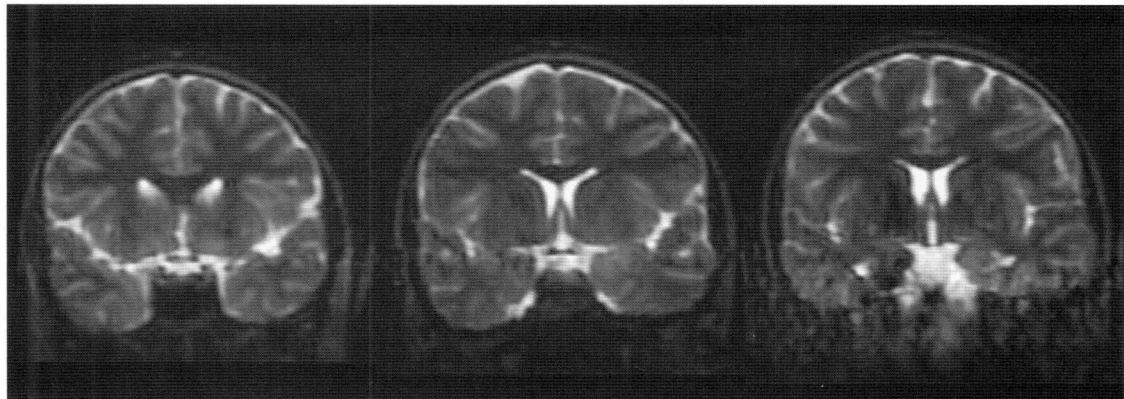

FIG. 4.15. T2 artefacts can occur, and can be a particular problem when interpreting subtle changes in the hippocampus and in the anterior temporal lobes. There is artifact that arises from the flow in the arteries at this level. This gives artifact from left to right across the temporal lobes in the phase encode direction. There is variation in the intensity of the tissue effects, but note that the contrast between the gray and white matter is maintained even in the presence of this artifact. This type of artifact should be easily recognizable and not confused with real signal change in the hippocampus.

Hippocampal Signal Hypointensity on T1-weighted Images

The use of a heavily T1-weighted sequence is, in our experience, a valuable sequence to study HS. Currently, despite the time and coverage issues, we often use inversion recovery as part of our epilepsy protocol as we believe it provides information not seen on our three-dimensional or other T1-weighted sequences (Fig. 4.17A). It would be reasonable though to only run this sequence if the hippocampus looks normal or equivocal on other sequences in the context

of a diagnosis of TLE. The atrophic hippocampus often demonstrates decreased signal with a dark appearance and this corresponds to the high signal on T2-weighted sequences (Fig. 4.17B). We have not found a major dissociation between T2 signal increase and T1 signal decrease and believe they show the same pathology but with sometimes different sensitivity. The inversion recovery sequence can be thought of as doing the job of increasing the sensitivity of T1 images for this feature of signal abnormality. One of the advantages of the sequence is that it gives excellent anatomical definition for assessment of atrophy at the same

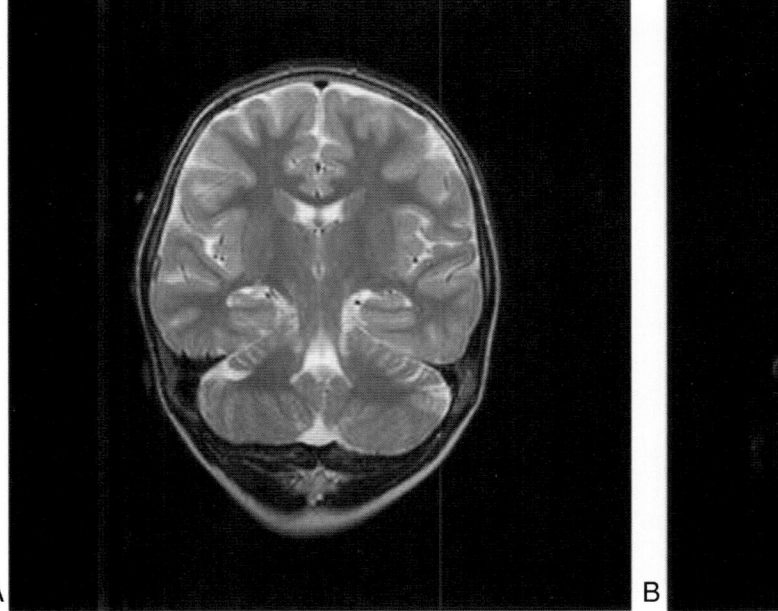
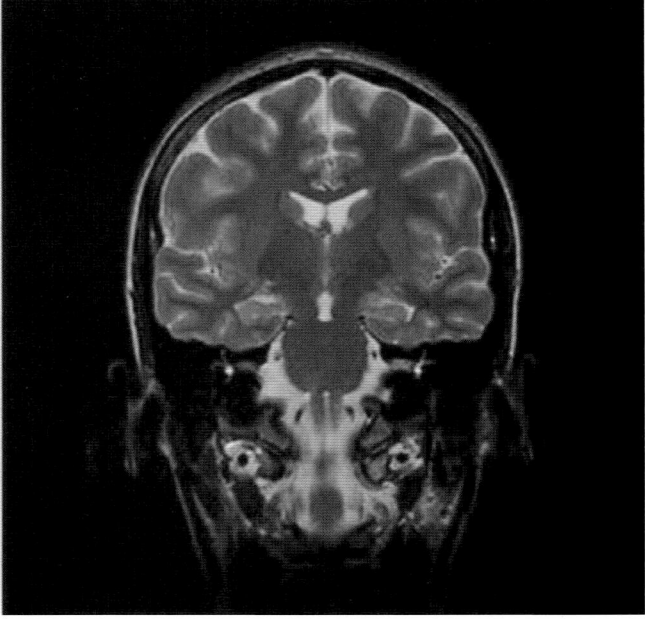

A B

FIG. 4.16. These images show examples of normal hippocampi on T2 weighted images in control subjects. In all there are small focal areas of increased signal. This represents fluid in the incompletely obliterated hippocampal fissure and is a normal finding. These small areas do not change the average T2 relaxation time in the hippocampus. These are normal variations and not pathological.

Continued

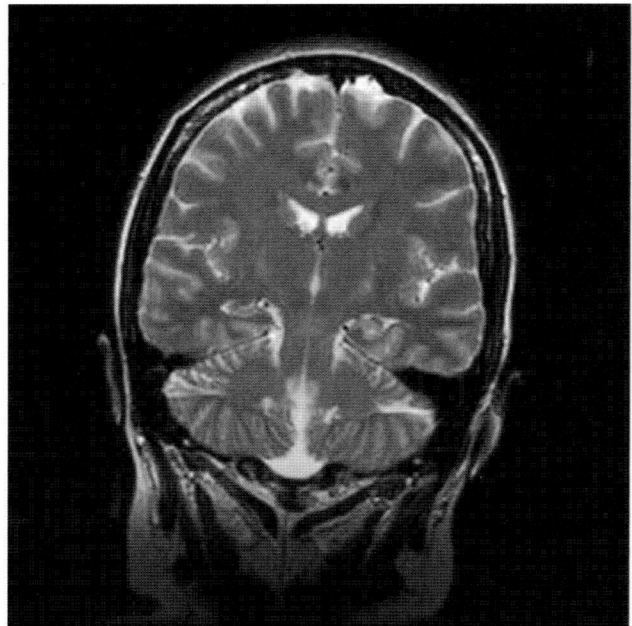

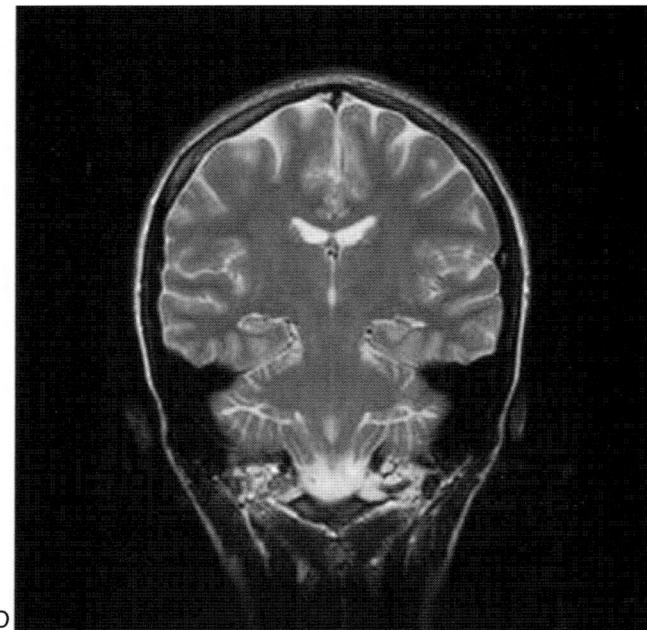

FIG. 4.16. *Cont.*

time as providing information about signal that is usually not present on typical T1 volume sequences.

The use of T1 and T2 contrast really achieves the same purpose. It is a means of identifying the fact that the tissue is abnormal in some way. In cases where there is abnormal morphology (atrophy) but apparently normal signal, such sequences may add valuable information. There seems little doubt that HS with atrophy and signal change is classic epileptogenic HS (Fig. 4.18). We often argue that atrophy without signal change on optimized images may indicate a nearby epileptogenic focus that is causing secondary change in the hippocampus rather than being a primarily epileptogenic

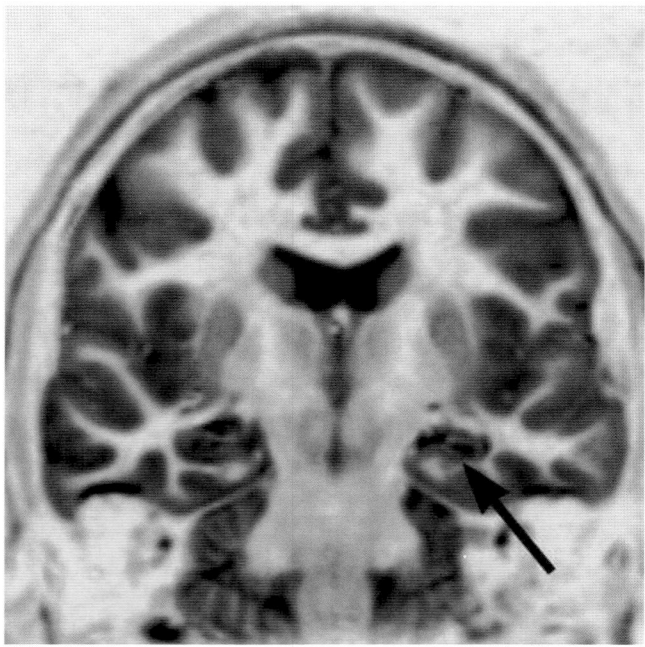

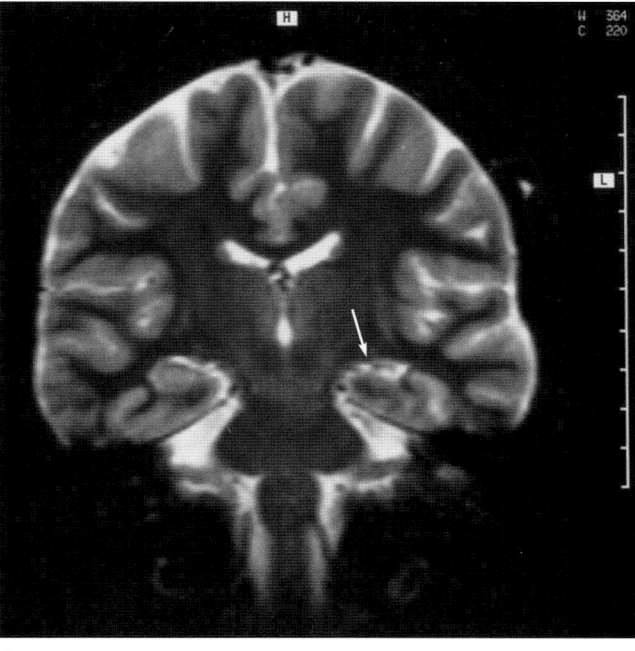

FIG. 4.17. A. Classical hippocampal sclerosis. This is a heavily T1-weighted (inversion recovery) coronal image that shows low-intensity signal from the left hippocampus (arrow). The abnormal signal appears in the center of the structure, in the atrophic hippocampal tissue surrounded by the alveus. Compare with contralateral hippocampus, which is normal in size but has some decreased signal in the CA1 and end-folium regions. **B.** T2-weighted coronal image showing high-intensity signal from the left hippocampus (arrow). The high signal is localized in the center of the structure, which is atrophic. Visually, comparing it with the contralateral hippocampus emphasizes these features.

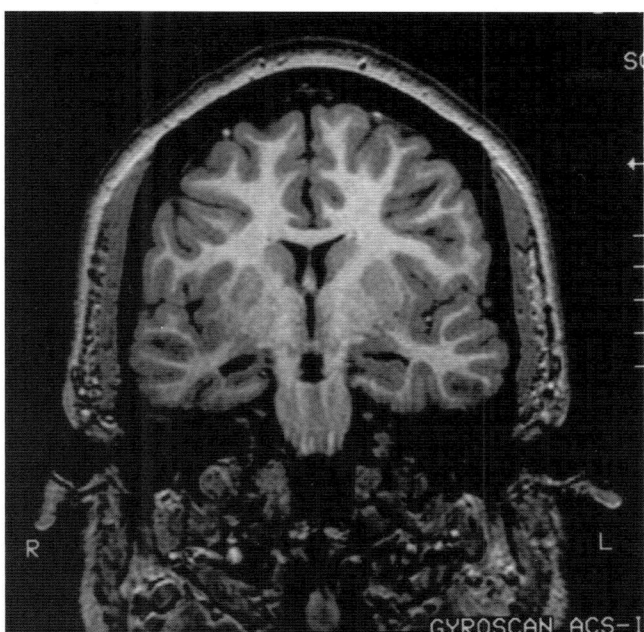

FIG. 4.18. Hippocampal sclerosis. Coronal image through the hippocampal body showing unequivocal right hippocampal atrophy. The right hippocampus is atrophic and flat when compared to the normal left side. The ipsilateral temporal horn is enlarged. Note that there is also right temporal neocortical atrophy and subtle signal change in the temporal white matter.

lesion. If the assessment of signal change in the hippocampus is insensitive then this distinction is clearly not possible. We interpret subtle quantitative signal change, which is not evident on visual inspection in the same way.

Changes in Morphology

Hippocampal Atrophy

Since the anatomy of the hippocampus and adjacent limbic structures is complex, one should use the appropriate imaging planes to correctly visualize these structures, as discussed above. It must be remembered that the hippocampus is like a sea-horse in shape, parts of it curving around the mesencephalon with a superior rostrocaudal angulation of approximately 30–35° (see Fig. 4.10C). In addition, each of its segments (as shown in Chapter 3 and Fig. 4.10, above) has a slightly different orientation: the head and tail are oriented more transversely while the body is more sagittal in orientation.

Using MRI, the assessment of the cross-sectional size of the hippocampus must be made in images obtained in the coronal axis that transects the hippocampus at right angles, known as the hippocampal axis (see Fig. 4.10). Using this angulation largely avoids partial volume effects, in particular in the posterior sections of the body and tail of the hippocampus. While assessment of epilepsy has adopted this coronal plane in most centers, axial imaging is usually

ignored. Axial images or reconstructions should also follow the long axis of the hippocampus, thus avoiding similar problems.

Visual assessment of hippocampal atrophy is the first feature that many radiologists use to assess the hippocampus. This feature was initially questioned because of its subtle nature, often being attributed to normal variation and head tilt in the scanner and variation in normal imaging (see Fig. 4.18). The MR era made many challenges to radiology: a new level of anatomical knowledge was needed and principles from plain film radiography, where subtle variations in side-to-side size could have many artifactual causes, meant that these subtle changes were cautiously and conservatively interpreted. The normal appearance of the hippocampus is shown in Figure 4.19.

Visual assessment of optimally oriented images enables this feature to be reliably recognized in most cases, and with high sensitivity (162, 175, 188, 193, 202, 204, 205). Volumetry confirms the presence of this atrophy (112, 116, 206–211) and is discussed in more detail below. Cases with predominantly unilateral atrophy and proven HS are shown in Figure 4.20.

The visual assessment appears to be almost as good as volume estimation of hippocampal size in detecting hippocampal atrophy in experienced hands. For some time, many centers relied on quantitative measurement of the hippocampus to assess hippocampal atrophy. This has had the effect of allowing calibration of the sensitivity of visual interpretation and centers such as ours do not use volume measurement for clinical purposes (212–220). Atrophy as a single feature of HS will be found in more than 80–85% of cases using optimized images and visual inspection alone (130, 221, 222).

While the pattern of posterior-to-anterior distribution of the volume loss in HS may be important in some cases, such as postictal psychosis (Fig. 4.21), in general the pattern of HS has not proven to be an important predictor of pathology subtype, clinical outcome or associated aetiology (207, 223, 224).

Loss of Definition of Internal Architecture of the Hippocampus (Internal Structure)

Normal internal morphologic structure of the hippocampus is produced by the alveus, the molecular cell layer of the dentate gyrus, and the pyramidal cell layer of the cornu ammonis, and can be seen on optimized coronal MR images. The hippocampus can be thought of as like a Swiss (jam or jelly) roll (Fig. 4.22), with its neuronal layers rolled up in the medial portion of the temporal lobe. In this analogy the neurons are the jam and the white matter is the sponge cake, as shown in the diagram and histologic section of the normal hippocampal internal structure (Fig. 4.23). These features can be clearly seen both in histologic sections and in optimized MR images (Fig. 4.24; see Figs. 4.17A and

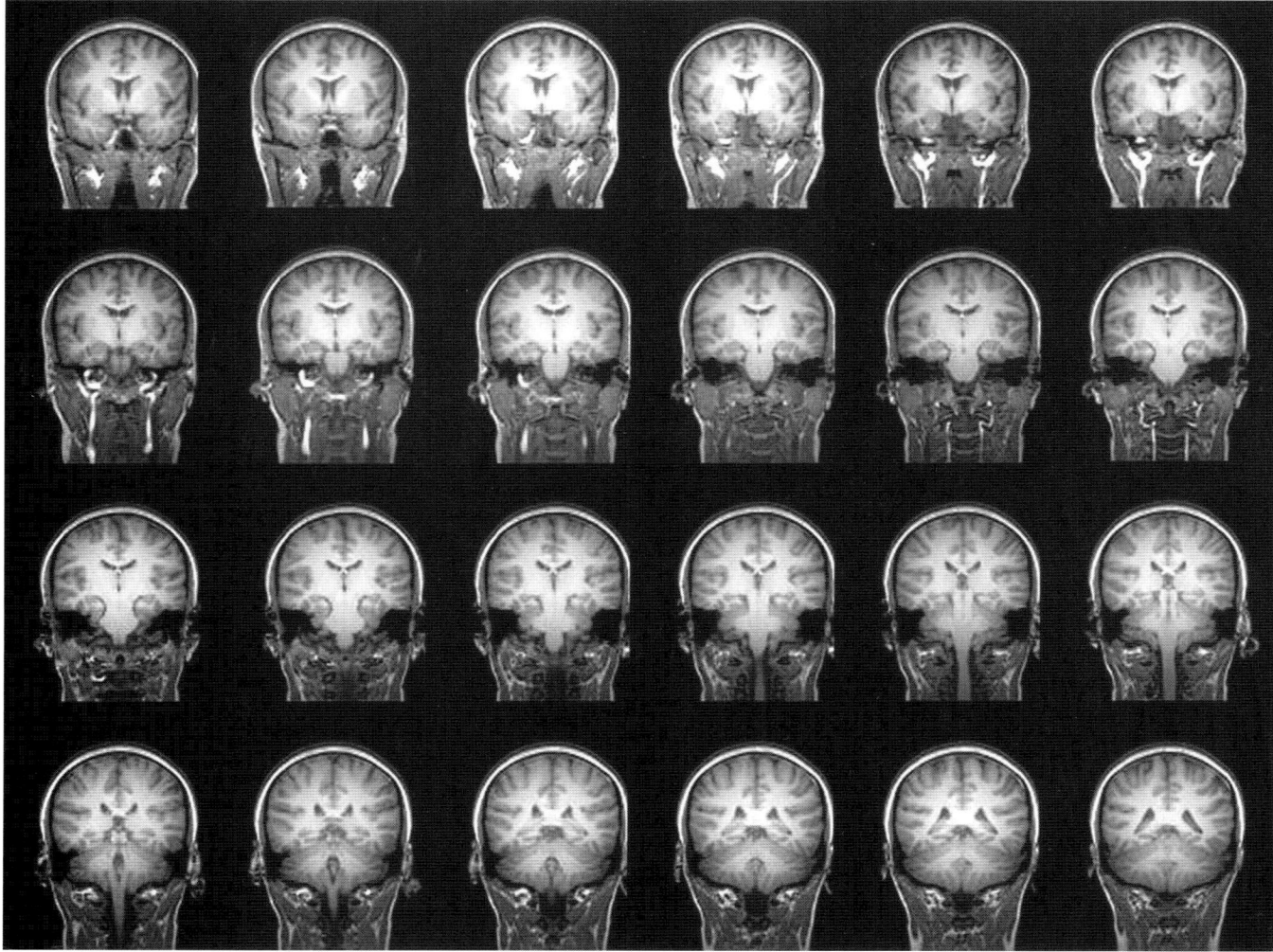

FIG. 4.19. A T1-weighted sequence through the whole length of the hippocampus in a normal subject (3 T, 250 FOV 512 × 256 slice 2 mm no gap FSPGR T_R14 TE2.8 T1500 Flip20°1nex). The expected symmetry of the hippocampus is seen.

Fig. 4.10, where the internal structure can be clearly seen in the contralateral hippocampus).

Special surface coils placed on the temporal lobe can increase signal-to-noise, and spatial resolution, and has been used to show these features (225). By comparing the features seen in histologic sections with these MR images, it is clear that we can see these internal features of the hippocampus in images optimized to demonstrate this (Figs 4.24, 4.25).

In HS, loss of this normal internal structure is a consequence of neuronal cell loss and replacement of normal anatomical layers with gliotic tissue (Fig. 4.26). It is difficult to describe this feature precisely, but once recognized it is important for confidence of diagnosis in cases where other features are only mildly abnormal. Inversion recovery images can be important because these images have good anatomical detail as well as contrast within the normal hippocampus; making it easier to see that it is lost (Fig. 4.27). There appears to be something in the hippocampal neuronal layers that has different T1 contrast from other areas of the cortex. It is our suggestion that this is the major reason that inversion recovery images have been considered helpful by

many clinicians. Along with the loss of this internal architecture may go increased signal in the central part of the hippocampus (see the left hippocampus in Fig. 4.27, on the right of the image).

Sometimes microarchitecture can be mistakenly assumed to be present because of the appearance of the alveus in less heavily contrast-weighted images (typical T1 volume sequences) as compared to the clearly abnormal hippocampus. It is important that one sees the tissue of the CA1 region before confidently saying that the internal architecture is preserved. The classical histologic features of HS are shown in Figure 4.28. This is a case where the atrophy is relatively minimal but signal abnormality and loss of internal structure give a clear diagnosis. In the absence of atrophy, dysplasia should be considered, but in this instance the internal features are those of HS.

In order to visualize the internal structure of the hippocampus (see Fig. 4.26), the requirements are for high spatial resolution, at the same time as good contrast (see Fig. 4.27). By increasing the number of pixels covering the region and dealing with the problem of signal-to-noise by lengthening

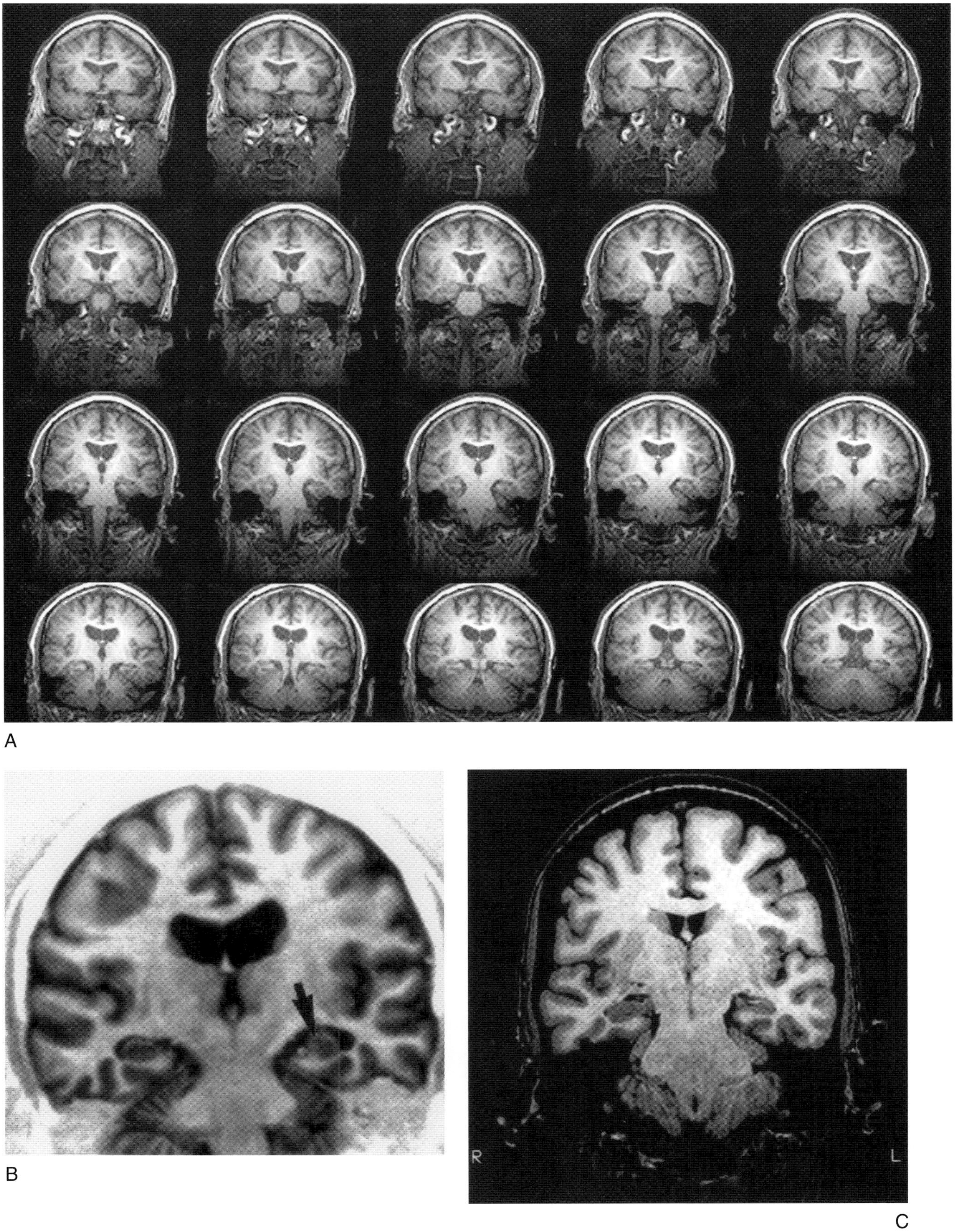

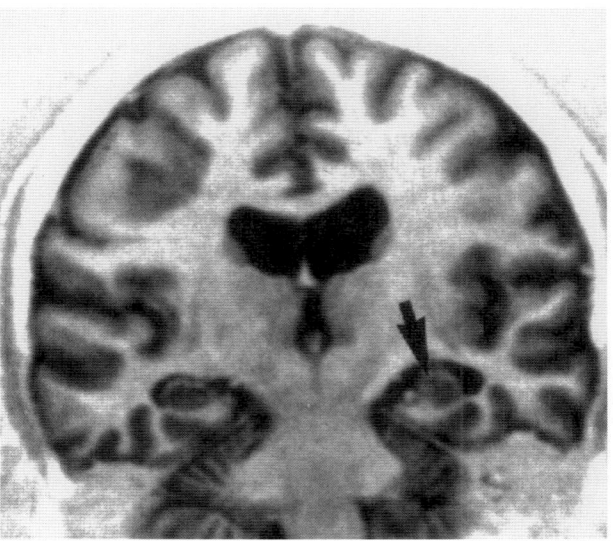

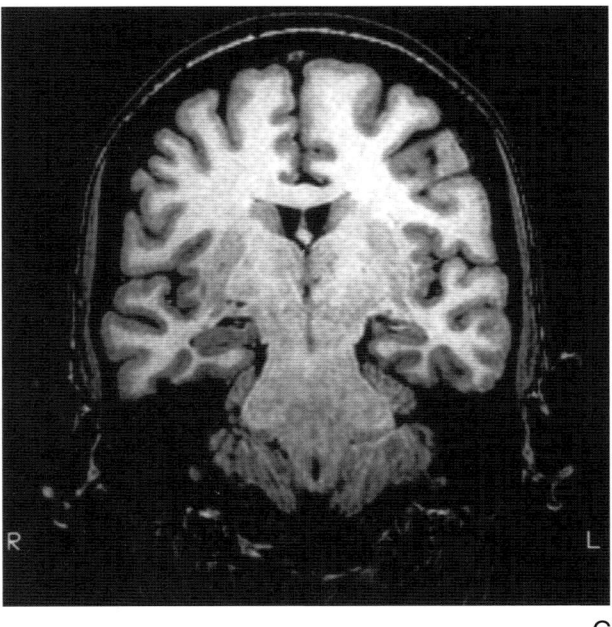

FIG. 4.20. A. T1-weighted sequence of the whole length of the hippocampus, showing left hippocampal sclerosis (right of image). There is also subtle atrophy of the left temporal lobe and widening of the sylvian fissure. This is comparable to the normal anatomy shown in Figure 4.19 with the same imaging parameters. B. Hippocampal sclerosis on the left (arrow). Note the subtle atrophy of the temporal lobe. In this case the sclerotic hippocampus is round in shape. C. Left hippocampal sclerosis with a flattened shape.

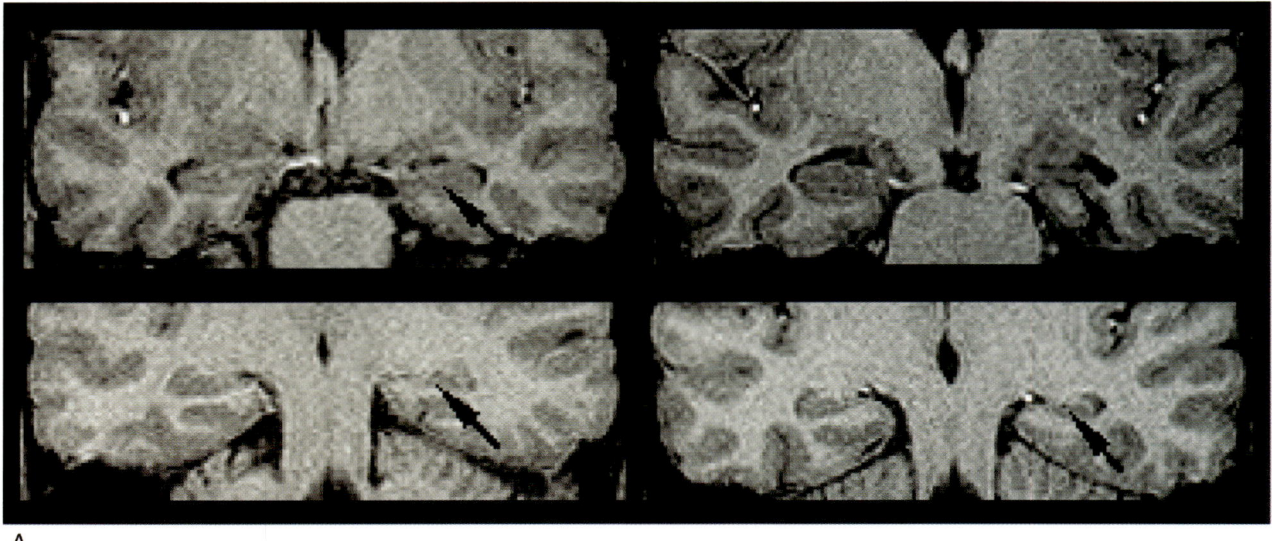

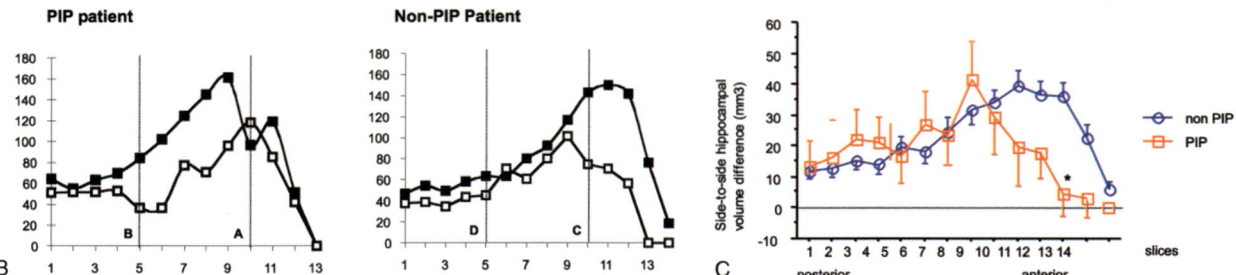

FIG. 4.21. A. Coronal MR slices of a patient with postictal psychosis (PIP; left sides) and a patient without postictal psychosis (right sides). Both patients have left-sided hippocampal sclerosis. The arrows point to the ipsilateral hippocampus. **B.** The graphs demonstrate the posterior-to-anterior distribution of the hippocampal volume of the same two patients. The ipsilateral (open squares) and contralateral side (black squares) are expressed as a function of the slice position. In the posterior hippocampus there is no difference in the degree of the atrophy (slices B and D). In the anterior hippocampus there is a relative hippocampal preservation in the patient with PIP (slice A) but a marked hippocampal atrophy in the patient without PIP (slice C). **C.** The graph shows the anterior-to-posterior distribution of the side-to-side difference in hippocampal volumes in PIP patients (squares) and non-PIP patients (circles). The bars represent SE. Side-to-side difference is calculated by subtracting the ipsilateral from the contralateral side at each slice position. A value of 0 means no difference between the two sides. Positive values indicate a smaller ipsilateral than contralateral volume (higher values reflect more ipsilateral 'volume deficit'). In the tail and body of the hippocampus (slices 1–8) there was no difference between the groups. However, in the anterior part there was less volume deficit in patients with PIP (12th slice; $p = 0.003$, Mann–Whitney U test). (With permission from Briellmann et al. 2000 (460).)

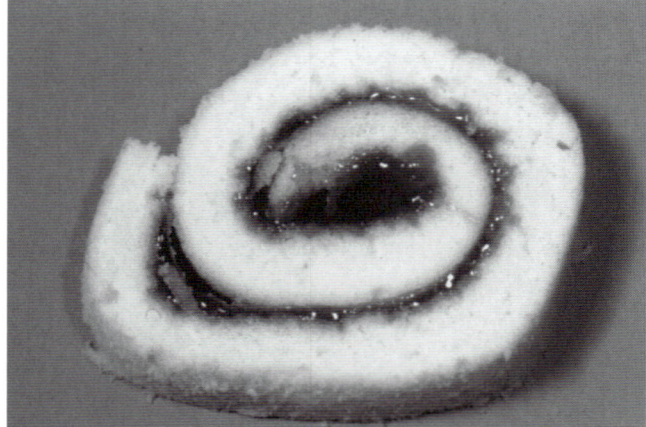

FIG. 4.22. The internal structure of the hippocampus consists of a three-layered cortex. The central layer contains the pyramidal neurons, equivalent to the jam in this 'Swiss' or 'jelly' roll. These layers curve around in the way shown in this analogy.

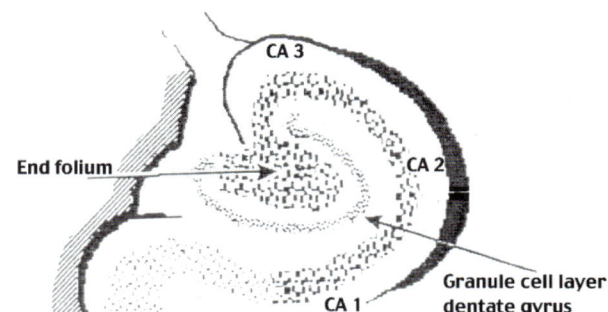

FIG. 4.23. Diagram of the normal hippocampus showing the pyramidal neurons of the various areas. The area labeled the end folium is also known as CA4. CA, cornu ammonis.

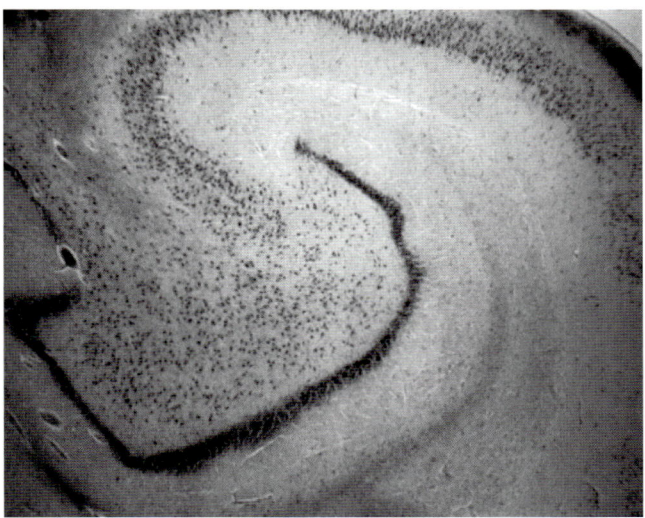

FIG. 4.24. High-powered photomicrograph showing the features shown in Figures 4.22 and 4.23 in a normal hippocampus. Hematoxylin and eosin stain.

the time of image acquisition, one can generate high-resolution images of the hippocampus (see Fig. 4.27). High field (3 T and above) imaging has greatly helped with this. Another alternative that gives higher signal to noise is the use of temporal surface coils.

We have found that recognition of normal internal structure is quite important in some cases where the features, such as T2 signal change and atrophy, are less prominent for visual assessment. Although it is not always possible to detect clearly the internal structure of the hippocampus on standard imaging, it is surprising how often it lends weight to the visual diagnostic confidence of normality of the hippocampus or HS. If doubt exists, reimaging with attention to spatial resolution and contrast can be helpful. As MR techniques and high field strength become more common it is likely that in the future this feature will be one of the most important for the diagnosis of hippocampal pathology. The gain in resolution will bring MR closer to what is seen on pathology.

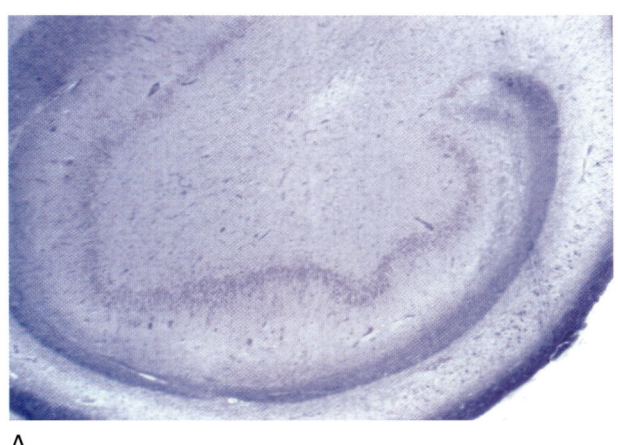

A

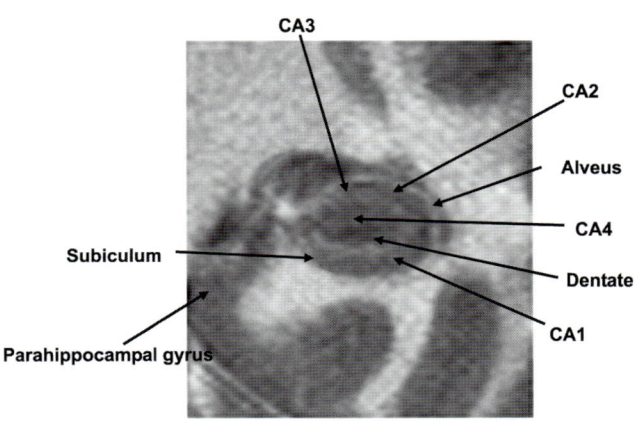

B

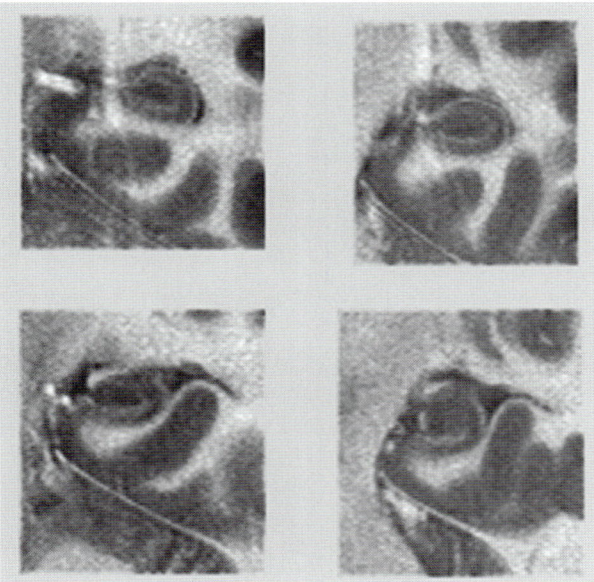

C

FIG. 4.25. A. Photomicrograph showing the classic features of hippocampal sclerosis, with loss of neurons and increased gliosis in the end folium and CA areas, with some sparing of the neurons in CA2. The splaying of the dentate granule cells is also visible when compared to a normal hippocampus (see Fig. 4.24). Hematoxylin and eosin stain. **B.** These histologic features can be seen using MR to show hippocampal internal structure (inversion recovery, 4 mm slice, TI 400, TR 3500). **C.** T1-weighted inversion recovery images showing four examples of normal hippocampi illustrating the hippocampal internal structure using MRI.

Continued

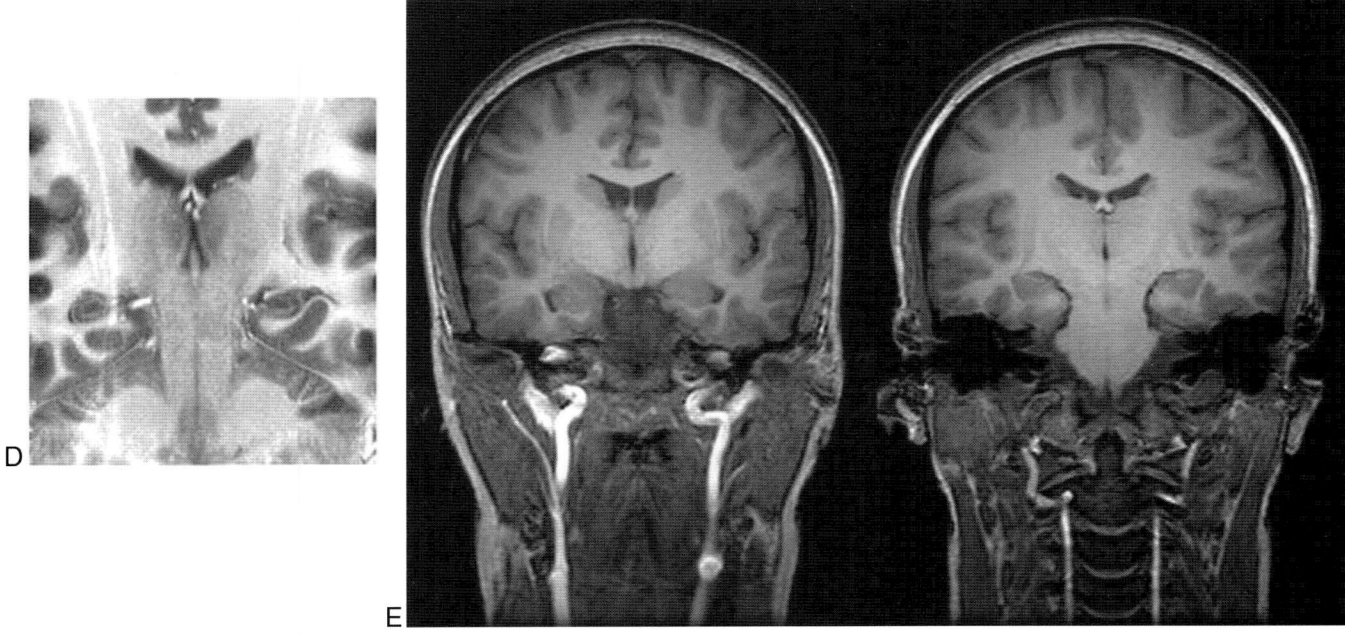

FIG. 4.25. *Cont.* **D, E.** Hippocampal internal structure (**D**) with a high-contrast (inversion recovery sequence) and (**E**) with an FSPGR sequence at high resolution. Note that the internal structure appears bland on these sequences; even though they are high-resolution, they do not have the strong T1 contrast that highlights these internal features. (**B** and **C** with permission from Jackson et al. 1993 (175).)

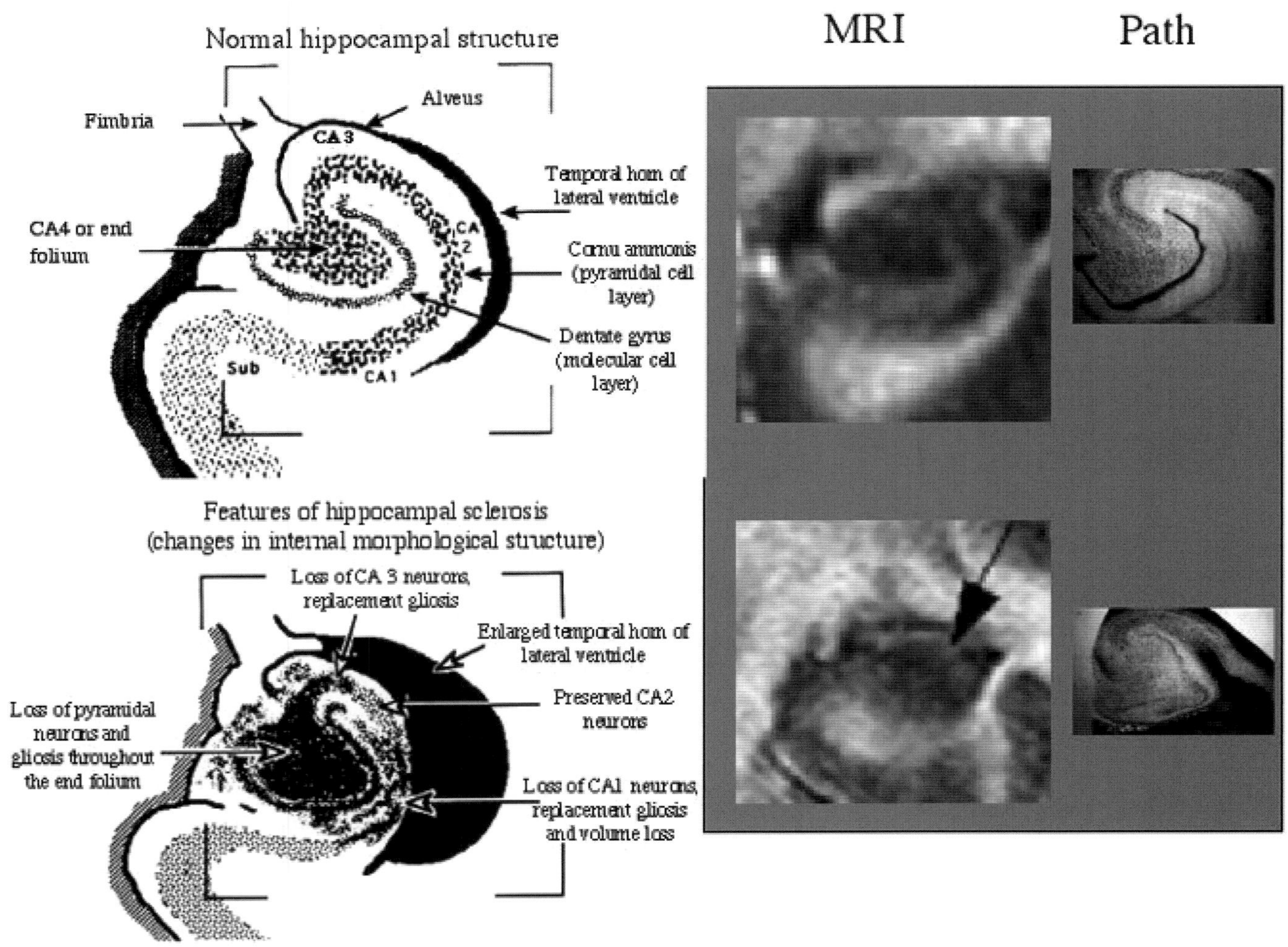

Normal hippocampal structure

MRI   Path

Fimbria

Alveus

CA 3

Temporal horn of
lateral ventricle

CA4 or end
folium

Cornu ammonis
(pyramidal cell
layer)

CA
2

Dentate gyrus
(molecular cell
layer)

Sub   CA1

Features of hippocampal sclerosis
(changes in internal morphological structure)

Loss of CA 3 neurons,
replacement gliosis

Enlarged temporal horn of
lateral ventricle

Loss of pyramidal
neurons and
gliosis throughout
the end folium

Preserved CA2
neurons

Loss of CA1 neurons,
replacement gliosis
and volume loss

FIG. 4.26. The left panels show in diagram form the features of the internal structure of the normal hippocampus (upper) and hippocampal sclerosis (lower panel). Examples of MRI at high resolution illustrating the internal features are shown in the middle panels. Equivalent histologic sections are shown in the right panels.

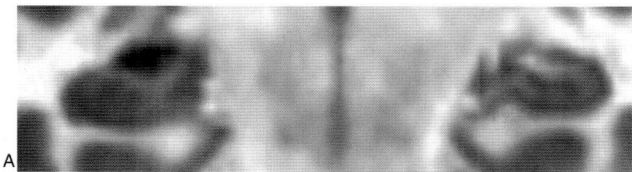

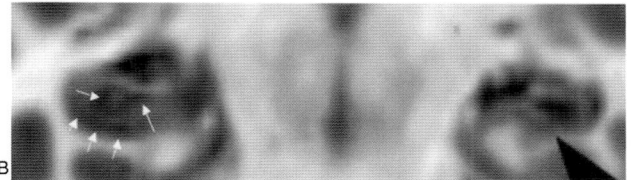

FIG. 4.27. Heavily T1-weighted inversion recovery sequence from a case of identical twins, one of whom had severe febrile convulsions and subsequent TLE, while the other had neither of these events. The affected twin is shown in the lower panel. There is clear atrophy and decreased signal in the left hippocampus(dark arrow), which is typical of hippocampal sclerosis. The contralateral right hippocampus maybe shows some decreased signal in the CA1 and end-folium regions (small light arrows) when compared to the normal twin. Note how similar is the subtle internal structure of this contralateral hippocampus in the two twins. (With permission from Jackson et al. 1998 (346).)

Visual Analysis of Images

Optimized imaging of the hippocampus and temporal lobe structures depends critically on image orientation and image sequences optimized to display the anatomy and signal abnormality of HS and temporal pathology (226). The hippocampus should be imaged in planes parallel and perpendicular to the hippocampus – now known as the hippocampal plane

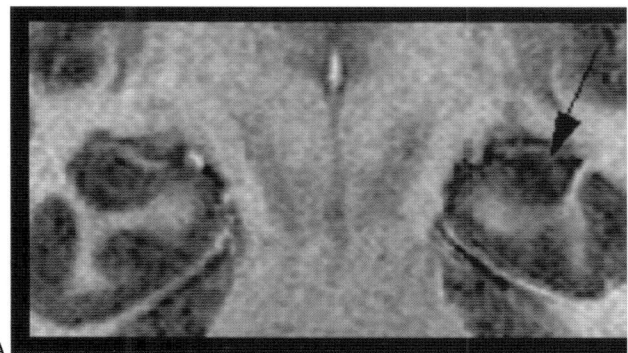

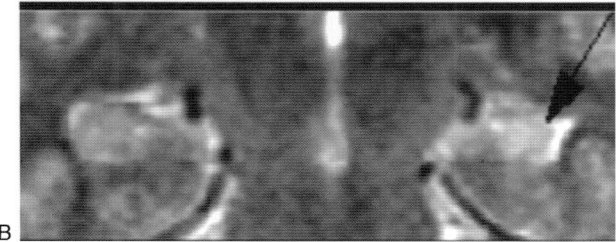

FIG. 4.28. A. Hippocampal sclerosis on the left (arrowed), without obvious atrophy. **B.** T2-weighted image. Note that the internal structure in the contralateral (right) hippocampus is more easily seen on the heavily T1-weighted IR sequence than the T2-weighted images.

(see Fig. 4.10). Assessing the hippocampus in other planes is not adequate (repetition, said above). Diagnosis depends on knowledge of both the normal and pathologic anatomy of the hippocampus (208, 226–229). These features can incorrectly be dismissed as 'normal variation', 'head tilt in the scanner', or 'occult partial volume effects'.

As with any subtle changes in radiology, there is a learning tendency to both 'undercall' this diagnosis and to 'overcall' it. In experienced hands, the visual diagnosis of HS is very reliable, and most centers that have such an experienced person usually rely on visual interpretation of images for clinical decision-making. Quantitative and special techniques remain useful for research and for evaluation of the 'MR-negative' TLE case where additional clues to subtle pathology may be found.

Visual Assessment of Contralateral and Bilateral Abnormality

For confident diagnosis of the degree of contralateral hippocampal abnormality, visual analysis is not so sensitive, and quantitative or advanced analysis methods are indicated. While there may be clues on visual analysis that there is contralateral minor hippocampal atrophy (see, for example, Fig. 4.28) and in some cases this can be suggested on sequences such as FLAIR, this is a very difficult visual diagnosis unless the atrophy is obvious and severe. The significance of minor contralateral abnormality in routine clinical practice is not yet clear in terms of long term seizure outcome or prediction of neurocognitive defects (230–234).

Quantitative Measurements of Hippocampal Sclerosis

As we have noted throughout the previous section, visual analysis is an excellent method of detecting HS if optimized images are acquired and the reporting specialist is expert in the interpretation of these images. There remain issues of what is the optimal method; for example, do we need high-resolution images to examine the hippocampal internal structure? What sequences are necessary, and how much imaging time is required? We have addressed all these issues above. Now we turn to quantitative measures of hippocampal pathology.

For many reasons it is useful to have a quantitative and objective number to describe pathology. A truly objective measurement would take the subjective skill level of the person reporting the pathology out of the list of variables we have to consider. Also, we can determine the degree of abnormality as a continuous variable. This is important for many research studies designed to unravel the neurobiology of many of these conditions, and may help us to understand normal functions.

On the other hand, subtle atrophy as determined by quantitative analysis cannot be simply assumed to have the same meaning as visually assessed atrophy and signal change.

Also, just because a measurement is reported as a number does not necessarily mean that it is a totally objective measurement or that a high degree of subjective skill is not needed for the acquisition of that number. Similarly, once a number is derived, we can become totally oblivious to the assumptions and compromises that went into acquiring that number, and mistakenly confuse it with objective reality. What this means, really, is that if you use numbers to make decisions, you need to know something about how they were acquired, what they mean, and what their limitations are. This is also true of such statistically based methods as voxel-based morphology and relaxometry (discussed below). In the context of temporal lobe epilepsy these numbers (hippocampal volumes and T2 relaxation times) are a means of reaching a diagnosis, and trying to standardize information and objectify the thresholds at which significant abnormality is diagnosed. As in all medical measurements, the clinical context and overall pattern are important.

To summarize, the MR features of HS are atrophy, an increased T2 and a decreased T1 signal, and disruption of the internal structure (175). The atrophy and signal change can be quantified. Quantitative MR protocols, including hippocampal volumetric studies (207, 218, 235–240) and T2 quantification (130, 241–243), are essential in research protocols and for selected clinical cases. These two measurements are complementary and allow a full description of the spectrum of HS (130, 244). Hippocampal atrophy correlates with neuronal cell loss, mainly in the CA1 hippocampal subfield (210, 245–247). The pathologic correlate of hippocampal T2 is gliosis, which most likely correlates with hippocampal T2 (136, 247).

Volumetrics

Since volume measurement of the hippocampus was first described, the technique has been widely used, with many modifications of technique that have become largely center specific. Despite this the principles and use have changed little since these early descriptions. With the advent of statistical approaches to analysis there have been enormous developments in advanced analysis methods of volume data, which are dealt with further in Chapter 8.

Jack et al. (235) first demonstrated in-vivo volume loss in the hippocampus in the context of epilepsy. Volume loss was soon seen as a sensitive and specific indicator of HS in the clinical context of epilepsy (112, 116, 161, 163, 206–211, 245, 248, 249). Hippocampal volume estimates permitted definition of minor volume asymmetries in these patients and also gave confidence to reporting specialists when making visual judgments. The detection of bilateral atrophy remains a problem for studies of this type, which generally compare the two sides. Absolute measures have a large inherent variability due to biological and measurement reasons. The range of normal hippocampal volumes is large, and because of this absolute volumes are not a reliable measure of pathology, particularly of mild degrees of abnormality. Test–retest and interobserver variation in absolute volumes can also be up to 7%. This is only slightly better at high field strengths (250).

Because of the relative anisotropy of the hippocampus, slices 3 mm thick or less are probably necessary for accurate estimation of hippocampal volume (207). Van Paeschen showed that a sampling strategy of one in every three slices is accurate to the degree required for the diagnosis of HS (130, 218, 247, 250–252). Volumetry is a simple, reliable method of detecting hippocampal asymmetries that can be carried out in almost all centers with little or no advanced image processing or technical expertise. In centers with excellent expertise in visual assessment of optimized images acquired for the purpose of assessing the hippocampus, the sensitivity from visual diagnosis is such that volumetric assessment usually adds little. Without this expertise, volumes are a very sensitive means of detecting hippocampal abnormality. There are some pitfalls, however, and we will discuss these now.

Because of the large range of variation in normal hippocampi, both within series and between different groups (often using slightly different techniques), absolute abnormality is difficult to define. The correction of hippocampal volume for total intracranial volume is a useful method of improving the usefulness of volume measurements. Corrections for influence of height, gender, body mass, and age have also been suggested. Females have smaller hippocampi than males and this is largely corrected by correcting for total brain size (253). Hippocampal volumes have also been shown to change with the effects of seizures that affect that temporal lobe (254, 255). Thus volumes may reflect the original pathology as well as the effects of seizures projecting to the temporal lobe. Subtle abnormalities may only reflect seizure effects and should not be used on their own to infer the site of seizure origin.

The basic finding is that the side of hippocampal volume loss as measured by side-to-side asymmetry, in the context of intractable epilepsy, correlates with both the presence of HS as found in the post resection specimen and the side of seizure onset.

An important group of patients is those in whom the findings are more difficult: those with marginal MR abnormalities that approach the limits of normal variation. Spencer and colleagues (211) investigated a population with difficult-to-localize epilepsy (but not difficult MRI findings) and found, even in this group, that volume measurements of the hippocampus were 75% sensitive to and 64% specific for medial temporal seizure onset as recorded with intracranial electrodes. This was the most useful of all noninvasive localizing tests in their patient group.

The ability of a quantitative method to measure the degree of hippocampal asymmetry enables the comparison of the degree of pathology to the degree of memory impairment postoperatively (112, 210, 256) and to outcome following temporal lobe surgery (257).

Hippocampal Boundaries

For the actual technique of hippocampal volume measurement, the estimation of the hippocampal boundaries is an important issue (Fig. 4.29). Jack (258) pointed out that even the difference between including the pixels under the drawn boundary and excluding those pixels under the drawn boundary can make a difference of up to 30% in total hippocampal volume estimation. It is the surface pixels that create the greatest variation, and unfortunately the hippocampus has a large surface-to-volume ratio. Because of this, the exact boundary of the hippocampus can make a large difference in the total estimated volume, and the variation and placement of this region between observers can sometimes be great. Similarly, the test–retest measurement in the same observer can differ considerably until considerable skill is acquired in the use of the technique.

The normal variation of volume measurements of the hippocampus also depends on the subjective drawing of the boundary of the hippocampus in multiple slices. This is a problem for the comparison of hippocampal volumes across centers. Not all centers define the boundaries of the hippocampus in the same way, and this can have a considerable difference in estimating total hippocampal volume. For example, Jack (258) defined the boundaries of the hippocampus in the coronal plane to be the *inplane* boundaries and the *anterior posterior* boundaries. The areas to be included are the CA1–CA4 sectors of the hippocampus, the dentate gyrus, and the subiculum. This includes the pyramidal cell outflow tracts (the alveus) and uses this as a high-contrast boundary of the hippocampus.

In the body and tail regions of the hippocampus, the boundaries of the hippocampus are easily determined, being defined by CSF in the temporal horn, CSF in the carotid fissure, and CSF in the uncal and ambient cisterns. Inferiorly, the gray–white matter junction between the subiculum and white matter of the parahippocampal gyrus is also easy to define. The boundary between the hippocampus and the subiculum where it is continuous with that of the parahippocampal gyrus is a more subjective issue (259–264). Jack's studies used the boundary as the line from the angle formed by the most medial extent of both the subiculum cortex and the parahippocampal cortex (see Chapter 3). It is important to have an understanding of the issues involved in defining the boundaries of the hippocampus (161).

In the head of the hippocampus (pes hippocampi), the distinction of the head of the hippocampus from the overlying amygdala may be more difficult. In some cases it may be easier to make this determination than in others. For example, if the uncal recess of the temporal horn is patent this can provide a superior landmark for the head of the hippocampus. Otherwise the thin line formed by the alveus, which divides the fused hippocampus and amygdala, can also usually be distinguished and used as a boundary. In some cases, however, neither of these landmarks is easily seen, and a straight horizontal line is sometimes drawn between a mid portion of the ambient gyrus medially and the most superior medial portion of the temporal horn laterally.

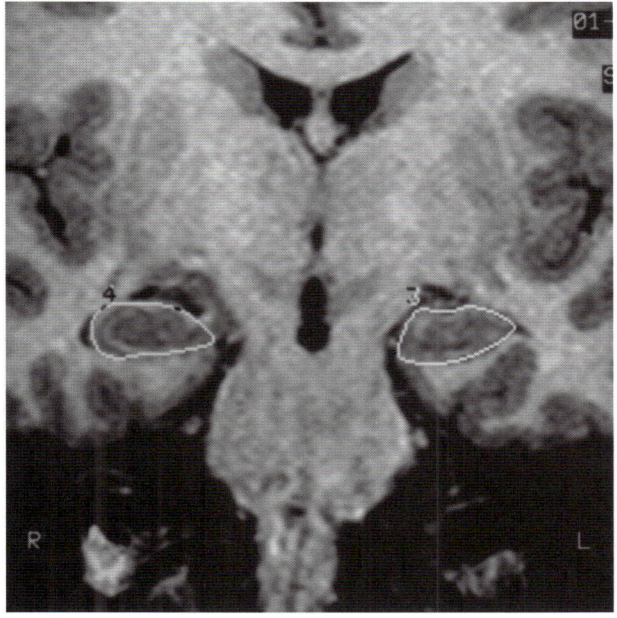

A

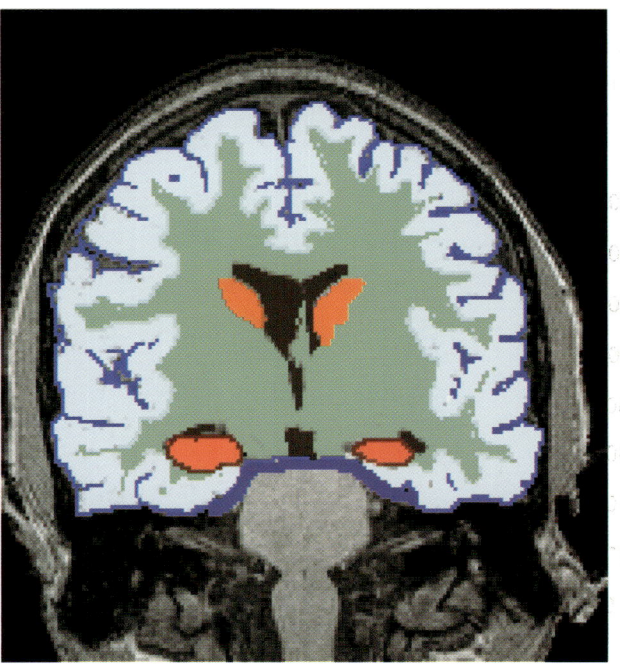

B

FIG. 4.29. Volumetric measurements of the hippocampus. **A.** Manual outlining of the hippocampus, which is usually done in the coronal plane. **B.** Semi-automated segmentation of gray and white matter structures can be achieved with segmentation algorithms, although some manual completion in the mesial temporal regions is usually required. This image shows the results of such segmentation.

In their study, the intralimbic gyrus (the portion of the dentate and Ammon's horn in the posterior uncus) is included in the measurement of hippocampal volume. The choroid plexus is excluded.

The definition of the anterior-posterior borders is also important. In the posterior extent, the coronal section on which the crus of the fornix is seen in full profile can be used to define the posterior boundary of the volume assessment. It is estimated that this includes approximately 90–95% of the total hippocampal volume (161). Other groups have addressed this problem and solved it in different ways. For example, in the studies from Yale (211), only a strictly defined 2.5 cm segment of the hippocampus is included, and the region of the hippocampal head beneath the amygdala is excluded, as is the more posterior hippocampus. This allows a less subjective determination of the anterior and posterior boundaries but suffers from several problems, including the fact that only a portion of the hippocampus is assessed.

The majority of studies have used coronal images for drawing the hippocampal boundaries because of the clear definition of the hippocampal boundaries in this orientation. It is, of course, possible to use any imaging plane. The sagittal plane has been used (see Fig. 4.10), and it has been argued that it is easier to distinguish the amygdala from the hippocampus in this plane. The data can be represented by the cross-sectional area of the hippocampus in each slice (Fig. 4.30). This gives an almost axial view of the length of the hippocampus (compare with Fig. 4.10).

Accuracy and Reproducibility of Volumetric Studies

Given the adoption of any specific technique, the accuracy and reproducibility of the test must be estimated. This will depend on machine factors, as well as on subjective factors of placement of the hippocampal boundaries. In the early studies, Jack (235, 265) reported the limit on accuracy to be within 0.1 cm³, while Cook et al. (207, 266) showed an accuracy of more than 98% for volume measurements of phantom objects. This most probably reflects the inherent issues of accuracy of the MR technology.

Much more important, however, is the intraobserver variability. Jack initially reported that the variation of hippocampal volume and measurement for experienced individuals varied from 1.9% to 4% (208). In Jack's study the interobserver variation was 14%. Using three-dimensional volumetric images, a 1.2% intraobserver variability and a 3.4% interobserver variability has been cited (163). Cook (207) estimated that a minimum of 10–12 coronal slices (this corresponds to a slice thickness of 3 mm) is necessary in order to reduce the error of hippocampal volume measurements to below 5%. Later studies have been consistent with this.

These data demonstrate that hippocampal volume estimates can be made with a high degree of reproducibility within experienced centers. Sadly, the greatest potential benefit of a quantitative technique – collection of large numbers of patients across many centers to assess major issues about pathogenesis and secondary damage – has never materialized because of issues of standardization. This is largely because the measurements of hippocampal volume, as implemented, have been very site- and user-specific.

The actual numeric produced by volume measurements is dependent on:

- imaging slice thickness
- selection of anterior and posterior anatomic boundaries
- orientation of the plane of acquisition
- whether or not the imaging data have been interpolated in-plane prior to tracing
- the method implored for counting the boundary pixels under the trace
- the subjective inplane boundary tracing
- the error of the measurement
- the population studied.

Sensitivity and Specificity of Hippocampal Volumetrics

Hippocampal volume changes have been found in a number of other disorders, including dementia (267–269), schizophrenia (270–276), amnesias (277, 278), and even rarely in normal individuals (142, 279).

T2 Relaxometry

The classical MR features of HS include reduced hippocampal volume, increased signal intensity on T2-weighted imaging, and disturbed internal architecture (188, 280). Methods to quantify volume changes on MR images were quickly introduced and widely used (257, 281, 282)

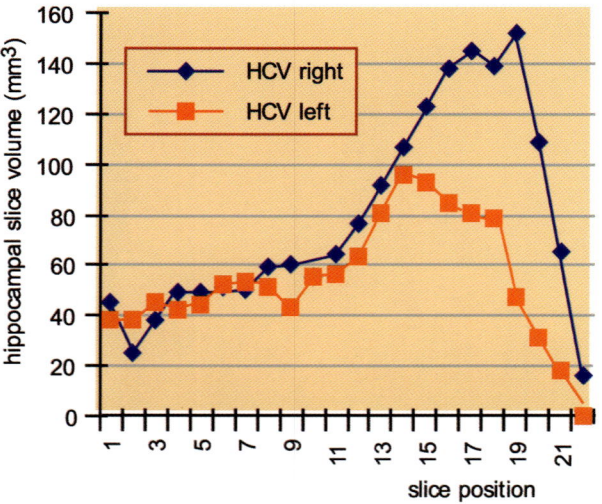

FIG. 4.30. If the cross-sectional area of the hippocampus is plotted as a function of slice position, the volume distribution of the hippocampus can be plotted. In this example there is clear atrophy of the anterior hippocampus on the left.

and are discussed above. The development of T2 relaxometry for the MR assessment of epilepsy was fostered by the observation of increased signal on T2-weighted images in the hippocampus of patients with HS and the desire to have a quantitative and rapid measure of hippocampal abnormality that was objective and standardizable across centers. T2 relaxometry was introduced in 1993 as a quantitative measurement tool of tissue pathology in the hippocampal gray matter (177). This quantitative measurement is an objective means of determining the frequency and severity of T2 abnormality and enables the detection of bilateral pathology. Since its introduction, the technique of T2 relaxometry has been used by many centers. Other indications than HS have been added and technical improvements have been made.

In our experience, the measurement of T2 values within the hippocampus is a robust and reliable objective measurement of hippocampal pathology, providing a means of assessing the hippocampus that is as good as the most skilled visual interpretation of hippocampal abnormality in optimized scans (162, 188, 241). Hippocampal T2 quantification has the ability to detect very mild, bilateral, and progressive hippocampal abnormalities. Moreover, hippocampal T2 values can be interpreted in terms of hippocampal pathology even when the other hippocampus is incomplete or distorted, such as when a lesion is present or following temporal lobe surgery.

Technical Considerations in Acquiring T2 Relaxation Times

Method of Acquiring T2 Relaxation Time Measurement

The acquisition that enables the measurement of T2-relaxometry time is a multiple spin-echo sequence (Fig. 4.31). Several T2-weighted images are acquired at different echo times and in each voxel the resultant values are fitted with an exponential decay curve to estimate the T2 decay rate of the imaged tissue. For a 16-echo CPMG sequence, as initially suggested (241), 16 separate spin-echo images are taken for each slice at echo times (T_E) ranging from 22 ms to 256 ms. This range was chosen somewhat empirically as it proved to give precise values in normal subjects. The intensity of the image decreases for all structures as the T_E becomes longer. If the intensity of signal is plotted as a function of time, then the time constant of this decay is proportional to the T2 relaxation time. This decay can be assessed for every pixel in the image.

In a T2 map the gray scale of each pixel equals the T2 relaxation time or T2 value of this pixel. On the T2 map, the T2 value of an anatomical structure can be measured by placing a region of interest over this region and measuring the mean T2 relaxation time within this region of interest (Fig. 4.31A, lower right panel). It is of importance that this region is placed fully within the anatomical structure to

avoid partial volume effects. The acquisition plane may further help to avoid partial volume effects. Best results are obtained with T2 maps and structural imaging acquired in a plane orthogonal to the long axis of the hippocampus.

T2 relaxation times are easy to acquire and postacquisition processing to calculate T2 maps from the data takes only a few minutes (Fig. 4.31B). The necessary acquisition and processing software is available on most commercial imaging systems. However, an accurate knowledge of the normal and pathologic anatomy is required for placement of the region of interest.

Developments in T2-relaxometry Methods

The initial description of a technique to measure T2 values in patients with HS was based on a multi-echo sequence with 16 echoes with a T_E between 22 and 262 ms (177). The sequence had an acquisition time of approximately 10 min. Measurements of the hippocampal T2 relaxation times in normal subjects were precise (99–106 ms) and showed minimal interobserver variation (241). It was highlighted at that time that the technique, although precise and allowing the objective diagnosis of hippocampal pathology without the need for comparison with the contralateral hippocampus, did not necessarily measure accurately the actual physical quantity of T2 relaxation time. The technique was precise and reproducible, which are the most important qualities for such a diagnostic test. Instrumental variation may mean that the actual normal control range could vary between centers and techniques. The use of percentage change compared to normal values allows cross-institutional comparisons despite different absolute values.

Subsequent methodologic work focused on the ideal number of echoes, shorter acquisition times, and improved accuracy of the measurement. Stimulated echoes are unwanted contributions to the signal in multiple echo sequences (90°–180°–180°– …) and arise from coherence pathways that arise from the conjunction of multiple refocusing pulse trains (with more than two pulses). Modification of the pulse sequence using optimized refocusing pulses or phase cycling techniques can reduce the effects of these unwanted signal pathways.

Several alternatives have been explored in relation to the number of echoes used to obtain the decay curve. Some groups have suggested the implementation of a dual-echo acquisition (199, 243, 283). The two T_E used are usually around 30–40 ms and 100–120 ms. However, the disadvantage of using just two echoes is that the two data points only allow a linear fit and thus may deliver less precise measurements. In one study, using echo times of 80 ms and the mean hippocampal T2 values demonstrate a small range of variation in the 20 controls studied and clearly abnormal values in patients with HS (244). This suggests that the technique is robust enough to detect hippocampal abnormalities even with a simplified acquisition method.

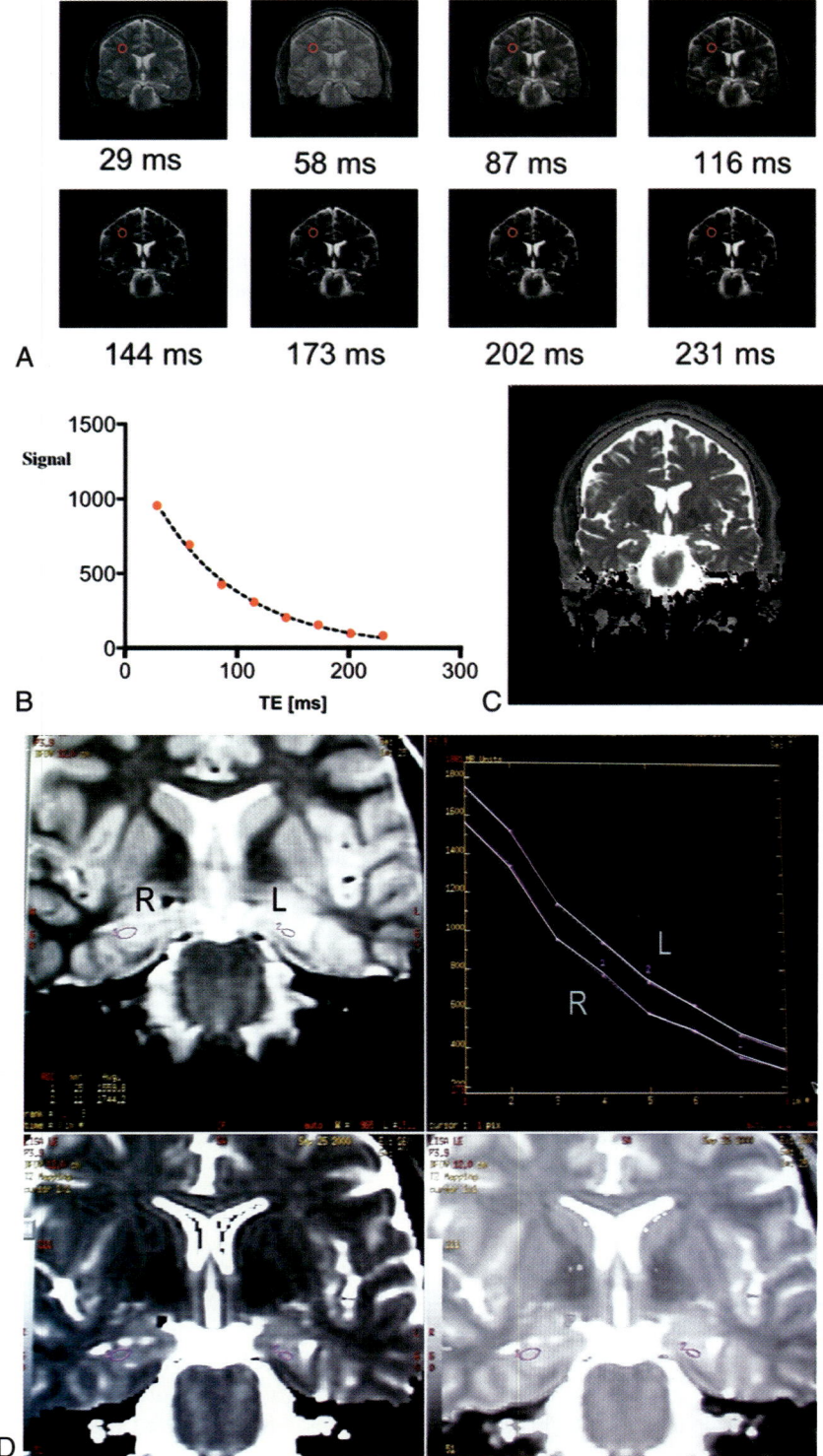

FIG. 4.31. Measurement of T2-relaxometry times T2 relaxometry was acquired with a CPMG sequence with eight images per location (T_E 29–231 ms, T_R 5000 ms) on a 3 T GE LX Horizon scanner (Milwaukee, USA). **A.** All eight acquired images are shown, with echo times between 29 and 231 ms, on one slice at the level of the hippocampus. Note the changing brightness of the images, reflecting the T2 decay. In the region within the red circle, the signal was measured on each image. This decay is shown graphically in **B.** The signal intensity is highest for the images with the lowest T_E. **C.** The T2 map, where the gray scale of each pixel equals the T2 relaxation time. The measurement of the T2-relaxation time can be performed on these calculated T2 maps, using software such as the proprietary GE software package (Functool®). A T2-weighted coronal slice through the hippocampus can be used to identify the region of interest (ROI), corresponding to the second image acquired with a T_E of 58 ms. **D.** An example with left hippocampal sclerosis. Top left: the T2-weighted image; top right: the measured T2 decay curves; bottom: the calculated T2 map.

Methodologic studies, however, suggest that a multi-echo sequence has advantages (284). This is especially important with the consideration of the non-monoexponential characteristics of signal decay in tissue. The different contributions of signal decay in a voxel include different degrees of myelination of white matter and also gray matter and CSF. Use of a simple monoexponential fit in these cases is, therefore, an unrealistic model for such data. However, unless echo trains with large numbers of echoes (≥16) are used (284), a fit to a single exponential is more robust and is, therefore, the most common analysis procedure.

Over the past few years, many centers have been using scanners with increased magnetic field strengths of 3 T and above. The increased signal-to-noise ratio at the higher field strength can be used to significant advantage in improving the time efficiency and image quality of imaging protocols. As a consequence, quantification of brain volumes or of structures within the brain should become more accurate at higher field strength, thus reducing the standard deviation in the measurement results (250, 285). The parameter that is quantified by the T2 relaxometry technique is largely independent of magnetic field strength. The measured T2 relaxation times of known tissues types depend somewhat on the sequence used and, therefore, optimization of the acquisition has a greater influence than the field strength on the final images (286).

We suggest that at least an eight-echo T2-relaxometry sequence is optimal (287). In addition, advances have been made in the fitting procedure for T2 quantification and for the statistical analysis of deviations of the resulting T2 maps from control distributions (287). The power of the T2-relaxometry method has been suitably enhanced, thereby improving the chances of detecting more subtle effects. Furthermore, the combination of modified fitting and statistical analysis procedures used in this study will remove the component of the subjectivity of relaxometry data analysis.

Concordance: Do More Investigations Help?

In the past, concordance was sensibly used to solve what can be considered to be a signal-to-noise problem. This means that when no piece of data is definitive in telling, for example, which temporal lobe is abnormal, then several pieces of suggestive evidence all pointing in the same direction can be used to improve the certainty that one of other temporal lobe is primarily involved in seizure genesis. Conversely when one piece of information is definitive, for example when HS is clearly present on one side, then multiple tests for laterality add no information unless they suggest that the seizures are not originating from that hippocampus, or that there are multiple foci of epileptogenesis (288).

Discordance now primarily serves as a warning that the problem of understanding the pathogenesis of seizures in an individual patient has not been solved by our major information (e.g. finding HS). Studies need to determine what is necessary and sufficient information prior to offering surgical removal of an abnormal area of the brain as a treatment for epilepsy. It is our guess that no formula will work in all cases and the answer will be to understand the mechanism of seizure generation in each patient. More studies will be required in some cases than in others.

PATHOPHYSIOLOGY OF HIPPOCAMPAL SCLEROSIS AND ASSOCIATED TEMPORAL LOBE EPILEPSY

Observing Hippocampal Sclerosis Development

Acute Changes in Patients with Epilepsy Progressing to Hippocampal Sclerosis

The presence of short-term, seizure-associated changes is an important issue. There is debate about whether seizures cause damage to the brain or whether all or a portion of the abnormalities seen in the brains of patients with epilepsy are due to pre-existing factors. A change in T2 relaxometry after a seizure would favor the idea that seizure-associated damage can occur. An early study suggested that recent seizures do not influence T2 values (289). In this study of 63 patients with chronic epilepsy, four patients were scanned a second time after a recent complex partial or secondary generalized seizure. There was no change of the T2 values after the seizure.

However, several other reports have shown an acute increase in T2-signal after a brain injury such as status epilepticus, together with an increase in hippocampal volume (Fig. 4.32) (290–293). Experimental models provide evidence that T2-time acutely increases after kainate injection, reflecting cytotoxic edema (294). A gradual resolution of the high T2 signal may occur, reflecting resolution of the edema. If there is no evolution into HS, and acute electroencephalographic abnormalities resolve, T2-signal may normalize, as has been shown in some case reports (295, 296). However, several other cases have demonstrated the evolution into HS, with the typical MR features of hippocampal volume loss and T2 signal increase visible weeks to months after the acute insult (291, 297). Some examples of progression of the hippocampal changes are shown in Figures 4.33–4.35.

Information on pathologic changes is not always available and is therefore very important if given. Two reports show histopathologic results on patients who had acute T2-relaxometry changes within the region that was later microscopically assessed. One report describes a child who died 44 days after a refractory status epilepticus. Histopathology showed neuronal necrosis and gliosis in CA1, CA3, and dentate gyrus. Another child underwent a temporal lobectomy for seizure control 38 months after a prolonged febrile convulsion. Histopathology again showed the typical HS features of focal neuron loss and gliosis.

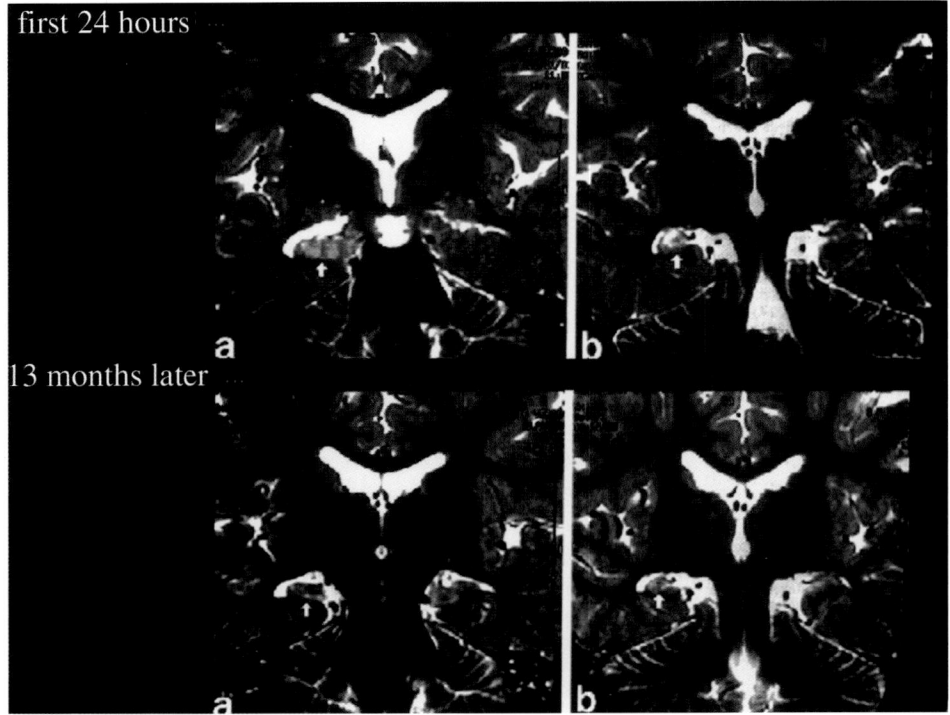

FIG. 4.32. Progression of hippocampal sclerosis after a prolonged seizure. (With permission from Nohria et al. 1994 (358).)

Whereas the studies reported above consist of case reports or small series, one recent report assessed a series of 35 children (298). All had MR investigations within 5 days of a generalized status epilepticus. Quantitative assessments included T2 relaxometry and hippocampal volumetry. T2 relaxation time was elevated in patients with prolonged febrile convulsions compared with control subjects when they were scanned within 2 days of the acute event, whereas no difference in the T2-values were found in patients examined 3–5 days after the event. These findings are consistent with another series in children, scanned within 14 days of the event (299). In this series, T2 relaxometry findings showed no abnormalities.

The development of HS, although most frequently observed in young children, has also been described in adults. It has been observed after severe seizures in adulthood (297), after a series of brief seizures (see Fig. 4.33) (300), in the context of other focal pathology such as cavernous angioma and neurocysticercosis (301), and also after domoic acid intoxication (302). The last report suggests that the human hippocampus is vulnerable to kainate receptor excitotoxicity and provides strong evidence for a supporting role of excitotoxic injury in epileptogenesis. These observations suggest that T2-signal increase occurring shortly after a seizure, associated with increased volume, reflects cell edema. This abnormality can evolve into HS, in which T2-signal increase is again increased but now associated with reduced volumes. This chronic change in T2-value increase may reflect gliosis, as outlined below.

Retrospective quantitative MRI studies have addressed the issue of progression of HS due to seizures, and suggested that seizure activity may (303, 304) or may not (305, 306) be associated with progressive hippocampal volume loss. Wieshmann et al. (291) and O'Brien et al. (307) described two patients with HS and progressive hippocampal volume loss on repeat MR imaging associated with frequent secondary generalized seizures. In a prospective study of patients with newly diagnosed partial epilepsy and a repeat MRI scan 1 year after the first MRI, one patient was observed with bilateral hippocampal atrophy and normal hippocampal T2s, who had significantly increased hippocampal T2s with no measurable further hippocampal volume loss on follow-up 7 months later. These hippocampal changes were associated with daily seizures and frequent secondary generalization (308).

Chronic Changes in the Hippocampus in Patients with Epilepsy

The original observation of increased hippocampal T2 relaxometry was made in patients with refractory temporal lobe epilepsy (241). This report recorded that the side of the seizure origin was ipsilateral to the hippocampal T2 abnormality when the abnormality was unilateral. When there were bilateral abnormalities with one side more abnormal than the other, the side of seizure origin also always correlated with the more abnormal hippocampal T2 signal.

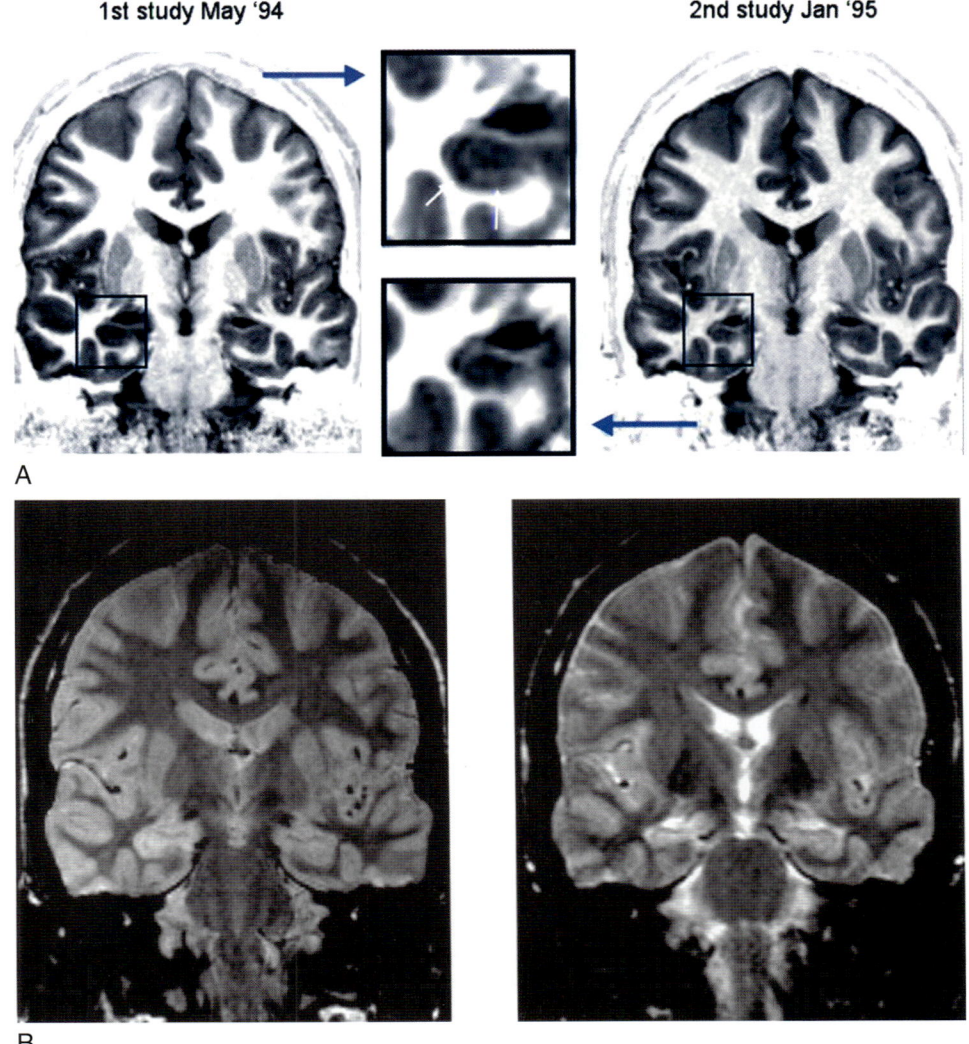

1st study May '94

2nd study Jan '95

A

B

FIG. 4.33. A. Progression of hippocampal sclerosis: IR study. The patient was a 25-year-old man who presented with 3 × tonic–clonic seizures. Note the internal architecture of the hippocampus (arrows), clearly seen in the first study but absent in the second, and atrophy of the hippocampus in the second, present in the first study. **B.** This adult with recent-onset TLE had imaging that was considered normal (left panel); 18 months later, after three tonic–clonic seizures there is clear hippocampal sclerosis in the right hippocampus. Increased signal was present in the first study. (**A.** With permission from Jackson et al. 1999 (297).)

T2 relaxometry abnormalities correctly lateralized 70% of all patients with intractable partial epilepsy, regardless of the localization of seizure onset. Some 30% were not confidently lateralized but no case was lateralized incorrectly. The patients with abnormal contralateral hippocampal T2 values in addition to the ipsilateral marked abnormality may represent the bilateral hippocampal abnormalities described in pathology studies of HS (126, 127, 309) and in volumetric studies of hippocampal volumes (207, 258, 310, 311).

Several studies later confirmed the initial description of hippocampal signal increase patients, quantified by T2 relaxometry, in the ipsilateral hippocampus of patients with refractory TLE (130, 199, 231, 232, 283, 312–315). Based on our experience, the signal increase in the ipsilateral hippocampus in a patient with HS can be expected to be about 15–20%. For identification of severely sclerotic hippocampi,

detection of signal increase is as sensitive by visual assessment on the T2-weighted images (316). However, T2 relaxometry allows quantification of subtle abnormalities, for example in the contralateral hippocampus or in other brain structures. Furthermore, T2 relaxometry may be used to classify the severity of HS and thus allows assessment of whether different subtypes of HS exist and are correlated with different clinical manifestations.

Grading of HS Severity

Since the introduction of MR into the investigation of epilepsy patients, there have been attempts to classify the degree of hippocampal abnormalities on the basis of the change in the T2 signal (317). Based on our experience,

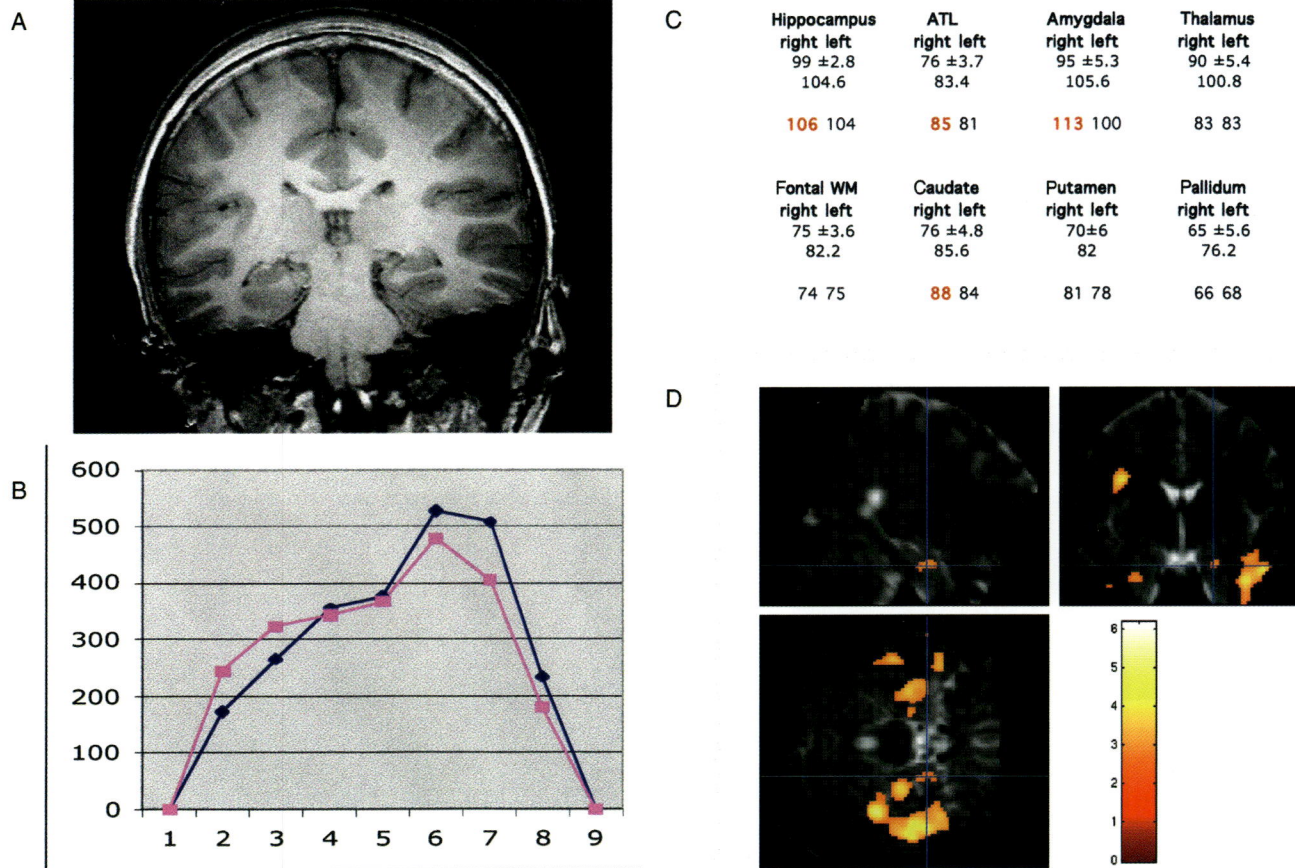

A

B

C

Hippocampus right left	ATL right left	Amygdala right left	Thalamus right left
99 ±2.8	76 ±3.7	95 ±5.3	90 ±5.4
104.6	83.4	105.6	100.8
106 104	**85** 81	**113** 100	83 83

Fontal WM right left	Caudate right left	Putamen right left	Pallidum right left
75 ±3.6	76 ±4.8	70±6	65 ±5.6
82.2	85.6	82	76.2
74 75	**88** 84	81 78	66 68

D

FIG. 4.34. High-field investigations in a 9-year-old boy with MR-negative epilepsy. The EEG suggests a right temporal lobe seizure focus, the clinical symptomatology suggests involvement of the amygdala. **A.** Coronal T21-weighted image at the level of the hippocampi (left side). There is no side-to-side asymmetry or signal change of this structure. This is confirmed by hippocampal volumetry. **B.** Posterior-to-anterior distribution of the hippocampal volume (right side blue, left side purple). The volumes of the right (2143 mm³) and left hippocampus (2060 mm³) were not different from each other or from controls. C. T2 relaxation time measurements in the same case. There was a subtle increase in the signal in the right hippocampus, amygdala, anterior temporal lobe white matter, and caudate, consistent with a seizure focus in the right hemisphere. **D.** Voxel-based analysis of the same patient, compared to a series of 25 control subjects. Areas with significant signal increase as compared to the control group are highlighted. They include both temporal lobes, predominantly on the right, affecting the anterior temporal lobe white matter and the mesial temporal structures. (Courtesy of Dr Gaby Pell, Brain Research Institute, Melbourne, Australia.)

slightly increased hippocampal T2-values may indicate that the seizure focus is not within this hippocampus but may be extrahippocampal in the ipsilateral temporal lobe, extratemporal, or in the contralateral hippocampus. Alternatively, hippocampal T2-signal increase not quite reaching the degree expected for classical HS may reflect mild HS with only relatively mild histopathologic cell abnormalities. It is unlikely that the hippocampus is damaged in such a way that either 50% of neurons are lost (a common definition of HS) (182) or no damage has occurred; hippocampal damage is more likely to be a continuum, with definite HS being that level of damage which can unequivocally be detected visually by neuropathologists. Figure 4.34 shows the MR investigation of a child with the clinical features of mesial temporal lobe epilepsy, following a past history of a prolonged febrile convulsion. Whereas his conventional MR investigation was not conclusive, measurement of volumes,

T2-signal change, and MRS metabolites strongly suggest presence of a left mesial temporal abnormality.

The presence of HS can be suggested if hippocampal T2 values are higher than 2 SD above the mean value in controls. In our populations, an abnormal increase of T2-relaxometry value was diagnosed if the measured value was increased for more than 9%. The values of the ipsilateral hippocampal T2 relaxometry can be used to classify the severity of HS into mild HS (T2 values between 9% and 15% above normal), moderate, classical HS (T2 values between 16% and 25% above normal) and severe, classical HS (T2 >25% above normal). In a series of 37 patients, 8 patients would have been classified as mild, 14 as moderate, and 15 as severe using this classification scheme (318).

Based on the T2-relaxometry values it is not possible to distinguish whether a mild increase in hippocampal T2 values reflects mild HS or mild seizure-associated damage.

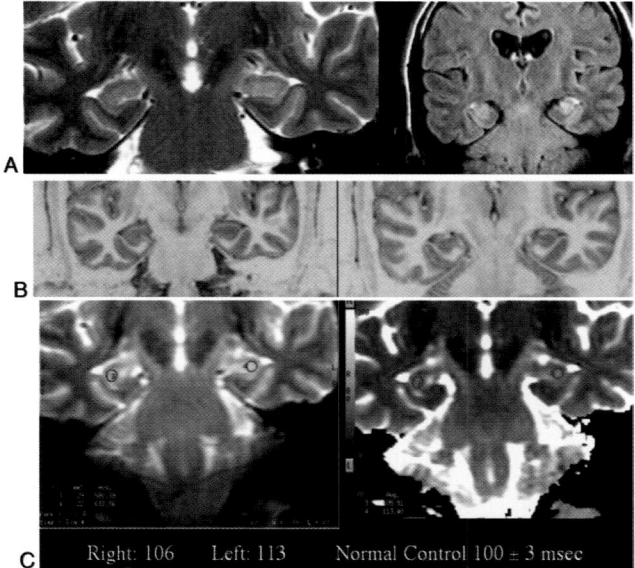

FIG. 4.35. Hippocampal signal increase without hippocampal atrophy. This young man had refractory temporal lobe epilepsy. Electroclinical features suggested mesial temporal left seizure onset. MR imaging was performed on a 3 T GE LX Horizon scanner (Milwaukee, USA). MR investigation showed increased signal in the left hippocampus, visible on T2-weighted and FLAIR images (**A**). However, the internal structure of the hippocampus is intact, visible on the IR images (**B**), and the hippocampal volume is not reduced (visible on all imaging modalities). Volumetric measurements of the hippocampus confirmed values within the range of healthy controls, without significant asymmetry between the two sides. T2 relaxometry confirmed increased T2 signal in the left hippocampus (**C**). T2-relaxometry acquisition and analysis was performed as described in Figure 4.1. A standard left temporal lobectomy was performed. Histology showed minimal neuronal cell loss but extensive gliosis; no diagnosis of hippocampal sclerosis was made. The patient had a postoperative reduction in seizure frequency but did not become seizure-free.

The hippocampus and the other mesial temporal structures are connected to many other brain areas and it is possible that the hippocampus is involved in seizure spread, arising from seizures originating in other brain regions.

Correlation of Hippocampal T2-signal Increase with Hippocampal Volume Deficit

In contrast to elaborate volumetric assessment, the measurement of T2 relaxometry is a quick technique and can be implemented in large studies and measured routinely by the radiographer or reporting radiologist (319). The measured value of both hippocampal volume and the T2 time are inversely correlated with each other (218, 247, 318, 320). The inverse correlation between T2 signal and hippocampal volumes is present in the ipsilateral hippocampus but not in the contralateral hippocampus (318). This indicates that a marked volume loss is associated with a significant increase in T2 relaxation time, or in other words that an atrophic

hippocampus corresponds to a brighter signal in an individual T2-weighted image.

Whereas it is true in general that volume loss mirrors signal increase, there are exceptions to this rule. Some refractory TLE patients have only minimal volume loss but T2 signal increase (see, for example Fig. 4.28) (232, 321), whereas others have normal T2-relaxometry values but hippocampal volume loss (130). Histopathologic examination showed marked gliosis but no neuron cell loss. In unselected patients with refractory TLE, up to 15% do not have detectable hippocampal atrophy on MRI. A recent study evaluated whether T2 relaxometry could identify hippocampal pathology in patients with normal hippocampal volumes on volumetry. It compared 11 TLE patients without atrophy with 14 TLE patients with unilateral atrophy (232). All TLE patients with hippocampal atrophy and 9/11 (82%) patients with normal MRI had abnormally high hippocampal T2 values ipsilateral to the epileptic focus, which was defined based on history, video-EEG, and surgical response. It was concluded that hippocampal T2 mapping provided evidence of hippocampal damage in the majority of patients with intractable TLE without hippocampal volume loss on MRI (232).

Pathologic Correlates of Increased Hippocampal T2 Signal

Hippocampal sclerosis, as defined by Margerison and Corsellis, consists of atrophy of the hippocampal formation associated with neuron cell loss and gliosis in CA1, CA3, and the granule cell layer of the dentate gyrus (CA4), with relative sparing of the CA2 region (126). Quantification of neuronal density in the different hippocampal subfields has been consistently reported (92, 322, 323), and the reduction of neuron cell counts in HS patients is well recognized.

The MR features of HS are well described and include volume decrease and T2-weighted signal increase for MRI. It is established that hippocampal volumes reflect neuron cell counts (206, 210, 245, 324). In contrast, the pathologic–anatomic correlate of increased signal on T2-weighted images is still controversial. It has been suggested that signal change reflects unspecific increased concentration and mobility of water (294). This can be found in edema (286), demyelination (325), or gliosis (326). In patients with refractory TLE, T2 signal increase in the temporal white matter has been suggested to reflect myelin abnormalities (discussed further below) (252, 327) or edema (252), whereas hippocampal signal increase has been suggested to reflect gliosis (280).

Two studies have quantitatively assessed the relationship between T2 relaxometry and glial cell numbers in different hippocampal subfields (247, 313). One suggested that volume loss was associated with neuronal cell loss and gliosis in different hippocampal regions (CA1, CA2, CA3, and hilus), whereas the T2-signal increase was associated only with damage in CA1 and hilus (247). This study used neuron/glial ratios and the direct contribution of neuron and glial cells could not be inferred. The other study analyzed cell ratios and absolute cell counts in patients with refractory TLE (313). A stepwise regression analysis suggested that the ipsilateral hippocampal volume was predicted best by the neuron cell count in the dentate gyrus ($p = 0.005$, $r = 0.4$). Hippocampal T2 time, on the other hand, was predicted best by the glial cell count in the dentate gyrus ($p = 0.01$, $r = 0.4$). Thus, T2-weighted signal increase in the hippocampus was mainly influenced by gliosis in the dentate gyrus, a region where a high proportion of glial cells show abnormal activity.

Correlation of Hippocampal T2-signal Increase with Clinical Findings

There is still debate as to whether T2-signal changes remain stable once HS has become established. There is evidence for progressive change with ongoing seizure activity (253, 304). This progression may be more easily seen in terms of volume deficits than T2 relaxometry (253). However, some reports have found a correlation of the T2-signal increase with the duration of the epilepsy, suggesting progressive change of T2 abnormalities as well (312).

Hippocampal Sclerosis in the Absence of Epilepsy

The MR features of HS can also rarely be found in subjects without any history of seizures, although this is controversial. In an unselected series of patients having an MR scan of the brain for other reasons than epilepsy, some indication of hippocampal abnormalities was found in 14% (29 of 204 subjects) (141). Some 9% had hippocampal atrophy only, 1% had T2 signal abnormalities only, and 4% met the criteria for both (141). However, there were major flaws in this study. Some forms of TLE with HS may have a genetic background. First-degree relatives of patients with familial mesial temporal lobe epilepsy were studied (142); volumetric studies showed hippocampal atrophy in 34% of 52 individuals. Increased T2 signal and/or abnormal internal structure were found in 14 of these 18 individuals. These two reports indicate that MRI evidence of HS is not necessarily associated with epilepsy and may occur in individuals who have never had seizures.

Hippocampal Sclerosis with Incomplete Magnetic Resonance Features

Hippocampal sclerosis without hippocampal atrophy has also been described (321, 130). In some cases the underlying pathology is typical HS and in some cases with similar imaging findings gliosis appears to be the major histologic

finding in the hippocampus (Fig. 4.35). High signal in a hippocampus that does not show atrophy is not typical of HS. Similarly, atrophy without signal change requires explanation. The primary epileptogenic focus may not be in that hippocampus or the other hippocampus might be abnormal. In either case, atrophy without signal change on optimized images should be a reason for further thoughts.

Hippocampal Sclerosis and Memory Function

Particular interest has found the relationship between quantitative measures of hippocampal disease, including T2 relaxometry and memory function (233, 234, 315, 328). Jack argues the usefulness of T2 relaxometry in predicting the postoperative outcome in regard to verbal memory (329). Interestingly, one study found that increased hippocampal T2 signal was associated with memory ability independent of MRI-determined hippocampal atrophy. This suggests that quantitative T2 relaxometry is an independent predictor of verbal memory outcome (234). We also assessed a group of 31 TLE patients (25 left, 6 right) with unilateral HS (233). Principal components analysis of preoperative memory data resulted in two factors. The arbitrary forms of verbal recall correlated with left hippocampal T2 values, while semantic forms of verbal recall did not. This study suggests that abnormalities in the left hippocampus are related more to the acquisition of arbitrary associates than to semantically structured material (233).

Quantitative Extrahippocampal Abnormality in Patients with Epilepsy

The vast majority of quantitative MR studies using T2 relaxometry are focused on the hippocampus in patients with pathologically proven HS. Changes in other areas have also been documented. Amygdaloid changes were assessed in a study of 29 patients with newly diagnosed and 54 patients with chronic temporal lobe epilepsy. In the newly diagnosed patients, the mean amygdaloid volume did not differ from that in controls. The mean T2 relaxation time in newly diagnosed or chronic patients did not differ from each other or from control values. However, unilateral T2 time of the amygdala was prolonged in 12% (171). T2-weighted signal abnormalities have also been observed in the anterior temporal lobe of TLE patients (252, 330), although their etiology and relevance is not known. We have recently observed T2 relaxometry changes outside the ipsilateral hippocampus of patients with HS, affecting the subcortical structures. These observations suggest that the structural signal abnormality in HS is not restricted to the seizure focus but may affect other areas such as the amygdala and the anterior temporal lobe, contralateral hippocampus, or even more distant areas such as subcortical structures. All these areas may be involved in the spread of the seizure activity.

Can Mesial Temporal Abnormality Reflect Nonepileptogenic Secondary Damage?

Sensitivity has increased in imaging techniques. When sensitivity is poor, it is likely that the abnormalities detected are major and likely to be causative for the epilepsy syndrome. There is increasing evidence that seizures themselves may cause detectable abnormalities as techniques improve. If this is so, then merely the detection of abnormality may not define the epileptogenic area even though it is likely to reflect something important about the seizures. For example it is not certain whether MRS abnormalities detected in the absence of any imaging lesion (331, 332) represent the cause or the effects of seizures (333). This issue of the secondary effects of seizures is dealt with in more detail later in this chapter.

HIPPOCAMPAL DYSPLASIA

Hippocampal dysplasia is a nonspecific term that is used to mean a developmental abnormality of the hippocampus (see Chapter 6 for a full discussion of malformations of cortical development). In this context it is defined by the presence of distinct architectural and cellular abnormalities in the hippocampus. Although there is debate as to what the role of development is in the origins of HS, we do not include HS as dysplasia. We include hippocampal dysplasia here because of the imaging issues, which are similar to HS. The major importance of hippocampal dysplasia is that it can be a major cause of determining the incorrect side for HS. That is, the smaller hippocampus is often considered to represent HS. This can be easily done if sequences without strong T1 or T2 contrast are obtained, or when the size of the hippocampus (atrophy) is the sole feature of HS that is used diagnostically. When dysplasia increases the size of the hippocampus, the normal hippocampus can be diagnosed as HS (Fig. 4.36). We have seen this happen on a number of occasions when insufficient attention has been given to the signal characteristics and internal structure as features of an abnormal hippocampus.

These cases are usually diagnosed preoperatively with optimized imaging demonstrating the morphology and signal characteristics of the hippocampus (Figs. 4.36–4.38). There is a range of underlying microscopic abnormalities seen in the resected hippocampi (Fig. 4.39).

TEMPORAL LOBE OTHER THAN THE HIPPOCAMPUS

Sclerosis of the Amygdala

Although most of the attention has been given to the hippocampus, we must not forget that the amygdala (as well as the temporal pole and entorhinal cortex) is also involved in the pathologic process in mesial temporal sclerosis (9, 88,

115, 127). The amygdala sits on top of the hippocampal head at the level of the anterior commissure and it can be problematic to separate the hippocampal head from the lateral amygdaloid nucleus at that level (226). As pointed by Jack et al. (208, 265), disarticulating the uncus, amygdala, and hippocampus anteriorly sometimes requires arbitrary judgments. Using qualitative three-dimensional studies, atrophy of the amygdala can be diagnosed (161, 163). However, atrophy of the amygdala is uncommon without concomitant hippocampal atrophy.

The majority of quantitative MR studies using T2 relaxometry are focused on the hippocampus in patients with pathologically proven HS. Changes in other areas, particularly the amygdala, have also been documented (165–167, 171, 172, 178, 236, 334). Amygdaloid changes were assessed in a study of 29 patients with newly diagnosed and 54 patients with chronic temporal lobe epilepsy. In the newly diagnosed patients, the mean amygdaloid volume did not differ from that in controls. The mean T2 relaxation time in newly diagnosed or chronic patients did not differ from each other or from control values. However, unilateral T2 time of the amygdala was prolonged in 12% (171).

We have proposed that the amygdala can be best seen in tilted axial images in which clear separation of the hippocampus and amygdala is possible (Fig. 4.40), together with the standard coronal images (see top row of Fig. 4.19). Visual diagnosis of amygdaline sclerosis has proven to be very difficult except in rare cases. Because of the difficulty of using manual volume-based measurements, one effective way to assess the amygdala is with quantitative methods such as T2 relaxometry and volumetry (165–167, 171, 172, 178, 236, 334).

Parahippocampal Gyrus Abnormalities

Other indirect features of mesial sclerosis commonly seen in these patients are the presence of parahippocampal gyrus atrophy and sometimes signal change. These changes are difficult to visualize but with optimized images one can evaluate the presence of thinning of the underlying white matter and blurring of the gray/white matter pattern. This usually depends on having images that assess signal change well (Fig. 4.41).

Similarly, changes of the collateral white matter, which is located between the hippocampus and the collateral sulcus, are occasionally seen (245). In some cases, abnormality of the parahippocampal white matter can be the only clue to the origin of seizures. Seizures originating in the parahippocampal region can mimic many different epilepsy syndromes, most probably because of the patterns of spread from this area. Typically they present as ipsilateral temporal lobe seizures. Sometimes the seizures can first appear in the contralateral (normal) temporal lobe, as in the patient shown in Figure 4.41. This can be a cause of disconcordant findings and poor outcome in MRI-negative TLE, as the EEG findings point to the incorrect side and the imaging features are

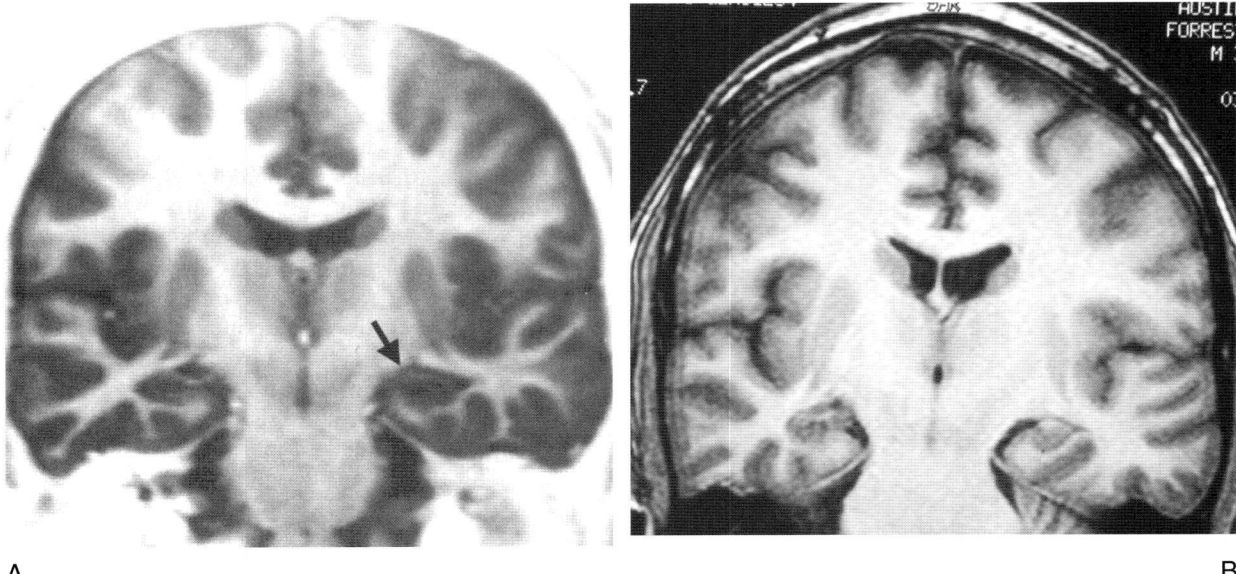

A

B

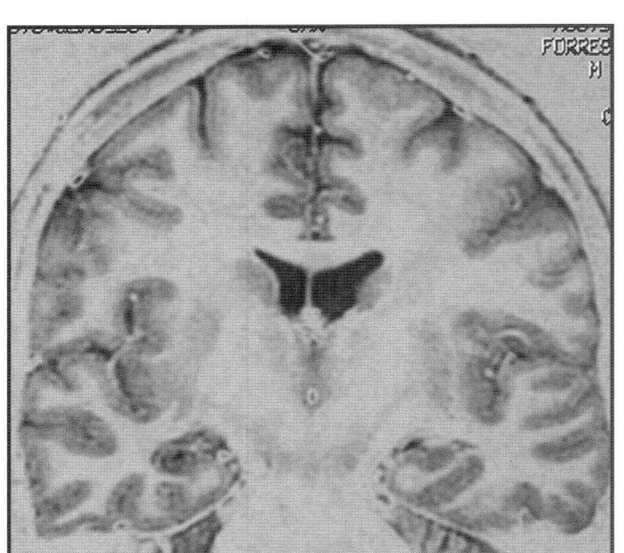

C

FIG. 4.36. A. The left hippocampus is abnormal, with abnormal signal and increased size. Sometimes, if images that assess hippocampal signal are not acquired, this can be mistaken for hippocampal atrophy on the normal side. The histologic diagnosis after surgical resection was left hippocampal dysplasia. **B.** The right hippocampus is of normal size but has disrupted internal structure. After resection this was hippocampal dysplasia but no hippocampal sclerosis, despite seizure origin in the right mesial temporal region. **C.** This is the same case as in **B**. On inversion recovery images, there is abnormal signal seen in the right hippocampus. The abnormal signal is in the CA1 and end folium and appears more localized than in the T1-weighted 3D volume study (**B**). There was hippocampal dysplasia but no definite neuronal loss to suggest HS. These focal changes may represent signal change in the sectors of the hippocampus involved in seizures. Compare this to Figures 4.27, which was the hippocampus contralateral to the seizure focus, and 4.33, where this pattern was seen prior to progression to hippocampal sclerosis.

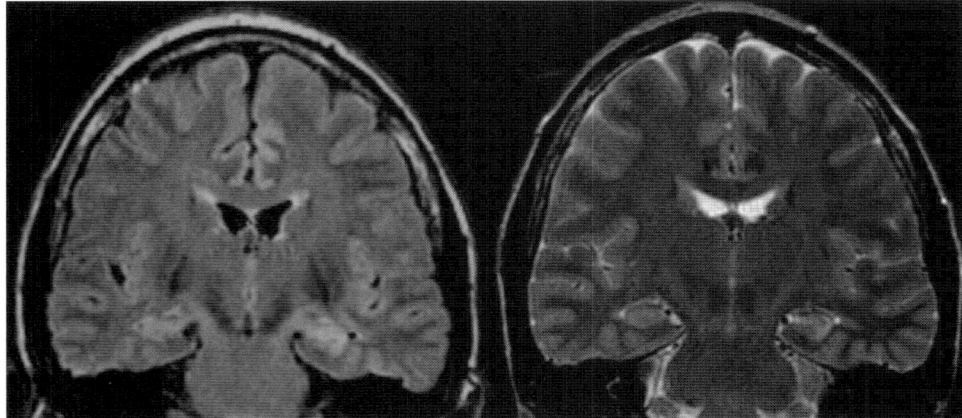

FIG. 4.37. Hippocampal malformation with increased hippocampal volume and signal: This 30-year-old man has frequent day and night time seizures, which are refractory to antiepileptic medication. During a typical seizure, he stands still and picks at his clothes for a duration between 30 seconds and 10 minutes. He has a borderline IQ. MR imaging was performed on a 3 T GE LX Horizon scanner (Milwaukee, USA). On the left is a slice through the hippocampus acquired with a FLAIR sequence. Note the increased signal in the region of the left hippocampus. The right image shows a slice through the hippocampus acquired with a T2-weighted sequence. Note the increased signal in the region of the left hippocampus. In contrast to hippocampal sclerosis, there is no atrophy, but volume increase. Hippocampal T2 relaxometry was within normal limits on both sides; the measurement was taken in the body of the hippocampus. However, the measurement on the left side was slightly higher than on the right side (right 95 ms, left 104 ms, normal >107 ms).

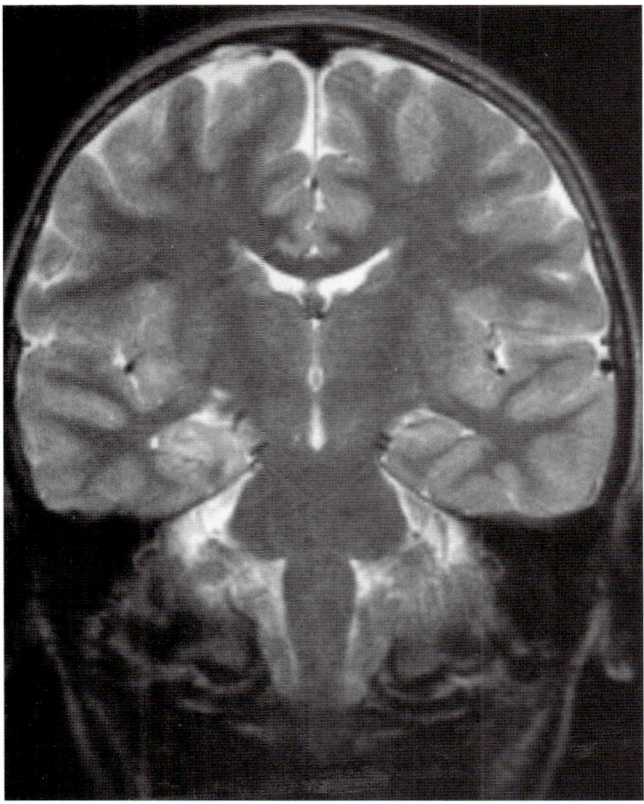

FIG. 4.38. Increased signal in the larger right hippocampus and extending into the parahippocampal gyrus. This is a foreign tissue lesion that included focal hippocampal dysplasia on histological examination.

considered subtle, possibly due to artifacts of the sort shown in Figure 4.15.

Seizures can also spread to the parietal region, as was the case with the patient shown in Figure 4.42. In this case parietal resection was performed, based on intracranial monitoring. Subsequently, and after recognition of abnormality in the parahippocampal region in the MR images, posteriorly inserted electrodes confirmed the origin in the parahippocampal gyrus. Resection of this area led to freedom from seizures and the patient has been seizure-free and off medications for more than 5 years. We believe that posterior parahippocampal lesions, like occipital lesions, mimic seizures arising in other locations in patients with intractable epilepsy. This area should be carefully evaluated in MRI-negative patients as the abnormality can be subtle.

DUAL PATHOLOGY: EXTRAHIPPOCAMPAL PATHOLOGY ASSOCIATED WITH HIPPOCAMPAL SCLEROSIS

The definition of dual pathology is the presence of an extrahippocampal structural lesion and hippocampal pathology in the same patient (+HS). The exact incidence of dual pathology in temporal lobe epilepsy is difficult to ascertain but it

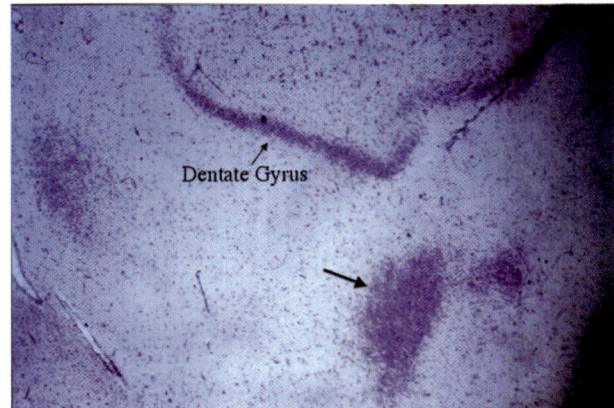

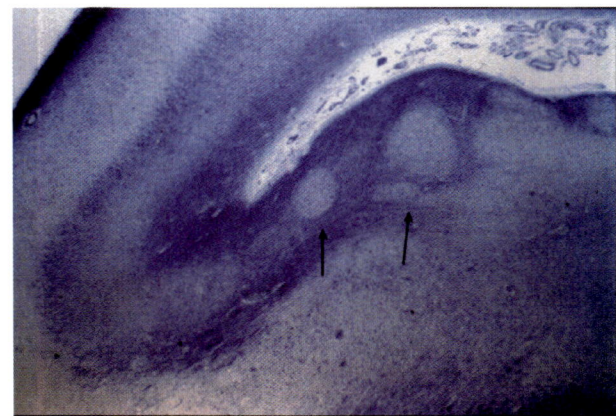

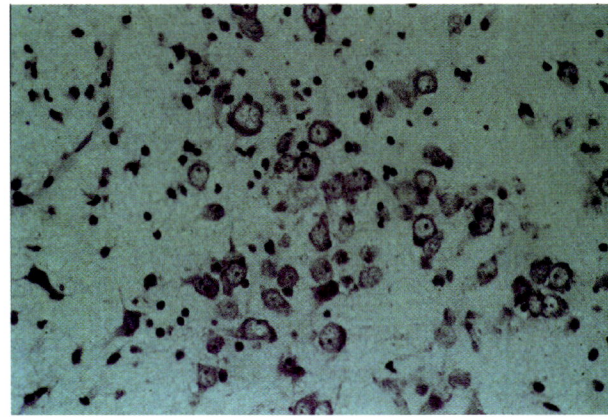

FIG. 4.39. A. Photomicrograph showing hippocampal dysplasia with a collection of abnormal cells (large arrow) in the hippocampus peripheral to the dentate gyrus (labeled) in the striatum lacunosum moleculare/radiata. **B.** Photomicrograph showing mesial temporal dysplasia with abnormal structure of cellular and sparse areas in the entorhinal region. This area normally has an unusual microarchitecture, but this structure is abnormal. **C.** Hippocampal dysplasia where there are abnormal cells in the hippocampus.

is common in MR imaging series and is usually on the same side as the HS (Table 4.3).

In pathology series there are difficulties associated with surgical and pathologic sampling and histologic classification. Bruton reported dual pathology in 7.2% of cases in the Maudsley series (127) but in many ways pathologic

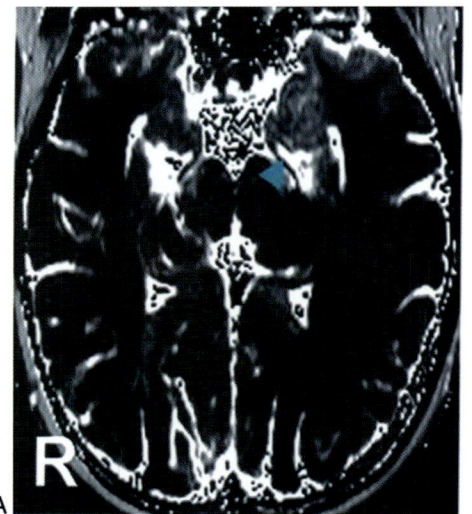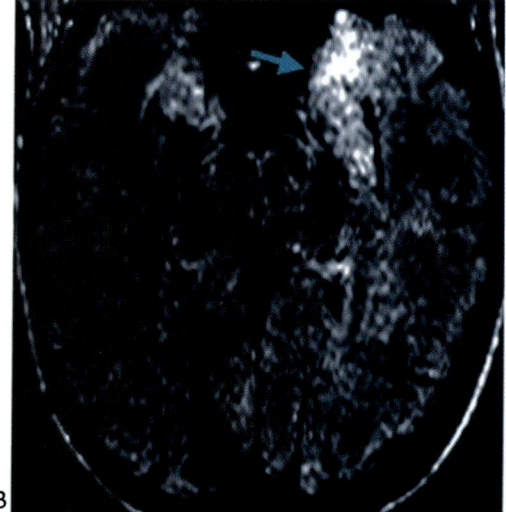

FIG. 4.40. Amygdala sclerosis: abnormal signal can be seen in the mesial temporal region and primarily involving the amygdala. Because of the architecture of the amygdala, abnormality in signal is often the clue to focal abnormality. (Courtesy of Wim Van Paesschen (166).)

assessment is a poor way to assess the presence of additional lesions when only resected specimens are available for analysis. The majority demonstrated HS associated with 'foreign' or 'alien' tissue lesions, developmental lesions, or trauma. Babb et al. (90, 91) reported a 20% incidence of dual pathology in temporal lobe specimens and Levesque et al. (335) reported an incidence of 30.3% among 178 patients who underwent temporal lobe resections. For practical reasons this must be an underestimate of the true incidence.

Levesque et al. found that hippocampal cell loss was less common in dual pathology than in patients without extrahippocampal pathology. The distribution and severity of hippocampal damage was associated with the type of pathology. The hamartoma and glioma groups had the least cell loss and the heterotopia group had the most severe loss. The presence of mild changes prompted the authors to propose that extrahippocampal pathology could produce, by a similar mechanism to kindling, damage to the hippocampus. Despite the attractiveness of this hypothesis, Kim et al. (336) did not find hippocampal cell loss in patients with temporal lobe gliomas, pointing out that these lesions are epileptogenic on their own.

In dual pathology the best surgical results are obtained when both HS and the second lesion are removed (262, 337–339). Failure to render a patient with HS seizure-free after anterior temporal lobectomy may be due to the presence of a cortical dysplasia that was not detected on standard MR imaging (340). There are a number of cases in all surgical series that date back to the pre-MR era, in which unrecognized and unsuspected second pathologies are subsequently found, often on the side of the resection (e.g. insular developmental malformations, as in Fig. 4.43, and a more subtle example of insular gyral abnormality, in Fig. 4.44). There is no doubt that HS exists in these cases and that they have TLE.

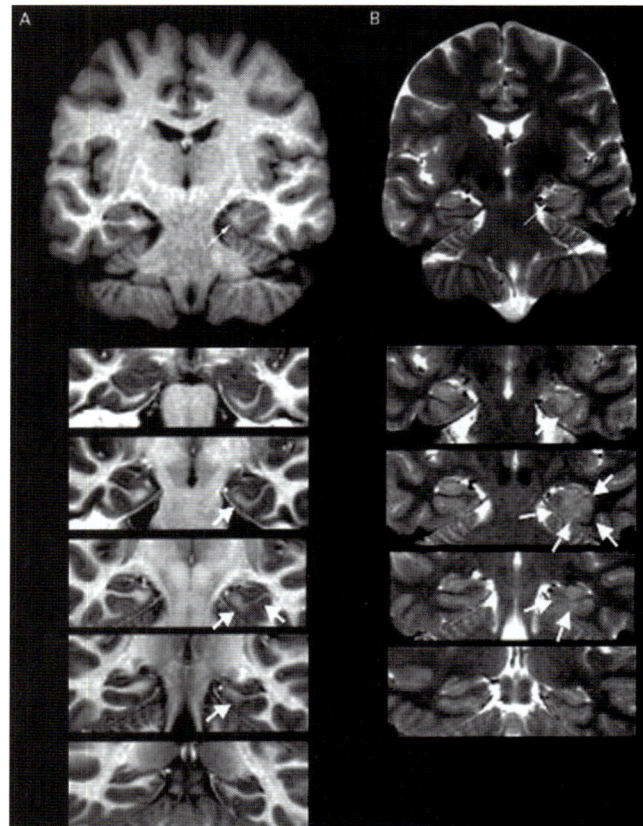

FIG. 4.41. These images show the problem of parahippocampal epilepsy. The clinical syndrome was mesial temporal epilepsy. Bilateral depth electrodes were implanted and the seizures appeared to arise from the right mesial region. After recognition of the abnormal parahippocampal region on the left (arrows), this region was eventually resected, with an excellent outcome. Some simple partial seizures persist but the majority of complex partial seizures resolved.

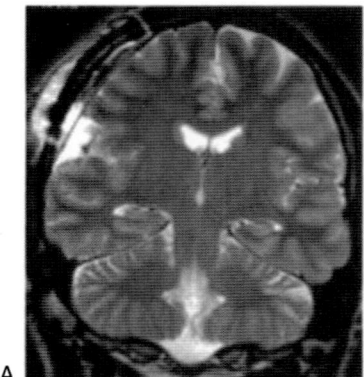

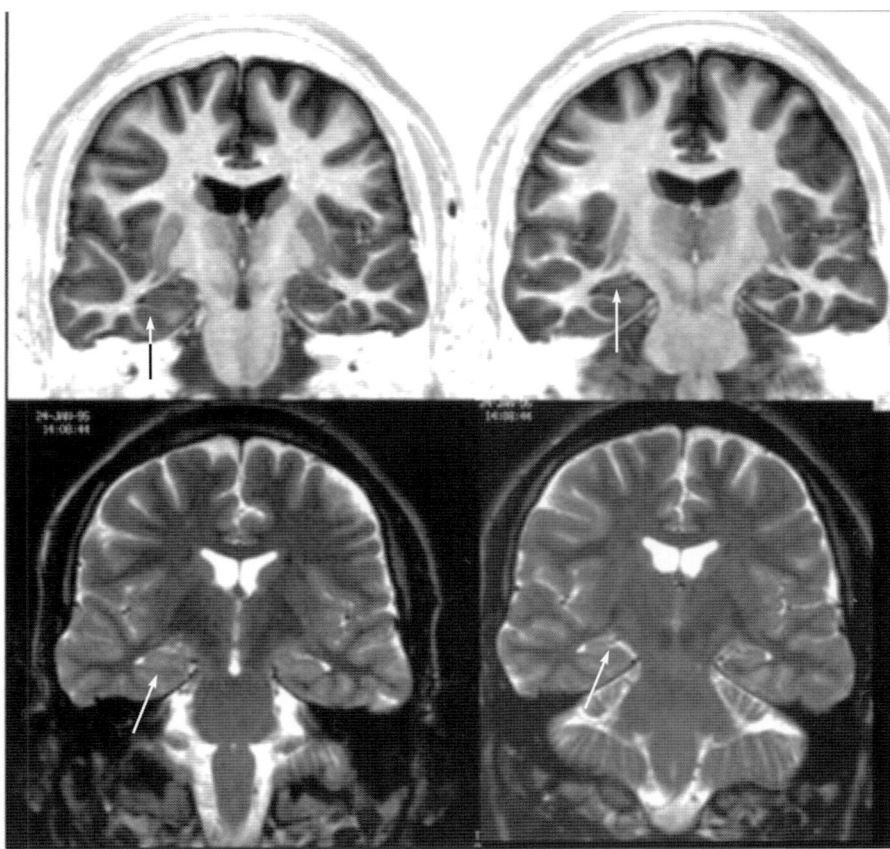

FIG. 4.42. This patient had complex partial seizures and was extensively investigated with intracranial monitoring and supported by ictal spect; a focus was found in the right parietal region. Resection of this (**A**) did not improve his seizures. Signal change in the parahippocampal gyrus was noted on subsequent investigations (**B**). Note the loss of clarity in the white matter of the parahippocampal region (arrows). Depth electrodes in the parahippocampal region confirmed this as the origin of seizures. The patient has been seizure free for 5 years following resection of the right medial temporal region. This is an example of parahippocampal epilepsy, which can mimic seizures from many other regions, including the parietal and contralateral temporal regions.

The development of new MRI techniques and postprocessing protocols enable us to detect these subtle malformations (341, 342) with ever greater sensitivity (Chapter 8). As discussed above, the increasing problem is to determine whether the abnormalities in addition to the HS are part of the same injury that is represented by the hippocampal sclerosis (HS+) or a pre-existing and separate abnormality that may be important in the pathogenesis and seizure generation (+HS). The HS and second pathology are typically on the same side – suggesting a possible reason for predominantly unilateral HS (see Table 4.3).

There are also many MR examples of progression of lesions and development of HS after seizures from another source, as for example in Figure 4.45. Here, a swollen hippocampus without atrophy was seen on initial imaging when the patient presented with status epilepticus from the cavernoma bleed. As can be seen in the figure, classic HS evolved. This is dual pathology in which the temporal relationship

Table 4.3. Unilateral Hippocampal Sclerosis and the Side of the Extrahippocampal Lesion (see 461, 462)

	Raymond et al. 1994	Li et al. 1997 (338)	Ho et al. 1998	A & RMC
Ipsilateral to hippocampal hippocampal sclerosis	3	9	11	23
Bilateral extrahippocampal lesion	5	3	0	5
Contralateral	1	0		

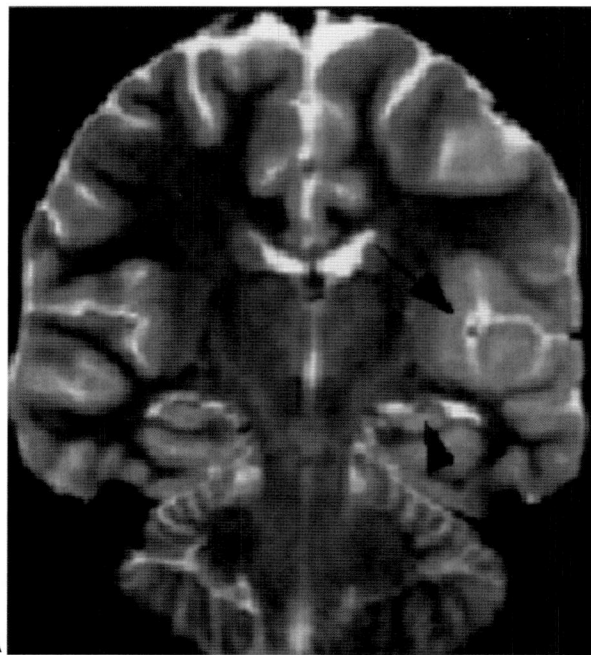 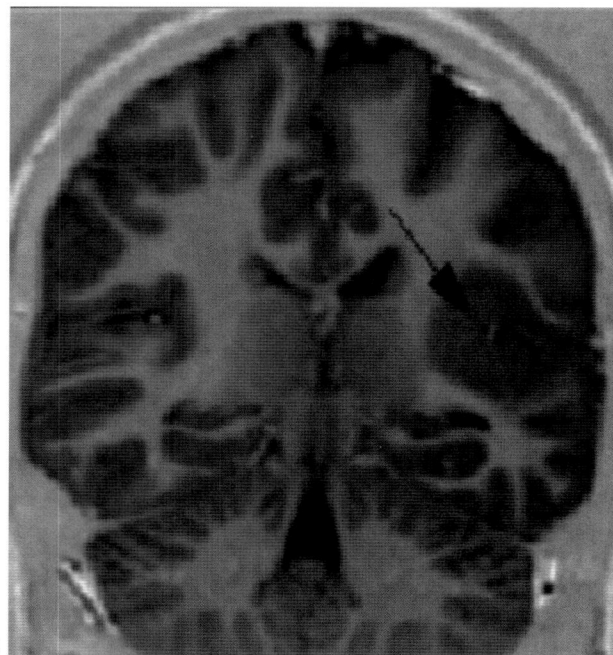

FIG. 4.43. Dual pathology with periventricular polymicrogyria (arrowed) with thickening of the gray matter on the side ipsilateral to hippocampal sclerosis (arrowhead in **A**).

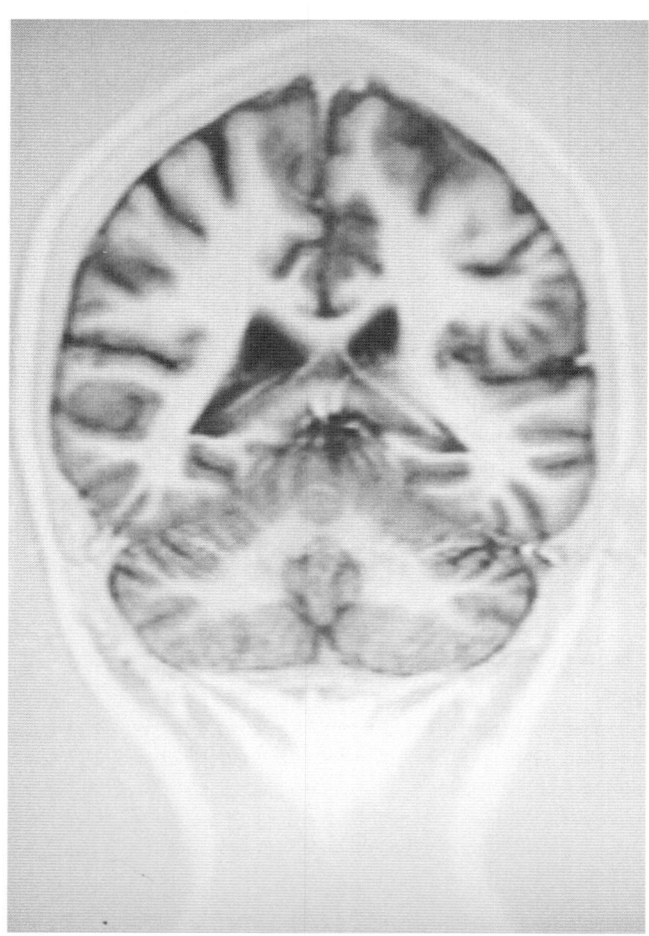

FIG. 4.44. Dual pathology with multiple small gyri in the frontal operculum ipsilateral to hippocampal sclerosis.

between the initial event and the subsequent HS can be documented. There is no longer any doubt that this sequence is not uncommon and that epileptogenic HS can be secondary to such an injury, even though we often see examples (Fig. 4.46) where the causal mechanism is unknown. Of course this does not mean that all HS is acquired in this manner (see below).

The most extreme example of a condition that may appear to have significant extrahippocampal abnormality is the hemiplegia, hemiatrophy, and epilepsy (HHE) syndrome (Fig. 4.47). From talking to older epileptologists, it appears that this syndrome is less common than it used to be. One reason might be that prolonged seizures in childhood are more readily and aggressively treated. We do not really consider this to be dual pathology, as it is likely that the HS and the other abnormality are part of the same injury (HS+).

ANTERIOR TEMPORAL LOBE SIGNAL AND VOLUME CHANGES ASSOCIATED WITH HIPPOCAMPAL SCLEROSIS (HS+)

Over 30 years ago, Falconer and Corsellis noted that HS was part of a continuum of abnormalities found in the temporal lobe, stating that "the process, although mainly affecting the mesial gray matter in the temporal lobe may spread widely throughout the lobe leading to generalized atrophy and gliosis of both cortex and white matter" (12). Likewise, surgeons have frequently noted macroscopic

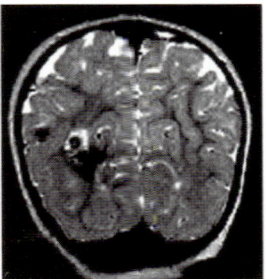

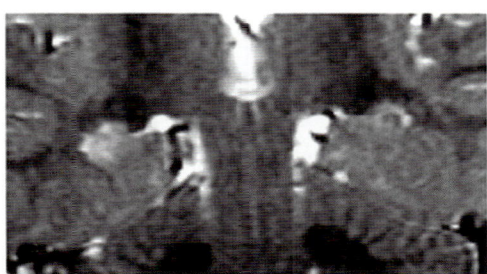
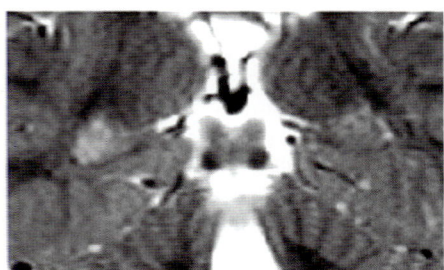

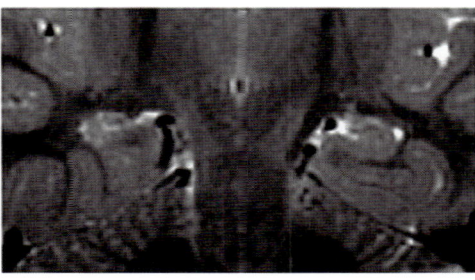
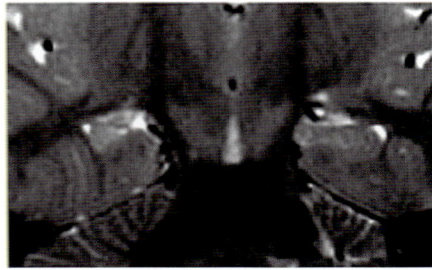

FIG. 4.45. This patient had familial cavernous angiomas and had a single seizure lasting 45 minutes at 13 months of age. Postictal left-sided weakness occurred for 24 hours after the seizure. Complex partial seizures began at age 2.5 and progressed to 2 seizures/day typical of TLE. The top image shows the nonhippocampal lesion, suggesting a cavernous angioma that has bled. The top row of images were taken at 13 months, 24 hours after the prolonged seizure, and show increased hippocampal signal but no atrophy. The bottom row of images were acquired 13 months later when complex partial seizures of temporal type began. The patient now has typical right hippocampal sclerosis. (Courtesy of Simon Harvey, Royal Children's Hospital, Melbourne, Australia.)

changes in the temporal lobe, especially in the superior temporal gyrus, and have often noted an abnormal consistency of the temporal lobe specimen.

Magnetic resonance studies show that abnormality in the anterior temporal lobe is common in patients with HS (Fig. 4.48) (138, 252, 327, 343, 344). Like the initial observations in HS, anterior temporal lobe changes have often been incorrectly attributed to artifacts caused by partial voluming, flow or field inhomogeneity (see Fig. 4.15). These changes are exclusively on the side ipsilateral to the seizure focus and there are no similar changes in control cases imaged in an identical fashion, mixed with the patient scans and reported in a blinded fashion (252). The main possibilities that have been assumed as an explanation were either gliosis of the anterior temporal white matter, or developmental abnormalities such as ectopic neurons, which

are known to be more frequent in patients with HS (345). Ho et al. (345) assumed that all cases had the same abnormality as the few in which histopathology was available. Subsequent detailed studies of this abnormality show that this is not the case (252, 327) and this abnormality should not be interpreted as having the same significance as dual pathology. It now seems clear that these changes reflect a persistent immature state (or a failure of postnatal development including myelination) of the anterior temporal lobe.

Magnetic Resonance Imaging Features of Anterior Temporal Lobe Abnormalities

Anterior temporal lobe (AT) signal abnormality consists of increased T2 signal and decreased T1 signal within the

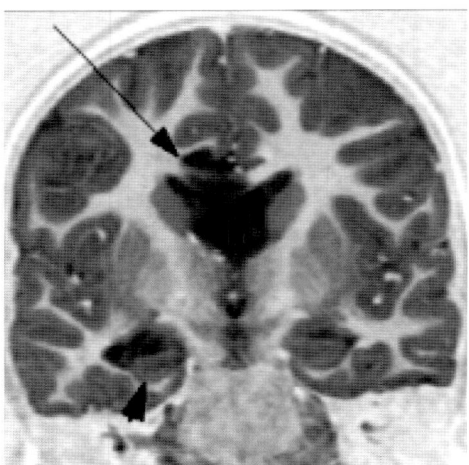
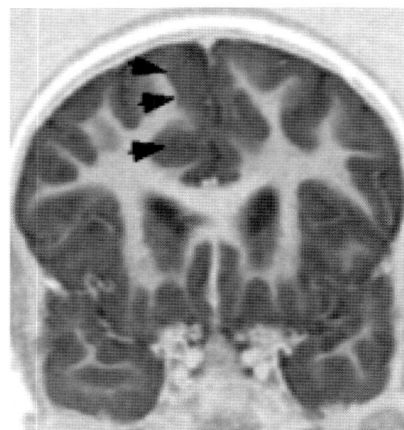

FIG. 4.46. This patient had seizure onset at the age of 9 years following normal development to that stage. The seizures were complex partial with no focal features, Neuropsychology showed diffuse abnormality with verbal IQ 83, performance IQ 58. The EEG showed interictal high-amplitude slow waves over the right hemisphere. Quantitative evaluation of the hippocampus showed bilateral abnormality, marked and sclerotic on the right (T2 left 112, right 121. Normal <108). The long arrow shows an unusual destructive lesion in the medial frontal region with loss of the corpus callosum. Further anteriorly, there is thickened cortex suggesting a malformation of cortical development. The arrowhead indicates hippocampal sclerosis.

affected anterior temporal lobe white matter (Fig. 4.49) (330). This is often associated with atrophy (Fig. 4.50). These findings commonly result in reduced definition of the gray–white matter boundary and apparent shrinkage of the white matter core of the temporal pole on protein-density (PD)- and T2-weighted images. These changes are most easily identified as predominantly white matter signal change but, on the inversion recovery sequence, abnormal signal can often be appreciated in the cortical gray matter as well as

in the white matter. These changes can be seen on all pulse sequences using careful windowing but, when subtle, they are most readily appreciated on T2- and PD-weighted images (Fig. 4.51).

Mitchell (252) reported the frequency of ipsilateral AT abnormality in patients with intractable TLE to be 58%, and 64% in the group with HS. This is similar to the 71% reported by Meiners et al. in their smaller group (327). However, these changes are not exclusive to HS, as identical

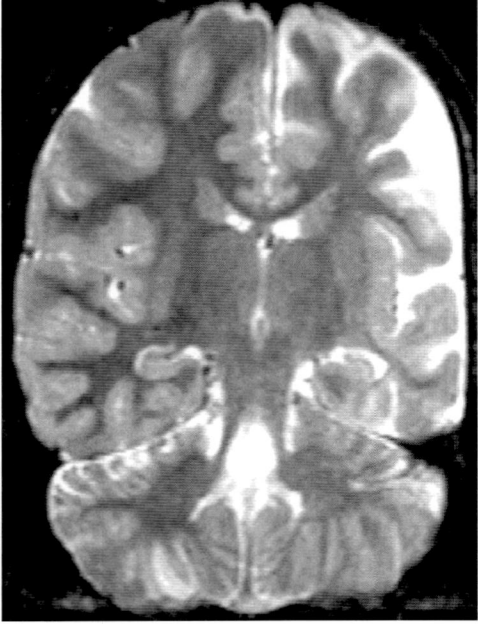
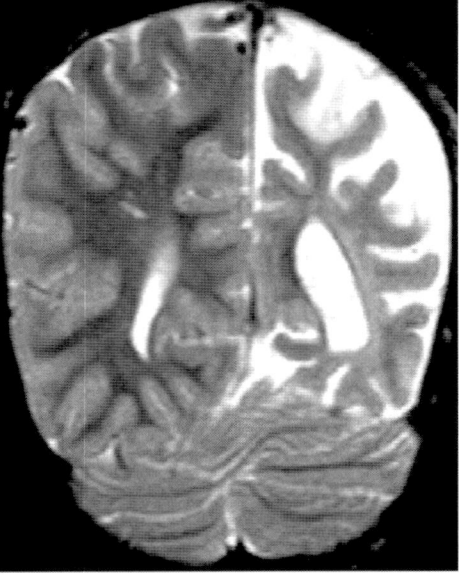

FIG. 4.47. This patient had congenital right body hemiplegia and seizures with an onset at the age of 6 weeks. There were simple partial and complex partial events. Development was delayed. There is marked loss of tissue in the entire left hemisphere, and an abnormal hippocampus on that side, interpreted as hippocampal sclerosis.

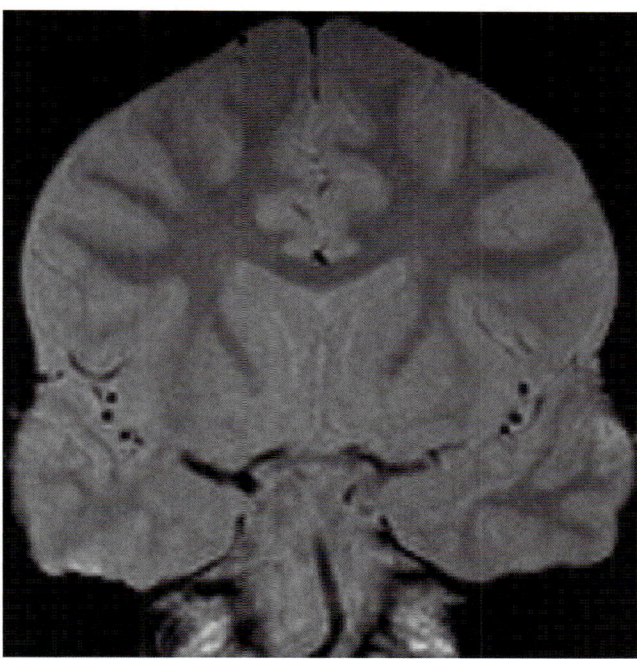

FIG. 4.48. Changes in the anterior temporal lobe are seen on the right side. The features are increased T2-weighted signal in the white matter and loss of clarity of the gray–white matter junction. Although these features can be seen in malformations of cortical development, this is not the explanation in cases such as this. Proton density image.

changes were seen in isolation, and in two patients with cavernous hemangioma in Mitchell's series. One other patient with abnormalities eventually proved to be due to Rasmussen's encephalitis also had similar changes. Therefore, while the major association is with HS, this anterior temporal abnormality occurs in the broader context of intractable TLE, with various underlying pathologies.

Pathology correlations of these findings

The surgically resected temporal lobe specimens from patients with intractable TLE have a number of abnormalities not seen in normal controls. The major pathologic findings are listed in Table 4.4. Pathologic findings include degenerative changes, which might be encountered in normal aging brains, minor dysplastic or microdysgenesic changes, and inflammatory changes. Degenerative findings include dilated perivascular spaces, accumulation of corpora amylacea, and fibrous thickening of the leptomeninges. The most commonly encountered microdysgenesic change is an apparent increase in white matter neurons. Histopathologic quantitation studies have suggested that this is a real phenomenon, although volume changes in the resected temporal lobes may account for at least some of the apparent increase. In the cortex, the frequency of very minor abnormalities, such as the occurrence of medium- or large-sized neurons in the molecular layer, is increased in specimens from epileptic patients compared with normal controls. Minor inflammatory changes are also commonly found, usually consisting of small numbers of perivascular macrophages and lymphocytes in the subarachnoid space and the white matter itself.

All these minor changes are equally common whether AT change is present on MR scans or not. There is no difference in the frequency, or severity of these histologic findings between the MR groups. Molecular layer gliosis and minor inflammatory changes were very different in both patient groups when compared to the control groups, but this did not differentiate cases with anterior temporal MR abnormality from the MR-negative ones. A possible interpretation of these MR changes has been the presence of minor dysplastic or developmental abnormalities in the AT lobe. Minor microdysgenesis appears to be more frequent in patients with TLE than in controls but their presence equally in frequency and severity in the two groups appears to exclude microdysgenesis as the cause of the visible AT change.

To simply interpret these AT changes as developmental abnormality in the sense of a pre-existing pathologic process separate to the HS is incorrect. Diffuse gliosis would agree with the established explanations of high T2-weighted signal reflecting gliosis in HS. Quantitation of glial cell counts support the observation of Falconer and Corsellis (12) that there is gliosis in the temporal lobes of these patients when compared to controls. However, there is no difference between the AT and non-AT group in the density of glial cell nuclei in the

Table 4.4. Histopathologic findings in the Anterior Temporal Lobe (252)

Finding (n = 42)	AT signal change (n = 25)	No AT signal change (n = 17)	Controls (n = 11)
Dilated perivascular spaces	3	4	3
Corpora amylacea	12	7	2
Prominent white matter neurons	22	15	4
Molecular layer gliosis	25	17	0
Minor inflammatory change	22	13	1
Oligodendroglial cell clusters	2	1	0

AT, anterior temporal lobe.

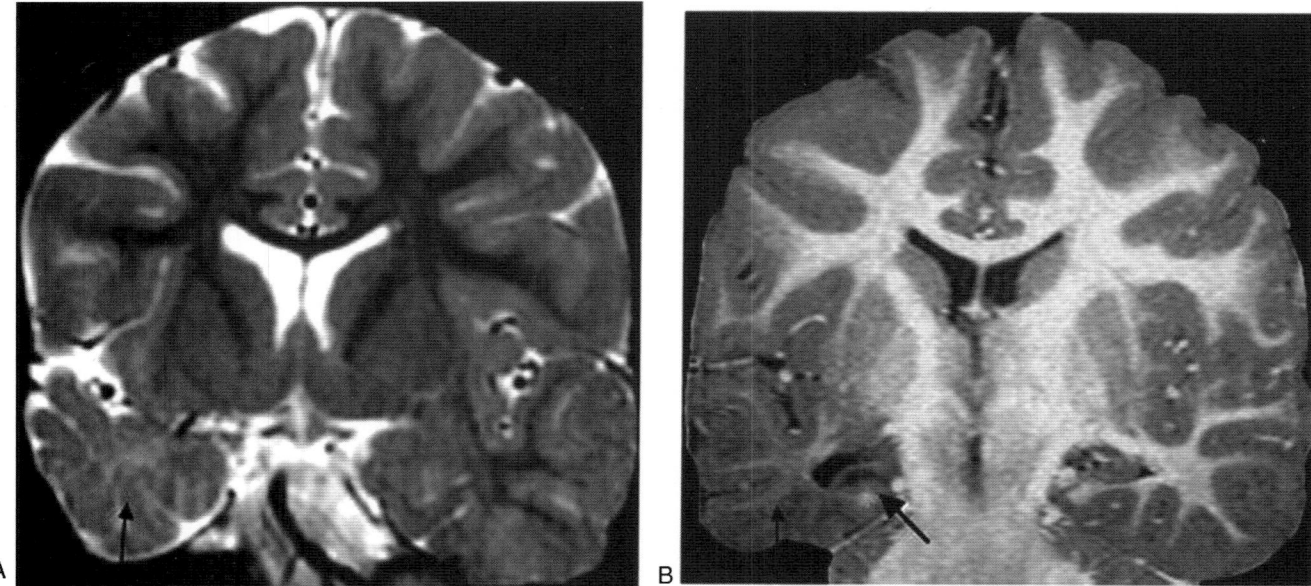

FIG. 4.49. This is a severe example of signal change in the anterior temporal lobe and temporal pole. The T2-weighted image (**A**) shows high signal in the temporal white matter, in this case even greater than the gray matter (long arrow). The heavily T1-weighted IR sequence (**B**) shows decreased signal in temporal white matter. Abnormal signal is also in the atrophic hippocampus and was proved to be typical hippocampal sclerosis. There was no developmental abnormality in the resected temporal lobe.

temporal white matter. In common with Mitchell's study, no convincing pathologic abnormality was observed in Meiners's reports (327, 330, 343) of these findings.

In the absence of gliosis or minor dysplasia as an explanation of these MRI findings, it is tempting to attribute them to defective myelination, failure of myelination, or loss of myelin, due either to seizures or to an early childhood event.

Abnormal temporal lobe myelination is unlikely to be the whole explanation, as the signal change involves the cortical gray matter in some cases. We now believe these changes are due to an arrest in development of the temporal lobes and persistence of immature cell types (465) and myelin. The immature temporal lobe does indeed look remarkably like the changes we describe (Fig. 4.52).

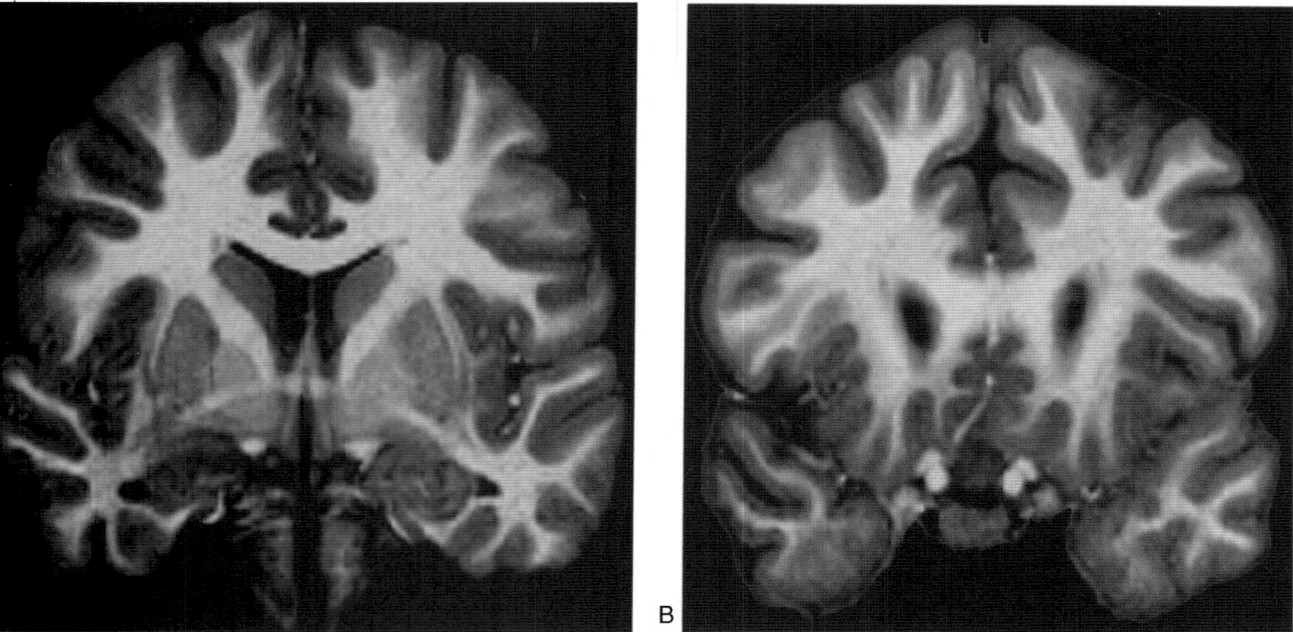

FIG. 4.50. This is a subtle example of anterior temporal lobe abnormality seen on heavily T1-weighted IR images. Careful examination of the white matter shows decreased signal in the right temporal lobe core (**A**). There is also subtle atrophy, particularly of the superior and middle temporal gyrus on the right (**B**). The left image shows abnormal signal in the mesial gray matter, which is more obviously in the hippocampal body.

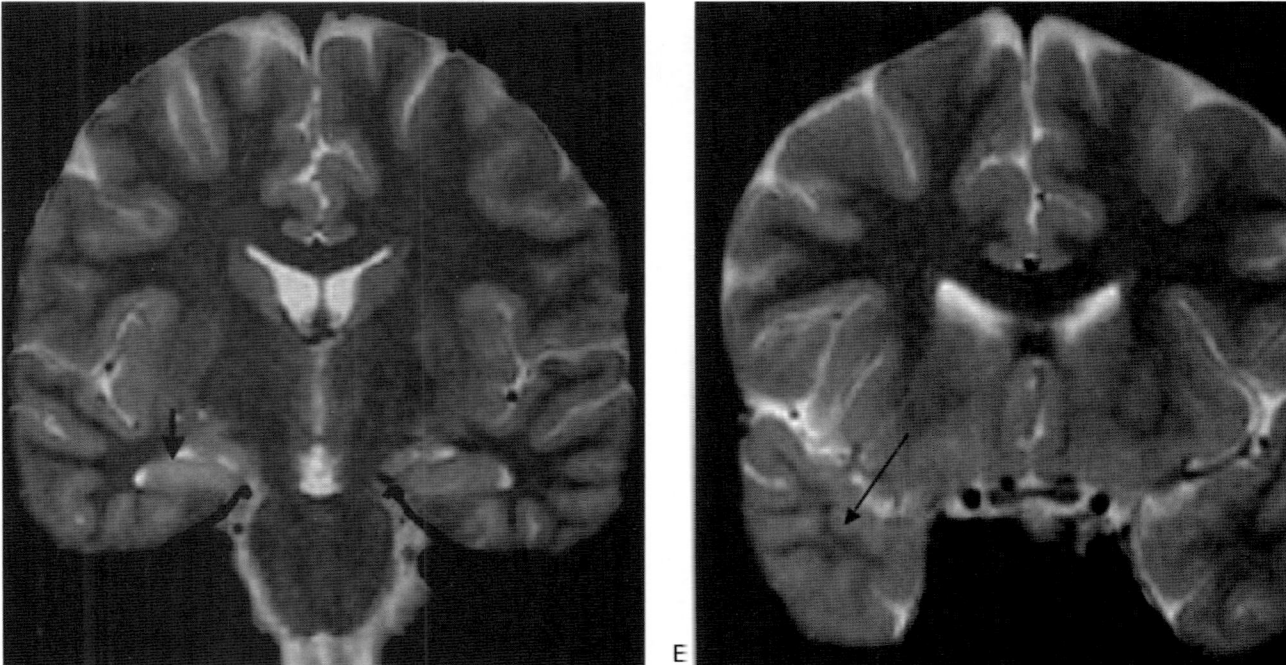

FIG. 4.51. Subtle changes in the anterior temporal lobe seen on T2-weighted images. The left image shows increased signal in a small hippocampal head consistent with hippocampal sclerosis (short arrow). The anterior temporal lobe white matter core is poorly defined compared to the contralateral side (long arrow, **B**).

The anterior temporal lobe abnormality is present in children with the same frequency as adults (about 66% of cases with HS), suggesting that it is not the consequence of long-standing seizures (138). It is the arrested myelination that most probably gives these signal changes. Atrophy, on the other hand, is likely to be a combination of arrest of growth and secondary damage from seizures. The temporal pole is the last part of the cortex to fully develop and myelination and other developmental changes occur here up to 80 months after birth.

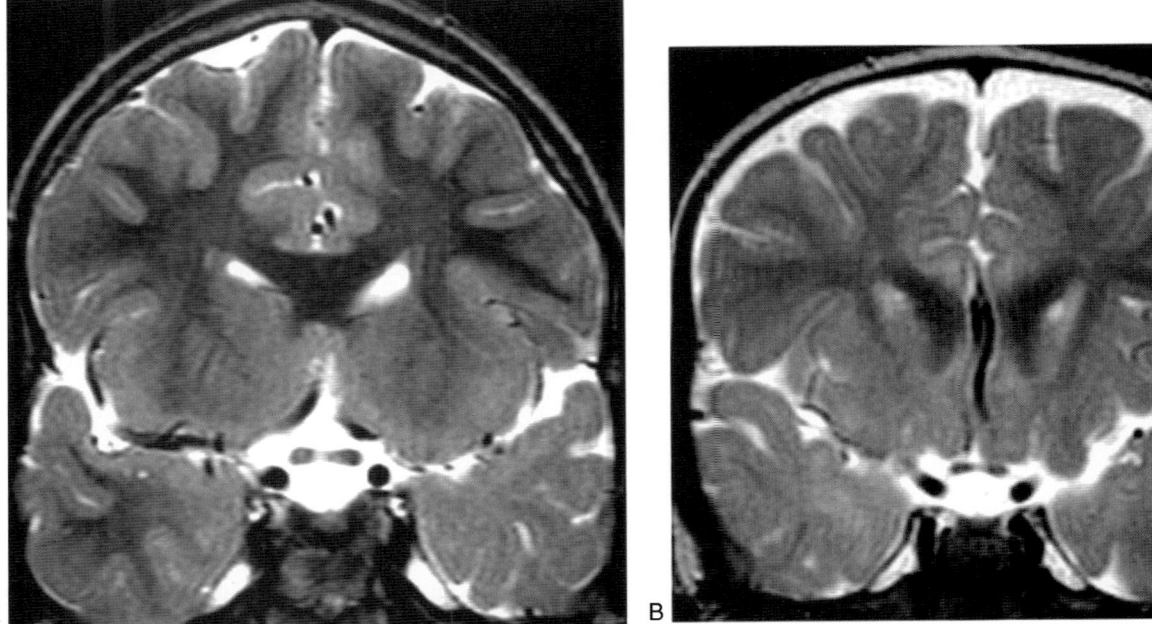

FIG. 4.52. A. A 10-year-old boy with TLE and definite and classical HS on the left side. The anterior temporal lobe shows marked signal change similar to that see in Figure 4.49. This extends through the temporal lobe and can involve the insula, as in this case. **B.** A normal 12-month-old boy. Note the similarity of this normal developmental stage with the persistent features in our patient with HS and TLE.

The finding, in a children cohort, that an initial precipitating event before the age of 2 almost always leads to this change, suggests that the injury that causes hippocampal damage causes changes in the immature AT that arrests its development. There is no correlation between the presence of AT changes on MRI and length of seizure history or age of onset of epilepsy. There is no difference in seizure-free outcome between the groups with and without AT changes. The temporal pole is virtually the last area of the brain to mature, and this may make it vulnerable to the effects of seizures.

In the patients with HS, there is an association between AT signal abnormality and the severity of HS as determined by a higher T2-relaxation time within the hippocampus. Severity of insult as a cause of this change is supported by the significant twofold increase in the incidence of febrile convulsions in the patients with AT changes.

There appears to be few consequences of anterior temporal abnormality (138, 252). Neuropsychologic findings appear to be identical in patients with and without this, seizure outcome is the same, and postoperative memory deficit in left-sided operations was the same in both groups (138, 252). Overall it seems that the AT MR changes do not determine functionality of tissue.

One must always be careful not to assume that all anterior temporal changes in signal are due to the same process; other causes must be recognized. True developmental abnormality, if severe, can give this appearance (Fig. 4.53).

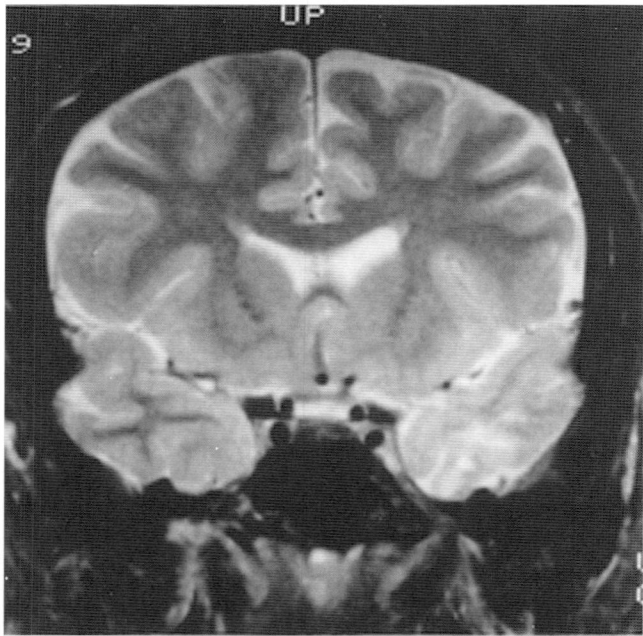

FIG. 4.53. An example of a focal cortical dysplasia, which can give a similar appearance in the anterior temporal lobe. Coronal T2 image showing increased signal from the left temporal lobe, which has a more focal distribution than is the case for the more diffuse anterior temporal lobe change. No mass effect is seen.

HOW IMAGING HAS HELPED UNDERSTANDING OF THE EPILEPTOGENIC PROCESSES IN TEMPORAL LOBE EPILEPSY

The Origins of Hippocampal Sclerosis

Some facts about HS are undoubted. The histopathologic and MR features of this lesion have been recognized and are well described. The epileptogenic properties of this lesion have also been investigated. There is a broad consensus that HS is epileptogenic and that removal of this structure has a high chance of rendering the patient seizure-free. The clinical pattern of the epilepsy associated with HS has been described, and there has been some controversy about whether the clinical features are distinct enough to call TLE with HS a specific syndrome. The major controversy in HS, however, relates to the etiology of this lesion. Several possibilities have been discussed in the literature:

- HS is an acquired, epileptogenic lesion
- HS is a developmental, epileptogenic lesion
- HS is a combination of several factors.

Types of Hippocampal Sclerosis that can be Defined with Magnetic Resonance Methods

The features of volume loss, signal change, and abnormal morphology are now well recognized. Volume loss with abnormal signal within the hippocampus probably does not have the same meaning as volume loss alone. Similarly, HS in the context of another distinct lesion may need to be interpreted differently. Also, abnormalities are often not confined to the hippocampus, or even solely to the epileptogenic temporal lobe (346). We might ask: Why is HS typically unilateral? Why is 'dual pathology' so common? Why are there regional abnormalities? Why after successful surgery is there late seizure recurrence?

If we summarize the findings in the brain that are detectable by MR imaging methods (see Fig. 4.4), we can recognize that at least three major subgroups exist (see Table 4.2). This first two of these seem to fit with the basic concepts we have of essentially classical HS. These are:

- *Classical HS.* In this case HS with volume loss and signal change is the sole lesion. As we have discussed, increasing sophistication of analysis and imaging demonstrates a range of other abnormality in the brain of these patients (e.g. see Fig. 4.35)
- *HS+.* In this situation there is identified abnormality in addition to HS, but the abnormality is not a definitely different lesion (such as temporal pole white matter signal abnormality, temporal lobe, or hemisphere atrophy)

The findings that are typical on MR studies in these first two categories are summarized in Table 4.2. If all patients with HS are considered, rather than only those who come to surgical resection, then the observations divide into the asymmetric HS cases and the symmetric HS cases. The latter can be seen in children with very bad seizures and syndromes other than TLE. These children may have a very poor intellectual and life prognosis and are best known to pediatricians where intellectual and milestone gains are lost with every bout of bad seizures. The mechanism of damage is easier to understand in these cases, with seizures being postulated to cause neuroexcitotoxic release of neurotransmitters or other substances, and the damage occurring to the most vulnerable areas (see Fig. 4.4 and Table 4.2), although it may include other areas to a lesser extent (318). The individuals most affected may have a high vulnerability to damage via unknown, possibly genetic mechanisms (347–349). See also the model presented below, and the discussion of secondary damage from seizures.

+HS, Where Hippocampal Sclerosis is Present in Addition to Another Clearly Identified Lesion (Such as a Focal Tumor or Definite Dysplasia)

This group is the well-known 'dual pathology' problem in epilepsy. We do not include nonspecific white matter signal changes as part of this, as this only sometimes represents true dual pathology such as dysplasia (252). In cases that have a predominantly unilateral or asymmetric nature, the condition is easier to understand if we assume that the hippocampal damage is initiated by a seizure that persists beyond a neurotoxic threshold in one temporal lobe because of a focal abnormality (Fig. 4.54) in that hemisphere. This is supported by an analysis of the side of an extrahippocampal lesion and the side of HS (see Table 4.2).

It is tempting to suggest that all unilateral HS cases without dual pathology may be hiding some undetected focal

abnormality but the evidence for this does not exist in all cases. In some examples a focal microscopic abnormality might be present in the resection specimen and we would consider these to be +HS. In cases such as the one shown in Figure 4.44, the sequence of events has been proved by MRI observations to occur in this way. In some cases the seizure may not have an underlying structural abnormality, such as a febrile seizure. More important here might be the structures that maintain and prolong the seizure. When seizures are prolonged, the vulnerable structures may be affected by supraphysiologic release of excitatory neurotransmitters. This mechanism might be lateralizing if there is a priming event. If the seizures are prolonged and involve vulnerable structures in their mechanism of maintenance and spread, then damage may be diffuse, with the most vulnerable structures being most affected (Fig. 4.55). One can postulate that there are many factors, such as immune response, synaptic release of neurotransmitter, blood flow response, and many others that may be important in the threshold at which damage occurs (Fig. 4.56).

It is clear that not all abnormalities currently labeled HS are the same thing. HS, like congestive cardiac failure, is not a diagnosis but a pathologic endpoint for a number of different processes that need to be diagnosed. Increasing sophistication in understanding these differences will lead to better understanding of the process of epileptogenesis, and treatment correctly tailored to each patient. Determining whether the patient has +HS or HS+ or some hippocampal abnormality such as dysplasia that includes some features of HS is critical in correct treatment and preventing late seizure recurrence (349, 350). It is likely that, when HS exists, it is the most highly epileptogenic lesion and may mask the presence of another pathology with lesser epileptogenicity until surgical resection is performed.

Two ways in which seizures might cause lateralised HS and damage

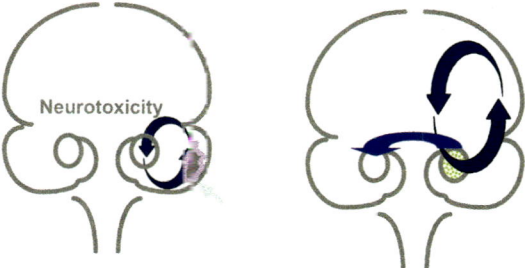

FIG. 4.54. Persistence of an epileptic seizure in one temporal lobe due to abnormality, in this case in the cortex (left). Once hippocampal sclerosis is present, the areas of maximal seizure spread are suggested in the right panel. This process could represent two stages of damage, the first to establish hippocampal sclerosis and the second that accounts for the other areas of damage seen with hippocampal sclerosis (HS+).

Bilateral symmetric hippocampal damage

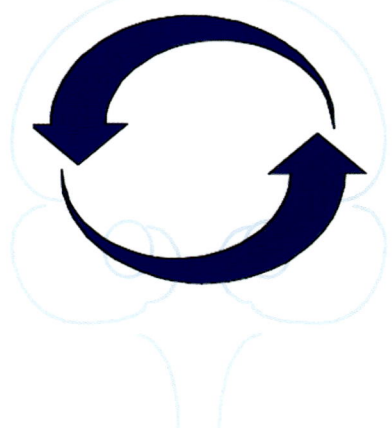

FIG. 4.55. In cases where there is bilateral symmetric hippocampal damage, seizures may involve the whole brain with no specific focality. Bilateral hippocampal damage may be because of a severe seizure or vulnerable brain.

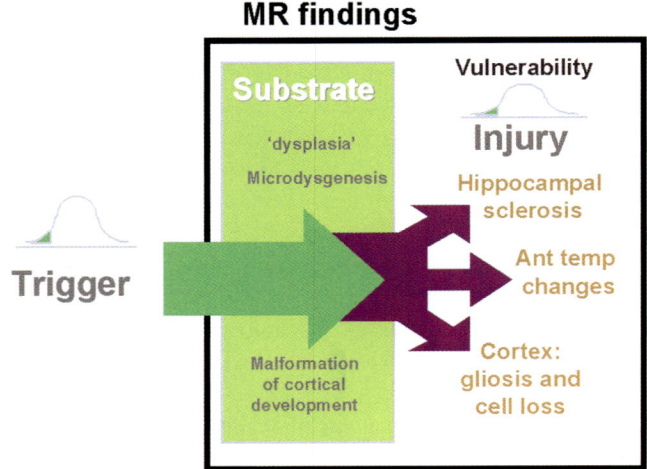

FIG. 4.56. The elements that may be important in the genesis of hippocampal sclerosis and the MR findings in this condition. There needs to be a trigger to the first seizure: this can include a genetic background and environmental factors (such as a fever). The 'bell' curve is intended to suggest that only some of the population will be affected in this way. This trigger than acts on the brain substrate to cause injury. The 'MR findings' in the brain may be a combination of pre-existing development and injury. The 'bell' curve suggests that there may be a distribution of individual vulnerability to a given seizure load, with some individuals having more damage from supraphysiologic release of neurotransmitters than others. This may include factors such as the response to inflammation.

Evidence of Initial Precipitating Insults in Patients with Hippocampal Sclerosis

Patients with chronic, refractory TLE associated with HS often report a significant event that happened several months or years prior to the onset of the habitual seizures. Overall, 60–80% of HS patients have had such an initial precipitating injury. The most common initial precipitating injury is prolonged febrile convulsions during infancy or early childhood (48). Complicated febrile convulsions have been reported in around 50% of cases of HS (94, 98, 130, 150, 155, 351). Other factors that are typically regarded as risk factors for epilepsy are severe perinatal events (documented intraventricular hemorrhage, skull fracture, severe birth asphyxia defined as failure to establish spontaneous respiration within 20 minutes of birth, Apgar 0–3 at 5 min, or umbilical artery pH <7.0), severe postnatal head injury (documented coma for >2 h, documented contusion, or cerebral hemorrhage), significant cerebral infection (documented viral encephalitis, bacterial meningitis, or cerebral abscess), stroke (intracerebral hemorrhage or major cerebral infarction), and cerebral tumour (48, 155). However, these risk factors have been associated with a variety of types of epilepsy and may not all be a risk factor for the development of HS.

This is in contrast to domoic acid intoxication, a glutamic acid analog, which causes a limbic status epilepticus, specifically causing hippocampal damage and HS, with development of TLE (302). Further, minor risk factors have often

been associated with epilepsy, such as prematurity, low birthweight, mild head injuries, and uncomplicated febrile seizures. However, there is no scientific proof that they predispose to HS or epilepsy.

Evidence for Hippocampal Sclerosis as an Acquired, Subsequently Epileptogenic Lesion

The presence of an initial precipitating insult suggests an acquired etiology of HS. It is thought that these early events could damage the hippocampal tissue, so that after some reorganization process, this tissue could then become epileptogenic. A major proportion of the patients with antecedent events have had a prolonged febrile convulsion. In humans, it has been proposed that there is a critical period (up to 5 years) when the hippocampus is susceptible to damage from prolonged seizures (352–354). It has been supposed that the adult human hippocampus is resistant to these changes except in special cases such as domoic acid poisoning (302). This may suggest that a prolonged seizure early in life may be particularly likely to induce a cascade of events leading to HS.

Indeed, several recent MRI studies have shown that prolonged (febrile) convulsions can damage the hippocampus acutely, with progressive changes to HS in the following months (297, 355, 356). VanLandingham et al. (357) performed MRI scans in 15 infants with focal complicated febrile convulsions and 12 infants with generalized febrile convulsions. In four of the 15 infants with focal complicated febrile convulsions, acute hippocampal damage was found, characterized by an increased hippocampal T2 signal and volume, consistent with edema. Follow-up MRI in two infants showed progression to HS.

Long duration of seizures appears to be a major determinant of hippocampal damage and development of HS (351). Nohria et al. (358) reported a single case, which demonstrates that the signal change and atrophy of the hippocampus did not precede the episode of status that occurred in their child. Tien et al. (129) also report a study of the hippocampus in five children presenting with status epilepticus and no previous history of an epilepsy disorder. In two patients with a long follow-up, hippocampal atrophy developed in the later imaging.

Wieshmann (356) reported bilateral increased T2 signal in an adult after prolonged generalized seizures. Hippocampal atrophy was present bilaterally at 2 months and progressive bilateral atrophy subsequently occurred. This is further evidence that hippocampal injury secondary to seizures can occur in an adult human. Van Paesschen (359) followed new-onset epilepsy patients with T2 relaxometry of the hippocampus over a 1-year period and found that hippocampal injury, as measured by T2, progressed in one patient with daily seizures. It has also been observed that hippocampal injury can occur in patients who have had encephalitis or meningitis and is seen as subtle bilateral hippocampal volume loss (360).

Animal experiments have delivered similar results. Hippocampal neuronal loss can be induced in animals by seizure activity or subconvulsive electrical stimulation in the amygdala, hippocampus, and other structures (361–363), even in the absence of hypoxia (155, 352, 353, 364). This suggests that excitotoxicity is an important mechanism of the neuronal damage in the hippocampus.

In stroke, where hypoxia and hypoperfusion are the cause of tissue damage, glutamate neurotoxicity as well as the ischaemia leads to much of the neuronal damage (365). A mechanism like this has also been postulated in epilepsy (366). This is the basis for neuroprotective agents being trialed early in the course of stroke. Excess glutamate release occurs in seizures, and its action on N-methyl D-aspartate (NMDA) receptors leading to calcium influx, and a subsequent cascade of intracellular events leading to cell death, is hypothesized to be a cause of neuronal damage in HS (367, 368). The regions of the hippocampus that are typically affected in HS patients (CA1 and CA4) have a high density of NMDA receptors.

The Process of Epileptogenesis After an Initial Precipitating Event

There is usually an interval between the initial precipitating event and the onset of habitual seizures (155). This interval has been called the silent or latent period. During this interval, the epileptogenic lesion may develop, suggesting that HS is, at least in the beginning, a progressive and dynamic disease (48, 124). The age at initial injury has been reported to be inversely correlated with the latent interval (155). In two independent quantitative MRI studies using a combination of hippocampal volumetry and T2 mapping, age at onset of the habitual epilepsy correlated inversely with the extent of hippocampal damage, i.e. patients with bilateral severe HS had the earliest age of onset of TLE and patients with normal hippocampi the latest (130, 244). Further, the amount of hippocampal damage correlated with the number of secondary generalized seizures during the patient's life time. This could mean that the extent of hippocampal damage during the initial precipitating injury determines the duration of the latent interval and the severity of the habitual epilepsy, i.e. Sloviter's dentate lamellar hypothesis (369).

There is also indication that the silent interval could be influenced by genetic factors (370). In an animal model of HS and TLE, however, severity of epilepsy was determined only by the shortness of the latent period, regardless of duration of status epilepticus and the amount of hippocampal damage (371). This could mean that the amount of hippocampal damage is secondary to the severity of epileptic seizures.

Unanswered Questions With the Model of Acquired Etiology

Overall, these reports give compelling evidence for the development of HS after an initial precipitating insult, for an acquired etiology of HS. This evidence is particularly strong for the effects of prolonged febrile convulsions. Nevertheless, it is still not clear whether these observed cases represent a common pattern or whether they are exceptional cases. There are several still unanswered questions: There are still a significant number of patients with chronic epilepsy and HS in whom, even after most careful inspection of all childhood records, no precipitating events can be detected. HS is typically unilateral, whereas the febrile convulsions appear to be generalized; it is not clear why one hippocampus should be more vulnerable to the damaging effects of the early seizure.

Evidence that Hippocampal Sclerosis Might be a 'Developmental' Lesion

A pre-existing hippocampal abnormality could be a risk factor for the development of febrile convulsions and HS. Fernández and colleagues (372) performed MRI studies in 23 members of two families. Of these, 13 had a history of febrile convulsions and two of TLE. The two patients with TLE (those with the longest and most numerous febrile convulsions) had left HS. Eleven patients with febrile convulsions and no TLE and six asymptomatic persons had small left hippocampal volumes. In one family, mainly the hippocampal heads were affected and in the other family the hippocampal body. A pre-existing inherited unilateral hippocampal abnormality, which appears to be causally related to the febrile convulsions, could explain why HS is often unilateral.

Genetic predisposition may play a role in the pathogenesis of HS, which traditionally has not been regarded to have a major genetic contribution (349). HS in familial TLE may be under-reported (373). Corey et al. (374) reported a genetic predisposition for status epilepticus. Kanemoto et al. (375) reported a strong association of a polymorphism in the interleukin-1β gene in patients with TLE and HS compared with nonepileptic controls and patients with TLE and no HS. Interleukin-1β is a proinflammatory cytokine that modulates neurotoxic neurotransmission and prolongs kainate-induced seizures by enhancing glutamatergic neurotransmission (347). This genetic predisposition, therefore, could predispose to the development of HS after febrile convulsions.

Evidence that Hippocampal Sclerosis is a Combination of Several Factors

The origins of HS are not simple (44, 349). The MRI data provide a greater understanding of what causes HS. It becomes increasingly clear that there are a number of factors that are important in the pathogenesis of HS. Much is now known and consensus occurs on many points. We think that a framework is useful in solving the remaining puzzle understanding the factors that are important in the development of HS (Fig. 4.56).

Clearly HS occurs as a consequence of a cascade of events in individuals of differing genetic makeup. The susceptibility to an initiating event such as febrile seizures will vary in the population. A single seizure in someone who has had a prolonged febrile convulsion may have different consequences from a seizure in an individual who has not had this (priming). Increasing evidence suggests that the damage threshold for each individual may be different. MR has given us the opportunity to understand many of these factors in each of our patients. Contributions from genetic assessment will no doubt add more of the missing pieces (349).

We think that some factor leads to the first seizure. This may be a developmental abnormality, a foreign tissue lesion, or subtle dysplasia (even sometimes in the hippocampus). For a seizure to be prolonged, it involves a circuit. The hippocampus is likely to be critically involved in this circuit (see Fig. 4.54). In some cases seizures may involve the whole brain and both hippocampi, and lead to bilateral symmetrical disease (see Fig. 4.55). In cases where one hemisphere leads for some reason, such as the presence of focal pathology, only one hippocampus may be involved in sustaining the seizure (see Fig. 4.54).

There are clearly factors in the individual that determine the degree of damage that occurs as a consequence of such sustained seizure activity. It may be the inflammatory response, the persistence of activity at the synapse, or the release and reuptake of glutamine that is important. Whatever factors are important, it is clear that some individuals experience more 'damage' from seizures than others who apparently have the same insult. Understanding the genetics of these individuals is likely to give further insights into this process.

Outcome After Temporal Lobe Resection of Hippocampal Sclerosis

Two-thirds of patients with HS are rendered seizure-free after anterior temporal lobectomy (19, 112, 350, 376–379) and there has been little change in this figure over time or across centers (Fig. 4.57). The single most important predictor of good outcome after anterior temporal lobectomy is the presence of unilateral HS on MRI (124, 380). Patients with unilateral HS and scalp interictal epileptic discharges concordant with location of ictal onset have an excellent surgical outcome in 94%. On the other hand, only 60% of patients with unilateral HS and bitemporal EEG changes have a good surgical outcome (380).

In the case of HS, there is a continuing incidence of seizures that occur even after many years of seizure freedom. The cause of this is not known in all cases. Sometimes incomplete resection of the hippocampus might be the cause. In some patients we are aware of, another, usually developmental, lesion has been found on repeat investigation with advanced MR investigations. These are almost always ipsilateral to the temporal resection but not always in

the temporal lobe. If one considers that at least 30% of HS cases will have 'macroscopic' dual pathology, one can speculate that there might be two epileptogenic lesions in these patients – the HS, which is intractable and has been treated by the resection, and another less epileptogenic lesion that may have had a part in the pathogenesis of the epilepsy and can independently cause seizures every few years. It is chastening, when we see cases such as this, to realize that what appeared to be straightforward TLE with mesial onset at the time of surgery can be found to have another possibly significant lesion that we were unable to detect at the time.

Mesial Temporal Lobe Epilepsy with Hippocampal Sclerosis: a Syndrome?

Mesial TLE with HS as its cause is not recognized in the classification of epileptic syndromes (3) (see Chapter 1). It is nonetheless an important entity that has a special significance because of the potential for surgical cure of a psychosocially and medically disabling illness.

If there is a syndrome deserving special attention, it is the following. Patients have an increased familial incidence of febrile convulsions in early childhood. Typically, patients have a history of complicated febrile seizures during the first years of life. After a silent period lasting from 3 to 20 years, patients develop complex partial seizures. At first, seizures may be controlled on anticonvulsants, but with time, intractable seizures become the dominant feature. The clinical symptoms include visceral and experiential auras, with other auras less commonly seen. The patients often report an aura followed by arrest of activity and clouding of consciousness. Oroalimentary and manual automatisms followed by contralateral dystonic posturing of the upper extremity are often present. Postictal confusion with dysphasia (dominant hemisphere) are also prominent.

Neurologic evaluation usually reveals no focal neurologic findings, although studies have reported facial asymmetries in patients with mesial temporal sclerosis (381). Material specific memory deficits can sometimes be detected using sophisticated neuropsychologic testing, particularly when the epilepsy arises in the dominant hemisphere.

Electroencephalographic studies demonstrate interictal sharp and slow wave activity from the anterior temporal regions. Interictal activity is usually increased during stage 1 sleep and may become bilateral with slow sleep stages. Ictal scalp recordings usually show lateralizing rhythmic theta activity, and with intracranial recordings focal discharges originating in the hippocampus and amygdala are commonly seen.

Imaging features include the classical MRI abnormalities described in this chapter and functional studies (PET and SPECT) demonstrate metabolic and blood flow pattern abnormalities showing lateralized defects involving the abnormal temporal lobe (chapter PET and SPECT).

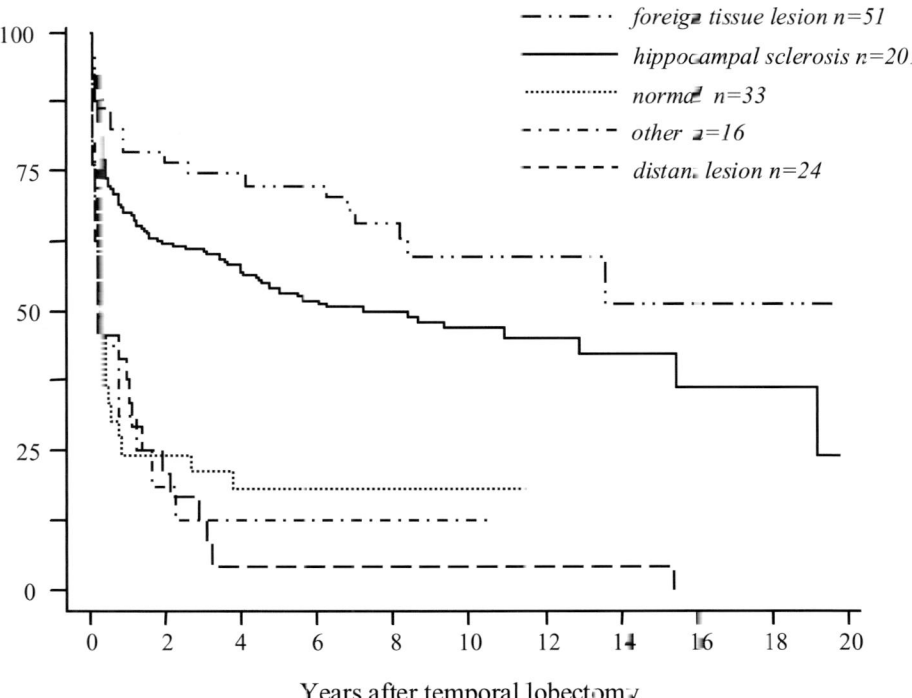

FIG. 4.57. Actuarial analysis of temporal lobectomy outcome by preoperative MRI diagnosis. McIntosh AM, Kalnins RM, Mitchell LA, Fabinyi GCA, Briellmann RS, Berkovic SF. Temporal lobectomy: long term seizure outcome, late recurrence and risks for seizure recurrence. *Brain* 2004; 127:2018–2030.

Recognition of this syndrome is of great importance since it is clear that surgical treatment is the most appropriate therapeutic intervention in many of these patients.

These issues have been discussed recently by the ILAE commission, which we recommend as additional reading.

FOREIGN TISSUE LESIONS

Detailed analysis of MRI images has revealed a high percentage of abnormalities that can be detected in the brains of patients with intractable partial epilepsy. This is to be expected. Partial epilepsy either has a focal area that is the origin of the seizures (see Chapter 1) or the seizures themselves may affect areas involved in seizures. MR techniques can now detect these

Apart from mesial temporal sclerosis, other epileptogenic lesions commonly seen in the temporal lobes of patients with epilepsy include tumors, vascular malformations, developmental lesions, etc. In this group we have classified different tumors and vascular lesions. In general, these lesions constitute approximately 10–15% of the abnormalities found at pathology in surgical series (12, 90, 91, 95, 127, 162, 188, 382–386). Mathieson (95) reported the pathologic findings in 503 patients operated at the MNI between 1961 and 1970. Of the 503, 301 (60%) had temporal lobe resections. Gliomas were present in 13% of specimens whereas vascular malformations were observed in

only six patients. Bruton, in his review from the Maudsley series, reported alien or foreign tissue lesions in 38 (15%) out of 249 cases of temporal lobe resection (127). This group included specimens with ganglioglial, neuronoglial, glial, vascular, and oligodendroglial lesions.

Neoplasms

Astrocytic Tumors

Bruton reported that astrocytic tumors constituted 3.6% of the total sample of patients and 18% of those with alien lesions. These lesions may present as discrete masses or as more extensive lesions. Interestingly, Bruton reported that most cases were pathologically localized and involved the parahippocampal gyrus and the amygdala. The histologic type consisted of predominantly fibrillary astrocytomas but protoplasmic type astrocytic tumors were also observed. It is difficult to compare the present and long-term behavior of these lesions with the data reported by Mathieson and Bruton. In their series, patients were often diagnosed at surgery whereas at present any patient who has this type of lesion will be operated without delay (387–391).

Magnetic resonance imaging is able to detect these lesions in almost all cases if the appropriate imaging sequences are carried out. Although the sensitivity of MRI is almost 100%, its specificity has not paralleled its sensitivity. However, the information provided by MRI regarding intrinsic tissue characteristics in neoplasms, and in particular among gliomas, is important and should be exploited fully. A variety of nondifferentiating features are present, the most consistent being the presence of a mass lesion with signal inhomogeneity (392, 393). Variable MRI presentations will include high signal on T1- and T2-weighted images or isosignal on T1 images but high signal on T2 images. Solid as well as cystic components may be present with variable signal from the cystic components (Fig. 4.58). In most cases, the signal arising from the cystic formation may be isointense with CSF on all sequences; short T_R/T_E, long T_R/short T_E, and long T_R/long T_E (394). However, not uncommonly neoplastic cysts may have higher signal than CSF on long T_R/short T_E images because of the presence of high protein content on the cavity (Table 4.5).

The most frequent type of astrocytoma is the fibrillary type (390, 395). This tumor comprises about 75% of hemispheric astrocytomas of adults. In children, they are usually localized to the brain stem. Histologically, these tumors manifest diffuse cellular heterogeneity and are consistent in nature. Pleomorphic xanthoastrocytomas can also occur in these patients (Fig. 4.59) MRI usually demonstrates homogenous masses but cystic lesions may also be seen (Figs 4.58, 4.60). Calcifications are present in 20% of cases. The location is variable with cortical lesions reported in a number of patients but extension into the white matter is common.

Conversely, small lesions involving the mesial structures can be detected (Fig. 4.61).

Although highly anaplastic tumors or glioblastomas are the most frequent in this group, for obvious reasons they do not constitute a significant number of those patients referred with intractable epilepsy (390). In some occasions, we have seen patients with small lesions and intractable epilepsy who, at pathology, demonstrate lower-grade gliomas but subsequently evolved into more aggressive tumors (Fig. 4.62).

Pilocystic astrocytomas are more frequent in children. Most commonly these tumors are located in the diencephalon but occasionally may be present in the cerebral hemispheres (395, 396). These lesions on MRI differ from the fibrillary tumors in being sharply demarcated. They also are often lobular in nature. The lesions tend to be hypointense on T1 images whereas they are highly hyperintense on long T2 sequence (Fig. 4.63). In contrast to fibrillary astrocytomas, contrast enhancement is present and may be marked and is due to the prominent vascularity of these lesions. Edema is rare and calcifications are not seen (Fig. 4.64) (393, 396).

Xanthoastrocytomas usually occur in the first decade of life, with most patients having a favorable course. Cystic components are more common in this tumor. Histologically, moderate cellular pleomorphism is present and mononuclear infiltrates are common. This tumor is usually located in the temporal or parietal regions.

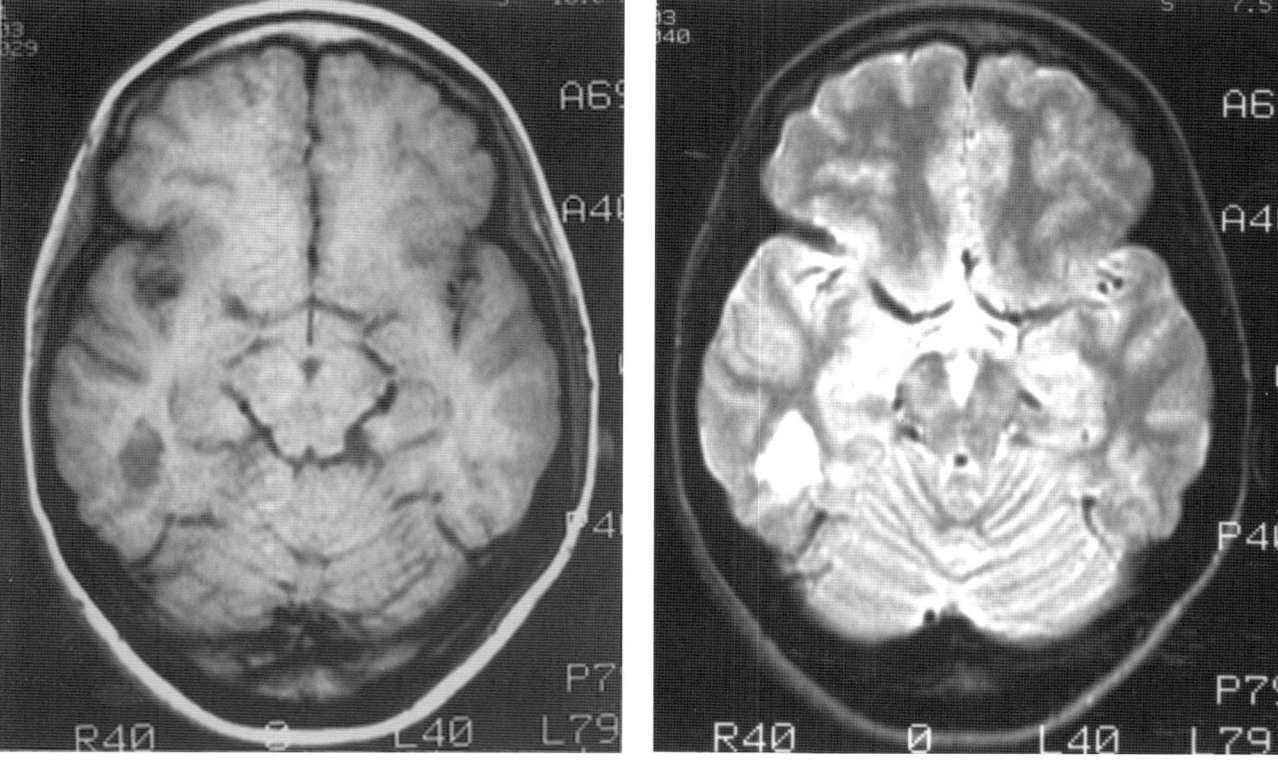

A   B

FIG. 4.58. Fibrillary astrocytoma in a patient with intractable seizures. **A.** Axial T1 (600/20) MR image shows small hypointense lesion in the right posterior temporal region without mass effect. **B.** T2 (2500/80) image shows increased signal from the lesion.

Table 4.5. MRI Characteristics of Astrocytic Neoplasms

	Fibrillary	Pilocystic	Anaplastic	Gliomatosis
Common sites	Cerebral hemisphere (adult)	Cerebral hemisphere (adult)	Cerebral hemisphere (adult)	Cerebral hemisphere (adult)
Signal changes	Homogeneous intensity	Cystic Demarcated	Heterogeneous	Ill defined
Contrast	Variable	Common dense	Common irregular	Uncommon

Oligodendrogliomas

Oligodendrogliomas are histologically characterized by the presence of compact groups of large, rounded cells with empty cytoplasm (Fig. 4.65). In almost half the cases, the tumors are mixed with glial components. Calcifications are frequent, with calcium deposits in the intrinsic blood vessels (393, 397–399). These tumors are less frequent than astrocytomas and also infrequent in our experience in patients referred for intractable epilepsy. In Bruton's series, oligodendroglioma only represented 2.4% of the total population. Interestingly, these lesions are located in most cases within the temporal lobe and tend to involve the amygdala. The uncus and parahippocampal gyrus are also frequently involved, both on pathology and on MRI, with sparing of the middle and inferior temporal convolutions. The underlying white matter, however, is often infiltrated by the tumor.

Magnetic resonance imaging often reveals heterogeneous masses located superficially in the frontal lobes but also more mesially in the temporal regions. Cystic components and hemorrhages may be seen within the masses. Calcifications are more frequent than in astrocytomas and can be difficult to detect with conventional spin-echo techniques. Gradient-echo sequences are more sensitive for the detection of calcifications. Mild to moderate enhancement has been reported in half the patients but edema is rarely

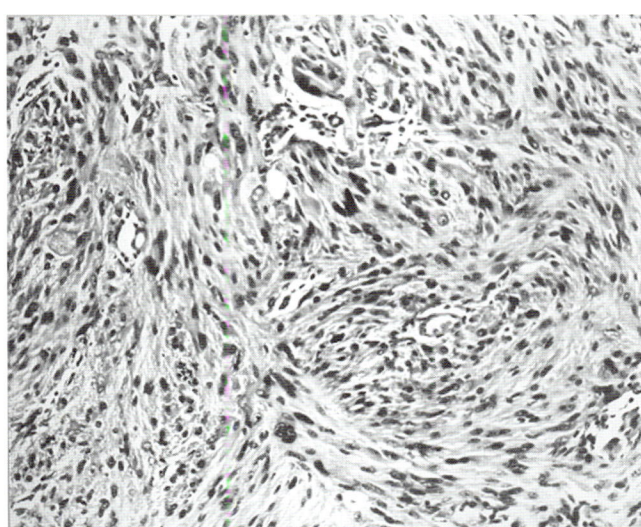

FIG. 4.59. Pleomorphic xanthoastrocytoma. Long-standing intractable temporal lobe seizures. Palisading pattern with astrocytic proliferation (hematoxylin and eosin, ×200).

observed (Fig. 4.66). The most typical features differentiating oligodendromas from fibrillary astrocytomas are the heterogeneity, the presence of calcifications, and the superficial location (393, 400).

Mixed Glial Lesions

Mixed glial lesions were reported by Bruton in 5.2% of patients and were the most frequent type of alien tissue lesion (Fig. 4.67). Calcifications are often present. The age of seizure onset appeared to differ from the other lesions, with seizures beginning at an early age in most patients. These tumors are predominantly seen in young patients (under age 14) (176, 385, 401). Tampieri et al. (402) reported that 17 of 19 of their patients presented with seizures before the age of 16. According to Bruton, gangliogliomas and ganglioglial lesions are common in the temporal lobe, representing approximately 10% of lesions in this group. In fact, compared with other neoplasms, gangliogliomas are usually found in the temporal lobes.

There are controversial issues regarding the proper classification of these lesions. The histologic features resemble a mixed glial abnormality with giant nerve cells, resembling ganglion cells, but in some cases a mixed astrocytic component can be seen (Fig. 4.68). In some lesions, there is a paucity of glial cells with a predominance of ganglion cells. These lesions are sometimes classified as gangliocytomas (403). Calcification is also common. Similarly to other possible developmental lesions, gangliogliomas tend to spare the lateral temporal neocortex, with primary involvement of the mesial structures.

Magnetic resonance imaging often demonstrates a *solid mass lesion* in the temporal lobe. At times a partially cystic component may be present (Fig. 4.68). The cystic component has been observed in 25–30% of patients. Inhomogeneous signals on T1 and high signal on T2 images or high signal in both T1 and T2 sequences can be seen. Isointense signal on T1 and inversion recovery sequences can be observed in some patients. Calcifications may be present and may be detected using gradient-echo images. Pathology may show binucleated cytoplasmic changes (Fig. 4.69).

Dysembryoplastic Neuroepithelial Tumors

Dysembryoplastic neuroepithelial tumors (DNET) (404, 405) have become an important cause of intractable partial

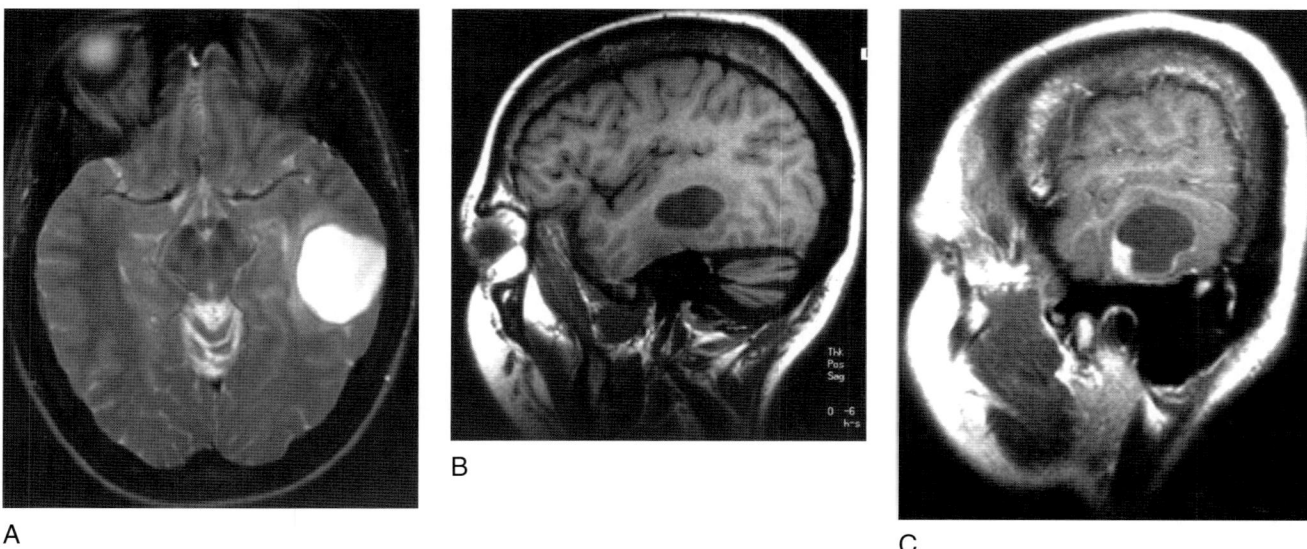

FIG. 4.60. Astrocytoma, cystic type, in patient with a 10-year history of partial seizures. **A.** Axial T2 MR image showing a high signal intensity with minimal mass effect but no edema. **B.** Sagittal T1 image showing a cystic cavity with a signal slightly less hypointense than CSF. **C.** Gadolinium shows partial enhancement of the wall.

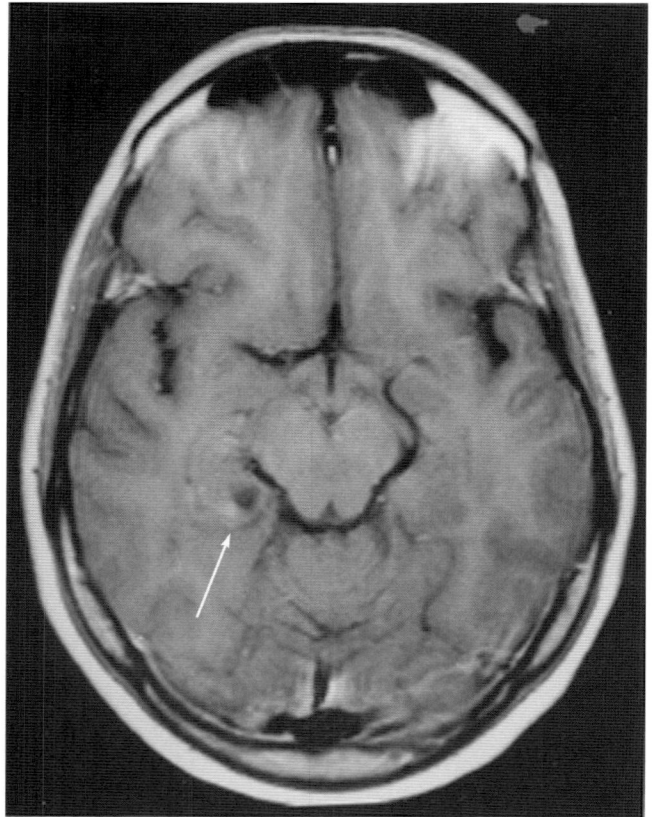

FIG. 4.61. Astrocytoma in a patient with long-standing complex partial seizures. Axial (550/15) gadolinium study shows a small hypointense lesion in the right posterior hippocampus. Minimal enhancement is noticed (arrow).

seizures. These tumors are commonly seen in young patients who present with intractable seizures. They constitute approximately 10% of all tumors removed in patients with intractable epilepsy. In fact, Daumas-Duport and colleagues reported that, among their 265 patients operated for intractable seizures between 1964 and 1983, 20 had DNET tumors.

The tumors are usually located in the temporal region. Daumas-Duport and colleagues (404, 405) reported that, in their series, 62% of tumors were in the temporal region, whereas the frontal lobe was involved in 30% of patients and very few individuals had parietal occipital tumors. Microscopically, these tumors are obvious at the cortical surface. Cystic formation is uncommon. The tumors usually involve both gray and white matter. Microscopically, they are characterized by a high degree of cellular pleomorphism with multiple cell types, including astrocytes, oligodendrocytes, and neurons. Prior to the relatively recent recognition of this as a distinct pathologic entity, many of these lesions were labeled as oligoastrocytomas. In many of these lesions, regions of glial neuronal elements are primarily based in the center of the lesions with areas of nodular foci and areas of cortical dysplasia in the margins of the glial neuronal elements.

Daumas-Duport considered these lesions to be benign because of their excessive proliferation of cells, long-standing chronic symptomatology, and lack of evidence of tumor recurrence after resection. In addition, the possible embryologic origin of these lesions is based on the presence of mixed population of cells and their location (temporal and frontal).

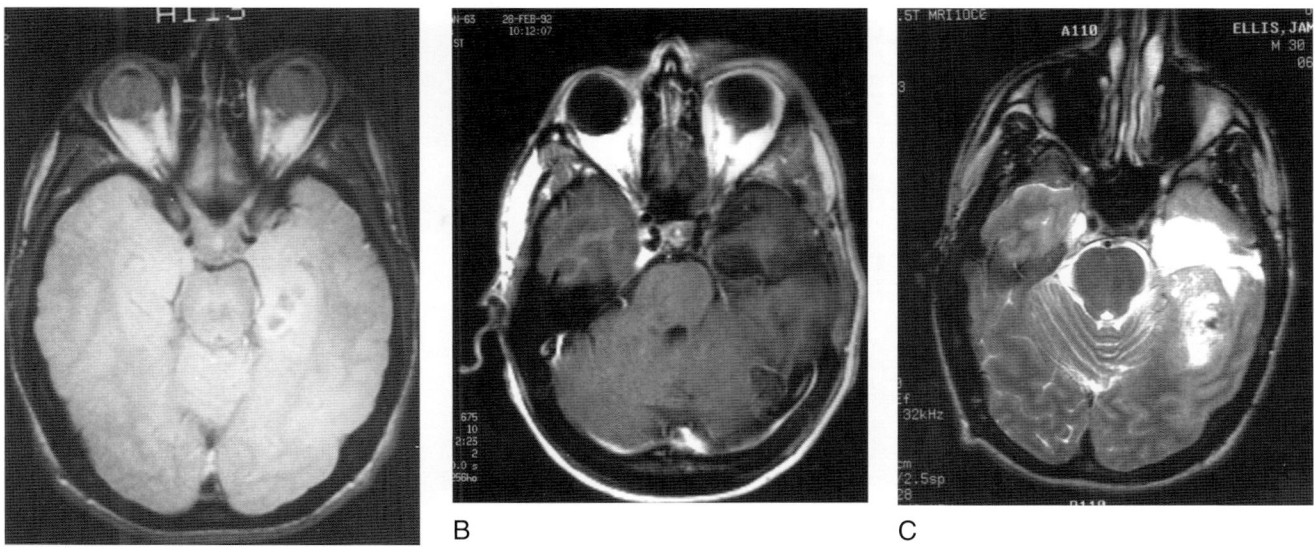

FIG. 4.62. Evolution of a tumor in a young patient with intractable partial seizures of 2 years' duration. The CT findings were negative. **A.** First MR image: axial (2000/30) study shows a heterogeneous lesion on the left mesial temporal region. Calcifications were present. Pathologic examination demonstrated oligodendroglioma. **B.** Follow-up MR image (675/10) 1 year after surgery. The patient was seizure-free and not receiving medication. **C.** Follow-up MR image 2 years after initial surgery. Headaches had developed. An abnormal signal was detected with a lesion in the posterior temporal lobe. Biopsy revealed an anaplastic astrocytoma.

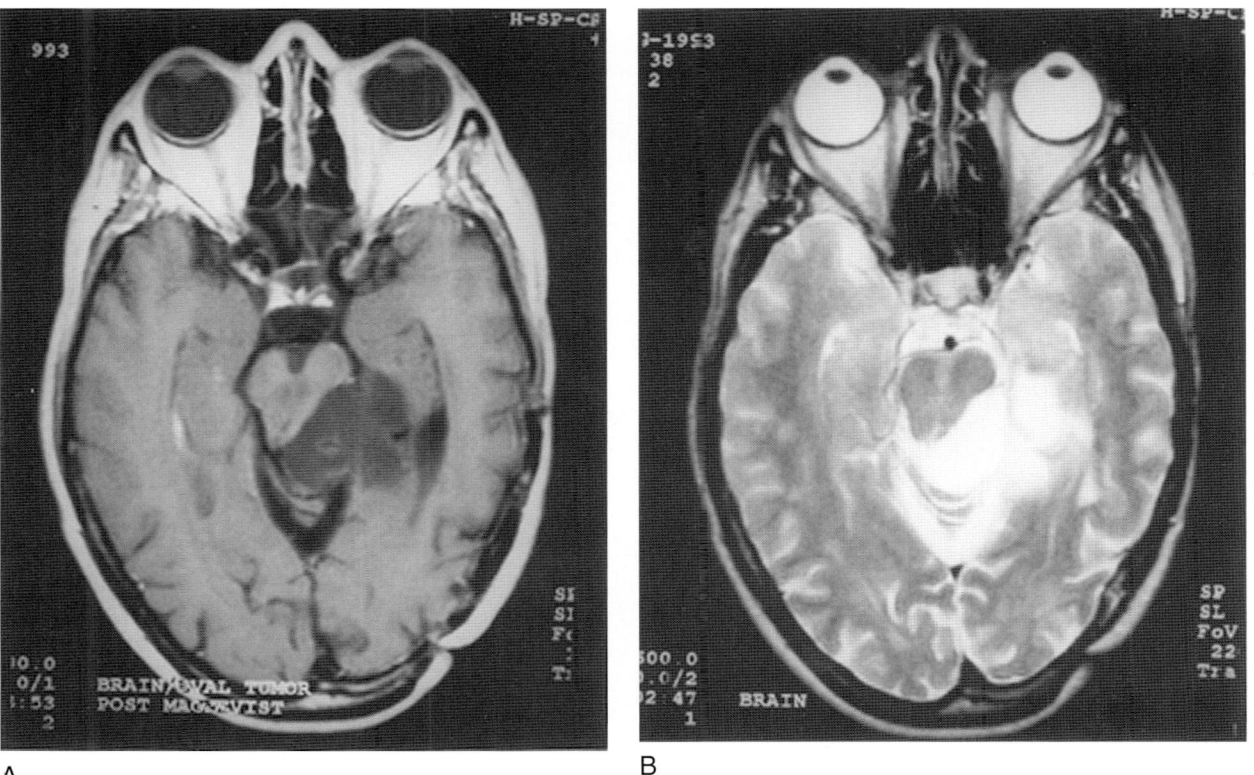

FIG. 4.63. Pilocystic astrocytoma. **A.** Axial MRI (600/15) with contrast shows hypointense lesion involving the posterior temporal lobe with a mass effect on the brain stem. No enhancement is noted. **B.** T2 axial MRI (3,600/90) demonstrates a high signal similar to cerebrospinal fluid.

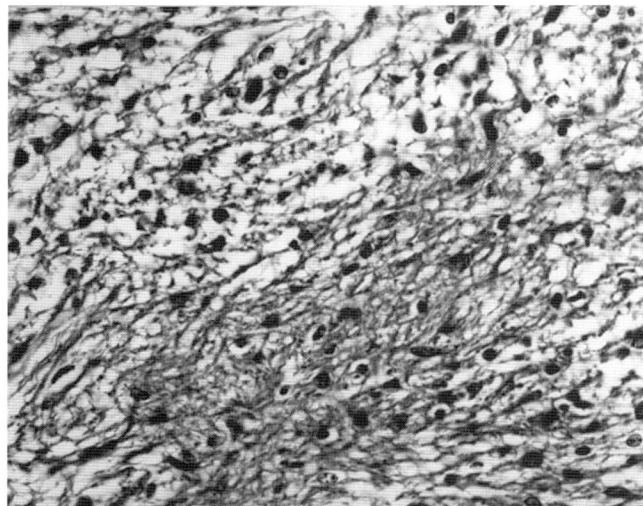

FIG. 4.64. The histologic type is pilocystic astrocytoma. Mildly pleomorphic astrocytic nuclei with hair-like processes in a multicystic background (hematoxylin and eosin, ×200).

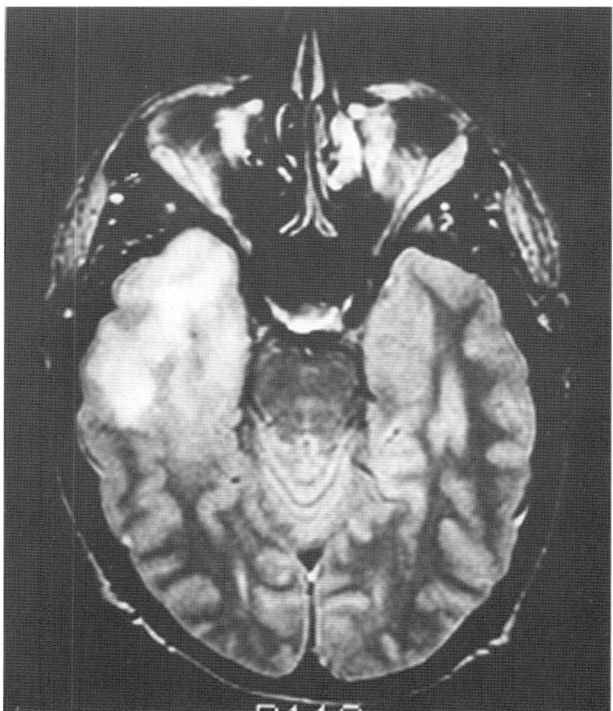

A

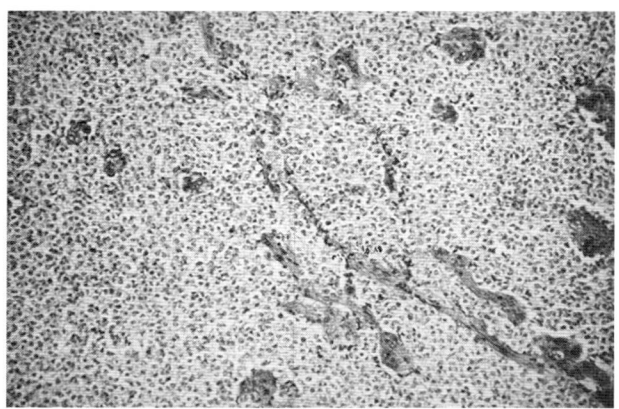

A

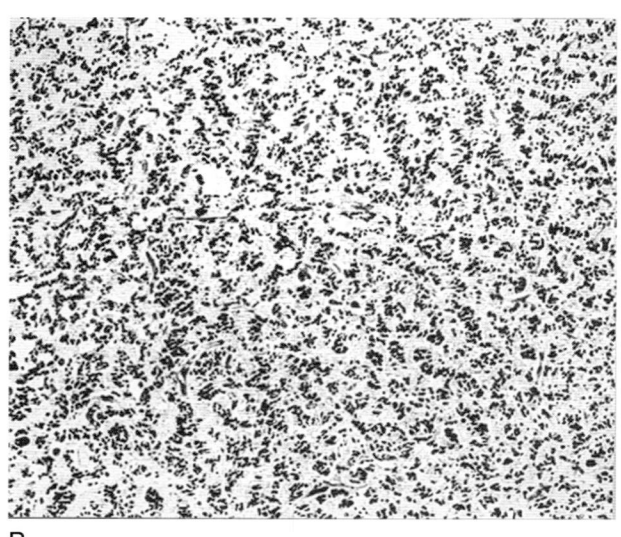

B

FIG. 4.65. The histologic type is oligodendroglioma. **A.** A typical pattern was found of a highly cellular and compact collection of regular spherical nuclei and clear cytoplasm without neurologic fibers (×200). **B.** Nuclear palisading pattern can be seen in some cases (hematoxylin and eosin, ×l00).

B

FIG. 4.66. Oligodendroglioma in a patient with partial seizures. **A.** Axial MR (3000/30) study shows a high signal abnormality over the right temporal lobe with prominent involvement of the white matter. **B.** Coronal MRI (2500/90) demonstrates white/gray matter involvement.

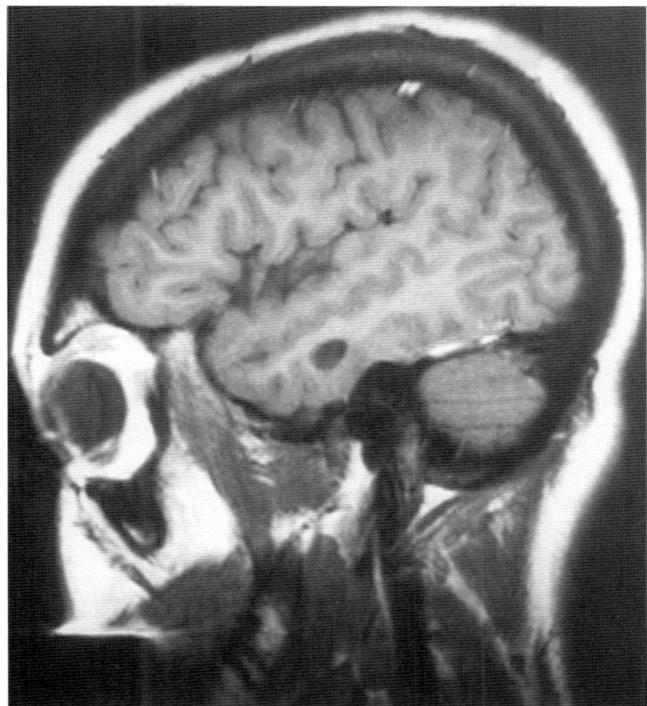

FIG. 4.67. Oligoastrocytoma in a patient with intractable partial complex seizures since age 4. Sagittal view demonstrates the cystic lesion. The CT findings were normal.

The clinical characteristics include seizures in 85% of patients before the age of 15 years. The seizures are disabling and drug-resistant in the majority of patients.

Imaging findings in patients with DNET tumors are quite characteristic. Koeller and Dillon (386) reported six cases of

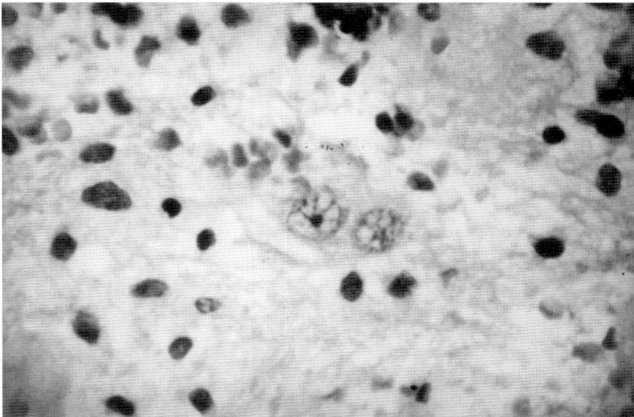

FIG. 4.69. Histologic type ganglioglioma. Magnification demonstrates binucleated cytoplasm changes typical of this tumor (hematoxylin and eosin, ×250).

DNET tumors. Five of the six were located in the temporal lobe, while one patient had an occipital lobe lesion. On CT scan, the lesions are hypodense and do not enhance with contrast. CT scans have been reported to be normal in some patients with abnormal MRIs. The lesions on MRI usually are well localized and hypointense on T1 images (Fig. 4.70). The lesions are usually hyperintense to gray matter on T2-weighted images. Enhancement is very uncommon, but has been reported. Although these lesions do not have edema and may resemble a benign cyst, increased signal intensity on proton density images should suggest the presence of a

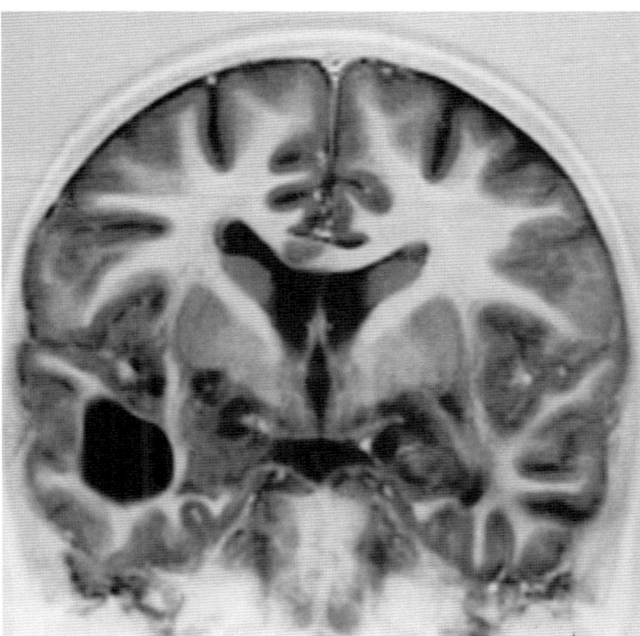

FIG. 4.68. Ganglioglioma. intractable seizures in a young patient. Coronal IR study shows left cystic cavity with signal isointense to cerebrospinal fluid. Note tumor location and primary white matter involvement.

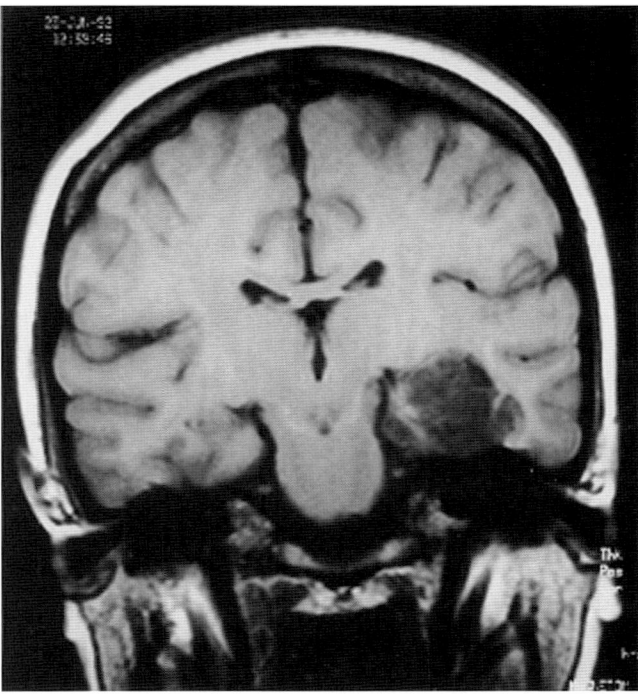

FIG. 4.70. Dysembryoplastic neuroepithelial tumor. Axial and coronal MRI (630/15) studies showing hypointense lesion in the left temporal lobe. On the axial image, the lesion appears to be slightly irregular in the center.

more complex lesion. Calcifications are less common when compared to calcifications in gangliogliomas. In most cases involving the temporal lobes, mesial and mesial plus temporal neocortical involvement is observed. The MR characteristics, although not pathognomonic of this condition, should strongly suggest the underlying abnormality (406–411).

Metastatic Disease

Metastatic spread of tumor to the brain is relatively common (412). Cerebral metastases comprise approximately 20% of brain neoplasms. A variety of neurologic symptoms are present in these patients. Seizures are the presenting symptom in approximately 30% of patients with cerebral metastasis. Metastasis have fairly stereotyped localization (gray-white matter junction) and often have peripheral edema. These lesions are easy to identify using enhanced and non-enhanced MRI. We will not discuss these lesions further since they are not associated with chronic intractable epilepsy in isolation.

Vascular Malformations

Although seizures and epilepsy are frequent presentations of vascular malformations of the brain, these lesions are less common (1–2%) among the alien lesions in patients with intractable epilepsy referred to epilepsy surgery. These abnormalities are less frequent in the temporal lobes compared to other regions.

Vascular malformations are a heterogenous group of lesions not only from the pathologic viewpoint but also as concerns the mechanisms associated with epilepsy (413–418). These malformations can be divided into arteriovenous malformations, cavernous angiomas, capillary telangiectasia, and venous angiomas (414, 419, 420). Capillary telangiectasias and venous angiomas are rarely associated with chronic seizures disorders and will not be discussed in detail.

Arteriovenous Malformations

Arteriovenous malformations (AVM) are the most common of the vascular malformations. Supratentorial involvement is seen in almost 80% of patients and usually the location follows the territory of the middle cerebral artery. In adults, the most common initial symptom is intracranial hemorrhage or seizures. Larger AVMs appear to present more commonly with seizures rather than hemorrhage. It is difficult to estimate the actual incidence of AVMs in the temporal lobes of patients with intractable epilepsy. Mathieson reported six such cases in the MNI series, being most frequent in the temporal lobes (95, 415, 416, 419). However, this may be related to patient selection and the type of referral for surgery.

Pathologically, AVMs are formed by a cluster of vessels with intermixed hemoglobin derivatives and adjacent gliosis. Brain tissue is usually not present between the vessels and mass effect is uncommon unless there has been previous bleeding. Angiography demonstrates arteriovenous shunting with tortuous feeding arteries and draining veins, although rarely an AVM may be thrombosed and angiographically occult.

On MRI, AVMs have typical features consistent with the underlying pathology. Dilated vascular structures with void signal are usually observed on spin-echo sequences arising from the abnormally dilated vessels. High signal may appear with gradient-echo techniques and it is related to the presence of slow flow in the venous phase. Adjacent gliosis or previous hemorrhage can be detected without difficulty and may be important in the generation of the epilepsy (Fig. 4.71).

The pathophysiology underlying chronic seizures in patients with AVMs is complex and is discussed below. Treatment decisions are made on the basis of potential bleeding from the lesion. Although no studies have been reported, differences between surgery, embolization, or radiation do not appear to influence seizure control except for complete lesion excision (421). Resection of the AVM and surrounding gliotic tissue may be needed in some cases, but no controlled studies are available.

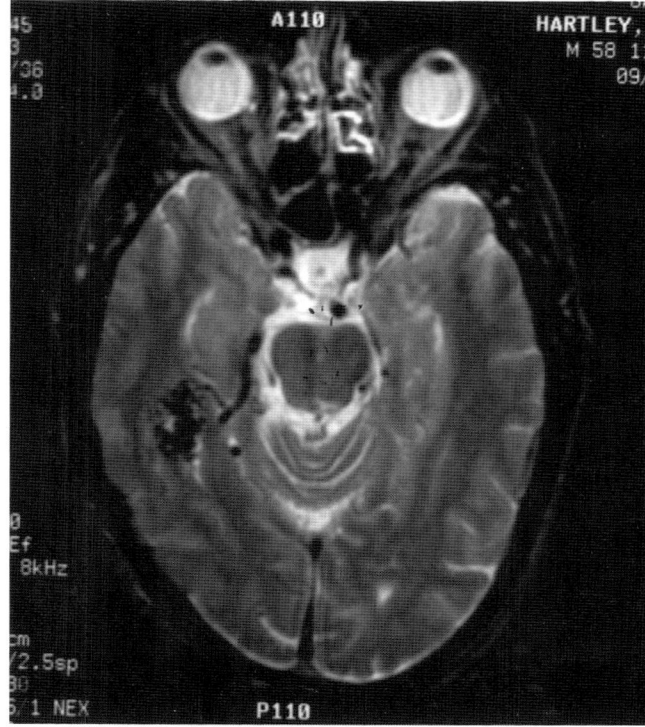

FIG. 4.71. An arteriovenous malformation. Axial (3000/78) image shows typical imaging features of arteriovenous malformation with feeding vasculature. The patient presented with frequent partial complex seizures.

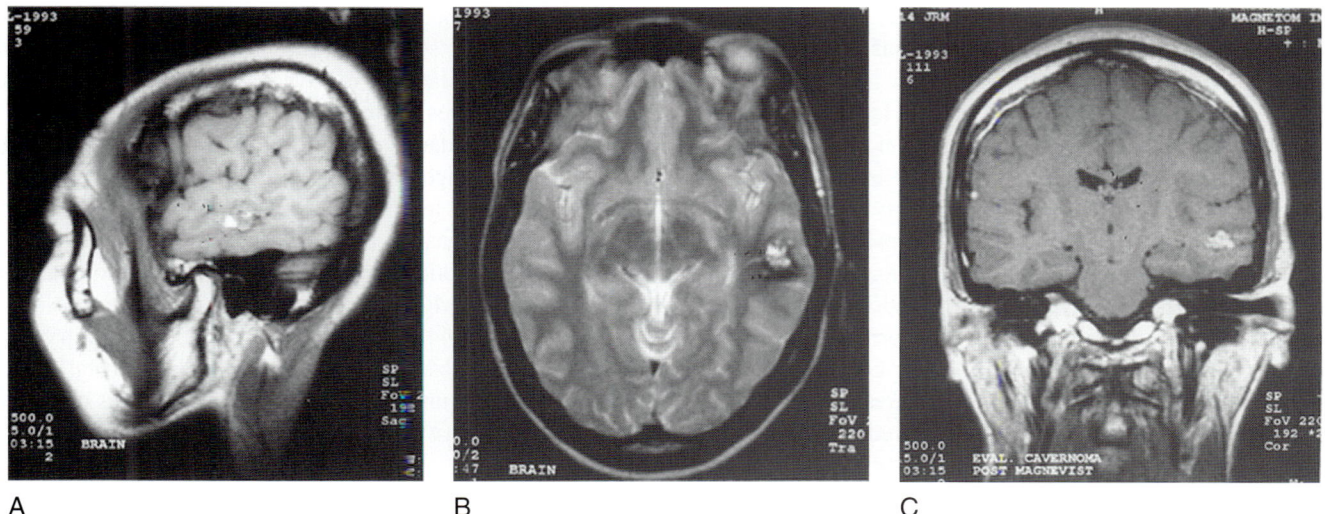

FIG. 4.72. Cavernous angioma in a patient with complex partial seizures. **A.** Sagittal (500/15) magnetic resonance image shows increased signal abnormality from the left mid-temporal region. **B.** Axial (3600/90) image demonstrates reticulated pattern typical of cavernous angioma with hypointense signal surrounding it. **C.** Coronal (500/15) image with gadolinium shows no enhancement.

Cavernous Angiomas

Cavernous angiomas constitute a distinct vascular malformation. In the majority of patients with intractable seizures, cavernous angiomas constitute the most common vascular abnormality (414, 420, 422–425). Autosomal dominant transmission has been reported in some families (426). These lesions are often microscopically typical, showing a honeycomb of vascular spaces with blood. No arteries or veins are seen in these lesions. Hemorrhages and calcification are common and, in 25–40% of individuals, the lesions may be multiple. The surrounding tissue is gliotic and contains haemosiderin-laden macrophages, suggesting previous hemorrhage. This is extremely important in view of experimental data indicating a close association between epileptogenicity and Fe^{2+}-induced injury.

The MRI features of cavernous angiomas are fairly stereotypical (Fig. 4.72). The lesions have a reticulated central core with mixed signals indicating blood byproducts of different stages. Within the core, methemoglobin appears as high signals, often intermixed with lower signals. Typically, a complete rim of hypointensity surrounds the central core. This rim is usually hypointense on both long and short echoes, with marked hypointensity in the longer echo. These lesions are void of mass effect or surrounding edema. These features are typical and should allow the diagnosis without difficulties.

Cavernous angiomas often demonstrate chronic hemorrhage with reactive angiogenesis. These lesions tend to bleed more frequently in females during the middle decade of life. Excision in cases with intractable epilepsy is necessary but may be complicated by the presence of multiple lesions in some patients (Fig. 4.73).

Venous angiomas are probably the most common vascular malformation but rarely associated to chronic epilepsy.

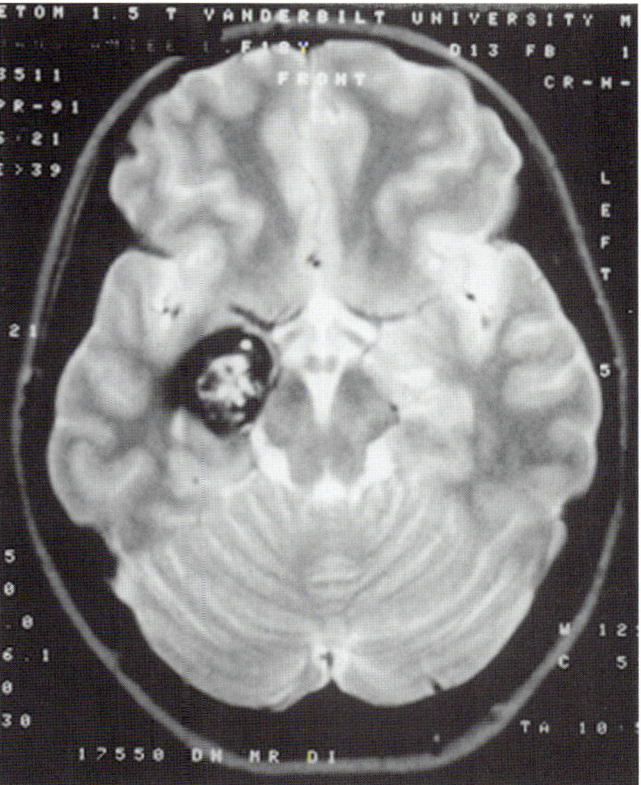

FIG. 4.73. Multiple cavernous angiomas. T2 axial image shows well-defined lesion in the right mesial temporal region. Presurgical investigations revealed that the lesion was responsible for the seizures. Excision resulted in seizure-free outcome (Courtesy of Dr B. Abou-Khalil, Vanderbilt University, Nashville, TN).

These lesions are characterized by parenchymal abnormal venous formation with absence of normal cortical venous drainage (422). Capillary telangiectasias are characterized by abnormal proliferation of capillaries with normal parenchyma. These lesions are coincidental but may be associated to other epileptogenic vascular malformations.

The pathogenic mechanisms of epilepsy in patients with vascular malformations are complex and probably multifactorial. Cortical EEG recordings during surgery have demonstrated epileptiform activity in cortex adjacent to AVMs. Intracellular recordings have shown abnormal spontaneous bursting indicating hyperexcitability with normal inhibition (144). The possibility of epileptogenic activation or kindling at a distance also needs to be considered (427). Several reports have documented mesial temporal pathology in some patients with extrahippocampal vascular lesions (424) and, therefore, it is likely that independent epileptogenic foci may be present in some patients.

In addition to the above potential mechanisms, another important neurochemical mechanism should be mentioned. Experimental data strongly supports the epileptogenicity of hemosiderin–iron-induced damage (428–430). Application of iron solutions in the cerebral cortex is a model for partial epilepsy (429). Iron decreases glutamate reuptake and inhibits glutamine synthetase, thus creating a propensity for seizures. In addition, iron has been implicated in the production of free radicals and lipid peroxides that can alter calcium influx, intracellular second messengers, and excessive glutamate and aspartate release (431, 432). Finally, alterations in blood supply and steal phenomenon producing chronic ischemia may have a role in some of these patients (417, 433).

Post-traumatic Lesions

Cranial injuries are recognized as an important cause of epileptic seizures (434–438). Approximately half a million head injuries per year occur in the United States alone. Although the prevalence of post-traumatic epilepsy is not high, the large number of patients affected by brain injuries makes this cause very important (434).

The incidence of post-traumatic epilepsy varies depending on the type of injury (penetrating versus nonpenetrating) and whether seizures occur early during the first week after injury or later (late-onset epilepsy). The incidence of early seizures ranges from 2.1% to 15% depending on multiple factors.

Affecting the temporal lobes, in particular, are cortical contusions. Cortical contusions affect the superficial gray matter and often in the acute phase are associated with hemorrhages. Contusions involve the temporal lobes in approximately 45% of cases, with frontal lobe involvement reported in 30% of individuals (439–441). Lesions above the petrous bone are more common. In addition, temporopolar injuries are also common and may not be associated with other lesions (Figs 4.74, 4.75). The prevalence of bilateral temporal lesions is common but the exact incidence is unknown. Another type of insult is the one associated with indirect injury to the mesial temporal structures caused by acute edema and partial uncal herniation. We have studied some patients who developed seizures in this situation. Although at surgery there was clear damage to the mesial structures with old hemorrhagic changes, the only abnormality found on the MRI was hippocampal atrophy.

Magnetic resonance imaging features consist of hemorrhagic foci or gliotic changes involving both the cortical and at times the underlying white matter depending on the time after injury (442–445). In some cases, frank destruction of the parenchyma is observed, with residual gliosis (Fig. 4.76). Herniation of the uncus may be seen in some cases of severe trauma.

Other Pathology

Less frequent pathologic abnormalities have been reported in patients with temporal lobe epilepsy. These include hamartomas, gliotic nodules, fibroglial lesions, meningiomatosis, developmental cysts, and other unusual conditions (Figs 4.79–4.83) (19, 95, 127, 162, 384, 446).

Abnormalities due to infectious and inflammatory disorders such as Rasmussen's encephalitis can also occur. This can be a surprisingly difficult diagnosis to make. In the early course of these patients, one usually is concerned with focal cortical dysplasia, and the signal change can be attributed to the secondary effects of seizures. Even when focal encephalitis is the cause of the seizures, some of the signal change can be due to secondary effects of seizures (Fig. 4.84).

SECONDARY DAMAGE FROM SEIZURES

Seizures can induce acute, transient changes in brain structure. Patients with established epilepsy often have chronic, permanent changes in brain structure. A few reports document the evolution from an acute seizure-associated change to the pattern of abnormalities typically seen in chronic patients, such as HS. As HS is intrinsically epileptogenic, these reports suggest that, in some circumstances, a prolonged seizure initiates events that lead to an epileptogenic lesion.

Histopathologic Evidence of Seizure-associated Damage

The presence of seizure-associated damage has been documented in the histopathologic literature on animals and humans (for review see reference 447). In experimental studies, neuronal damage was most extensive in animals experiencing generalized convulsive status epilepticus, but was also found to a lesser degree after single short seizures. Neurons show selective vulnerability to the effects of status epilepticus; the hippocampus is particularly vulnerable. Several factors have been associated with the cascade of

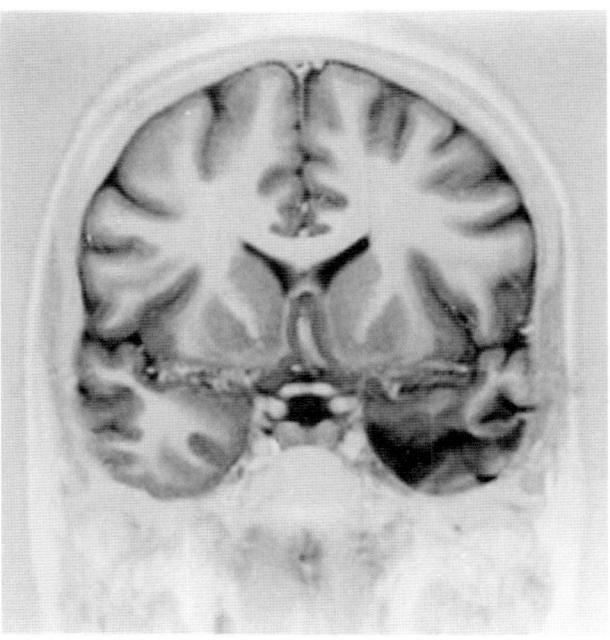

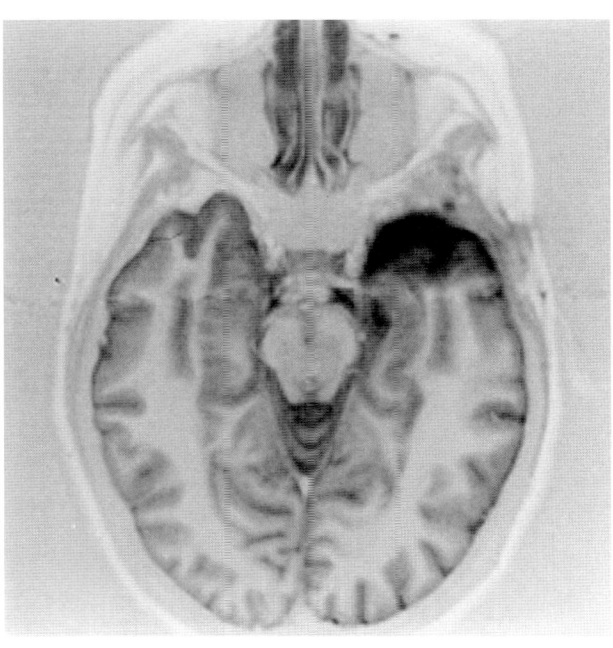

A   B

FIG. 4.74. Post-traumatic epilepsy (coronal heavily T1-weighted IR study). **A.** Coronal image shows destruction of parenchyma involving the left anterior temporal pole. **B.** Axial image demonstrates the extent of the abnormality in this plane.

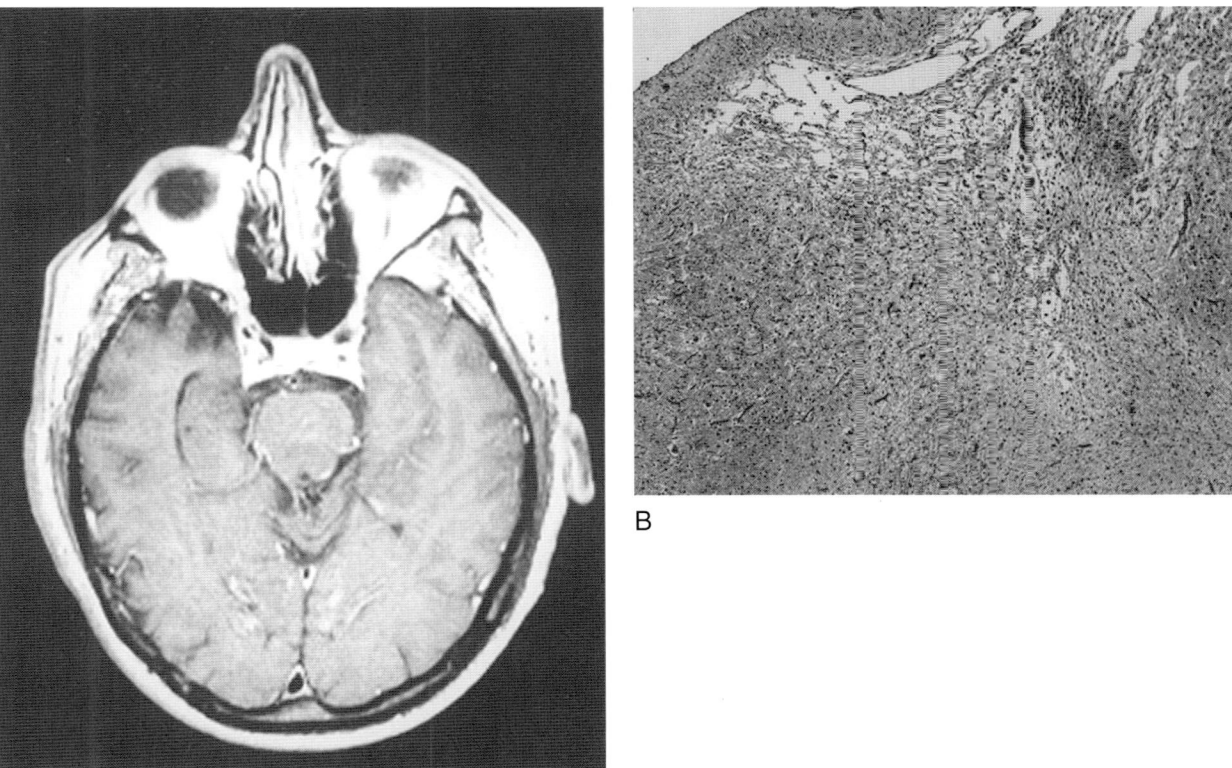

A

B

FIG. 4.75. Post-traumatic epilepsy. The patient fell down while inebriated, and intractable partial seizures developed 6 months later. **A.** MRI shows destruction of the right temporal pole. **B.** Pathologic section demonstrates contusion. Molecular layer spared with underlying rarefaction and tissue loss (hematoxylin and eosin, × 100).

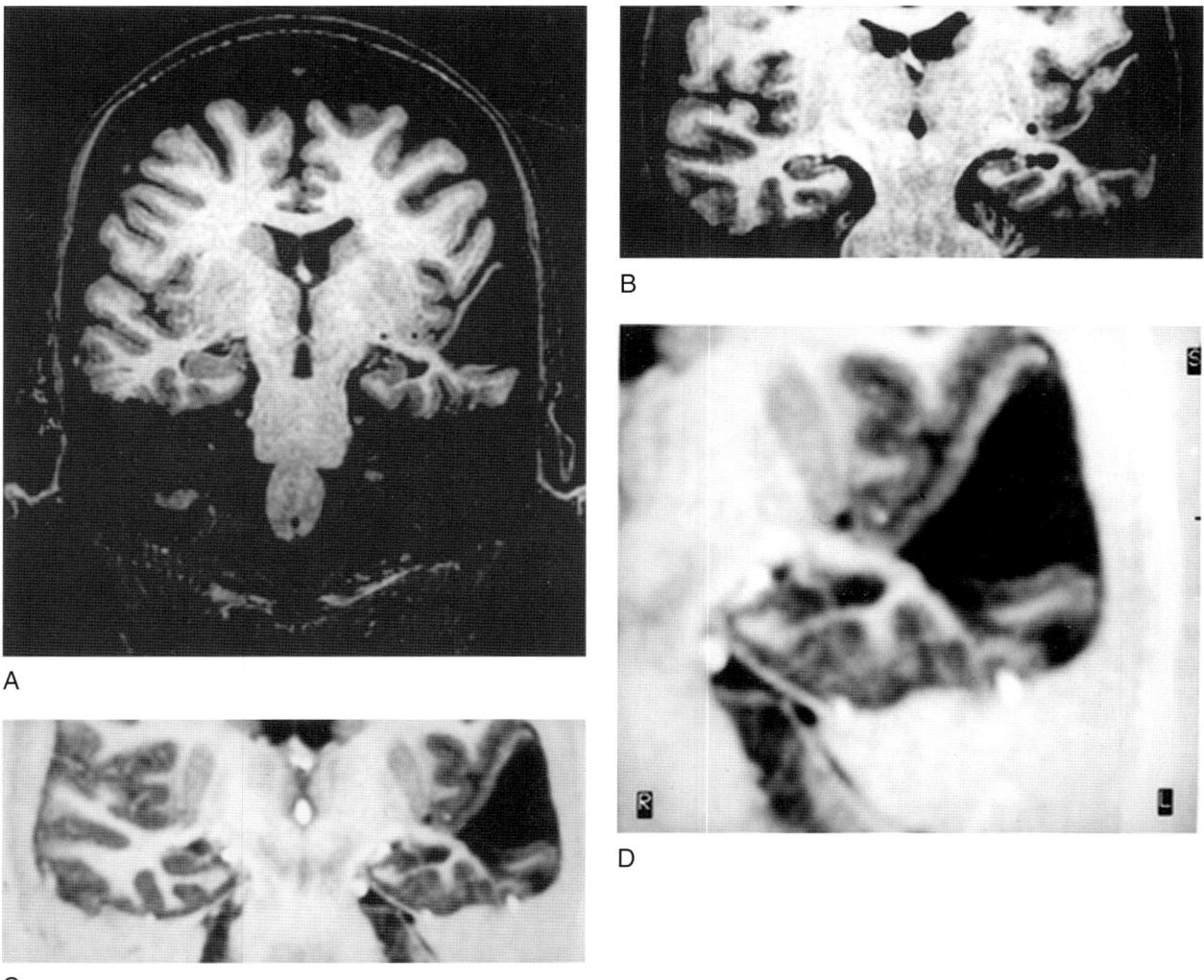

FIG. 4.76. The results of presumed temporal lobe trauma affecting the lateral left temporal neocortex. There is co-existent left hippocampal sclerosis. **A, B.** The coronal images show developmental malformation involving the superior temporal gyrus. In **B**, abnormal left hippocampus and temporal neocortex are observed. **C, D.** The IR sequences demonstrate that the hippocampus has an abnormal signal.

changes leading to neuronal death, such as the neurotoxic effects of excitatory neurotransmitters, particularly glutamate, and failure of ion pumps, particularly the Ca^{2+} pumps (447).

Histologic changes in the early stage after a seizure are characterized by cytotoxic cell edema, later after a seizure appear neuronal loss, reactive gliosis, and aberrant synaptic reorganization of surviving cells (448). These changes may lead to increased excitability of the affected area and result in an epileptogenic lesion. The epileptogenic process is complex and may depend on the loss of inhibitory neurons, so that the remaining cells are disinhibited and hyperexcitable. Aberrant recurrent excitatory connections between normally unconnected cells may be initiated (447). In humans, widespread neuronal loss and reactive gliosis in the hippocampus, amygdala, thalamus, and cerebellum were observed in previously healthy patients who died in status epilepticus (449).

Overall, these histopathologic studies document seizure-associated damage. However, they can only assess

post-mortem changes at a single time-point. MRI is non-invasive, and serial imaging allows examination of the temporal evolution of seizure-associated changes.

Magnetic Resonance Evidence of Seizure-associated Injury

Several MR sequences have been shown to be sensitive to acute seizure-induced changes (for review see reference 197). The initiation of cytotoxic edema restricts the free diffusion of water in the reduced volume of the extracellular space. This can be detected as an increase in the signal intensity of diffusion-weighted images or quantitatively by a reduction in the diffusivity (a parameter that reflects the freedom of diffusion). The subsequent progression to vasogenic edema will result in swelling of the extracellular space in the affected area. The volume change can be detected and measured on high-resolution anatomical sequences. The change in the environment of extracellular

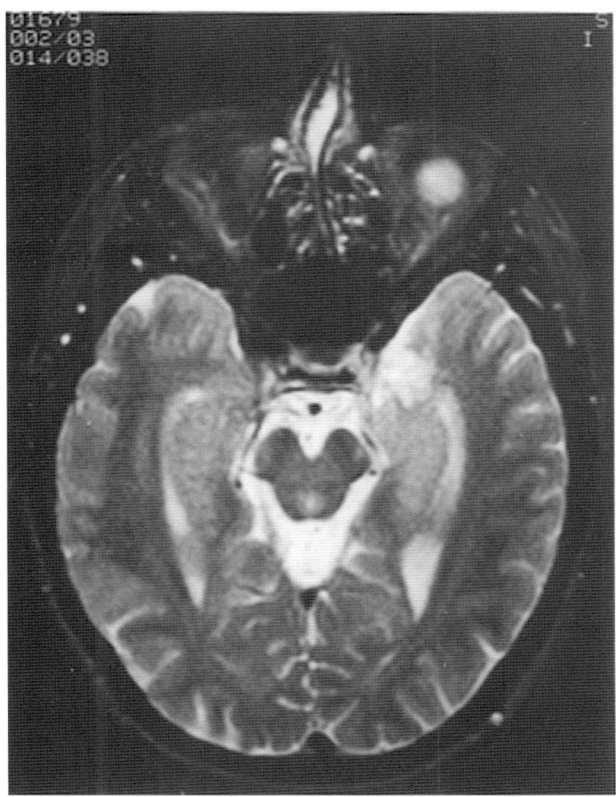

A

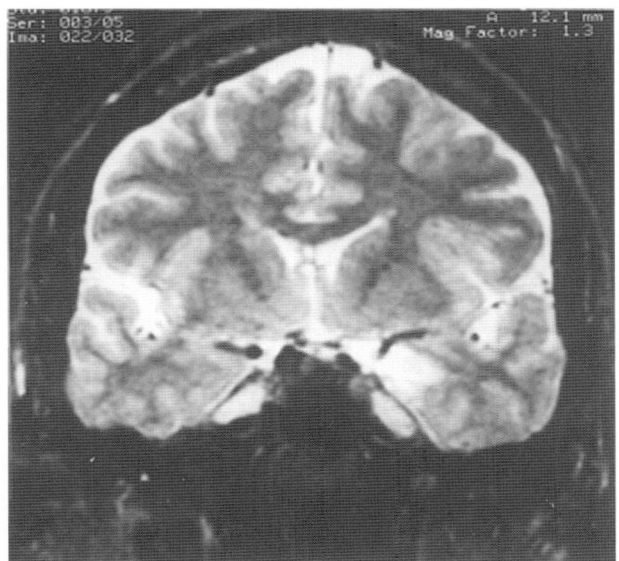

B

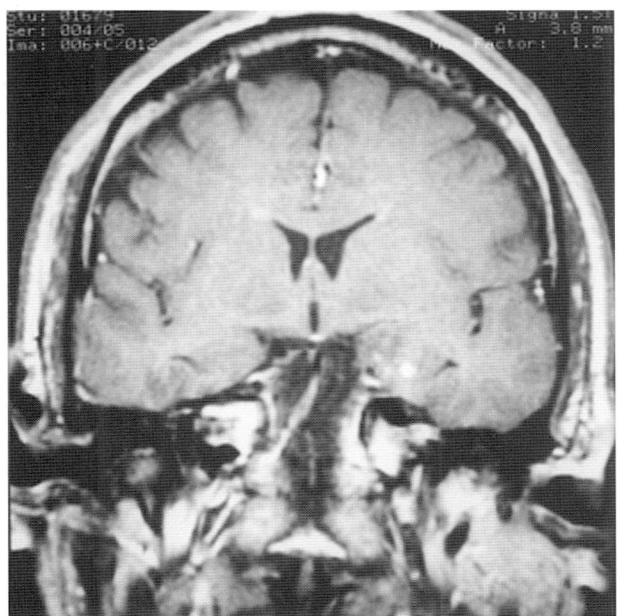

C

FIG. 4.77. Hamartoma. **A.** Axial (3000/100) MRI shows a high-intensity signal from the left anterior mesial region, probably in the uncus. **B.** Coronal (2500/90) image demonstrates the lesion in the uncus. **C.** Coronal (700/29) image with gadolinium showing minimal enhancement. The patient had a 25-year history of simple and complex partial seizures. Surgery effectively rendered the patient seizure-free.

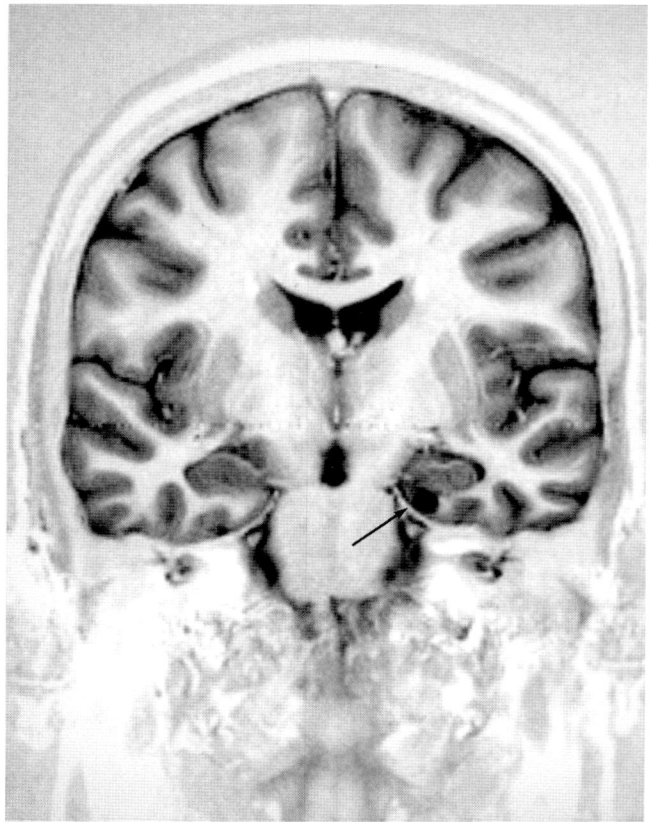

FIG. 4.78. Hamartoma in a patient with intractable epilepsy. After resection, this appeared to be a densely gliotic nodule (arrow). This patient had previously had an anterior temporal lobectomy without knowledge of this lesion. This image is after operation at the back edge of the anterior temporal resection. The first operation did not influence seizures. The second operation, which removed only this lesion, led to seizure freedom. This suggests that it, or the nearby tissue, was highly epileptogenic. Coronal IR sequence shows a small hamartoma in the left parahippocampal gyrus. The signal intensity is significantly lower than that of gray matter, having some characteristics of fluid (high T2, low T1, but isodense PD). Note that the hippocampal formations are symmetric bilaterally, which suggests the absence of dual pathology (hippocampal sclerosis).

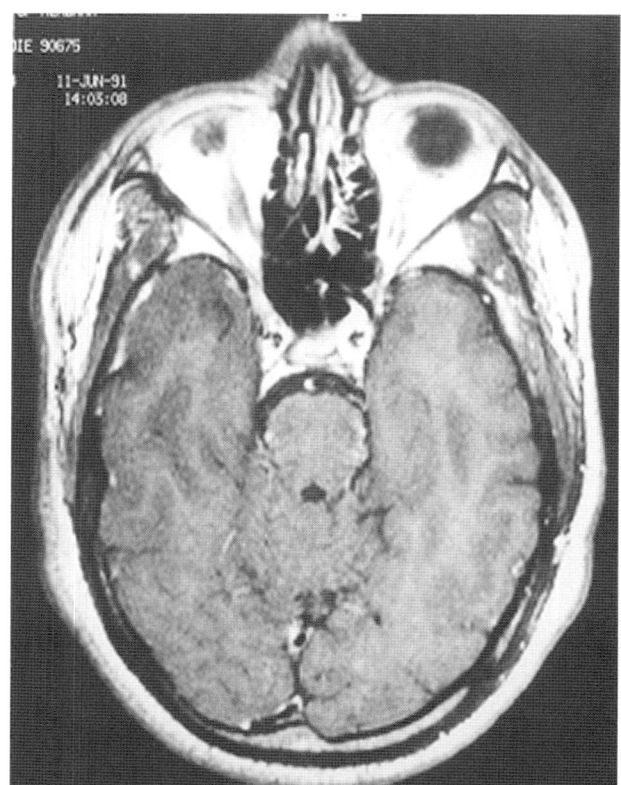

A

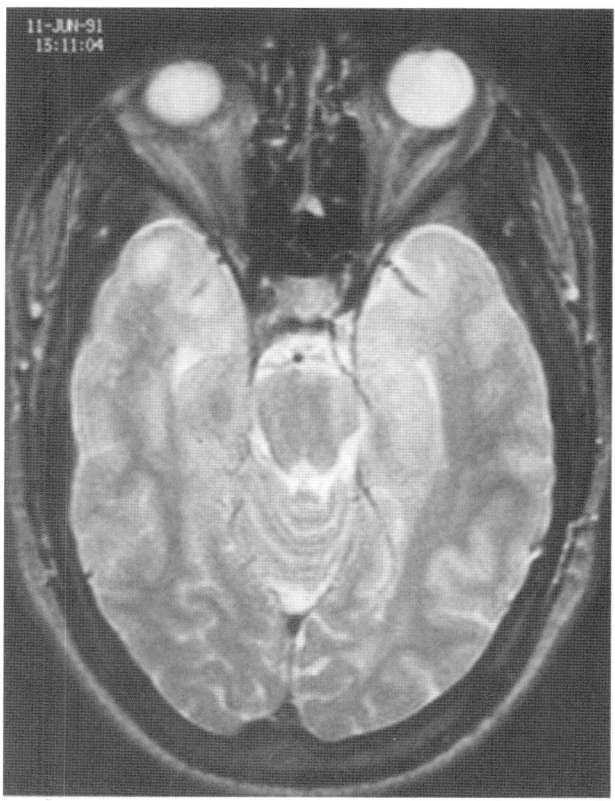

B

FIG. 4.79. Temporal lobe fibrodysplasia in a 12-year-old male with intractable partial seizures. **A.** Axial T1 image shows abnormal right temporal pattern. Compare with the left temporal lobe. **B.** Axial image (2200/67) demonstrates a high signal abnormality from the same region.

water can be detected as an increase in the T2 relaxation time and as a further change in the diffusivity of free water. Acute changes in tissue metabolism are accessible by MR spectroscopy.

There are several case reports (356, 358, 450–452) and a few studies of small groups of patients (298, 453–456) that document the ability of MR to detect acute seizure-associated changes. They consist of focal swelling, T2-weighted hyperintensity (453), and focal reduction in diffusivity (455, 456). These effects were consistently observed after status epilepticus but appear to be less robust after single, short seizures (457). These patient data are confirmed by numerous animal MR studies of acute seizure-associated changes (294). Postictal changes in NA, but also other proton metabolites, particularly lactate, have been described and the exciting potential they suggest means that we are only at the beginning of uncovering the basis of epilepsy and its effects on the brain. These techniques are presented in subsequent chapters of this volume.

The issue is increasingly how to interpret and use these findings. Sensitivity is such that we can no longer simply assume that a detected abnormality means we have found the epiletogenic lesion. The sensitivity of these technologies challenges our understanding of the biology of epilepsy and its effects on the whole brain of humans. In turn, detection of abnormalities have to be interpreted in terms of all of the wide range of pathologic processes associated with epilepsy as well as the normal processes of brain reorganization and compensation for seizures.

When the first edition of this book was written 9 years ago the amazing expansion of MR into all areas of brain function was just beginning. Now it is perhaps paradoxical that our biologic understanding of all of these new data is just commencing. MR findings are changing our view of epilepsy. The range of abnormalities seen in patients even with simple HS is large, and often not only in the seizure focus. The challenge now is to use these tools to understand the pathogenesis of HS so that preventative strategies and early treatments become effective.

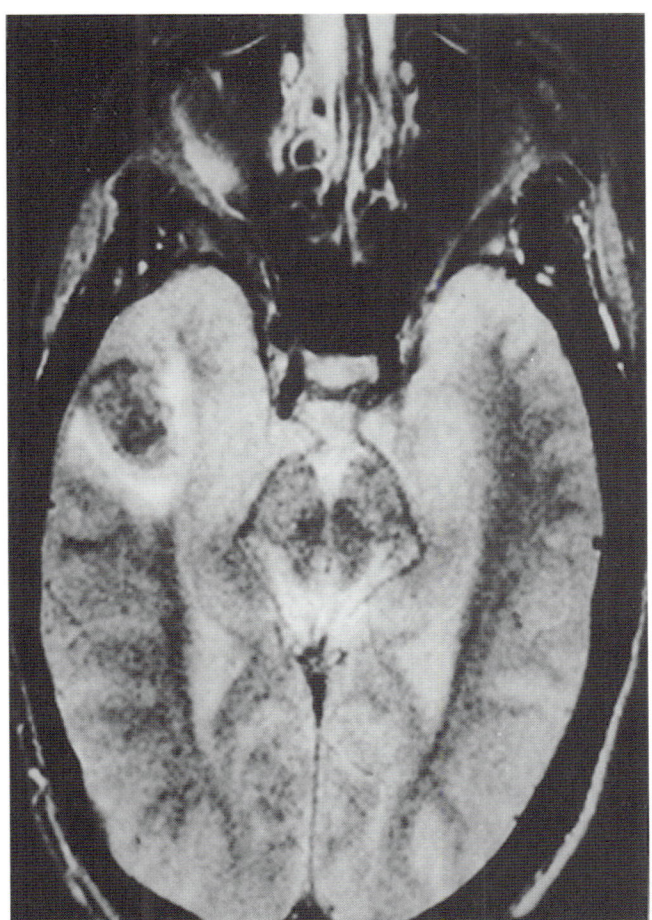

FIG. 4.80. Meningioangiomatosis. Axial T2 image shows a heterogeneous calcified lesion with a surrounding high-intensity signal from the capsule.

in a few other human proton MRS studies (458), whereas phosphorus MRS has gained almost no attention for its potential in the investigation of postictal changes. We have observed dramatic postictal changes in energy-dependent metabolites (see Fig. 4.3). Phosphorus MRS certainly has the sensitivity to detect such changes, as demonstrated by physiologic neuronal activity in humans inducing subtle fluctuations in PCr (459).

SUMMARY

While often, in the past, no cause could be identified for many cases of intractable partial epilepsy, it is now becoming clear that a large proportion of adults and children with partial epilepsy have defined brain abnormalities visualized on appropriate optimized imaging. Advances in image analysis techniques and in MR technologies continues to push to boundaries of sensitivity of the detection of epilepsy-related brain abnormalities from gross macroscopic structural changes as seen on imaging to functional metabolic and neurophysiologic abnormalities. New techniques

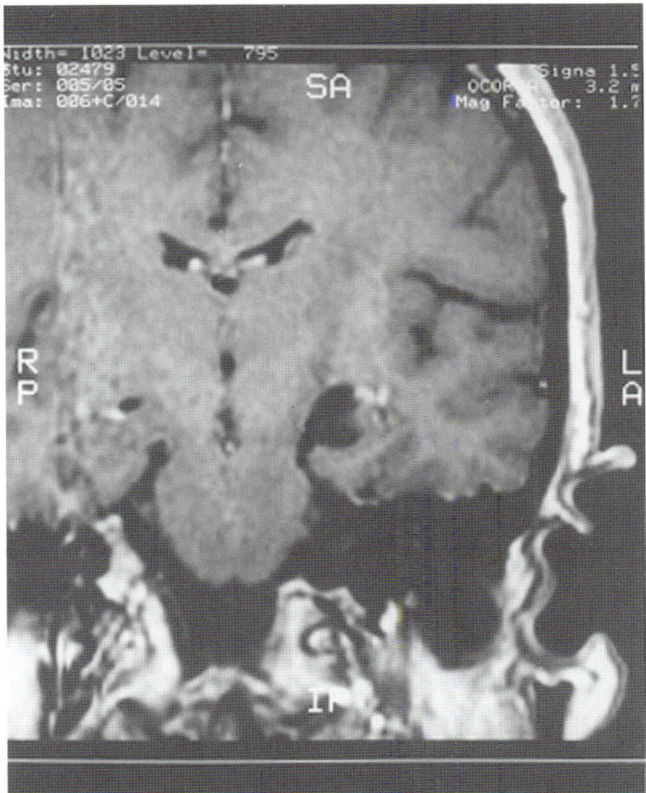

FIG. 4.81. Developmental mesial temporal cyst in a woman with infrequent seizures and depression. Coronal image with gadolinium shows no enhancement.

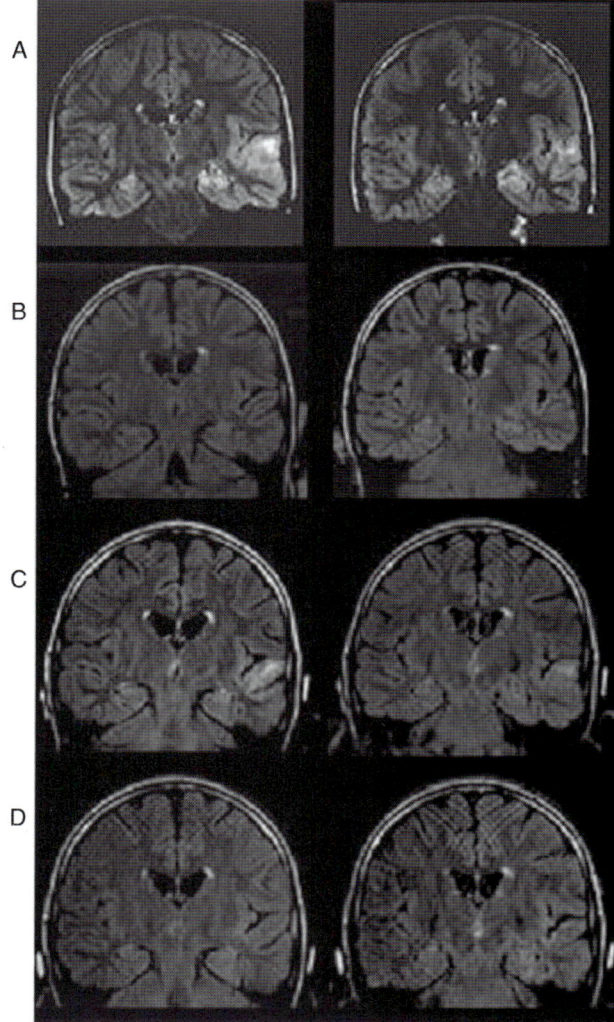

FIG. 4.82. Rasmussen's encephalitis with variable appearance related to seizure activity. Coronal FLAIR images. **A.** The initial imaging with status epilepticus. There is signal change in the left temporal lobe including the hippocampus, with an emphasis in the superior temporal gyrus. **B.** Repeat imaging 11 months later, showing mild increase of signal in the left hippocampus, but the signal change has largely returned to normal. **C.** With recurrent status epilepticus 20 months after the original presentation, there is again focal increased signal in the left superior temporal gyrus. **D.** Two months later this signal change has again resolved. Because of the possibility of a focal abnormality in the superior temporal gyrus, this was resected and Rasmussen's encephalitis was confirmed on histopathologic examination of the resected specimen. Wellard RM, Briellmann RS, Wilson JC, Kalnins RM, Federico P, Scheffer IE, et al. Longitudinal study of MRS metabolites in Rasmussen's encephalitis. *Brain* 2004; 127:1302–1312, by permission of Oxford University Press.

ACKNOWLEDGMENT

We should like to thank Claire Jennings for all her hard work on this chapter.

REFERENCES

1. Volpe J. Neurology of the newborn, 4th ed. Philadelphia, PA: Elsevier Health Sciences, 2001.

2. Gloor P. The temporal lobe and limbic system. New York: Oxford University Press, 1997.

3. Commission on Classification and Terminology of the International League Against Epilepsy. A revised proposal for the classification of epilepsy and epileptic syndromes. *Epilepsia* 1989;30:268–278.

4. Engel J Jr, Williamson PD, Wieser HG. Mesial temporal lobe epilepsy. In: Engel J Jr, Pedley TA, eds. Epilepsy: a comprehensive textbook. Philadelphia, PA: Lippincott-Raven, 1998:2417–2426.

5. Williamson PD, Engel J Jr, Munari C. Anatomic classification of localization-related epilepsies. In: Engel J Jr, Pedley TA, eds. Epilepsy: A Comprehensive Textbook. Philadelphia, USA: Lippincott-Raven Publishers, 1998:2405–2416.

6. Burgerman RS, Sperling M, French J, et al. Comparison of mesial versus neocortical onset temporal lobe seizures: neurodiagnostic findings and surgical outcome. *Epilepsia* 1995;36:662–670.

7. Walczak T. Neocortical temporal lobe epilepsy: characterising the syndrome. *Epilepsia* 1995;36:633–635.

8. Pacia SV, Devinsky O, Perrine K, et al. Clinical features of neocortical temporal lobe epilepsy. *Ann Neurol* 1996;40:724–730.

9. Gloor P, Olivier A, Quesney LF, et al. The role of the limbic system in experimental phenomena of temporal lobe epilepsy. *Ann Neurol* 1982; 12:129–144.

10. Gupta AK, Jeavons PM, Hughes RC, Covanis A. Aura in temporal lobe epilepsy: clinical and electroencephalographic correlation. *J Neurol Neurosurg Psychiatry* 1983;46:1079–1083.

11. Taylor DC, Lochery M. Temporal lobe epilepsy: origin and significance of simple and complex auras. *J Neurol Neurosurg Psychiatry* 1987;50:673–681.

12. Falconer MA, Serafetinides EA, Corsellis JAN. Etiology and pathogenesis of temporal lobe epilepsy. *Arch Neurol* 1964;10:233–240.

13. Glaser G. Natural history of temporal lobe-limbic epilepsy. In: Engel J, ed. Surgical treatment of the epilepsies. New York: Raven Press, 1987.

14. Engel J Jr. Seizures and epilepsy. Philadelphia, PA: Davis, 1989.

15. Gastaut H, Broughton R. Epileptic seizures. Springfield, IL: Charles C Thomas, 1972.

16. Dreifuss FE. Proposal for revised clinical and electroencephalographic classification of epileptic seizures. *Epilepsia* 1981;22:489–501.

17. Bancaud J. Clinical presentation of temporal epileptic seizures. *Rev Neurol Paris* 1987;143:392–400.

18. Delgado-Escueta AV, Walsh GO. Type I complex partial seizures of hippocampal origin: excellent results of anterior temporal lobectomy. *Neurology* 1985;35:143–154.

19. Duncan JS, Sagar HJ. Seizure characteristics, pathology, and outcome after temporal lobectomy. *Neurology* 1987;1987:405–409.

20. Hauser WA. The natural history of temporal lobe epilepsy. In: Luders H, ed. Epilepsy surgery. New York: Raven Press, 1991:133–141.

21. Hopkins IJ, Klug GL. Temporal lobectomy for the treatment of intractable complex partial seizures of temporal lobe origin in early childhood. *Dev Med Child Neurol* 1991;33:26–31.

22. Jensen I. Temporal lobe epilepsy. With special reference to surgical results, neuropathology, and social conditions. Copenhagen: Forlag, 1977.

23. Karlov VA. Temporal epilepsy starting at the ages of 6 to 12 and 12 to 16. *Zh Nevropatol Psikhiatr Im S S Korsakova* 1988;88:37–41.

24. Wieser HG. Human limbic seizures: EEG studies, origin, and patterns of spread. In: Meldrum BS, Ferrendelli JA, Wieser HG, eds. Anatomy of epileptogenesis. London: John Libbey, 1988:127–138.

25. Williamson PD, Spencer DD, Spencer SS, et al. Complex partial seizures of frontal lobe origin. *Ann Neurol* 1985;18:497–504.

26. Williamson PD. Frontal lobe seizures. Problems of diagnosis and classification. *Adv Neurol* 1992;57:289–309.

27. Veilleux F, Saint-Hilaire JM, Giard N, et al. Seizures of the human medial frontal lobe. *Adv Neurol* 1992;57:245–256.

28. Takeda A, Inaguma J, Shimizu A. Complex partial seizures of frontal lobe origin. *J Jpn Epilepsy Soc* 1985;3:24–30.

29. Karbowski K, Vassella F, Pavlincova E, Nielsen J. Psychomotor seizures in infancy and early childhood. *EEG EMG Z Elektroenzephalogr Elektromyogr Verw, Geb* 1988;19:30–34.

30. Bancaud J, Bonis A, Munair C, et al. Localizing value of the clinical manifestations of the partial seizures. *Acta Neurochir* 1984;33:7–15.

31. Quesney LF. Clinical and EEG features of complex partial seizures of temporal lobe origin. *Epilepsia* 1986;27:S27–S45.

32. So N, Gloor P, Quesney LF, et al. Depth electrode investigations in patients with bitemporal epileptiform abnormalities. *Ann Neurol* 1989; 25:423–431.

33. Olivier A, Gloor P, Quesney LF, Andermann F. The indications for and the role of depth electrode recording in epilepsy. *Appl Neurophysiol* 1983;46:33–36.

34. Engel J, Driver MV, Falconer MA. Electrophysiological correlates of pathology and surgical results in temporal lobe epilepsy. *Brain* 1975; 98:129–156.

35. Engel J Jr. Surgical treatment of the epilepsies, 2nd ed. New York: Raven Press, 1993.

36. Engel J Jr. Localization of the epileptogenic lesion. In: Engel J Jr, ed. Surgical treatment of the epilepsies. New York: Raven Press, 1987:76.

37. Cendes F, Andermann F, Gloor P, et al. Relationship between atrophy of the amygdala and ictal fear in temporal lobe epilepsy. *Brain* 1994; 117:739–746.

38. Kotagal P. Seizure symptomatology of temporal lobe epilepsy. In: Luders H, ed. Epilepsy surgery. New York: Raven Press, 1991:143–156.

39. Palmini A, Gloor P. The localizing value of auras in partial seizures: a prospective and retrospective study. *Neurology* 1992; 42:801–808.

40. Holmes MD, Kelly K, Theodore WH. Complex partial seizures. Correlation of clinical and metabolic features. *Arch Neurol* 1988;45: 1191–1193.

41. Sperling MR, Lieb JP, Engel J Jr, Crandall PH. Prognostic significance of independent auras in temporal lobe seizures. *Epilepsia* 1989;30: 322–331.

42. Jackson JH. Observations on the anatomical, physiological, pathological investigations of epilepsies. West Riding Lunatic Asylum Rep 1873; 3:315.

43. Jackson JH. A study of convulsions. *Trans St Andrews Med Grad Assoc* 1870;3:162–207.

44. Gowers WR. Epilepsy and other chronic convulsive disorders. New York: William Wood, 1885.

45. Aicardi J. Epilepsy in children. New York: Raven Press, 1986.

46. Blume WT. Clinical profile of partial seizures beginning at less than four years of age. *Epilepsia* 1989;30:813–819.

47. Ciarmatori C. Epilepsy and involuntary movements during wakefulness and sleep: comparison between two clinical cases studied by video-EEG analysis. *Boll Lega Ital Epilessia* 1988;63(61–62).

48. French JA, Williamson PD, Thadani VM, et al. Characteristics of medial temporal lobe epilepsy: I. Results of history and physical examination. *Ann Neurol* 1993;34:774–780.

49. Luna D, Dulac O, Plouin P. Ictal characteristics of cryptogenic partial epilepsies in infancy. *Epilepsia* 1989;30:827–832.

50. Lüders HO, Engel J Jr, Munari C. General principles. In: Engel J Jr, ed. Surgical treatment of the epilepsies, 2nd ed. New York: Raven Press, 1993.

51. Kotagal P, Luders H, Morris HH, et al. Dystonic posturing in complex partial seizures of temporal lobe onset: A new lateralizing sign. *Neurology* 1989;39:196–201.

52. Ciarmatori C. Dystonic seizures and psychomotor epilepsy: a clinical case studied by video-EEG. *Boll Lega Ital Epilessia* 1989;67 (141–144).

53. Kodama K. [MRI in patients with temporal lobe epilepsy: correlation between MRI findings and clinical features]. *Seishin Shinkeigaku Zasshi* 1992;94:26–57.

54. Fois A, Tomaccini D, Balestri P, et al. Intractable epilepsy: etiology, risk factors and treatment. *Clin EEG* 1988;19:68–73.

55. Abou-Khalil B, Andermann E, Andermann F, et al. Temporal lobe epilepsy after prolonged febrile convulsions: excellent outcome after surgical treatment. *Epilepsia* 1993;34:878–883.

56. Meletti S, Cantalupo G, Stanzani-Maserati M et al. The expression of interictal, preictal, and postictal facial-wiping behavior in temporal lobe epilepsy: a neuro-ethological analysis and interpretation. *Epilepsy Behav* 2003;4:635–643.

57. Leutmezer F, Baumgartner C. Postictal signs of lateralizing and localizing significance. *Epileptic Disord* 2004;4:43–48.

58. Wennberg R. Postictal coughing and nose rubbing coexist in temporal lobe epilepsy. *Neurology* 2001;56:133–134

59. Hirsch LJ, Lain AH, Walczak TS. Postictal nosewiping lateralizes and localizes to the ipsilateral temporal lobe. *Epilepsia* 1998;39:991–997.

60. Geyer JD, Payne TA, Faught E, Drury I. Postictal nose-rubbing in the diagnosis, lateralization, and localization of seizures. *Neurology* 1999; 52:743–745.

61. Sperling MR, Engel J Jr. Electroencephalographic recording from the temporal lobes: a comparison of ear, anterior temporal, and nasopharyngeal electrodes. *Ann Neurol* 1985; 7:510–513.

62. Devinsky O, Sato S, Kufta CV, et al. Electroencephalographic studies of simple partial seizures with subdural electrode recordings. *Neurology* 1989;39:527–533.

63. Rose DF, Sato S, Smith PD, et al. Localization of magnetic interictal discharges in temporal lobe epilepsy. *Ann Neurol* 1987;22:348–354.

64. Rougier A. Ratio of stereoelectroencephalographic elements between and during epileptic seizures: effect on result of cortectomy. *Rev Neurol Paris* 1987;143:437–442.

65. Nuwer MR. Frequency analysis and topographic mapping of EEG and evoked potentials in epilepsy. *Electroencephalogr Clin Neurophysiol* 1988;69:118–126.

66. Meador KJ, Loring DW, Huh K, et al. Spectral analysis of sphenoidal evoked potentials predicts epileptic focus. *Epilepsia* 1988;29:434–439.

67. Theodore WH, Holmes MD, Dorwart RE, et al. Complex partial seizures: cerebral structure and cerebral function. *Epilepsia* 1986;27: 576–582.

68. Williamson PD, French JA, Thadani VM et al. Characteristics of medial temporal lobe epilepsy: II. Interictal and ictal scalp electroencephalography, neuropsychological testing, neuroimaging surgical results, and pathology. *Ann Neurol* 1993;34:781–787.

69. Bancaud J. Surgery of epilepsy based on stereotactic investigations – the plan of the SEEG investigations. *Acta Neurochir* 1980;30: 25–34.

70. Blom S, Flink R, Hetta J, et al. Interictal and ictal activity recorded with subdural electrodes during preoperative evaluation for surgical treatment of epilepsy. *J Epilepsy* 1989;2:9–20.

71. Weiser HG, Engel J Jr, Williamson PD, et al. Surgically remedial temporal lobe syndromes. In: Engel J Jr, ed. Surgical treatment of the epilepsies, 2nd ed. New York: Raven Press, 1993.

72. Sperling MR, O'Connor MJ. Comparison of depth and subdural electrodes in recording temporal lobe seizures. *Neurology* 1989;39: 1497–1504.

73. Uetsuhara K, Asakura T. Epileptogenic focus and MRI – the study of MRI and EEG of no relation to epileptogenic focus. *Jpn J Psychiatry Neurol* 1989;43:389–392.

74. Forsgren L, Fagerlund M, Zetterlund B. Electroencephalographic and neuroradiological findings in adults with newly diagnosed unprovoked seizures. *Eur Neurol* 1991;31:61–67.

75. Mattioli GL, Bernardini E, Cilio R, Arpino C. EEG vectorial analysis contribution to early lesional epilepsy. *Boll Lega Ital Epilessia* 1989; 67(199–202).

76. Baldy MM, Rondouin G, Duval E, et al. Spectral analysis and topographic mapping of interictal basal EEG activity in partial epilepsies. *Epilepsies* 1989;1:234–243.

77. Novak GP. The electroencephalogram in the diagnosis of epilepsy. *Child Hosp Q* 1989;1:247–252.

78. Munari C. Stereo-EEG exploration for 'temporal' lobe epilepsies. *Boll Lega Ital Epilessia* 1988;63(17–19).

79. Quirk JA, Smith SJM, Fish DR, Cook MJ. Correlation between interictal EEG and MRI evidence of hippocampal sclerosis. *Epilepsia* 1993;34:138.

80. Sloviter RS, Pedley TA. Subtle hippocampal malformation: importance in febrile seizures and development of epilepsy. *Neurology* 1998;50.

81. Wieser HG, Yasargil MG. Selective amygdalohippocampectomy as a surgical treatment of mesiobasal limbic epilepsy. *Surg Neurol* 1982;17:445–457.

82. Montplaisir J, Laverdiere M, Saint HJM, et al. A study of epileptic patients investigated with depth electrodes during sleep. *Union Med Can* 1985;114:1019–1020.

83. Goldring S, Gregorie EM. Surgical management of epilepsy using epidural recordings to localize the seizure focus. Review of 100 cases. *J Neurosurg* 1984;60:457–466.

84. Spencer SS, Spencer DD, Williamson PD, Mattson R. Combined depth and subdural electrode investigation in uncontrolled epilepsy. *Neurology* 1990;40:74–79.

85. Spencer SS, So NK, Engel J Jr, et al. Depth electrodes. In: Engel J Jr, ed. Surgical treatment of the epilepsies, 2nd ed. New York: Raven Press, 1993:359–376.

86. Van VC, Debets R, Van HA, et al. Combined use of subdural and intracerebral electrodes in preoperative evaluation of epilepsy. *Neurosurgery* 1990;26:93–101.

87. Hausser HC, Bancaud J. Gustatory hallucinations in epileptic seizures. Electrophysiological, clinical and anatomical correlates. *Brain* 1987;110:339–359.

88. Hudson LP, Munoz DG, Miller L, et al. Amygdaloid sclerosis in temporal lobe epilepsy. *Ann Neurol* 1993;33:622–631.

89. Bogerts B, Lieberman JA, Ashtari M, et al. Hippocampus–amygdala volumes and psychopathology in chronic schizophrenia. *Biol Psychiatry* 1993;33:236–246.

90. Babb TL, Brown WJ. Pathological findings in epilepsy. In: Engel J Jr, ed. Surgical treatment of the epilepsies. New York: Raven Press, 1987:511–540.

91. Babb TL, Pretorius JK. Pathological substrates of epilepsy. In: Wylie E, ed. The treatment of epilepsy: principles and practice. Philadelphia, PA: Lea & Febiger, 1993:55–70.

92. Babb TL, Brown WJ, Pretorius J, Lieb JP. Temporal lobe volumetric cell densities in temporal lobe epilepsy. *Epilepsia* 1984;25:729–740.

93. Cavenagh EC, Hart BL, Rose D. Association of linear sebaceous nevus syndrome and unilateral megalencephaly. *Am J Neuroradiol* 1993;14:405–408.

94. Falconer MA. Mesial temporal (Ammon's horn) sclerosis as a common cause of epilepsy: aetiology, treatment and prevention. *Lancet* 1974;2:767–770.

95. Mathieson G. Pathology of temporal lobe foci. In: Penry JK, Daly DD, eds. Complex partial seizures and their treatment. New York: Raven Press, 1975:163–185.

96. Matsuda K, Mihara T, Tottori T, et al. Neuropathology of hippocampus of intractable temporal lobe epilepsy. *Jpn J Psychiatry Neurol* 1988;42:648–650.

97. Meencke HJ, Veith G. Hippocampal sclerosis in epilepsy. In: Luders H, ed. Epilepsy surgery. New York: Raven Press, 1991:705–715.

98. Sagar SJ, Oxbury JM. Hippocampal neuron loss in temporal lobe epilepsy: correlation with early childhood convulsions. *Ann Neurol* 1987;22:334–340.

99. Engel J Jr, Brown WJ, Kuhl DE, et al. Pathological findings underlying focal temporal lobe hypometabolism in partial epilepsy. *Ann Neurol* 1982;12:518–528.

100. Sano K, Malamud N. Clinical significance of sclerosis of the cornu ammonis. *Arch Neurol Psychiatr* 1953;70:40–53.

101. Jay V, Becker LE, Otsubo H et al. Pathology of temporal lobectomy for refractory seizures in children. Review of 20 cases including some unique malformative lesions. *J Neurosurg* 1993;79:53–61.

102. Fried I, Kim JH, Spencer DD. Hippocampal pathology in patients with intractable seizures and temporal lobe masses. *J Neurosurg* 1992;76:735–740.

103. Meldrum BS, Corsellis JAN. Epilepsy. In: Adams JH, Corsellis JAN, Duchen LW, eds. Greenfields neuropathology. London: Edward Arnold, 1984:921–950.

104. Wilson SJ, Bladin PF, Saling MM. Paradoxical results in the cure of chronic illness: the 'burden of normality' as exemplified following seizure surgery. *Epilepsy Behav* 2004;5:13–21.

105. Wilson SJ, Bladin PF, Saling MM, et al. The longitudinal course of adjustment after seizure surgery. *Seizure* 2001;10:165–172.

106. Wilson S, Bladin P, Saling M. The 'burden of normality': concepts of adjustment after surgery for seizures. *J Neurol Neurosurg Psychiatry* 2001;70:649–656.

107. Wilson SJ, Saling MM, Lawrence J, Bladin PF. Outcome of temporal lobectomy: expectations and the prediction of perceived success. *Epilepsy Res* 1999;36:1–14.

108. Bladin PF, Wilson SJ, Saling MM, et al. Outcome assessment in seizure surgery: the role of postoperative adjustment. *J Clin Neurosci* 1999;6:313–318.

109. Berkovic SF, McIntosh AM, Jackson GD, Bladin PF. Visual analysis of MRI predicts outcome of temporal lobectomy. *Epilepsia* 1993;34:145.

110. Drake J, Hoffman HJ, Kobayashi J, et al. Surgical management of children with temporal lobe epilepsy and mass lesions. *Neurosurgery* 1987;21:792–797.

111. Engel J Jr. Modern approaches to surgical treatment of epilepsy. *Boll Lega Ital Epilessia* 1990;71(53–59).

112. Jack CRJ, Sharbrough FW, Cascino GD, et al. Magnetic resonance image-based hippocampal volumetry: correlation with outcome after temporal lobectomy. *Ann Neurol* 1992;31:138–146.

113. Kawamura H, Amano K, Tanikawa T, et al. Surgical treatment of temporal lobe epilepsy – long-term follow-up and alteration of EEGs after resection of anterior temporal lobe. *Folia Psychiatr Neurol Jpn* 1982;36:263–265.

114. Meyer FB, Marsh WR, Laws EJ, Sharbrough FW. Temporal lobectomy in children with epilepsy. *J Neurosurg* 1986;64:371–376.

115. Rasmussen TB. Surgical treatment of complex partial seizures: results, lessons, and problems. *Epilepsia* 1983.

116. Cahan LD, Engel Jr. J. Surgery for epilepsy: a review. *Acta Neurol Scand* 1986;73:551–560.

117. Engel J Jr, Van Ness PC, Rasmussen TB, Ojemann LM. Outcome with respect to seizures. In: Engel J Jr, ed. Surgical treatment of the epilepsies, 2nd ed. New York: Raven Press, 1993:609–621.

118. Rougier A, Dartigues JF, Duche B, et al. Longitudinal analysis of the results in 60 cortical resections. *Epilepsies* 1989;1:301–309.

119. So N, Olivier A, Andermann F, et al. Results of surgical treatment in patients with bitemporal epileptiform abnormalities. *Ann Neurol* 1989;25:432–439.

120. Clusmann H, Schramm J, Kral T, et al. Prognostic factors and outcome after different types of resection for temporal lobe epilepsy. *J Neurosurg* 2002;97:1131–1141.

121. Antel SB, Li LM, Cendes F, et al. Predicting surgical outcome in temporal lobe epilepsy patients using MRI and MRSI. *Neurology* 2002;58:1505–1512.

122. Kral T, Kuczaty S, Blumcke I, et al. Postsurgical outcome of children and adolescents with medically refractory frontal lobe epilepsies. *Childs Nerv Syst* 2001;17:595–601.

123. Salanova V, Markand O, Worth R, et al. Presurgical evaluation and surgical outcome of temporal lobe epilepsy. *Pediatr Neurol* 1999;20:179–184.

124. Jeong SW, Lee SK, Kim KK, et al. Prognostic factors in anterior temporal lobe resections for mesial temporal lobe epilepsy: multivariate analysis. *Epilepsia* 1999;40:1735–1739.

125. Corsellis AN. The incidence of ammons horn sclerosis. *Brain* 1957;80:193–203.

126. Margerison JH, Corsellis JAN. Epilepsy and the temporal lobes: a clinical electrographic and neuropathological study of the brain in epilepsy, with particular reference to the temporal lobes. *Brain* 1966;89:499–530.

127. Bruton CJ. The neuropathology of temporal lobe epilepsy. Oxford: Oxford University Press, 1988.

128. Gates JR, Cruz, Rodriguez R. Mesial temporal sclerosis: pathogenesis, diagnosis, and management. *Epilepsia* 1990.

129. Tien RD, Felsberg GJ, Campi de Castro C, et al. Complex partial seizures and mesial temporal sclerosis: evaluation with fast spin-echo MR imaging. *Radiology* 1993;189:835–842.

130. Van Paesschen W, Connelly A, King MD, et al. The spectrum of hippocampal sclerosis: a quantitative magnetic resonance imaging study. *Ann Neurol* 1997;41:41–51.

131. Sommer W. Erkrankung des Ammonshorns als ätiologisches Moment der Epilepsie. *Arch Psychiatr Nervenkr* 1880;10:631–675.

132. Bouchet C, Cazauvieilh R. De l'epilepsie consideree dans ses rapports avec l'alienation mentale. *Arch Gen Med* 1825;9:510–542.

133. Peiffer J. Probleme der Krampfschädigung beim Menschen. *Epilepsie* 1988;88:257–267.

134. Peiffer J. Morphologische Aspekte der Epilepsien. Berlin: Springer, 1963.

135. Scott RC, Gadian DG, Cross JH, et al. Quantitative magnetic resonance characterization of mesial temporal sclerosis in childhood. *Neurology* 2001;56:1659–1665.

136. Briellmann RS, Kalnins RM, Berkovic SF, Jackson GD. Hippocampal pathology in refractory temporal lobe epilepsy: T2-weighted signal change reflects dentate gliosis. *Neurology* 2002;58:265–271.

137. Cross JH, Jackson GD, Neville BGR, et al. Early detection of abnormalities in partial epilepsy using magnetic resonance. *Arch Dis Child* 1993;69:104–109.

138. Mitchell A, Harvey S, Coleman L, et al. Anterior temporal changes in children with hippocampal sclerosis: an effect of seizures on the immature brain? *Am J Neuroradiol* 2003;24:1670–1677.

139. Sztriha L, Gururaj AK, Bener A, Nork M. Temporal lobe epilepsy in children: etiology in a cohort with new-onset seizures. *Epilepsia* 2002;43:75–80.

140. Harvey AS, Berkovic SF, Wrennall JA, Hopkins IJ. Temporal lobe epilepsy in childhood: clinical, EEG, and neuroimaging findings and syndrome classification in a cohort with new-onset seizures. *Neurology* 1997;49:960–968.

141. Benbadis SR, Wallace J, Reed Murtagh F. MRI evidence of mesial temporal sclerosis in subjects without seizures. *Seizure* 2002;11:340–343.

142. Kobayashi E, Li LM, Lopes-Cendes I, Cendes F. Magnetic resonance imaging evidence of hippocampal sclerosis in asymptomatic, first-degree relatives of patients with familial mesial temporal lobe epilepsy. *Arch Neurol* 2002;59:1891–1894.

143. During M, Spencer DD. Extracellular hippocampal glutamate and spontaneous seizure in the conscious human brain. *Lancet* 1993;341:1607–1610.

144. Choi DW, Rothman SM. The role of glutamate neurotoxicity in hypoxic ischemic neuronal death. *Ann Rev Neurosci* 1990;13:171–182.

145. Meyerhoff JL, Koller KJ, Walczak DD, Coyle JT. Brain regional levels of N-acetyl aspartylglutamate NAAG: the effect of kindled seizures. *Brain Res* 1985;346:392–396.

146. Kauppinen RA, Williams SR. Nondestructive detection of glutamate by ^{1}H NMR spectroscopy in cortical brain slices from the guinea pig: evidence for changes in delectability during severe anoxic insults. *J Neurochem* 1991;57:1136–1144.

147. Koller JK, Zaczek R, Coyle JT. N-acetyl-aspartyl-glutamate: regional levels in rat brain and the effects of brain lesions as determined by a new HPLC method. *J Neurochem* 1984;43:1136–1142.

148. Blakeley RD, Coyle JT. The neurology of N-acetyl aspartylglutamate. *Int Rev Neurobiol* 1988;30:39–99.

149. Brancati A, D'Arcangelo P. Effects evoked by pentamethylenetetrazol-induced seizures upon N-acetyl aspartate and N-acetyl aspartatyl-glutamate levels in different regions of the rat neuraxis. *Life Sci* 1990;48:2229–2232.

150. Cendes F, Andermann F, Dubeau F, et al. Early childhood prolonged febrile convulsions, atrophy and sclerosis of mesial structures, and temporal lobe epilepsy: An MRI volumetric study. *Neurology* 1993;43:1083–1087.

151. Holmes GL. Do seizures cause brain damage? *Epilepsia* 1991;32:S14–S28.

152. Kuks JBM, Cook MD, Fish DR, et al. Hippocampal sclerosis in epilepsy and childhood febrile seizures. *Lancet* 1993;342:1391–1394.

153. Resnick TJ. Evaluation of children for epilepsy surgery. *Int Pediatr* 1988;3:136–142.

154. Sutula T, Cascino G, Cavazos J, et al. Mossy fiber synaptic reorganization in the epileptic human temporal lobe. *Ann Neurol* 1989;26:321–330.

155. Mathern GW, Babb TL, Vickrey BG, et al. The clinical–pathogenic mechanisms of hippocampal neuron loss and surgical outcomes in temporal lobe epilepsy. *Brain* 1995;118:105–118.

156. Mathern GW, Adelson PD, Cahan LD, Leite JP. Hippocampal neuron damage in human epilepsy: Meyer's hypothesis revisited. *Prog Brain Res* 2002;135:237–251.

157. Agosti R, Yasargil G, Egli M, et al. Neuropathology of a human hippocampus following long-term treatment with vigabatrin: lack of microvacuoles. *Epilepsy Res* 1990;6:166–170.

158. Dutar P, Nicoll RA. Pre- and postsynaptic GABA receptors in the hippocampus have different pharmacological properties. *Neuron* 1988;1:585–591.

159. Davenport CJ, Brown WJ, Babb TL. Sprouting of GABAergic and mossy fiber axons in dentate gyrus following intrahippocampal kainate in the rat. *Exp Neurol* 1990;109:180–190.

160. Olivier A, Tanaka T, Andermann F. Reoperations in temporal lobe epilepsy. *Epilepsia* 1988;29:678.

161. Watson C, Andermann F, Gloor P, et al. Anatomic basis of amygdaloid and hippocampal volume measurement by magnetic resonance imaging. *Neurology* 1992;42:1743–1750.

162. Kuzniecky R, De La Sayette V, Ethier R, et al. Magnetic resonance imaging in temporal lobe epilepsy: pathological correlations. *Ann Neurol* 1987;22:341–347.

163. Cendes F, Andermann F, Gloor P, et al. MRI volumetric measurement of amygdala and hippocampus in temporal lobe epilepsy. *Neurology* 1993;43:719–725.

164. Cendes F, Andermann F, Gloor P, et al. Atrophy of mesial structures in patients with temporal lobe epilepsy: cause or consequence of repeated seizures? *Ann Neurol* 1993;34:795–801.

165. Van Paesschen W, King MD, Duncan JS, Connelly A. The amygdala and temporal lobe simple partial seizures: a prospective and quantitative MRI study. *Epilepsia* 2001;42:857–862.

166. Van Paesschen W, Connelly A, Johnson CL, Duncan JS. The amygdala and intractable temporal lobe epilepsy: a quantitative magnetic resonance imaging study. *Neurology* 1996;47:1021–1031.

167. Bernasconi N, Bernasconi A, Caramanos Z, et al. Mesial temporal damage in temporal lobe epilepsy: a volumetric MRI study of the hippocampus, amygdala and parahippocampal region. *Brain* 2003;126:462–469.

168. Blume WT. Epilepsy: advances in management. *Eur Neurol* 1997;38:198–208.

169. Ho SS, Consalvo D, Gilliam F, et al. Amygdala atrophy and seizure outcome after temporal lobe epilepsy surgery. *Neurology* 1998;51:1502–1504.

170. Salmenpera T, Kalviainen R, Partanen K, Pitkanen A. Hippocampal and amygdaloid damage in partial epilepsy: a cross-sectional MRI study of 241 patients. *Epilepsy Res* 2001;46:69–82.

171. Kalviainen R, Salmenpera T, Partanen K, et al. MRI volumetry and T2 relaxometry of the amygdala in newly diagnosed and chronic temporal lobe epilepsy. *Epilepsy Res* 1997;28:39–50.

172. Lambert MV, Brierley B, Al-Sarraj S, et al. Quantitative magnetic resonance imaging of the amygdala in temporal lobe epilepsy – clinico-pathological correlations (a pilot study). *Epilepsy Res* 2003;53:39–46.

173. DeLong GR, Heinz ER. The clinical syndrome of early-life bilateral hippocampal sclerosis. *Ann Neurol* 1997;42:11–17.

174. Jackson GD, Berkovic SF, Connelly A, et al. Four diagnostic criteria for the MRI diagnosis of hippocampal sclerosis. In: Book of abstracts,

Society for Magnetic Resonance Medicine, 1992. Berlin: Society for Magnetic Resonance Medicine, 1992.

175. Jackson GD, Berkovic SF, Duncan JS, Connelly A. Optimizing the diagnosis of hippocampal sclerosis using magnetic resonance imaging. *Am J Neurorad* 1993;14:753–762.

176. Kuzniecky R, Murro A, King D, et al. Magnetic resonance imaging in childhood intractable partial epilepsies: Pathologic correlations. *Neurology* 1993;43:681–687.

177. Jackson GD, Connelly A, Duncan JS, et al. Detection of hippocampal pathology in intractable partial epilepsy: increased sensitivity with quantitative magnetic resonance T2 relaxometry. *Neurology* 1993;43:1793–1799.

178. Bartlett PA, Richardson MP, Duncan JS. Measurement of amygdala T2 relaxation time in temporal lobe epilepsy. *J Neurol Neurosurg Psychiatry* 2002;73:753–755.

179. Consalvo D, Giobellina R, Silva W, et al. [Mesial temporal sclerosis syndrome in adult patients]. *Medicina (B Aires)* 2000;60:165–169.

180. Mohamed A, Wyllie E, Ruggieri P, et al. Temporal lobe epilepsy due to hippocampal sclerosis in pediatric candidates for epilepsy surgery. *Neurology* 2001;56:1643–1649.

181. Commission on Neuroimaging of the International League Against Epilepsy. Guidelines for neuroimaging evaluation of patients with uncontrolled epilepsy considered for surgery. *Epilepsia* 1998;39:1375–1376.

182. Commission on Neuroimaging of the International League Against Epilepsy. Recommendations for neuroimaging of patients with epilepsy. *Epilepsia* 1997;38:1255–1256.

183. Kuzniecky R, Jackson GD. Magnetic resonance in epilepsy. New York: Raven Press, 1995.

184. Holmes MD, Miles AN, Dodrill CB, et al. Identifying potential surgical candidates in patients with evidence of bitemporal epilepsy. *Epilepsia* 2003;44:1075–1079.

185. Boling W, Olivier A. The current state of epilepsy surgery. *Curr Opin Neurol* 1998;11:155–161.

186. Jackson GD, Duncan JS. MRI neuroanatomy: a new angle on the brain. Edinburgh: Churchill Livingstone, 1996.

187. Jackson GD, Berkovic SF, Duncan JS, Connelly A. Optimizing the diagnosis of hippocampal sclerosis using magnetic resonance imaging. *Am J Neuroradiol* 1993;14:753–762.

188. Jackson GD, Berkovic SF, Tress BM, et al. Hippocampal sclerosis can be reliably detected by magnetic resonance imaging. *Neurology* 1990;40:1869–1875.

189. Schorner W, Meencke HJ, Felix R. Temporal-lobe epilepsy: comparison of CT and MR imaging. *AJR* 1987;149:1231–1239.

190. Sostman HD, Spencer DD, Gore JC, et al. Preliminary observations of magnetic resonance imaging in refractory epilepsy. *Magnetic Resonance Imaging* 1984;2:301–306.

191. Rougier A, Biset JM, Kien P, et al. MRI and surgery of epilepsy. *Neurochirurgie* 1988;34:188–193.

192. Laster DW, Penry JK, Moody DM, et al. Chronic seizure disorders: contribution of MR imaging when CT is normal. *Am J Neuroradiol* 1985;6:177–180.

193. Berkovic SF, Ethier R, Robitaille Y, et al. Magnetic resonance imaging of the hippocampus: II. mesial temporal sclerosis. *Epilepsia* 1986;27:612.

194. Takanashi J, Sugita K, Fujii K, Niimi H. MR evaluation of tuberous sclerosis: increased sensitivity with fluid-attenuated inversion recovery and relation to severity of seizures and mental retardation. *Am J Neuroradiol* 1995;16:1923–1928.

195. Jack CR Jr, Rydberg CH, Krecke KN, et al. Mesial temporal sclerosis: diagnosis with fluid-attenuated inversion-recovery versus spin-echo MR imaging. *Radiology* 1996;199:367–373.

196. Bradley WG, Shey RB. MR imaging evaluation of seizures. *Radiology* 2000;214:651–656.

197. Briellmann RS, Pell GS, Wellard RM, et al. MR imaging of epilepsy: state of the art at 1.5T and potential of 3T. *Epileptic Disord* 2003;5:3–20.

198. Meiners LC, van Gils AD, De Kort G, et al. Fast fluid-attenuated inversion recovery (FLAIR) compared with T2-weighted spin-echo in the magnetic resonance diagnosis of mesial temporal sclerosis. *Invest Radiol* 1999;34:134–142.

199. Woermann FG, Steiner H, Barker GJ, et al. A fast FLAIR dual-echo technique for hippocampal T2 relaxometry: first experiences in patients with temporal lobe epilepsy. *J Magn Reson Imaging* 2001;13:547–552.

200. Wieshmann UC, Free SL, Everitt AD, et al. Magnetic resonance imaging in epilepsy with a fast FLAIR sequence. *J Neurol Neurosurg Psychiatry* 1996;61:357–361.

201. Bergin PS, Fish DR, Shorvon SD, et al. FLAIR imaging in partial epilepsy: improving the yield of MRI. *Epilepsia* 1993;34:121.

202. Kuzniecky R, Suggs S, Gaudier J, Faught E. Lateralization of epileptic foci by MRI in temporal lobe epilepsy. *J Neuroimaging* 1991;1:163–167.

203. Ryvlin P, Cinotti L, Froment JC, et al. Metabolic patterns associated with non-specific magnetic resonance imaging abnormalities in temporal lobe epilepsy. *Brain* 1991;114:2363–2383.

204. Berkovic SF, Andermann F, Olivier A, et al. Hippocampal sclerosis in temporal lobe epilepsy demonstrated by magnetic resonance imaging. *Ann Neurol* 1991;29:175–182.

205. Jackson GD, Duncan JS, Connelly A, Austin SJ. Increased signal in the mesial temporal region on T2 weighted MRI; a quantitative study of hippocampal sclerosis. *Neurology* 1991;41(Suppl 1):170–171.

206. Cascino GD, Jack CR Jr, Parisi JE, et al. Magnetic resonance imaging – based volume studies in temporal lobe epilepsy: pathological correlations. *Ann Neurol* 1991;30:31–36.

207. Cook MJ, Fish DR, Shorvon SD, et al. Hippocampal volumetric and morphometric studies in frontal and temporal lobe epilepsy. *Brain* 1992;115:1001–1015.

208. Jack CJ, Gehring DG, Sharbrough FW, et al. Temporal lobe volume measurement from MR images: accuracy and left-right asymmetry in normal persons. *J Comput Assisted Tomography* 1988;12:21–29.

209. Jack CJ, Sharbrough FW, Marsh WR. Use of MR imaging for quantitative evaluation of resection for temporal lobe epilepsy. *Radiology* 1988;169:463–468.

210. Lencz T, McCarthy G, Bronen RA, et al. Quantitative magnetic resonance imaging in temporal lobe epilepsy: relationship to neuropathology and neuropsychological function. *Ann Neurol* 1992;31:629–637.

211. Spencer SS, McCarthy G, Spencer DD. Diagnosis of medial temporal lobe seizure onset: relative specificity and sensitivity of quantitative MRI. *Neurology* 1993;43:2117–2124.

212. Lemieux L, Liu RS, Duncan JS. Hippocampal and cerebellar volumetry in serially acquired MRI volume scans. *Magn Reson Imaging* 2000;18:1027–1033.

213. Bilir E, Craven W, Hugg J, et al. Volumetric MRI of the limbic system: anatomic determinants. *Neuroradiology* 1998;40:138–144.

214. Lawson JA, Cook MJ, Bleasel AF, et al. Quantitative MRI in outpatient childhood epilepsy. *Epilepsia* 1997;38:1289–1293.

215. Kilpatrick C, Cook M, Kaye A, et al. Non-invasive investigations successfully select patients for temporal lobe surgery. *J Neurol Neurosurg Psychiatry* 1997;63:327–333.

216. Chee MW, Low S, Tan JS, et al. Hippocampal volumetry with magnetic resonance imaging: a cost-effective validated solution. *Epilepsia* 1997;38:461–465.

217. Breier JI, Leonard CM, Bauer RM, et al. Quantified volumes of temporal lobe structures in patients with epilepsy. *J Neuroimaging* 1996;6:108–114.

218. Van Paesschen W, Sisodiya S, Connelly A, et al. Quantitative hippocampal MRI and intractable temporal lobe epilepsy. *Neurology* 1995;45:2233–2240.

219. Luby M, Spencer DD, Kim JH, et al. Hippocampal MRI volumetrics and temporal lobe substrates in medial temporal lobe epilepsy. *Magn Reson Imaging* 1995;13:1065–1071.

220. Jack CR Jr, Theodore WH, Cook M, McCarthy G. MRI-based hippocampal volumetrics: data acquisition, normal ranges, and optimal protocol. *Magn Reson Imaging* 1995;13:1057–1064.

221. Vadillo J, Noya M. [Differential diagnosis of the epilepsies]. *Neurologa* 1996;11(Suppl 4):13–21.

222. Van Paesschen W, Sisodiya S, Connelly A, et al. Quantitative hippocampal MRI and intractable temporal lobe epilepsy. *Neurology* 1995;45:2233–2240.

223. Briellmann RS, Kalnins RM, Hopwood MJ, et al. TLE patients with postictal psychosis: mesial dysplasia and anterior hippocampal preservation. *Neurology* 2000;55:1027–1030.

224. Li LM, Caramanos Z, Cendes F, et al. Lateralization of temporal lobe epilepsy (TLE) and discrimination of TLE from extra-TLE using pattern analysis of magnetic resonance spectroscopic and volumetric data. *Epilepsia* 2000;41:832–842.

225. Tsuruda J, Ojeman G, Holmes M, Alvord E. Comparison of clinical features, histology and high resolution fast spin MRI using a phased coil in patients undergoing surgery for temporal lobe epilepsy. *Epilepsia* 1993;34:36.

226. Duvernoy HM. The human hippocampus. Munich: Bergmann Verlag, 1988.

227. Bronen RA, Cheung G. MRI of the temporal lobe: normal variations, with special reference toward epilepsy. *Magn Reson Imaging* 1991;9:501–507.

228. Bronen RA, Cheung G. MRI of the normal hippocampus. *Magn Reson Imaging* 1991;9:497–500.

229. Bronen RA, Cheung G. Relationship of hippocampus and amygdala to coronal MRI landmarks. *Magn Reson Imaging* 1991;9:449–457.

230. Baxendale SA, van Paesschen W, Thompson PJ, et al. The relationship between quantitative MRI and neuropsychological functioning in temporal lobe epilepsy. *Epilepsia* 1998;39:158–166.

231. Namer I, Waydelich R, Armspach JP, et al. Contribution of T2 relaxation time mapping in the evaluation of cryptogenic temporal lobe epilepsy. *Neuroimage* 1998;7:304–313.

232. Bernasconi A, Bernasconi N, Caramanos Z, et al. T2 relaxometry can lateralize mesial temporal lobe epilepsy in patients with normal MRI. *Neuroimage* 2000;12:739–746.

233. Wood AC, Saling MM, O'Shea MF, et al. Components of verbal learning and hippocampal damage assessed by T2 relaxometry. *J Int Neuropsychol Soc* 2000;6:529–538.

234. Wendel JD, Trenerry MR, Xu YC, et al. The relationship between quantitative T2 relaxometry and memory in nonlesional temporal lobe epilepsy. *Epilepsia* 2001;42:863–868.

235. Jack CJ, Bentley MD, Twomey CK, Zinsmeister AR. MR imaging-based volume measurements of the hippocampal formation and anterior temporal lobe: Validation studies. *Radiology* 1990;176:205–209.

236. Cendes F, Andermann F, Gloor P, et al. MRI volumetric measurement of amygdala and hippocampus in temporal lobe epilepsy. *Neurology* 1993;43:719–725.

237. Kuks JB, Cook MJ, Fish DR, et al. Hippocampal sclerosis in epilepsy and childhood febrile seizures. *Lancet* 1993;342:1391–1394.

238. Trenerry MR, Jack CR Jr, Ivnik RJ, et al. MRI hippocampal volumes and memory function before and after temporal lobectomy. *Neurology* 1993;43:1800–1805.

239. Kim JH, Tien RD, Felsberg GJ, et al. MR measurements of the hippocampus for lateralization of temporal lobe epilepsy: value of measurements of the body vs the whole structure. *AJR* 1994;163:1453–1457.

240. Free SL, Bergin PS, Fish DR, et al. Methods for normalization of hippocampal volumes measured with MR. *Am J Neuroradiol* 1995;16:637–643.

241. Jackson GD, Connelly A, Duncan JS, et al. Detection of hippocampal pathology in intractable partial epilepsy: increased sensitivity with quantitative magnetic resonance T2 relaxometry. *Neurology* 1993;43:1793–1799.

242. Grunewald RA, Jackson GD, Connelly A, Duncan JS. MR detection of hippocampal disease in epilepsy: factors influencing T2 relaxation time. *Am J Neuroradiol* 1994;15:1149–1156.

243. Duncan JS, Bartlett P, Barker GJ. Technique for measuring hippocampal T2 relaxation time. *Am J Neuroradiol* 1996;17:1805–1810.

244. Woermann FG, Barker GJ, Birnie KD, et al. Regional changes in hippocampal T2 relaxation and volume: a quantitative magnetic resonance imaging study of hippocampal sclerosis. *J Neurol Neurosurg Psychiatry* 1998;65:656–664.

245. Bronen RA, Cheung G, Charles JT, et al. Imaging findings in hippocampal sclerosis: correlation with pathology. *Am J Neuroradiol* 1991;12:933–940.

246. Lee N, Tien RD, Lewis DV, et al. Fast spin-echo, magnetic resonance imaging-measured hippocampal volume: correlation with neuronal density in anterior temporal lobectomy patients. *Epilepsia* 1995;36:899–904.

247. Van Paesschen W, Revesz T, Duncan JS, et al. Quantitative neuropathology and quantitative magnetic resonance imaging of the hippocampus in temporal lobe epilepsy. *Ann Neurol* 1997;42:756–766.

248. Ashtari M, Barr WB, Schaul N, Bogerts B. Three-dimensional fast low-angle shot imaging and computerized volume measurement of the hippocampus in patients with chronic epilepsy of the temporal lobe. *Am J Neuroradiol* 1991;12:941–947.

249. Watson C. Volumetric MRI in patients with extratemporal structural lesions. *Epilepsia* 1993;34:128.

250. Briellmann RS, Syngeniotis A, Jackson GD. Comparison of hippocampal volumetry at 1.5 tesla and at 3 tesla. *Epilepsia* 2001;42:1021–1024.

251. Van Paesschen W, Revesz T, Sisodiya S, et al. Quantitative neuropathology and quantitative magnetic resonance imaging of the hippocampus of patients with intractable temporal lobe epilepsy. *Epilepsia* 1995;36(Suppl 3):S96.

252. Mitchell LA, Jackson GD, Kalnins RM, et al. Anterior temporal abnormality in temporal lobe epilepsy: a quantitative MRI and histopathologic study. *Neurology* 1999;52:327–336.

253. Briellmann RS, Berkovic SF, Jackson GD. Men may be more vulnerable to seizure-associated brain damage. *Neurology* 2000;55:1479–1485.

254. Briellmann RS, Newton MR, Wellard RM, Jackson GD. Hippocampal sclerosis following brief generalized seizures in adulthood. *Neurology* 2001;57:315–317.

255. Briellmann RS, Berkovic SF, Syngeniotis A, et al. Seizure-associated hippocampal volume loss: a longitudinal magnetic resonance study of temporal lobe epilepsy. *Ann Neurol* 2002;51:641–644.

**256. Trenerry MR, Jack CR Jr, Ivnik RJ, et al. MRI hippocampal volumes and memory function before and after temporal lobectomy. *Neurology* 1993;43:1800–1805.

257. Cascino GD, Jack CR Jr, Parisi JE, et al. MRI in the presurgical evaluation of patients with frontal lobe epilepsy and children with temporal lobe epilepsy: pathologic correlation and prognostic importance. *Epilepsy Res* 1992;11:51–59.

258. Jack C. MRI-based hippocampal volume measurements in epilepsy. *Epilepsia* 1994;35(Suppl 6):14–19.

**259. Watson C, Andermann F, Gloor P, et al. Anatomic basis of amygdaloid and hippocampal volume measurement by magnetic resonance imaging. *Neurology* 1992;42:1743–1750.

260. Watson C, Cendes F, Fuerst D, et al. Specificity of volumetric magnetic resonance imaging in detecting hippocampal sclerosis. *Arch Neurol* 1997;54:67–73.

261. Watson C, Nielsen SL, Cobb C, et al. Medial temporal lobe heterotopia as a cause of increased hippocampal and amygdaloid MRI volumes. *J Neuroimaging* 1996;6:231–234.

262. Li LM, Cendes F, Andermann F, et al. Surgical outcome in patients with epilepsy and dual pathology. *Brain* 1999;122:799–805.

263. Fuerst D, Shah J, Shah A, Watson C. Hippocampal sclerosis is a progressive disorder: a longitudinal volumetric MRI study. *Ann Neurol* 2003;53:413–416.

264. Fuerst D, Shah J, Kupsky WJ, et al. Volumetric MRI, pathological, and neuropsychological progression in hippocampal sclerosis. *Neurology* 2001;57:184–188.

265. Jack CJ, Twomey CK, Zinsmeister AR, et al. Anterior temporal lobes and hippocampal formations: normative volumetric measurements from MR images in young adults. *Radiology* 1989;172:549–554.

266. Cook MJ, Fish DR, Shorvon SD, et al. Bilateral hippocampal atrophy: volumetric MRI assessment. *Epilepsia* 1993;34:136.

267. Wang L, Swank JS, Glick IE, et al. Changes in hippocampal volume and shape across time distinguish dementia of the Alzheimer type from healthy aging. *Neuroimage* 2003;20:667–682.

268. Morys J, Bobek-Billewicz B, Dziewiatkowski J, et al. Changes in the volume of temporal lobe structures related to Alzheimer's type dementia. *Folia Neuropathol* 2002;40:47–56.

269. Steffens DC, Payne ME, Greenberg DL, et al. Hippocampal volume and incident dementia in geriatric depression. *Am J Geriatr Psychiatry* 2002;10:62–71.

270. Szeszko PR, Goldberg E, Gunduz-Bruce H, et al. Smaller anterior hippocampal formation volume in antipsychotic-naive patients with first-episode schizophrenia. *Am J Psychiatry* 2003;160:2190–2197.

271. Pegues MP, Rogers LJ, Amend D, et al. Anterior hippocampal volume reduction in male patients with schizophrenia. *Schizophr Res* 2003;60:105–115.

272. Keshavan MS, Dick E, Mankowski I, et al. Decreased left amygdala and hippocampal volumes in young offspring at risk for schizophrenia. *Schizophr Res* 2002;58:173–183.

273. Seidman LJ, Faraone SV, Goldstein JM, et al. Left hippocampal volume as a vulnerability indicator for schizophrenia: a magnetic resonance imaging morphometric study of nonpsychotic first-degree relatives. *Arch Gen Psychiatry* 2002;59:839–849.

274. Shenton ME, Gerig G, McCarley RW, et al. Amygdala–hippocampal shape differences in schizophrenia: the application of 3D shape models to volumetric MR data. *Psychiatry Res* 2002;115:15–35.

275. Velakoulis D, Stuart GW, Wood SJ, et al. Selective bilateral hippocampal volume loss in chronic schizophrenia. *Biol Psychiatry* 2001;50:531–539.

276. Wood SJ, Velakoulis D, Smith DJ, et al. A longitudinal study of hippocampal volume in first episode psychosis and chronic schizophrenia. *Schizophr Res* 2001;52:37–46.

277. Isaacs EB, Vargha-Khadem F, Watkins KE, et al. Developmental amnesia and its relationship to degree of hippocampal atrophy. *Proc Natl Acad Sci USA* 2003;100:13060–13063.

278. Squire LR, Amaral DG, Press GA. Magnetic resonance imaging of the hippocampal formation and mammillary nuclei distinguish medial temporal lobe and diencephalic amnesia. *J Neurosci* 1990;10:3106–3117.

279. Benbadis SR, Tatum WO, Murtagh FR, Vale FL. MRI evidence of mesial temporal sclerosis in patients with psychogenic nonepileptic seizures. *Neurology* 2000;55:1061–1062.

280. Jackson GD, Berkovic SF, Duncan JS, Connelly A. Optimizing the diagnosis of hippocampal sclerosis using magnetic resonance imaging. *Am. J. Neuroradiol* 1993;14:753–762.

281. Bartzokis G, Mintz J, Marx P, et al. Reliability of in vivo volume measures of hippocampus and other brain structures using MRI. *Magn Reson Imaging* 1993;11:993–1006.

282. Cascino GD, Jack CR Jr, Hirschorn KA, Sharbrough FW. Identification of the epileptic focus: magnetic resonance imaging. *Epilepsy Res Suppl* 1992.

283. Okujava M, Schulz R, Ebner A, Woermann FG. Measurement of temporal lobe T2 relaxation times using a routine diagnostic MR imaging protocol in epilepsy. *Epilepsy Res* 2002;48:131–142.

284. Whittall KP, MacKay AL, Li DK. Are mono-exponential fits to a few echoes sufficient to determine T2 relaxation for in vivo human brain? *Magn Reson Med* 1999;41:1255–1257.

285. Levy-Reis I, Casasanto DJ, Gonzalez JB, et al. Cortical reorganization in linear nevus sebaceous syndrome: a multimodality neuroimaging study. *J Neuroimaging* 2000;10:225–228.

286. Barnes D, McDonald WI, Johnson G, et al. Quantitative nuclear magnetic resonance imaging: characterisation of experimental cerebral oedema. *J Neurol Neurosurg Psychiatry* 1987;50:125–133.

287. Pell GS, Briellmann RS, Waites AB, et al. Voxel-based relaxometry: a new approach for analysis of T2 relaxometry changes in epilepsy. *Neuroimage* 2004;21:707–713.

288. Adam C, Clemenceau S, Semah F, et al. [Strategy of evaluation and surgical results in medial temporal lobe epilepsy]. *Rev Neurol (Paris)* 1997;153:641–651.

289. Grunewald RA, Jackson GD, Connelly A, Duncan JS. MR detection of hippocampal pathology in epilepsy: factors influencing T2 relaxation time. *Am J Neuroradiol* 1994;15:1149–1156.

290. Nohira V, Lee N, Tien RD, et al. Magnetic resonance imaging evidence of hippocampal sclerosis in progression: a case report. *Epilepsia* 1994;35:1332–1336.

291. Wieshmann UC, Woermann FG, Lemieeux L, et al. Development of hippocampal atrophy: a serial magnetic resonance imaging study in a patient who developed epilepsy after generalized status epilepticus. *Epilepsia* 1997;38:1238–1241.

292. Henry TR, Drury I, Brunberg JA, et al. Focal cerebral magnetic resonance changes associated with partial status epilepticus. *Epilepsia* 1994;35:35–41.

293. VanLandingham KE, Heinz ER, Cavazos JE, Lewis DV. Magnetic resonance imaging evidence of hippocampal injury after prolonged focal febrile convulsions. *Ann Neurol* 1998;43:413–426.

294. Bouilleret V, Nehlig A, Marescaux C, Namer IJ. Magnetic resonance imaging follow-up of progressive hippocampal changes in a mouse model of mesial temporal lobe epilepsy. *Epilepsia* 2000;41:642–650.

295. Cox JE, Mathews VP, Santos CC, Elster AD. Seizure-induced transient hippocampal abnormalities on MR: correlation with positron emission tomography and electroencephalography. *Am J Neuroradiol* 1995;16:1736–1738.

296. Chan S, Chin SS, Kartha K, et al. Reversible signal abnormalities in the hippocampus and neocortex after prolonged seizures. *Am J Neuroradiol* 1996;17:1725–1731.

297. Jackson GD, Chambers BR, Berkovic SF. Hippocampal sclerosis: development in adult life. *Dev Neurosci* 1999;21:207–214.

298. Scott RC, Gadian DG, King MD, et al. Magnetic resonance imaging findings within 5 days of status epilepticus in childhood. *Brain* 2002;125:1951–1959.

299. Grunewald RA, Farrow T, Vaughan P, et al. A magnetic resonance study of complicated early childhood convulsion. *J Neurol Neurosurg Psychiatry* 2001;71:638–642.

300. Briellmann RS, Newton MR, Wellard RM, Jackson GD. Hippocampal sclerosis following brief generalized seizures. *Neurology* 2001;57:315–317.

301. Kobayashi E, Guerreiro CA, Cendes F. Late onset temporal lobe epilepsy with MRI evidence of mesial temporal sclerosis following acute neurocysticercosis: case report. *Arq Neuropsiquiatr* 2001;59:255–258.

302. Cendes F, Andermann F, Carpenter S, et al. Temporal lobe epilepsy caused by domoic acid intoxication: evidence for glutamate receptor-mediated excitotoxicity in humans. *Ann Neurol* 1995;37:123–126.

303. Saukkonen A, Kalviainen R, Partanen K, et al. Do seizures cause neuronal damage? A MRI study in newly diagnosed and chronic epilepsy. *Neuroreport* 1994;6:219–223.

304. Tasch E, Cendes F, Li LM, et al. Neuroimaging evidence of progressive neuronal loss and dysfunction in temporal lobe epilepsy. *Ann Neurol* 1999;45:568–576.

305. Cendes F, Andermann F, Dubeau F, et al. Early childhood prolonged febrile convulsions, atrophy and sclerosis of mesial structures, and temporal lobe epilepsy: an MRI volumetric study. *Neurology* 1993;43:1083–1087.

306. Trenerry MR, Jack CR Jr, Sharbrough FW, et al. Quantitative MRI hippocampal volumes: association with onset and duration of epilepsy, and febrile convulsions in temporal lobectomy patients. *Epilepsy Res* 1993;15:247–252.

307. O'Brien TJ, So EL, Meyer FB, et al. Progressive hippocampal atrophy in chronic intractable temporal lobe epilepsy. *Ann Neurol* 1999;45:526–529.

308. Van Paesschen W, Duncan JS, Stevens JM, Connelly A. Longitudinal quantitative hippocampal magnetic resonance imaging study of adults with newly diagnosed partial seizures: one-year follow-up results. *Epilepsia* 1998;39:633–639.

309. Babb TL. Bilateral pathological damage in temporal lobe epilepsy. *Can J Neurol Sci* 1991;18(4 Suppl):645–648.

310. Barr WB, Ashtari M, Schaul N. Bilateral reductions in hippocampal volume in adults with epilepsy and a history of febrile seizures. *J Neurol Neurosurg Psychiatry* 1997;63:461–467.

311. Martin RC, Sawrie SM, Knowlton RC, et al. Bilateral hippocampal atrophy: consequences to verbal memory following temporal lobectomy. *Neurology* 2001;57:597–604.

312. Kälviäinen R, Salmenperä T, Partanen K, et al. Recurrent seizures may cause hippocampal damage in temporal lobe epilepsy. *Neurology* 1998;50:1377–1382.

313. Briellmann RS, Kalnins RM, Berkovic SF, Jackson GD. Hippocampal pathology in refractory temporal lobe epilepsy: T2-weighted signal change reflects dentate gliosis. *Neurology* 2002;58:265–271.

314. Namer IJ, Bolo NR, Sellal F, et al. Combined measurements of hippocampal N-acetyl-aspartate and T2 relaxation time in the evaluation of mesial temporal lobe epilepsy: correlation with clinical severity and memory performances. *Epilepsia* 1999;40:1424–1432.

315. Kalviainen R, Partanen K, Aikia M, et al. MRI-based hippocampal volumetry and T2 relaxometry: correlation to verbal memory performance in newly diagnosed epilepsy patients with left-sided temporal lobe focus. *Neurology* 1997;48:286–287.

316. Achten E, Boon P, De Poorter J, et al. An MR protocol for presurgical evaluation of patients with complex partial seizures of temporal lobe origin. *Am J Neuroradiol* 1995;16:1201–1213.

317. Heinz ER, Crain BJ, Radtke RA, et al. MR imaging in patients with temporal lobe seizures: correlation of results with pathologic findings. *Am J Neuroradiol* 1990;11:827–831.

318. Briellmann RS, Jackson GD, Kalnins R, Berkovic SF. Hemicranial volume deficits in patients with temporal lobe epilepsy with and without hippocampal sclerosis. *Epilepsia* 1998;39:1174–1181.

319. Briellmann RS, Jackson GD, Mitchell LA, et al. Occurrence of hippocampal sclerosis: is one hemisphere or gender more vulnerable? *Epilepsia* 1999;40:1816–1820.

320. Pitkänen A, Laakso M, Kälviäinen R, et al. Severity of hippocampal atrophy correlates with the prolongation of MRI T2 relaxation time in temporal lobe epilepsy but not in Alzheimer's disease. *Neurology* 1996;46:1724–1730.

321. Jackson GD, Kuzniecky RI, Cascino GD. Hippocampal sclerosis without detectable hippocampal atrophy. *Neurology* 1994;44:42–46.

322. Lee DH, Gao FQ, Rogers JM, et al. MR in temporal lobe epilepsy: analysis with pathologic confirmation. *Am J Neuroradiol* 1998;19:19–27.

323. Babb TL, Lieb JP, Brown WJ, et al. Distribution of pyramidal cell density and hyperexcitability in the epileptic human hippocampal formation. *Epilepsia* 1984;25:721–728.

324. Lee JW, Reutens DC, Dubeau F, et al. Morphometry in temporal lobe epilepsy. *Magn Reson Imaging* 1995;13:1073–1080.

325. Barkhof F, van Walderveen M. Characterization of tissue damage in multiple sclerosis by nuclear magnetic resonance. *Philos Trans R Soc Lond B Biol Sci* 1999;354:1675–1686.

326. Barnes D, McDonald WI, Landon DN, Johnson G. The characterisation of experimental gliosis by quantitative nuclear magnetic resonance imaging. *Brain* 1988;111:83–94.

327. Meiners LC, Witkamp TD, de Kort GA, et al. Relevance of temporal lobe white matter changes in hippocampal sclerosis. Magnetic resonance imaging and histology. *Invest Radiol* 1999;34:38–45.

328. Baxendale SA, Van Paesschen W, Thompson PJ, et al. The relation between quantitative MRI measures of hippocampal structure and the intracarotid amobarbital test. *Epilepsia* 1997;38:998–1007.

329. Jack CR Jr. Hippocampal T2 relaxometry in epilepsy: past, present, and future. *Am J Neuroradiol* 1996;17:1811–1814.

330. Meiners LC, Valk J, Jansen GH, Luyten PR. Magnetic resonance of epilepsy: three observations. In: Shorvon SD, Fish DR, Andermann F, et al, eds. Magnetic resonance scanning and epilepsy. New York: Plenum Press, 1994:79–82.

331. Achten E, Deblaere K, De Wagter C, et al. Intra- and interobserver variability of MRI-based volume measurements of the hippocampus and amygdala using the manual ray-tracing method. *Neuroradiology* 1998;40:558–566.

332. Connelly A, Van Paesschen W, Porter DA, et al. Proton magnetic resonance spectroscopy in MRI-negative temporal lobe epilepsy. *Neurology* 1998;51:61–66.

333. Fujii M, Akimura T, Ozaki S, et al. An angiographically occult arteriovenous malformation in the medial parietal lobe presenting as seizures of medial temporal lobe origin. *Epilepsia* 1999;40:377–381.

334. Salmenpera T, Kalviainen R, Partanen K, et al. MRI volumetry of the hippocampus, amygdala, entorhinal cortex, and perirhinal cortex after status epilepticus. *Epilepsy Res* 2000;40:155–170.

335. Levesque M, Nakasato N, Vinters H, Babb T. Surgical treatment of limbic epilepsy associated with extrahippocampal lesions: the problem of dual pathology. *J Neurosurg* 1991;75(364–370).

336. Kim J, Guimaraes P, Shen M, Masukawa L. Hippocampal neuronal density in temporal lobe epilepsy with and without gliomas. *Acta Neuropathol* 1990;80:41–45.

337. Cascino GD, Jack CR Jr, Parisi JE, et al. Operative strategy in patients with MRI-identified dual pathology and temporal lobe epilepsy. *Epilepsy Res* 1993;14:175–182.

338. Li LM, Cendes F, Watson C, et al. Surgical treatment of patients with single and dual pathology: relevance of lesion and of hippocampal atrophy to seizure outcome. *Neurology* 1997;48:437–444.

339. Cendes F, Li LM, Andermann F, et al. Dual pathology and its clinical relevance. *Adv Neurol* 1999;81:153–164.

340. Sisodiya SM, Moran N, Free SL, et al. Correlation of widespread preoperative magnetic resonance imaging changes with unsuccessful surgery for hippocampal sclerosis. *Ann Neurol* 1997;41:490–496.

341. Sisodiya SM, Free S, Fish DR, Shorvon SD. Novel magnetic resonance imaging methods for quantifying changes in the cortical ribbon in patients with epilepsy. *Adv Neurol* 1999;81:81–87.

342. Bastos AC, Comeau RM, Andermann F, et al. Diagnosis of subtle focal dysplastic lesions: curvilinear reformatting from three-dimensional magnetic resonance imaging. *Ann Neurol* 1999;46:88–94.

343. Meiners LC, van der Grond J, van Rijen PC, et al. Proton magnetic resonance spectroscopy of temporal lobe white matter in patients with histologically proven hippocampal sclerosis. *J Magn Reson Imaging* 2000;11:25–31.

344. Ryvlin P, Coste S, Hermier M, Mauguiere F. Temporal pole MRI abnormalities in temporal lobe epilepsy. *Epileptic Disord* 2002;(4 Suppl 1):S33–S39.

345. Ho SS, Kuzniecky RI, Gilliam F, et al. Temporal lobe developmental malformations and epilepsy: dual pathology and bilateral hippocampal abnormalities. *Neurology* 1998;50:748–754.

346. Jackson GD, McIntosh AM, Briellmann RS, Berkovic SF. Hippocampal sclerosis studied in identical twins. *Neurology* 1998;51:78–84.

347. Vezzani A, Conti M, De Luigi A, et al. Interleukin-1 beta immunoreactivity and microglia are enhanced in the rat hippocampus by focal kainate application: functional evidence for enhancement of electrographic seizures. *J Neurosci* 1999;19:5054–5065.

348. Briellmann RS, Jackson GD, Torn-Broers Y, Berkovic SF. Twins with different temporal lobe malformations: schizencephaly and arachnoid cyst. *Neuropediatrics* 1998;29:284–288.

349. Berkovic SF, Jackson GD. The hippocampal sclerosis whodunit: enter the genes. *Ann Neurol* 2000;47:557–558.

350. Berkovic SF, McIntosh AM, Kalnins RM, et al. Preoperative MRI predicts outcome of temporal lobectomy: an actuarial analysis. *Neurology* 1995;45:1358–1363.

351. Maher J, McLachlan RS. Febrile convulsions: is seizure duration the most important predictor of temporal lobe epilepsy? *Brain* 1995;118:1521–1528.

352. Mathern GW, Leite JP, Pretorius JK, et al. Children with severe epilepsy: evidence of hippocampal neuron losses and aberrant mossy fiber sprouting during postnatal granule cell migration and differentiation. *Brain Res Dev* 1994;78:70–80.

353. Mathern GW, Babb T, Leite JP, et al. The pathogenic and progressive features of chronic human hippocampal epilepsy. *Epilepsy Res* 1996;26:151–161.

354. Shinnar S. Prolonged febrile seizures and mesial temporal sclerosis. *Ann Neurol* 1998;43:411–412.

355. Nohira V, Lee N, Tien RD, et al. Magnetic Resonance Imaging Evidence of Hippocampal Sclerosis in Progression: a case report. *Epilepsia* 1994;35:1332–1339.

356. Wieshmann UC, Woermann FG, Lemieux L, et al. Development of hippocampal atrophy: a serial magnetic resonance imaging study in a patient who developed epilepsy after generalized status epilepticus. *Epilepsia* 1997;38:1238–1241.

357. VanLandingham KE, Heinz ER, Cavazos JE, Lewis DV. Magnetic resonance imaging evidence of hippocampal injury after prolonged focal febrile convulsions. *Ann Neurol* 1998;43:413–426.

358. Nohria V, Lee N, Tien RD, et al. Magnetic resonance imaging evidence of hippocampal sclerosis in progression: a case report. *Epilepsia* 1994;35:1332–1336.

359. Van Paesschen W, Duncan JS, Stevens JM, Connelly A. Longitudinal quantitative hippocampal magnetic resonance imaging study of adults with newly diagnosed partial seizures: one-year follow-up results. *Epilepsia* 1998;39:633–639.

360. Free SL, Li LM, Fish DR, et al. Bilateral hippocampal volume loss in patients with a history of encephalitis or meningitis. *Epilepsia* 1996;37:400–405.

361. Bertram EH, D. LM, Lenn NJ. The hippocampus in experimental chronic epilepsy: a morphometric analysis. *Ann Neurol* 1990;27:43–48.

362. Castiglioni AJ, Peterson SL, Sanabria EL, Tiffany CE. Structural changes in astrocytes induced by seizures in a model of temporal lobe epilepsy. *J Neurosci Res* 1990;26:334–341.

363. Cavazos JE, Sutula TP. Progressive neuronal loss induced by kindling: a possible mechanism for mossy fiber synaptic reorganization and hippocampal sclerosis. *Brain Res* 1990;527:1–6.

364. Meldrum BS. In vivo and in vitro models of epilepsy and their relevance to man. In: Meldrum BS, Ferrendelli JA, Wiesere HG, eds. Current problems in epilepsy 6: Anatomy of epileptogenesis. London: John Libbey, 1988.

365. Scheinberg P. The biologic basis for the treatment of acute stroke. *Neurology* 1991;41:1867–1873.

366. Mathern GW, Price G, Rosales C, et al. Anoxia during kainate status epilepticus shortens behavioral convulsions but generates hippocampal neuron loss and supragranular mossy fiber spouting. *Epilepsy* Res 1998;30:133–151.

367. Schwartzkroin PA. Basic mechanisms of epileptogenesis. In: Wylie E, ed. The treatment of epilepsy: principles and practice. Philadelphia, PA: Lea & Febiger, 1993:83–98.

368. Sutula TP. Experimental models of temporal lobe epilepsy: new insights from the study of kindling and synaptic reorganization. *Epilepsia* 1990;31(Suppl 3):S45–S54.

369. Sloviter RS. The functional organisation of the hippocampal dentate gyrus and its relevance to the pathogenesis of temporal lobe epilepsy. *Ann Neurol* 1994;35:640–654.

370. Briellmann RS, Torn-Broers Y, Busuttil BE, et al. APOE ε4 genotype is associated with an earlier onset of chronic temporal lobe epilepsy. *Neurology* 2000;55:435–437.

371. Pitkanen A, Nissinen J. What predicts the development of epilepsy after status epilepticus? *Epilepsia* 2000;41(Suppl.):57.

372. Fernandez G, Effenberger O, Vinz B, et al. Hippocampal malformation as a cause of familial febrile convulsions and subsequent hippocampal sclerosis. *Neurology* 1998;50:909–917.

373. Cendes F, Lopes Cendes I, et al. Familial temporal lobe epilepsy: a clinically heterogeneous syndrome. *Neurology* 1998;50:554–557.

374. Corey LA, Pellock JM, Boggs JG, et al. Evidence for a genetic predisposition for status epilepticus. *Neurology* 1998;50:558–560.

375. Kanemoto K, Kawasaki J, Miyamoto T, et al. Interleukin (IL)1β, IL-1α, and IL-1 receptor antagonist gene polymorphisms in patients with temporal lobe epilepsy. *Ann Neurol* 2000;47:571–574.

376. Kim JH, Tien RD, Felsberg GJ, et al. Fast spin-echo MR in hippocampal sclerosis: correlation with pathology and surgery. *Am J Neuroradiol* 1995;16:627–636.

377. Thadani VM, Williamson PD, Berger R, et al. Successful epilepsy surgery without intracranial EEG recording: criteria for patient selection. *Epilepsia* 1995;36:7–15.

378. Arruda F, Cendes F, Andermann F, et al. Mesial atrophy and outcome after amygdalohippocampectomy or temporal lobe removal. *Ann Neurol* 1996;40:446–450.

379. Salanova V, Markand O, Worth R. Longitudinal follow-up in 145 patients with medically refractory temporal lobe epilepsy treated surgically between 1984 and 1995. *Epilepsia* 1999;40:1417–1423.

380. Radhakrishnan K, So EL, Silbert PL, et al. Predictors of outcome of anterior temporal lobectomy for intractable epilepsy: a multivariate study. *Neurology* 1998;51:465–471.

381. Cascino GD, Luckstein R, Sharbrough FW, Jack CR Jr. Facial asymmetry, hippocampal pathology, and remote symptomatic seizures: A temporal lobe epileptic syndrome. *Neurology* 1993;43:725–727.

382. Matsuda K, Yagi K, Mihara T, et al. MRI lesion and epileptogenic focus in temporal lobe epilepsy. *Jpn J Psychiatry Neurol* 1989;43:393–400.

383. Meyer A, Falconer NA, Beck E. Pathological findings in temporal lobe epilepsy. *J Neurol Neurosurg Psychiatry* 1954;17:276–285.

384. Jay V, Becker LE, Otsubo H, et al. Pathology of temporal lobectomy for refractory seizures in children: review of 20 cases including some unique malformative lesions. *J Neurosurg* 1993;79:53–61.

385. Johanson JH, Rekate HL, Roesmann U. Gangliogliomas: pathological and clinical correlation. *J Neurosurg* 1981;54:58–63.

386. Koeller KK, Dillon WP. Dysembryoplastic neuroepithelial tumors: MR appearance. *Am J Neuroradiol* 1992;13:1319–1325.

387. Fried I, Spencer DD. Glial tumors and vascular malformations associated with intractable seizures: differences in surgical outcome. *Epilepsia* 1993;34:78.

388. Kishikawa H, Ohmoto T, Nishimoto A. Brain tumor with seizures in children. *Brain Develop Tokyo* 1980;12:19–26.

389. Russell DS, Rubinstein LJ. Pathology of tumors of the nervous system, 5th ed. Baltimore, MD: Williams & Wilkins, 1989.

390. Burger PC. Malignant astrocytic neoplasms: classification, pathologic anatomy and response to treatment. *Semin Oncol* 1986;13:16.

391. Graux P, Frigard B, Merlier LB. Tumoral epilepsy. *Rev Geriat* 1983;8:213–214.

392. Kos BO, Brant-Zawadzki M, Kucharczyk W, et al. Cystic intracranial lesions: magnetic resonance imaging. *Radiology* 1985;155:363–369.

393. Atlas SW, Grossman RI, Hackney DB, et al. Calcified intracranial lesions: detection with gradient-echo-acquisition rapid MR imaging. *Am J Neuroradiol* 1988;9:253–259.

394. Atlas SW, Grossman RI, Gomori JM, et al. Hemorrhagic intracranial malignant neoplasms: spin-echo MR imaging. *Radiology* 1987;164:71–77.

395. Earnest F, Kelly PJ, Scheithauer BW, et al. Cerebral astrocytomas: histopathologic correlation of MR and CT contrast enhancement with stereotact biopsy. *Radiology* 1988;166:823–827.

396. Lee Y, Van Tassel P, Bruner JM, et al. Juvenile pilocytic astrocytomas: CT and MR characteristics. *Am J Neuroradiol* 1989;10:363–370.

397. Wee AS, Parent AD, Ashley RA. Pathologic findings in brains of patients with focal epileptic seizures who had a craniotomy procedure. *J Miss State Med Assoc* 1990;31:219–221.

398. Mork SJ, Lindegaard JF, Halvonsen TB, et al. Oligodendroglioma: incidence and biological behavior in a defined population. *J Neurosurg* 1985;63:881–889.

399. Roberts M, German WJ. A long term study of patients with oligodendrogliomas. Follow-up of 50 cases, including Dr Harvey Cushing's series. *J Neurosurg* 1966;24:697–700.

400. Lee Y, Tassel PV. Intracranial oligodendrogliomas: imaging findings in 35 untreated cases. *Am J Neuroradiol* 1989;10:119–127.

401. Denierre B, Stinchnoth FA, Hori A, Spoerri O. Intracerebral gangliogliomas. *J Neurosurg* 1986;65:177–182.

402. Tampieri D, Moumdjian R, Melanson D, Ethier R. Intracerebral gangliogliomas in patients with complex partial seizures: CT and MR imaging findings. *Am J Neuroradiol* 1991;12:749–755.

403. Altman NR. MR and CT characteristics of gangliocytoma: a rare cause of epilepsy in children. *Am J Neuroradiol* 1988;9:917–921.

404. Daumas-Duport C, Scheithauer BW, Chodkiewicz JP, et al. Dysembryoplastic neuroepithelial tumor: a surgically curable tumor of young patients with intractable partial seizures. *Neurosurgery* 1988;23:545–556.

405. Daumas-Duport C. Dysembryoplastic neuroepithelial tumours. *Brain Pathol* 1993;3:283–295.

406. D'Incerti L. Morphological neuroimaging of malformations of cortical development. *Epileptic Disord* 2003;5(Suppl 2):S59–S66.

407. Park JY, Suh YL, Han J. Dysembryoplastic neuroepithelial tumor. Features distinguishing it from oligodendroglioma on cytologic squash preparations. *Acta Cytol* 2003;47:624–629.

408. Prayson RA, Frater JL. Cortical dysplasia in extratemporal lobe intractable epilepsy: a study of 52 cases. *Ann Diagn Pathol* 2003;7:139–146.

409. Luyken C, Blumcke I, Fimmers R, et al. The spectrum of long-term epilepsy-associated tumors: long-term seizure and tumor outcome and neurosurgical aspects. *Epilepsia* 2003;44:822–830.

410. Vaquero J, Zurita M, Oya S, Coca S. Dysembryoplastic neuroepithelial tumor or dysembryoplastic cortical neurocytoma? *J Neurooncol* 2003;62:359–360.

411. Fernandez C, Girard N, Paz Paredes A, et al. The usefulness of MR imaging in the diagnosis of dysembryoplastic neuroepithelial tumor in children: a study of 14 cases. *Am J Neuroradiol* 2003;24:829–834.

412. Vieth RG, Odom GL. Intracranial metastases and their neurosurgical treatment. *J Neurosurg* 1965;23:375–383.

413. Penfield W. The evidence for a cerebral vascular mechanism in epilepsy. *Ann Intern Med* 1933;7:303–310.

414. Seifert V, Trost HA, Dietz H. Cavernous angiomas of the supratentorial compartment. *Zentralbl Neurochir* 1989;50:89–92.

415. Leblanc R, Feindel W, Ethier R. Epilepsy from cerebral arteriovenous malformations. *Can J Neurol Sci* 1983;10:91–95.

416. Fortuna A, Ferrante L, Mastronardi L, et al. Cerebral cavernous angioma in children. *Child's Nerv Syst* 1989;5:201–207.

417. Batjer HH, Devous MD, Seibert GB, et al. Intracranial arteriovenous malformation: contralateral steal phenomena. *Neurol Med Chir (Tokyo)* 1989;29:401–406.

418. Piepgras D, Sundt T, Ragoowansi A, Stevens L. Seizure outcome in patients with surgically treated cerebral arteriovenous malformations. *J Neurosurg* 1993;79:5–11.

419. Trussart V, Berry I, Manelfe C, et al. Epileptogenic cerebral vascular malformations and MRI. *J Neuroradiol* 1989;16:273–284.

420. Lechevalier B, Houtteville JP. [Intracranial cavernous angioma]. *Rev Neurol (Paris)* 1992;148:173–179.

421. Awad IA, Rosenfeld J, Ahl J, et al. Intractable epilepsy and structural lesions of the brain: mapping, resection strategies, and seizure outcome. *Epilepsia* 1991;32:179.

422. Tannier C, Pons M, Treil J. Cerebral venous angiomas. Twelve cases and a review of the literature. *Rev Neurol* 1991;147:356–363.

423. Hardjasudarma M. Cavernous and venous angiomas of the CNS neuroimaging. *J Neuroimag* 1991;1:191–196.

424. Awad IA, Robinson JR. Cavernous malformations and epilepsy. In: Awad IA, Barrow DL, eds. Cavernous malformations. Park Ridge, IL: American Association of Neurological Surgeons, 1993:49–64.

425. Robinson JR, Awad IA. Clinical spectrum and natural course. In: Awad IA, Barrow DL, eds. Cavernous Malformations. Park Ridge, IL: American Association of Neurological Surgeons, 1993:25–36.

426. Requena I, Arias M, Lopez IL, et al. Cavernomas of the central nervous system: clinical and neuroimaging manifestations in 47 patients. *J Neurol Neurosurg Psychiatry* 1991;54:590–594.

427. Morrell F. Secondary epileptogenesis in man. *Arch Neurol* 1985;42:318–335.

428. Willmore LJ, Sypert GW, Munson JB. Recurrent seizures induced by cortical iron injection: a model of posttraumatic epilepsy. *Ann Neurol* 1978;4:329–336.

429. Willmore LJ, Sypert GW, Munson JV, Hurd RW. Chronic focal epileptiform discharges induced by injection of iron into rat and cat cortex. *Science* 1978;200:1501–1503.

430. Willmore LJ, Hiramatsu M, Kochi H, Mori A. Formation of superoxide radicals, lipid peroxides and edema after FeCl3 injection into rat isocortex. *Brain Res* 1983;277:393–396.

431. Willmore LJ. Post-traumatic epilepsy: cellular mechanisms and implications for treatment. *Epilepsia* 1990;31:S67–S73.

432. Triggs WJ, Willmore LJ. In vivo lipid peroxidation in rat brain following intracortical Fe^{2+} injection. *J Neurochem* 1984;42:976–980.

433. Constantino A, Vintners HV. A pathogenic correlate of the 'steal' phenomenon in a patient with cerebral arteriovenous malformation. *Stroke* 1986;17:103–106.

434. Hardman JM. The pathology of traumatic brain injuries. In: Thompson RA, Green JR, eds. Complications of nervous system trauma: advances in neurology 22. New York: Raven Press, 1979:15–50.

435. Holbourn AHS. The mechanics of brain injuries. *Br Med Bull* 1945;3:147–149.

436. Choi KG, Choi IS, Kim JS, Kim KW. A clinical study of adult-onset seizure disorder. *J Korean Med Assoc* 1986;29:189–197.

437. Jennett WB. Epilepsy and acute traumatic intracranial hematoma. *J Neurol Neurosurg Psychiatry* 1975;38:378–381.

438. Jennett WB. Epilepsy after non-missile head injuries, 2nd ed. London: Heinemann, 1975.

439. Gentry LR, Godersky JC, Thompson B, Dunn VD. Prospective comparative study of intermediate-field MR and CT in the evaluation of closed head trauma. *Am J Neuroradiol* 1988;9:91–100.

440. Gentry LR, Godersky JC, Thompson B. MR imaging of head trauma: review of the distribution and radiopathologic features of traumatic lesions. *Am J Neuroradiol* 1988;9:101–110.

441. French BN, Dublin AB. The value of computerized tomography in the management of 1000 consecutive head injuries. *Surg Neurol* 1977;7:171–183.

442. Lipper MH, Kishore PRS, Enas GG, et al. Computed tomography in the prediction of outcome in head injury. *Am J Neuroradiol* 1985;6:7–10.

443. Levin HS, Handel SF, Goldman AM, et al. Magnetic resonance imaging after 'diffuse' nonmissile head injury. *Arch Neurol* 1985;42:963–968.

444. Groswasser Z, Reider-Groswasser I, et al. Magnetic resonance imaging in head injury patients with normal late computed tomography scans. *Surg Neurol* 1987;27:331–337.

445. Atlas SW, Mark AS, Grossman RI, Gomori JM. Intracranial hemorrhage: gradient-echo MR imaging at 1.5T: comparison with spin-echo imaging and clinical application. *Radiology* 1988;168:803–807.

446. Theodore WH, Katz D, Kufta C, et al. Pathology of temporal lobe foci: Correlation with CT, MRI, and PET. *Neurology* 1990;40:797–803.

447. Wasterlain CG, Fujikawa DG, Penix L, Sankar R. Pathophysiological mechanisms of brain damage from status epilepticus. *Epilepsia* 1993;34:S37–S53.

448. Sloviter RS. Status epilepticus-induced neuronal injury and network reorganization. *Epilepsia* 1999;40(Suppl 1):S34–S39; discussion S40–S41.

449. Fujikawa DG, Itabashi HH, Wu A, Shinmei SS. Status epilepticus-induced neuronal loss in humans without systemic complications or epilepsy. *Epilepsia* 2000;41:981–991.

450. Chang LB, Lirng JF, Teng MM, et al. Sequential MRI studies of a patient with complex partial status – a case report. *Kaohsiung J Med Sci* 2001;17:633–637.

451. Hisano T, Ohno M, Egawa T, et al. Changes in diffusion-weighted MRI after status epilepticus. *Pediatr Neurol* 2000;22:327–329.

452. Lazeyras F, Blanke O, Perrig S, et al. EEG-triggered functional MRI in patients with pharmacoresistent epilepsy. *J Magn Reson Imaging* 2000;12:177–185.

453. Meierkord H, Wieshmann U, Niehaus L, Lehmann R. Structural consequences of status epilepticus demonstrated with serial magnetic resonance imaging. *Acta Neurol Scand* 1997;96:127–132.

454. Perez ER, Maeder P, Villemure KM, et al. Acquired hippocampal damage after temporal lobe seizures in 2 infants. *Ann Neurol* 2000;48:384–387.

455. Kim JA, Chung JI, Yoon PH, et al. Transient MR signal changes in patients with generalized toncoclonic seizure or status epilepticus: periictal diffusion-weighted imaging. *Am J Neuroradiol* 2001; 22:1149–1160.

456. Diehl B, Najm I, Ruggieri P, et al. Postical diffusion-weighted imaging for the localization of focal epileptic areas in temporal lobe epilepsy. *Epilepsia* 2001;42:21–28.

457. Hufnagel A, Weber J, Marks S, et al. Brain diffusion after single seizures. *Epilepsia* 2003;44:54–63.

458. Lazeyras F, Blanke O, Zimine I, et al. MRI, H-MRS, and functional MRI during and after prolonged nonconvulsive seizure activity. *Neurology* 2000;55:1677–1682.

459. Sappey-Marinier D, Calabrese G, Fein G, et al. Effect of photic stimulation on human visual cortex lactate and phosphates using ^{1}H and ^{31}P magnetic resonance spectroscopy. *J Cereb Blood Flow Metab* 1992;12:584–592.

460. Briellmann RS, Kalnins RM, Hopwood MJ, et al. Postical psychosis in TLE: microdysplasia and anterior hippocampal preservation. *Neurology* 2000;55:1027–1030.

461. Ho SS, Kuzniecky RI, Gillian F, Faugnt E, Morawetz R. Temporal lobe developmental malformations and epilepsy: dual pathology and bilateral hippocampal abnormalities. *Neurology* 1988;50(3): 748–754.

462. Raymond AA, Fish DR, Stevens JM, Cook MJ, Sisodiya SM, Snorvon SD. Association of hippocampal sclerosis with cortical dysgenesis in patients with epilepsy. *Neurology* 1994;44(10):1841–1845.

463. McIntosh AM, Kalnins RM, Mitchell LA, Fabinyi GCA, Briellmann RS, Berkovic SF. Temporal lobectomy: long term seizure outcome, late recurrence and risks for seizure recurrencee. *Brain* (in press).

464. ILAE Commission Report: Mesial temporal lobe epilepsy with hippocampal sclerosis. Compiled by HG Wieser for the ILAE Commission of Neurosurgery of Epilepsy. *Epilepsia* 2004;45(6): 695–714.

465. Blumcke I, Thom M, Wiestler OD. Ammon's horn sclerosis: a maldevelopmental disorder associated with temporal lobe epilepsy. *Brain Pathol* 2002; 12:199–211.

CHAPTER 5

Extra-Temporal Lobe Epilepsy

Ruben I. Kuzniecky and Graeme D. Jackson

"The clonic movements frequently spread so slowly and remain to one segment so long that it is possible to study them carefully."

Gordon Holmes, 1927

INTRODUCTION

Epilepsies arising from extratemporal lobe structures encompass a wide variety of clinico-electrophysiologic entities. Some are focal in nature while others are hemispheric or more diffuse in nature. We recognize the limitations of grouping these various syndromes and entities under this chapter but, from an imaging perspective, they share a number of common characteristics. In this chapter, we first discuss the MRI findings in patients with localization related epilepsies arising from the frontal lobes. In the second section, we discuss epilepsies arising from the occipitoparietal region.

FRONTAL LOBE EPILEPSY

Clinical Aspects

In humans, the frontal lobes are the largest of the lobes, weighting approximately 510 g (50% of the whole brain weight). The frontal lobes are anatomically complex, with a sizable part of them located in the mesial and inferior surfaces of the brain (Fig. 5.1). In addition to their anatomic characteristics, there are many rapidly conduction pathways connecting the various parts of the frontal lobe (1, 2).

Frontal lobe epilepsies are less well understood compared with temporal lobe seizures and in general they remain a major clinical challenge (3–5). It has been estimated that of the 1.5–2 million patients with epilepsy in the United States, at least 50% have frontal lobe seizures and epilepsies and, of those, 250 000 are incapacitated because of medical intractability. In contrast to temporal lobe epilepsy, frontal lobe seizures are more difficult to define clinically and electrographically. This is the result of often unusual clinical

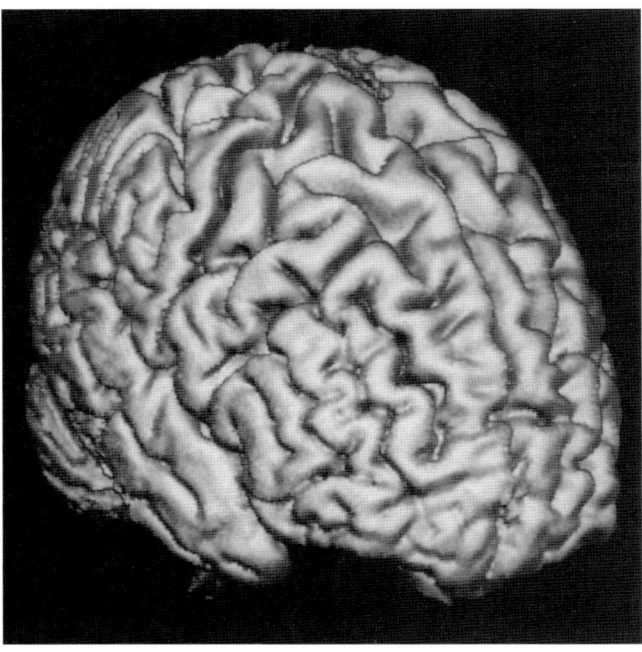

FIG. 5.1. Surface reconstruction demonstrating the right cerebral hemisphere, primarily frontal and temporal lobes.

177

behaviors associated with frontal lobe seizures and the difficulties associated with routine investigation methods, including EEG analysis, and the fact that lesions are less commonly detected in many patients with frontal lobe epilepsy.

Frontal Lobe Syndromes

Multiple investigators have attempted to classify clinical syndromes in frontal lobe epilepsy. The work of several investigators, in particular Bancaud and Tailarach, is based on defining the anatomic–electrographic-clinical state during frontal lobe seizures. Using this approach, Bancaud and others (2), as well as Williamson et al. (4, 6), have proposed the use of an original anatomic subdivision of the frontal lobes to study these epilepsies. This subdivision has identified seven anatomic areas in the frontal lobes that are perhaps associated with distinctive clinical syndromes. The area regions are as follows:

- Rolandic area
- Inferior frontal
- Intermediate medial frontal
- Intermediate dorsolateral frontal
- Cingulate gyrus
- Supplementary motor area
- Frontopolar
- Orbitofrontal.

As reported by Bancaud et al. (2), this approach has the advantage of partially responding to the needs of an anatomic classification but does not consider the dynamic nature of seizures. Furthermore, the rapid spread of seizures in frontal lobe patients and the presence of silent areas makes this more difficult to justify. Nevertheless, this approach is a starting point to understand these complex behavioral and electrographic seizure patterns.

Seizures From the Rolandic Area (Areas 4 and 6)

Seizures arising from the rolandic region are common among patients with frontal lobe epilepsy. Among the 210 patients reported by Bancaud et al. (2), 53 had seizures arising from this region. The semiology of seizures arising from this area consists of either focal or brief clonic motor events, jacksonian motor seizures (7) and, less commonly, other symptoms. On some occasions, specific epileptic patterns such as epilepsia partialis continua, or syndromes such as Rasmussen's encephalitis (8), seem to be primarily localized to this anatomic region.

Seizures from the rolandic region can be subclassified according to clinical and electrographic data. Chauvel et al. have subclassified these seizures into five groups depending on the localization of the EEG abnormality (3). Seizures arising from the premotor area often consist of tonic posturing, usually involving the upper limb, and are usually unilateral, although bilateral activity can be observed. Versive movements of the eyes occur infrequently and are usually contralateral to the electrical discharge. Analyzing this data, however, it becomes obvious that very likely, the ictal behavior is related to electrical discharges spreading to the supplementary motor area. Therefore, it is very likely that seizures arising from the premotor area may often manifest themselves as seizures of the supplementary motor area (9–11).

The second group consists of motor seizures corresponding to discharges in the lateral part of the motor and premotor areas. In this group, the ictal symptomatology again is complex and, since the number of patients is very small, conclusions regarding the clinical behavior resulting from these lesions are difficult to make. In contrast, seizures arising from the primary motor area (area 4) are very common. Most patients have contralateral hemiparesis or infantile hemiplegia (12). Clinical correlations demonstrate clonic activity in 85% of the seizures, being purely clonic in almost 50% of cases. Clonic and tonic activity can also be observed in some patients. Analysis of the distribution of clonic activity reveals that preferential involvement of the upper extremity, and often the fingers, is common. Quick spread to involve the whole limb or the same side of the body is often observed. Interestingly, Chauvel noted that, in some patients, primarily tonic activity followed the clonic discharges (3).

Seizures arising from the mesial part of the motor and premotor cortex can be seen in approximately 25% of this population. The semiology of the seizures often suggests bilateral activation. Complex symmetric posturing of both arms and legs is common. Compared with motor seizures arising from the lateral primary motor areas, unilateral clonic activity is seldom present. It is possible, as described above, that the majority of the manifestations in these patients are related to discharges involving the supplementary motor area. Finally, motor seizures corresponding to widespread discharges to the motor and premotor areas manifest, as would be expected, with bilateral tonic or clonic activity.

Inferior Frontal Gyrus Seizures

Seizures from the posterior portion of the inferior frontal gyrus may affect the nondominant or dominant hemisphere. Nondominant involvement usually is manifested by speech arrest and tonic contractions or isolated clonic activity in the contralateral and sometimes in the homolateral muscles of the angle of the mouth (2). Swallowing and salivation are common, especially, if the discharge propagates to the operculum (13–16). Autonomic symptoms such as tachycardia or respiratory distress are also observed in some patients. Conversely, when the seizure discharge affects the dominant hemisphere, aphasia and dysarthria are very prominent (17–20). Contralateral facial motor deficits are also common. The speech disturbances in the nondominant cerebral hemisphere is usually related to motor phonatory difficulties.

Seizures From the Intermediate Medial Frontal Region

The semiology of these seizures is difficult to ascertain when analyzing different studies. It is unclear whether most of the clinical manifestations are the result of propagation of ictal discharges to the intermediate frontal regions or whether the discharges are originating in that region and producing the ictal behavior. In most cases, the manifestations of seizures either arising or primarily involving the mesial frontal regions excluding the cingulate gyri consist of marked motor phenomena with contralateral head and eye deviation, tonic elevation of one or both arms, and contralateral clonic movements of the arms and face with frequent secondary generalization (21–24). However, speech and movement arrest, and complex and simple automatisms have also been reported. In our own experience, patients with medial frontal seizures sometimes develop marked tonic motor activity as well as autonomic symptoms during their attacks.

Intermediate Dorsal Lateral Frontal Seizures

As with other types of frontal lobe seizure, epileptic discharges emanating from the dorsal lateral intermediate frontal region are difficult to characterize because the discharges usually spread very rapidly in multidirectional pathways. As reported by Bancaud et al. (1, 25), tonic adversive eye and head turning is one of the most frequent clinical manifestations of seizures arising in this area. Subsequent face and arm motor involvement and visual hallucinations and illusions have also been reported. Forced thinking and complex postural manifestations are also seen in some patients (26).

An aura is seldom present in patients with dorsal lateral frontal lobe seizures. Dizziness and a cephalic aura are common. Quesney et al. (27–29) reported auras in 40% of these patients. Aphasia and arrest of activity are also common with dominant hemisphere involvement (17, 30–32). Unconscious, as well as conscious, head turning is also common in these patients.

Cingulate Gyrus Seizures

Ictal discharges primarily involving the anterior cingulate region usually begin with intense fright, screaming, and vigorous and aggressive verbalization. Autonomic symptoms, as well as partial awareness, are also present. In our experience, vegetative symptoms are frequent with marked respiratory, cardiovascular, and digestive disturbances (13, 33, 34). This is probably related to distal spread of the initial discharge. Integrated and complicated behavior, sometimes in the form of agitation, can be seen. Unilateral tonic or bilateral tonic activity can be seen and probably relates to activation of adjacent structures such as the supplementary motor areas (35–40).

Supplementary Motor Seizures

Typical semiology of this seizure type consists of tonic movements of the contralateral limb and at times activation of the ipsilateral limb or foot. Dilatation of the eyes and tonic posturing are common at the beginning of the event. Postural patterns involving the contralateral arm and hand, followed by tonic activity and vocalization or speech arrest, may be seen. Urinary incontinence with posterior spread may occur without loss of consciousness (9–11, 23, 41–46). These seizures are relatively easy to recognize and tend to occur in clusters, particularly at night. Most patients retain awareness of their surroundings.

Frontopolar Seizures

Frontal polar seizures are difficult to investigate because the clinical manifestations are very hard to characterize and to date no clear syndrome has been identified. In most of the reported studies, eye opening and staring with loss of contact is one of the first clinical manifestations. Total amnesia and complex gestural behavior have also been reported. The clinical manifestations are probably related to the rapid spread of ictal activity to the cerebral hemispheres and subcortical structures.

Orbitofrontal Seizures

Orbital frontal seizures constitute another fascinating type of frontal lobe seizure. Bancaud et al. reported olfactory hallucinations as well as visceral sensory symptoms in 18 patients with this seizure type (2). Autonomic phenomena, including changes in heart rate, apnea, and thermoregulatory disorders, have also been reported. It is likely, however, that most of the clinical symptomatology observed in seizures arising from the orbital frontal cortex is the result of ictal propagation. Munari et al. (47), in a detailed analysis of nine patients, concluded that in most cases the ictal discharge was silent and that the clinical manifestations only occurred after involving in general the temporal lobe, the cingulate gyrus, or the lateral temporal structures.

Clinical Summary

We have attempted to summarize the clinical behavior and correlate this with specific anatomic areas. However, as previously reported, frontal lobe seizures are often less likely to be anatomically linked to a single structure within the frontal lobes. Advances in noninvasive neuroimaging techniques, in particular functional MR and ictal single-positron-emission computed tomography (SPECT), may indeed be extremely helpful in trying to define and correlate more accurately symptoms and anatomic structures within the frontal lobes. The presence of a lesion on MRI needs to be carefully analyzed with the clinical behavior, electrophysiologic data, and the results of other investigations. Table 5.1 summarizes some of the clinical information in frontal lobe seizures.

TABLE 5.1. *Topographic Distribution of Frontal Lobe Epilepsy (210 Patients)*

Area of seizure onset	Patients (n)
Areas 4 and 6	53
Inferior frontal	18
Intermediate medial frontal	39
Intermediate dorsolateral frontal	25
Anterior cingulate	16
Frontopolar	14
Orbitofrontal	18
Opercular–insular	27

Data from Bancaud et al.[2]

Pathology and Magnetic Resonance Imaging of Frontal Lobe Epilepsy

An analysis of frontal lobe epilepsy surgical series is most insightful in its relationship to the underlying pathology in patients with this type of seizure. In the most comprehensive review, Mathieson (48) reviewed 180 cases of nontumoral or vascular specimens from patients undergoing frontal lobe resections.

The histopathologic diagnosis was classified in four major groups with meningocerebral cicatrix in the largest one, being found in 33.3% of patients. Among these patients, post-traumatic pathology was the predominant etiology (67.2%). Infections and other causes were less frequent. Post-traumatic neuronal loss and gliosis were observed in 13.5% of the population. Cortical dysgenesis, which grouped both cortical dysplasia and tuberous sclerosis, accounted for 15.5% of cases and contusions related to trauma were seen in 11% of specimens. In the group of nonspecific neuronal loss and gliosis, trauma, infections, and previous neurosurgical procedures were the most frequent etiologic factors found. However, it is important to point out that, in a large percentage of patients with neuronal loss and gliosis, no clear etiology was found as the cause of seizures.

Among the patients reported by Mathieson (48) in a general epilepsy pathology study, frontal lobe pathology was present in 47 of the 503 cases. However, multilobe lesions, as well as frontal temporal lesions, were present in another 100 patients. Among those with histologic lesions related to trauma, seven had frontal lobe pathology, whereas nine had post-frontal and temporal lobe pathology. A review of the Montreal series reveals that the majority of patients had tumors whereas post-traumatic lesions and cortical developmental malformations followed in incidence. Among those with frontotemporal lobe pathology, cortical neuronal loss and post-traumatic lesions were the most prevalent. Interestingly, patients with central lobe lesions predominantly had gliomas on pathology, whereas vascular malformations and other type of minor lesion were encountered in a few patients. One should keep in mind, however, that this series is based on pathologic material from selected patients and therefore may not be representative of the actual incidence of these different lesions in patients with frontal lobe epilepsy. We believe that MRI has the ability to provide this information noninvasively these days, but prospective studies and large populations are needed.

Post-Traumatic Pathology

As stated above, cranial injuries are an important cause of chronic epilepsy, in particular among patients with frontal lobe epilepsy (49–57). In most studies, head traumas have been divided into missile versus nonmissile injuries. Missile injuries result in penetrating cranial cerebral trauma with focal brain damage and hemorrhages. In contrast, nonmissile injuries usually are more likely to produce widespread brain injury. Further subclassifications, including the presence of intracranial hemorrhage or penetrating lesions through the dura, have been used (52, 58).

The exact frequency of these lesions is rather homogeneous when one analyzes the incidence of post-traumatic lesions in epilepsy surgical series. However, there is an obvious bias towards those patients who ultimately have resections. In addition, one of the problems regarding frequency, is whether early epileptic attacks are considered in the overall picture.

It is important to comment on some of the factors that may influence seizures. According to Jennett and others (53, 54, 59), the incidence of post-traumatic seizures appears to be greater in children younger than 5 years than in older patients. Jennett (53, 54, 59) found an incidence of 9.4% in the younger group compared to 3.3% in children age 6–15. The incidence in those aged 46 and above was in the range of 1.5%. As with early studies, the incidence of epilepsy appears to increase significantly when post-traumatic amnesia lasts longer than 24 hours. Obviously, the presence of severe head injuries will correlate with an increased incidence of epilepsy. Another associated factor is the presence of skull fractures and their location. In the frontoparietal region the incidence is of 8.3% compared to occipital fractures, where the incidence was 2.3%.

One of the most significant correlations is the presence of intracranial hematomas and seizures. There appeared to be no major differences between the presence of subdural and intracerebral hematomas with respect to seizures. Interestingly, most patients with intracranial hematomas developed seizures well beyond the first 24 hours and not before. Another factor influencing late onset of epilepsy is the severity of injury. According to Caveness (60, 61), 34% of patients with missile injuries developed epilepsy compared with only 7.5% of those with nonmissile injuries. In addition, the site of injury for both types of injury appears to increase the rate of epilepsy. Injuries involving the parietal region and the central motor cortex are highly associated with seizures, with up to 50% of patients developing seizures from injuries in those areas. In patients with residual aphasia, seizures occurred in 86% of patients (60, 61).

Other interesting data includes the results from the penetrating head injury studies. Among the 525 patients studied in the Vietnam veterans study, 241 had frontal lobe injuries. It is noteworthy that the percentage of patients with frontal lobe lesions who had seizures was 41% and of those who had nonfrontal lobe lesions 51%. The investigators also found that patients with frontal lobe lesions who had seizures were more likely to have generalized convulsions than those with nonfrontal lesions. Clinically, no correlation was found between the frontal and nonfrontal groups, except that those who had retrograde amnesia immediately following head injury were more likely to have frontal lobe seizures.

The reviewers also correlated specific areas of the frontal lobe and their association with the incidence of epilepsy. They found that orbitofrontal lesions were associated with epilepsy in 44% of cases. Other frontal lobe lesions were associated with an incidence of approximately 21%. According to Jennett, frontal lobe fractures appeared to be more likely to lead to epilepsy. In his large series, 34.4% of patients with frontal fractures developed epilepsy as opposed to 24% with temporal parietal injuries.

The pathologic findings in post-traumatic epilepsy may vary and will depend on the type of trauma sustained (56, 62–65). Penetrating injuries produce fibroangiomatous meningeal cortical scarring at different depths in the brain parenchyma. These cortical lesions consist of gliosis and neuronal damage, as well as small hematomas (Fig. 5.2). Closed head injuries may produce leptomeningeal fibrosis.

Having summarized the type of lesions and the pathogenic mechanisms underlying brain injury, we should address some of the clinical correlates of these lesions. The clinical manifestations of the epileptic attacks in patients with post-traumatic epilepsy depend on the location and extent of spread of the ictal activity (59). Focal sensory seizures are extremely common in patients with parietal lesions and, as stated above, these type of seizures are common in patients with post-traumatic epilepsy. Involvement of the precentral motor strip results in focal motor seizures and, as reported

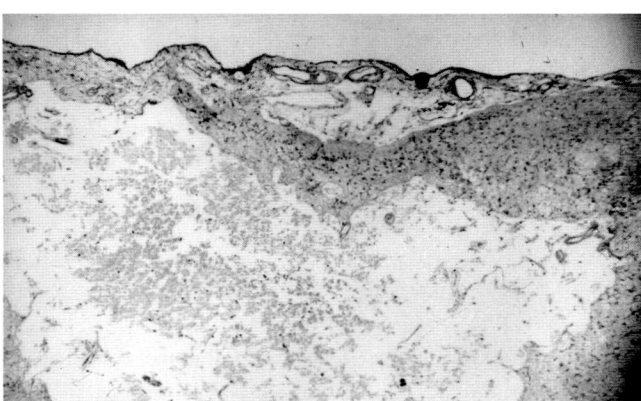

FIG. 5.2. Pathologic specimen demonstrating fibromeningeal cortical scarring with destruction of underlying cortex (hematoxylin and eosin, ×100).

by previous investigators, this is an area that frequently gives rise to epileptic attacks (59). In most patients, partial seizures with or without secondary generalization will occur. The frequency of seizures, however, varies considerably between patients. When one analyzes the focality of these lesions, it is often difficult to exactly localize the presence of the epileptogenic area. This is often related to the fact that these patients may have bilateral lesions or multifocal lesions while seizures appear to be originating from one location.

Imaging and MRI findings in patients with post-traumatic epilepsy are variable (57, 66–69). The changes are dependent on the type and location of the lesion. Parenchymal lesions in the form of contusions are quite characteristic and have been described in Chapter 4. These contusions are often in the superficial gray matter, and in the acute stage they may be associated with hemorrhages (65). Severe trauma can lead to underlying tissue cavitation and encephalomalacia with, commonly, bilateral asymmetric lesions involving the frontal lobes. Bilateral frontal lesions may be seen in patients with severe injuries. The frontopolar regions, as well as the orbitofrontal regions, are often affected (Fig. 5.3). Frontal lobe lesions, which tend to lie just above the cribriform plate and the planum sphenoidale, are common..

T1-weighted images are useful for diagnosis but fluid-attenuated inversion recovery (FLAIR) sequences are more sensitive in detecting bilateral pathology, in particular lesions in proximity to the ventricles (Fig. 5.4). As hemosiderosis and blood byproducts are common, one should carefully seek these changes. A number of MR sequences may be more appropriate at certain times depending on the maturation of these lesions. In chronic conditions, T1-weighted images often reveal most of the pathology but FLAIR images are very sensitive to gliosis and white matter changes, making them extremely useful in the detection of subtle abnormalities (Fig. 5.5).

Mass-related lesions such as subdural and epidural hematomas and intraventricular hemorrhages may be seen in some patients. Intracerebral hematomas are usually seen in the acute phase and are located in the frontotemporal regions (70). They usually involve the white matter and basal ganglia and may be associated with skull fractures. Other pathology, including subarachnoid hemorrhages, vascular dissections, and lacerations, may occur but has little impact on the management of patients with chronic epilepsy.

Neoplasms

As stated in Chapter 4, frontal lobe neoplastic lesions are present in patients who are referred to surgery for intractable epilepsy (71–73). However, fewer patients with long-standing neoplasms are seen because of the high sensitivity of MRI in diagnosing these lesions early in the disease process.

Among the 503 patients reported by Mathieson, fewer than 10% (48) had frontal lobe neoplasms. Gliomas were present

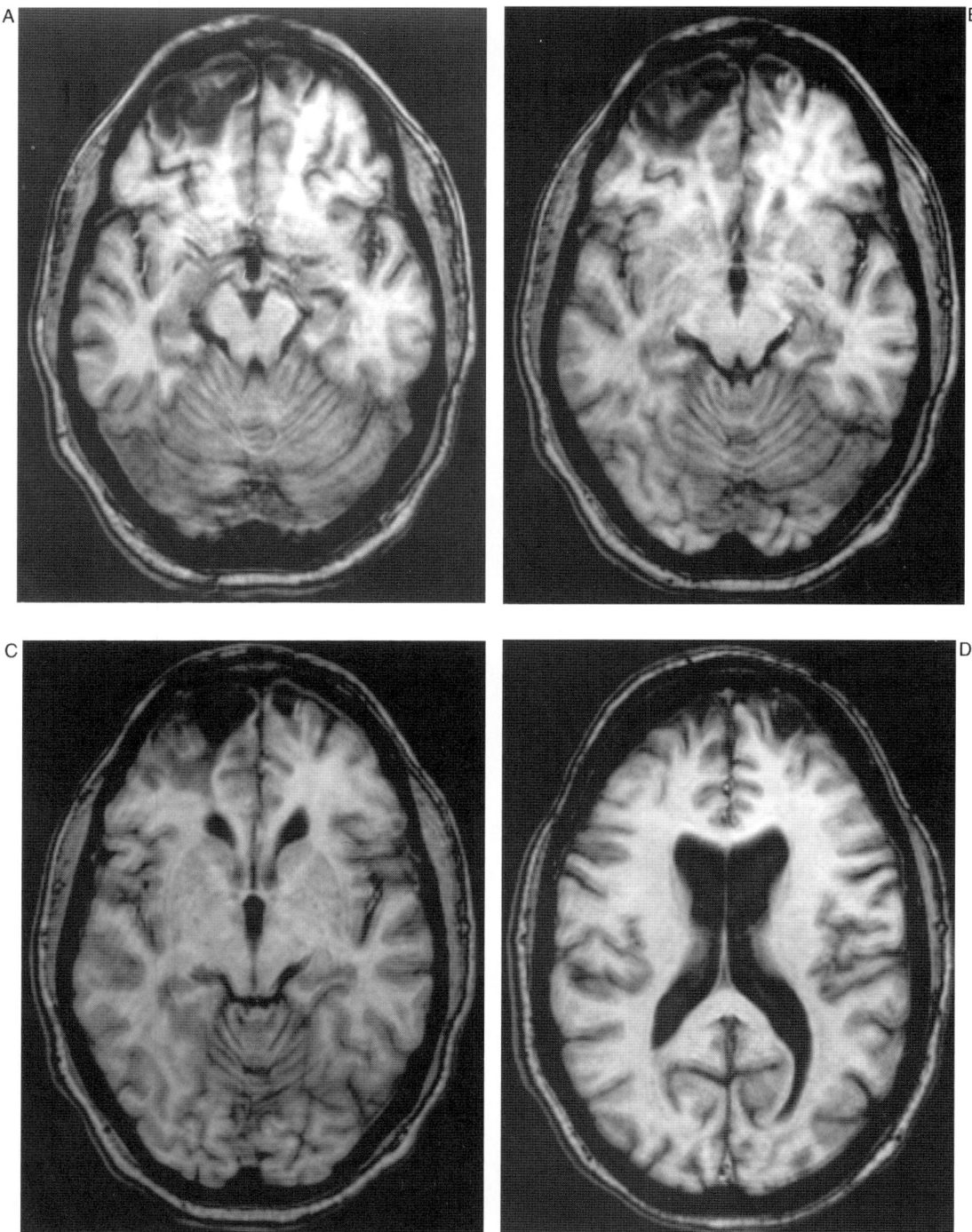

FIG. 5.3. Posttraumatic epilepsy. The patient was a 28-year-old man who sustained severe head injury in a motor vehicle accident. Primarily left frontal lobe seizures recorded on surface electroencephalogram. **A–D.** Axial T1-weighted images (30/6) showing bilateral encephaloclastic lesions involving frontal lobes with destruction of white matter. Mild ventriculomegaly is noted.

in 12 (15%) of patients in this series and, although Mathieson did not describe the exact subtype of glioma, most of them were probably low-grade astrocytomas. In contrast, Leblanc et al. from the same center reported an incidence of 35%, albeit some patients did not have chronic epilepsy (74). In spite of advances in imaging, in particular MRI, the incidence of the lesions in frontal lobe epilepsy patients appears to

be stable. This is partially related to the fact that, with new onset of seizures and the presence of such a lesion, the patients are now referred for surgical intervention before the development of chronic seizures. Therefore, it is difficult to estimate what is the true incidence of these lesions in patients with frontal lobe epilepsy. It is clear, however, that focal neoplastic lesions have been ruled out with MRI

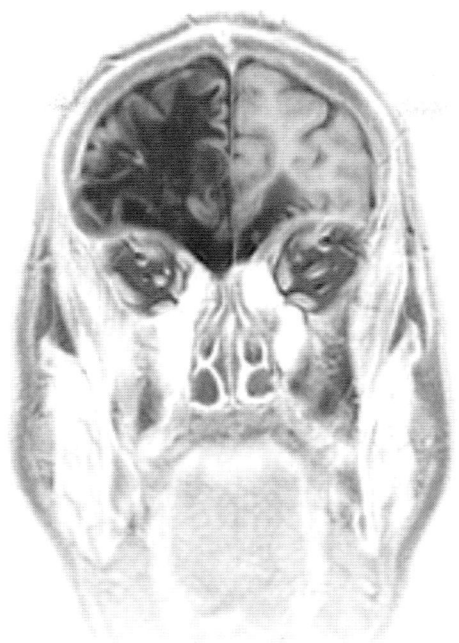

A

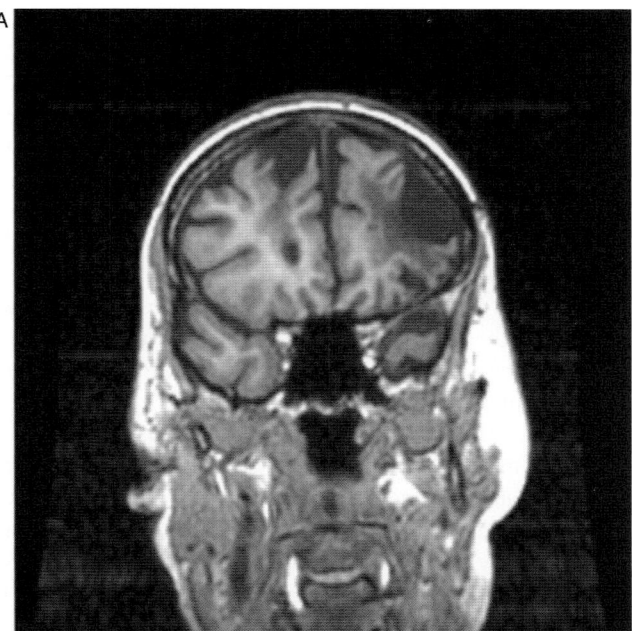

A

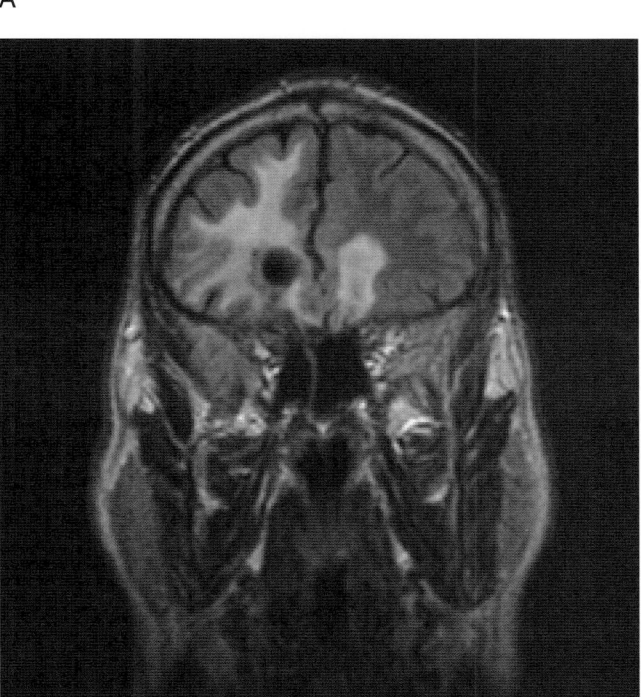

B

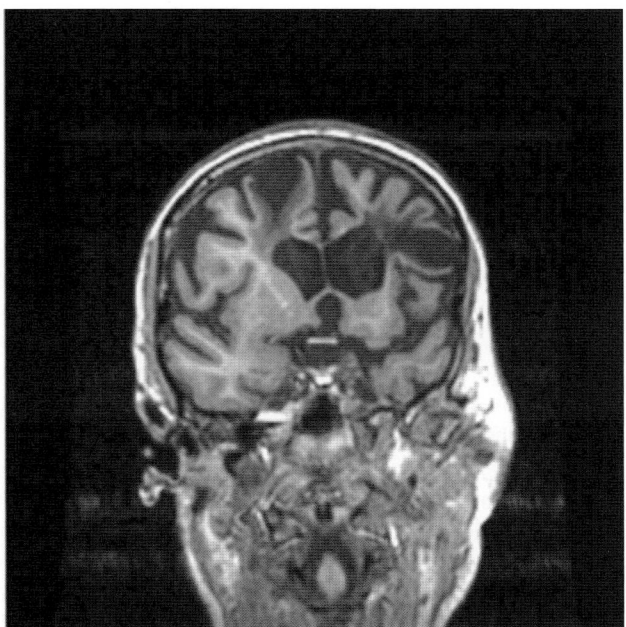

B

FIG. 5.4 A. Coronal reverse T2-weighted image showing a large area of encephalomalacia involving the right frontal lobe with destruction of underlying white matter. The left frontal lesion is much smaller and inferior. **B.** Coronal FLAIR image posterior to main frontal lobe lesion showing extensive signal abnormalities involving frontal regions bilaterally.

FIG. 5.5 Posttraumatic epilepsy. The patient was a 32-year-old woman with intractable epilepsy and cognitive dysfunction. **A, B.** Coronal T1-weighted images through frontal lobes showing a large area of encephalomalacia of the left frontal lobe. Contralateral changes are more subtle. Note ipsilateral left hemisphere atrophy.

in the majority of patients referred to tertiary epilepsy centers.

The histologic characteristics of neoplastic processes involving the frontal lobes are similar to those described in Chapter 4 for temporal lobe epilepsy. Glial tumors appear to be more frequent in this location. In contrast, oligodendrogliomas, dysembryoplastic neuroepithelial tumors, and gangliogliomas appear to be more frequent in the temporal lobes in the context of patients with intractable epilepsy (75).

As noted, the most common neoplasm is low-grade astrocytoma (76–80). The location of these tumors is variable within the frontal regions. Although not aggressive tumors, they can be infiltrative and may involve gray and white matter. Histologically, they have hypercellularity and minimal pleomorphism. Necrosis and vascular proliferation are usually not present.

Magnetic resonance imaging features of neoplasms in the frontal lobe follow the characteristics described in other chapters (76–80). MRI is more sensitive than computed tomography (CT) in the detection of these lesions, with CT being positive in only 45–55% of cases. Astrocytomas usually present with abnormal mass lesions. On T2-weighted images, high intensity signal is observed (see Fig. 5.6). On T1 images, the signal may be isointense or hypointense with respect to the gray matter. Contrast enhancement is usually seen with more aggressive tumors.

Oligodendrogliomas may have very similar MR features with little mass effect unless anaplastic changes are present (81–84). Calcifications may be present but are more frequent in older patients. These tumors are usually well defined and edema is extremely rare (Fig. 5.7). Enhancement is seen in less than 25% of cases (Fig. 5.7B). Other tumoral lesions, such as gangliogliomas and dysembryoplastic tumors, may occur in the frontal regions but are less frequent compared to temporal lobe tumors. Refer to Chapter 4 for a review of these neoplasms.

Vascular Lesions

Vascular lesions, including typical arteriovenous malformations and cavernous angiomas, follow the same characteristics as described in other chapters. Frontally located arteriovenous malformations are of variable size and distribution. In most cases, when the lesions are large, patients are most likely to be referred for treatment of the vascular malformation as opposed to epilepsy (85–87). When the lesions are small, and in many cases have been there for several years, patients may have a history of intractable epilepsy. MR is the imaging technique of choice in the investigation of patients with vascular lesions, since CT may only reveal calcifications with or without other abnormalities (Fig. 5.8). Signal void changes secondary to hemosiderin are observed from around the lesions and the presence of previous hemorrhage can be detected (Fig. 5.9).

Magnetic resonance angiography is also useful since it can provide information regarding the vascular supply and venous drainage of arteriovenous malformations, but in general angiography is done in most patients prior to treatment.

In contrast to arteriovenous malformations, cavernous angiomas are a common cause of intractable seizures and are frequent in the frontal lobes (85–87). We have studied several patients who had the diagnosis of calcified lesions by CT scan in which MRI clearly demonstrated the typical features of a cavernous angioma characterized by the presence of a T2-weighted reticulated core of mixed intensity surrounded by a rim of decreased signal intensity. These lesions often are localized in the premotor areas and may be surgically accessible (Fig. 5.10). In some patients, multiple

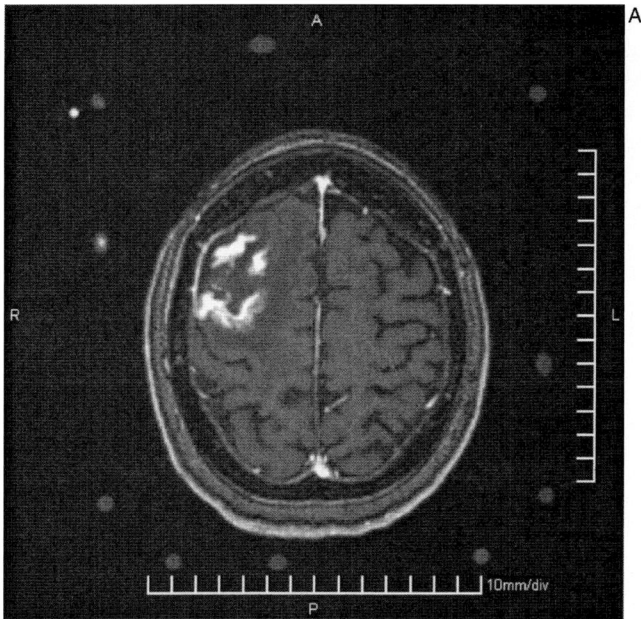

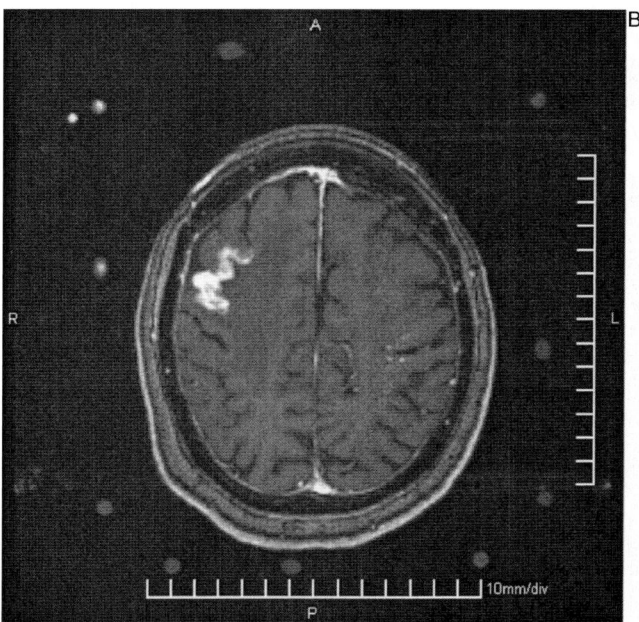

FIG. 5.6. Frontal lobe malignant astrocytoma. **A, B.** T1-weighted images demonstrating gyral enhancement with associated perilesional edema.

lesions may be present. In those circumstances, it is important to determine which lesion is responsible for the patient's seizures if surgery is indicated for epilepsy. However, in some patients, more than one cavernous angioma need to be surgically targeted at times.

Malformations of Cortical Development

Malformations of cortical development are now recognized as causing frontal lobe epilepsy in many patients with

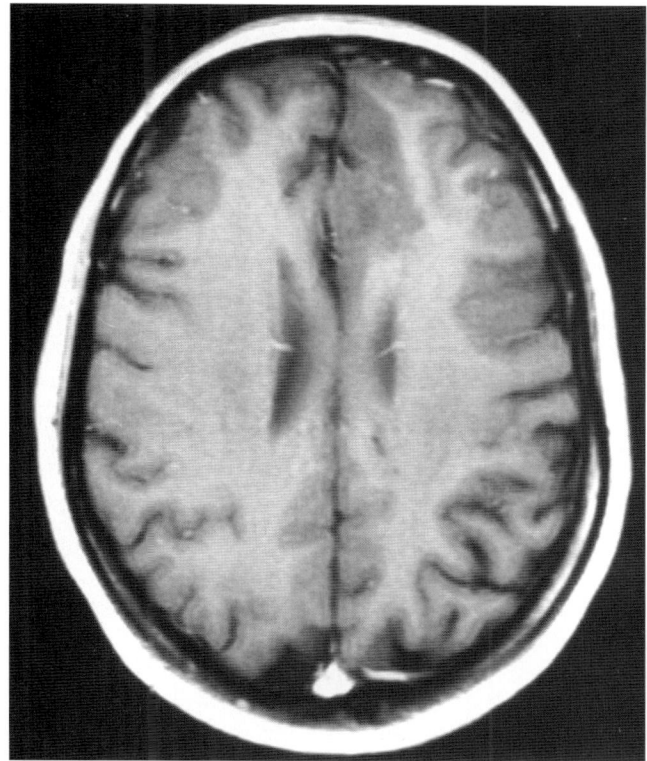

A

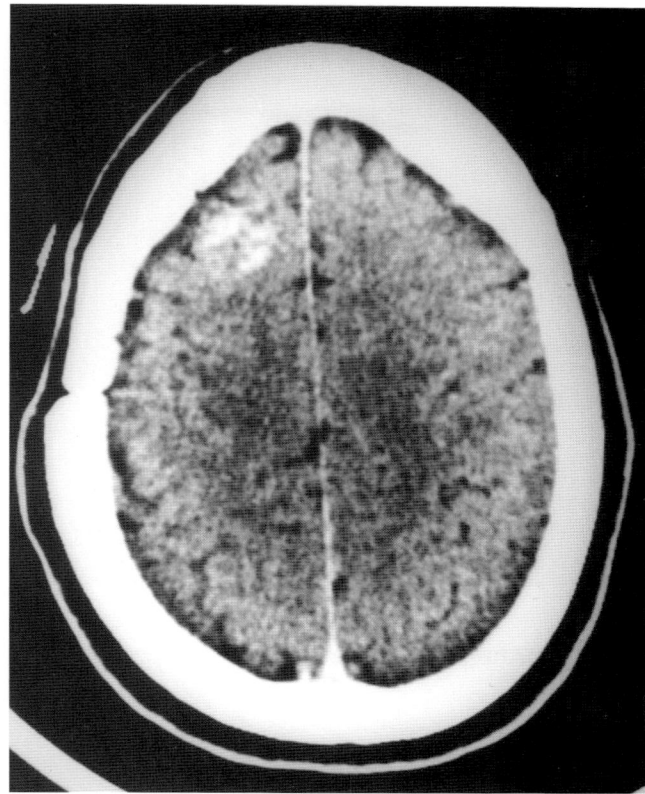

FIG. 5.8. Axial CT scan showing area of calcification involving frontal lobe in a patient with cavernous angioma and intractable epilepsy.

or without intractable seizures. These lesions are described in Chapter 7. Because of the importance of these developmental focal lesions, we have expanded this section further to include other examples of focal developmental lesions. In this section we expand on focal dysplasia, transmantle dysplasia, and developmental tumors. For further details see Chapter 7.

Clinical and Anatomic Features

Developmental focal lesions of the frontal lobe are common. These primarily include focal cortical dysplasia or Taylor's focal cortical dysplasia, focal transmantle dysplasia, focal subcortical heterotopia, and other less common malformations. Previous studies have demonstrated that 50–60% of focal developmental lesions are localized to the frontal lobes (88–92). In a recent study, we described frontal as well as central abnormalities in 19/44 cases (92). In most patients with frontal lobe lesions, tumors as well as cortical dysplasia were found. In those with frontal lobe seizures, the lesions were located near the parasagittal regions, involving the mesial frontal convexity and the cingulate gyrus or the precentral motor and the postcentral sensory cortex. In a previous study, we demonstrated the presence of these lesions in the sensory motor cortex in association with focal myoclonus (88).

An important and interesting feature is that, in extratemporal lobe focal cortical dysplasia, the central and pericentral cortex is often the site of the malformations. In a review

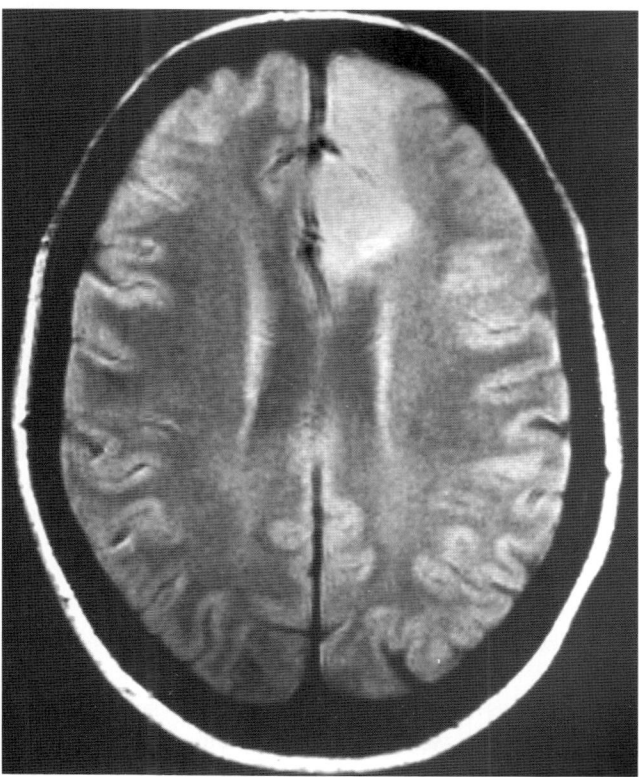

B

FIG. 5.7. Anaplastic oligodendroglioma. **A.** Axial T1-weighted (500/15) showing left mesial frontal lobe hypointense abnormality with mild edema involving mesial frontal area. **B.** Axial image (2200/22) showing homogeneous increased signal from tumor.

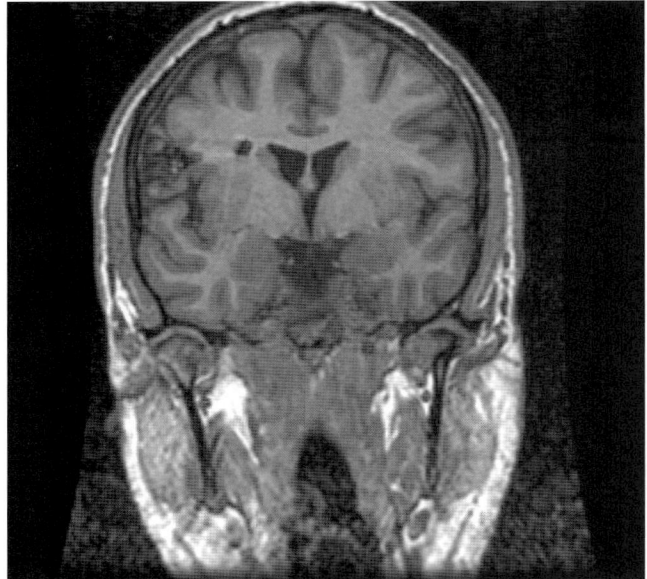

A

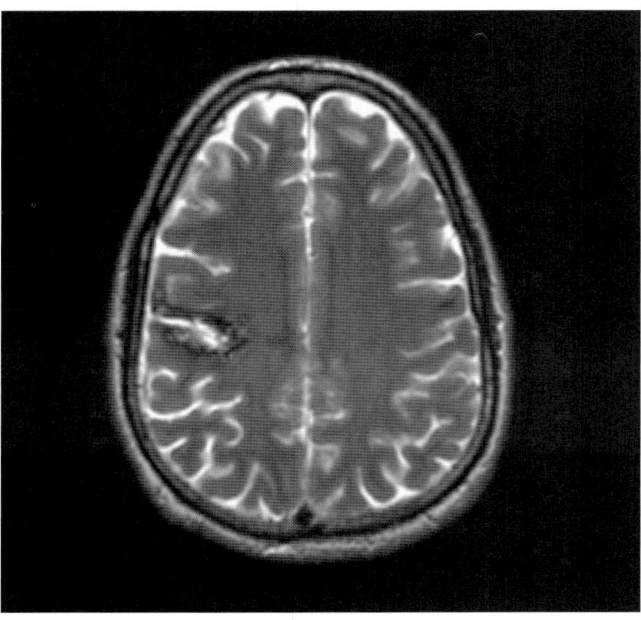

B

FIG. 5.9. A. Coronal T1-weighted image showing hypodense area of abnormality in the deep white matter. In addition, a less defined area of abnormality with signal changes suggestive of hemosiderin is observed in the lateral frontal area. **B.** T2-weighted axial image demonstrating hemosiderin deposition around lesion.

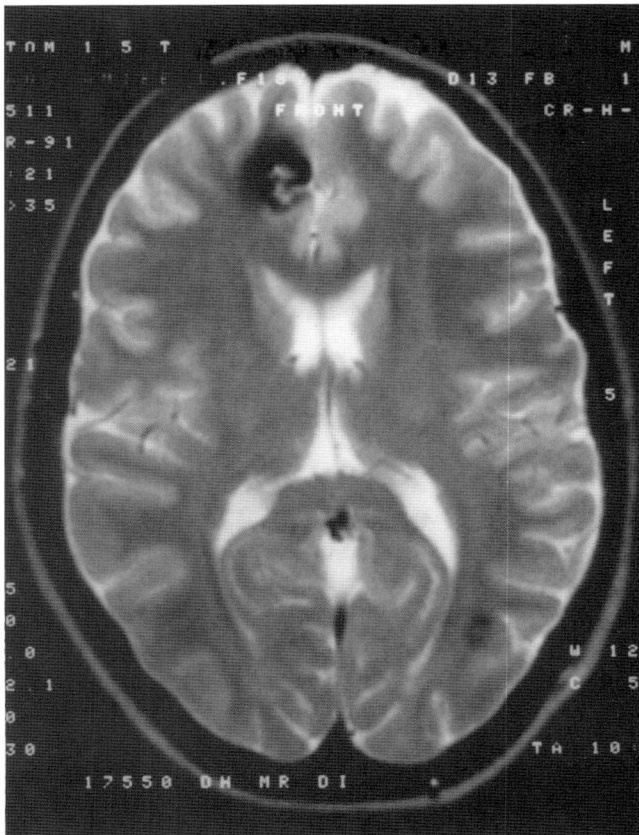

FIG. 5.10. Cavernous angiomas. T2-weighted axial image showing two lesions, a right frontal and a left parietal lobe. The frontal lobe lesion has evidence of larger hemosiderin deposition. The patient had multiple lesions but a unifocal seizure onset. (Courtesy of Dr Abou-Khalil, Nashville, TN.)

of children undergoing surgery for intractable epilepsy, six out of 13 patients with extra-temporal-lobe dysplasia demonstrated lesions in the central cortex (93–95). These are often subtle, with minor degrees of cortical thickening and abnormal gyration in this region. In our experience, these lesions are often not detected if not carefully evaluated. It is not surprising that these lesions are most likely to be located in the central region. The central localization stem from the known propensity of the motor and sensory cortex to developmental lesions. As pointed out in Chapter 7, the high incidence of polymicrogyria and schizencephaly in this region is related to the ischemic nature of these lesions (96). It is likely, therefore, that cortical dysplastic lesions are the direct result of limited ischemia affecting these regions of the cerebral cortex during a specific period during development.

Following the central area localization, the frontal regions appear to be the most likely site of these malformations. There is no clear distribution within the frontal lobes, but our impression is that in many patients, the lesions involve the parasagittal frontal regions as opposed to the orbital-frontal or dorsal-lateral convexity. However, this impression is based on our own experience and maybe bias.

Focal Cortical Dysplasia with Balloon Cells

Experience indicates that focal cortical dysplasia (FCD), and in particular typical FCD with balloon cells (Taylor's type FCD), can be detected by MRI studies. CT may not reveal abnormalities unless associated calcifications are seen in some patients. The use of high-resolution studies with inversion recovery sequences should allow improved recognition of these lesions.

These developmental abnormalities are characterized as described above by the presence of abnormal gyration with abnormal underlying T2 signal from the white matter and

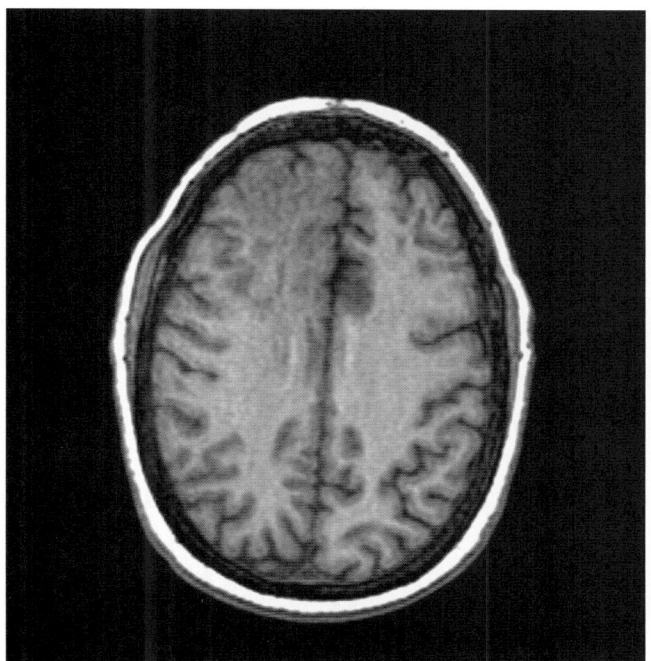

FIG. 5.11 Cortical lobar dysplasia. Axial T1-weighted image showing large right frontal abnormality involving precentral frontal lobe. The lesion involves a large area of the frontal convexity. The gyri are flat and poorly defined.

poor distinction between white and gray matter architecture (37, 97–103) (Fig. 5.11). In many of these individuals, however, the lesions are very small and may be easily undetected. In fact we believe that in up to 50% of patients these lesions had been missed by referring physician.

Focal cortical dysplasia may be circumscribed or may extend beyond one gyrus, or may involve a large portion of a gyrus or area of the frontal lobe (Fig. 5.12) (92, 103–109). One may also classify FCD lesions into those involving the crest of the gyri versus the bottom of the gyrus (bottom-of-sulcus FCD; Fig. 5.13). Histologic examination of these lesions reveals a spectrum of changes consistent with cortical disorganization. Type I lesions with cortical dyslamination but without any giant neurons may be seen at the periphery of the lesions while, in the core of the abnormalities, abnormal cellular distribution, large neurons, and giant astrocytes may be seen.

These abnormalities may be better defined using inversion recovery sequences, which improve the differentiation between white and gray matter. In addition, the signal intensity from the abnormal gray matter may be lower using this sequence, probably representing abnormal cellular organization. FLAIR sequences are particularly sensitive to the transmantle changes observed in Taylor's classic focal cortical dysplasia (see Chapter 7). When the lesions are suspected, surface coils may help in the detection of these lesions, since they improve signal-to-noise ratio (Fig. 5.14). A number of studies have reported improved detection rates with surface coils. However, placement of a surface coil demands either suspicion of a lesion or a well-defined electro-clinical syndrome to guide placement.

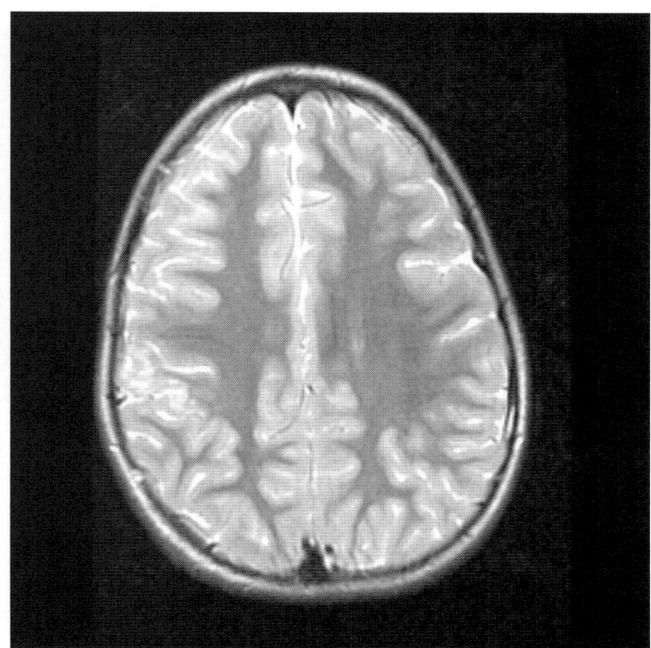

A

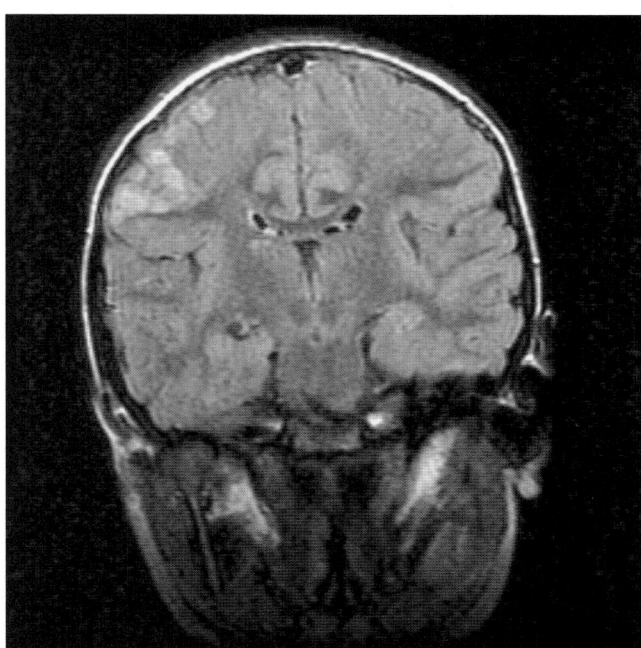

B

FIG. 5.12 Focal cortical dysplasia. **A.** Axial T2-weighted image showing subtle changes in the right central region. **B.** FLAIR coronal image showing abnormal signal from cortical surface. Note that the abnormality involves cortical mantle and gyrus entirely.

Focal Transmantle Dysplasia

Focal transmantle dysplasia, a type of FCD, consists of a streak or column of abnormal cells that extends from the ependyma to the pial surface, but the pathologic appearance is similar to FCD with balloon cells. Although quite recently described in the literature, experience suggest that this is not

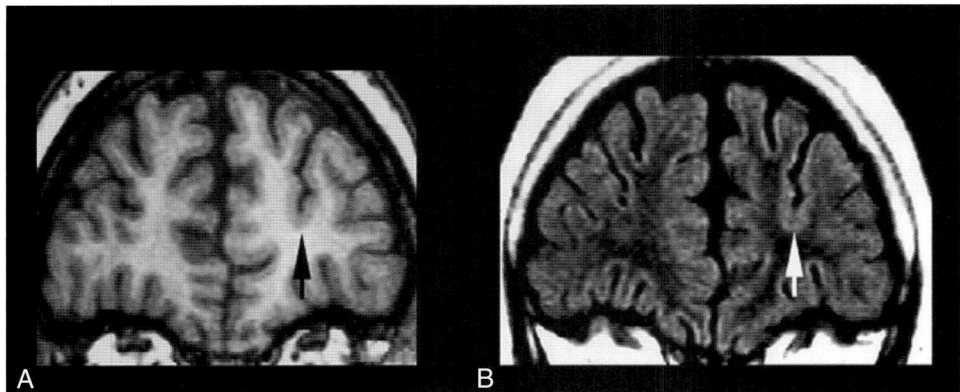

FIG. 5.13. Bottom-of-sulcus focal cortical dysplasia. Coronal T1-weighted (**A**) and FLAIR (**B**) images demonstrating focal abnormality. The lesion is very small and has slight increased signal at the bottom of the sulcus. The patient has been seizure-free since receiving a frontal lobe resection.

a rare condition (110). Diagnosis is based on the imaging features, which consist of cortical thickening associated with a streak from the pial surface to the ventricular wall well visualized on T2-weighted or FLAIR sequences. In some patients, the column of abnormal cells is thick and can be visualized on T1-weighted images (Fig. 5.15). The clinical and EEG features are similar to those of patients with FCD.

Conclusions

Magnetic resonance imaging is sensitive in the detection of pathology associated with epilepsy in patients with frontal lobe seizures. Definition of clinical patterns in frontal lobe epilepsy may be important, since exploration of the frontal lobes is difficult for the reasons already discussed. Once the clinical diagnosis of frontal lobe seizures has been reached, the MR imaging protocol should be tailored to search for small structural abnormalities.

A number of new imaging analysis techniques, as discussed by Bernasconi, may be advantageous because they can provide further diagnostic and objective information in some patients. This is important in view of the complexity of gyral patterns in the frontal lobes.

OCCIPITOPARIETAL LOBE EPILEPSY

Clinical Aspects

The occipital and parietal lobes are anatomically localized in the posterior quadrants of the hemispheres. The parietal lobes are situated in the middle and superior part of the hemispheres while the occipital lobes are posteriorly located above the cerebellum. The anatomic division between the occipital and parietal lobes is not clearly distinguished but most anatomist agree that the posterior margin is formed by the perpendicular sulcus. Both lobes have a lateral and mesial surface with the calcarine fissure in the mesial occipital

region. The striate cortex is contained in this region, corresponding to Brodmann's area 17. Association visual cortex include areas 18 and 19. For further anatomic details, refer to Chapter 3 and other sources.

Occipital and parietal lobe seizures are less frequent than partial seizures originating from the temporal and frontal lobes (111–114). The approximate frequency is unknown, since epidemiologic studies in general have not attempted anatomic localization. However, previous data and clinical experience suggest that occipital and parietal lobe epilepsy may constitute approximately 10% of the partial epilepsies (111–114).

Among the occipital epilepsies, symptomatic and benign forms have been described. The benign form of this epilepsy is classified within the benign childhood epilepsies (115) and is characterized by visual auras followed by motor seizures. EEG abnormalities over the occipital regions consist of high-amplitude spike-wave complexes occurring only with eyes closed. This condition appears less homogenous than benign rolandic epilepsy (116). In addition, a benign form of seizures with parietal lobe EEG foci has been described in children but a clear syndrome has not been defined. Conversely, it is likely that the majority of cases of parietal and occipital lobe at least in adults are symptomatic in nature (117–121). Based on surgical series and clinical experience, these epilepsies constitute fewer than 5% of the cases operated at epilepsy centers.

Although several clinical syndromes have been described with epilepsies arising from the temporal and frontal lobe regions, less frequent symptomatic syndromes have been identified in patients with occipital or parietal lobe epilepsy. One example is the syndrome of bilateral occipitoparietal polymicrogyria (122). However, patients with occipital lobe epilepsy manifest specific clinical symptoms. In contrast, patients with parietal lobe epilepsy do not share common distinctive clinical symptoms. We will first describe the clinical manifestations of occipital and parietal lobe seizures and then discuss both these localized seizure disorders in the context of pathology and MRI.

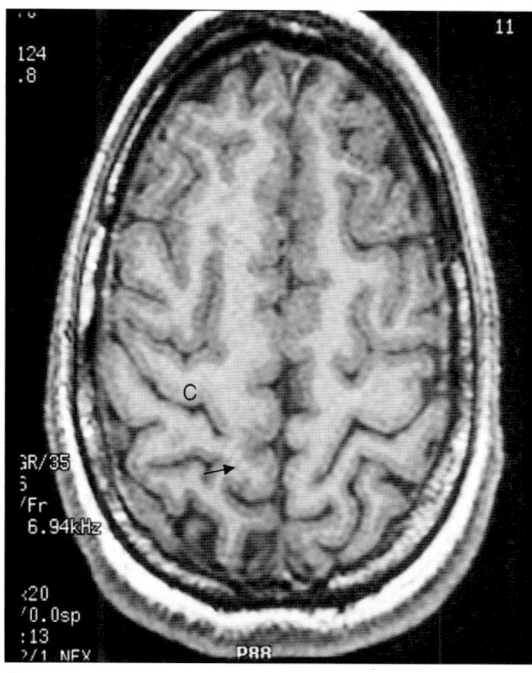

A

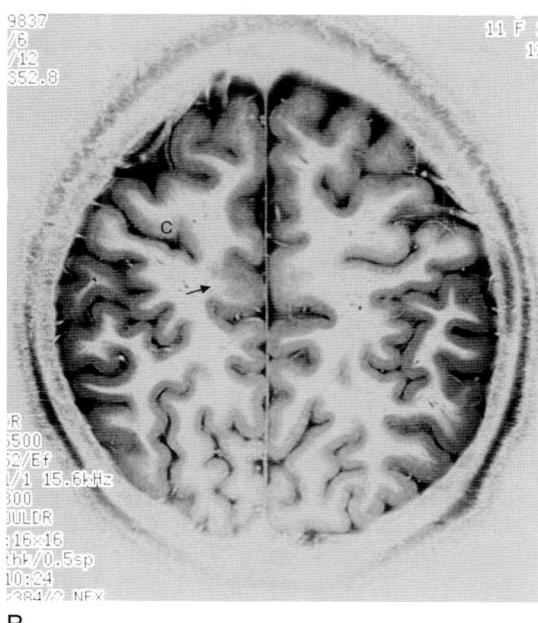

B

FIG. 5.14 Surface coil study in a patient with frontal lobe seizures. **A.** Axial SPGR images in the head coil were interpreted as normal. Even in retrospect, it is difficult to detect the region of cortical dysgenesis (arrow) medial to the central sulcus (C). **B.** Inversion recovery image (video inverted) using the phased array surface coil demonstrates blurring of the gray–white junction and thickening of the cortex (arrow) involving the posterior paracentral lobule, posterior-medial to the central sulcus (C). (Courtesy Dr R. Bronen, Yale University.)

Occipital Lobe Epilepsy

Clinically, occipital lobe seizures are most commonly manifested by visual auras and ocular movements. Review of major series indicate that visual auras are reported in approximately 47–73% of patients with occipital lobe

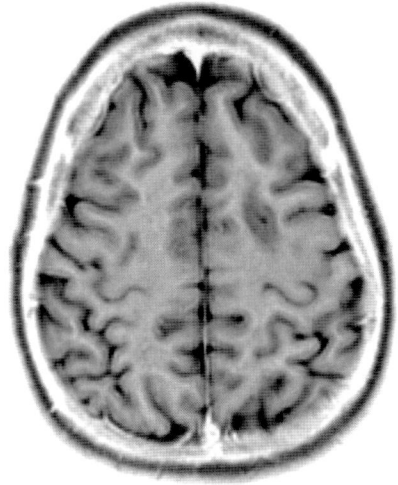

A

B

FIG. 5.15 Focal transmantle dysplasia. **A.** Axial inverted T2-weighted image showing minor sulcal abnormality in the left precentral area. **B.** Coronal FLAIR showing signal changes with typical radial pattern extending from ventricular wall to abnormal cortical region.

epilepsy. In a recent report, Williamson et al. (111) described 25 patients with occipital lobe epilepsy studied retrospectively. Of the 25 patients, 15 reported elementary visual hallucinations consisting of colored or white lights, or reported changes in the contralateral visual field. Interestingly, ictal amaurosis was reported by 10 of the 25 patients. In other studies, the frequency of visual extinction has been in the order of 40%. Other patients also report eye-pulling sensations or moving sensations within the eyes. Other signs of occipital lobe seizures consist of rapid bilateral blinking, eye-fluttering or eye deviation with or without head deviation which, in most cases, is contralateral to the seizure focus. In another study, Blume et al. (123) reported 19 patients with occipitoparietal lobe seizures. Visual elementary symptoms were present in

11 of 19 patients. However, six patients in his series never reported any visual changes with seizure onset.

In addition, many patients with occipital seizures, after their initial seizure symptom (aura), manifest temporal lobe behavior, whereas a small number may demonstrate frontal lobe seizure symptomatology. This is the result of infrasylvian seizure spread, which, in most patients, is towards the temporal region. Infrasylvian spread, either lateral or medial through the inferior longitudinal fasciculus, usually results in features suggestive of temporal lobe seizures with automatisms, posturing, and visual hallucinations. Medial spread through the superior longitudinal fasciculus usually produces asymmetric tonic posturing, whereas lateral suprasylvian spread usually produces contralateral clonic activity or sensory changes.

Parietal Lobe Epilepsy

Clinical semiology in parietal lobe epilepsy is more difficult to study (124–127). The incidence of proven seizure foci in the parietal lobe, in most series, is very small. Auras may not be present or may be difficult to interpret. Apart from patients with the expected classical somatosensory semiology, other symptoms include vertigo, complex visual hallucinations, and body movement sensations. Interestingly, most reports also stress the fact that up to 50% of patients with parietal lobe epilepsy do not have any localizing warnings. Williamson et al. (126) reported that only seven of 11 patients with parietal lobe seizures manifested any auras and most these were somatosensory in nature. Importantly, somatosensory auras were not always contralateral to the seizure focus.

Classic studies have indicated that parietal lobe seizures may induce vertigo and complex visual hallucinations. However, Williamson and Blume did not report this in their patient population (123, 126). In contrast to occipital lobe seizures, parietal lobe epilepsy usually produces very few reliable findings to help identify the seizure focus. Clinical behavior with seizure spread usually depends on the pattern of extra parietal or occipital activation. In most cases, the symptomatology will depend on suprasylvian activation with supplementary motor or other frontal lobe symptomatology. Similarly, patients with seizures of parietal lobe origin with secondary spread to mesial temporal regions have been reported. In contrast to the above findings, Rasmussen reported that most patients with parietal regional epilepsy had either unilateral motor or sensory phenomena or other symptoms. Only 10% of patients in his series failed to show any significant localizing features.

Pathology of Occipitoparietal Epilepsy

As stated above and contrary to temporal and frontal lobe epilepsy, occipital or parietal lobe resections are less common. Among the 503 pathologic specimens from the Mathieson series, 16 had parietal lobe resections and five had occipital lobe resections (48). In his series, parietal lesions included tumors, vascular malformations, tuberous sclerosis, and miscellaneous lesions. Occipital lobe pathology was evenly distributed between no abnormalities and the presence of gliomas or ulegyria. Rasmussen reported 132 patients who received surgery of the parietal regions between 1930 and 1973 (128). One-third of these patients had tumors or vascular malformations encompassing 35% of the total series lesions. Postnatal or perinatal trauma or anoxia constituted another 60% of the lesions, while postinflammatory brain meningocicatrix and miscellaneous causes were responsible for the remaining 5%. Similarly, occipital lobe pathology was less likely related to tumors than is the case with parietal lobe lesions. Rasmussen reported 25 such cases between 1931 and 1972 and only two had tumors while the rest had other lesions. Meningocerebral cicatrix and traumatic pathology were observed in 22% of patients.

In more recent series, including Blume's and Williamson's (123, 126), perinatal insult was common in many of the patients with occipitoparietal lesions. On pathology, cortical developmental abnormalities were found in some patients, whereas tumors and vascular malformations were seen in the others. In Williamson's series, most patients had hamartomas or grade I astrocytomas on the parietal lobe, whereas on the occipital lobe, 40% of patients had low-grade tumors or hamartomas. Encephalomalacia and perinatal lesions were also observed in some patients.

Imaging Findings

Most reported series antedate the use of MRI. Therefore, very limited data is presently available on the sensitivity of MRI in the detection of lesions in patients with occipitoparietal epilepsy. Previous series using CT scanning revealed a low yield of abnormalities in patients with occipitoparietal epilepsy.

One common detectable imaging finding is the presence of occipital horn enlargement. Occipital horn dilatation, either unilateral or bilateral, can be detected in some patients. Unfortunately, occipital horn dilatation, although useful, has in general provided limited localizing value. This is because the epileptogenic focus in some of these patients may be localized to the occipital pole, mesial occipital region, or the lateral occipitoparietal convexity. MRI is superior in these patients because it can demonstrate the presence of parenchymal abnormalities responsible for seizure generation in association with ventricular dilatation.

Blume et al. (123) reported abnormalities in seven of his 19 patients. Atrophic lesions, tumors, vascular abnormalities, and megalencephaly were reported. Most patients in their series had CT scans and not MRIs. In many of these cases, however, radiologic abnormalities were more extensive in some patients, being hemispheric in four but always unilateral to the same occipitoparietal foci. In contrast, Williamson reported that all patients in their series with parietal lobe epilepsy had lesions detected by neuroimaging techniques (123). However, in six of his patients the lesions were not detected at the time of initial evaluation or prior to the introduction of high-resolution MRI. In his occipital lobe series, 19 of the 25 had MRIs and 15 of the 19 patients had circumscribed focal lesions in the occipital lobe detected by MRI. However, since most of the patients had tumors or vascular malformations, it is not surprising that MRI was highly sensitive and yielded positive results in the majority of patients in this selected series.

Our experience is similar to the one reported by Williamson and Blume (123, 126). Patients with occipitoparietal epilepsy may demonstrate abnormalities on MRI studies that are either neoplastic, developmental, or vascular in origin. This selection bias may reflect the difficulties encountered in the investigation of patients with this type of localized epilepsy who do not have structural lesions. However, recent experience at many centers suggests that occipital epilepsy is often associated with developmental or perinatal pathology such as polymicrogyria, focal dysplasia, anoxia, or ulegyria.

Tumors

Tumors in these regions follow similar MRI features as described in previous chapters (77, 78, 129). Low-grade astrocytomas were commonly reported in previous studies but more recent experience has been modified by the advent of MRI and early detection of lesions upon seizure onset. Nevertheless, low-grade astrocytomas and oligodendrogliomas are common abnormalities (Figs 5.16, 5.17). The

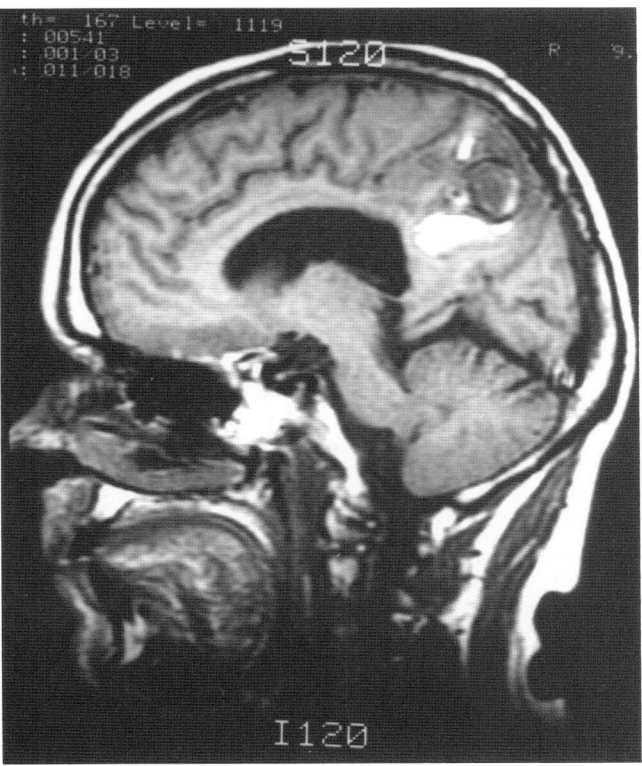

A

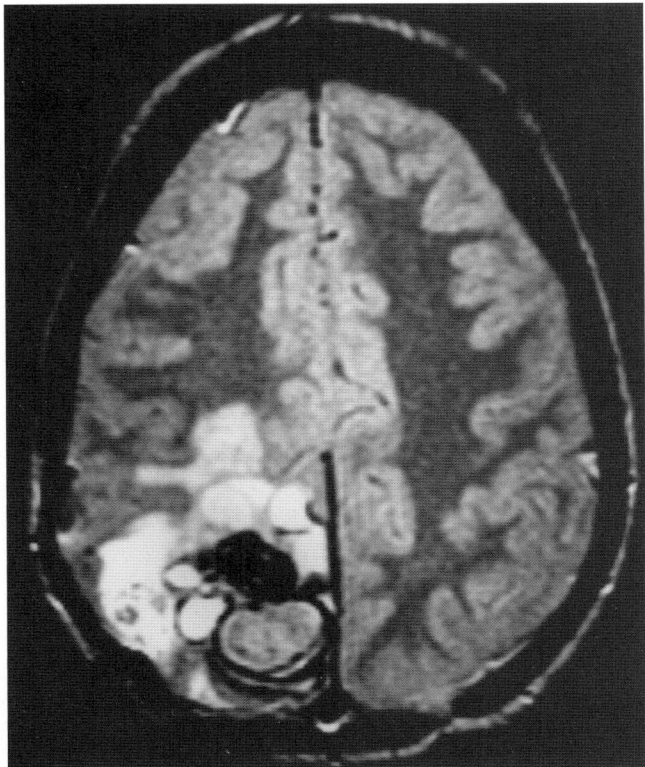

B

FIG. 5.17. Malignant paraganglioma. **A.** Sagittal MRI demonstrates mixed signal changes and involvement of mesial parietal region. **B.** Axial image showing right posterior parietal lesion with multiple tissue complexity including calcified tissue.

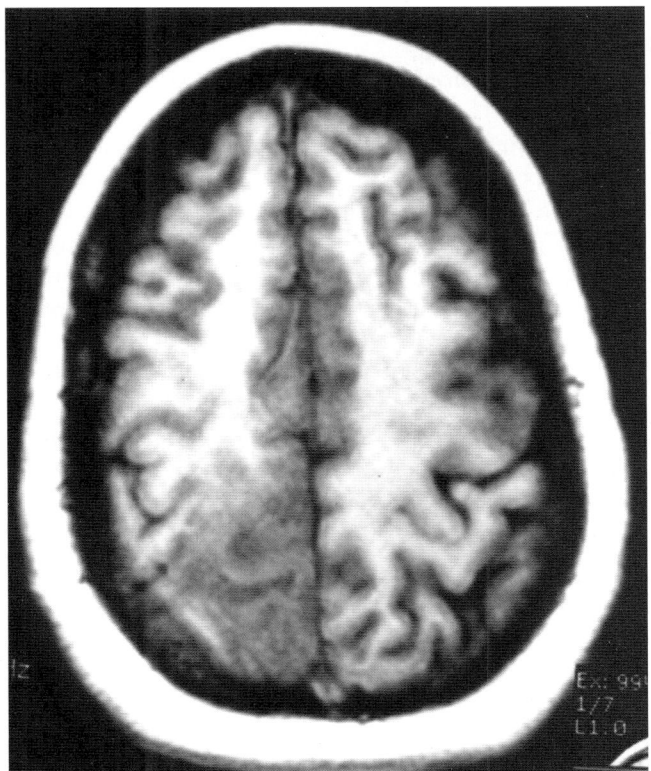

FIG. 5.16 Occipitoparietal oligodendroglioma. Axial T1-weighted (21/5) showing hypointense abnormality with gyral changes and edema.

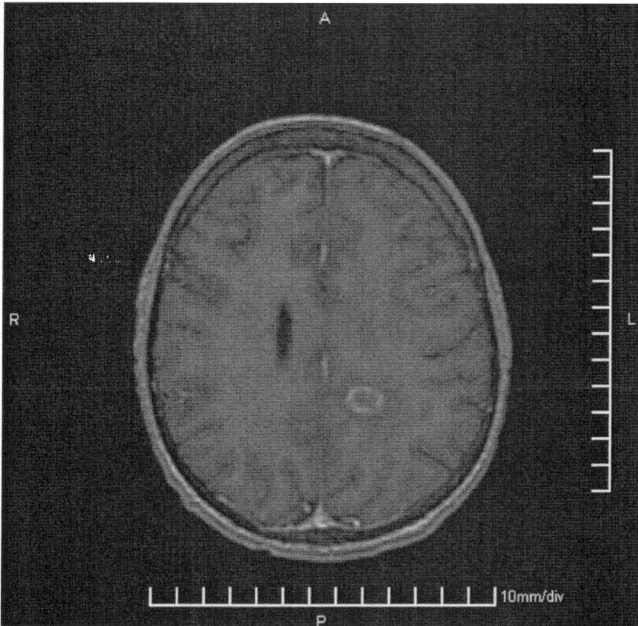

FIG. 5.18. Metastatic lesion. T1-weighted axial image with GAD showing ring-enhancing lesion in the deep gray/white matter parietal area. Mild edema is seen on the white matter around the lesion.

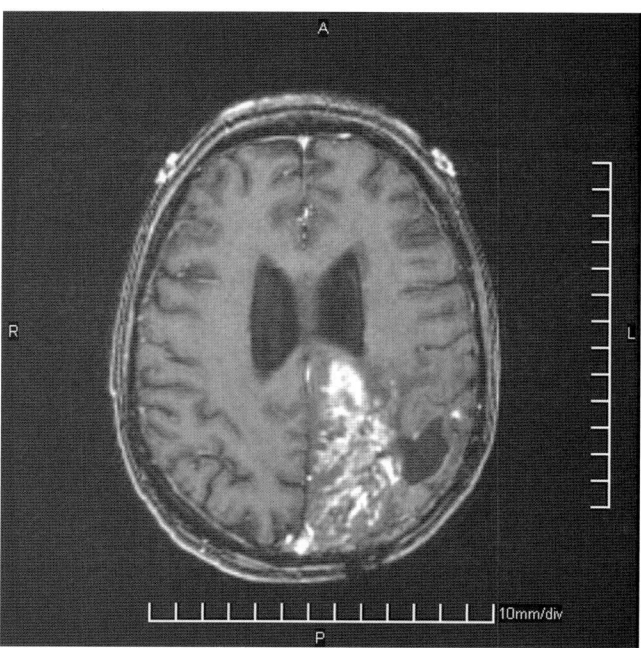

FIG. 5.20. T1-weighted axial image. Heterogeneous lesion with calcifications and contrast enhancement. Postoperative changes are seen laterally. Pathology revealed anaplastic astrocytoma.

role of gadolinium has been described before and is similar to its role in other foreign-tissue lesions. The imaging features of these tumors are described in previous chapters. More aggressive neoplasms may also present with seizures or may lead to intractable epilepsy (Figs 5.18–5.20). An important issue in certain patients relates to the location of these lesions, in particular when the calcarine fissure or the

angular gyrus is involved (130). Accurate identification of the lesions and their relation to these structures prior to surgery is important to prevent the possibility of postoperative visual field or language defects. Stereotactic lesionectomy may play an important role in these cases (76, 129, 131–133).

Congenital Acquired and Developmental Lesions

In this group, we include in-utero developmental pathology and perinatal acquired injuries. In our own surgical experience, the majority of patients demonstrate prenatal or perinatal injuries. Porencephalic cyst formation may be localized to the posterior cortex, in particular to the parietal regions (134–136). The mechanisms underlying these lesions have been described before. These abnormalities are of variable size and location and may be single or multiple. The presence of multiple lesions in some patients may raise difficult clinical questions regarding the localization of the epileptogenic focus or whether multiple epileptogenic foci are present (Fig. 5.21). Focal damage to the sulcus depth may result in ulegyria. This pathology is described in Chapter 6.

Occipital horn dilatation, either unilateral or bilateral, can be detected in some patients. Its presence may be useful but in many patients its significance is unclear. Etiologies are variable. The presence of unilateral dilatation may be indicative of regional epileptogenesis in some patients, in particular in those with prenatal or perinatal etiologies. The presence of unilateral occipital ventricular enlargement may be associated with periventricular cortical pathology of different degrees and types, or may not be specific at all.

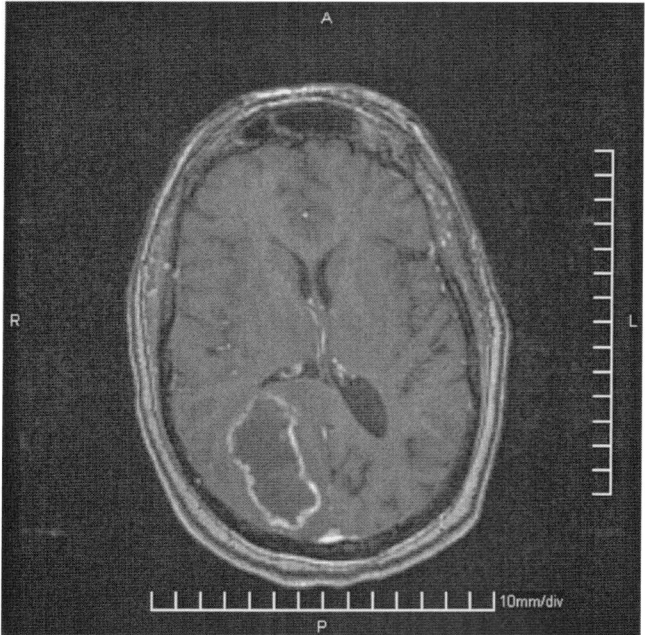

FIG. 5.19. T1-weighted axial contrast study demonstrating a large ring enhancing lesion in the occipitoparietal region. The core is hypointense and on histology demonstrates necrosis. Pathology consistent with high-grade astrocytoma.

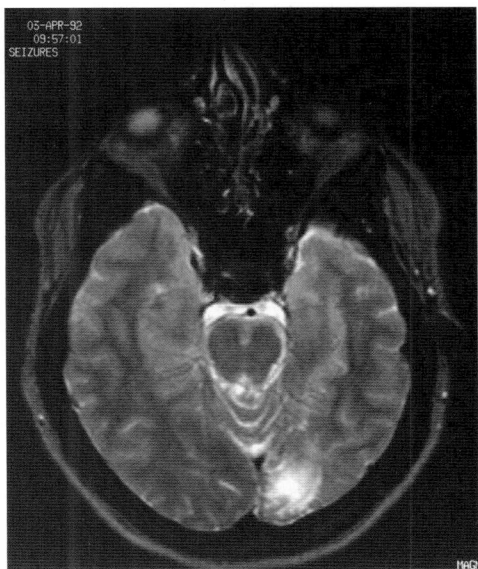

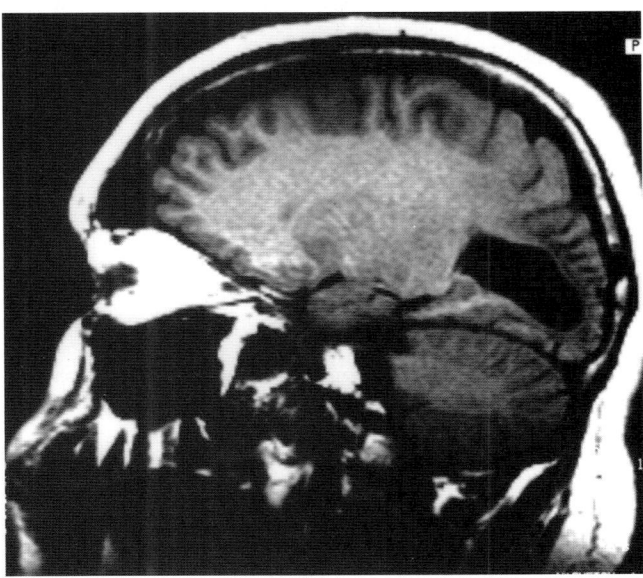

B

FIG. 5.21. Perinatal injury. **A.** Axial T2-weighted image showing high signal changes from occipital lobe with underlying atrophy. **B.** Sagittal T1-weighted image showing occipital lobe dilatation and encephalomalacia. Note microgyria in the underlying cortex.

In our experience it is difficult to use this particular finding as more than a guide to the hemispheric lateralization of the epileptic focus (Fig. 5.22).

Prenatal developmental lesions, such as focal dysplasia, can be detected in the occipital or parietal lobes and may involve the mesial as well as the lateral convexity (Fig. 5.23), but are less common than in the frontal lobes. However, polymicrogyria involving the parietal or occipital lobes has been described in various syndromes of bilateral polymicrogyria and may be genetic in origin. The MRI features are similar to the ones described in other chapters, with thin gyri and poor white/gray matter configuration. Occipital horn

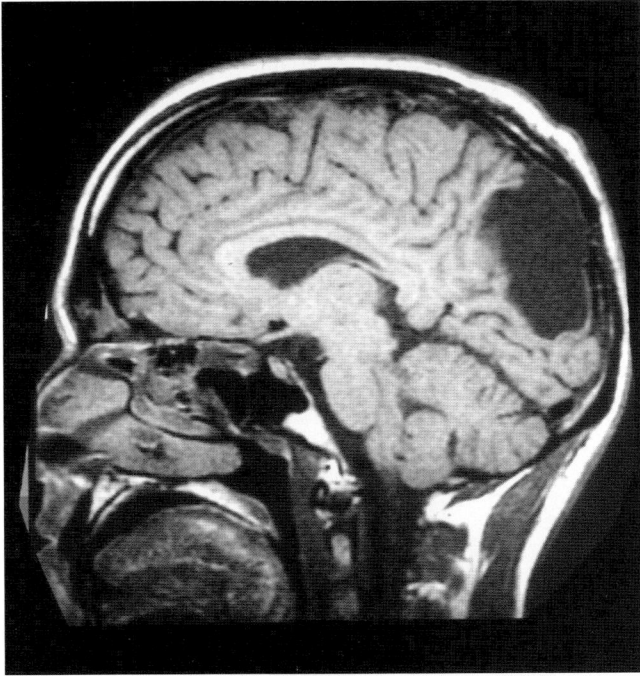

FIG. 5.22. Porencephaly following intraparenchymal hemorrhage at birth. Sagittal T1-weighted image showing cystic formation. Patient has occipital lobe seizures preceded by elementary visual aura.

dilatation may be present unilaterally in some of these patients. Other developmental lesions such as schizencephaly may be localized to the same region and are discussed in other chapters (137–140).

Specific abnormalities such as ulegyria or Sturge–Weber angiomatosis are usually localized to the posterior temporal, parietal, and occipital regions or may be fairly localized in some individuals to the occipital lobe. These conditions are described in more detailed under Chapter 6.

Vascular Malformations

Vascular malformations can occur in the parietal and occipital lobes (86, 141, 142). The MR imaging characteristics are well described in previous chapters and in the literature. Arteriovenous malformations may be small and should be carefully sought in some patients. Cavernous angiomas are also found in the posterior cortex but in our experience are less frequently seen than in other regions.

Conclusions

The clinical, as well as the surgical experience, suggests that epilepsies arising from the occipitoparietal regions are difficult to localize from the clinical and EEG viewpoint. It is likely that many of these patients are not selected for surgery because of poor localizing clinical and laboratory features. In most reported cases, structural lesions have been found on pathology in the occipitoparietal cortex,

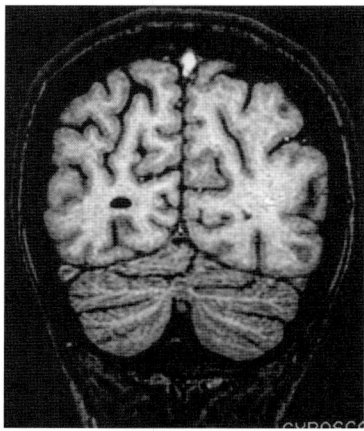

A

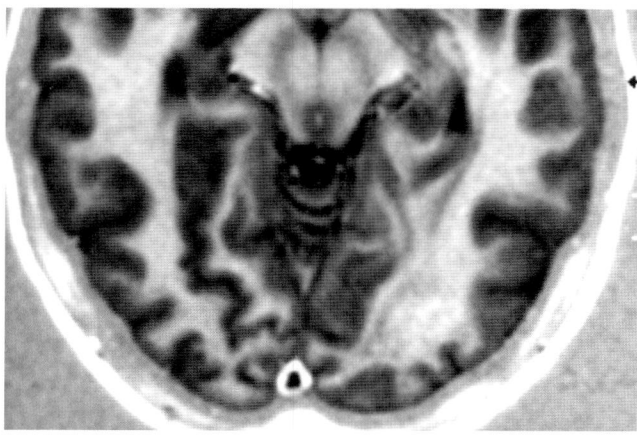

B

FIG. 5.23. Cortical dysplasia. Occipital lobe. **A.** Coronal T1-weighted image demonstrating abnormal left occipitoparietal anatomy. The occipital horn is asymmetric and the overall anatomy of the region is abnormal. **B.** Axial IR demonstrating abnormal gray/white matter pattern in the same region.

underscoring the fact that in previous years a selection bias existed towards those with structural lesions. However, recent experience suggests that many patients with these abnormalities and more subtle lesions can now be detected with MRI. Further experience and larger series are needed in this respect.

REFERENCES

1. Bancaud J, et al. Localizing value of the clinical manifestations of the partial seizures. *Acta Neurochir* 1984;33:7–15.
2. Bancaud J, Talairach J. Clinical semiology of frontal lobe seizures. *Adv Neurol* 1992;57:3–57.
3. Chauvel P et al. Somatomotor seizures of frontal lobe origin. *Adv Neurol* 1992;57:185–230.
4. Williamson PD. Frontal lobe epilepsy. Some clinical characteristics. *Adv Neurol* 1995;66:127–150.
5. Williamson PD. Frontal lobe seizures. Problems of diagnosis and classification. *Adv Neurol* 1992;57:289–309.
6. Williamson PD, et al. Complex partial seizures of frontal lobe origin. *Ann Neurol* 1985;18:497–504.
7. Jackson JH. Observations on the anatomical, physiological, pathological investigations of epilepsies. *West Riding Lunatic Asylum Rep* 1873;3:315.
8. Rasmussen T, Olszewski J, Lloyd-Smith D. Focal seizures due to chronic localized encephalitis. *Neurology* 1958;6:435–445.
9. Laich E, et al. Supplementary sensorimotor area epilepsy. Seizure localization, cortical propagation and subcortical activation pathways using ictal SPECT. *Brain* 1997;120:855–864.
10. Bass N, et al., Supplementary sensorimotor area seizures in children and adolescents. *J Pediatr* 1995;126:537–544.
11. Ebner A, et al. SSMA area seizures and ictal SPECT. In: Luders H, ed. Supplementary sensorimotor area. Philadelphia, PA: Lippincott-Raven, 1996:363–368.
12. Aicardi J. Diseases of the nervous system in childhood. London: MacKeith Press, 1992.
13. Haussser HC, Bancaud J. Gustatory hallucinations in epileptic seizures. Electrophysiological, clinical and anatomical correlates. *Brain* 1987;110:339–359.
14. Schlaug G., et al. Ictal motor signs and interictal regional cerebral hypometabolism. *Neurology* 1997;49:341–350.
15. Bittar RG, Ptito A, Reutens DC. Somatosensory representation in patients who have undergone hemispherectomy: a functional magnetic resonance imaging study. *J Neurosurg* 2000;92:45–51.
16. Shuper A, Stahl B, Mimouni M. Transient opercular syndrome: a manifestation of uncontrolled epileptic activity. *Acta Neurol Scand* 2000;101:335–338.
17. Kudo T., et al. [Postictal aphasia and its generating mechanism in 3 patients with localization-related epilepsy]. *Seishin Shinkeigaku Zasshi* 1993;95:125–150.
18. Kirshner HS, et al. Aphasia secondary to partial status epilepticus of the basal temporal language area. *Neurology* 1995;45:1616–1618.
19. Abou-Khalil B., et al. Global aphasia with seizure onset in the dominant basal temporal region. *Epilepsia* 1994;35:1079–1084.
20. Chung P.W., et al. Nonconvulsive status epilepticus presenting as a subacute progressive aphasia. *Seizure* 2002;11:449–454.
21. Chand RP. Ipsilateral motor seizures. *Austr New Zealand J Med* 1986;16:234–235.
22. Abou-Khalil B., et al. Inhibitory motor seizures: correlation with centroparietal structural and functional abnormalities. *Acta Neurol Scand* 1995;91:103–108.
23. Ikeda A., et al. Asymmetric tonic seizures with bilateral parietal lesions resembling frontal lobe epilepsy. *Epileptic Disord* 2001;3:17–22.
24. Bonelli SB, Baumgartner C [Frontal lobe epilepsy–clinical seizure seminology]. *Wien Klin Wochenschr* 2002;114:334–340.
25. Bancaud J. Surgery of epilepsy based on stereotactic investigations – the plan of the SEEG investigations. *Acta Neurochir* 1980;30:25–34.
26. Gloor P, et al. The role of the limbic system in experimental phenomena of temporal lobe epilepsy. *Ann Neurol* 1982;12:129–144.
27. Quesney LF, Constain M, Rasmussen T. Seizures from the dorsolateral frontal lobe. *Adv Neurol* 1992;57:233–244.
28. Quesney LF, et al. Frontal lobe epilepsy – a field of recent emphasis. *Am J EEG Technol* 1990;30:177–193.
29. Quesney LF, et al. The clinical differentiation of seizures arising in the parasagittal and anterolaterodorsal frontal convexities. *Arch Neurol* 1990;47:677–679.
30. Zentner J, et al. Functional results after resective procedures involving the supplementary motor area. *J Neurosurg* 1996;85:542–549.
31. Von Manitius-Robeck, S, Pauli E, Stefan H. Periictal speech as function of the age of cerebral damage. *Adv Neurol* 1999;81:183–187.
32. Janszky J, et al. Automatisms with preserved responsiveness and ictal aphasia: contradictory lateralising signs during a dominant temporal lobe seizure. *Seizure* 2003;12:182–185.
33. Sturm K, et al. Autonomic seizures versus syncope in 18q-deletion syndrome: a case report. *Epilepsia* 2000;41:1039–1043.
34. Stefan H, et al. [Goose flesh and cold sensation. Symptoms of visceral epilepsy]. *Nervenarzt* 2002;73:188–193.

35. Fried I, et al. Functional organization of human supplementary motor cortex studied by electrical stimulation. *J Neurosci* 1991;11:3656–3666.

36. Ikeda A, et al. 'Supplementary motor area (SMA) seizure' rather than 'SMA epilepsy' in optimal surgical candidates: a document of subdural mapping. *J Neurol Sci* 2002;202:43–52.

37. Gondo K, et al. Reorganization of the primary somatosensory area in epilepsy associated with focal cortical dysplasia. *Dev Med Child Neurol* 2000;42:839–842.

38. Wieshmann UC, Niehaus L, Meierkord H. Ictal speech arrest and parasagittal lesions. *Eur Neurol* 1997;38:123–127.

39. Atkinson DS Jr, et al. Midsagittal corpus callosum area, intelligence, and language dominance in epilepsy. *J Neuroimaging* 1996;6:235–239.

40. Morioka T, et al. Functional mapping of the sensorimotor cortex: combined use of magnetoencephalography, functional MRI, and motor evoked potentials. *Neuroradiology* 1995;37:526–530.

41. Mihara T, et al. Surgical strategies for patients with supplementary sensorimotor area epilepsy. The Japanese experience. *Adv Neurol* 1996;70:405–414.

42. Wyllie E, Bass NE. Supplementary sensorimotor area seizures in children and adolescents. *Adv Neurol* 1996;70:301–308.

43. Laich E, et al. Supplementary sensorimotor area epilepsy: seizure localization, cortical propagation and subcortical activation pathways using ictal SPECT. *Brain* 1997;120:855–864.

44. King D, Smith J. Supplementary sensorimotor area epilepsy in adults. In: Luders H, ed. Supplementary sensorimotor area. Philadelphia, PA: Lippincott-Raven, 1996:285–291.

45. Morris HH. Supplementary motor seizures. In: Wyllie E, ed. The treatment of the epilepsies. Philadelphia, PA: Lea & Febiger, 1993: 541–546.

46. Penfield W, Welch K. The supplementary area in the cerebral cortex of man. *Arch Neurol Psychiatr* 1951;66:289–317.

47. Munari C, Bancaud J. Electroclinical symptomatology of partial seizures of orbital frontal origin. *Adv Neurol* 1992;57:257–265.

48. Mathieson G. Pathology of temporal lobe foci. In: Penry JK, Daly DD, eds. Complex partial seizures and their treatment. New York: Raven Press, 1975:163–185.

49. Sempere AP, et al. First seizure in adults: a prospective study from the emergency department. *Acta Neurol Scand* 1992;86:134–138.

50. Aminoff MJ, Simon RP. Status epilepticus. Causes, clinical features and consequences in 98 patients. *Am J Med* 1980;69:657–666.

51. Janz D. Prognosis and prevention of traumatic epilepsy. *Rev Chil Neuro Psiquiatr* 1985;23:46–55.

52. Willmore LJ. Post-traumatic epilepsy: cellular mechanisms and implications for treatment. *Epilepsia* 1990;31:S67–S73.

53. Jennett WB. Epilepsy and acute traumatic intracranial hematoma. *J Neurol Neurosurg Psychiatry* 1975;38:378–381.

54. Jennett WB, Lewin W. Traumatic epilepsy after closed head injuries. *J Neurol Neurosurg Psychiatry* 1960;23:295–301.

55. Ng KK, Ng PW, Tsang KL. Clinical characteristics of adult epilepsy patients in the 1997 Hong Kong epilepsy registry. *Chin Med J (Engl)* 2001;114:84–87.

56. Jabbari B, et al. Intractable epilepsy and mild brain injury: incidence, pathology and surgical outcome. *Brain Inj* 2002;16:463–467.

57. Mazzini L, et al. Posttraumatic epilepsy: neuroradiologic and neuropsychological assessment of long-term outcome. *Epilepsia* 2003;44:569–574.

58. Mironenko TV, Zubov PG. [Clinico-neurophysiological correlations in post-traumatic epilepsy]. *Lik Sprava* 2002:63–67.

59. Jennett WB. Epilepsy after non-missile head injuries, 2nd ed. London: William Heinemann, 1975:179.

60. Caveness WF, et al. The nature of posttraumatic epilepsy. *J Neurosurg* 1979;50:545–553.

61. Caveness WF. Onset and cessation of fits following craniocerebral trauma. *J Neurosurg* 1963;20:570–583.

62. Hardman JM. The pathology of traumatic brain injuries. In: Thompson RA, Green JR, eds. Complications of nervous system trauma. Advances in neurology 22. New York: Raven Press, 1979:15–50.

63. Wieshmann UC, et al. Blunt-head trauma associated with widespread water-diffusion changes. *Lancet* 1999;353:1242–1243.

64. Makarov A, Sadykov EA, Kiselev VN. [Posttraumatic epilepsy: diagnosis and clinical variety]. *Zh Nevrol Psikhiatr Im S S Korsakova* 2001;101:7–11.

65. Aotsuka A, et al. [Punch drunk syndrome due to repeated karate kicks and punches]. *Rinsho Shinkeigaku* 1990;30:1243–1246.

66. Groswasser Z, et al. Magnetic resonance imaging in head injury patients with normal late computed tomography scans. *Surg Neurol* 1987;27:331–337.

67. Wilberger JE, Deeb Z, Rothfus W. Magnetic resonance imaging in cases of severe head injury. *Neurosurgery* 1987;20:571–576.

68. Levin HS, et al. Magnetic resonance imaging after 'diffuse' nonmissile head injury. *Arch Neurol* 1985;42:963–968.

69. Rao TH, Libman RB, Patel M. Seizures and 'disappearing' brain lesions. *Seizure* 1995;4:61–65.

70. Miller DJ, Steinmetz M, McCutcheon IE. Vertex epidural hematoma: surgical versus conservative management: two case reports and review of the literature. *Neurosurgery* 1999;45:621–624.

71. Cabantog AM, Bernstein M. Complications of first craniotomy for intra-axial brain tumour. *Can J Neurol Sci* 1994;21:213–218.

72. Cascino GD. Neuroimaging in neocortical epilepsies: structural magnetic resonance imaging. *Adv Neurol* 2000;84:377–389.

73. Cascino GD. Structural neuroimaging in partial epilepsy. Magnetic resonance imaging. *Neurosurg Clin N Am* 1995;6: 455–464.

74. Leblanc R, Rasmussen T. Cerebral seizures and brain tumors. *Handbook Clin Neurol* 1974;15:295–301.

75. Whittle IR, et al. Dysembryoplastic neuroepithelial tumour with discrete bilateral multifocality: further evidence for a germinal origin. *Br J Neurosurg* 1999;13:508–511.

76. Britton JW, et al. Low-grade glial neoplasms and intractable partial epilepsy: efficacy of surgical treatment. *Epilepsia* 1994;35:1130–1135.

77. Jay V, Becker LE. Surgical pathology of epilepsy: a review. *Pediatr Pathol* 1994;14:731–750.

78. Stieber VW. Low-grade gliomas. *Curr Treat Options Oncol* 2001;2:495–506.

79. Cascino GD. Epilepsy and brain tumors: implications for treatment. *Epilepsia* 1990;31(Suppl 3):S37–S44.

80. Glantz MJ, et al. Identification of early recurrence of primary central nervous system tumors by [18F]fluorodeoxyglucose positron emission tomography. *Ann Neurol* 1991;29:347–355.

81. Mork SJ, et al. Oligodendroglioma: incidence and biological behavior in a defined population. *J Neurosurg* 1985;63:881–889.

82. Rizk T, et al. Cerebral oligodendrogliomas in children: an analysis of 15 cases. *Childs Nerv Syst* 1996;12:527–529.

83. Daumas-Duport C, et al. Oligodendrogliomas. Part I: Patterns of growth, histological diagnosis, clinical and imaging correlations: a study of 153 cases. *J Neurooncol* 1997;34:37–59.

84. Lee Y, Tassel PV. Intracranial oligodendrogliomas: imaging findings in 35 untreated cases. *Am J Neuroradiol* 1989;10:119–127.

85. Trussart V, et al. Epileptogenic cerebral vascular malformations and MRI. *J Neuroradiol* 1989;16:273–284.

86. Griffiths PD, et al. Cerebellar arteriovenous malformations in children. *Neuroradiology* 1998;40:324–31.

87. Essig M, et al. Arteriovenous malformations: assessment of gliotic and ischemic changes with fluid-attenuated inversion-recovery MRI. *Invest Radiol* 2000;35:689–694.

88. Kuznieecky R, et al. Focal cortical myoclonus and rolandic cortical dysplasia: clarification by MRI. *Ann Neurol* 1988;23:317–325.

89. Kuznieecky R, et al. Cortical dysplasia in temporal lobe epilepsy: magnetic resonance imaging correlations. *Ann Neurol* 1991;29:293–298.

90. Kuznieecky R, et al. Temporal Lobe developmental malformations and hippocampal sclerosis: epilepsy surgical outcome. *Neurology* 1999; 52:479–484.

91. Kuznieecky R, Jackson G. Neuroimaging in epilepsy. In: Magnetic resonance in epilepsy. New York: Raven Press, 1995:27–48.

92. Kuzniecky R, et al. Frontal and central lobe focal dysplasia: clinical, EEG and imaging features. *Dev Med Child Neurol* 1995;37:159–166.

93. Barkovich AJ. Malformations of neocortical development: magnetic resonance imaging correlates. *Curr Opin Neurol* 1996;9: 118–211.

94. Barkovich AJ, Kuzniecky RI, Dobyns WB. Radiologic classification of malformations of cortical development. *Curr Opin Neurol* 2001;14:145–149.

95. Barkovich AJ. Pediatric neuroimaging, 2nd ed. New York: Raven Press, 1995:668.

96. Barkovich A, et al. Classification system for malformations of cortical development: update 2001. *Neurology* 2001;57:2168–2178.

97. Mackay MT, et al. Malformations of cortical development with balloon cells: clinical and radiologic correlates. *Neurology* 2003;60: 580–587.

98. Urbach H, et al. Focal cortical dysplasia of Taylor's balloon cell type: a clinicopathological entity with characteristic neuroimaging and histopathological features, and favorable postsurgical outcome. *Epilepsia* 2002;43:33–40.

99. Montenegro MA, et al. Focal cortical dysplasia: improving diagnosis and localization with magnetic resonance imaging multiplanar and curvilinear reconstruction. *J Neuroimaging* 2002;12:224–230.

100. Matsuda K, et al. Neuroradiologic findings in focal cortical dysplasia: histologic correlation with surgically resected specimens. *Epilepsia* 2001;42(Suppl 6):29–36.

101. Lee SK, et al. Neuroimaging findings of cortical dyslamination with cytomegaly. *Epilepsia* 2001;42:850–856.

102. Lee BC, et al. MRI of focal cortical dysplasia. *Neuroradiology* 1998;40:675–683.

103. Kuzniecky RI, Magnetic resonance imaging in developmental disorders of the cerebral cortex. *Epilepsia* 1994;35(Suppl 6): S44–S56.

104. Otsubo H, et al. Focal cortical dysplasia in children with localization-related epilepsy: EEG, MRI, and SPECT findings. *Pediatr Neurol* 1993;9:101–107.

105. Raymond A, et al. Abnormalities of gyration, heterotopias, tuberous sclerosis, focal cortical dysplasia, microdysgenesis, dysembryo-plastic neuroepithelial tumor and dysgenesis of the archicortex in epilepsy. Clinical, EEG and neuroimaging features in 100 adult patients. *Brain* 1995;118:629–660.

106. Aso K, Nakashima S, Watanabe K. [Neuronal migration disorders and epilepsy]. *No To Hattatsu* 1997;29:129–133.

107. Sheth RD, Gutierrez AR, Riggs JE. Rolandic epilepsy and cortical dysplasia: MRI correlation of epileptiform discharges. *Pediatr Neurol* 1997;17:177–179.

108. Gomez-Anson B, et al. Imaging and radiological-pathological correlation in histologically proven cases of focal cortical dysplasia and other glial and neuronoglial malformative lesions in adults. *Neuroradiology* 2000;42:157–167.

109. Leventer RJ, et al. Clinical and imaging features of cortical malformations in childhood. *Neurology* 1999;53:715–722.

110. Barkovich AJ, et al. Focal transmantle dysplasia: a specific malformation of cortical development. Neurology 1997;49:1148–1152.

111. Williamson PD, et al. Occipital lobe epilepsy: clinical characteristics, seizure spread patterns, and results of surgery. *Ann Neurol* 1992; 31:3–13.

112. Gilliam F, Wyllie E. Ictal amaurosis: MRI, EEG, and clinical features. *Neurology* 1995;45:1619–1621.

113. Huott AD, Madison DS, Niedermeyer E. Occipital lobe epilepsy: a clinical and electroencephalographic study. *Eur Neurol* 1974;11: 325–339.

114. Salanova V, et al. Occipital lobe epilepsy: electroclinical manifestations, electrocorticography, cortical stimulation and outcome in 42 patients treated between 1930 and 1991. *Brain* 1992; 115:1655–1680.

115. Van den Hout B, et al. Seizure semiology of occipital lobe epilepsy in Children. *Epilepsia* 1997;38:1118–1191.

116. Kramer U, et al. Benign childhood epilepsy with centrotemporal spikes: clinical characteristics and identification of patients at risk for multiple seizures. *J Child Neurol* 2002;17:17–91.

117. Kuzniecky R. Symptomatic occipital lobe epilepsy. *Epilepsia* 1998;39(Suppl 4):S24–S31.

118. Olivier A, Boling W Jr. Surgery of parietal and occipital lobe epilepsy. *Adv Neurol* 2000;84:533–575.

119. Gokcay A, et al. Occipital epilepsies in children. *Eur J Paediatr Neurol* 2002;6:261–268.

120. Kaneko Y. [Symptomatic occipital lobe epilepsy]. *Ryoikibetsu Shokogun Shirizu* 2002;37:50–53.

121. Ambrosetto G, Antonini L, Tassinari CA. Occipital lobe seizures related to clinically asymptomatic Coeliac disease in adulthood. *Epilepsia* 1992;33:476–481.

122. Guerrini R, et al. Bilateral parietoccipital polymicrogyria and epilepsy. *Ann Neurol* 1997;41:65–73.

123. Blume WT, Whiting SE, Girvin JP. Epilepsy surgery in the posterior cortex. *Ann Neurol* 1991;29:638–645.

124. Lawn N, et al. Occipitoparietal epilepsy, hippocampal atrophy, and congenital developmental abnormalities. *Epilepsia* 2000;41:1546–1553.

125. Sveinbjornsdottir S, Duncan JS. Parietal and occipital lobe epilepsy: a review. *Epilepsia* 1993;34:493–521.

126. Williamson PD, et al. Parietal lobe epilepsy: diagnostic considerations and results of surgery. *Ann Neurol* 1992;31:193–201.

127. Ho S, et al. Parietal lobe epilepsy: Clinical features and seizure localization by ictal SPECT. *Neurology* 1994;44:2277–2284.

128. Rasmussen TB. Surgical treatment of complex partial seizures: results, lessons, and problems. *Epilepsia* 1983;24(Suppl 1):S65–S76.

129. Lombardi D, Marsh R, de Tribolet N. Low grade glioma in intractable epilepsy: lesionectomy versus epilepsy surgery. *Acta Neurochir Suppl (Wien)* 1997;68:70–74.

130. Smith KA, Spetzler RF. Supratentorial-infraoccipital approach for posteromedial temporal lobe lesions. *J Neurosurg* 1995;82:940–944.

131. Cascino G, et al. Long-term follow-up of stereotactic lesionectomy in partial epilepsy: predictive factors and electroencephalographic results. *Epilepsia* 1992;33:639–644.

132. Siegel AM, et al. Pure lesionectomy versus tailored epilepsy surgery in treatment of cavernous malformations presenting with epilepsy. *Neurosurg Rev* 2000;23:80–83.

133. Casazza M, et al. Lesionectomy in epileptogenic temporal lobe lesions: preoperative seizure course and postoperative outcome. *Acta Neurochir Suppl (Wien)* 1997;68:64–69.

134. Pasternak JF, Mantovani JF, Volpe JJ. Porencephaly from periventricular intracerebral hemorrhage in a premature infant. *Am J Dis Child* 1980;134:673–675.

135. Ho S, et al. Congenital porencephaly: MR features and relationship to hippocampal sclerosis. *Am J Neuroradiol* 1998;19:135–141.

136. Carreno M, et al. Intractable epilepsy in vascular congenital hemiparesis: clinical features and surgical options. *Neurology* 2002;59:129–131.

137. Cakirer S, et al. MR imaging in epilepsy that is refractory to medical therapy. *Eur Radiol* 2002;12:549–558.

138. Denis D, et al. Schizencephaly: clinical and imaging features in 30 infantile cases. *Brain Dev* 2000;22:475–483.

139. Morioka T, et al. [Schizencephaly: clinical and MRI features]. *No To Shinkei* 1999;51:938–944.

140. Packard AM, Miller VS, Delgado MR. Schizencephaly: correlations of clinical and radiologic features. *Neurology* 1997;48:1427–1434.

141. Leblanc R, Feindel W, Ethier R. Epilepsy from cerebral arteriovenous malformations. *Can J Neurol Sci* 1983;10:91–95.

142. Chen JS, Ilsen PF. Parieto-occipital arteriovenous malformation. *Optometry* 2002;73:477–491.

CHAPTER **6**

MRI in Special Conditions Associated with Epilepsy

Ruben I. Kuzniecky and Graeme D. Jackson

"Attacks bear a certain degree of affinity to epilepsy ... without coming up to the description of it.... The convulsion is not always universal, being sometimes confined to one half of the muscular system, and scarcely passing over the median line."

J.C. Prichard, 1822

INTRODUCTION

The epilepsies have various underlying etiologies, some of which are acquired and can be detectable using modern imaging techniques. Some of these entities are acquired, whereas others may be genetic. These pathologies may include lesions that occupy small areas or may involve, at times, an entire lobe, a hemisphere, or may be multifocal or diffuse in nature. In this chapter, instead of following the anatomic approach, we describe a number of specific conditions and syndromes where epilepsy is a prominent part of the clinical condition. Some of these conditions are characterized by unilateral hemispheric or diffuse abnormalities that have not been dealt with specifically in other chapters and, on the other hand, some are focal in nature and have been described in other chapters in more detail. This chapter by definition does not include all potential conditions associated with epilepsy, but we will highlight what we believe are a number of important entities.

The epileptic conditions described in this chapter can result from multiple mechanisms and etiologies. A classification of these disorders is beyond the scope of this chapter. Depending on the time of injury, these injuries may be divided into prenatal, perinatal, or postnatal in nature. According to their histologic basis, they can be classified into developmental, neoplastic, ischemic, inflammatory, or infectious. A classification based on the etiologic factors responsible for each condition will include some of the histologic changes described before but other etiologies such as trauma may be included in the classification. In this chapter we will describe some of these conditions, in particular those associated with epilepsy and how MRI may help in the diagnosis and management of these patients. In this chapter we include stroke and related vascular conditions, two distinct congenital malformations (Sturge–Weber syndrome and hypothalamic hamartomas), and infectious diseases associated with epilepsy.

VASCULAR OR ISCHEMIC INJURY

Vascular injury can be associated with epilepsy by a number of entirely different mechanisms. These include ischemia, infarction, and hemorrhage. Importantly, the age at time of the vascular insult has a significant impact on the mechanisms involved in injury and development of epilepsy. In this section we emphasize vascular injuries to the developing brain since they are more commonly associated with the development of epilepsy.

Ischemia in a young developing brain can occur prenatally, perinatally, and postnatally. The lesions can produce unilateral or bilateral, regional or widespread hemispheric pathology. Commonly these injuries are extensive and involve large parts of one hemisphere. These lesions can be classified according to the time of injury, by the gross morphologic features, and by their histologic characteristics. Most authorities classify these lesions as prenatal, perinatal and postnatal (1–4).

Prenatal injuries usually present with cavity lesions of the full thickness of the hemispheric wall, which represents

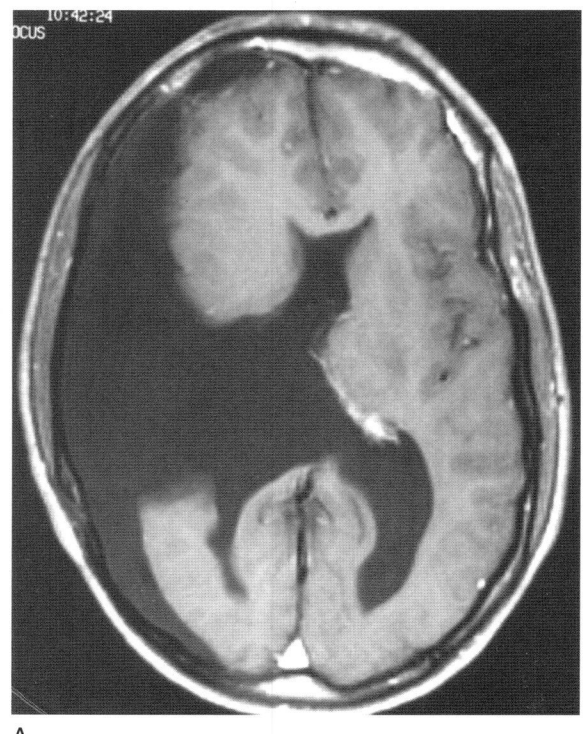

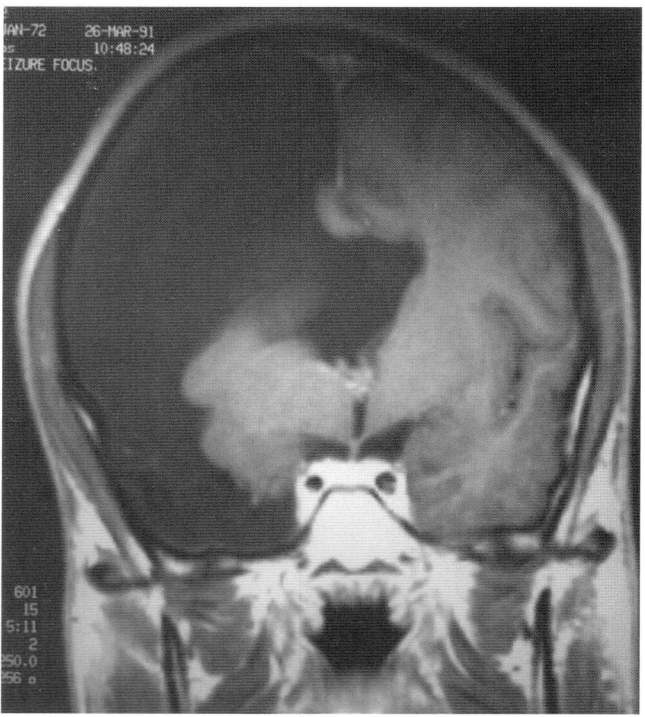

B

FIG. 6.1 Prenatal infarction. **A.** Axial T1 image showing large cavity involving the right hemisphere in the distribution of the middle cerebral artery. Possible occlusion at the proximal level of the right middle cerebral artery. **B.** Coronal image showing large cavity with remaining frontal pole. The patient had intractable partial seizures of right occipital lobe origin.

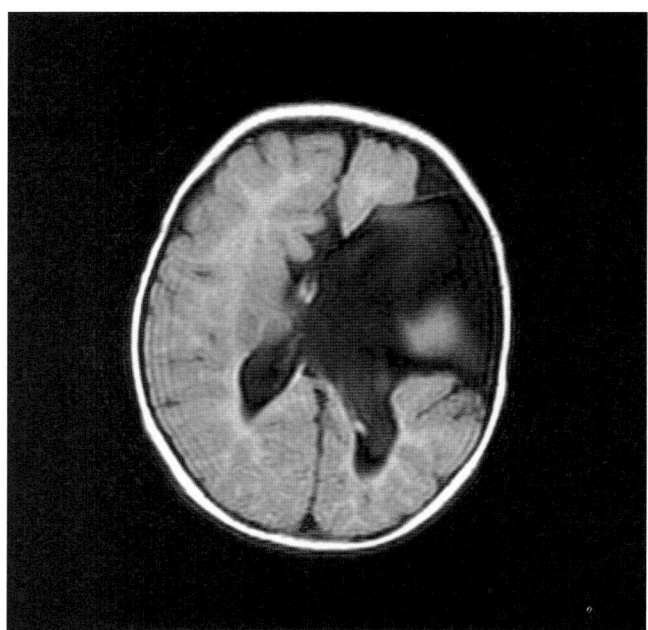

FIG. 6.2 Prenatal infarction and partial seizures. Axial T1 image showing a large cavity involving the right frontal temporal region. The frontal medial and occipital regions are spared, indicating involvement of the middle cerebral artery.

destruction or injury of the cerebral tissue during early development (4). In some cases, the injuries are severe enough to cause massive destruction of an hemisphere, while in other cases the injury is more restricted in nature (Figs 6.1, 6.2).

Porencephaly

One of the most common forms of prenatal hemispheric lesion is porencephaly (4). A few familial cases have been reported, raising questions about the possible genetic base in some individuals (5). Porencephalic cysts communicate with the ventricles, with the subarachnoid space, or with both (Fig. 6.3). These lesions are secondary to circumscribed hemispheric necrosis that occurs in utero or before the cerebral hemisphere is formed (2). The mechanism underlying these lesions is usually ischemia or resolution of an intracerebral hemorrhage related to occlusion of a major cerebral artery (6). Neonatal hemorrhages may give rise to these lesions after reabsorption and can be large or small in size (Fig. 6.4) (7–11). The developmental origin of these lesions is clear in view of the minimal gliosis and the commonly associated changes in the adjacent cortex, which demonstrates developmental abnormalities (12). Cyst formation in the neonatal brain is the direct result of poor collateral circulation and the lack of a strong astrocytic response. As opposed to pure porencephalic lesions, encephaloclastic lesions in the terminal phase of the pregnancy do not alter the gyral development and usually produce irregular defects in the lesions. Encephaloclastic lesions are usually related to periventricular infarcts or to infarcts in early childhood (13).

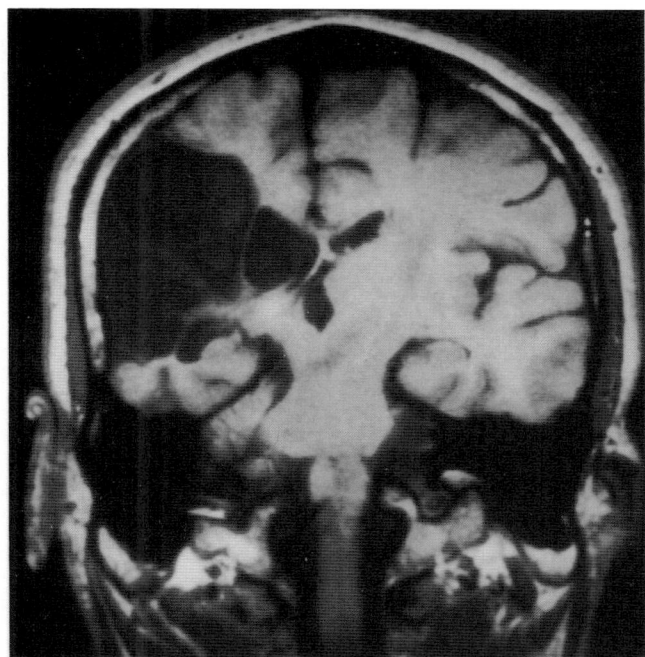

FIG. 6.3 Coronal MRI demonstrating a large cavity involving the left frontal central temporal region associated with a left middle cerebral artery infarction. The cavity is communicating with the ventricle and has the same signal as cerebrospinal fluid. Cavitations are observed, indicating late injury.

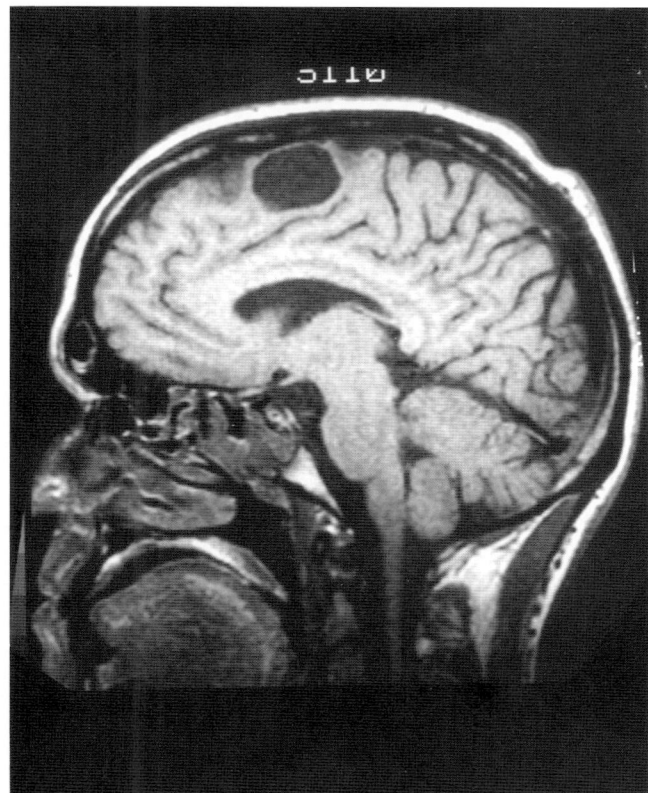

FIG. 6.4 Small cystic cavity secondary to a neonatal intraparenchymal bleed. The patient developed intractable epilepsy in childhood. T1-weighted images show evidence of a well defined cystic cavity in the mesial frontal region.

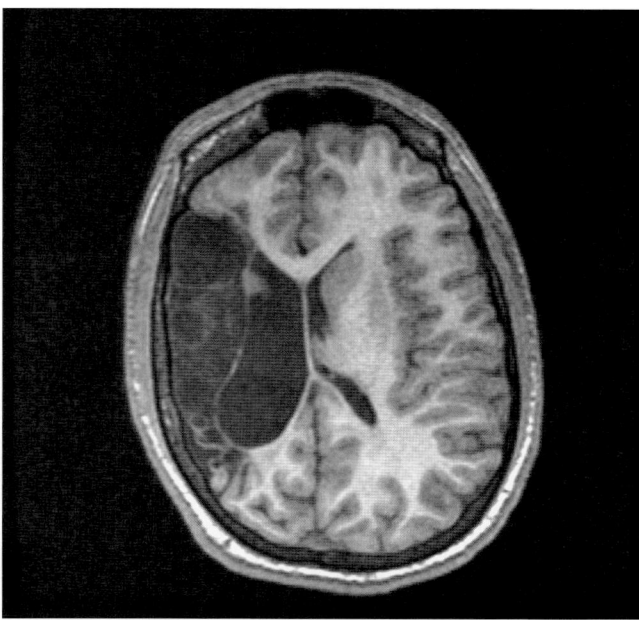

FIG. 6.5 Perinatal ischemic stroke. T1-weighted axial images. Large porencephalic cyst involving the territory of the middle cerebral artery. Seizures were of widespread onset, involving the entire hemisphere.

Porencephaly is commonly bilateral, but may be unilateral and is usually localized to the perisylvian region. The defect is usually covered by a thin arachnoid membrane without mass effect. The cysts are not lined by ependyma and their surface is gliotic. These lesions may communicate with the ventricle or may be separated from it by a thin layer of tissue (Fig. 6.5). As stated above, many of these lesions manifest changes in the adjacent cortex, which may be polymicrogyria in some cases (14–16). In other patients, the adjacent gyri are also abnormal but do not demonstrate polymicrogyria. However, cases of porencephalic cysts with polymicrogyria have been well documented (4).

Autopsy series in neonates have demonstrated *cerebral infarcts* in up to 5% of patients. The histologic changes are similar to those found in infarcts in adults and the findings are consistent with events that occur in utero. It is possible that, in the majority of these cases, embolization is the cause. These patients often have congenital heart conditions and will manifest other symptoms at birth. In those children who survive, focal seizures are often the presenting event. A large study examining more than 500 infants at autopsy (17) reported an incidence of 5.4% of cerebral infarcts. In that study, the authors found that arterial occlusion with embolization was a major causative agent in neonates. Many of the patients who survived had focal neurologic deficit with porencephaly, hemiplegia, and motor retardation. In general, one can state that infarcts occurring early in fetal-life will produce cortical neuronal cell loss and cytoarchitectonic abnormalities with polymicrogyria. Infarcts in the late uterine phase may resemble those of adults. They are

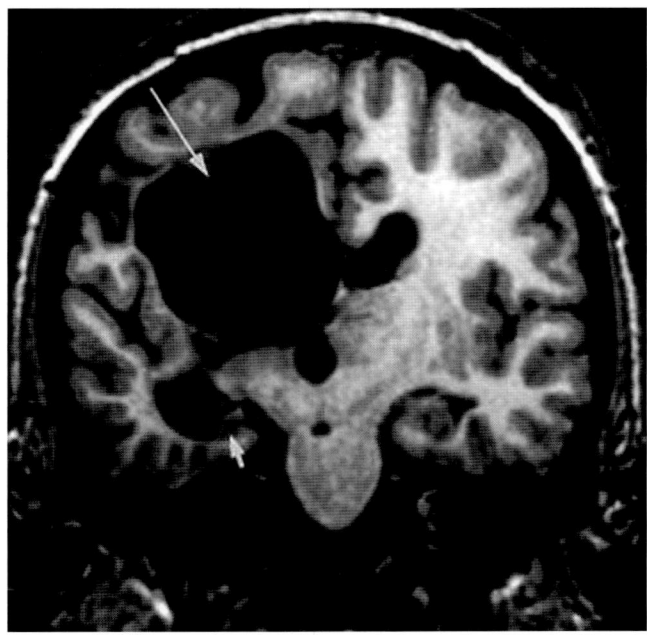

A

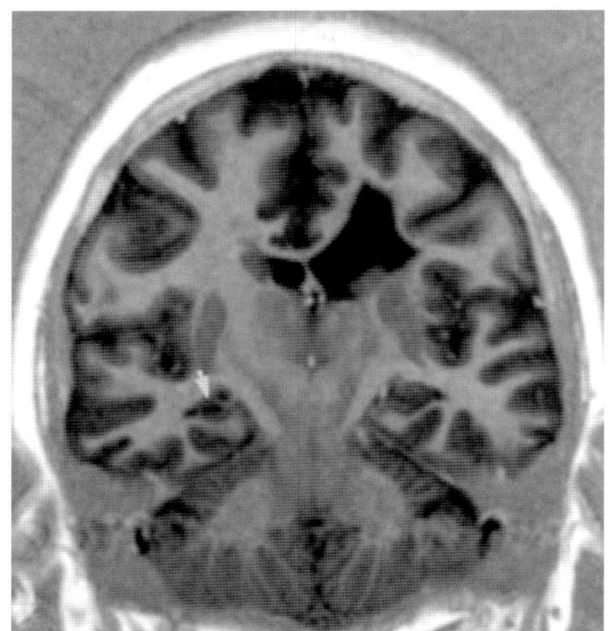

B

FIG. 6.6 A. Congenital porencephaly and intractable epilepsy. T1-weighted coronal image shows a large cystic cavity (arrow). In addition, note evidence of ipsilateral hippocampal atrophy typical of hippocampal sclerosis (arrowhead). **B.** Porencephaly and intractable epilepsy with contralateral hippocampal sclerosis (arrow).

characterized by formation of a cavity with varying degree of phagocytes and astrocytosis.

Perinatal and postnatal occlusive diseases are usually characterized pathologically by the presence of severe cortical necrosis and hemorrhages of the cortical and subcortical white matter. Friede reported that, in neonates, most acute cerebral

infarcts of arterial origin are hemorrhagic in nature (4, 18). Interestingly, many of these children do not manifest any epileptic activity during the early and acute phase of their illness but, if they survive, they usually go on to develop hemiparesis or hemiplegia and focal seizures, as well as variable cognitive dysfunction. MRI shows unilateral lesions, variable in size and location but usually in the territory of the middle cerebral arteries. In addition, hemorrhages may result in general ventricular dilatation and hydrocephalus in some patients (8, 19).

Periventricular infarcts are related to anoxia during the perinatal period (20–23). Although fairly typical, in some patients they may be associated with focal ischemic lesions or ulegyria (3, 13). The clinical features are not further described.

Although porencephaly is common in children with epilepsy, it is not necessarily the cause of seizures (24). Recent data suggest, in fact, that most patients with hemispheric porencephaly and seizures have temporal lobe epilepsy secondary to mesial temporal sclerosis that can be detected with optimized techniques (Fig. 6.6). The presence of mesial temporal sclerosis is usually ipsilateral to the porencephaly but it can be contralateral as well (Fig. 6.6B). Volumetric studies have shown however, that patients with porencephaly often have bilateral asymmetric or symmetric hippocampal atrophy. The significance of these findings is twofold: first, the detection of mesial temporal sclerosis in a given patient with extratemporal porencephaly may indicate localization of the epileptic focus to the mesial temporal region. Second, the presence of mesial temporal sclerosis in this context requires careful evaluation for subtle contralateral hippocampal atrophy. Third, ischemic injury may produce focal as well as widespread pathology, with some areas more vulnerable than others.

Ulegyria

A less common perinatal injury, ulegyria, or atrophic sclerosis, was first described in 1899 by Bressler (25). Although ulegyria is considered a hallmark of birth injury, the pattern of damage is not exclusive to infancy. Histologically, ulegyria is characterized by vacuolization, chromatolysis, and neuronal drop-out. There is usually no evidence of vascular occlusion (26–28). With time there is massive proliferation of glial and blood vessels and macrophages. These lesions are usually in the sulci and tend to spare the crowns of the convolutions. The degree of change is variable and, in the most severe lesions, the entire cortex may be destroyed at the bottom of the sulci. Laminar necrosis occurs most often in the third cortical layer (4).

Ulegyria is usually distributed in the arterial border zones. The preferential perisulcal distribution may result from perfusion defects associated with hypotension. Venous drainage impairment may contribute to the particular distribution. The lesions are usually unilateral and may extend through

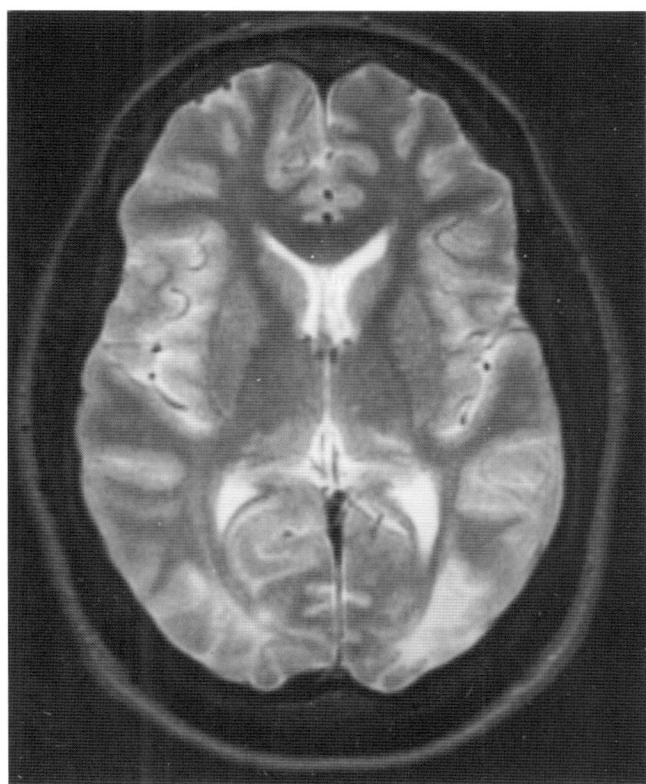

FIG. 6.7 Ulegyria; partial seizures. Axial MR T2-weighted image demonstrating high-intensity signal from the right posterior parietal occipital region. The high-intensity signal appears to involve the white matter with a typical distribution at the arterial border zone. Right posterior resection confirmed the diagnosis.

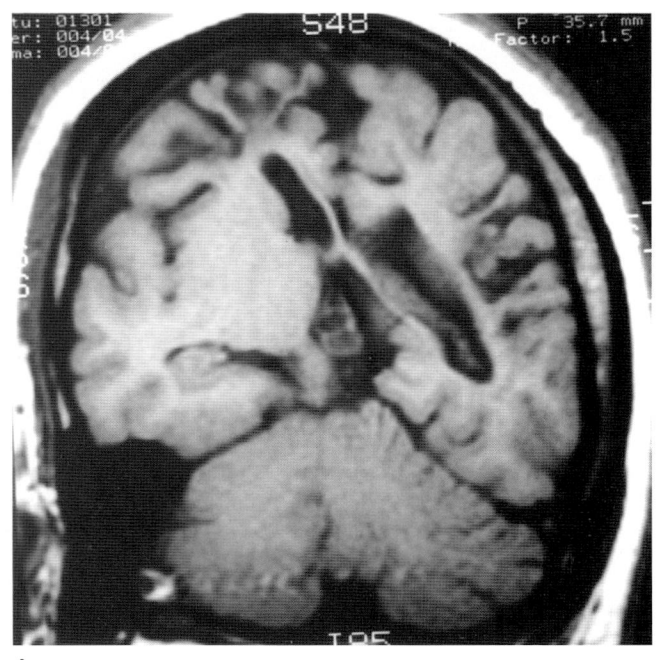

A

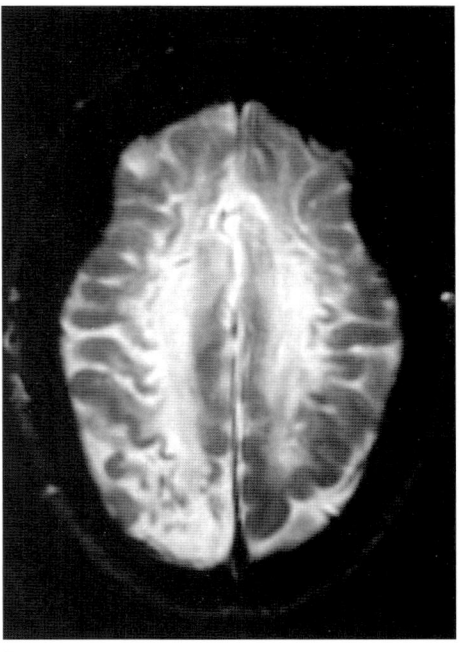

B

FIG. 6.8 Diffuse prenatal anoxia. Coronal axial image showing diffuse cerebral atrophy with prominent cortical thinning and ventricular asymmetry. Axial T2-weighted images show microgyria and diffuse cerebral atrophy.

one hemisphere but bilateral lesions have also been reported. In some cases, porencephalic cyst formation and adjacent ulegyria can been observed. Figure 6.7 demonstrates a case of ulegyria of the occipital parietal region associated with intractable partial seizures. The MRI features often can be recognized because of the location and the presence of T2 high signal changes (as seen in infarcts) in the cortico/white matter regions.

Having described some of the pathologic features of these injuries we should briefly mention that the mechanisms responsible for injury are diverse. Embolization in children with congenital heart anomalies is common. Other causes of embolization in neonates include patent ductus, placental vessel thrombosis, and sepsis. Thrombosis may be related to trauma, coagulopathy, infection, and polycythemia. Hypoxia and hypotension are rarely responsible for unilateral hemispheric lesions but it can occur.

Among patients with diffuse nonspecific anoxic injuries and epilepsy, we have attempted to classify some of these cases according to the possible underlying time and type of injury. In many, pre- and perinatal injuries appear to be common. As with unilateral vascular-related injuries, bilateral pathology may be detected in some children. In-utero malformations resulting from perfusion failures may result

in cortical migration and postmigration disorders associated with changes that appear to be postnatal as well. Intrauterine ischemia may result in a variety of injuries depending on the offending agent, the time of injury, and other related factors. Perinatal anoxic insults resulting in extensive and diffuse cortical and subcortical injuries are commonly observed (Fig. 6.8).

ISCHEMIC STROKE AND EPILEPSY

Incidence

Stroke is one of the most frequent causes of seizures in adulthood (29–34). The incidence of epilepsy in older individuals is dramatically increasing because of the total increase in the elderly population. Since the prevalence of cerebrovascular disease increases with age, it is expected that both of these conditions will become more frequent with time.

Although the frequency of seizures after stroke is variously estimated at 4–14%, the data is based on retrospective studies with variable follow-up, often without computed tomographic (CT) confirmation of the lesion. Often included were patients with arteriovenous malformations, brain-stem strokes, subarachnoid hemorrhage, or a previous history of seizures or epilepsy. Therefore, earlier data were less reliable.

The most comprehensive study is the stroke after seizures study (SASS). The study enrolled 1897 patients and found an overall incidence of seizures of 8.9%, with chronic epilepsy a sequela in only 2.5%. However, the mean follow-up was only 9 months. Previous studies indicated that patients with hemorrhagic stroke were at significantly greater risk of seizures (20% per year) compared with patients with ischemic stroke (14% per year), particularly in the first few days after stroke onset.

The frequency of epilepsy as a late sequela of stroke has been estimated previously at 3–10%, with a higher risk after late-onset than early-onset seizures. In SASS, epilepsy occurred in 2.5% of patients (up to 9 months) overall but was present in approximately half of those with late-onset seizures after ischemic stroke and in all patients with late-onset seizures after hemorrhagic stroke. After controlling for other clinical variables, late-onset seizures were identified as an independent risk factor (with a 12-fold increase) only for epilepsy after ischemic stroke. In another study, 81% of the patients who had seizures after the second week from onset of the stroke develop epilepsy while seizures during the first 2 weeks led to epilepsy in only 6% of patients.

Seizures are a more common accompaniment of hemorrhagic rather than ischemic stroke (35–37). Bladin et al. found the incidence of seizures to be 10.6% among 265 patients with intracerebral hemorrhage versus 8.6% among 1632 with ischemic stroke. In another prospective series, seizures occurred in 4.4% of 1000 patients, including 15.4% with lobar or extensive intracerebral hemorrhage, 8.5% with subarachnoid hemorrhage, 6.5% with cortical infarction, and 3.7% with hemispheric transient ischemic attacks. A seizure was the presenting feature of intracranial hemorrhage in 30% of 1402 patients.

Location and Seizures

Cortical location is among the most reliable risk factors for poststroke seizures, although controversial data exist. Poststroke seizures were more likely to develop in patients with larger lesions involving multiple lobes of the brain than in those with single lobar involvement (30, 32, 38–41). However, any stroke, including those with only subcortical involvement, may occasionally be associated with seizures. Earlier studies, relying on less sensitive neuroimaging techniques, may not have detected concomitant small cortical lesions that could cause ictal activity. In addition, the only clinical predictor for seizures after ischemic stroke is the severity of the initial neurologic deficit. Greater initial stroke severity or stroke disability predicted seizures. By contrast, in the Oxfordshire Community Stroke Project, only 3% of 225 patients who were independent 1 month after a stroke experienced a seizure between 1 month and 5 years.

The lobar site is considered to be the most epileptogenic location in patients with intracerebral hemorrhage. In a series of 123 patients (40), seizure incidence was highest with bleeding into lobar cortical structures (54%), low with basal ganglionic hemorrhage (19%), and absent with thalamic hemorrhage. Caudate involvement of the basal ganglia and temporal or parietal involvement within the cortex predicted seizures. Hemorrhage due to cerebral venous thrombosis also commonly presents with seizures. Parenchymal, often cortical, hemorrhage resulting from local venous congestion is the likely cause of seizure activity.

Magnetic resonance imaging findings in stroke and epilepsy are well recognized and are not described in detail here since the imaging features are not different from those seen in patients without seizures or epilepsy. Diffusion-weighted MRI and new perfusion techniques are able to detect ischemia earlier and may be of help in investigating stroke and epilepsy.

STURGE–WEBER SYNDROME

This syndrome is described under this chapter in view of the vascular and progressive nature of the lesions, even though we recognize that it is developmental in origin. The Sturge–Weber syndrome or encephalotrigeminal angiomatosis is one of the neurocutaneous syndromes first described by Sturge in 1879 (42). This condition is considered to be a sporadic noninherited abnormality but few familiar cases have been reported.

Clinical Features

Clinical features include the presence of a facial vascular nevus in the territory of the trigeminal nerve, in conjunction with a variety of cerebral manifestations. This include partial seizures, cognitive deficits, hemiparesis or hemiplegia, hemianopsia, buphthalmos, and glaucoma. Seizures are recorded in over 90% of patients and, in general, the more the seizures the more the developmental disorder and hemiparesis. However, the variation in severity of the epilepsy

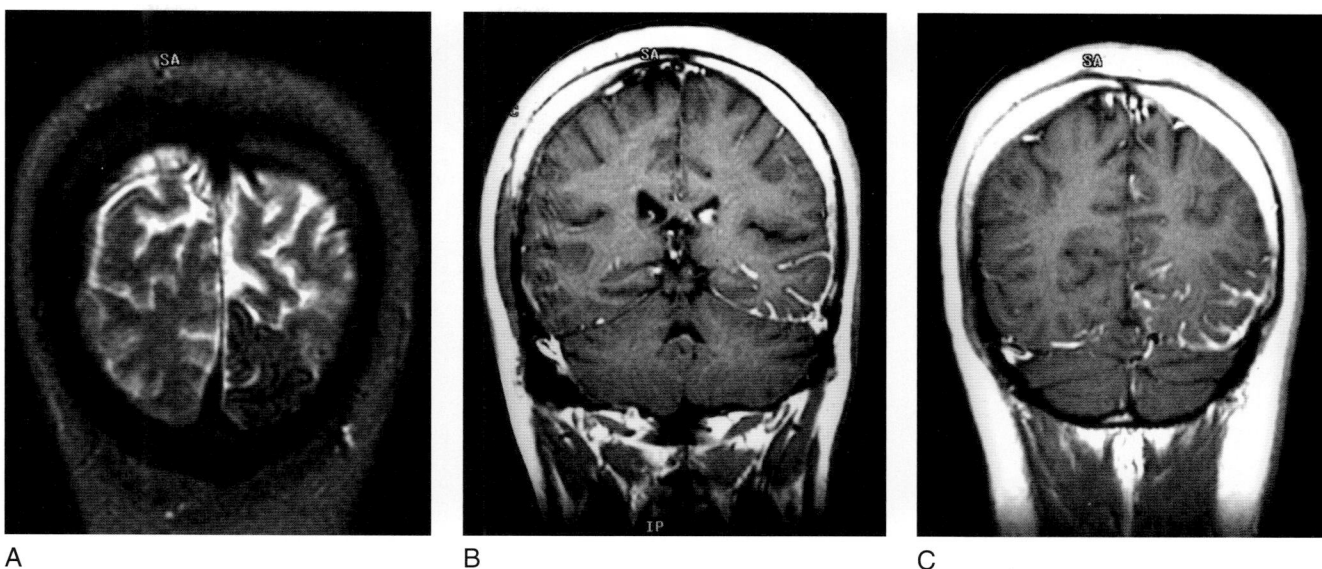

FIG. 6.9 Sturge–Weber syndrome. **A.** Coronal spin-echo 2800–90 demonstrates gyri with calcifications over the left occipital region. Hypointensity is marked on long T_R/T_E images. **B, C.** Two consecutive coronal images on the same patient using gadolinium (500–13). Note enhancement of pial angiomatosis over the temporal occipital region.

related to Sturge–Weber syndrome is great and not all patients have seizures or intractable epilepsy (43).

Intracranial abnormalities in this syndrome consist of venous angiomatosis of the leptomeninges. The meningeal abnormality is usually found in the anterior lateral occipital lobe, with variable extension into the posterior temporal and parietal regions. In most cases the intracranial lesion is ipsilateral to the nevus but contralateral and bilateral lesions have been described. In addition, the *forme fruste* of the syndrome has been described in some patients, with the presence of angiomatosis in the cerebral cortex but no evidence of skin lesions. Calcifications are progressive, are seen in older patients, and are usually adjacent to the leptomeningeal abnormality. Histologic analysis reveals that these calcifications have a pericapillary distribution, usually in the fourth layer of the cerebral cortex, and are thought to be related to hypoxia.

Imaging Findings

Radiologic investigations in these patients have been useful since 1922 when Weber first noted the characteristic intracranial calcification in skull X-rays. CT scan is also useful in the diagnosis of this condition. Cerebral atrophy, sinus hypertrophy, intracranial calcifications, and abnormal choroid plexus prominence are detected with CT scans. In addition, enlarged internal cerebral veins may be seen in some of these individuals with associated absence of superficial cortical veins overlying the areas of cerebral atrophy.

Magnetic resonance imaging investigations in patients with Sturge–Weber syndrome are extremely useful for the diagnosis (44–48). Both short-echo and long T_R/T_E studies should be done. In addition, gradient-echo sequences are useful in the detection of calcifications (47). On MRI, there are usually diffuse calcifications involving the cortex of the brain, which is commonly in the occipital or occipital-parietal temporal region (as discussed above; Fig. 6.9). However, rarely the angiomatosis may be localized to the frontal region, as demonstrated in Figure 6.10. In the region of calcifications, spin-echo MR images often show hypointensity indicating the presence of deposited iron rather than calcifications. There is usually cortical atrophy in the involved site, especially in the areas of calcifications. Gradient-echo sequences are helpful for demonstrating the presence of microcalcifications. In younger children, the calcifications may be absent and the only abnormality may be the presence of atrophy and small gyri. These features may be related to iron content in the vessels. Choroid plexus angiomas are usually well demonstrated and abnormal venous drainage can also be studied with MRI.

Contrast enhancement appears to be relatively useful in the study of these malformations. According to several investigators, contrast-enhanced MRI may reveal abnormalities in some patients in which the standard T1 techniques may not (47, 49).

Magnetic resonance imaging in the investigation of patients with Sturge–Weber syndrome is important for several reasons. First, the extent of calcifications and angiomatosis can be well demarcated with MRI. This is of extreme importance if the patient is a candidate for surgical

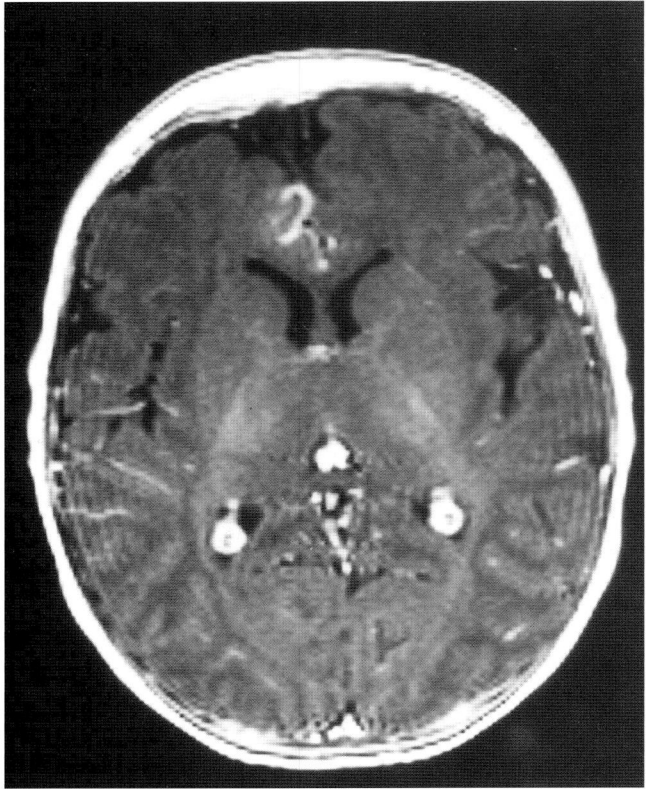

FIG. 6.10 Sturge–Weber syndrome. Axial enhanced MRI study in a 2-month-old child with intractable focal seizures. Atrophy and abnormal enhancement is noted with gadolinium. (Courtesy of Dr B. Abou-Khalil, Vanderbilt University, Nashville, TN.)

intervention for intractable epilepsy. Secondly, in cases in which the skin lesions may be absent (*forme fruste* of Sturge–Weber syndrome), the diagnosis of the condition can be made. Figure 6.11 demonstrates such an example. This patient had no skin lesions; neurologic examination was normal, and the cause of seizures unknown prior to MR examination. MRI demonstrated typical findings confirmed at surgery and pathology (Fig. 6.12).

Finally, MR investigations may provide more information about the vascular supply, and the venous drainage of these malformations in patients who are considered for surgery.

HYPOTHALAMIC HAMARTOMAS AND GELASTIC SEIZURES

Gelastic epilepsy was first described in 1957. Gelastic seizures are an uncommon epileptic seizure type, with laughter as the main ictal manifestation. They typically occur in association with hypothalamic hamartomas but laughter may also occur in complex partial seizures of frontal or temporal lobe origin. Hypothalamic hamartoma with gelastic seizures is recognized in patients with epilepsy

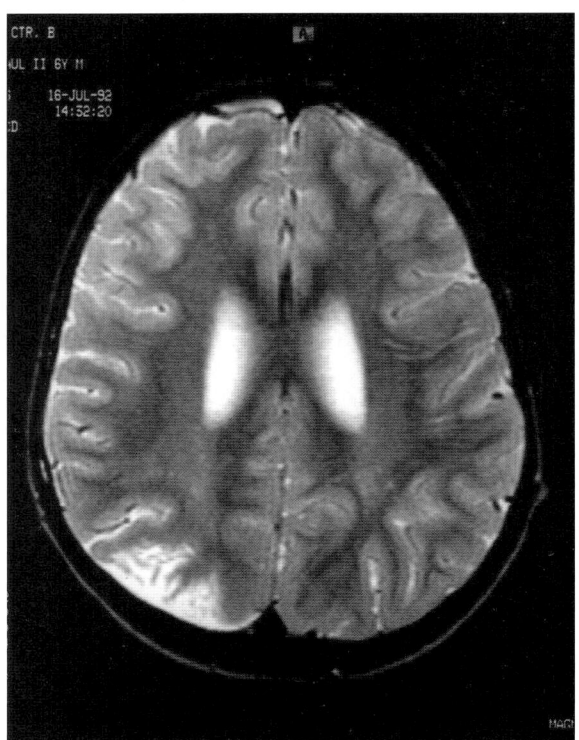

A

B

FIG. 6.11 *Forme fruste* of Sturge–Weber syndrome. **A.** Axial T2-weighted image showing cortical atrophy and hyperintense signal from the right occipital region. **B.** Axial 600–15 images with gadolinium demonstrating enhancement of cortical abnormality. Enhancement shows very clearly the extent of the abnormality.

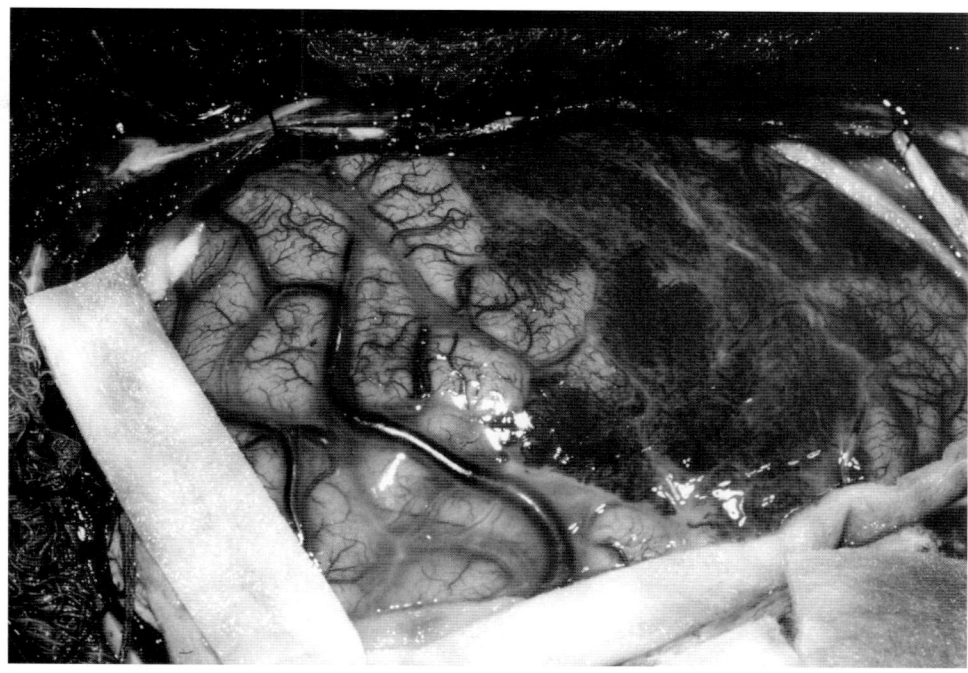

FIG. 6.12 Intraoperative photograph on patient shown in Figure 6.11. Pial angiomatosis is clearly demonstrated over the right occipital cortex. (Courtesy of Dr. B. Abou-Khalil, Vanderbilt University, Nashville, TN.)

as a very particular syndrome. Seizures usually begin in infancy or childhood and often consist of laughing attacks. Most patients, however, develop other seizure types with time, ranging from partial complex seizures to drop attacks. Associated features include precocious puberty and behavioral problems, and in some patients progressive cognitive and social deterioration has been documented (50, 51). The ictal laugh is usually mechanical and most commonly occurs as the initial behavioral change. Seizure frequency is variable, with some individuals having few seizures while others experience up to 200 seizures per day. Cognitive testing shows mental retardation or borderline intelligence in most patients. Aggressive and violent behavior is common (52–59).

Electroencephalographic (EEG) abnormalities are commonly bitemporal or multifocal. Most commonly, interictal discharges are localized in the temporal or frontal lobes or are hemispheric. Ictal EEG studies are seldom clearly focal in nature (52–59). However, ictal single-positron-emission computed tomography (SPECT) has clearly shown the exact origin of the ictus and has led to surgical intervention with dramatic results in most treated patients.

Hypothalamic hamartomas have been classified in several ways. Valdueza et al. (56) developed a classification system based on topographic and clinical data and correlated the surgical risk with the type. Pedunculated hamartomas are classified under types 1a and 1b while sessile hamartomas are classified as type 2a or 2b. There are clinical correlations to the different subtypes, with type 1 usually associated with precocious puberty whereas the others are associated with epilepsy.

More recently, Arita et al. (60) classified these lesions into two types on the basis of MRI findings. The parahypothalamic type, in which the hypothalamic hamartoma is attached to the floor of the third ventricle or is on a peduncle, is associated with precocious puberty. The intrahypothalamic type, in which the hypothalamic hamartoma is enveloped by the hypothalamus and distorts the third ventricle, is commonly associated with gelastic epilepsy, with or without precocious puberty, mental retardation, and behavioral problems. The sessile or intrahypothalamic types of hypothalamic hamartomas, which have a prominent intraventricular component, are most strongly associated with gelastic epilepsy, perhaps because of the hypothalamic distortion and close connection to the thalamus (Fig. 6.13). The size of hypothalamic hamartomas may also be a determinant of clinical manifestations, with large lesions often associated with gelastic epilepsy.

These results suggest that classification of hypothalamic hamartomas into these two categories based on MR findings results in a clear correlation between symptoms and the subsequent clinical course.

Magnetic resonance imaging is the imaging method of choice for detecting the hamartomas and planning surgery (54, 60–64). The size of the hamartomas is variable, and they may be pedunculated or sessile as described above. They are localized in the tuber cinereum and, using multiplanar imaging, the lesions can be detected as hyperintense on T2 images or isointense with gray matter on T1 sequences (Fig. 6.13). On inversion recovery (IR) images the hamartomas have low signal intensity. Sagittal images are often

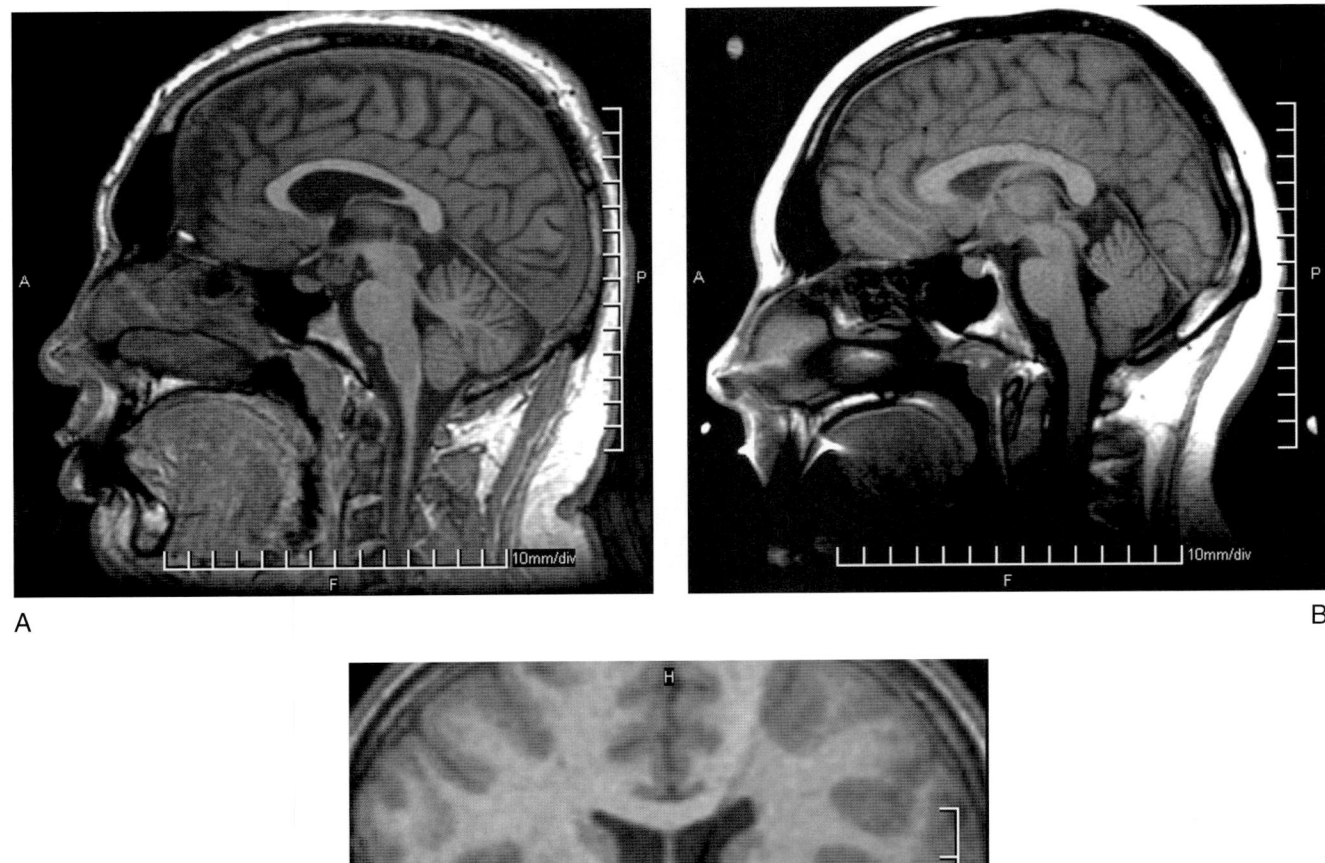

FIG. 6.13 Hypothalamic hamartoma. **A.** Sagittal T1-weighted image showing a large hamartoma extending inferiorly and anteriorly. No other abnormalities are observed. **B.** In this other patient, the hamartoma is attached to the mamillary bodies. **C.** Coronal T1-weighted image of another patient with hypothalamic hamartoma. In this case, the lesion is much smaller and is totally intraventricular (III ventricle). There is attachment to the mamillary body on the left.

the best for screening purposes. The most important differential diagnosis includes glioma. The absence of growth is a critical imaging feature that differentiates both lesions.

The history of hypothalamic hamartoma and its treatment is a fascinating one in terms of the origin of seizures. Neurosurgical intervention often resulted in poor outcome. Led by nonfocal or false lateralizing EEG findings, the possibility of occult cerebral dysgenesis, and the high morbidity of traditional neurosurgical treatment of hypothalamic

hamartomas, physicians were reluctant to intervene. These factors, plus unsuccessful cortical resections and corpus callosotomy, in fact, discourage surgical treatment. However, evidence to support the intuitive concept that gelastic seizures and other seizure types arise in hypothalamic hamartomas has led to surgical or radiosurgical treatments now being used to remove, injure, or disconnect hypothalamic hamartomas in patients with intractable epilepsy, with excellent results.

INFECTIOUS/INFLAMMATORY CONDITIONS

Infectious and postinfectious disorders are common antecedents in patients with epilepsy. However, the underlying injury after these conditions is either focal (abscess) or widespread in nature. We will first address one particular condition, possibly postinfectious and immune-related, predominantly unilateral hemispheric, and associated with intractable epilepsy. Abscess and other infectious disorders are described later on in this chapter.

Rasmussen's Encephalitis

One of the most devastating unilateral epileptic conditions is the syndrome of chronic encephalitis of Rasmussen (65–67). This syndrome, first described in 1958, is characterized by a slowly progressive neurologic hemisyndrome and severe focal seizures. The syndrome, which occurs worldwide, has now been reported in the literature in more than 300 patients.

Clinical Features

The clinical features consist of early-onset partial seizures which usually start after the age of 1 and before the age of 14. Some 85% of patients develop seizures before the age of 10 years. Perinatal and postnatal courses are usually normal in these patients.

Up to 50% of patients report a history of an infectious or inflammatory episode before the onset of the syndrome. This has been reported to occur 1–6 months prior to the onset of epilepsia partialis continua. The illness is usually reported to be a nonspecific upper respiratory infection. Some patients have had measles encephalitis prior to the chronic illness. Although focal motor seizures are the main epileptic semiology in this syndrome, up to 30% of patients present with generalized tonic–clonic convulsions. Up to 25% of patients develop simple partial seizures and another 25% may develop complex partial seizures. Interestingly, up to 20% of patients may present with status epilepticus as the first manifestation of their epilepsy (68).

The main seizure type is partial motor seizures. These occur in 75% of patients and tend to persist throughout the clinical course. They tend to involve exclusively one side of the body, in particular the arm and, less frequently, the leg and face. Focal seizures with secondary generalization may occur in up to 40% of patients. Complex partial seizures with motionlessness, followed by motor involvement of the side of the body, are also seen in some patients. The frequency of seizures in this condition is great. Patients without epilepsia partialis continua have frequent attacks with more than one focal motor seizure per hour. Epilepsia partialis continua is one of the most common clinical seizure patterns in this condition and is reported in up to 60% of

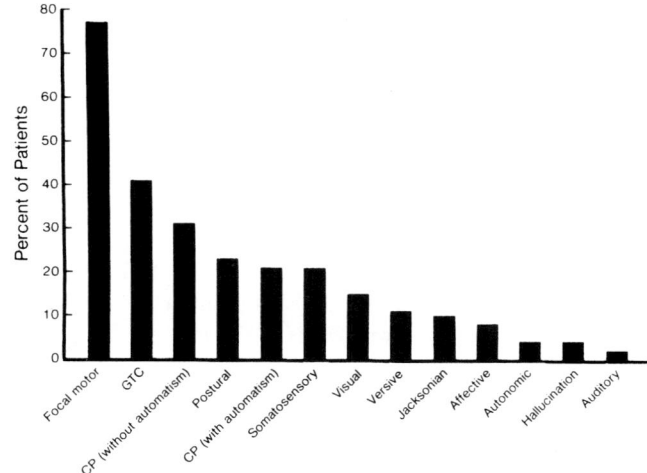

FIG. 6.14 Clinical seizure types and relative frequency among patients with Rasmussen's encephalitis. (With permission from Andermann 1991.[68])

patients. Generalized convulsive status epilepticus is seen in up to 20%. Figure 6.14 demonstrates the relative frequency of each seizure pattern in a population of patients with Rasmussen's encephalitis.

The clinical course in this condition is relentless and progressive deterioration in most patients. Seizure frequency and severity appears to increase with time but this is variable. Hemiparesis gradually becomes apparent 3 months to 10 years after the onset of the epilepsy. This is the case in most individuals. With time, continuous deterioration and progressive hemiparesis develops until the patient loses almost complete use of his/her limbs, with associated partial visual field defect (Fig. 6.15). In most cases, seizures tend to decrease somewhat in the late part of the illness. Progressive mental deterioration, dysphasia, and toxicity from medications account for the devastating neurologic sequelae of

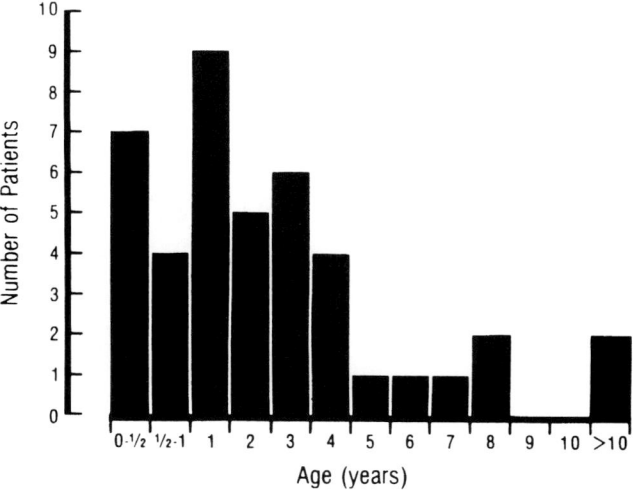

FIG. 6.15 Time from seizure onset to the development of hemiparesis in patient's with Rasmussen's encephalitis (*n* = 42). (With permission from Andermann 1991.[68])

this syndrome. Prior to surgical intervention, all patients have a mild to severe hemiparesis with more than 80% also developing cognitive deterioration, visual field changes, dysphasia, and other behavioral problems (69–71).

Electroencephalographic Findings

Electrographic investigations usually reveal the presence of abnormal background activity with asymmetric slow wave activity in almost 90% of patients. Polymorphic delta activity and a combination of polymorphic delta and intermittent bilateral rhythmic delta activity is seen in all patients. Interictal epileptiform discharges are recorded in most patients and consist of multiple independent foci, usually lateralized to one hemisphere. However, bilateral, multiple independent discharges may be seen over both hemispheres in up to 30% of patients. If one is able to follow the electrographic changes through the year, one can also observe evidence of progressive deterioration of the EEG background activity with also the appearance of low amplitude activity from the damaged hemisphere. These changes are the direct result of the continuous and relentless burn-out phenomenon that occurs in these patients (72).

Neuropathologic Aspects

Chronic encephalitis, which is the hallmark of this condition, refers to a persistent inflammatory response of the brain to an unknown pathologic factor. The pathologic features of chronic encephalitis are well known. In the acute phase of the disease, chronic encephalitis is characterized by the presence of microglial nodules with neuronophagia and perivascular chronic inflammation (Fig. 6.16). The microglial nodules tend to be found near the perivascular cuffs with small lymphocytes and monocytes (65, 73–79). Spongiosis is mostly observed in association with inflammatory changes and is variable. These changes are primarily

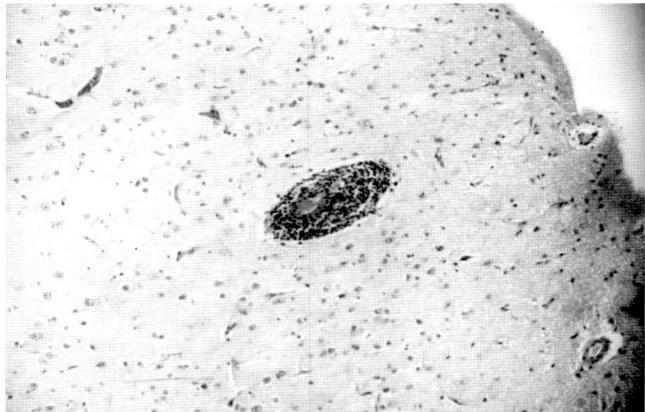

FIG. 6.16 Chronic Rasmussen's encephalitis. Intensive lymphomonocytic perivascular chronic inflammation in a patient with a 2-year history of Rasmussen's (hematoxylin and eosin stain ×100).

seen in the cortical mantle and the white matter appears to be involved very seldom. Within the cortex, multifocal neuronal loss is frequently seen and predominates on the superficial and intermediate cortex. There are usually abundant, bizarre, hypertrophic astrocytes and areas of collapse merge with cavities with large amounts of perivascular lymphocytes. In a few patients, granulomatous inflammatory changes and absence of microglial nodules in neuronophagia have been reported.

Although the morphologic substrate of chronic encephalitis is in itself nonspecific, the distribution, spread, and evolution of the inflammatory changes are quite definitive and specific for Rasmussen's encephalitis. As pointed out by Robitaille et al., this disorder is predominantly a cortical disease with unpredictable patchy regional distribution and it is overwhelming unilateral in the cerebral hemispheres without involvement of the cerebellar structures (65, 73).

Although the histologic features are very similar to an inflammatory postviral disorder, viral inclusions are not observed. In addition, immunocytochemical studies using multiple viral antigens have yielded negative results. Although a recent report using in-situ hybridization reported a correlation between chronic encephalitis and cytomegalovirus (80), this has not been confirmed at other laboratories (50). More recent studies by McNamara have suggested that high titers of antibodies against glutamate receptors (GluR) give rise to an autoimmune hypothesis for Rasmussen's encephalitis. It has been proposed that, in some of these patients, circulating antibodies reach the brain to interact with subunit 3 of [alpha]-amino-3-hydroxy-5-methyl-4-isoxazole propionic acid glutamate receptors (GluR3). This is supported by the finding that some of the rabbits immunized with synthetic fragments of the extracellular portion of GluR3 developed recurrent seizures and neuropathologic alterations similar to those observed in patients with Rasmussen's encephalitis. However, the possibility that other autoantibodies might be involved cannot be ruled out. It is also possible that anti-GluR3 antibody generation is only the epiphenomenon of a more complex and intriguing disease process, and this must be investigated by determining whether these antibodies are also present in other autoimmune or viral diseases, or in patients with other types of severe drug-resistant epilepsy (81).

Imaging Studies

Imaging studies have been carried out in patients with chronic encephalitis since the 1940s. Skull radiography and pneumoencephalography reveal the presence of unilateral atrophy and progressive atrophy with increased ventricular size in patients with this condition. With pneumoencephalography, gradual and progressive unilateral cerebral atrophy can be recorded (65).

With the advent of CT scan, hemiatrophy could be observed directly (77, 82, 83). In most cases, the process of

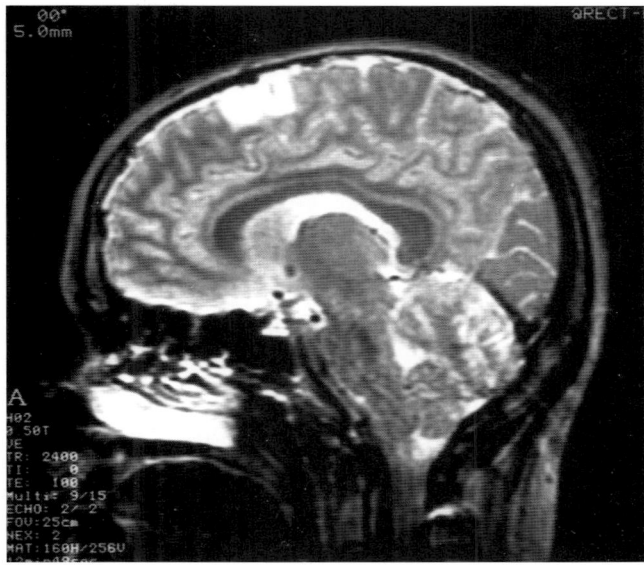

A

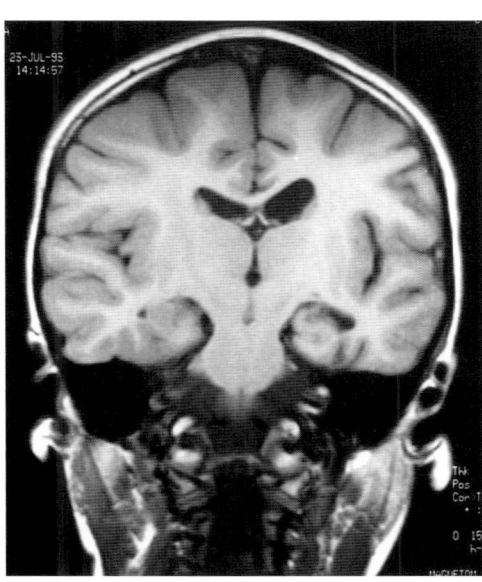

B

FIG. 6.17 Early Rasmussen's encephalitis. **A.** Sagittal spin-echo 2400–100 image showing high-intensity signal from the premotor frontal region in a patient with a 6-month history of focal motor seizures. **B.** Coronal T1 image demonstrating minimal left hemispheric atrophy involving cortical, as well as subcortical white matter in another patient with Rasmussen's. Note involvement of the temporal and lateral horns. In addition, the hippocampus in the affected hemisphere is atrophic.

atrophy begins in the temporal insular region and causes enlargement of the temporal horn and sylvian fissure. With the advent of MRI, better resolution and anatomic definition of this condition can be achieved. MRI is more sensitive than CT in detecting early changes (82–90). MRI examinations early in the condition may demonstrate high-intensity signals from the cortex or minimal cortical atrophy (Fig. 6.17). This is related to gliosis and inflammation. With progression of the illness, hemiatrophy and increased T2 signal are

observed from the cortical regions. The temporal horn can be enlarged, usually unilaterally, and progressive changes can be seen in the affected hemisphere.

The hallmarks of the MRI findings in this condition are, however, the presence of progressive unilateral changes similar to those seen with pneumoencephalography (Fig. 6.18). In the last stages of the condition, massive unilateral ventricular enlargement with frank destruction of the cortical surface is observed (Fig. 6.19). We believe that, in the context of a classical clinical presentation (e.g. a child with epilepsia partialis continua and progressive hemiparesis), and in the presence of unilateral ventricular enlargement with cortical and white matter T2-weighted changes on MRI, a diagnosis of this condition can be made with certainty. In addition, the absence of any other abnormality on MRI, such as a developmental malformation, which may occasionally present with the same symptomatology, confirms the diagnosis.

The use of a phase-mapping MR technique for detection of brain perfusion changes has been described in one patient with epilepsia partialis continua and may be another potentially interesting application of MR technique in this syndrome (92). In addition, MR spectroscopy can unequivocally identify reductions in NAA in the affected hemisphere in a widespread fashion – something not seen in any other epileptic condition. Furthermore, MR spectroscopy can quantify progressive reductions in NAA, which again are the hallmark of this condition (93).

Common Central Nervous System Infections and Epilepsy

Central nervous system (CNS) infections are common and are notable for their diversity (94–98). Seizures in CNS infections are common and may occur in acute, subacute, and chronic meningitis and encephalitis diseases, as well as in patients with infectious occupying lesions. Many of these conditions, however, present with seizures during the acute phase of the illness, whereas chronic seizures, or epilepsy, may not occur in many patients. As with CT scanning, MRI has replaced any other imaging procedure in patients screened for possible CNS infection and inflammation. MRI can detect lesions and complications from infections such as ischemia, infarctions, hemorrhage, or extra-axial fluid collections. In this section we discuss the role of MRI in patients with CNS infections and the potential utility in the investigation of patients with seizures.

Viral Infections

Most viral infections of the CNS involve the meninges, as in aseptic meningitis, or may cause a mild clinical syndrome of meningoencephalitis (99). Viral infections of the CNS have a broad spectrum and range from benign conditions

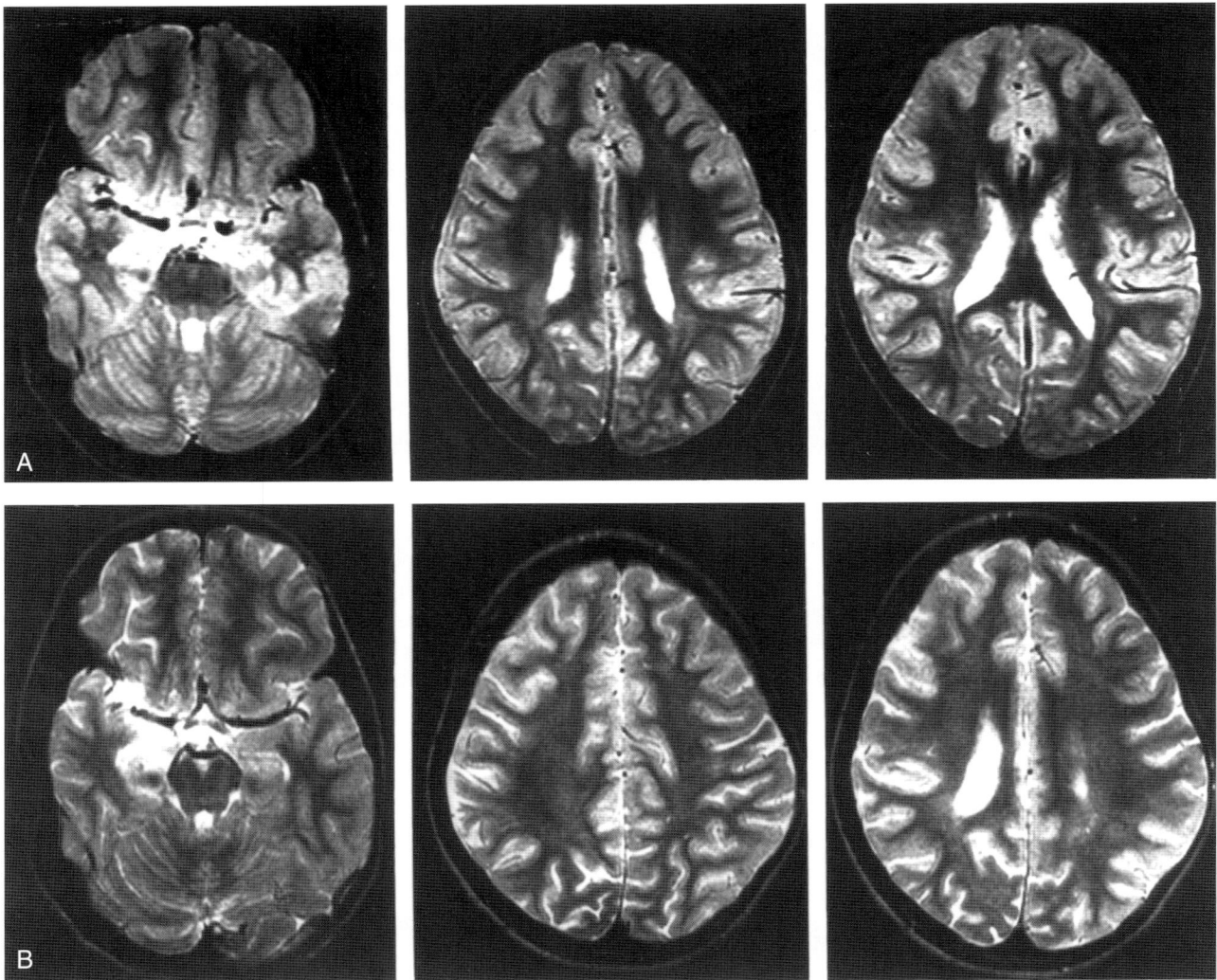

FIG. 6.18 Rasmussen's encephalitis. Axial images through the brain in the same patient – a 4-year-old child with epilepsia partialis continua. Progressive changes were seen over a 16-month period after the onset of seizures. **A.** MR study performed at the onset of epilepsia partialis continua. No abnormalities were noted. Increased signal from the cerebrospinal fluid (CSF) and artifact is noted over the temporal regions. **B.** MRI carried out 6 months after seizure onset demonstrating right temporal horn and right lateral horn enlargement. CSF appears to be a little more prominent over the right hemisphere.

Continued

(aseptic meningitis) to the degenerative diseases of the CNS that are presumed to be of viral origin. It is estimated that the incidence of viral leptomeningitis with infection of the CNS is in the range of 60 000 cases in the United States. The most common causes are herpes simplex virus (HSV) and rabies. In most viral infections the route of access is the hematogenous pathway. The neuronal and the olfactory routes of access are also implicated.

Seizures are common in patients with herpes simplex encephalitis, occurring in approximately 40% of patients in the acute phase (94). The exact mechanism of epileptogenesis is not entirely clear. Some have suggested that HSV produces changes in excitatory neurons while others have reported changes in excitatory neurotransmitter glutamate release following infection.

In general, the pathologic changes with viral encephalitis are those of neuronal degeneration and inflammation. There is often edema and hemorrhages, as well as necrosis, especially with HSV. Pathologic studies in HSV encephalitis reveal inflammation, congestion, and hemorrhages on gross pathology. Microscopically there is capillary congestion and petechiae. Perivascular cuffing becomes prominent in the second and third week of infection. Glial nodules are also common. Necrosis and inflammation with diffuse perivascular mononuclear cell infiltrates become the more typical changes at a later stage. Intranuclear inclusions are also characteristic and may be present in 50% of patients.

Diagnosis of herpes simplex encephalitis includes alteration in cognitive function, abnormal CSF findings, and absence of bacterial or fungal infection and focal abnormalities by either clinical, electrographic, or imaging studies. CSF studies should include polymerase-chain-reaction (PCR) analysis of the cerebrospinal fluid for viral DNA. PCR is positive within 24 hours after the onset of symptoms

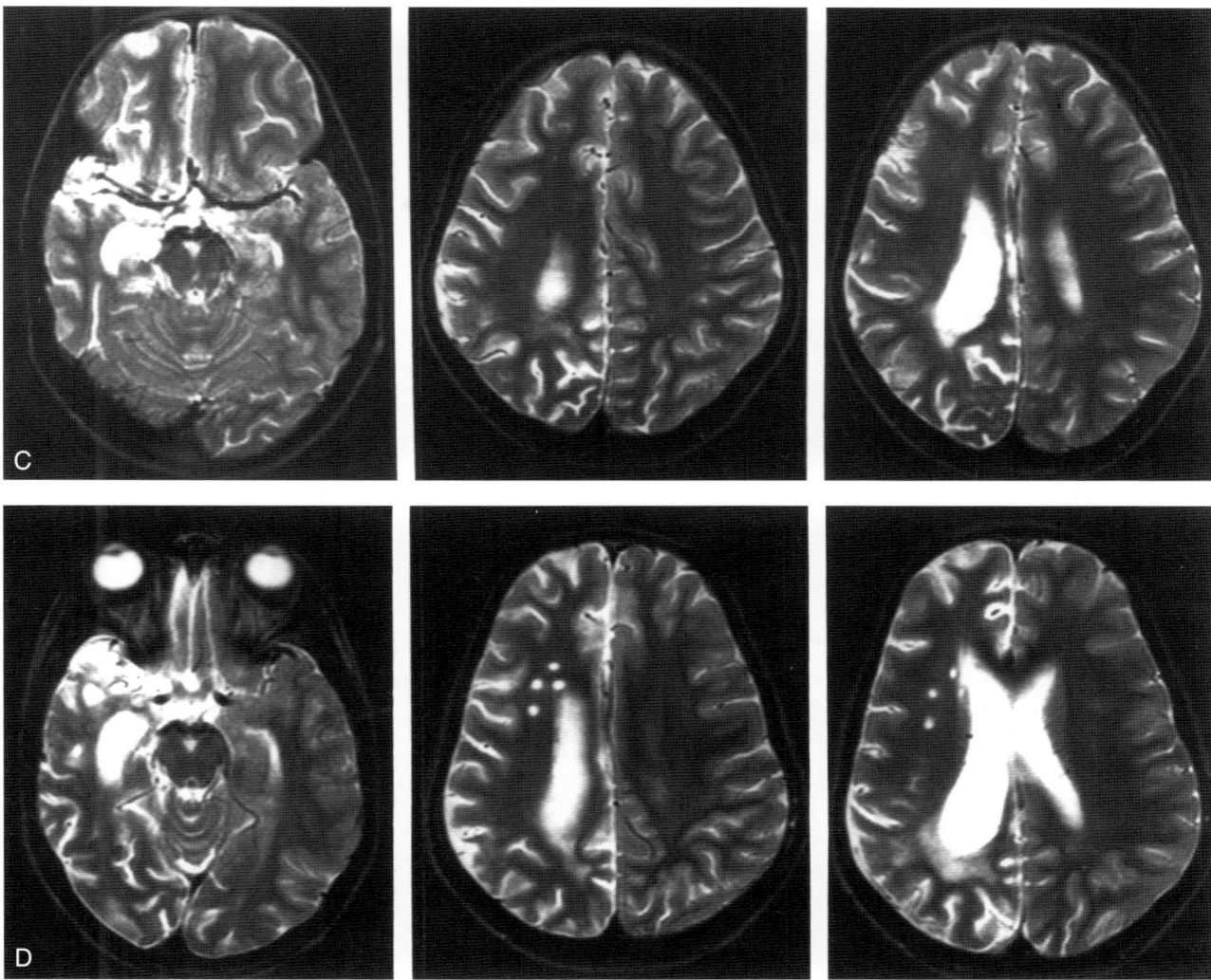

FIG. 6.18 *Cont.* **C.** MR carried out 12 months after the initial symptoms. Note the increased size of the right ventricle. **D.** MRI performed 16 months after the seizure onset. Note increased unilateral ventricular dilatation and white matter changes. The increased signal from the left anterior temporal region is secondary to a biopsy.

and remains positive during the first week of therapy. Comparisons of PCR of the cerebrospinal fluid with biopsy of the brain have revealed that PCR has a sensitivity of 98% and a specificity of 94–100% for detecting HSV DNA. Thus, the diagnostic power of PCR for HSV approximates that of temporal lobe biopsy.

Computed tomography scanning was demonstrated to be useful in the detection of pathology in herpes (100). MRI has been demonstrated to be more sensitive in the detection of early changes in patients with HSV encephalitis than CT (94, 101–103). Studies have demonstrated areas of hyperintensity in the temporal lobes with variable mass effect. Foci of subacute hemorrhage have also been noted and can be detected using spin-echo techniques. Diffusion-weighted MRI can detect early changes in HSV encephalitis but may not be distinct from ischemia. However, the clinical presentation should make the diagnosis possible.

Imaging findings in patients with other types of acute viral infection, including cytomegalovirus, may show subcortical calcifications and hydrocephalus in patients who have acquired the disease in utero. Other forms of viral encephalitis may have nonspecific imaging findings during the acute phase. One of the rare forms is subacute sclerosing panencephalitis caused by measles virus. In this condition, the clinical, EEG, and immunologic investigations make the diagnosis, but MRI has demonstrated periventricular white matter lesions, as well as cortical atrophy in some patients. Lesions are usually bilateral and asymmetric. Other viral illnesses include Creutzfeldt–Jakob disease, acute disseminated encephalomyelitis, and other uncommon viral diseases. Most of these conditions, however, have other neurologic symptoms and signs and chronic epilepsy, per se, does not appear to be an issue of importance in view of all the other neurologic deficits.

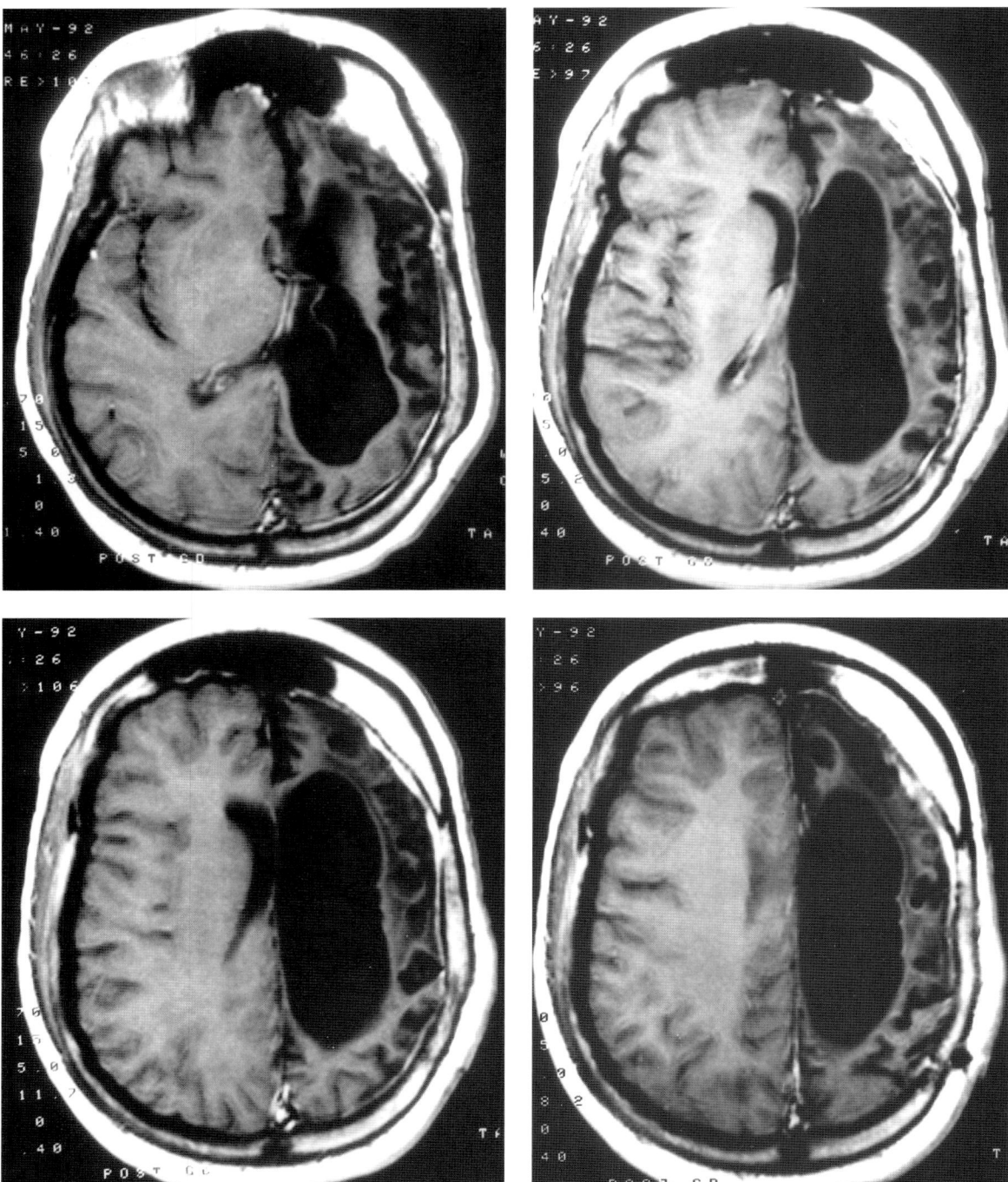

FIG. 6.19 Rasmussen's encephalitis. End-stage disease. Axial MRI 700/15 consecutive images. Note the extensive hemispheric atrophy and frank destruction of cortical and white matter. Massive ventricular dilatation is present. (Courtesy of Dr A. Abou-Khalil, Vanderbilt University, Nashville, TN.)

Bacterial Infections

Bacterial infections of the CNS are common, with approximately 25 000 cases of bacterial meningitis occurring annually in the United States. About 70% of cases occur in children less than 5 years of age with a relative frequency distribution dependent on age (95). Gram-negative bacilli, principally *Escherichia coli* and, less commonly, *Pseudomonas* sp. and group B streptococci, are a major cause of this type of meningitis during the neonatal period. *Haemophilus influenzae* and *Neisseria meningitidis* are the major causes among children beyond the age of 1 month. In adults, meningococci and pneumococci are the most common organisms.

Seizures occur in up to 40% of children with acute bacterial meningitis, usually during the first three days of illness (104, 105) Focal neurologic deficits may also occur and will depend on other related issues. Bacterial infections can produce either abscess formation, which can be pathologically described as a localized, yet poorly demarcated area of parenchymal softening with necrosis and vascular congestion, and perivascular inflammation.

Spin-echo MR images may show early changes as areas of increased signal intensity surrounded by edema (105). On short TI images these areas become isointense or slightly hypointense to normal brain parenchyma. Gadolinium enhancement, in general, is minimum at that stage. When the focus of cerebritis progresses to abscess formation then necrosis will occur in the center of the lesion (Fig. 6.20). At that point, imaging studies will show a well defined lesion that is encircled by a capsule. The center of the lesion is usually localized near the gray–white matter junction in the distribution of the anterior or middle cerebral artery, most commonly in the frontal and parietal lobes. Cerebellar abscesses are less common.

On MR images, the signal intensity from the center of the abscess is usually related to necrosis, with decreased signal compared to the brain parenchyma around it. The capsule, in general, has a higher-intensity signal. The signal intensity from the capsule has been attributed to hemorrhage or collagen, or perhaps to paramagnetic substances related to fibrocytosis from macrophages. Ring enhancement of the abscess occurs with gadolinium. Figure 6.20 demonstrates a bacterial abscess with pre- and postcontrast enhancement.

The detection of postabscess lesions in patients with intractable partial seizures is of great importance. MRI can accurately demonstrate the location and extension of the cavity that usually results after the acute treatment of these conditions. As demonstrated in Figure 6.21, the location of these lesions is variable and may extend with evidence of cortical as well as subcortical destruction. The lesions can be well defined and amenable to surgical resection (Fig. 6.22).

Septic emboli are a possible complication of acute bacterial infections. In general, this complication is more common in intravenous drug abusers, patients with bacterial endocarditis, or young patients with cyanotic congenital heart diseases. In most cases, the septic emboli will result in infarctions that have very similar characteristics on MRI to those seen in patients without infections, especially if they involve major cerebral arteries. Multiple small lesions may be seen in some patients with mycotic aneurysms and tend to be localized to the gray–white matter junction.

Extra-axial lesions, such as subdural or epidural collections, may also occur in patients with CNS bacterial infections. These will not be discussed further because they are usually associated with acute illnesses and usually have little relevance to patients with chronic epilepsy.

Tuberculosis

Tuberculosis of the CNS is not uncommonly associated with seizures (106, 107). The frequency of CNS tuberculosis, especially in other countries than the United States, is significant. In the acute phase, tuberculous meningitis may

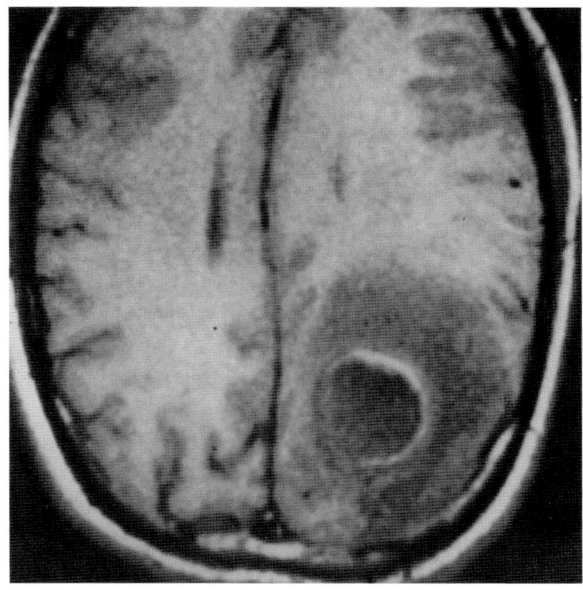

A

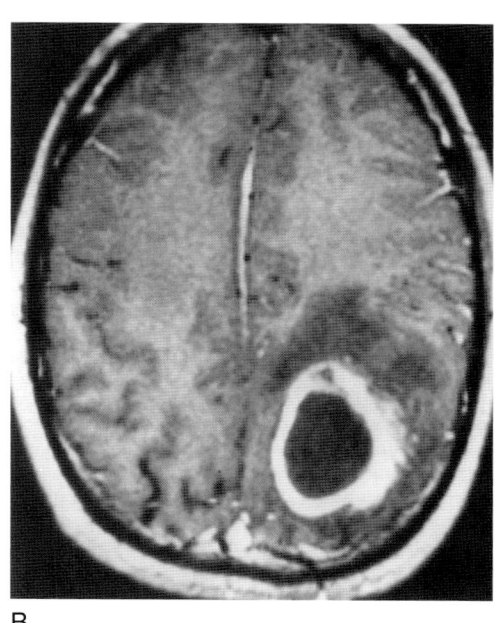

B

FIG. 6.20 Bacterial abscess. **A.** Axial MRI demonstrating a left parietal mass lesion with surrounding edema and mild hyperintense rim and hypointensity. **B.** Postcontrast scan showing marked ring enhancement.

present with seizures in up to 20% of children and 15% of adults. Seizures may correlate with the presence of a focal lesion such as a granuloma or tuberculoma. MRI can demonstrate distention of the subarachnoid space, which can be seen in patients with early tuberculous meningitis. Basilar enhancement with contrast can be seen and is attributed to meningeal inflammation.

Tuberculomas can be located anywhere in the cerebral hemispheres or cerebellum. In addition, there may be subarachnoid, subdural, or epidural involvement. Intraparenchymal granulomas are located at the gray–white matter

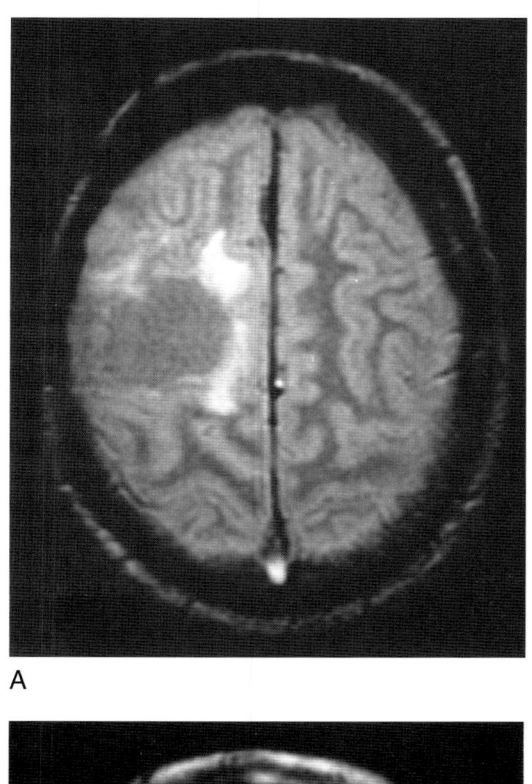

A

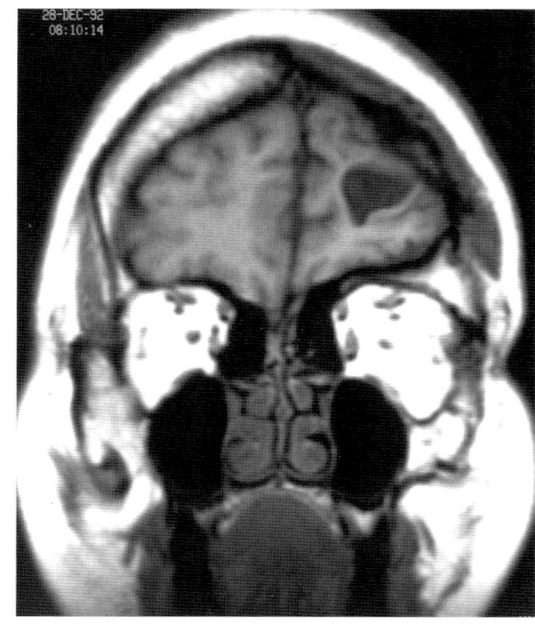

A

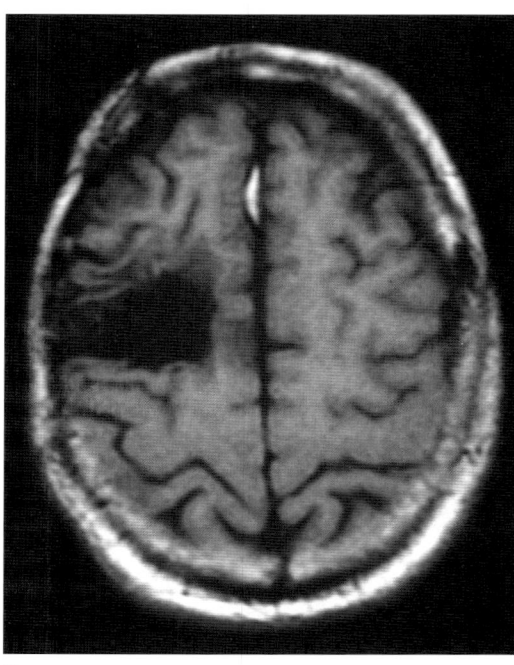

B

FIG. 6.21 Postabscess cavity with extensive gliosis in a patient with intractable partial seizures. **A.** T2-weighted images showing gliosis around the cavity. **B.** T1-weighted axial image showing the cavity following surgical intervention.

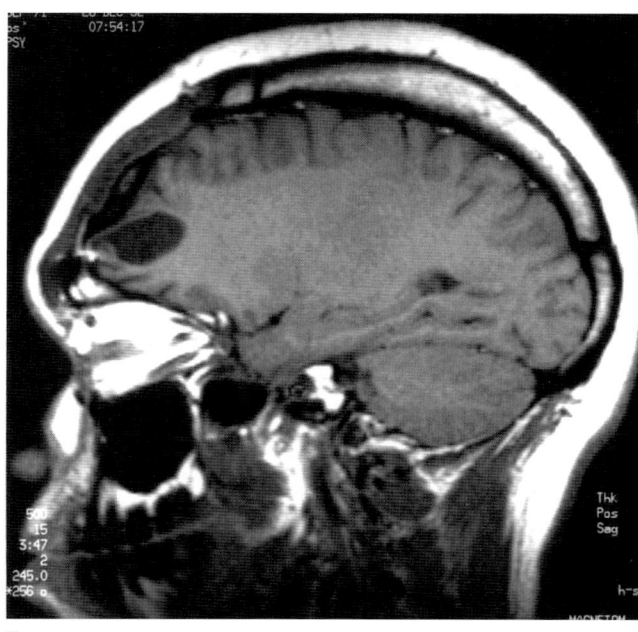

B

FIG. 6.22 Frontal lobe epilepsy. **A**, **B**. MRI images of the residual cavity with smooth walls following dental infection with a secondary brain abscess.

junction, usually in the periventricular regions. Edema is usually minimal when compared with a bacterial abscess. In most cases, tuberculomas have a isointense signal intensity on short T_R images, although signal hyperintensity on long spin-echo sequences may be observed (Fig. 6.23). This may be related to the histologic characteristics of the tuberculoma. In the acute phase, intravenous gadolinium will usually demonstrate intense nodular or ring-like enhancement. Central caseation

necrosis usually is seen as hypointense or isointense on all sequences. Early complications, such as infarctions, may be detected better with MRI. Calcifications, which are uncommon, may be detected with the use of special techniques (108).

Fungal Infections

Fungal infections may present as space-occupying lesions and may include infections such as aspergillosis, mucormycosis, candidiasis, and cryptococcosis. These conditions

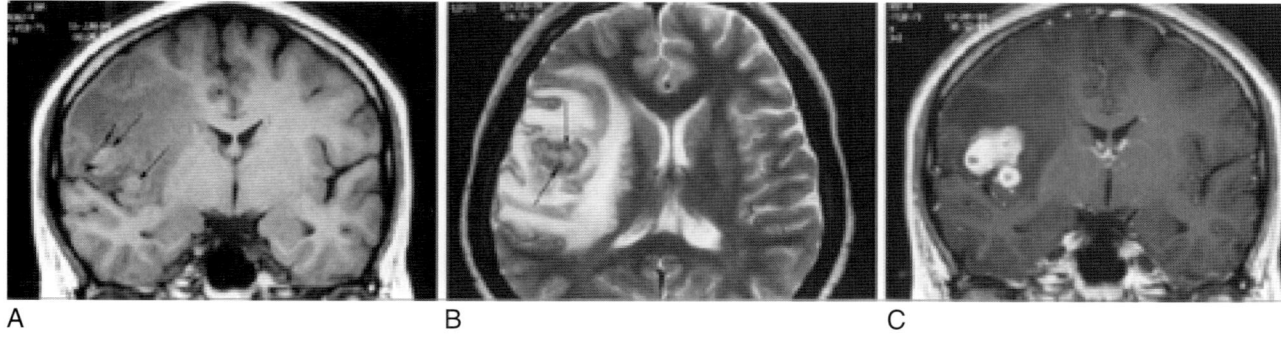

FIG. 6.23 Tuberculoma. **A.** T1-weighted coronal image showing two hyperintense rims relative to gray matter with hypointense rim (short arrow) and central hypointensity in the frontal lobe. **B.** T2-weighted axial image showing heterogeneous intensity with hypointensity foci in the mass with edema. **C.** Gadolinium-enhanced coronal image showing multiple ring enhancement areas with hyperintense/hypointense rims. (With permission from Kim et al. 1995.[123])

are very rare and seldom present with chronic epilepsy without other stigmata of the disease. We will not therefore discuss them.

Parasitic Infections

Toxoplasmosis is a relatively common infection (74, 97, 109). It is usually benign and usually produces lymphadenopathy with or without fever. In immunocompromised patients, however, it can cause diffuse focal encephalitis. The congenital form produces severe brain injury with diffuse focal lesions. Often this will result in focal calcifications in young children. In immunocompromised patients, especially those with AIDS, toxoplasmosis usually presents with multiple lesions. The lesions can be located in the subcortical as well as the cortical regions. A distinctive feature is the absence of a capsule. MRI is more sensitive than CT scanning in detecting the presence of new and old lesions. On long spin-echo techniques, the lesions have variable intensity. They may be hyper-, iso- or hypointense and may be seen as multiple foci. Enhancement with gadolinium produces typical ring or nodular hyperintensity in active lesions.

Most of the *Toxoplasma* lesions are subcortical and, if located in the cerebral hemispheres, are localized to the gray–white matter junction. These lesions are uncommon as the cause of chronic epilepsy and will not be discussed further.

Helminthic Infections

More than 20 species of helminth can invade or involve the CNS. These include cestodes (cysticercosis, coenurosis, cystic hydatid disease, and sparganosis), nematodes (eosinophilic meningitis, trichinosis, strongyloidiasis) and trematodes (schistosomiasis, paragonimiasis). These diseases are common in certain regions and may be an important cause of epilepsy in some countries, especially in Latin America (110–115). In fact, a recent study indicates that cysticercosis is the most common cause of epilepsy in Peru and has been

recognized as the major cause of seizures in endemic areas of Brazil and Mexico (111). When the eggs of *Taenia solium* are ingested by humans, they hatch in the intestine, where the primary larvae are formed. This larva penetrates the intestinal mucosa and then spread through the blood to different systems, including the brain.

Neurocysticercosis develops when the larva develops within the brain. Neurocysticercosis can be localized in the CNS in different regions including the brain parenchyma, meninges, and intraventricular space, and may have more than one location in some patients. The cysticercus is a vesicular larva, usually measuring between 5 and 20 mm in diameter. When the larvae is alive, the cyst formation is clear, but when the larvae dies the cyst becomes turbid and gelatinous.

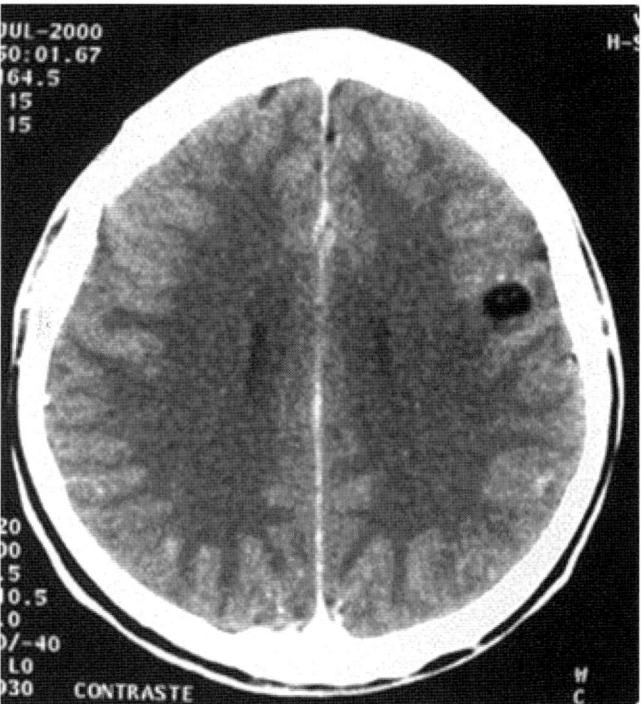

FIG. 6.24 Cysticercosis. CT scan demonstrating a small, low-density cystic lesion in the frontal lobe without edema. This image is typical of a living cysticercus. (With permission from Garcia and Brutto, 2003.[124])

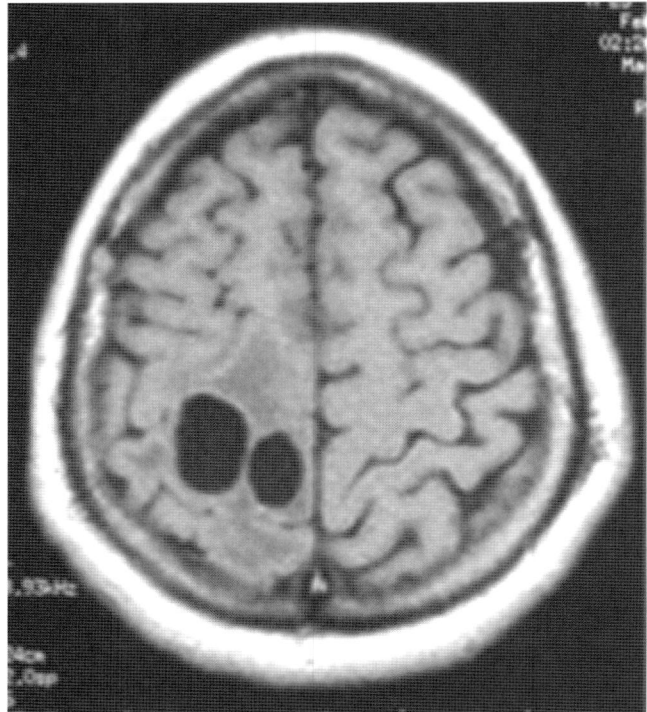

A

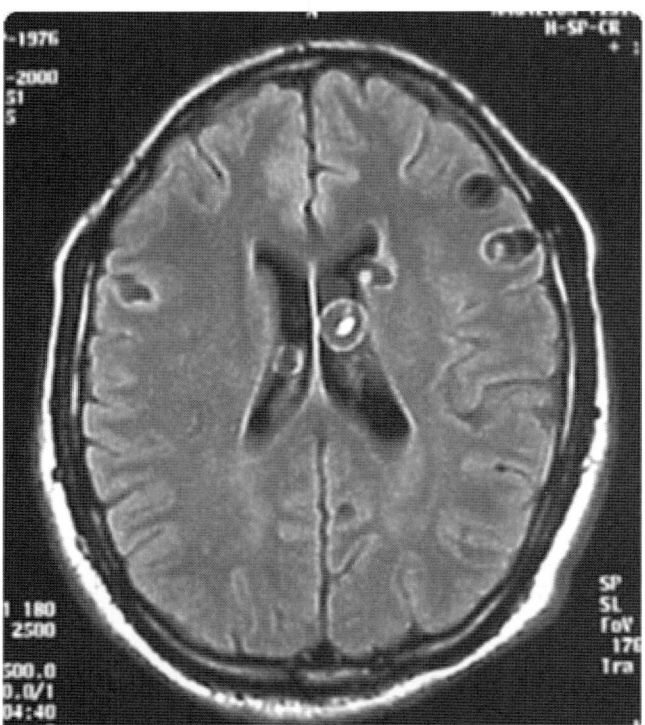

B

FIG. 6.25 A. Cysticercosis. MRI scan without contrast demonstrates a few small, low-density cystic lesions in the frontal lobe with mild edema. **B.** Intraventricular and parenchymal cysticercosis. Fluid-attenuated inversion recovery (FLAIR) images show high-intensity signal from a cyst representing a scolex. (With permission from Garcia and Brutto, 2003.[124])

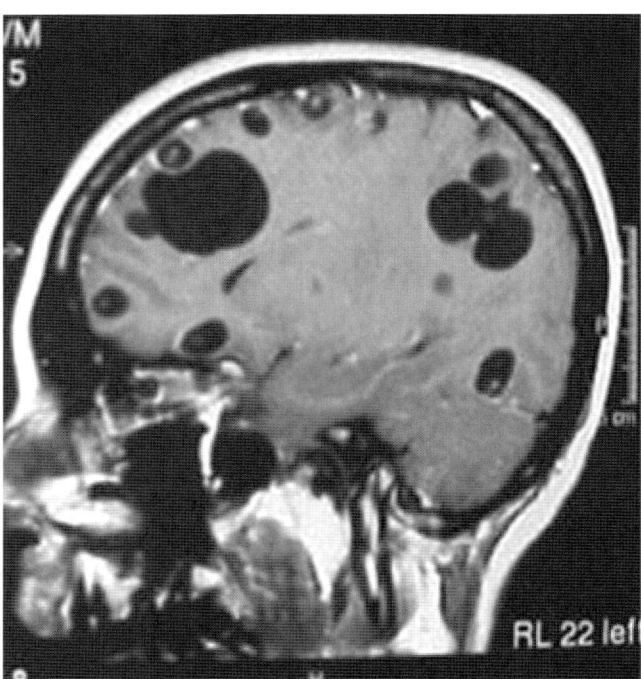

FIG. 6.26. Cysticercosis. T1-weighted with gadolinium. Multiple cysts are observed through the brain with different characteristics. The scolex is visualized in some cysts. (With permission from Garcia and Brutto, 2003.[124])

The location of the lesion is variable. In a recent study, 54% of patients were found to have intraventricular cysts without associated parenchymal cysts. Parenchymal cysts were seen in 69% of patients and usually involved the gray–white matter junction (Fig. 6.24) and could be detected using CT. Fewer than 50% of patients present with parenchyma cysts alone: the rest will have a combination of intraventricular and parenchymal cysts, which can be readily detected with MRI (Fig. 6.25).

Using MRI, the changes due to cyst degeneration become very clear (110, 114, 116–119). With degeneration, the increased signal intensity of the fluid on T1- and proton-density-weighted sequences can be seen. This is related to T1 shortening the effects of increased protein solution. Contrast enhancement with gadolinium has been used but has been found to be only relatively informative. Chang et al. (120) found that enhancement usually occurred in patients in whom the precontrast MRI findings had showed active inflammation secondary to cyst degeneration. In only a minority of cases was there any enhancement in patients who had no degeneration (120) (Fig. 6.26).

Magnetic resonance imaging studies have also been carried out in patients pharmacologically treated for neurocysticercosis (121). Increases in signal intensity and appearance of edema are usually observed as early as 24 hours following treatment. These changes are related to gradual cyst degeneration. Cysts also appear to have a variable response to the drug in their rate of disappearance. MRI with conventional imaging sequences may be less sensitive than CT scan in the detection of calcification in cysticercosis. However, using appropriate sequences, microcalcifications can be detected.

Other helminthic infections, such as echinococcosis, are less common as the cause of chronic intractable epilepsy (122). Echinococcosis may present with large brain cysts that are not associated with edema or ring enhancement. Multiple cysts can occur and usually the presence of these abnormalities on CT or MRI is pathognomonic of this condition.

The remaining infections are extremely rare and will not be discussed further since they do not present a common cause of intractable epilepsy.

SUMMARY

Magnetic resonance imaging is valuable in the study of specific disorders associated with epilepsy. It is important to recognize some of the typical imaging findings in these patients since proper diagnosis will result in adequate treatment. For example, evidence of progressive unilateral MRI hemispheric atrophy in a patient with epilepsia partialis continua and progressive hemiparesis, is almost always associated with Rasmussen's encephalitis. Knowledge of the MRI features may avoid biopsies and other unnecessary diagnostic procedures in these patients.

Vascular injuries and developmental malformations are an important cause of chronic epilepsy. Detection of these lesions is important not only because it may be crucial for surgical intervention but because the surgical outcome may in part be related to the presence of pathology and the extent of viable resection. MRI can provide much of this information in many patients.

Finally, detection of specific pathologic entities is important in patients with seizures and in those with medically intractable epilepsy. Evidence of extensive injury by MRI (atrophy, white matter changes, diffuse encephalomalacia) may be important for surgical planning and for overall outcome. Similarly, as with hypothalamic hamartomas, detecting a lesion should give pause to those attending to patients with epilepsy: the lesion is linked to the epilepsy until proved otherwise.

REFERENCES

1. Aicardi J. Diseases of the nervous system in childhood. London: MacKeith Press, 1992.
2. Barth PG. Prenatal clastic encephalopathies. *Clin Neurol Neurosurg* 1984;86:65–75.
3. Norman RM. Neuropathological findings in acute hemiplegia in childhood. In: Acute hemiplegia in childhood, ed. R. Mitchell. London: Heinemann, 1962.
4. Friede RL. Developmental neuropathology. Heidelberg: Springer-Verlag, 1989.
5. Berg RA, Aleck KA, Kaplan AM. Familial porencephaly. *Arch Neurol* 1983;40:567–569.
6. Pasternak JF, Mantovani JF, Volpe JJ. Porencephaly from periventricular intracerebral hemorrhage in a premature infant. *Am J Dis Child* 1980;134:673–675.
7. Dykes FD, et al. Intraventricular hemorrhage: a prospective evaluation of etiopathogenesis. *Pediatrics* 1980;66:42–49.
8. Hill A. Ventricular dilation following intraventricular hemorrhage in the premature infant. *Can J Neurol Sci* 1983;10:81–85.
9. Scher MS, et al. Intraventricular hemorrhage in the full-term neonate. *Arch Neurol* 1982;39:769–772.
10. Tarby TJ, Volpe JJ. Intraventricular hemorrhage in the premature infant. *Pediatr Clin North Am* 1982;29:1077–1104.
11. Allan WC, Volpe JJ. Periventricular-intraventricular hemorrhage. *Pediatr Clin North Am* 1986;36:47–63.
12. Dekaban A. Large defects in cerebral hemispheres associated with cortical dysgenesis. *J Neuropathol Exp Neurol* 1965;24:512–530.
13. Norman RM, Urich H, Woods GE. The relationship between prenatal porencephaly and the encephalomalacias of early life. *J Ment Sci* 1958;104:758–771.
14. Bordarier C, Robain O, Ponsot G. Bilateral porencephalic defect in the newborn after injection of Benzol during pregnancy. *Brain Dev* 1991;13:126–129.
15. Barkovich A, et al. Normal maturation of the neonatal and infant brain: MR imaging at 1.5T. *Radiology* 1988;166:173–180.
16. Barkovich AJ, Gressens P, Evrard P. Formation, maturation, and disorders of brain neocortex. *Am J Neuroradiol* 1992;13:423–446.
17. Barmada MD, Moossy J, Shuman RM. Cerebral infarcts with arterial occlusion in neonates. *Ann Neurol* 1979;6:495–502.
18. Goddard-Finegold J. Periventricular, intraventricular hemorrhages in the premature newborn. Update on pathologic features, pathogenesis, and possible means of prevention. *Arch Neurol* 1984;41:766–771.
19. Hill A, Rozdilsky B. Congenital hydrocephalus secondary to intra-uterine germinal matrix/intraventricular hemorrhage. *Dev Med Child Neurol* 1984;26:524–527.
20. De Reuck J, Chattha AS, Richardson EP. Pathogenesis and evolution of periventricular leukomalacia in infancy. *Arch Neurol* 1972;27:229–236.
21. Dubowitz LMS, Bydder GM, Mushin J. Developmental sequence of periventricular leukomalacia. Correlation of ultrasound, clinical, and nuclear magnetic resonance functions. *Arch Dis Child* 1985;60:349–355.
22. Grunnet MD. Periventricular leukomalacia complex. *Arch Pathol Lab Med* 1979;103:6–10.
23. Leviton A, Gilles FH. Acquired perinatal leukoencephalopathy. *Ann Neurol* 1984;16:1–8.
24. Kuzniecky RI, Knowlton RC. Neuroimaging of epilepsy. *Semin Neurol* 2002;22:279–88.
25. Bresler J. Klinische und pathologisch-anatomische Beitrage zur Mikrogyrie. *Arch Psychiatr Nervenkr* 1899;31:566–573.
26. Norman MG. On the morphogenesis of ulegyria. *Acta Neuropathol* 1981;53:331–332.
27. Myers RE. Atrophic cortical sclerosis associated with status marmoratus in a perinatally damaged monkey. *Neurology* 1969;19:1177–1188.
28. Norman RM. Atrophic sclerosis of the cerebral cortex associated with birth injury. *Arch Dis Child* 1944;19:111–121.
29. Kotila M, Waltimo O. Epilepsy after stroke. *Epilepsia* 1992;33:495–498.
30. Olsen TS, Hogenhaven H, Thage O. Epilepsy after stroke. *Neurology* 1987;37:1209–1211.
31. Shinton RA, et al. The frequency of epilepsy preceding stroke: case controlled study in 230 cases. *Lancet* 1987;1:11–12.
32. Gupta SR. Postinfarction seizures. A clinical study. *Stroke* 1988;19:1477–1481.
33. Cocito L, Favale E, Reni L. Epileptic seizures in cerebral arterial occlusive disease. *Stroke* 1982;13:185–195.
34. Louis S, McDowell F. Epileptic seizures in nonembolic cerebral infarction. *Arch Neurol* 1967;17:414–418.

35. Faught E, Peters D. Seizures in intracerebral haemorrhages. *Epilepsia* 1984;25:666.

36. Berger AR, Lipton RB, Lesser ML. Early seizures following intracerebral hemorrhage: implications for therapy. *Neurology* 1988; 38:1363–1365.

37. Cocito L, et al. Epileptic seizures heralding intracerebral hemorrhage. *Stroke* 1994;25:2292–2293.

38. Fish DR, et al. The natural history of late-onset epilepsy secondary to vascular disease. *Acta Neurol Scand* 1989;80:524–526.

39. Lancman ME, et al. Risk factors for developing seizures after a stroke. *Epilepsia* 1993;34:141–143.

40. Kilpatrick CJ, et al. Epileptic seizures in acute stroke. *Arch Neurol* 1990;47:157–160.

41. Luhdorf F, Jensen LK, Plesner A. Etiology of seizures in the elderly. *Epilepsia* 1986;27:458–463.

42. Sturge WA. A case of partial epilepsy apparently due to a lesion of one of the vaso-motor centers of the brain. *Trans Clin Soc Lond* 1879;12:162–167.

43. Aicardi J. Epilepsy in children. New York: Raven Press, 1986.

44. Miranda Mallea J, et al. [Sturge–Weber syndrome: experience with 14 cases]. *An Esp Pediatr* 1997;46:138–142.

45. Adamsbaum C, et al. Accelerated myelination in early Sturge–Weber syndrome: MRI-SPECT correlations. *Pediatr Radiol* 1996;26:759–762.

46. Chamberlain MC, Press GA, Hesselink JR. MR imaging and CT in three cases of Sturge–Weber syndrome: prospective comparison. *Am J Neuroradiol* 1989;10:491–496.

47. Wasenko J, et al. The Sturge–Weber syndrome: comparison of MR and CT characteristics. *Am J Neuroradiol* 1989;11:131–134.

48. Maria BL, et al. High prevalence of bihemispheric structural and functional defects in Sturge–Weber syndrome. *J Child Neurol* 1998;13:595–605.

49. Elster A, Chen M. MRI of Sturge–Weber syndrome: role of GD-DTPA and gradient-echo techniques. *Am J Neuroradiol* 1990;11:685–689.

50. Boggs JG, et al. Frequency of potentially ictal patterns in comatose ICU patients. *Epilepsia* 1994;35:135.

51. Cascino GD, et al. Gelastic seizures and hypothalamic hamartomas: evaluation of patients undergoing chronic intracranial EEG monitoring and outcome of surgical treatment. *Neurology* 1993;43:747–750.

52. Gaggero R, et al. [Epilepsy with laughing seizures, hypothalamic hamartoma and precocious puberty. Contributions of MRI, computed EEG topography (CET) and ambulatory EEG (A-EEG)]. *Minerva Pediatr* 1991;43:801–810.

53. Deonna T, Ziegler AL. Hypothalamic hamartoma, precocious puberty and gelastic seizures: a special model of 'epileptic' developmental disorder. *Epileptic Disord* 2000;2:33–37.

54. Debeneix C, et al. Hypothalamic hamartoma: comparison of clinical presentation and magnetic resonance images. *Horm Res* 2001;56: 12–18.

55. Kuzniecky R, et al. Intrinsic epileptogenesis of hypothalamic hamartoma and gelastic epilepsy. *Ann Neurol* 1997;44:60–67.

56. Valdueza JM, et al. Hypothalamic hamartomas: with special reference to gelastic epilepsy and surgery. *Neurosurgery* 1994;34:949–958.

57. Striano S, et al. Gelastic epilepsy: symptomatic and cryptogenic cases. *Epilepsia* 1999;40:294–302.

58. Striano S, et al. Small hypothalamic hamartomas and gelastic seizures. *Epileptic Disord* 2002;4:129–133.

59. Boyko OB, et al. Hamartomas of the tuber cinereum: CT, MR, and pathologic findings. *Am J Neuroradiol* 1991;12:309–314.

60. Arita K, et al. The relationship between magnetic resonance imaging findings and clinical manifestations of hypothalamic hamartoma. *J Neurosurg* 1999;91:212–220.

61. Boyko O, et al. Hamartomas of the tuber cinereum: CT, MR, and pathologic findings. *Am J Neuroradiol* 1991;12:309–314.

62. Kuzniecky R, et al. Intrinsic epileptogenesis of hypothalamic hamartomas in gelastic epilepsy. *Ann Neurol* 1997;42:60–67.

63. Meiners LC, et al. MR contribution in surgery of epilepsy. *Eur Radiol* 1999;9:493–507.

64. Valdueza J, et al. Hypothalamic hamartomas: with special reference to gelastic epilepsy and surgery. *Neurosurgery* 1994;34:949–958.

65. Rasmussen T, Olszewski J, Lloyd-Smith D. Focal seizures due to chronic localized encephalitis. *Neurology* 1958;6:435–445.

66. Rasmussen T. Further observations on the syndrome of chronic encephalitis and epilepsy. *Appl Neurophysiol* 1978;41:1–12.

67. Aguilar MJ, Rasmussen T. Role of encephalitis in pathogenesis of epilepsy. *Arch Neurol* 1960;2:663–676.

68. Andermann F, ed. Chronic encephalitis and epilepsy. In: Andermann F, ed. Rasmussen's syndrome. Boston, MA: Butterworth-Heinemann, 1991.

69. Aguilar Rebolledo F, et al. [Rasnmussen syndrome. 7 years' follow-up. Aspects related to cerebral plasticity in epilepsy]. *Rev Invest Clin* 2002;54:209–217.

70. Chinchilla D, et al. Reappraisal of Rasmussen's syndrome with special emphasis on treatment with high doses of steroids. *J Neurol Neurosurg Psychiatry* 1994;57:1325–1333.

71. Farrell MA, et al. Neuropathologic findings in cortical resections (including hemispherectomies) performed for the treatment of intractable childhood epilepsy. *Acta Neuropathol (Berl)* 1992;83: 246–259.

72. So NK, Gloor P. Electroencephalographic and electrocorticographic findings in chronic encephalitis of the Rasmussen type. In: Andermann, F, ed. Chronic encephalitis and epilepsy: Rasmussen's syndrome. Boston, MA: Butterworth-Heinemann, 1991:37–45.

73. Robitaille Y. Neuropathologic aspects of chronic encephalitis. In: Andermann, F, ed. Chronic encephalitis and epilepsy: Rasmussen's syndrome. Boston, MA: Butterworth-Heinemann, 1991:79–110.

74. Thomas WB. Inflammatory diseases of the central nervous system in dogs. *Clin Tech Small Anim Pract* 1998;13:167–78.

75. Velkey I, Lombay B. [Rasmussen syndrome]. *Orv Hetil* 1993;134: 2653–2656.

76. Wainwright MS, et al. Human herpesvirus 6 limbic encephalitis after stem cell transplantation. *Ann Neurol* 2001;50:612–619.

77. McLachlan RS, et al. Rasmussen's chronic encephalitis in adults. *Arch Neurol* 1993;50:269–274.

78. Kalinina LV, et al. [Rasmussen's chronic progressive focal encephalitis]. *Zh Nevropatol Psikhiatr Im S S Korsakova* 1996;96: 21–25.

79. Jay V, et al. Chronic encephalitis and epilepsy (Rasmussen's encephalitis): detection of cytomegalovirus and herpes simplex virus 1 by the polymerase chain reaction and in situ hybridization. *Neurology* 1995;45:108–117.

80. Farrell MA, et al. Cytomegalovirus and Rasmussen's encephalitis. *Lancet* 1991;337:1551–1552.

81. McNamara JO, et al. Evidence for glutamate receptor autoimmunity in the pathogenesis of Rasmussen encephalitis. *Adv Neurol* 1999; 79:543–550.

82. Velkey I, Lombay B. Neuroimaging of Rasmussen's encephalitis. *Pediatr Radiol* 1993;23:487–488.

83. Tien RD, et al. Rasmussen's encephalitis: neuroimaging findings in four patients. *AJR* 1992;158:1329–1332.

84. Yacubian EM, et al. Neuroimaging findings in Rasmussen's syndrome. *J Neuroimaging* 1997;7:16–22.

85. Nakasu S, et al. Serial magnetic resonance imaging findings of Rasmussen's encephalitis–case report. *Neurol Med Chir (Tokyo)* 1997;37:924–928.

86. Ishibashi H, et al. Multimodality functional imaging evaluation in a patient with Rasmussen's encephalitis. *Brain Dev* 2002;24:239–244.

87. Aguilar Rebolledo F, et al. [SPECT-^{99m}Tc-HMPAO in a case of epilepsia partialis continua and focal encephalitis]. *Rev Invest Clin* 1996;48:199–205.

88. Peretti P, et al. Magnetic resonance imaging in partial epilepsy of childhood. Seventy-nine cases. *J Neuroradiol* 1989;16:308–316.

89. Chiapparini L, et al. Diagnostic imaging in 13 cases of Rasmussen's encephalitis: can early MRI suggest the diagnosis? *Neuroradiology* 2003;45:171–183.

90. Granata T, et al. Rasmussen's encephalitis: early characteristics allow diagnosis. *Neurology* 2003;60:422–425.
91. Kuzniecky R, Powers R. Epilepsia partialis continua due to cortical dysplasia. *J Child Neurol* 1993;8:93–96.
92. Fish DR, et al. Use of magnetic resonance imaging to identify changes in cerebral blood flow in epilepsia partialis continua. *Magn Reson Med* 1988;8:238–240.
93. Cendes F, et al. Imaging of axonal damage in vivo in Rasmussen's syndrome. *Brain* 1995;118:753–758.
94. Whitley RJ, Schlitt M. Encephalitis caused by herpesviruses, including B virus. In: Durack DT, ed. Infections of the central nervous system. New York: Raven Press, 1991:41–86.
95. Roos KL, Tunkel AR, Scheld WM. Acute bacterial meningitis in children and adults. In: Durack DT, ed. Infections of the central nervous system. New York: Raven Press, 1991:335–409.
96. Cameron MD, Durack DT. Helminthic infections of the central nervous system. In: Durack DT, ed. Infections of the central nervous system. New York: Raven Press, 1991:825–850.
97. Dukes CS, Luft BJ, Durack DT. Toxoplasmosis of the central nervous system. In: Durack DT, ed. Infections of the central nervous system. New York: Raven Press, 1991:801–815.
98. Nakazaki S, et al. Toxoplasmic encephalitis in patients with acquired immunodeficiency syndrome–four case reports. *Neurol Med Chir (Tokyo)* 2000;40:120–123.
99. Asher DM. Slow viral infections of the human nervous system. In: Durack DT, ed. Infections of the central nervous system. New York: Raven Press, 1991:145–166.
100. Zimmerman RD, et al. CT in the early diagnosis of herpes simplex encephalitis. *AJR* 1980;134:61–66.
101. Tolly TL, Wells RG, Sty JR. MR features of fleeting CNS lesions associated with Epstein–Barr virus infection. *J Comput Assist Tomogr* 1989;13:665–658.
102. Bourgeois M, et al. Reactivation of herpes virus after surgery for epilepsy in a pediatric patient with mesial temporal sclerosis: case report. *Neurosurgery* 1999;44:633–635.
103. Wolf RW, et al. Atypical herpes simplex encephalitis presenting as operculum syndrome. *Pediatr Radiol* 1999;29:191–193.
104. Marks WJ Jr, Garcia PA. Management of seizures and epilepsy. *Am Fam Physician* 1998;57:1589–600:1603–1604.
105. Sempere AP, et al. First seizure in adults: a prospective study from the emergency department. *Acta Neurol Scand* 1992;86:134–138.
106. Farrar DJ, et al. Tuberculous brain abscess in a patient with HIV infection: case report and review. *Am J Med* 1997;102:297–301.
107. Modi G, et al. New onset seizures in HIV-infected patients without intracranial mass lesions or meningitis – a clinical, radiological and SPECT scan study. *J Neurol Sci* 2002;202:29–34.
108. Lorber J. Intracranial calcification following tuberculous meningitis in children. *Acta Radiol* 1958;50:204–210.
109. Horowitz SL, et al. CNS toxoplasmosis in acquired immunodeficiency syndrome. *Arch Neurol* 1983;40:649–652.
110. McCormick GF, Zee C, Heiden J. Cysticercosis cerebri. Review of 127 cases. *Arch Neurol* 1982;39:534–539.
111. Garcia HD, et al. Cysticercosis as a major cause of epilepsy in Peru. *Lancet* 1993;341:197–200.
112. Cardenas JC. Cysticercosis of the nervous system: pathologic and radiologic findings. *J Neurosurg* 1962;19:635–640.
113. Escobar A. The pathology of neurocysticercosis. In: Taveras JM, ed. Cysticercosis of the central nervous system. Springfield, IL: Charles C Thomas, 1983: 27–54.
114. Del Brutto OH. [Neurocysticercosis]. *Rev Neurol* 1999;29:456–466.
115. Carpio A, Escobar A, Hauser WA. Cysticercosis and epilepsy: a critical review. *Epilepsia* 1998;39:1025–1040.
116. Juhl ZK, Logager VB. [Subcutaneous cysticercosis and neurocysticercosis]. *Ugeskr Laeger* 2000;162:6691–6692.
117. Just M, et al. [MR tomography in parenchymatous neurocysticercosis]. *Radiologe* 1987;27:123–126.
118. Puri V, Gupta RK. Magnetic resonance imaging evaluation of focal computed tomography abnormality in epilepsy. *Epilepsia* 1991;32:460–466.
119. Santos IC, et al. Cysticidal therapy: impact on seizure control in epilepsy associated with neurocysticercosis. *Arq Neuropsiquiatr* 2000;58:1014–1020.
120. Chang KH, et al. The role of contrast-enhanced MR imaging in the diagnosis of neurocysticercosis. *Am J Neuroradiol* 1990;157:509–512.
121. Teitelbaum GP, et al. MR imaging of neurocysticercosis. *Am J Neuroradiol* 1989;153:857–866.
122. Gutierrez Y. Cysticercosis, coenurosis and sparganosis. Diagnostic pathology of parasitic infections with clinical correlations. Philadelphia: Lea & Febiger, 1990:432–459.
123. Kim TK, *et al.* Intracranial tuberculoma: comparison of MR with pathologic findings. *Am J Neuroradiol* 1995;16:1903–1908.
124. Garcia HH, Del Brutto O. Imaging findings in neurocysticercosis. *Acta Trop* 2003;87:71–78.

CHAPTER 7

Malformations of Cortical Development

A. James Barkovich

PRINCIPLES OF NORMAL CEREBRAL CORTICAL DEVELOPMENT

The development of the cerebral cortex is an extraordinarily complex process (1). There are many steps that are sequential in nature and necessary for the normal development of the cerebral cortex. In many ways we wonder how is it possible not to have more malformations or misdevelopment, given the many mechanisms and factors involved. The developmental process is summarized in Box 7.1.

The formation of the cortex begins with the appearance of the neural plate at around 18 days of gestation. Two days later, one can distinguish the three major divisions of the brain. Differentiation of the cerebral vesicles occurs at about day 33 of gestation. The hemispheres begin as a single layer of columnar epithelium. Once patterning has been established, one of the most critical processes of cortical development begins in the ventricular zone – proliferation of precursor cells that will eventually populate the cerebral cortex. Box 7.2 depicts the different stages of cortical cell population.

Cerebral cortical development consists of three major processes: cell proliferation, neuronal migration, and cortical organization.

Cell proliferation is the process that takes place in the germinal zones of the developing prosencephalon. Prior to neurogenesis, the pool of progenitor cells is expanded through a series of cell divisions in which both daughter cells re-enter the cell cycle as progenitors. Eventually, under the influence of signals that are not yet known, asymmetric division begins and gradually increases in proportion to symmetric division; neuroblasts (predominantly) and glial precursors are generated.

Neuronal migration requires the migrating neuroblasts to attach to radial glial cells that span the developing hemisphere from the germinal zone to the pia, migrate along the radial glial cells, and detach when they reach the proper layer of the developing cerebral cortex.

A number of proteins have been identified that play important roles in these steps, including filamin 1, which encodes an actin cross-linking phosphoprotein, which transduces ligand–receptor interactions on the cell surface to actin reorganization in the cytoskeleton. Such actin cross-linking plays an essential role in the locomotion of many cell types, such as migrating neurons. Without actin cross-linking, the growth cones of migrating neuroblasts cannot be extended along radial glia cells and neuronal migration cannot be initiated (2, 3).

BOX 7.1. Development of the Cerebral Cortex

- A stepwise process
- Some steps are sequential, some simultaneous
- Specific genes regulate specific steps
- Genes act cell-autonomously or as extrinsic signals

BOX 7.2. Different Stages of Cortical Cell Populations

- Specification of neural epithelium
- Patterning
- Proliferation
- Identity
- Migration-axon outgrowth, transmitter type
- Differentiation
- Adult function

The *LIS1* and doublecortin (*DCX*, *XLIS*) genes produce proteins that are postulated to have a role in the migration of the neuroblast along the radial glial cell. Depending on the gene and the type of mutation, the result may be pachygyria, lissencephaly, or band heterotopia (3). The topography of the malformation differs depending upon the affected gene (4), suggesting that the gene products differ either in function or location. Two other molecules, neureglin and astrotactin, have been identified as regulating the interactions between the migrating neuroblasts and the radial glial cells (5) in animal models. The effects of their mutations in humans have not been identified. Termination of neuroblast migration has been linked to the extracellular protein reelin and the cytoplasmic protein Mdab1, which is believed to transduce signals generated by putative reelin receptors ApoEr2 and VLDLr.

The mechanisms of cell migration and formation of the cortex are important in the conceptualization of the changes occurring during migration. The first wave of cells create an intermediate zone. Thereafter, these cells migrate further into the marginal zone to form the preplate. The second wave is a large one and begins in the 10–11th week. These waves end by the 16th week, when most cells have migrated. These cells form the vast majority of layers 2–6 of the cortex. Radial and non-radial migration takes place during this stage. By week 22, distinctive layers can be visualized (Fig. 7.1).

The molecular mechanisms involved in *cortical organization* are those of neurite extension, synaptogenesis, and neuronal maturation. The molecular mechanisms of these steps are slowly being elucidated.

As the separation of cortical development into stages of proliferation, migration and cortical organization forms a conceptual framework for genetic study (6) and pathologic analysis of cortical malformations, it seems logical to use this method as the primary feature by which to classify malformations based on neuroimaging features. Secondary features, based on topology, characteristics of white matter, known associated histologic characteristics, or associated cerebellar malformations, can then be used for further classification into more distinct categories. The classification is based on the stages of proliferation, migration, and organization (Box 7.3).

IMAGING OF MALFORMATIONS OF CEREBRAL CORTICAL DEVELOPMENT

Introduction

Malformations of cerebral cortical development are being discovered with increasingly greater frequency on imaging examinations of children with developmental delay and patients with epilepsy. Several studies have now shown that malformations of cortical development are the cause of 23–26% of intractable epilepsies in children and young adults (1, 2, 3–5), indicating that cortical malformations must be ruled out in essentially every pediatric patient with developmental delay or epilepsy. In addition, the fact that many malformations of cortical development are caused by chromosomal mutations (6–9) emphasizes the importance of counseling of parents of affected children.

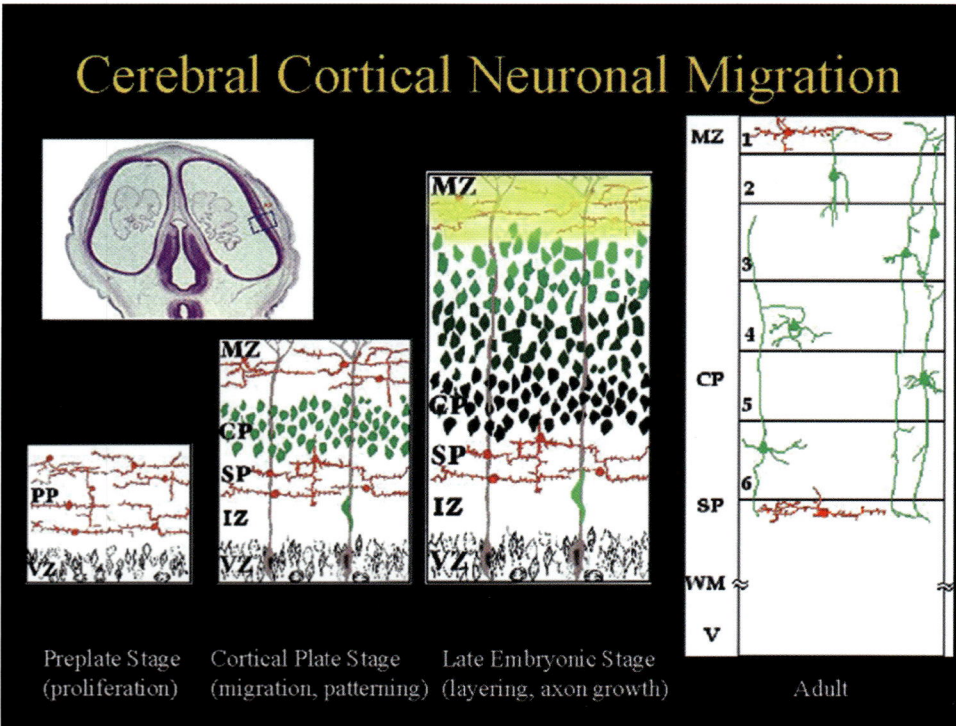

FIG. 7.1. Representation of the cellular stages of the cerebral cortex during development. (Courtesy of Dr C. Walsh, Boston, MA.)

BOX 7.3. Classification Scheme for Cortical Malformations

I. Malformations due to abnormal neuronal and glial proliferation or apoptosis
  A. Decreased proliferation/increased apoptosis – microcephalies
    1. Microcephaly with normal to thin cortex
    2. Microlissencephaly (extreme microcephaly with thick cortex)
    3. Microcephaly with polymicrogyria/cortical dysplasia
  B. Increased proliferation/decreased apoptosis (normal cell types) – megalencephalies
  C. Abnormal proliferation (abnormal cell types)
    1. Non-neoplastic
      a. Tuberous sclerosis
      b. Cortical dysplasia with balloon cells
      c. Hemimegalencephaly (HMEG)
    2. Neoplastic (associated with disordered cortex)
      a. DNET (dysembryoplastic neuroepithelial tumor)
      b. Ganglioglioma
      c. Gangliocytoma
II. Malformations due to abnormal neuronal migration
  A. Lissencephaly/subcortical band heterotopia spectrum
  B. Cobblestone complex
    1. Congenital muscular dystrophy syndromes
    2. Syndromes with no involvment of muscle
  C. Heterotopia
    1. Subependymal (periventricular)
    2. Subcortical (other than band heterotopia)
    3. Marginal glioneural
III. Malformations due to abnormal cortical organization (including late neuronal migration)
  A. Polymicrogyria and schizencephaly
    1. Bilateral polymicrogyria syndromes
    2. Schizencephaly (polymicrogyria with clefts)
    3. Polymicrogyria with other brain malformations or abnormalities
    4. Polymicrogyria or schizencephaly as part of multiple congenital anomaly/mental retardation syndromes
  B. Cortical dysplasia without balloon cells
  C. Microdysgenesis
IV. Malformations of cortical development, not otherwise classified
  A. Malformations secondary to inborn errors of metabolism
    1. Mitochondrial and pyruvate metabolic disorders
    2. Peroxisomal disorders
  B. Other unclassified malformations
    1. Sublobar dysplasia
    2. Others

As malformations of cortical development generally cause neocortical epilepsy, this chapter will start with a general discussion of imaging techniques in the assessment of patients with neocortical epilepsy. A discussion of specific malformations and their imaging characteristics will follow. As this title focuses on epilepsy, the chapter will omit discussion of complex syndromes that have cortical malformations as a component and focus on the malformations themselves.

Imaging Techniques

Proper imaging technique and a high index of suspicion are crucial for the identification of cortical malformations. MR is the initial imaging study of choice, as its high contrast resolution allows a much better analysis of the cerebral cortex than any other neuroimaging technique. Computed tomography (CT) misses cortical malformations in more than 30% of affected patients (10). If a cortical malformation is suspected to be the cause of epilepsy, the MR protocol should include:

- T1-weighted volumetric 3DFT spoiled gradient-echo sequences using 1.0 or 1.5 mm partition size (and reformatting in three orthogonal planes (11)) and
- T2-weighted 3DFSE volumetric acquisition (using 1.5 mm partition size and multiplanar reformation) or 2–3 mm spin-echo or fast spin-echo sequences in two planes (usually axial and coronal).

As subtle white matter abnormalities may give important clues to the presence of the cortical malformation (especially in focal balloon cell dysplasias), it is important to obtain a proton-density-weighted or a fluid-attenuated inversion recovery (FLAIR) sequence. These sequences, obtained using a standard quadrature head coil, are adequate in the vast majority of patients with macroscopic malformations of cortical development. If the malformation is small or subtle, imaging of the cortex using phased array surface coils dramatically improves the sensitivity of MR imaging, as it allows very high-resolution images to be obtained while maintaining high signal-to-noise (12). Advanced quantification techniques are discussed in Chapter 8.

Other MR techniques may be useful occasionally. Some evidence has been presented that proton MR spectroscopic imaging may be useful in localization of epileptogenic foci (13–15), although this technique is still at an early stage of development. Woermann *et al.* have shown abnormal metabolite levels in nearly 90% of patients with malformations of cortical development; however, the abnormalities were inconsistent, with the metabolite levels varying among patients (15). Li *et al.* have shown that the NAA:Cr ratio is reduced in malformations secondary to abnormal stem cell formation (in which the neurons are dysplastic), is variably normal or reduced in heterotopic gray matter (in which neurons are of variable maturity and have variably reduced synapses), and is normal in polymicrogyria (in which the neurons are mature) (16). This suggests that the low NAA values present in some cortical malformations result from dysplastic or immature neurons in the malformation.

Another MR technique, diffusion tensor imaging, has been used to show the presence of increased water motion in white matter underlying the cortical malformation and decreased anisotropy of the white matter compared with the same area of the brain in age-matched controls (17, 18). Although neither the diffusion changes nor the spectroscopic changes are specific for malformations of cortical development, they may be useful in localizing the region of abnormality such that reinvestigation with MR imaging (perhaps with surface coils) might better locate the lesion.

When the MR imaging study is normal in patients with electrically well defined epileptogenic foci, single-photon-emission CT (SPECT, Chapter 14) and positron-emission tomography (PET, Chapter 15) may be helpful in localizing very small foci of cortical dysplasia (19–24) and for focusing attention on specific parts of the brain for more detailed analysis on MR. In general, the PET studies use ^{18}F-fluoro-deoxyglucose or ^{11}C-flumazenil and the SPECT studies use ^{99m}Tc-HMPAO or ^{123}I-iodoamphetamine.

[18]F-fluorodeoxyglucose PET shows decreased uptake in regions of dysplastic cortex; the sensitivity and specificity for frontal lobe lesions can be improved dramatically (from 50% to >90%) when quantitative analysis with a region of interest template is used (9). [11]C flumazenil PET shows changes in gamma-amino butyric acid $(GABA)_A$/benzodi-azepine receptor binding; decreased ^{11}C flumazenil binding has been observed in patients with focal cortical dysgenesis (20); up to 72% of patients with partial epilepsy and normal conventional MR imaging studies have abnormalities on these studies (25). Ictal SPECT may be sensitive to extra-temporal foci of cortical dysplasia, especially in the frontal lobes (24, 26, 27). The timing of radionuclide injection is critical in ictal SPECT because variable and evolving patterns of perfusion may make localization much more difficult if the isotope is not administered as closely as possible to the time of seizure onset. Postictal studies are not reliable in localizing extratemporal foci (27).

Another compound, ^{11}C methionine, has also been shown to be useful in the detection of small cortical dysplasias by PET (28, 29). Increased uptake is seen in the dysplasia. The mechanism by which the ^{11}C methionine is concentrated in the area of the dysplasia is not known. As with [18]FDG PET, ^{11}C methionine PET is nonspecific and can be concentrated by tumors and abscesses as well as dysplasias.

Overall, however, MR imaging is the cornerstone of the imaging evaluation of malformations of cortical development (26). Even if the epileptogenic focus is identified by another technique, the focus must always be co-registered with an MR image before any intervention is planned. Therefore, this section will deal primarily with MR imaging.

MALFORMATIONS OF CORTICAL DEVELOPMENT

Malformations of cortical development are divided into three categories based upon the step at which cortical development was probably first disturbed:

- abnormal proliferation/apoptosis
- abnormal neuronal migration
- abnormal late migration/cortical organization (30).

They will be presented in this order. It should be noted that many malformations result from disturbance of more than one stage of development; these malformations are classified according to the first step that is disturbed. Although from an imaging perspective, the malformations of cortical developments can be divided into three major groups, there are a number of malformations that are yet to be classified appropriately and have been classified under a fourth group under the present classification scheme (see Box 7.3). It is clear that changes will occur in the coming years and that this classification will change to some degree.

Malformations Secondary to Abnormal Stem Cell Formation

Microcephaly with Simplified Gyral Pattern

Microcephaly with simplified gyral pattern (MSG) is the term that has been proposed to describe malformations in which children are born with a head circumferences of 3 or more SD below the norm and their imaging studies show too few gyri and abnormally shallow sulci (less than half the depth of normal sulci), and usually reduced volume of white matter (31, 32). It is postulated that children with MSG are microcephalic because of reduced proliferation of neurons and glia in the germinal zones; some cases may result from intrauterine injury or infection.

Affected patients are subdivided into six groups based upon the neonatal course and the neuroimaging findings; groups 5 and 6 are sometimes called microlissencephaly. The details of these groups are beyond the scope of this chapter. Most of the groups are characterized by neonatal encephalopathy and generalized seizures either during the neonatal period or in early infancy (31, 32). Imaging studies show a very small brain compared to head size on sagittal images. Axial images show sulci that are too few and too shallow (Fig. 7.2).

Focal Cortical Dysplasia with Balloon Cells (Focal Transmantle Dysplasia)

Although the term focal cortical dysplasia has been in use for many years, it has become evident that some dysplasias are composed only of dysplastic neurons, whereas others are composed of dysplastic neurons and large abnormal cells with large nuclei and abundant eosinophilic cytoplasm; the latter cells are called balloon cells. Balloon cell dysplasias are characterized by the presence of abnormal cells from the wall of the lateral ventricle to the cortex; this transmantle extent, which is usually visible on MR imaging studies, has resulted in the use of the term 'transmantle dysplasia' for these malformations (33). This malformation is also sometimes called '*forme fruste* tuberous sclerosis' because identical histologic findings are seen in the cortical hamartomas

When large regions of cortex are involved, patients may have motor (if precentral involvement) or sensory (if postcentral) disturbances. When only small regions of cortex are involved, affected patients may have normal neurologic examinations (33). Almost all affected patients have partial epilepsy, which typically becomes clinically apparent during the first decade of life, sometimes as early as the first few days of life (33). Most of these patients have epilepsy that is highly refractory to medication, secondary to the high intrinsic epileptogenicity of these lesions (35). Therefore, many such patients require surgical resection of the dysplasia if the epileptogenic focus can be found.

Magnetic resonance imaging studies have a characteristic appearance (33, 36–38). When the involved region of brain is large, the cortical gyral pattern will be abnormal, with broad gyri and large, irregular sulci (Fig. 7.3). Abnormal heterogeneous signal intensity extends radially inward from the cortex to the ventricular surface. The region of abnormal signal intensity contains some portions isointense to gray matter and other areas isointense to white matter; some patients have regions of abnormal hyperintensity, probably representing dysplastic white matter. The cortical–white matter junction is typically indistinct.

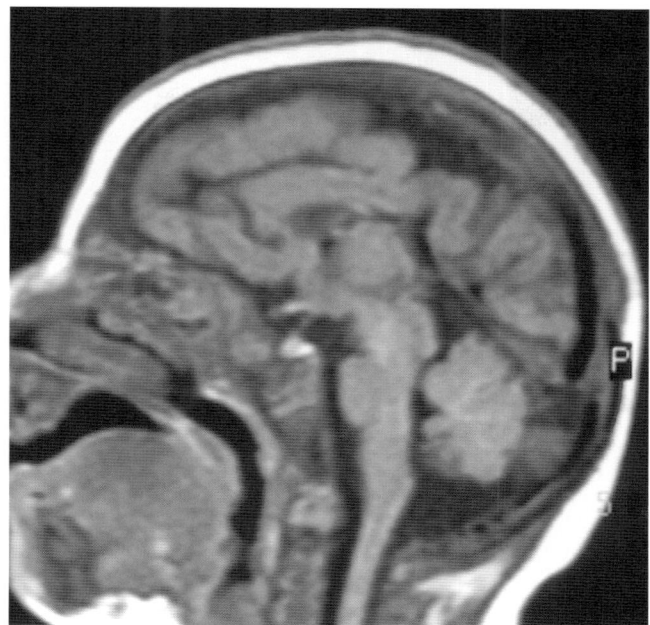

A

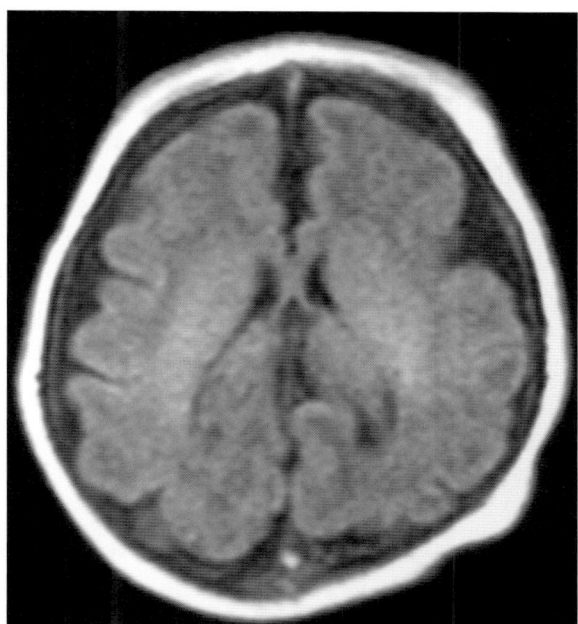

B

FIG. 7.2. Microcephaly with simplified gyral pattern. **A.** Sagittal T1-weighted image shows that the brain is much too small compared with the head size. **B.** Axial T1-weighted image shows that sulci are too few and too shallow.

of patients with tuberous sclerosis (34); therefore, all patients with radiologic or histologic findings of this malformation should be seen by a geneticist or child neurologist in order to be screened (skin, kidneys, heart, etc.) for tuberous sclerosis.

The presenting signs and symptoms of affected patients depend upon the size and location of the malformation.

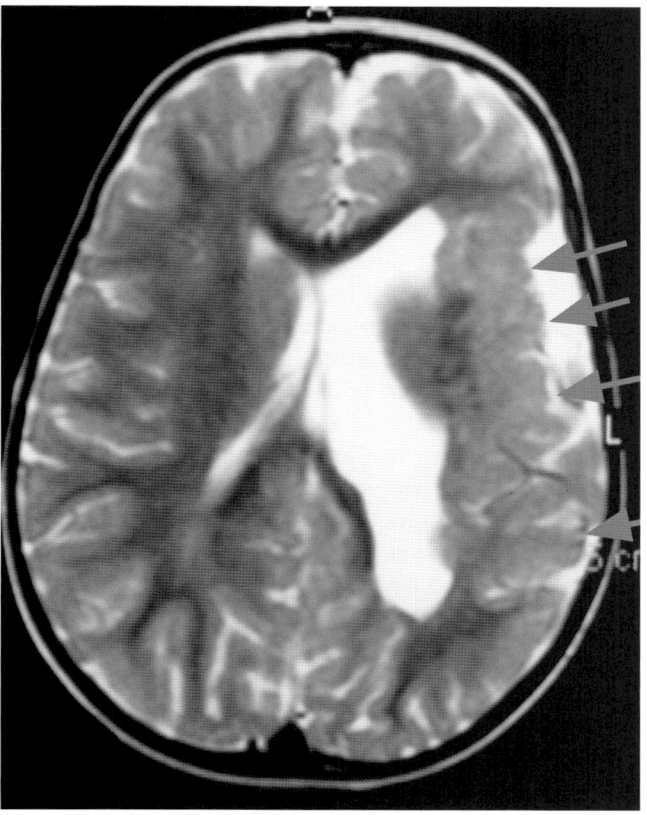

FIG. 7.3. Large transmantle dysplasia. Axial T2-weighted image showing thickened cortex (arrows) and an abnormal gyral pattern in the left perisylvian region. Reduced volume of white matter is seen beneath the abnormal cortex. Abnormal tissue is seen from the pia to the ependyma.

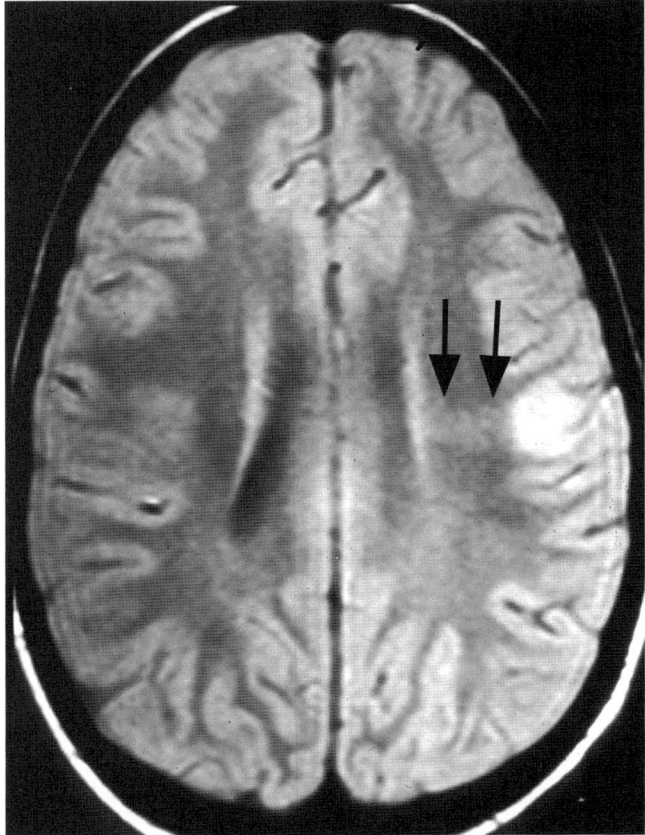

FIG. 7.4. Small transmantle dysplasia. Axial first-echo T2-weighted image showing focal cortical hyperintensity with a cone of abnormal hyperintensity (arrows) extending from the depth of the affected sulcus to the ventricular margin.

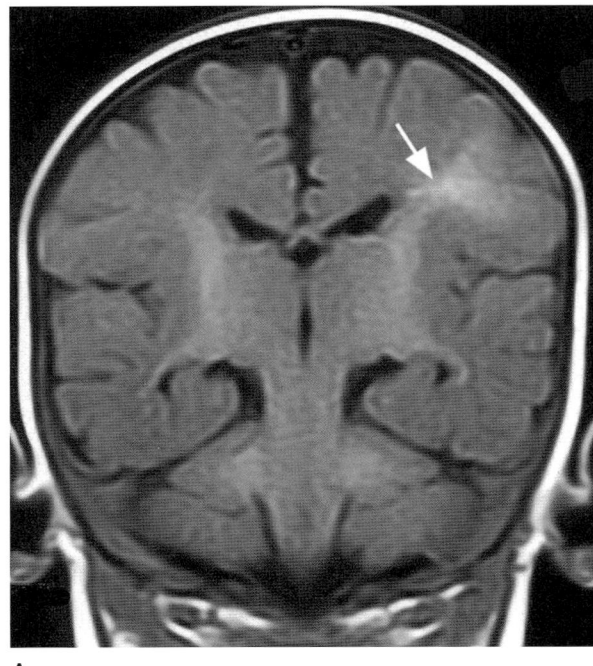

A

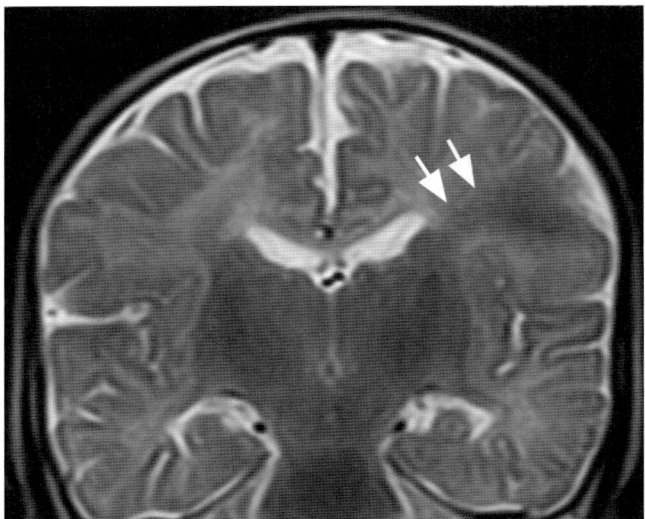

B

FIG. 7.5. Small transmantle dysplasia in an infant. Coronal T1-weighted (**A**) and T2-weighted (**B**) images show a cone-shaped area of hyper- (**A**) and hypointensity (**B**) (arrows) extending from the depth of the affected sulcus to the ventricular margin.

Smaller areas are much more difficult to detect. Most typically, one sees smaller lesions, with linear or curvilinear hyperintensity (relative to mature white matter), extending from the cortical–white matter junction to the ventricular surface (Fig. 7.4). Some of the affected cortex may also be hyperintense and, on occasion, T2 hyperintensity is seen extending for several millimeters along the cortical–white matter junction on one or both sides of the tract from the cortex to the ventricle; this is most easily seen if FLAIR is used and the proper imaging plane is chosen. The cortical–white matter junction will typically be blurred on high-resolution imaging. In neonates and infants, the tract extending from the cortex to the ventricle will look hyperintense on T1-weighted images and hypointense on T2-weighted images (Fig. 7.5). The relative intensity of the tract compared to the surrounding white matter gradually changes as the white matter matures. The use of phased-array surface coil imaging may be useful in detecting the smaller, more subtle foci (12, 33).

The few reports of proton MR spectroscopy in transmantle dysplasias suggest that there is a significant reduction of the NAA:Cr ratio compared with normal controls and with normal areas in the affected brain (13, 16).

Tuberous Sclerosis

Tuberous sclerosis is an autosomal dominant genetic disease that involves multiple organ systems. Mutations of two separate genes have been found to cause this disorder. The *TSC1* gene is localized to chromosome 9q34 (39, 40) and codes for a protein called hamartin, while the *TSC2* gene has been localized to chromosome 16p13.3 (41, 42) and codes for a protein called tuberin. Hamartin and tuberin interact physically in vivo, a fact that clarifies how mutations in two different genes result in the common phenotype (43, 44).

It appears that mutations of these two genes make up the vast majority of, if not all, cases of tuberous sclerosis (45–47).

Mutations of *TSC1* have been identified in relatively few (13–18%) patients. They are somewhat more common (15–50%) in familial cases than in sporadic cases (47). Few differences in the clinical phenotype have yet been noted in patients with one mutation as compared with the other (48). The new mutation rate is high; however, before concluding that an affected child is a new mutation, it is necessary to examine both parents thoroughly, including ultraviolet light examination, neuroimaging and, if possible, chromosomal analysis from multiple tissues, including germ cells (49, 50). A 2–3% risk of recurrence in future pregnancies remains even if both parents seem unaffected (49, 50).

Classically, tuberous sclerosis was characterized by the clinical triad of mental retardation, epilepsy, and characteristic skin lesions known as adenoma sebaceum (51). Recent experience has shown that half of affected patients have normal intelligence, only 75% have epilepsy, and almost any organ of the body can be affected (52). As a result, more sophisticated criteria for clinical diagnosis of the disorder have been established and are listed in Box 7.4. Increasing awareness of the condition and use of the new diagnostic criteria have resulted in a revision of the estimated incidence from approximately 1 in 100 000 patients (53) to 1 in 6000 live births (51, 54). No racial or sexual predilection has been detected.

Infantile spasms or myoclonic seizures that begin in infancy or early childhood are the presenting symptom of tuberous sclerosis in approximately 80% of patients. The infantile spasms evolve into other seizure types, most commonly symptomatic generalized epilepsy ($\approx$60%), partial epilepsy ($\approx$20%) or a mixture of partial and generalized epilepsy ($\approx$20%) (56). Affected patients can have nearly any type of seizure; therefore, the diagnosis of tuberous sclerosis should be considered in any child with epilepsy.

The incidence of cognitive impairment ranges from 45% to 82%; most recent publications suggest that the lower number is more accurate (51, 57). Among cognitively impaired patients, approximately two-thirds will be moderately to severely impaired and one-third only mildly to moderately affected. Patients with more than 10 cortical tubers seem to have a higher incidence of impaired cognition but this may be related to the higher incidence of epilepsy in this group (58). Patients who manifest seizures before the age of 5 are more likely to have cognitive impairment than those who develop seizures at a later age (51, 59).

Neuroimaging of Tuberous Sclerosis

On neuroimaging studies, three specific types of lesion are seen in patients with tuberous sclerosis: subependymal hamartomas, cortical/subcortical hamartomas, and subependymal giant cell tumors (60).

The *subependymal hamartomas* are typically small lesions that lie along the walls of the lateral ventricles,

---

BOX 7.4. Diagnostic Criteria for Tuberous Sclerosis Complex

MAJOR FEATURES
- Facial angiofibromas or forehead plaque
- Nontraumatic ungual or periungual fibromas
- Hypomelanotic macules (more than three)
- Shagreen patch (connective tissue nevus)
- Multiple retinal nodular hamartomas
- Cortical tuber*
- Subependymal nodule
- Subependymal giant cell astrocytoma
- Cardiac rhabdomyoma, single or multiple
- Lymphangioleiomyomatosis†
- Renal angiomyolipoma†

MINOR FEATURES
- Multiple randomly distributed enamel pits in dental enamel
- Hamartomatous rectal polyps‡
- Bone cysts§
- Affected first-degree relative
- Cerebral white matter radial migration lines*§
- Gingival fibromas
- Nonrenal hamartoma‡
- Retinal achromic patch
- 'Confetti' skin lesions
- Multiple renal cysts‡

Definite tuberous sclerosis complex – Either two major features, or one major plus two minor features
Probable tuberous sclerosis complex – One major plus one minor feature
Possible TSC – Either one major feature or two or more minor features

*When cerebral cortical dysplasia and cerebral white matter migration tracts occur together, they should be counted as one rather than two features of tuberous sclerosis.
†When both lymphangioleiomyomatosis and renal angiomyolipomas are present, other features of tuberous sclerosis should be present before a definite diagnosis is assigned.
‡Histologic confirmation is suggested.
§Radiologic confirmation is sufficient.
From Roach *et al.*, 1998 (55)

---

sometimes involving the walls of the third or fourth ventricles. Although the regions of ventricular wall around the foramina of Monroe are the most common sites, subependymal hamartomas can be seen in any part of the lateral ventricles, including the frontal horns, occipital horns, and temporal horns. They most commonly have an elliptical shape with the long axis of the ellipse being perpendicular to the long axis of the lateral ventricle.

Their appearance on neuroimaging studies varies with the age of the patient. In infants, subependymal hamartomas can be detected by ultrasonography, CT, or MR. Ultrasound shows the lesions as elliptical regions of hyperechogenicity that protrude into the lateral ventricles. They are more difficult to detect on CT in infants than in older children and adults, as they are not yet calcified. However, they can be seen on good-quality studies as elliptical lesions originating in the ventricular wall and protruding into the ventricular lumen. Administration of iodinated contrast shows variable enhancement.

Magnetic resonance imaging is the study of choice for the identification of subependymal hamartomas in neonates and infants, showing elliptical lesions that demonstrate short T1 and T2 relaxation times compared with the surrounding unmyelinated brain parenchyma (60, 61). Care should be taken not to misdiagnose these as small subependymal hemorrhages. Gradient-echo scans or CT will help to make this distinction, if necessary, as the hamartomas are isodense to surrounding brain parenchyma on CT (in contrast to hyperdensity of blood) and do not show any 'blooming' (apparent increase of size) on gradient echo images.

In older children and adults, the nodules change in their appearance. On CT, they become easier to see as they calcify; the number of calcified nodules increases with the increasing age of the patient (57). On MR, the white matter becomes isointense to the subependymal nodules as myelination proceeds; as a result, the nodules become slightly more difficult to see as discrete lesions and the irregularity of the ventricular wall becomes the most noticeable abnormality. If heavily calcified, the nodules may appear hypointense on T1-weighted images (62).

Giant cell tumors also are located in the wall of the lateral ventricle. These tumors differ from subependymal hamartomas by their size and their tendency to enlarge; their characteristic location and tendency toward enlargement usually result in a clinical presentation of hydrocephalus (62, 63). Their incidence in tuberous sclerosis is approximately 5–10% (51, 62). Histologically, subependymal lesions in patients with tuberous sclerosis appear to span a continuum between subependymal hamartomas and giant cell tumors; although some lesions are clearly in one category or the other, many lesions have histologic characteristics of both (51).

The neuroimaging appearance of giant cell tumors is one of a round-to-ovoid, often partially calcified, uniformly enhancing subependymal mass that is most commonly located near the foramina of Monroe but can be situated anywhere along a ventricular wall (Fig. 7.6). Thus, by a single neuroimaging study, it is not possible to distinguish a giant cell tumor from a subependymal hamartoma (60, 62). The only way to make the differentiation is to perform sequential studies – giant cell tumors show growth out of proportion to brain growth on sequential studies whereas hamartomas show growth proportional to that of the brain. In adults, hamartomas do not grow.

One other aspect of giant cell tumors warrants discussion: they rarely degenerate into invasive astrocytomas (51, 63, 64). Such degeneration should be suspected radiologically if the tumor is seen to invade the brain parenchyma (interstitial edema will typically be seen in the adjacent parenchyma), or if rapid enlargement is seen.

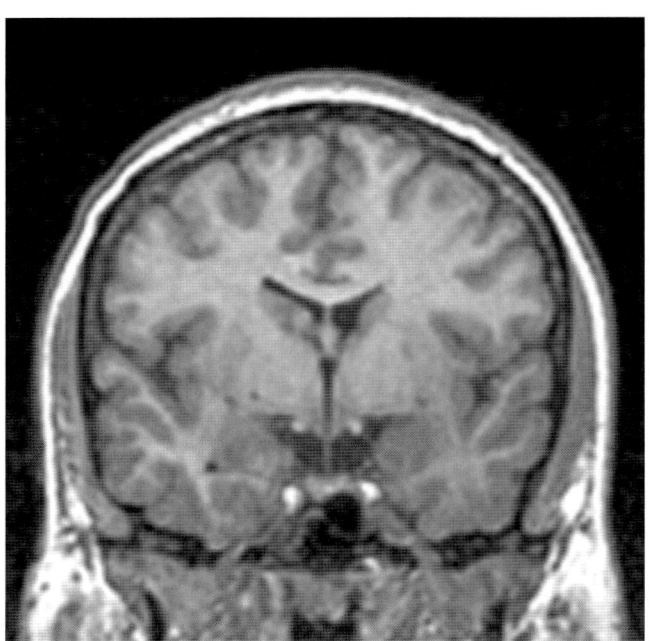

A

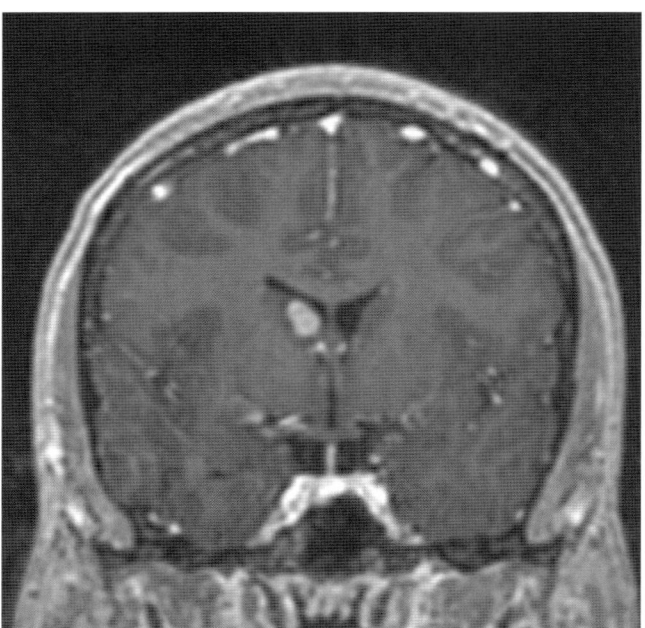

B

FIG. 7.6. Tuberous sclerosis complex. Coronal T1-weighted (**A**) and gadolinium T1-weighted (**B**) images showing evidence of a small subependymal giant cell astrocytoma in the foramen of Monroe.

The final cerebral lesion that is identified in tuberous sclerosis is the *cortical tuber*. These lesions are identical, by histology, neuroimaging, and clinical manifestations, to focal cortical dysplasia with balloon cells, described above (65). They vary widely in number, with any particular patient having as few as one or as many as 30 (51, 66). They are most common in the cerebral hemispheres but may occur in the cerebellum as well.

On CT, they appear in children as foci of low attenuation, typically expanding a gyrus and extending a variable distance into the underlying white matter (60). Some of the lesions calcify (the precise percentage is not known) and, when they do, they often shrink such that the overlying cortex is drawn centrally, creating a cortical 'dimple'.

On MR, the appearance of the lesions varies with the maturity of the brain (61, 62, 67, 68). In unmyelinated infant brains, the lesions are hyperintense to both gray and white matter on T1-weighted images and hypointense to white matter on T2-weighted images. Although the lesions appear to be primarily subcortical, at this age it is easy to see a curvilinear central extension of the lesion extending centrally towards the ventricular surface. As the white matter myelinates, the appearance of the lesions changes. Ultimately, they are seen as hyperintense lesions compared with surrounding white matter on T2-weighted and FLAIR images and they may be isointense or slightly hypointense compared with surrounding white matter on T1-weighted images (61, 62, 68). The central extension of the lesions becomes much more difficult to see as the brain myelinates; use of magnetization transfer to diminish the T1 shortening effect of the myelin (69) or FLAIR to increase sensitivity to the slight signal alterations (70, 71) may help to identify this finding (Fig. 7.7). Calcified cortical tubers sometimes appear bright on T1-weighted images (60), while degenerated tubers may show mild enhancement; such enhancement should not be misinterpreted as malignant degeneration, which is extraordinarily rare (60).

Two other lesions that should be briefly mentioned in tuberous sclerosis are *parenchymal cysts* and *vascular lesions*. An unknown percentage of patients with tuberous sclerosis have cyst-like structures, most commonly periventricular, in the cerebral hemispheric white matter. Their clinical significance is uncertain (72). The vascular lesions are usually arterial aneurysms, which can develop anywhere in the arterial system, including the cerebral vasculature (72–76). Cerebral aneurysms appear to involve children disproportionately; definitive conclusions await further studies.

Hemimegalencephaly (Unilateral Megalencephaly)

The term hemimegalencephaly describes a hamartomatous overgrowth of all or part of a cerebral hemisphere with defects in neuronal proliferation, migration, and organization within the affected hemisphere (77–81). The heterogeneous imaging (78, 80, 82) and pathologic (81, 83, 84) appearances suggest that several different disorders are included under this heading. The brain can be affected in isolation or can be associated with hemihypertrophy of part or all of the ipsilateral body. Affected patients typically have macrocephaly at birth and in early infancy; they present with an intractable seizure disorder that begins at a very early age (usually before the first birthday), hemiplegia, and severe developmental delay (78, 80, 81, 83). A high incidence of hemimegalencephaly seems to occur in patients with the epidermal nevus syndrome (85–87). Other associated conditions include Proteus syndrome (sometimes considered a

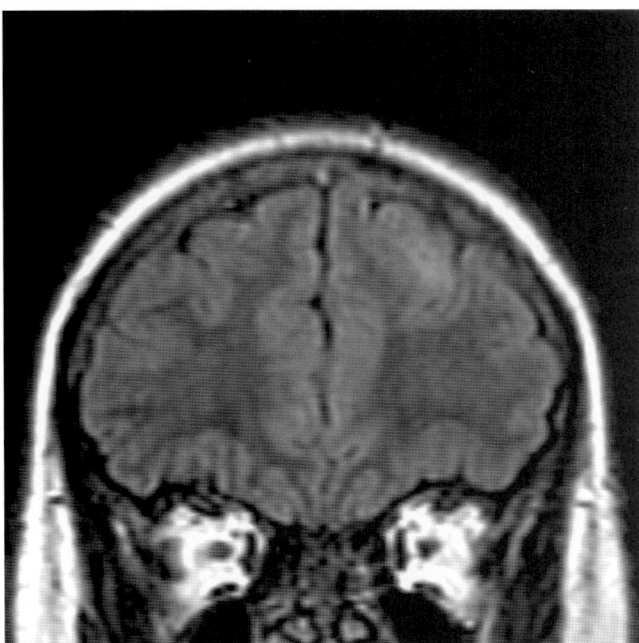

A

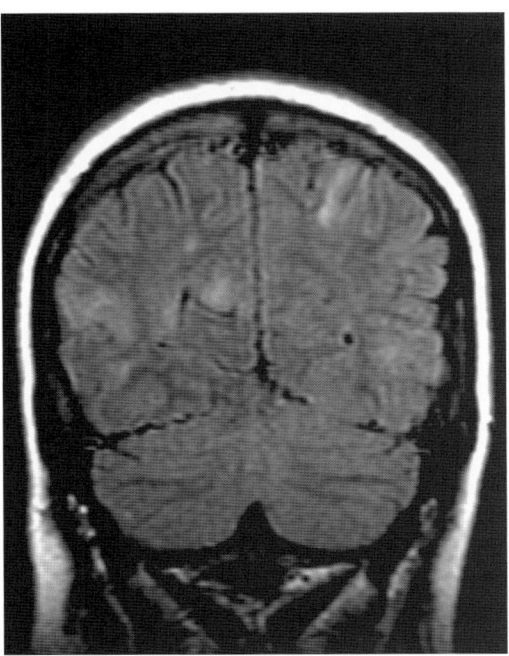

B

FIG. 7.7. Tuberous sclerosis complex. Both A and B are coronal FLAIR images showing evidence of multiple high signal lesions typical of hamartomas. Not all the lesions are epileptogenic in nature, although by MRI there is no distinction between them.

form of epidermal nevus syndrome (88–90)), unilateral hypomelanosis of Ito (91), neurofibromatosis type I (92), and tuberous sclerosis (93).

On CT and MR, the involved hemisphere appears moderately to markedly enlarged (Fig. 7.8). The cortex is typically dysplastic, with broad gyri, shallow sulci, and cortical thickening; however, the gyral pattern may appear grossly normal or may be frankly agyric. In many patients, the usually sharp

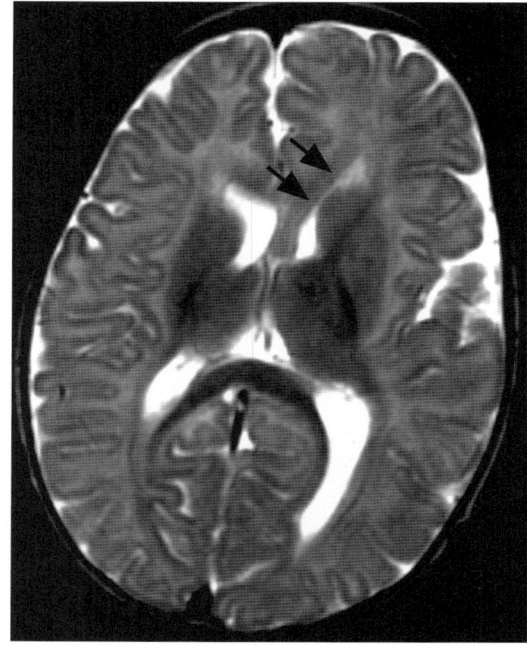

A

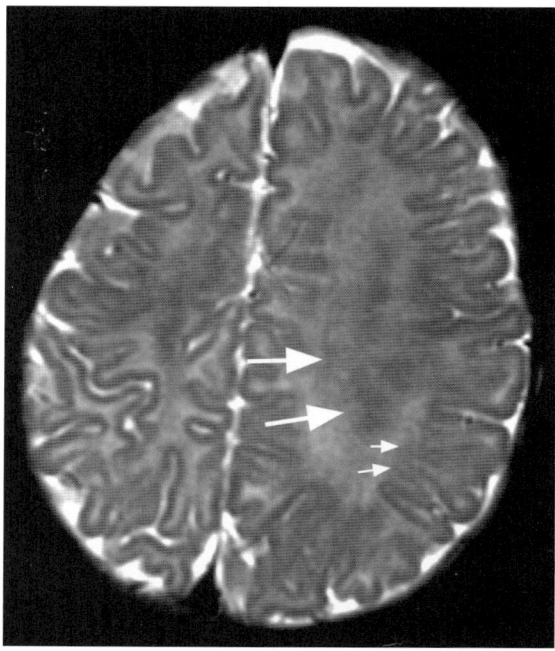

B

FIG. 7.8. Hemimegalencephaly. Axial T2-weighted images at two levels show that the left hemisphere is abnormally enlarged. **A.** At the level of the lateral ventricles, the left lateral ventricle is large and the left frontal horn is abnormally straight (black arrows). **B.** At the level of the centrum semiovale, abnormal signal is seen in the white matter (large arrows), the perirolandic gyral pattern is abnormal, and there is blurring of the cortical-white matter junction (small arrows).

it is enlarged, usually in proportion to the enlargement of the affected hemisphere, with the frontal horn being abnormally straight and pointing superiorly and anteriorly (78). In occasional patients, however, the ipsilateral ventricle is small (82). Rarely, the affected portion of the brain has a bizarre, hamartomatous appearance (78, 80); in this situation, the malformation is recognized by the characteristic enlargement of the affected brain and ipsilateral ventricle.

It is important to recognize that the radiologic appearance of the brain may change over time. Wolpert *et al.* reported a patient in whom the affected hemisphere atrophied during the first year of life and was smaller than the contralateral (normal) hemisphere when imaged at age 1 year (94). An analogous change was seen on SPECT imaging, where the tracer uptake in the affected hemisphere diminished over time (95). We have seen reduction in hemispheric size of affected patients after episodes of status epilepticus. The affected portion of the hemisphere has little function in these patients save for acting as a seizure focus; indeed, [18]FDG PET scans show markedly reduced glucose uptake in affected regions (96). Anatomic hemispherectomy, functional hemispherectomy, or hemidecortication may, therefore, be indicated if the seizure disorder is intractable and the contralateral hemisphere is normal (97, 98).

Malformations Secondary to Abnormal Neuronal Migration

Lissencephaly

The term lissencephaly means 'smooth brain' and refers to a paucity of gyral and sulcal development on the surface of the brain. *Agyria* is defined as an absence of gyri on the surface of the brain and is synonymous with 'complete lissencephaly,' whereas *pachygyria* is defined as the presence of a few broad, flat gyri and is used interchangeably with the term 'incomplete lissencephaly.'

In the past, patients with overmigration of neurons and associated congenital muscular dystrophy were classified as type II lissencephaly, later called cobblestone lissencephaly. The latest classification system (30) no longer classifies the cortical malformation associated with congenital muscular dystrophy as a lissencephaly; instead it is called cobblestone cortex. However, other new types of lissencephaly have been identified, including lissencephaly due to mutation of *RELN*[8] and a type of lissencephaly associated with agenesis of the corpus callosum and ambiguous genitalia (99). More types are sure to be found.

Classical Lissencephaly (the Agyria–Pachygyria Complex)

Children with classical lissencephaly almost always have global developmental delay and seizures, although the age of onset and severity of the clinical syndrome may vary depending upon the severity of the cortical malformation (100–102).

border between the cortex and the subcortical white matter may blur or disappear altogether (78, 80). The white matter is of abnormally low signal on CT and usually shows heterogeneous signal intensity on MR studies, representing heterotopia and dysplastic neurons and glia. The configuration of the ipsilateral lateral ventricle is usually quite characteristic;

Some patients with classical lissencephaly have a defect of the *LIS1* gene at locus 17p13.3 (103–105). A subset of the group with chromosome 17 mutations has characteristic facies and is classified as having the *Miller–Dieker syndrome* (102, 106).

Other patients with classical lissencephaly (currently estimated to be about 20% (107)) have mutations of the *DCX* (also called *XLIS*) gene at chromosome Xq22.3–q23 (*X-linked lissencephaly* (108)); these patients are typically boys whose mothers have band heterotopia (109, 110). Both these genes are believed to code for proteins that are important in the assembly of microtubules within migrating neurons (111); it is postulated that microtubule assembly is critical for neuronal cell bodies to follow the leading processes during the process of migration. Affected mothers have the same mutation of the X chromosome as do their offspring with X-linked lissencephaly (6). Many patients with band heterotopia have a significantly reduced number of sulci and gyri (112) and are better classified as having incomplete lissencephaly.

About 75% of patients with lissencephaly have mutations of either 17p13.3 or Xq22.3–23 (107), meaning that about one quarter of lissencephaly patients have other mutations; this is not surprising in view of the many genes that are involved in normal neuronal migration. With time, mutations of other chromosomal loci that are involved in neuronal migration will undoubtedly be found to underlie other cases of classical lissencephaly.

Children with *LIS1*-linked lissencephaly and those with *DCX*-linked lissencephaly have similar neurologic syndromes. Those with complete classical lissencephaly are typically hypotonic at birth, gradually developing appendicular and oropharyngeal spasticity as their nervous system matures (100, 113). Children with incomplete lissencephaly have less severe motor abnormalities and hypotonia (100). Infantile spasms are common in severely affected infants. The development of medically refractory epilepsy at a very early age, with increasingly complex seizure disorders over time, is characteristic. Systemic anomalies, particularly those of the ears, eyes, heart, and kidney, are present in the more severely affected patients (100, 102, 106, 114, 115).

Most patients in this group have areas of both agyria and pachygyria, i.e. incomplete lissencephaly. In patients with chromosome 17 mutations, the areas of agyria are most frequently parieto-occipital in location while the pachygyric areas are more common in the frontal and temporal regions (100, 113, 116). Some patients with lissencephaly have more severe pachygyria or agyria in the frontal lobes; most of these patients seem to have mutations of Xq22.3–23. Microscopically, the cerebral cortex is composed of a thin outer layer of neurons, a cell-sparse zone, and a thick inner layer of neurons. The inner layer of neurons is thought to represent young neurons that were prematurely stopped during their migration to the cortex. Alternatively, the arrest of neuronal migration may reflect some abnormality of the fetal ependyma (117, 118). Whatever the cause, the last phase of neuronal migration to the cerebral cortex is impaired.

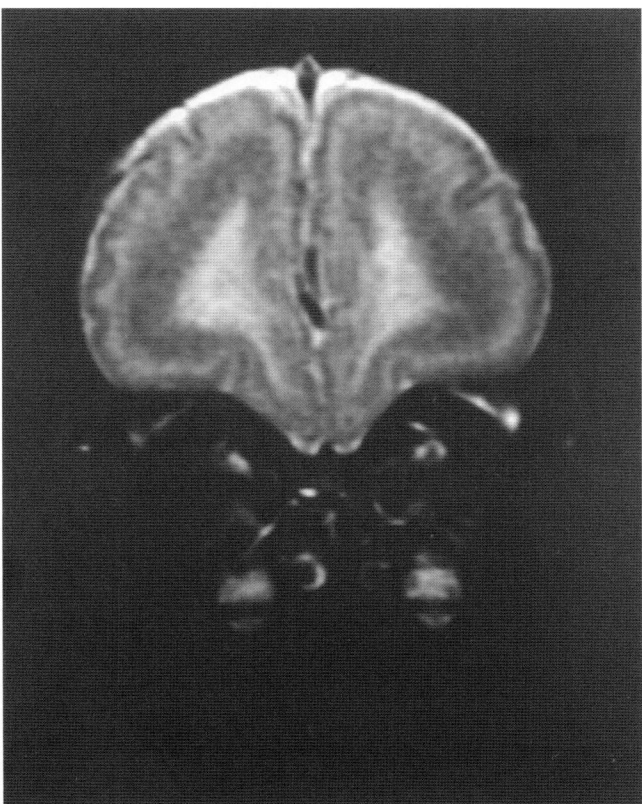

FIG. 7.9. Lissencephaly (agyria). Notice the smooth cortex and the cell-sparse layer between a thin outer cortex and a deep layer of partially migrated neurons.

Imaging studies of patients with complete classical lissencephaly reveal a smooth brain surface with diminished white matter and shallow, vertically oriented, sylvian fissures (79, 100, 102, 113, 119, 120). A thin outer cortical layer is separated from a thick deeper cortical layer by a zone of white matter (the 'cell-sparse zone') that seems to myelinate normally (Fig. 7.9). The gross appearance of the brain resembles that of the fetus prior to 23 or 24 gestational weeks when sulci normally begin to form. The cerebrum has been described as having a figure-of-eight appearance on axial images as a result of the shallow, vertical sylvian fissures. In cases of severe lissencephaly, sagittal images may show callosal hypogenesis. The ventricular trigones and occipital horns are enlarged, mostly because of underdevelopment of the calcarine sulci (113). The brain stem often appears small.

Incomplete lissencephaly, in which areas of pachygyria are present together with areas of agyria or areas of normal brain, is much more common than complete lissencephaly. Areas of pachygyria also have a thickened cortex, but broad gyri and shallow sulci are present. Pachygyria can be distinguished from polymicrogyria when thin-section, high-resolution images are obtained (121). In pachygyria, the cortical–white matter junction is smooth and, in some cases, a layer of normal white matter can be detected in the cell-sparse zone. In polymicrogyria, the cortical–white matter junction is always irregular (121).

Pachygyria can be focal or diffuse. When focal, it is almost always bilateral and typically posterior in patients

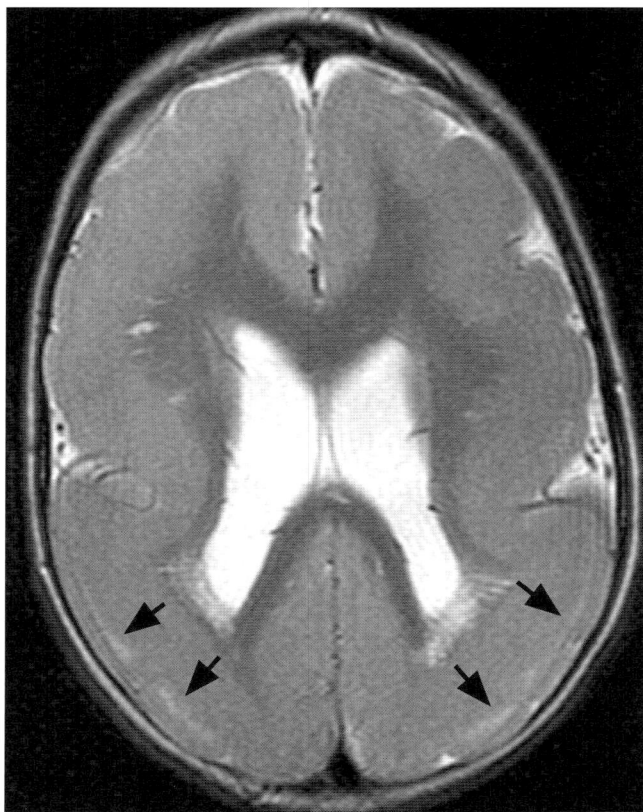

FIG. 7.10. Incomplete lissencephaly associated with a *LIS1* mutation. Pachygyria is present in the anterior frontal lobes, while agyria is present in the posterior frontal and parietal lobes. Note the presence of a cell-sparse layer (arrows) in the agyric region.

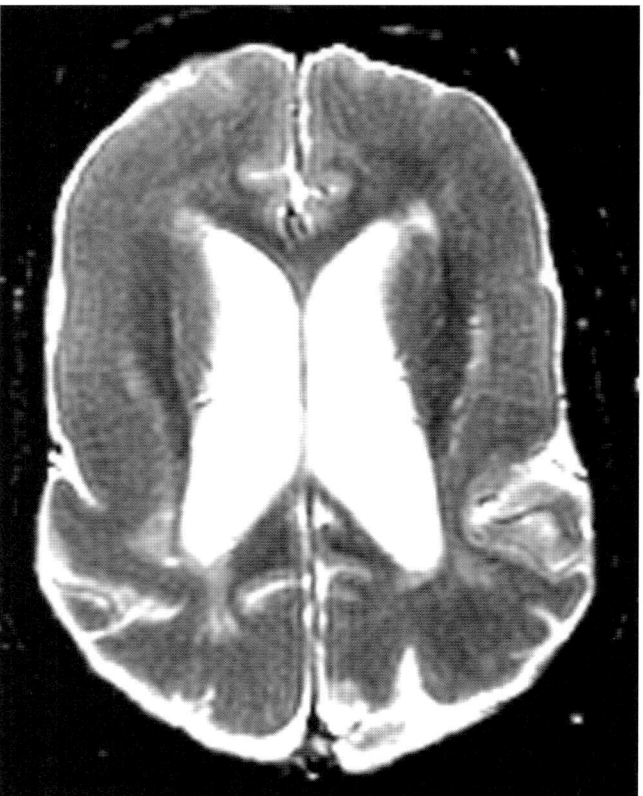

FIG. 7.11. Incomplete lissencephaly associated with a *DCX* mutation. Agyria is present in the frontal lobes, while pachygyria is seen in the parietal and occipital lobes.

with *LIS1* mutations. When diffuse, it is often associated with regions of agyria and is typically more severe in the parieto-occipital region of the brain (and least severe in the frontal and temporal lobes) in *LIS1* mutations (Fig. 7.10). The mid- to posterior frontal lobes are most severely affected in *DCX*-linked pachygyria (Fig. 7.11). When patients have classical lissencephaly with more severe involvement in the anterior cerebrum than in the posterior cerebrum, a good family history should be obtained. Band heterotopia may be found in some female family members if there is family history of seizures.

A subgroup of patients with lissencephaly have cerebellar hypoplasia (122, 123). This appears to be a heterogeneous group of disorders with differing patterns of inheritance, different patterns of lissencephaly, and different patterns of cerebellar hypoplasia or dysplasia. Patients with *LIS1*, *DCX*, and *RELN* mutations can have cerebellar hypoplasia (8, 122, 123). With *LIS1* and *DCX* mutations, the cerebellum is usually only mildly hypoplastic and the hypoplasia probably results from the fact that the same ligands and processes that are involved in neuronal migration in the cerebrum are also at work in the cerebellum. Therefore, it is not yet clear that the classification of lissencephaly with cerebellar hypoplasia should be classified as a separate malformation syndrome. However, some cases of lissencephaly have quite

dramatic cerebellar hypoplasia, such as those with *RELN* mutations (8). Therefore, it is possible that those patients with severe cerebellar hypoplasia may represent a distinct group.

Lissencephaly Secondary to RELN Mutation

The *RELN* gene codes for a protein called reelin, which seems to be important in the dissociation of migrating neurons from radial glial cells (8). When reelin is abnormal, therefore, migration of neurons to their final destination in the cerebral and cerebellar cortex is impaired (124). Affected patients suffer from cognitive impairment and epilepsy. Imaging studies of affected patients show pachygyria, with an abnormally thick cortex (usually about 8 mm), but no cell-sparse zone is seen, differentiating this anomaly from classical lissencephaly. In addition, the corpus callosum is thin, the pons is small, and the cerebellum is quite small and shows a complete absence of lobulation (8). The appearance is quite striking.

X-Linked Lissencephaly with Agenesis of the Corpus Callosum and Ambiguous Genitalia

Lissencephaly with callosal agenesis and ambiguous genitalia (99) is caused by mutation of the homeobox gene *ARX*, located at chromosome Xp22; the mutation prevents

GABA-ergic interneurons from migrating to the cerebral cortex from the medial ganglionic eminence. Other mutations of the same gene can cause X-linked infantile spasms and X-linked mental retardation. Affected patients are typically abnormal from birth. They are microcephalic and manifest refractory epilepsy from the time of birth, and possibly prenatally. Temperature regulation is abnormal and the children are often hypothermic. Few developmental milestones are reached. Death typically occurs during the first decade of life. Imaging studies show frontal pachygyria, with slightly thickened cortex, and parieto-occipital agyria with cortical thickness of 5–10 mm (Fig. 7.12). No cell-sparse zone is seen. The corpus callosum may be completely absent or hypogenetic, with resultant enlargement of the trigones and temporal horns of the lateral ventricles. The brain stem and cerebellum appear normal.

Cobblestone Cortex (Associated with Congenital Muscular Dystrophies)

Cobblestone malformations of the cortex are essentially all associated with congenital muscular dystrophies. It is likely that the mutated protein has a role in terminating neuronal migration at the external glial limitans during brain development in addition to functioning in muscle contraction in the mature child. The three main disorders in this group are the Walker–Warburg syndrome, muscle–eye–brain disease of Santavuori, and Fukuyama's congenital muscular dystrophy (FCMD).

Walker–Warburg Syndrome

Walker–Warburg syndrome is the name given to a condition in which patients have cobblestone cortex, hypomyelination, congenital hydrocephalus, hypotonia, and severe congenital ocular dysplasia (persistent hypoplastic primary vitreous, congenital glaucoma or microphthalmos, optic nerve hypoplasia (125)); occipital cephaloceles are present in about half (114, 119, 126–128). Affected patients are obviously abnormal at birth, manifesting hypotonia that is usually profound and unchanging, in addition to the ocular abnormalities and the progressive macrocephaly. Most patients show complete lack of psychomotor development and die in the first year of life secondary to recurrent aspiration and respiratory illnesses.

On imaging studies, patients with Walker–Warburg syndrome have a thickened cortex with only a few shallow sulci, microphthalmia (which may be unilateral or bilateral), hydrocephalus, callosal hypogenesis, and profound hypomyelination (129, 130). The appearance of the cortex is quite distinctive, with an irregular gray–white matter junction (Fig. 7.13), possibly reflecting the extension of bundles of disorganized cortical neurons into the underlying white matter (119); this is the characteristic imaging appearance of

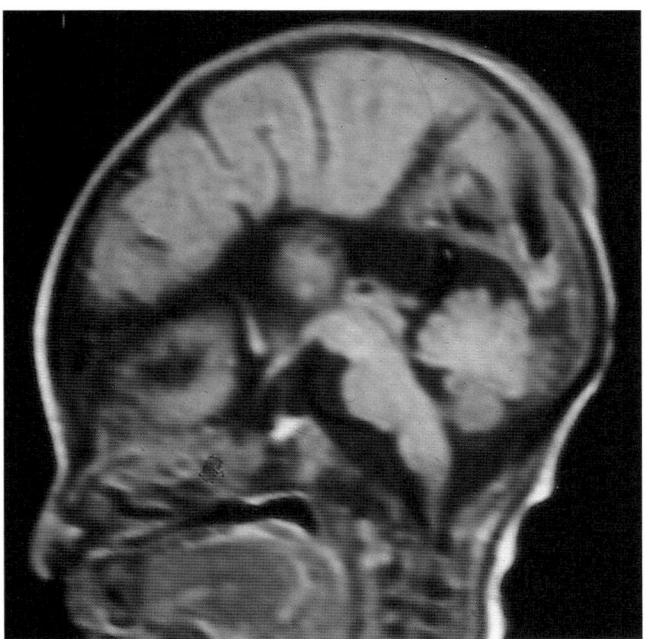

A

B

FIG. 7.12. X-linked lissencephaly with agenesis of the corpus callosum and ambiguous genitalia. **A.** Sagittal T1-weighted image showing absence of the corpus callosum and an abnormal gyral pattern in the cerebral hemispheres. **B.** Axial T1-weighted image showing nearly normal cortical thickness with a few shallow sulci anteriorly but nearly complete agyria with thickened cortex in the parietal and occipital lobes.

cobblestone cortex. These bundles of neurons are separated by fibroglial vascular tissue that extends from the cerebral white matter through the cerebral cortex into the subarachnoid space, which is obliterated by this tissue. The posterior fossa is also distinctive, with marked pontine hypogenesis, an enlarged quadrigeminal plate, and a distinctive dorsal 'kink'

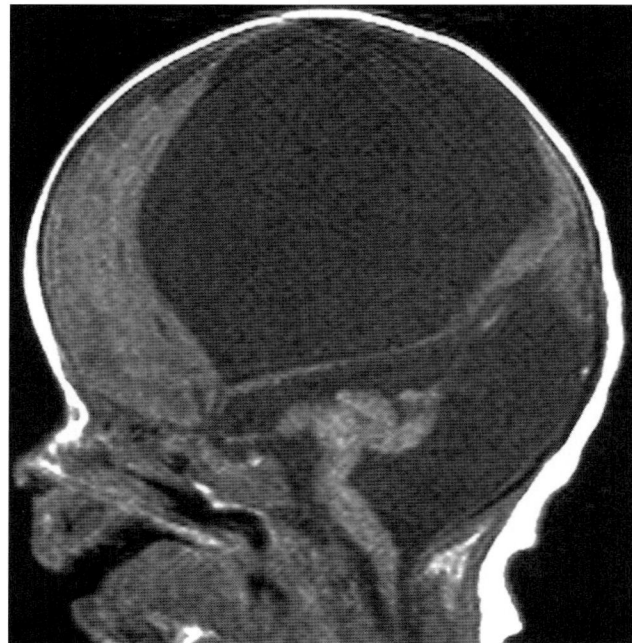

A

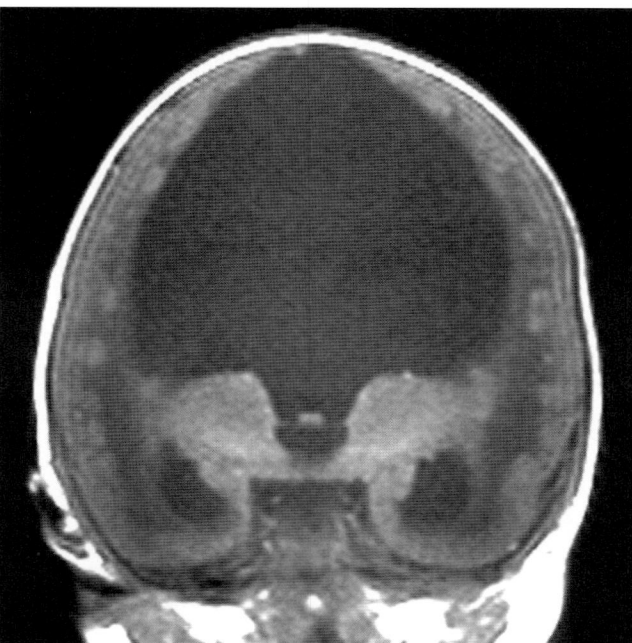

B

FIG. 7.13. Walker–Warburg syndrome. **A.** Sagittal T1-weighted image showing hydrocephalus. In addition, the pons is small, the quadrigeminal plate is dysplastic, and the brain stem is kinked at the pontomesencephalic junction. **B.** Coronal T1-weighted image showing the abnormal cerebrum with hypomyelination and bundles of dysplastic neurons in the cerebral cortex, causing an irregular cortical–white matter junction.

at the mesencephalic-pontine junction (Fig. 7.13), vermian hypoplasia, and small, dysplastic cerebellar hemispheres. Ocular imaging findings include ocular asymmetry, secondary to congenital microphthalmos or congenital glaucoma (with resultant buphthalmos), and vitreous and

subretinal hemorrhages. The hemorrhages are better seen by ophthalmoscopy than by imaging.

Fukuyama Congenital Muscular Dystrophy

Fukuyama congenital muscular dystrophy is a condition seen primarily in children of Japanese ancestry (131, 132). It is a genetic disorder, with affected patients having mutations of the *FCMD* gene at chromosome 9q31–33 (133). Affected children present with hypotonia and severe developmental delay; seizures develop during the first year of life in about half of affected individuals. Analysis of serum shows elevated creatine kinase level; this elevation typically leads to a muscle biopsy, which shows changes consistent with muscular dystrophy (131, 132, 134, 135). Patients with FCMD have dysplasias of the retina that lead to myopia, nystagmus, and chorioretinal degeneration (136) but the clinical manifestations are less severe than the ocular anomalies of muscle–eye–brain disease and Walker–Warburg syndrome.

Although CT shows an abnormal brain in patients with FCMD, MR is the study of choice to show all the abnormalities. Within the cerebral cortex, three types of abnormality are seen pathologically (137). Of these, two are detected by imaging: unlayered polymicrogyria, which is seen primarily in the frontal lobes, and cobblestone cortex, which is largely temporo-occipital (135). The frontal polymicrogyria is seen as irregularity of the cortical surface and cortical-white matter junction (Fig. 7.14A). The temporo-occipital cobblestone cortex is thick, with a smooth outer surface (Fig. 7.14A) but a slightly irregular inner surface. In addition, deep to the inner surface of the cortex, separated from the cortex by a layer of white matter, partly contiguous nodules of cortex can be identified on high-resolution scans.

Patients with FCMD also have dysplasia of the cerebellar cortex, which is manifest on imaging studies as dysplastic folia with subcortical cysts. These cysts tend to be located in the dorsal midportion of the cerebellar hemisphere, particularly in the superior semilunar lobule (Fig. 7.14C) (134). On histology, the cysts are found to have leptomeningeal tissue in their lumens and a molecular layer of nearly normal cerebellar tissue lining their walls, suggesting that they may have formed from subarachnoid spaces that were engulfed by overmigration of cerebellar cortical neurons (134, 138).

The other major finding on imaging studies of FCMD is delayed myelination. The abnormal white matter is hypodense on CT and shows prolonged T1 and T2 on MR. Of note, when myelination does occur, it begins in the subcortical white matter and extends centrally (135) in a pattern completely opposite to that of normal development.

Muscle–Eye–Brain Disease

Muscle–eye–brain disease is another disorder that has a cobblestone cortex as one of its main features. This disorder

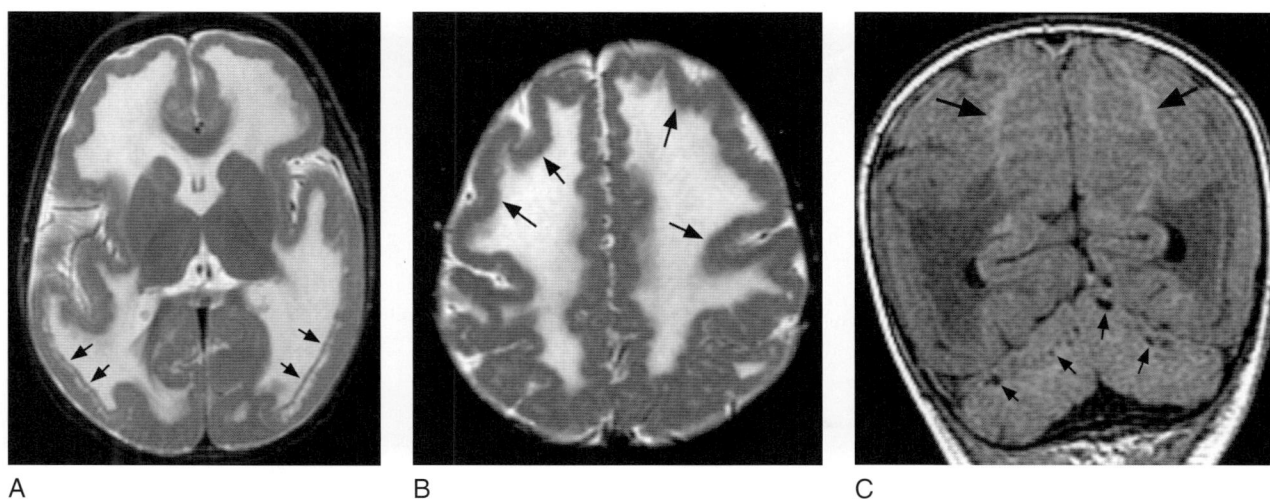

A   B   C

FIG. 7.14. Fukuyama congenital muscular dystrophy. **A.** Axial T2-weighted image showing the occipital cobblestone cortex, which is thick with a smooth outer surface but a slightly irregular inner surface. In addition, deep to the inner surface of the cortex, separated from the cortex by a layer of white matter, partly contiguous nodules of cortex (arrows) can be identified on high-resolution scans. Myelination (manifest as hypointensity on T2-weighted images) is almost completely missing in this 10-month-old infant. **B.** Axial T2-weighted image at a higher level showing polymicrogyria of the frontal lobes (arrows). **C.** Coronal T1-weighted image showing the characteristic cortical cysts in the cerebellar hemispheres (smaller arrows). In addition, note the subcortical myelination (hyperintensity of the white matter, large arrows) in the absence of deep white matter myelination.

is described primarily in patients from Finland. Patients with muscle–eye–brain disease have features similar to Walker–Warburg syndrome and FCMD, but the severity of involvement is intermediate between the other two diseases (139, 140). The disease has been linked to mutations of chromosome 1p32–34 (141).

In infancy and early childhood, affected children are hypotonic and have impaired vision (manifest as impaired visual fixation) from birth; epilepsy is common and mental retardation is usually severe (140). Spasticity typically begins to develop after age 5 years (140). Pathologic examination of the cerebral cortex reveals abnormal convolutions with a granular (cobblestone) surface to the cerebral cortex. A limited area of agyria may be seen on the occipital convexity. Light microscopy shows resemblance to the cortex in Walker–Warburg syndrome and FCMD in that irregular bundles of myelinated axons penetrate the cortex from the white matter and gliovascular strands cut through the cortex from the pia and separate the cortex into irregular neuronal clusters (142). No horizontal lamination or vertical columns of neurons can be identified. Similar gliovascular strands penetrate the cerebellar cortex, which is dysplastic and shows cysts similar to those in FCMD (142).

Neuroimaging of patients with muscle–eye–brain disease reveals diffusely abnormal cerebral cortex, which is thickened (anteriorly more than posteriorly) with decreased number and depth of sulci. The cortex–white matter junction may be irregular (Fig. 7.15). Myelination is delayed, and regions of T2 hyperintensity may remain within the cerebral hemispheres (Fig. 7.15) even after myelination is completed. In addition, the ventricles are large, the sylvian fissures are wide, the septum pellucidum is absent, the corpus callosum is dysplastic or hypoplastic, the pons and cerebellum are

hypoplastic (Fig. 7.16), and cerebellar cortical cysts are identified (143). Thus, the imaging appearance has features similar to the Walker–Warburg syndrome and FCMD.

Heterotopia

Gray matter heterotopia are collections of nerve cells in abnormal locations secondary to arrest of radial migration of neurons. (Note that the word heterotopia is plural; the singular form of the noun is heterotopion.) Patients with heterotopic gray matter almost always present with a seizure disorder (144–146). For the purposes of clinical evaluation and prognostication, it is useful to divide heterotopia into three groups:

- subependymal heterotopia;
- focal subcortical heterotopia;
- band heterotopia (double cortex) (146, 147).

Subependymal Heterotopia

In most affected patients, subependymal heterotopia are asymmetric, few in number, and largely confined to the trigones and the temporal and occipital horns of the lateral ventricles; these may be isolated or associated with other brain anomalies such as the Chiari II malformation, cephaloceles, or agenesis of the corpus callosum. A smaller number of patients have a large number of heterotopic nodules that completely or nearly completely line the walls of the lateral ventricles; these are sometimes called diffuse subependymal heterotopia (148).

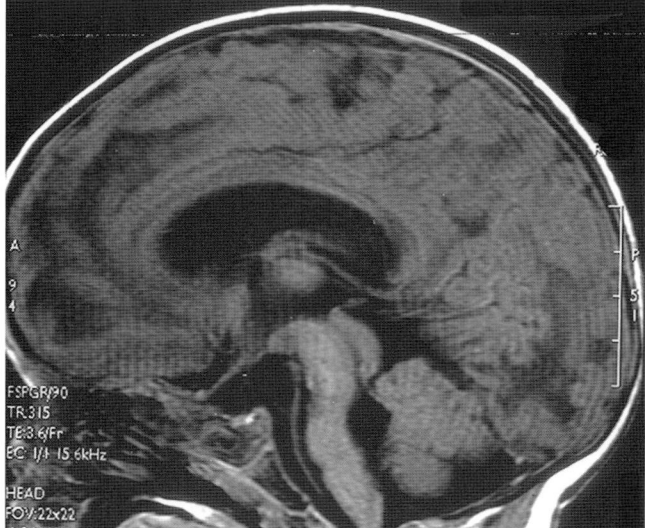

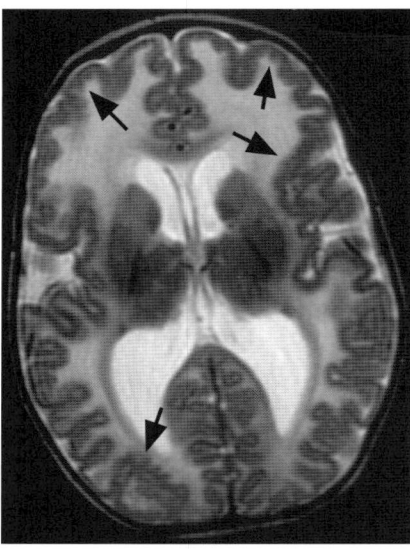

B

FIG. 7.15. Muscle–eye–brain disease. **A.** Sagittal T1-weighted image showing that the corpus callosum, pons, and cerebellum are hypoplastic. Cerebellar dysplasia, similar to that in Fukuyama congenital muscular dystrophy, is seen on axial and coronal images. **B.** Axial T2-weighted image showing diffusely abnormal cerebral cortex, which is thickened (anteriorly more than posteriorly) with decreased number and depth of sulci. The cortex–white matter junction is irregular (arrows) in multiple regions. Myelination is delayed.

It is likely that mutations of several genes can cause subependymal heterotopia (149) but the one that has been identified is the *FLN1* gene at chromosome Xq28 (150–152). The gene product, filamin-1, is a cytoplasmic structural protein that is anchored to cell surface receptors and has actin-binding domains that link the cell surface to the F-actin cytoskeleton; it is also involved in the formation of filapodia (153). The mechanism by which cell migration is impaired is unknown but is postulated to be impaired migration of immature neurons from the germinal zone due to

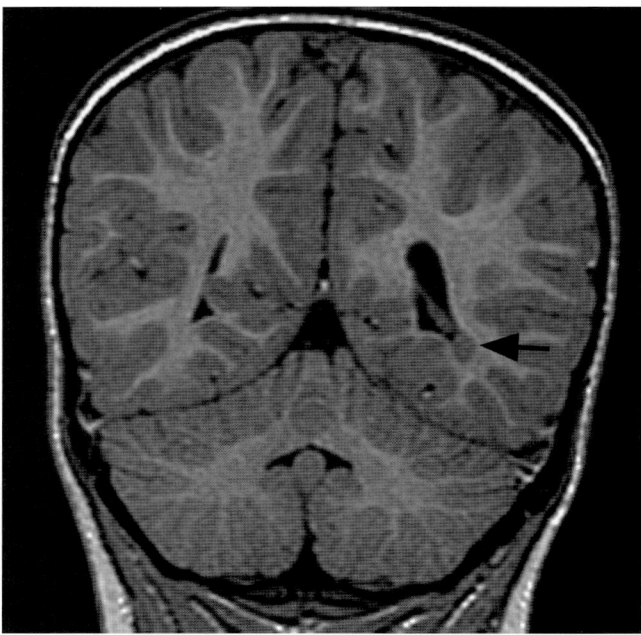

FIG. 7.16. Subependymal heterotopion. Coronal T1-weighted image showing a nodule of gray matter (arrow) in the inferior aspect of the left ventricular trigone.

these changes in the actin cytoskeleton and, perhaps, the inability of the nucleus to follow the leading process of the cell away from the germinal zone (153, 154).

Patients with isolated heterotopia (those without other brain or visceral anomalies) usually manifest mild clinical symptoms, with normal development, normal motor function, and onset of seizures during the second decade of life. Seizures are typically mixed partial complex and tonic–clonic (146, 151, 152) and may emanate from the heterotopia, the hippocampus, or both (155). Girls with X-linked subependymal heterotopia often have a large cisterna magna (144, 150, 156). Boys with syndromic subependymal heterotopia may have associated cortical malformations, syndactyly, ear abnormalities, and severe mental retardation (150).

Imaging studies reveal subependymal heterotopia as smooth, ovoid nodules that are isointense with gray matter on all imaging sequences (Fig. 7.17). The long axis of the nodule is parallel to the adjacent ventricular wall. The heterotopia may be considered cells in residual germinal matrix, perhaps persisting because of a defect in apoptosis; they are located in the wall of the ventricle and may be seen to protrude into the ventricular lumen.

Subependymal heterotopia due to *FLN1* mutations vary in configuration depending on what part of the filamen-1 protein is affected by the mutation and how severely protein function is impaired (149, 157). Although most patients with mutation of this gene show diffuse subependymal heterotopia lining the walls of the bodies of the lateral ventricles (Fig. 7.17), some with (relatively mild) local missense mutations may show only a few bilateral peritrigonal subependymal heterotopia (157).

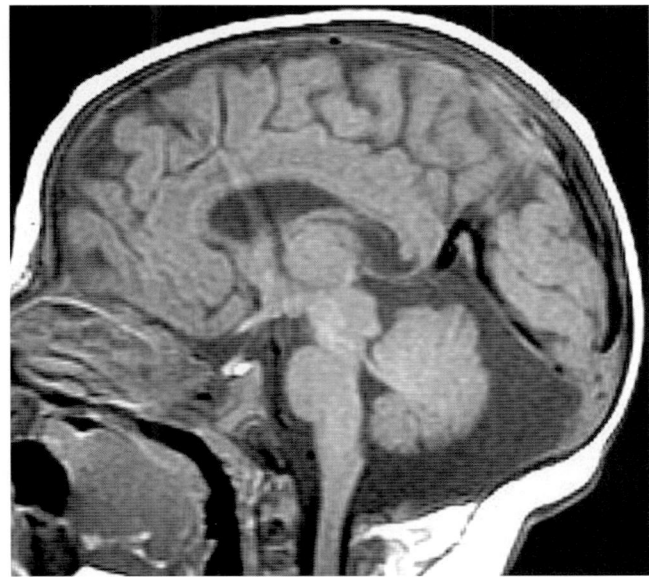

A

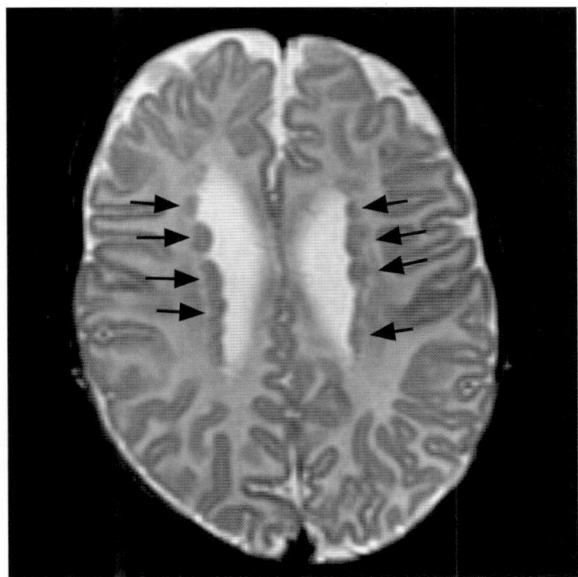

B

FIG. 7.17. Diffuse subependymal heterotopia in an infant with *FILN1* mutation. **A.** Sagittal T1-weighted image showing a large cisterna magna. **B.** Axial T2-weighted image showing multiple nodules of gray matter (arrows) lining the walls of the lateral ventricles.

Focal Subcortical Heterotopia

Patients with focal subcortical heterotopia have variable motor and intellectual disturbances, depending upon the size of the heterotopion and the effect on the overlying cortex (147, 158). Children with bilateral, large, thick subcortical heterotopia usually have moderate to severe developmental delay and motor dysfunction, whereas those with large unilateral heterotopia have hemiplegia and less severe (if any) mental retardation; children with small or thin unilateral subcortical heterotopia may have normal motor function and normal development (146, 158). Although exact numbers are not

known, it seems that most affected patients eventually develop epilepsy, usually during the first or second decades (146, 158). Some early reports suggest that surgical resection may be useful in patients with subcortical heterotopia and medically refractory epilepsy (159).

On neuroimaging, focal subcortical heterotopia appear as large, somewhat heterogeneous masses that are isointense to cortical gray matter on all sequences. They sometimes appear as multinodular gray matter masses and other times appear to be composed of swirling, curvilinear bands of gray matter. The portion of the hemisphere that is affected is almost always small, and the cortex overlying the heterotopion is thin, with shallow sulci, an appearance resembling polymicrogyria (Fig. 7.18).

Because the white matter in the affected portion of the cerebrum is reduced, the heterotopion may appear to exert a mass effect on the adjacent ventricle or the interhemispheric fissure and may thus be mistaken for tumor. Further scrutiny of the images, however, will show that the affected hemisphere is small and that the apparent mass effect is actually distortion of the hemisphere caused by the dysplasia. Thus, heterotopia can be differentiated from tumors, which will enlarge the affected hemisphere and, other than compression from mass effect, have a normal overlying cortex. Other important features in distinguishing heterotopia from tumors

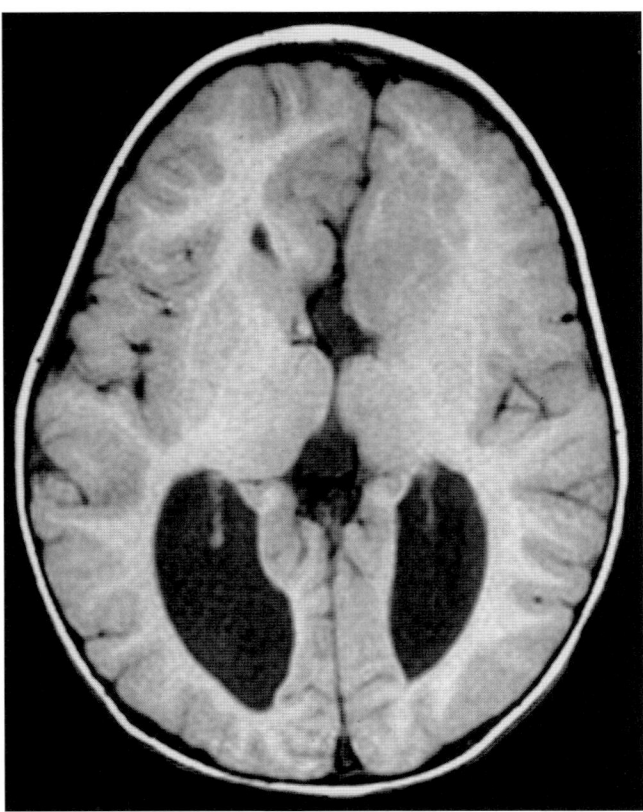

FIG. 7.18. Subependymal heterotopia. Axial T1-weighted image showing a large cluster of gray matter in the left frontal lobe, extending from the frontal horn to the cingulate gyrus. The left frontal lobes is small and the left frontal cortex has shallow sulci. The corpus callosum is absent.

are the lack of surrounding edema, isointensity with gray matter on all imaging sequences, and absence of enhancement after administration of contrast agents (79, 145, 146).

Associated brain anomalies are common; callosal agenesis or hypogenesis is present in about 70%, and the ipsilateral basal ganglia are dysplastic in >70% (158). Subcortical heterotopia will sometimes contain vessels or fluid, which, after close examination, are seen to be cerebrospinal fluid and vessels coursing in from the cerebral cortex (160).

Marsh et al. (161) reported that proton spectroscopy of heterotopia shows elevated creatine and choline with normal NAA. Li et al. found that the NAA:Cr ratio is variable, ranging from normal to low compared with age-matched normal controls (16).

Band Heterotopia (Double Cortex)

Patients with band heterotopia (112, 162), also called 'double cortex'(163, 164), may present for medical evaluation at any age, although they usually present in childhood with developmental delay of variable severity and mixed seizure disorders (112, 163, 164). Several authors have described patients who are normal except for relatively mild seizure disorders (109, 112, 163).

The overwhelming female preponderance (>90) is consistent with most cases resulting from mutations of the *DCX* (also called doublecortin) gene (6, 165), located on chromosome Xq22.3–q23 (108). Doublecortin is an intracellular phosphoprotein that binds and stabilizes microtubules and promotes microtubule assembly (111, 166, 167). Patients affected sporadically may have truncation or missense (single amino acid substitution) mutation, whereas most familial cases show missense mutations (168). Rarely, male patients with band heterotopia have been described (112, 169); most of these have missense mutations of *LIS1* (170) or somatic mosaicism, a condition in which some, but not all, neurons have the mutation of *DCX* (171). One case report revealed band heterotopia associated with trisomy 9p; however this patient had multiple other anomalies and mutation of Xq22.3–q23 was not ruled out (172).

On imaging, band heterotopia appear as homogeneous bands of gray matter that are situated between the lateral ventricles and the cerebral cortex and separated from both by a layer of normal-appearing white matter (Fig. 7.19). The overlying cortex may have normal or increased thickness; sulci are shallow. The heterotopia may be difficult to detect in the myelinated brain unless sequences that strongly contrast gray and white matter are used. Band heterotopia may be complete or partial (109, 173); when partial, the frontal lobes seem to be preferentially involved in *DCX* mutations, while the parietal lobes are affected in *LIS1* mutations (170, 174). In some patients, a second layer of heterotopia is present in the temporal lobe (112).

The severity of cortical anomaly seems to be related to the thickness of the band heterotopia; i.e., the thicker the band of heterotopic gray matter, the more shallow the sulci in the

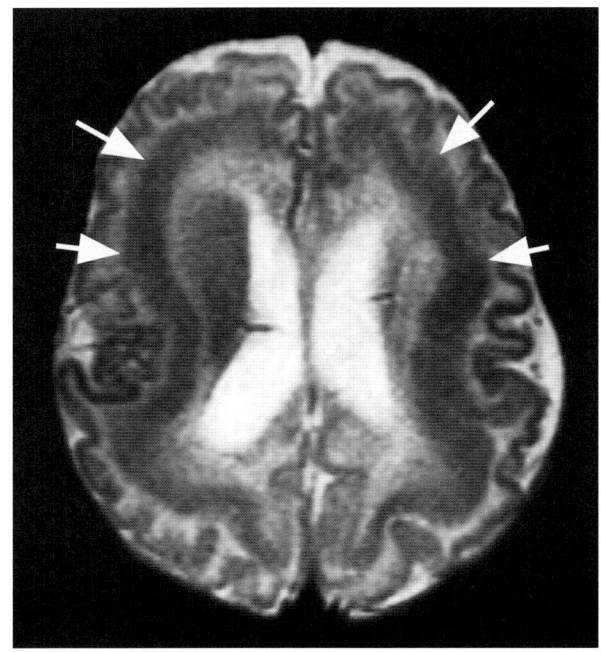

A

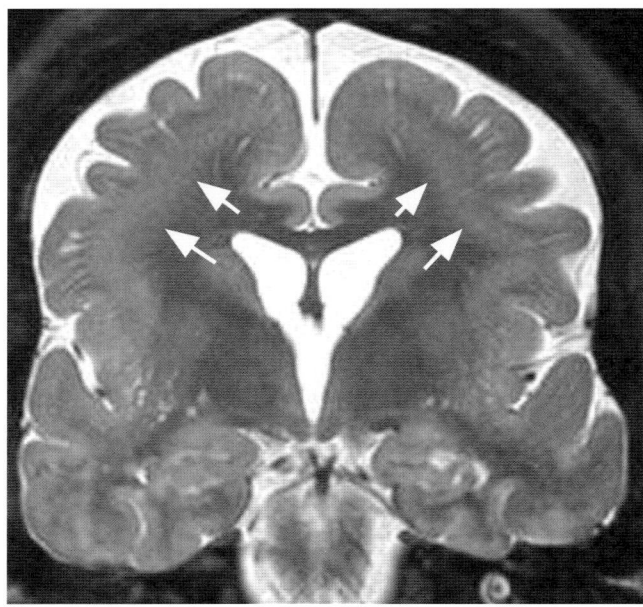

B

FIG. 7.19. Band heterotopia. **A.** Axial T2-weighted image in a neonate showing a circumferential band (arrows) that is thicker anteriorly than posteriorly. The cortical sulci are abnormally shallow. **B.** Coronal T2-weighted image in a 30-year-old woman with epilepsy showing that the band (arrows) is more difficult to appreciate in the myelinated brain.

overlying cortex (112). The more anomalous the cortex, the worse the clinical prognosis for epilepsy (112). Foci of T2 prolongation may be seen in the cerebral white matter; the presence of these foci is associated with a poor motor outcome (112). When imaged in a neonate, the band may be mistaken for myelinating white matter; identification of the cell-sparse zone between the band and the cortex, in addition to the shallow sulci, will help to make this differentiation easier.

When studied by PET using [^{18}F]-fluorodeoxyglucose, band heterotopia are found to have a glucose uptake that is similar to (175, 176) or greater than (177) normal cortex. This finding contrasts with the hypometabolism found in cortical dysplasias (see next section) and in most epileptogenic foci. Morell et al. (178) have found epileptiform discharges emanating from the band, suggesting that it is the source of the seizure activity in affected patients. Pinard et al. have found increased blood flow to the portion of the band that underlies the motor cortex using BOLD imaging (179). This combination of findings suggests that the band may have substantial communications with the rest of the brain and may send out projection fibers to communicate with the body.

Other Types of Heterotopia

Some heterotopia have configurations that do not fit into the three major groups. These include subependymal linear or laminar heterotopia, which are smooth linear regions of heterotopia that line the ependymal wall of the lateral ventricle, and 'ribbon' heterotopia (Fig. 7.20), curvilinear undulations of heterotopic gray matter in the deep, periventricular white matter. At present, the subependymal linear heterotopia are classified simply as subependymal heterotopia and ribbon heterotopia are classified as subcortical heterotopia. The clinical phenotypes and genetics of these particular entities are not well known at present.

Malformations Secondary to Abnormal Cortical Organization

Polymicrogyria

In polymicrogyria, the neurons reach the cortex but distribute abnormally, resulting in the formation of multiple small gyri; thus, it is a disorder of neuronal organization (30). Polymicrogyria has a range of histologic appearances, all having in common a derangement of the normal six-layered lamination of the cortex (119); thus, it may be considered a cortical dysplasia. However, the term cortical dysplasia is generally applied to smaller foci of abnormal cortical lamination that contain dysplastic neurons (180). Therefore, the term polymicrogyria, which is a well-established descriptive term, seems appropriate if one recognizes that this is probably the end result of a number of different causes.

Patients with polymicrogyria may present with developmental delay, focal neurologic signs and symptoms, or epilepsy, depending upon the portion(s) of brain involved. The condition may be associated with congenital cytomegalovirus infection, in utero ischemia (181, 182), or chromosomal mutations (mutations of Xq28, 16q12.2–21, 1p36, and 22q11.2 have been identified (9, 183–187)). No difference in neurologic manifestations have been detected in

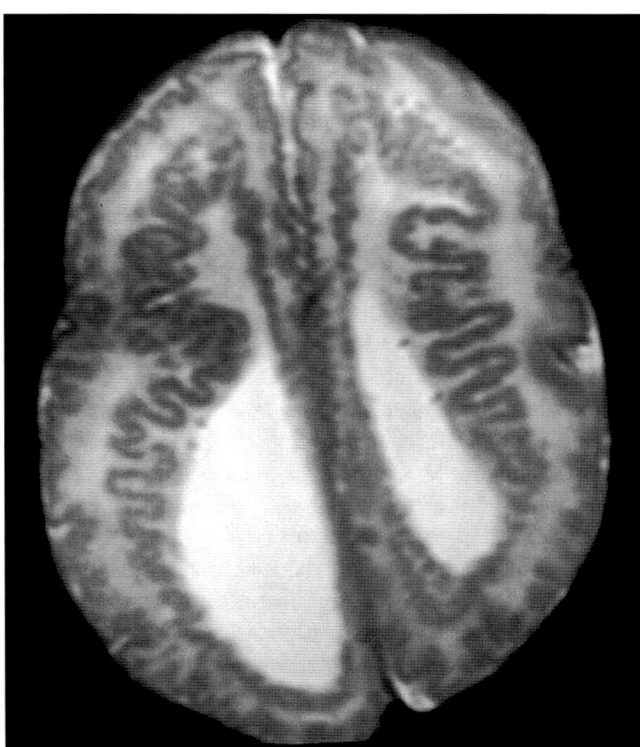

FIG. 7.20. Ribbon heterotopia. Axial T2-weighted image of a neonate showing an undulating ribbon of gray matter in the periventricular white matter. It is not clear whether this 'ribbon' is a variant of subcortical heterotopia or a separate entity.

patients who have polymicrogyria due to congenital infections versus other causes (188–190).

Because the presentations are so variable, the diagnosis may be made at any age, in infants or in septuagenarians who are undergoing imaging as part of a metastatic work-up. Questioning of older patients may reveal a history of congenital hemiplegia, epilepsy, or 'cerebral palsy'. The severity of the clinical presentation depends upon the extent of cortical involvement; bilateral involvement and involvement of more than half of a single hemisphere are poor prognostic indicators, portending moderate to severe developmental delay and significant motor dysfunction (190). The malformation may be focal, multifocal, or diffuse; it may be unilateral, bilateral and asymmetrical, or bilateral and symmetrical. The most common location is around the sylvian fissure (191), particularly the posterior aspect of the fissure; however, any cortical area, including the frontal, occipital, and temporal lobes, can be affected (119, 188, 190–192).

Syndromes Associated with Polymicrogyria

Several specific syndromes are associated with cerebral polymicrogyria. Kuzniecky et al. have described a syndrome of bilateral opercular polymicrogyria (congenital bilateral perisylvian syndrome), which may be sporadic or familial (187, 193, 194). The inheritance patterns of familial cases appear to be heterogeneous, suggesting that mutations of several different genes can cause this malformation (194); one location, on Xq28, has been identified (185). Sporadic cases typically present with a syndrome of developmental pseudobulbar palsy (oropharyngeal dysfunction and dysarthria, 100%), epilepsy (80–90%), mental retardation (50–80%), and, sometimes, congenital arthrogryposis (193, 195–198). Some patients present in infancy or early childhood with developmental delay (60%), poor palatal function (40%), hypotonia (30%), arthrogryposis (30%), and motor deficits (25%) (196, 199). Seizures (many clinical types) are present in 40–60% (196, 199, 200). Studies of familial cases of congenital bilateral perisylvian polymicrogyria show a lower incidence of these clinical manifestations (194), possibly because patients with minimal symptoms are more readily identified and examined.

Other syndromes of bilateral symmetrical polymicrogyria have been described (201). Several groups have described *bilateral symmetrical frontoparietal polymicrogyria* (202); a gene for this disorder has been identified at 16q12.2–21 (9). Affected patients show a characteristic syndrome of developmental delay in both cognitive and motor spheres, disconjugate gaze (typically esotropia), refractory seizures, and bilateral pyramidal and cerebellar signs (Dr Chris Walsh, personal communication). Guerrini *et al.* have described patients with *bilateral medial parietal-occipital polymicrogyria* (192, 203). In addition, cases of bilateral lateral parietal polymicrogyria and those with combinations of the above-mentioned patterns have been described; thus, it appears that any region of cortex may be involved by bilateral, symmetrical polymicrogyria (201).

Epilepsy syndromes can also be associated with polymicrogyria (188, 190, 192, 195, 200, 204). The epileptogenic focus is typically not within the dysplastic cortex itself but in the cortex adjacent to the polymicrogyria, known as the paramicrogyral zone (205). Studies in laboratory animals show increases in postsynaptic glutamate (excitatory) receptors and decreases in $GABA_A$ (inhibitory) receptors in the polymicrogyric cortex (205), factors that probably promote epileptogenesis. In addition, the polymicrogyric cortex appears to have fewer axonal connections with the rest of the brain (205). This lack of connections may be the reason why polymicrogyric cortex does not function normally and why seizures emanate from the paramicrogyral zone instead of the dysplastic cortex itself.

Imaging of Polymicrogyria

On MR imaging, polymicrogyria has two main appearances. The first is of a thin cortex (3 mm) with irregular inner and outer cortical margins (Figs 7.21, 7.22); this appearance is seen in the neonate or young infant with unmyelinated brain. The second pattern is that of a rather thick cortex (6–8 mm) with a variably irregular outer surface and an irregular inner surface (Figs 7.21, 7.22). As most patients with polymicrogyria are imaged after myelination has begun, the latter appearance is more common. With the second

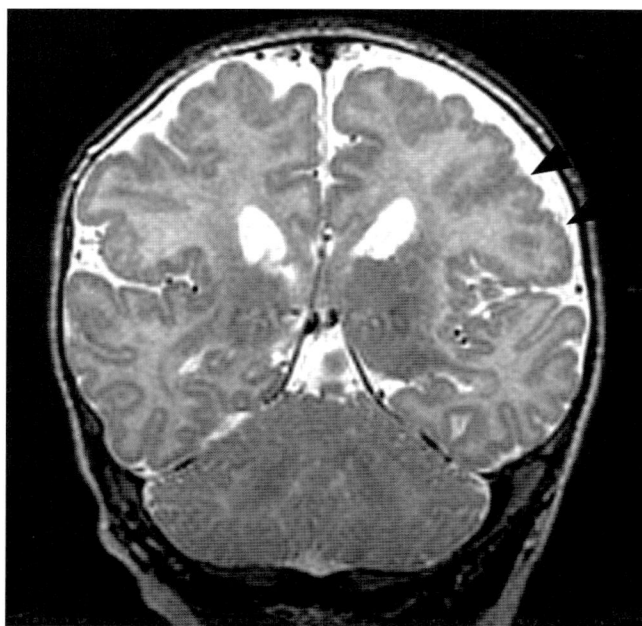

FIG. 7.21. Polymicrogyria in a 4-week-old infant. The cortex is thin and undulating.

pattern, the scan may show an irregularly bumpy surface or be paradoxically smooth because the outer cortical (molecular) layer fuses over the microsulci. In addition, the appearance may vary with the technique used to acquire the images; it may have the appearance of pachygyria, with broad, thickened gyri (79, 188, 190), or look normal if thick (5 mm or larger) sections are acquired or if the subcortical white matter is incompletely myelinated.

Thus, because the gyri are so small, polymicrogyria may be missed or misdiagnosed on routine spin-echo images.

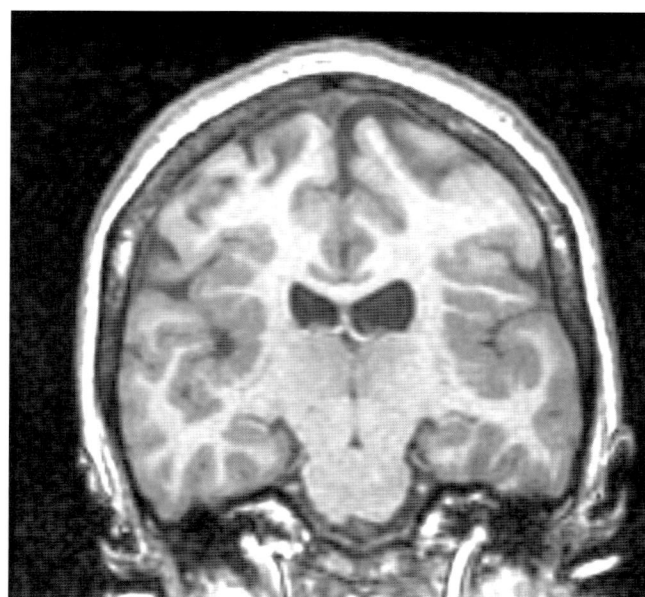

FIG. 7.22. T1-weighted images showing typical bilateral perisylvian polymicrogyria in a patient with CBPS. The abnormalities often extend beyond the opercular regions.

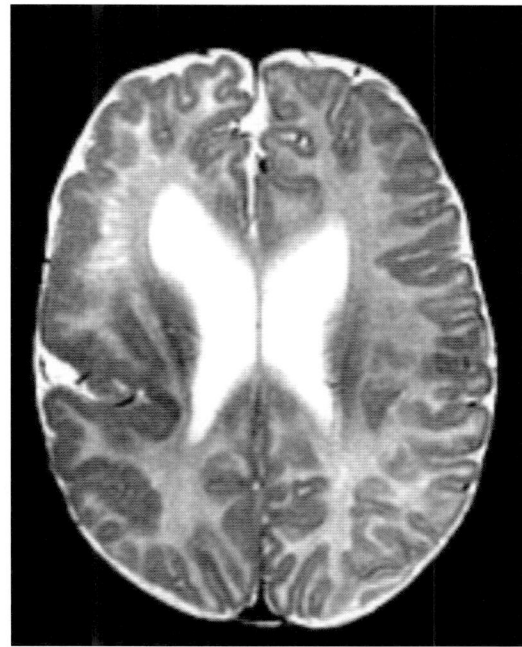

A

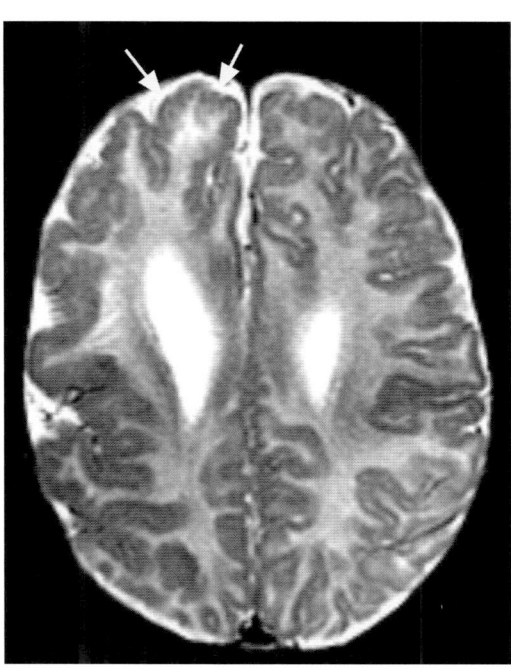

B

FIG. 7.23. Polymicrogyria in a 6-month-old infant with congenital hemiplegia, diagnosed as early hand preference. **A** is at the level of the lateral ventricles and **B** at the level of the centrum semiovale. Nearly the entire right frontal lobe is affected. Note the thin, undulating cortex in the prefrontal region of **B** (arrows). The white matter beneath the affected cortex is abnormally hyperintense, probably resulting from dilated perivascular spaces, and the ipsilateral lateral ventricle is enlarged.

Images with thin sections and optimal gray–white matter contrast (we use volume three-dimensional gradient-echo spoiled gradient acquisition (T1-weighted) and volume three-dimensional fast spin-echo (T2-weighted) images, both with ≤1.5 mm partition size) are obtained. Evaluation in

three planes is often necessary to detect irregularities of the gray–white matter junction, which are often the only evidence of dysplastic brain (121). The volume acquisitions can be displayed as two-dimensional images in any plane or as three-dimensional images, and can be used for stereotactic localization for surgical therapy.

Regions of polymicrogyria can be flat and congruent to the arc of normal cortex (Fig. 7.23A,B), or may extend centripetally, with the cortex appearing as if it were buckled or folded inward (Fig. 7.24). The affected cortex is usually isointense to normal cortex on imaging studies, unless it is calcified (≈5%). Polymicrogyria may be unilateral (≈40%) or bilateral (≈60%). The cortex surrounding the sylvian fissures is involved in approximately 80% of cases, with the frontal lobe being most commonly involved (≈70%), followed by parietal (63%), temporal (38%), and occipital (7%) lobes (191). The striate cortex, cingulate gyrus, hippocampus, and gyrus rectus are typically spared (191).

Abnormalities of the underlying white matter are common. Prolonged T2 relaxation time is present in the white matter underlying the dysplastic cortex in about 20–27% of patients (34, 190, 191, 206); recent studies suggest that these are dilated perivascular spaces (Fig. 7.25) (191). Finally, it is important to realize that anomalous venous drainage is common in areas of dysplastic cortex (207), seen in up to 51% (191). Large vessels are especially common in regions where there is a large infolding of thickened cortex. These are not vascular malformations and do not require angiography.

Proton MR spectroscopy seems to be normal in regions of polymicrogyria (16).

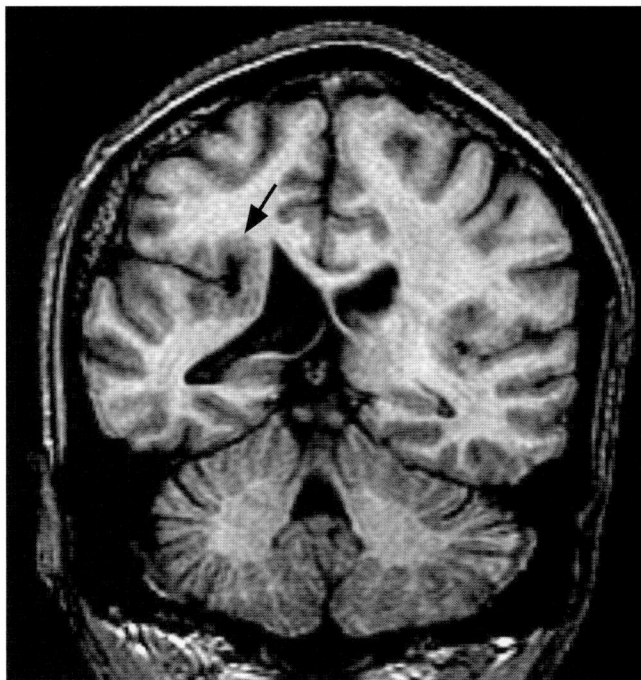

FIG. 7.24. Polymicrogyria in a 25-year-old woman with epilepsy. Abnormal infolding of cortex (arrow) indents the trigone of the right lateral ventricle. Note the irregular cortical–white matter junction.

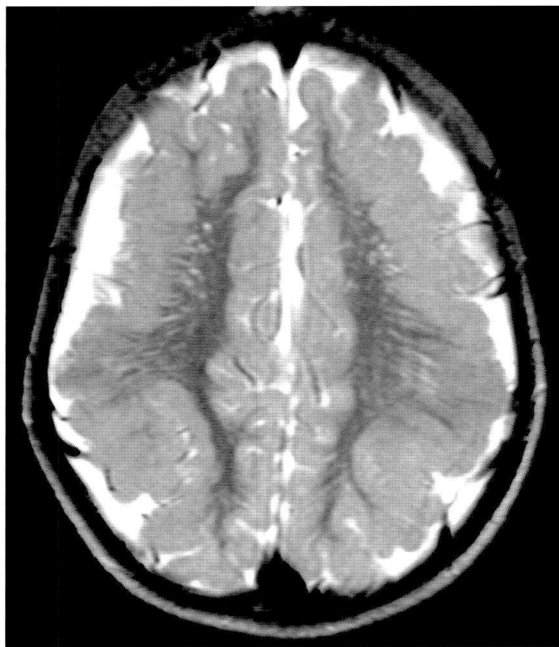

A

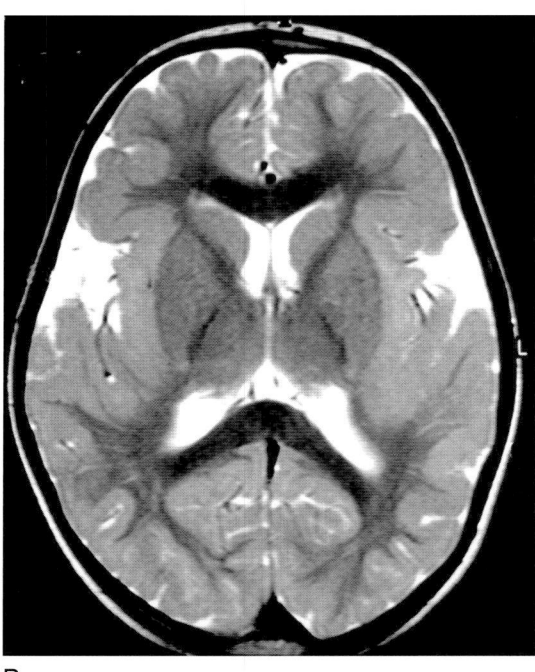

B

FIG. 7.25. Bilateral frontoparietal polymicrogyria. **A.** At the level of the centrum semiovale, polymicrogyria is seen in all of the frontal and parietal lobes visualized. Dilated perivascular spaces are seen in the underlying white matter. **B.** At the level of the basal ganglia, the opercula are seen to be enlarged and the insular cortex abnormally thickened.

Schizencephaly

The term schizencephaly describes gray-matter-lined clefts that extend through the entire cerebral hemisphere, from the lateral ventricle to the cortex (208, 209). Both genetic and acquired causes have been postulated, including in-utero transmantle injury (ischemic or infectious) during the middle portion of the second trimester. Other cases seem to be familial (210–212) and may be associated with mutations of the *EMX2* homeobox gene, located on chromosome 10q26 (210, 213), a gene expressed in the germinal matrix of the developing cerebral neocortex (214). For prognostic purposes, patients with schizencephaly are divided into those with unilateral (≈60%) and bilateral clefts (≈40%); the clefts are further divided into those with fused lips (closed lip schizencephaly, 15–20%) and those with separated lips (open lip schizencephaly) (215–218). The walls of clefts with fused lips appose one another directly, obliterating the cerebrospinal fluid space within the cleft at that point. Cerebrospinal fluid fills clefts with separated lips from the lateral ventricle to the subarachnoid spaces (208, 209, 217, 219).

It is thought that schizencephaly and polymicrogyria are similar entities. This is based on the fact that the clefts are lined by polymicrogyria and mechanistically schizencephaly is at the end of the spectrum in polymicrogyria. Whether this is the case in all patients is not known at present.

The severity of the affected patient's symptoms is related to the amount of involved brain (216, 217, 220, 221). Those patients with a single cleft with fused lips generally have epilepsy and, perhaps, a mild hemiparesis but are otherwise developmentally normal. Patients with unilateral clefts with separated lips are typically brought to medical attention because of macrocephaly and hemiparesis; ultimately, most develop epilepsy (>80%) and a mild to moderate developmental delay, depending upon the size and location of the cleft within the brain (215, 217, 220). Patients with bilateral clefts tend to be severely retarded with early onset of epilepsy, severe motor anomalies, and, frequently, blindness (216, 217, 220, 221). The blindness may relate to optic nerve hypoplasia, which is seen in up to one-third of patients with schizencephaly (222, 223). Some authors have noted that epilepsy is less common in bilateral than in unilateral schizencephaly (224). They speculate that the bilateral clefts may impair spread of the epileptic discharges. However, most reports suggest that seizures begin earlier and have worse outcome when clefts are bilateral (216, 220).

Imaging studies of schizencephaly show a full-thickness cleft through the affected hemisphere (Figs 7.26, 7.27); gray matter, typically characterized by a bumpy outer surface and an irregular gray–white matter junction, lines the cleft (79, 217, 219). This gray matter can extend into the ventricle and partially line the wall of the ventricle as heterotopic gray matter (see Fig. 7.27). Although any portion of the brain can be involved, the frontal horns and the anterior aspects of the temporal horns are relatively spared (218). The gyral pattern of the cortex adjacent to the cleft is usually abnormal (see Fig. 7.27), demonstrating sulci that radiate into the cleft.

Clefts with fused lips can be missed if the imaging plane is parallel to the plane of the cleft; therefore, imaging of patients who present with seizures or developmental delay should always be performed in at least two planes. Dysplastic cerebral cortex may be present in a 'mirror-image' location in

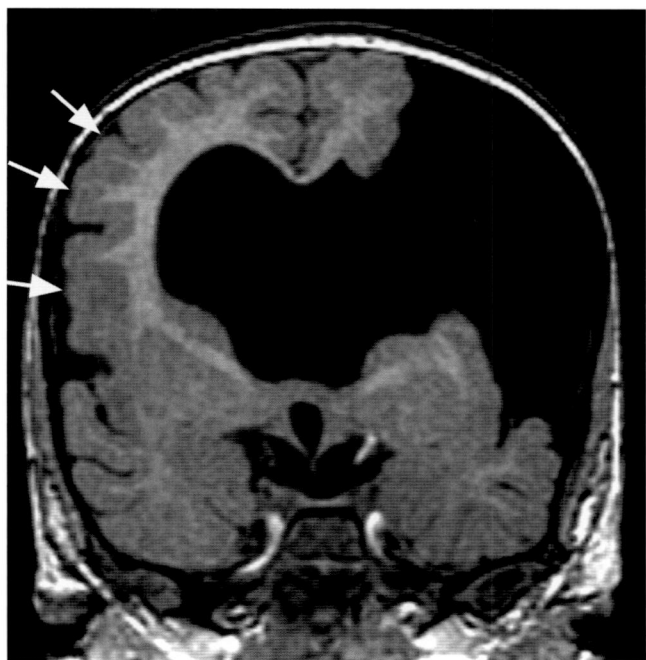

FIG. 7.26. Unilateral open-lip schizencephaly. Coronal T1-weighted image showing a large, gray matter lined communication between the left frontal horn and the subarachnoid space. Note the abnormally shallow sulci in the contralateral hemisphere (arrows).

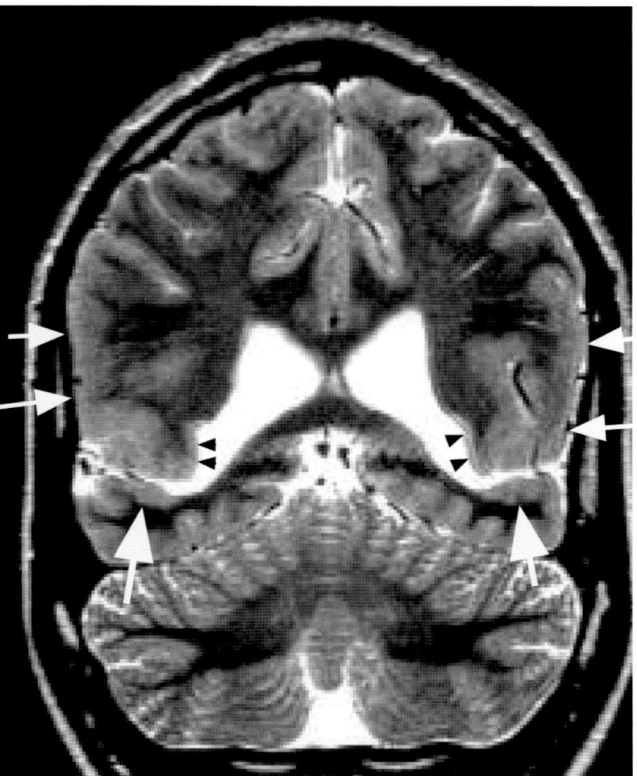

FIG. 7.27. Bilateral open lip schizencephaly. Coronal T2-weighted image showing bilateral horizontal small open-lip schizencephalies (large white arrows) extending from the ventricular trigones to the lateral surface of the hemispheres. The surrounding cortex (large white arrows) has an abnormal gyral pattern. Small areas of heterotopic gray matter (small black arrowheads) line the wall of the ventricles adjacent to the clefts.

the hemisphere contralateral to a unilateral schizencephaly in as many as 30% of patients, particularly when the schizencephaly is large and open-lipped (see Fig. 7.26) (190, 217, 218); thus, the contralateral hemisphere should always be scrutinized. The septum pellucidum is absent in about 70% of patients with schizencephaly (218) and is almost always absent when the clefts are bilateral; when unilateral, the septum is more commonly absent when the cleft is separated rather than fused.

Focal Cortical Dysplasia Without Balloon Cells

In focal cortical dysplasia without balloon cells, a focal abnormality of lamination is present in the cerebral cortex and, usually, the underlying white matter without the presence of balloon cells or of abnormal cells extending medially to the ventricular surface (180, 225–227). Patients with this type of focal cortical dysplasia almost always present with partial seizure disorders and normal neurologic examination.

The most common MR appearance, in my experience, is that of focal cortical thinning with hyperintensity of the underlying white matter, as if a previous ischemic injury has occurred. Frequently, the MR scan initially appears normal (228). Careful evaluation with thin sections and optimal gray matter-white matter contrast may show focal blurring of the cortical-white matter junction (229, 230); however, if dyslamination is the only abnormality, MR may be completely normal (228). A helpful finding may be a 'dimple' in the cortex, a focus where the size of the subarachnoid space

is focally increased (231). The relative signal intensity of dysplastic cortex and underlying white matter may change with age; therefore, serial MR studies may be necessary to find the focus in young infants (232). If the patients have refractory epilepsy or infantile spasms, PET scanning may aid in localizing the focus by showing local hypometabolism (23, 228).

Other Conditions Associated With Focal Cortical Dysplasia

Cortical dysplasia is often associated with other conditions. The best described of these conditions are neuronal–glial tumors (dysembryoplastic neuroepithelial tumors (233, 234) and gangliogliomas (235)) and mesial temporal sclerosis (236, 237). Discussion of these entities is beyond the scope of this chapter.

REFERENCES

1. Kuzniecky R, Murro A, King D, et al. Magnetic resonance imaging in childhood intractable partial epilepsy: pathologic correlations. *Neurology* 1993;43:681–687.

2. Wyllie E, Comair Y, Kotagal P, et al. Seizure outcome after epilepsy surgery in children and adolescents. *Ann Neurol* 1998;44:740–748.

3. Farrell MA, DeRosa M, Curran J, et al. Neuropathologic findings in cortical resections (including hemispherectomies) performed for the treatment of intractable childhood epilepsy. *Acta Neuropathol* 1992;83:246–259.

4. Frater JL, Prayson RA, Morris HH III, Bingaman WE. Surgical pathologic findings of extratemporal-based intractable epilepsy. A study of 133 consecutive resections. *Arch Pathol Lab Med* 2000; 124:545–549.

5. Pasquier B, Péoch M, Fabre-Bocquentin B, et al. Surgical pathology of drug-resistant partial epilepsy. A 10-year experience with a series of 327 consecutive resections. *Epileptic Disord* 2002;4:99–119.

6. Gleeson JG, Allen KA, Fox JW, et al. Doublecortin, a brain-specific gene mutated in human X-linked lissencephaly and double cortex syndrome, encodes a putative signaling protein. *Cell* 1998;92:63–72.

7. Fox JW, Lamperti ED, Eksioglu YZ, et al. Mutations in filamin 1 prevent migration of cerebral cortical neurons in human periventricular heterotopia. *Neuron* 1998;21:1315–1325.

8. Hong SE, Shugart YY, Huang DT, et al. Autosomal recessive lissencephaly with cerebellar hypoplasia (LCH) is associated with human reelin gene mutations. *Nature Genet* 2000;26:93–96.

9. Piao X, Basel-Vanagaite L, Straussberg R, et al. An autosomal recessive form of bilateral frontoparietal polymicrogyria maps to chromosome 16q12.2–21. *Am J Hum Genet* 2002;70:1028–1033.

10. Raymond AA, Fish DR, Sisodiya SM, et al. Abnormalities of gyration, heterotopias, tuberous sclerosis, focal cortical dysplasia, micro-dysgenesis, dysembryoplastic neuroepithelial tumor and dysgenesis of the archicortex in epilepsy: clinical, EEG and neuroimaging features in 100 adult patients. *Brain* 1995;118:629–660.

11. Barkovich AJ, Rowley HA, Andermann F. MR imaging in partial epilepsies: value of high resolution volumetric techniques. *Am J Neuroradiol* 1995;16:339–344.

12. Grant PE, Barkovich AJ, Wald LL, et al. High-resolution surface coil MR of cortical lesions in medically refractory epilepsy: a prospective study. *Am J Neuroradiol* 1997;18:291–301.

13. Kuzniecky R, Hetherington H, Pan J, et al. Proton spectroscopic imaging at 4.1 tesla in patients with malformations of cortical development and epilepsy. *Neurology* 1997;48:1018–1024.

14. Garcia PA, Laxer KD, van der Grond J, et al. Proton magnetic resonance spectroscopic imaging in patients with frontal lobe epilepsy. *Ann Neurol* 1995;37:279–281.

15. Woermann FG, McLean MA, Bartlett PA, et al. Quantitative short echo time proton magnetic resonance spectroscopic imaging study of malformations of cortical development causing epilepsy. *Brain* 2001; 124:427–436.

16. Li LM, Cendes F, Bastos AC, et al. Neuronal metabolic dysfunction in patients with cortical developmental malformations. A proton magnetic resonance spectroscopic imaging study. *Neurology* 1998;50: 755–759.

17. Eriksson SH, Rugg-Gunn FJ, Symms MR, et al. Diffusion tensor imaging in patients with epilepsy and malformations of cortical development. *Brain* 2001;124:617–626.

18. Rugg-Gunn FJ, Eriksson SH, Symms MR, et al. Diffusion tensor imaging of cryptogenic and acquired partial epilepsies. *Brain* 2001;124:627–636.

19. Swartz BE, Khonsari A, Brown C, et al. Improved sensitivity of [18]FDG-positron emission tomography scans in frontal and 'frontal plus' epilepsy. *Epilepsia* 1995;36:388–395.

20. Richardson MP, Koepp MJ, Brooks DJ, et al. Benzodiazepine receptors in focal epilepsy with cortical dysgenesis: an ^{11}C-Flumazenil PET study. *Ann Neurol* 1996;40:188–198.

21. Newton MR, Austin MC, Chan JG, et al. Ictal SPECT using [99]m-Tc-HMPAO: methods for rapid preparation and optimal deployment of tracer during spontaneous seizures. *J Nucl Med* 1993; 34:666–670.

22. Lee N, Radtke R, Gray L, et al. Neuronal migration disorders: positron emission tomography correlations. *Ann Neurol* 1994;35:290–297.

23. Chugani HT, Shields WD, Shewmon DA, et al. Infantile spasms: I. PET identifies focal cortical dysgenesis in cryptogenic cases for surgical treatment. *Ann Neurol* 1990;27:406–413.

24. Chiron C, Dulac O, Nuttin C, Depas G. Functional imaging in cortical dysplasia: SPECT. Philadelphia: Lippencott-Raven, 1996.

25. Richardson MP, Koepp MJ, Brooks DJ, Duncan JS. ^{11}C-flumazenil PET in neocortical epilepsy. *Neurology* 1998;51:485–492.

26. Fois A, Farnetani MA, Balestri P, et al. EEG, PET, SPET, and MRI in intractable childhood epilepsies: possible surgical correlations. *Child's Nerv Syst* 1995;11:672–678.

27. Newton MR, Berkovic SF, Austin MC, et al. SPECT in the localization of extra-temporal and temporal seizure foci. *J Neurol Neurosurg Psychiatry* 1995;59:26–30.

28. Sasaki M, Kuwabara Y, Yoshida T, et al. Carbon-11-methionine PET in focal cortical dysplasia: a comparison with fluorine-18-FDG PET and technetium-99m-ECD SPECT. *J Nucl Med* 1998;39:974–977.

29. Madakasira PV, Simkins R, Narayanan T, et al. Cortical dysplasia localized by [11C]methionine positron emission tomography: case report. *Am J Neuroradiol* 2002;23:844–846.

30. Barkovich AJ, Kuzniecky RI, Jackson GD, et al. Classification system for malformations of cortical development: Update 2001. *Neurology* 2001;57:2168–2178.

31. Barkovich AJ, Ferriero DM, Barr RM, et al. Microlissencephaly: a heterogeneous malformation of cortical development. *Neuropediatrics* 1998;29:113–119.

32. Dobyns W, Barkovich A. Microcephaly with simplified gyral pattern (oligogyric microcephaly) and microlissencephaly. *Neuropediatrics* 1999;30:105–106.

33. Barkovich AJ, Kuzniecky RI, Bollen AW, Grant PE. Focal transmantle dysplasia: a specific malformation of cortical development. *Neurology* 1997;49:1148–1152.

34. Palmini A, Andermann F, Olivier A, et al. Focal neuronal migration disorders and intractable partial epilepsy: results of surgical treatment. *Ann Neurol* 1991;30:750–757.

35. Palmini A, Gambardella A, Andermann F, et al. The human dysplastic cortex is intrinsically epileptogenic. In: Guerrini R, Andermann F, Canapicchi R, et al., eds. Dysplasias of cerebral cortex and epilepsy. Philadelphia, PA: Lippencott-Raven, 1996:43–52.

36. Bronen RA, Vives KP, Kim JH, et al. Focal cortical dysplasia of Taylor, balloon cell subtype: MR differentiation from low-grade tumors. *Am J Neuroradiol* 1997;18:1141–1151.

37. Urbach H, Scheffler B, Heinrichsmeier T, et al. Focal cortical dysplasia of Taylor's balloon cell type: a clinicopathological entity with characteristic neuroimaging and histopathological features, and favorable postsurgical outcome. *Epilepsia* 2002;43:33–40.

38. Marusic P, Najm IM, Ying Z, et al. Focal cortical dysplasias in eloquent cortex: functional characteristics and correlation with MRI and histopathologic changes. *Epilepsia* 2002;43:27–32.

39. Haines JL, Short MP, Kwiatkowski DJ, et al. Localization of one gene for tuberous sclerosis within 9q32–9q34, and further evidence for heterogeneity. *Am J Med Genet* 1991;49:764–772.

40. Harris RM, Carter NP, Griffithe B, et al. Physical mapping within the tuberous sclerosis linkage group in region 9q32-q34. *Genomics* 1993; 15:265–274.

41. Kandt RS, Haines JL, Smith M, et al. Linkage of an important gene locus for tuberous sclerosis to a chromosome 16 marker for polycystic kidney disease. *Nature Genet* 1992;2:37–41.

42. Consortium ECTS. Identification and characterization of the tuberous sclerosis gene on chromosome 16. *Cell* 1993;75:1305–1315.

43. Johnson M, Emelin J, Park S-H, Vinters, HV. Co-localization of TSC1 and TSC2 gene products in tubers of patients with tuberous sclerosis. *Brain Pathol* 1999;9:45–54.

44. Van Siegtenhorst M, Nellist M, Nagelkerken B, et al. Interaction between hamartin and tuberin, the TSC1 and TSC2 gene products. *Hum Mol Genet* 1998;7:1053–1057.

45. Dabora SL, Jozwiak S, Franz DN, et al. Mutational analysis in a cohort of 224 tuberous sclerosis patients indicates increased severity of TSC2,

compared with TSC1, disease in multiple organs. *Am J Hum Genet* 2001;68:64–80.

46. Jones A, Shyamsundar M, Thomas M, et al. Comprehensive mutation analysis of TSC1 and TSC2-and phenotypic correlations in150 families with tuberous sclerosis. *Am J Hum Genet* 1999;64:1305–1315.

47. MacCollin M, Kwiatkowski D. Molecular genetic aspects of the phakomatoses. *Curr Opin Neurol* 2001;14:163–169.

48. Webb DW, Osborne JP. Tuberous sclerosis. *Arch Dis Child* 1995;72: 471–474.

49. Rose V, Au K-S, Pollom G, et al. Germ-line mosaicism in tuberous sclerosis: how common? *Am J Hum Genet* 1999;64:986–992.

50. Griffiths PD, Martland TR. Tuberous sclerosis complex: the role of neuroradiology. *Neuropediatrics* 1997;28:244–252.

51. Gomez MR. Tuberous sclerosis complex, 3rd ed. New York: Oxford University Press, 1999.

52. O'Callaghan FJ, Osborne JP. Advances in the understanding of tuberous sclerosis. *Arch Dis Child* 2000;83:140–142.

53. Gomez MR. Tuberous sclerosis, 2nd ed. New York: Raven Press, 1988.

54. Ahlsen G, Gillberg IC, Lindblom R, Gillberg C. Tuberous sclerosis in western Sweden. A population study of cases with early childhood onset. *Arch Neurol* 1994;51:76–81.

55. Roach E, Gomez M, Northrup H. Tuberous sclerosis complex consensus conference: revised clinical diagnostic criteria. *J Child Neurol* 1998;13:624–628.

56. Fukushima K, Inoue Y, Fujiwara T, Yagi K. Long term course of West syndrome associated with tuberous sclerosis. *Epilepsia* 1998;39:51–54.

57. Kingsley DPE, Kendall BE, Fitz CR. Tuberous sclerosis: a clinico-radiological evaluation of 110 cases with particular reference to atypical presentation. *Neuroradiology* 1986;28:171–190.

58. Shepherd CW, Houser OW, Gomez MR. MR findings in tuberous sclerosis complex and correlation with seizure development and mental impairment. *Am J Neuroradiol* 1995;16:149–155.

59. Lagos JC, Gomez MR. Tuberous sclerosis: reappraisal of a clinical entity. *Mayo Clin Proc* 1967;42:26–49.

60. Barkovich A. The phakomatoses. In: Barkovich A, ed. Pediatric neuroimaging, 3rd ed. Philadelphia, PA: Lippincott Williams & Wilkins, 2000:383–442.

61. Baron Y, Barkovich AJ. MR imaging of tuberous sclerosis in neonates and young infants. *Am J Neuroradiol* 1999;20:907–916.

62. Braffman BH, Bilaniuk LT, Naidich TP, et al. MR imaging of tuberous sclerosis: pathogenesis of this phakomatosis, use of gadopentate dimeglumine, and literature review. *Radiology* 1992;183:227–238.

63. Tsuchida T, Kamata K, Kwamata M, et al. Brain tumors in tuberous sclerosis. *Child's Brain* 1981;8:271–283.

64. Morimoto K, Mogami H. Sequential study of subependymal giant cell astrocytoma associated with tuberous sclerosis. *J Neurosurg* 1986;65:874–877.

65. Mackay MT, Becker LE, Chuang SH, et al. Malformations of cortical development with balloon cells. Clinical and radiologic correlates. *Neurology* 2003;60:580–587.

66. Berg BO. Neurocutaneous disorders. In: Berg B, ed. Neurologic manifestations of pediatrics. Boston, MA: Butterworth-Heinemann, 1992:485–498.

67. Christophe C, Bartholome J, Blum D, et al. Neonatal tuberous sclerosis. US, CT, and MR diagnosis of brain and cardiac lesions. *Pediatr Radiol* 1989;19:446–448.

68. Christophe C, Sekhara T, Rypens F, et al. MRI spectrum of cortical malformations in tuberous sclerosis complex. *Brain Dev* 2000;22: 487–493.

69. Girard N, Zimmerman RA, Schnur R, et al. Magnetization transfer in the investigation of patients with tuberous sclerosis. *Neuroradiology* 1997;39:523–528.

70. Kato T, Yamanouchi H, Sugai K, Takashima S. Improved detection of cortical and subcortical tubers in tuberous sclerosis by fluid-attenuated inversion recovery MRI. *Neuroradiology* 1997;39:378–380.

71. Takanashi J, Sugita K, Fujii K, Niimi H. MR evaluation of tuberous sclerosis: increased sensitivity with fluid-attenuated inversion recovery and relation to severity of seizures and mental retardation. *Am J Neuroradiol* 1995;16:1923–1928.

72. Van Tassel P, Curé J, Holden KR. Cystlike white matter lesions in tuberous sclerosis. *Am J Neuroradiol* 1997;18:1367–1373.

73. Spangler WJ, Cosgrove GR, Moumdjian RA, Montes JL. Cerebral arterial ectasia and tuberous sclerosis. *Neurosurgery* 1997;40:191–194.

74. Smulewicz JJ, Tafreshi M. Angiographic changes in tuberous sclerosis. *Angiology* 1977;28:300–322.

75. Jones BV, Tomsick TA, Franz DN. Gugliemi detachable coil embolization of a giant midbasilar aneurysm in a 19 month old patient. *Am J Neuroradiol* 2002;23:1145–1148.

76. Lie JT. Cardiac, pulmonary, and vascular involvements in tuberous sclerosis. *Ann NY Acad Sci* 1991;615:58–70.

77. Fitz CR, Harwood-Nash DC, Boldt DW. The radiographic features of unilateral megalencephaly. *Neuroradiology* 1978;15:145–148.

78. Barkovich AJ, Chuang SH. Unilateral megalencephaly: Correlation of MR imaging and pathologic characteristics. *Am J Neuroradiol* 1990; 11:523–531.

79. Barkovich AJ, Chuang SH, Norman D. MR of neuronal migration anomalies. *Am J Neuroradiol* 1987;8:1009–1017.

80. Kalifa CL, Chiron C, Sellier N, et al. Hemimegalencephaly: MR imaging in five children. *Radiology* 1987;165:29–33.

81. Townsend JJ, Nielsen SL, Malamud N. Unilateral megalencephaly: Hamartoma or neoplasm? *Neurology* 1975;25:448–453.

82. Renowden SA, Squier M. Unusual magnetic resonance and neuro-pathological findings in hemimegalencephaly: report of a case following hemispherectomy. *Dev Med Child Neurol* 1994;36:357–369.

83. Manz HJ, Phillips TM, Rowden G, McCullough DC. Unilateral megalencephaly, cerebral cortical dysplasia, neuronal hypertrophy, and heterotopia: cytomorphometric, fluorometric cytochemical, and biochemical analyses. *Acta Neuropath (Berl)* 1979;45:97–103.

84. Bosman C, Boldrini R, Dimitri L, et al. Hemimegalencephaly. Histological, immunohistochemical, ultrastructural and cytofluorimetric study of six patients. *Child's Nerv Syst* 1996;12:765–775.

85. Sarwar M, Schafer M. Brain malformations in linear nevus sebaceous syndrome: an MR study. *J Comput Assist Tomogr* 1988;12:338–340.

86. Hager BC, Dyme IZ, Guertin SR, et al. Linear nevus sebaceous syndrome: megalencephaly and heterotopic gray matter. *Pediatr Neurol* 1991;7:45–49.

87. Pavone L, Curatolo P, Rizzo R, et al. Epidermal nevus syndrome: a neurologic variant with hemimegalencephaly, gyral malformation, mental retardation, seizures, and facial hemihypertrophy. *Neurology* 1991;41:266–271.

88. Happle R. How many epidermal nevus syndromes exist? A clinicogenetic classification. *J Am Acad Dermatol* 1991;25:550–556.

89. Griffiths PD, Welch R, Gardner-Medwin D, et al. The radiological features of hemimegalencephaly including three cases associated with proteus syndrome. *Neuropediatrics* 1994;25:140–144.

90. Dietrich RB, Glidden DE, Roth GM, et al. The Proteus syndrome: CNS manifestations. *Am J Neuroradiol* 1998;19:987–990.

91. Peserico A, Battistella PA, Bertoli P, Drigo P. Unilateral hypomelanosis of Ito with hemimegalencephaly. *Acta Paediatr Scand* 1988; 77:446–447.

92. Cusmai R, Curatolo P, Mangano S, et al. Hemimegalencephaly and neurofibromatosis. *Neuropediatrics* 1990;21:179–182.

93. Griffiths PD, Gardner S-A, Smith M, et al. Hemimegalencephaly and focal megalencephaly in tuberous sclerosis complex. *Am J Neuro-radiol* 1998;19:1935–1938.

94. Wolpert SM, Cohen A, Libenson M. Hemimegalencephaly: a longitudinal MR study. *Am J Neuroradiol* 1994;15:1479–1482.

95. Tagawa T, Otani K, Futagi Y, et al. Serial IMP-SPECT and EEG studies in an infant with hemimegalencephaly. *Brain Dev* 1994;16:475–479.

96. Hoffmann KT, Amthauer H, Liebig T, et al. MRI and F-18 fluorodeoxyglucose positron emission tomography in hemimegalen-cephaly. *Neuroradiology* 2000;42:749–752.

97. Villemure J-G. Hemispherictomy techniques: a critical review. In: Tuxhorn I, Holthausen H, Boenigk H, eds. Paediatric epilepsy

syndromes and their surgical treatment. London: John Lebbey, 1997:729–738.

98. King M, Stephenson J, Ziervogel M, et al. Hemimegalencephaly–a case for hemispherectomy? *Neuropediatrics* 1985;16:46–55.

99. Dobyns W, Berry-Kravis E, Havernick N, et al. X-linked lissencephaly with absent corpus callosum and ambiguous genitalia. *Am J Med Genet* 1999;86:331–337.

100. Aicardi J. The agyria-pachygyria complex: a spectrum of cortical malformations. *Brain Dev* 1991;13:1–8.

101. Warkany J, Lemire RJ, Cohen MM Jr. Mental retardation and congenital malformations of the central nervous system. Chicago, IL: Yearbook, 1981.

102. Dobyns WB. The neurogenetics of lissencephaly. *Neurol Clin* 1989;7:89–105.

103. Lo Nigro C, Chong CS, Smith AC, et al. Point mutations and an intragenic deletion in LIS1, the lissencephaly causative gene in isolated lissencephaly sequence and Miller–Dieker syndrome. *Hum Molec Genet* 1997;6:157–164.

104. Dobyns W, Elias E, Newlin A, et al. Causal heterogeneity in isolated lissencephaly. *Neurology* 1992;42:1375–1388.

105. Dobyns WB, Truwit CL. Lissencephaly and other malformations of cortical development. *Neuropediatrics* 1995;26:132–147.

106. Dobyns WB, Stratton RF, Greenberg F. Syndromes with lissencephaly. I: Miller–Dieker and Norman–Roberts syndromes and isolated lissencephaly. *Am J Med Genet* 1984;18:509–526.

107. Pilz DT, Matsumoto N, Minnerath S, et al. LIS1 and XLIS (DCX) mutations cause most classical lissencephaly, but different patterns of malformation. *Hum Molec Genet* 1998;7:2029–2037.

108. Ross ME, Allen KM, Srivastava AK, et al. Linkage and physical mapping of X-linked lissencephaly/SBH (*XLIS*): a gene causing neuronal migration defects in human brain. *Hum Mol Genet* 1997; 6:555–562.

109. Pinard JM, Motte J, Chiron C, et al. Subcortical laminar heterotopia and lissencephaly in 2 families: a single X-linked dominant gene. *J Neurol Neurosurg Psychiatr* 1994;57:914–920.

110. Dobyns WB, Andermann E, Andermann F, et al. X-linked malformations of neuronal migration. *Neurology* 1996;47:331–339.

111. Gleeson J, Lin P, Flanagan L, Walsh C. Doublecortin is a microtubule-associated protein and is expressed widely by migrating neurons. *Neuron* 1999;23:257–271.

112. Barkovich AJ, Guerrini R, Battaglia G, et al. Band heterotopia: correlation of outcome with MR imaging parameters. *Ann Neurol* 1994;36:609–617.

113. Barkovich AJ, Koch TK, Carrol CL. The spectrum of lissencephaly: report of ten cases analyzed by Magnetic Resonance Imaging. *Ann Neurol* 1991;30:139–146.

114. Dobyns WB, Kirkpatrick JB, Hittner HM, et al. Syndromes with lissencephaly. 2: Walker–Warburg and cerebral occular muscular syndromes and a new syndrome with Type 2 lissencephaly. *Am J Med Genet* 1985;22:157–195.

115. Garcia CA, Dunn D, Trevor R. The lissencephaly syndrome in siblings. *Arch Neurol* 1978;35:608–611.

116. Stewart RM, Richman DP, Caviness VS Jr. Lissencephaly and pachygyria: an architectonic and topographical analysis. *Acta Neuropathol* 1975;31:1–12.

117. Sarnat H. Role of the human fetal ependyma. *Pediatr Neurol* 1992;8:163–178.

118. Sarnat HB, Darwish HZ, Barth PG, et al. Ependymal abnormalities in lissencephaly/pachygyria. *J Neuropathol Exp Neurol* 1993; 52:525–541.

119. Barkovich AJ, Gressens P, Evrard P. Formation, maturation, and disorders of brain neocortex. *Am J Neuroradiol* 1992;13:423–446.

120. Zimmerman RA, Bilaniuk LT, Grossman RI. Computed tomography in migration disorders of human brain development. *Neuroradiology* 1983;25:257–263.

121. Raybaud C, Girard N, Canto-Moreira N, Poncet M. High-definition magnetic resonance imaging identification of cortical dysplasias:

micropolygyria versus lissencephaly. In: Guerrini R, Andermann F, Canapicchi R, et al., eds. Dysplasias of cerebral cortex and epilepsy. Philadelphia, PA: Lippencott-Raven, 1996:131–143.

122. Ross ME, Swanson K, Dobyns WB. Lissencephaly with cerebellar hypoplasia (LCH): a heterogeneous group of cortical malformations. *Neuropediatrics* 2001;32:256–263.

123. Dobyns WB, Truwit CL, Ross ME, et al. Differences in the gyral pattern distinguish chromosome 17-linked and X-linked lissencephaly. *Neurology* 1999;53:270–277.

124. D'Arcangelo G, Nakajima K, Miyata T, et al. Reelin is a secreted glycoprotein recognized by the CR-50 monoclonal antibody. *J Neurosci* 1997;17:23–31.

125. Gerding H, Gullotta F, Kuchelmeister K, Busse H. Ocular findings in Walker–Warburg syndrome. *Child Nerv Syst* 1993;9:418–420.

126. Walker AE. Lissencephaly. *Arch Neurol Psychiatry* 1942;48:13–29.

127. Warburg M, Heuer HE. Chorioretinal dysplasia-microcephaly-mental retardation syndrome. *Am J Med Genet* 1994;52:117.

128. Williams RS, Swisher CN, Jennings M, et al. Cerebro-ocular dysgenesis (Walker–Warburg syndrome): neuropathologic and etiologic analysis. *Neurology* 1984;34:1531–1541.

129. Rhodes RE, Hatten HP Jr, Ellington KS. Walker–Warburg syndrome. *Am J Neuroradiol* 1992;13:123–126.

130. Barkovich AJ. Neuroimaging manifestations and classification of congenital muscular dystrophies. *Am J Neuroradiol* 1998;19:1389–1396.

131. Fukuyama Y, Kawazura M, Haruna H. A peculiar form of congenital muscular dystrophy. Report of fifteen cases. *Paediatr Universit (Tokyo)* 1960;4:5–8.

132. Fukuyama Y, Osawa M, Suzuki H. Congenital progressive muscular dystrophy of the Fukuyama type – clinical, genetic, and pathological considerations. *Brain Dev* 1981;3:1–29.

133. Toda T, Segawa M, Nomura Y, et al. Localization of a gene for Fukuyama type congenital muscular dystrophy to chromosome 9q31–33. *Nat Genet* 1993;5:283–286.

134. Aida N, Yagishita A, Takada K, Katsumata Y. Cerebellar MR in Fukuyama congenital muscular dystrophy: polymicrogyria with cystic lesions. *Am J Neuroradiol* 1994;15:1755–1759.

135. Aida N, Tamagawa K, Takada K, et al. Brain MR in Fukuyama congenital muscular dystrophy. *Am J Neuroradiol* 1996;17:605–614.

136. Hino N, Kobayashi M, Shibata N, et al. Clinicopathological study on eyes from cases of Fukuyama type congenital muscular dystrophy. *Brain Dev* 2001;23:97–107.

137. Takada K, Nakamura H, Takashima S. Cortical dysplasia in Fukuyama congenital muscular dystrophy: a Golgi and angio-architectonic analysis. *Acta Neuropathol* 1988;76:170–178.

138. Takada K, Nakamura H. Cerebellar micropolygyria in Fukuyama congenital muscular dystrophy: observations in fetal and pediatric cases. *Brain Dev* 1990;12:774–778.

139. Santavuori P, Leisti J, Kruus S. Muscle, eye and brain disease: a new syndrome. *Neuropädiatrie (Suppl)* 1977;8:553–558.

140. Santavuori P, Somer H, Sainio K, et al. Muscle–eye–brain disease. *Brain Dev* 1989;11:147–153.

141. Cormand B, Avela K, Pihko H, et al. Assignment of the muscle–eye–brain disease gene to 1p32–34 by linkage analysis and homozygosity mapping. *Am J Hum Genet* 1999;64:126–135.

142. Haltia M, Leivo I, Somer H, et al. Muscle–eye–brain disease: a neuropathological study. *Ann Neurol* 1997;41:173–180.

143. Valanne L, Pihko H, Katevuo K, et al. MRI of the brain in muscle–eye–brain (MEB) disease. *Neuroradiology* 1994;36:473–476.

144. Raymond AA, Fish DR, Stevens JM, et al. Subependymal heterotopia: a distinct neuronal migration disorder associated with epilepsy. *J Neurol Neurosurg Psychiatry* 1994;57:1195–1202.

145. Smith AS, Weinstein MA, Quencer RM, et al. Association of heterotopic gray matter with seizures: MR imaging. *Radiology* 1988; 168:195–198.

146. Barkovich AJ, Kjos BO. Gray matter heterotopias: MR characteristics and correlation with developmental and neurological manifestations. *Radiology* 1992;182:493–499.

147. Barkovich AJ, Kuzniecky RI. Gray matter heterotopia. *Neurology* 2000;55:1603–1608.

148. Poussaint TY, Fox JW, Dobyns WB, et al. Periventricular nodular heterotopia in patients with filamin-1 gene mutations: neuroimaging findings. *Pediatr Radiol* 2000;30:748–755.

149. Sheen VL, Dixon PH, Fox JW, et al. Mutations in the X-linked filamin 1 gene cause periventricular nodular heterotopia in males as well as in females. *Hum Mol Genet* 2001;10:1775–1783.

150. Dobyns WB, Guerrini R, Czapansky-Beilman D, et al. Bilateral periventricular nodular heterotopia with mental retardation and syndactyly in boys: a new X-linked mental retardation syndrome. *Neurology* 1997;49:1042–1047.

151. Eksioglu YZ, Scheffer IE, Cardenas P, et al. Periventricular heterotopia: an X-linked dominant epilepsy locus causing aberrant cerebral cortical development. *Neuron* 1996;16:77–87.

152. Huttenlocher PR, Taravath S, Mojtahedi S. Periventricular heterotopia and epilepsy. *Neurology* 1994;44:451–455.

153. Pilz D, Stoodley N, Golden JA. Neuronal migration, cerebral cortical development, and cerebral cortical anomalies. *J Neuropath Exp Neurol* 2002;61:1–11.

154. Nikolic M, Chou MM, Lu W, et al. The p35/Cdk5 kinase is a neuron-specific Rac effector that ingibits Pak1 activity. *Nature* 1998;395:194–198.

155. Kothare SV, VanLandingham K, Armon C, et al. Seizure onset from periventricular nodular heterotopias: depth electrode study. *Neurology* 1998;51:1723–1727.

156. Oda T, Nagai Y, Fujimoto S, et al. Hereditary nodular heterotopia accompanied by mega cisterna magna. *Am J Med Genet* 1993;47:268–271.

157. Moro F, Carrozzo R, Veggiotti P, et al. Familial periventricular heterotopia: missense and distal truncating mutations of the *FLN1* gene. *Neurology* 2002;58:916–921.

158. Barkovich AJ. Subcortical heterotopia: a distinct clinico-radiologic entity. *Am J Neuroradiol* 1996;17:1315–1322.

159. Dubeau F, Tampieri D, Andermann E, et al. Periventricular and subcortical nodular heterotopia: comparison of clinical findings and results of surgical treatment. In: Guerrini R, ed. Dysplasias of cerebral cortex and epilepsy. Philadelphia, PA: Lippencott-Raven, 1996:395–406.

160. Barkovich AJ. Morphology of subcortical heterotopia: a magnetic resonance study. *Am J Neuroradiol* 2000;21:290–295.

161. Marsh L, Lim KO, Sullivan EV, et al. Proton magnetic resonance spectroscopy of a gray matter heterotopia. *Neurology* 1996;47:1571–1574.

162. Barkovich AJ, Jackson DE Jr., Boyer RS. Band heterotopia: a newly recognized neuronal migration anomaly. *Radiology* 1989;171:455–458.

163. Livingston JH, Aicardi J. Unusual MRI appearance of diffuse subcortical heterotopia or 'double cortex' in two children. *J Neurol Neurosurg Psychiatry* 1990;53:617–620.

164. Palmini A, Andermann F, Aicardi J, et al. Diffuse cortical dysplasia, or the 'double cortex' syndrome: the clinical and epileptic spectrum in 10 patients. *Neurology* 1991;41:1656–1662.

165. Des Portes V, Pinard JM, Billuart P, et al. A novel CNS gene required for neuronal migration and involved in X-linked subcortical laminar heterotopia and lissencephaly syndrome. *Cell* 1998;92:51–61.

166. Horesh D, Sapir T, Francis F, et al. Doublecortin, a stabilizer of microtubules. *Hum Molec Genet* 1999;8:1599–1610.

167. Gleeson JG, Walsh CA. Neuronal migration disorders: from genetic diseases to developmental mechanisms. *Trends Neurosci* 2000;23:352–359.

168. Gleeson J, Minnerath S, Fox J, et al. Characterization of mutations in the gene doublecortin in patients with double cortex syndrome. *Ann Neurol* 1999;45:146–153.

169. Ono J, Mano T, Andermann E, et al. Band heterotopia or double cortex in a male: bridging structures suggest abnormality of the radial glial guide system. *Neurology* 1997;48:1701–1703.

170. Pilz D, Kuc J, Matsumoto N, et al. Subcortical band heterotopia in rare affected males can be caused by missense mutations in DCX (XLIS) or LIS1. *Hum Molec Genet* 1999;8:1757–1760.

171. Kato M, Kanai M, Soma O, et al. Mutation of the doublecortin gene in male patients with double cortex syndrome: somatic mosaicism detected by hair root analysis. *Ann Neurol* 2001;50:547–551.

172. Federico A, Tomasetti, Zollino M, et al. Association of trisomy 9p and band heterotopia. *Neurology* 1999;53:430–432.

173. Franzoni E, Bernardi B, Marchiani V, et al. Band brain heterotopia. Case report and literature review. *Neuropediatrics* 1995;26:37–40.

174. Matsumoto N, Leventer RJ, Kuc JA, et al. Mutation analysis of the *DCX* gene and geneotype/phenotype correlation in subcortical band heterotopia. *Eur J Hum Genet* 2001;9:5–12.

175. Falconer J, Wada J, Martin W, Li D. PET, CT, and MRI imaging of neuronal migration anomalies in epileptic patients. *Can J Neurol Sci* 1990;17:35–39.

176. Miura K, Watanabe K, Maeda N, et al. MR imaging and positron emission tomography of band heterotopia. *Brain Dev* 1993;15:288–290.

177. De Volder AG, Gadisseux J-F, Michel CJ, et al. Brain glucose utilization in band heterotopia: synaptic activity of 'double cortex.' *Pediatr Neurol* 1994;11:290–294.

178. Morell F, Whisler W, Hoeppner T, et al. Electrophysiology of heterotopic gray matter in the 'Double Cortex' syndrome. *Epilepsia* 1992;33(Suppl 3):76.

179. Pinard J-M, Feydy A, Carlier R, et al. Functional MRI in double cortex: functionality of heterotopia. *Neurology* 2000;54:1531–1533.

180. Mischel PS, Nguyen LP, Vinters HV. Cerebral cortical dysplasia associated with pediatric epilepsy. Review of neuropathologic features and proposal for a grading system. *J Neuropath Exp Neurol* 1995;54:137–153.

181. Hallervorden J. Ueber eine Kohlenoxydvergiftung im Fetalleben mit Entwicklunsstorung der Hirnrinde. *Allg Z Psychiatr* 1949;124:289–298.

182. Barkovich AJ, Rowley HA, Bollen A. Correlation of prenatal events with the development of polymicrogyria. *Am J Neuroradiol* 1995;16:822–827.

183. Bingham PM, Lynch D, McDonald-McGinn D, Zackai E. Polymicrogyria in chromosome 22 deletion syndrome. *Neurology* 1998;51:1500–1502.

184. Kuzniecky R. Familial diffuse cortical dysplasia. *Arch Neurol* 1994;51:307–310.

185. Villard L, Nguyen K, Cardoso C, et al. A locus for bilateral perisylvian polymicrogyria maps to Xq28. *Am J Hum Genet* 2002;70:1003–1008.

186. Caraballo RH, Cers'simo RO, Mazza E, Fejerman N. Focal polymicrogyria in mother and son. *Brain Dev* 2000;22:336–339.

187. Borgatti R, Triulzi F, Zucca C, et al. Bilateral perisylvian polymicrogyria in three generations. *Neurology* 1999;52:1910–1913.

188. Guerrini R, Dravet C, Raybaud C, et al. Epilepsy and focal gyral anomalies detected by MRI: electroclinico-morphological correlations and follow-up. *Dev Med Child Neurol* 1992;34:706–718.

189. Barkovich AJ, Linden CL. Congenital cytomegalovirus infection of the brain: imaging analysis and embryologic considerations. *Am J Neuroradiol* 1994;15:703–715.

190. Barkovich AJ, Kjos BO. Non-lissencephalic cortical dysplasia: correlation of imaging findings with clinical deficits. *Am J Neuroradiol* 1992;13:95–103.

191. Hayashi N, Tsutsumi Y, Barkovich AJ. Polymicrogyria without porencephaly/schizencephaly. MRI analysis of the spectrum and the prevalence of macroscopic findings in the clinical population. *Neuroradiology* 2002;44:647–655.

192. Guerrini R, Dubeau F, Dulac O, et al. Bilateral parasagittal parietooccipital polymicrogyria and epilepsy. *Ann Neurol* 1997;41:65–73.

193. Kuzniecky R, Andermann F, Guerrini R. Congenital bilateral perisylvian syndrome: study of 31 patients. The congenital bilateral

perisylvian syndrome milticenter collaborative study. *Lancet* 1993;341:608–612.

194. Guerreiro MM, Andermann E, Guerrini R, et al. Familial perisylvian polymicrogyria: a new familial syndrome of cortical maldevelopment. *Ann Neurol* 2000;48:39–48.

195. Guerrini R, Dravet C, Raybaud C, et al. Neurological findings and seizure outcome in children with bilateral opercular macrogyric-like changes detected by MRI. *Dev Med Child Neurol* 1992;34:694–705.

196. Gropman AL, Barkovich AJ, Vezina LG, et al. Pediatric congenital bilateral perisylvian syndrome: clinical and MRI features in 12 patients. *Neuropediatrics* 1997;28:198–203.

197. Kuzniecky R, Andermann F, Tampieri D, et al. Bilateral central macrogyria: epilepsy, pseudobulbar palsy, and mental retardation – a recognizable neuronal migration disorder. *Ann Neurol* 1989;25:547–554.

198. Becker PS, Dixon AM, Troncoso JC. Bilateral opercular polymicrogyria. *Ann Neurol* 1989;25:90–92.

199. Rolland Y, Adamsbaum C, Sellier N, et al. Opercular malformations: clinical and MRI features in 11 children. *Pediatr Radiol* 1995;25:S2–S8.

200. Kuzniecky R, Andermann F, Guerrini R. The epileptic syndrome in the congenital bilateral perisylvian syndrome. CBPS Multicenter collaborative study. *Neurology* 1994;44:379–385.

201. Barkovich AJ, Hevner R, Guerrini R. Syndromes of bilateral symmetrical polymicrogyria. *Am J Neuroradiol* 1999;20:1814–1821.

202. Guerrini R, Barkovich A, Sztriha L, Dobyns W. Bilateral frontal polymicrogyria. *Neurology* 2000;54:909–913.

203. Guerrini R, Dulac O, Canapicchi R, et al. Epilepsie révélatrice d'une dysplasie corticale occipito-pariétale parasagittale bilatérale. *Epilepsies* 1994;6:131–139.

204. Guerrini R, Dravet C, Bureau M, et al. Diffuse and localized dysplasias of cerebral cortex: clinical presentation, outcome, and proposal for a morphologic MRI classification based on a study of 90 patients. In: Guerrini R, Andermann F, Canapicchi R, et al., eds. Dysplasias of cerebral cortex and epilepsy. Philadelphia, PA: Lippincott-Raven, 1996:255–269.

205. Jacobs K, Kharazia V, Prince D. Mechanisms underlying epileptogenesis in cortical malformations. *Epilepsy Res* 1999;36:165–188.

206. Palmini A, Andermann F, Olivier A, et al. Focal neuronal migration disorders and intractable partial epilepsy: a study of 30 patients. *Ann Neurol* 1991;30:741–749.

207. Barkovich AJ. Abnormal vascular drainage in anomalies of neuronal migration. *Am J Neuroradiol* 1988;9:939–942.

208. Yakovlev PI, Wadsworth RC. Schizencephalies. A study of the congenital clefts in the cerebral mantle. 1. Clefts with fused lips. *J Neuropathol Exp Neurol* 1946;5:116–130.

209. Yakovlev PI, Wadsworth RC. Schizencephalies. A study of the congenital clefts in the cerebral mantle. 2. Clefts with hydrocephalus and lips separated. *J Neuropathol Exp Neurol* 1946;5:169–206.

210. Granata T, Farina L, Faiella A, et al. Familial schizencephaly associated with EMX2 mutation. *Neurology* 1997;48:1403–1406.

211. Haverkamp F, Zerres K, Ostertun B, et al. Familial schizencephaly: further delineation of a rare disorder. *J Med Genet* 1995;32:242–244.

212. Robinson RO. Familial schizencephaly. *Dev Med Child Neurol* 1991;33:1010–1014.

213. Brunelli S, Faiella A, Capra V, et al. Germline mutations in the homeobox gene EMX2 in patients with severe schizencephaly. *Nature Genetics* 1996;12:94–96.

214. Gulisano M, Broccoli V, Pardini C, Boncinelli E. Emx1 and Emx2 show different patterns of expression during proliferation and differentiation of the developing cerebral cortex in the mouse. *Eur J Neurosci* 1996;8:1037–1050.

215. Packard AM, Miller VS, Delgado MR. Schizencephaly: correlations of clinical and radiologic features. *Neurology* 1997;48:1427–1434.

216. Miller GM, Stears JC, Guggenheim MA, Wilkening GN. Schizencephaly: a clinical and CT study. *Neurology* 1984;34:997–1001.

217. Barkovich AJ, Kjos BO. Schizencephaly: correlation of clinical findings with MR characteristics. *Am J Neuroradiol* 1992;13:85–94.

218. Hayashi N, Tsutsumi Y, Barkovich AJ. Morphological features and associated anomalies of schizencephaly in the clinical population: detailed analysis of MR images. *Neuroradiology* 2002; 44:418–427.

219. Barkovich AJ, Norman D. MR of schizencephaly. *Am J Neuroradiol* 1988;9:297–302.

220. Granata T, Battaglia G, D'Incerti L, et al. Schizencephaly: clinical findings. In: Guerrini R, ed. Dysplasias of the cerebral cortex and epilepsy. Philadelphia, PA: Lippencott-Raven, 1996:407–415.

221. Aniskiewicz AS, Frumkin NL, Brady DE, et al. Magnetic resonance imaging and neurobehavioral correlates in schizencephaly. *Arch Neurol* 1990;47:911–916.

222. Chuang SH, Fitz CR, Chilton SJ, et al. Schizencephaly: spectrum of CT findings in association with septo-optic dysplasia. In: Annual Meeting of the Radiological Society of North America, Washington, DC, 1984.

223. Barkovich AJ, Fram EK, Norman D. Septo-optic dysplasia: MR imaging. *Radiology* 1989;171:189–192.

224. Denis D, Chateil J-F, Brun M, et al. Schizencephaly: clinical and imaging features in 30 infantile cases. *Brain Dev* 2000;22:475–483.

225. Barkovich AJ, Kuzniecky RI, Dobyns WB, et al. A classification scheme for malformations of cortical development. *Neuropediatrics* 1996;27:59–63.

226. Meencke HJ, Janz D. The significance of microdysgenesis in primary generalized epilepsy: an answer to the considerations of Lyon and Gastaut. *Epilepsia* 1985;26:368–371.

227. Taylor DC, Falconer MA, Bruton CJ, Corsellis JAN. Focal dysplasia of the cerebral cortex in epilepsy. *J Neurol Neurosurg Psychiatry* 1971;34:369–387.

228. Kim S, Na D, Byun H, et al. Focal cortical dysplasia: comparison of MRI and FDG-PET. *J Comput Assist Tomogr* 2000;24:296–302.

229. Chan S, Chin SS, Nordli DR, et al. Prospective magnetic resonance imaging identification of focal cortical dysplasia, including the non-balloon cell subtype. *Ann Neurol* 1998;44:749–757.

230. Saint Martin C, Adamsbaum C, Robain O, et al. An unusual presentation of focal cortical dysplasia. *Am J Neuroradiol* 1995;16: 840–842.

231. Bronen R, Spencer D, Fulbright R. Cerebrospinal fluid cleft with cortical dimple: MR imaging marker for focal cortical dysgenesis. *Radiology* 2000;214:657–663.

232. Yagishita A, Arai N, Maehara T, et al. Focal cortical dysplasia: appearance on MR images. *Radiology* 1997;203:553–559.

233. Daumas-Duport C, Scheithauer BW, Chodkiewicz J-P, et al. Dysembryoplastic neuroepithelial tumor: a surgically curable tumor of young patients with intractable partial seizures. *Neurosurgery* 1988;23:545–556.

234. Daumas-Duport C. Dysembryoplastic neuroepithelial tumors. *Brain Pathol* 1993;3:283–295.

235. Prayson R, Khajavi K, Comair Y. Cortical architectural abnormalities and MIB1 immunoreactivity in gangliogliomas: a study of 60 patients with intracranial tumors. *J Neuropathol Exp Neurol* 1995;54: 513–520.

236. Raymond AA, Fish DR, Stevens JM, et al. Association of hippocampal sclerosis with cortical dysgenesis in patients with epilepsy. *Neurology* 1994;44:1841–1845.

237. Kuzniecky R, Garcia JH, Faught E, Morawetz RB. Cortical dysplasia in temporal lobe epilepsy: magnetic resonance imaging correlations. *Ann Neurol* 1991;29:293–298.

CHAPTER **8**

Structural Analysis Applied to Epilepsy

Andrea Bernasconi

INTRODUCTION

As has been made clear in previous chapters, in clinical practice the investigation and treatment of patients with epilepsy has been revolutionized by the advent of MRI. It has been demonstrated to be a reliable and accurate indicator of many of the pathologic findings underlying epilepsy. The use of MRI has resulted in a reduction in chronic intracranial electroencephalographic (EEG) monitoring at most epilepsy centers, especially in patients with lesional pathology. MRI has had a major impact in epilepsy surgery by helping to define cerebral structural damage and consequently in delineating the extent of the 'epileptogenic zone' (Chapter 1), i.e. the site of seizure onset. The close relation between structural lesions identified by MRI and the epileptogenic zone is demonstrated by favorable surgical outcome in patients with lesions as opposed to those with normal MRI.

Magnetic resonance imaging benefits from the ability to vary image acquisition and postprocessing parameters in order to study different types of anatomic and functional properties in the brain (Chapter 2). Techniques such as the volumetric acquisition of thin contiguous slices, three-dimensional (3D) reformatting and surface rendering have enhanced the ability of MRI to display brain anatomy and to visualize epileptogenic brain lesions. As opposed to visual MRI inspection, advanced image processing provides quantitative MRI analysis, which is likely to be of great aid in structural brain imaging.

Human epileptogenesis is clearly a complex functional process and its anatomic basis is poorly understood. Given the possibility that some of these functional changes may have a structural correlate, MRI could also play a pivotal role in elucidating the mechanisms underlying epileptogenesis. Advanced MR image analysis has great potential to improve our understanding of the basic mechanisms of, as well as for better defining indications for, surgery and improving outcome from this surgery.

The purposes of this chapter are to give an overview of some of the cutting edges in novel image analysis methods and their application to clinical research, and to indicate how these methods may allow us to approach new and relevant questions in clinical MRI research in epilepsy.

Understanding image processing involves a certain amount of technical knowledge. Some general concepts of MR image analysis will be discussed here. However, readers who would like to learn more details about the different methods should consult the papers listed in the references at the end of the chapter.

IMAGE ACQUISITION: THE IMPORTANCE OF VOLUMETRIC DATA ACQUISITION

Although MRI cannot provide histologic data directly (because of its low resolution), it can provide a surrogate measurement of pathologic processes that may underlie the epileptogenic process. Visual or quantitative assessment of hippocampal volume on volumetric 3D T1-weighted MRI, along with demonstration of signal change, has been demonstrated to be an accurate method for diagnosing hippocampal sclerosis. MR diagnosis has virtually replaced invasive EEG methods in most patients with temporal lobe epilepsy (TLE) in whom hippocampal sclerosis is the underlying major pathology.

The study of epilepsy arising from cortical abnormalities has been more limited in the past by difficulties of visualizing the cortical surface from conventional two-dimensional (2D) MRI slices, a challenge that is currently being met by advanced surface reconstruction techniques, volume rendering, and curvilinear modeling.

Adjusting time properties of the acquisition sequences, such as echo time and repetition time, provide contrast between brain tissues. A typical basic epilepsy MRI protocol comprises a T1-weighted volume acquisition, which may be reformatted in any orientation and used for volumetric measurements, along with proton-density, T2-weighted, fluid attenuated inversion recovery (FLAIR) and inversion recovery pulse sequence acquisitions. Images are obtained with adjacent slices that cover the entire brain with thin cuts usually oriented perpendicular to the long axis of the hippocampus.

The ideal MRI sequence for studying patients with epilepsy would be one that provides high spatial resolution, high contrast, and complete brain coverage, and does so in a short period of time. Unfortunately, these goals are mutually exclusive because of the inherent limitations imposed by MR physics (Chapter 2). In our experience, T1-weighted 3D gradient-echo technique, which provides exquisite anatomic detail and can be reconstructed to obtain high-quality volume imaging, gives us the best data for digital image processing.

Despite the improvement achieved by multiplanar reformatting, the complexity of brain anatomy limits, in some situations, the identification of subtle epileptogenic lesions. Curvilinear multiplanar reformatting (CMPR) of 3D MRI (1) offers an alternative to the conventional rectilinear visualization methods. In this technique, a series of curved slices

are automatically generated from an initial surface obtained by interactively delineating the contour of the hemispheric convexities (usually along the coronal plane; Fig. 8.1). The slices obtained are approximately symmetric, have an angle of incidence perpendicular to the inward folding gyri of the hemispheric convexities, and are generated at user-selected slice intervals depth levels. The thickness of the curves is usually 1 mm with a 1 mm interslice gap. This results in a symmetrical set of images of the cortex, which can be displayed as a 2D surface or 3D rendered image.

Curvilinear multiplanar reformatting can facilitate visual analysis by displaying multiple images that can be simultaneously displayed from identical viewing planes and examined in combination with conventional orthogonal MRI. Furthermore, the 3D viewing windows are linked so that 3D can be synchronously viewed in space (Fig. 8.2). The perpendicular orientation of the curved slices in relation to the gyri prevents the impression of artifactual cortical thickening by reducing volume averaging and obliquity of the slices in relation to the long axis of the gyrus. The utility of this method has been demonstrated by Bastos et al. (1), who studied five patients in whom conventional 2D and 3D MRI was initially considered normal. Subsequent studies using CMPR identified lesions in all patients. Four patients underwent surgery with histologic diagnosis of focal cortical dysplasia.

Curvilinear multiplanar reformatting provides a more realistic display of brain surface anatomy, which allows comparison between adjacent gyri and sulci and improves

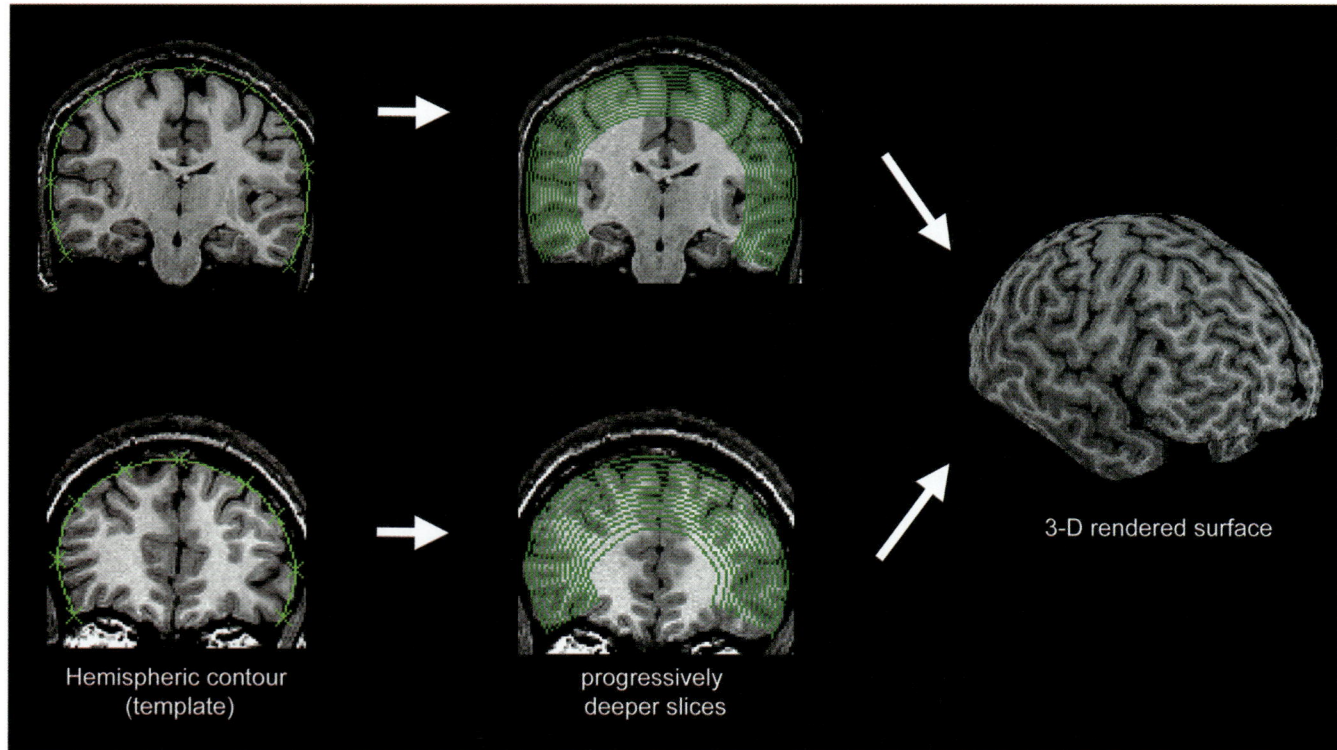

FIG. 8.1. Curvilinear multiplanar reformatting of three-dimensional MRI. A surface is obtained by manually delineating contour lines of the hemispheric convexities on several coronal sections. This surface will serve as a template for the generation of progressively deeper slices. The resultant surfaces may be displayed as a three-dimensionally rendered object.

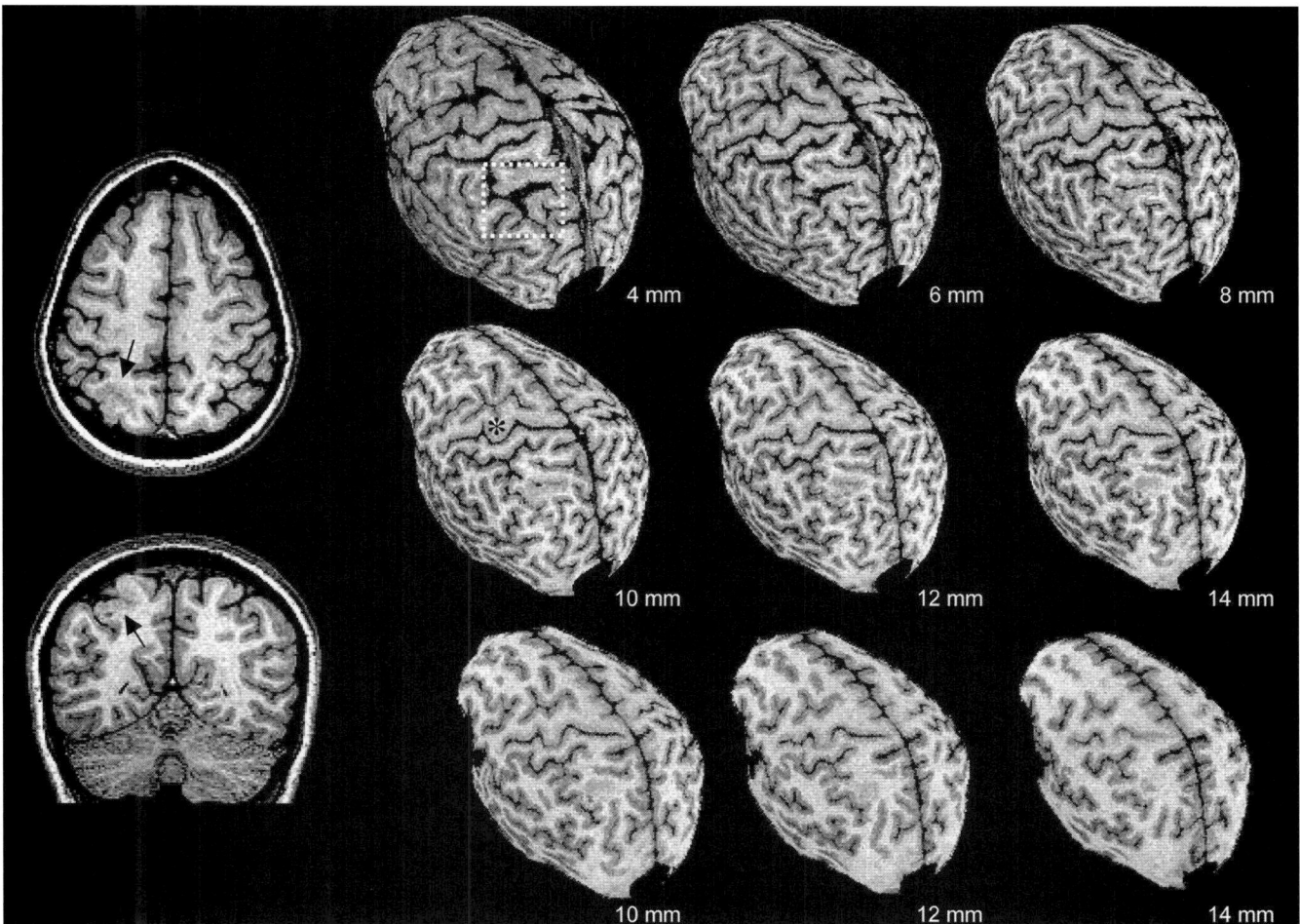

FIG. 8.2. Curvilinear multiplanar reformatting of three-dimensional MRI. Focal cortical dysplasia in the left parietal area. Axial and coronal view on orthogonal images (left) and nine curvilinear slices (right) at progressive depth are presented. On the 3D surface, the lesion is characterized mainly by a focal gyral abnormality with sulcal widening (dashed square). Deeper slices show cortical thickening and blurring of the gray–white matter transition in the lesional area. The asterisk (10 mm surface) indicates the anatomic location of the hand area.

anatomic localization of epileptogenic lesions with respect to functional areas. This is particularly useful in locating pivotal functional areas, such as the central sulcus and the pre- and postcentral gyri. However, the principle of CMPR applies typically to hemispheric convexities. Therefore, inspection of brain areas that have a more rectilinear shape, such as the parasagittal region, the insular cortex and the fronto- and temporobasal areas is best achieved when using conventional orthogonal and oblique planes (1). CMPR has been shown to be useful also in neurosurgical planning, by providing a better view of the position of subdural electrodes with respect to cortical anatomic landmarks compared to conventional orthogonal sections. Furthermore, visualization of subdural grids using CMPR does not require image fusion and thus avoids possible localization error associated with images registration (2).

An automated, data-driven method for curvilinear reconstruction has been implemented and applied to epilepsy. In this technique, the brain is first segmented from the 3D MRI using a region growing method with unsupervised threshold selection technique. The upper half of the segmented brain

is then extracted and fitted by a deformable surface model. This surface is finally interactively moved by the operator to visualize the desired curvilinear slice, which is projected on the screen as a 2D image that can fit the brain in three dimensions (3), as opposed to a cylindrical surface generated by interactive CMPR. The drawback of this method is a less realistic display of brain anatomy, which is unquestionably more difficult to assess on a 2D image than on multiple 3D rendered surfaces.

The main shortcoming of the above-mentioned conventional methodologies is that they rely on visual assessment of trained observers and are therefore subjective. Alternatively, quantitative image processing methods have the potential to help identify lesions that may be overlooked by conventional radiologic evaluation.

IMAGE PROCESSING: AN OVERVIEW

Image processing refers to quantitative analyses and/or algorithms applied to digital image data. It allows generation of 3D parametric maps and implies calculation of values that should be ultimately replicable and rater-independent. Image processing methods are becoming increasingly sophisticated and the tendency is to develop as much automation as possible. A common goal of image processing techniques applied to neuroimaging is to improve detection of abnormal brain tissue, including abnormalities that may not be readily recognizable by visual analysis alone.

It is important to bear in mind that the clinical input is determinant in deciding which image analysis method might be most useful to investigate specific brain pathologies. This can be done, for example, by modeling features described qualitatively during visual analysis of imaging data by expert observers. Also, there are some important aspects of image processing that should not be overlooked. Image quality is the most important factor in determining the reliability of the data produced by the image post-processing. The reproducibility of findings is another central issue.

The following aspects of image processing of 3D MRI will be discussed in this chapter: image pre-processing, tissue classification, shape analysis, voxel-based morphometry, cortical thickness measurements and texture analysis.

IMAGE PRE-PROCESSING

The necessary assumption of topologic correspondence across sets of data is satisfied by the broad anatomic information contained in 3D MRI. Registration, e.g. the alignment of images, is usually performed against some common reference (target) image. Because the choice of target should not bias the final result of registration, high-resolution large population averages are preferred (4).

An important concept for the analysis of multiple MRI data sets is the 'brain-based' coordinate system. For this purpose, we rely on a coordinate space (stereotaxic space) concept originally based on the atlas created by Talairach and Tournoux (5) for neurosurgical applications. This type of spatial normalization provides multiple advantages (6). First, this process (linear or nonlinear) allows adjusting for differences in total brain volume and brain orientation, and facilitates the identification of boundaries of brain structures by minimizing variability in slice orientation (4). Second, it provides a conceptual framework for the completely automated, 3D analysis across subjects. Third, it allows longitudinal and cross-sectional analysis. Stereotaxic registration is accomplished by the registration of one image to a target using an automated 3D image registration technique (4).

Low-frequency spatial intensity variations are primary source of errors in the computer-aided, quantitative analysis of MRI data. This artifact, often referred as RF inhomogeneity, is predominantly caused by electrodynamic interactions with subject and inhomogeneity of the RF receiver coil sensitivity (7). Therefore, algorithms have been created to automatically correct images for intensity non-uniformity due to radiofrequency inhomogeneity of the MR scanner and standardize intensity (8).

TISSUE CLASSIFICATION AND SEGMENTATION

Tissue classification refers to the differentiation of voxels within an MR image into tissue-based classes, such as gray matter (GM), white matter (WM), cerebrospinal fluid (CSF), and background. This procedure is usually based on the absolute MR intensity from one or more image types, since the above-mentioned classes have sufficiently different gray-level intensities on the MR-image histogram. Partial volume effects occur when more than one tissue class is present within a voxel at the resolution of the image. A classifier must then decide, based on a set of predefined rules, to which class the voxel belongs. Typically the context, or neighborhood, of a given voxel will be taken into consideration in the classification process (9, 10).

Tissue segmentation deals with the identification of specific anatomic structures. Segmentation of anatomic structures from large 3D MRI data sets represents a necessary yet difficult task in medical image analysis. The prototype of MRI-based segmentation used in epilepsy has been the manual volumetry of limbic structures, such as the hippocampus and the amygdala (see Duncan 1997 (11) for review). Past techniques measuring the hippocampus have focused on defining structures in a single two-dimensional plane (12–14). Because of the three-dimensional shape of the hippocampus, however, we have found great advantages in verifying hippocampal segmentation in coronal, sagittal, and transverse plain. Several studies have shown that these volumetric measurements are accurate and reproducible (15, 16). Initial studies performed by Jack and colleagues (13) indicated that volumetric analysis may reliably identify seizure origin in patients with TLE and there is now consensus that hippocampal atrophy detected by volumetric MRI is a reliable indicator of mesial temporal sclerosis in TLE patients (17–19).

Relatively little work has been done on quantitative imaging of extrahippocampal pathology, despite early pathologic studies, which suggested a more widespread involvement of the cortex in patients with epilepsy (20). Entorhinal cortex volumetry has been able to demonstrate structural abnormalities in the mesial temporal lobe, not only in patients with TLE and hippocampal atrophy on MRI (15, 21–23), but also in those with TLE and normal hippocampal volume (24). Preliminary studies have shown that abnormalities associated with TLE can lead to reduction of the hemicranial volume (25) and to specific structures such as the temporal neocortical GM and WM (22, 26–29), and the thalamus (30–32). Information provided by manual volumetric analysis of the hippocampus, amygdala, and entorhinal cortex can be routinely used in the clinical management of surgical candidates.

As discussed above, current volumetric MRI protocols for clinical research studies in epilepsy are based on manual segmentation of brain structures. This approach is time-consuming and requires great expertise in anatomy. In addition, manual segmentation introduces intra- and inter-observer variations in labeling strategy and makes often use of empirical guidelines for dealing with unclear anatomic borders. These factors apply particularly when dealing with the segmentation of neocortical areas.

Advanced imaging techniques for morphometry have been developed to try to overcome these limitations by using computational techniques to provide an objective assessment of brain structures. Some methods combine automated segmentation with some level of operator intervention. More recent programs aim to provide fully automated analytical tools, overcoming the variability and bias of interactive methods. The main problems faced are anatomic variability, nonhomogeneity of pixel values in a single tissue or structure, and the presence of blurred boundaries between different tissue types.

Different methods have been used to accomplish automatic segmentation, such as statistical pattern recognition techniques (33) and clustering algorithms (34, 35). More recently, there has been a massive proliferation of increasingly sophisticated methods that make use of artificial neural networks (6) and 3D model-based segmentation techniques (33, 36–52). A considerable advantage of deformable models is their ability to take into account global prior knowledge about the expected shape of the structure to be segmented and its variability. A detailed analysis of these methods is beyond the scope of this chapter. Many of the recent methods provide quite robust segmentation and labeling of brain structures, including the hippocampus, even in the presence of severe brain atrophy (46). Some methods have been validated by comparison of automatic segmentation with the results obtained by interactive expert segmentation (43, 47, 50).

Segmentation of the Hippocampus

Some general aspects of the automated hippocampal segmentation have been recently summarized by Shen and co-workers (50). The hippocampus is a small gray-matter structure that is adjacent to other gray-matter structures such as the amygdala and the parahippocampal region. Therefore, on MRI, the hippocampus has relatively low contrast and borders that are relatively difficult to identify along a significant portion of its surface. Moreover, the hippocampus has a high surface-to-volume ratio, and the hippocampal surface voxels are most difficult to define. These difficulties complicate the accurate automatic segmentation of the hippocampus.

To date three different approaches have been proposed for quantification of the hippocampal volumes: manual segmentation (discussed above), semi-automatic and fully automatic methods. A fully automated method for hippocampal segmentation would be ideal. However, conventional methods such as edge detection, thresholding, or region growing are not reliable due to the small size, low contrast, and apparent discontinuity of the edges of the hippocampus. One attempt proposed, which involves warping of an atlas to the individual MRI (53). may not generate accurate results because of its sensitivity to the imperfections involved with the registration and warping steps. Alternative methods use shape and boundary profile information (47) or an active

appearance-based technique (43) to guide the hippocampal segmentation. Semiautomatic methods may provide a more realistic approach for hippocampal segmentation because they combine a priori knowledge concerning hippocampal location, anatomic boundaries, and shape (45, 50, 54, 55).

Only a few attempts have been made to automatically segment the hippocampus in MRI data sets of patients with epilepsy. A preliminary study by Webb and colleagues (53) used a semi-automated method based on the analysis of image intensity differences between 15 TLE patients with hippocampal atrophy and 14 controls within a volume of interest (mask) centered on the hippocampus. The presence of an anomaly (in terms of intensity differences) in the mask region caused by encroachment of CSF or WM as a result of morphologic changes in the hippocampus (i.e. atrophy) formed the basis of the method for determining automatically hippocampal atrophy. Hippocampal atrophy could be detected only in 50% and 70% of the patients with manually determined atrophy in the right and left hippocampus, respectively. Because of the low sensitivity, the authors proposed to use this method as a screening tool obviating the need for time-consuming manual measurements in patients with clear-cut unilateral hippocampal atrophy.

Hogan and collaborators (56) verified the precision and reproducibility of hippocampal volumetric measurement using deformation-based segmentation in five patients with mesial temporal sclerosis. The overall percentage overlap between automated and manual segmentations was about 70%. This semi-automatic method required manual determination of global and hippocampus-specific landmarks, which provided an initial condition for the intensity-matching algorithm by roughly aligning the patient and control images. Furthermore, results in this study showed a greater variability in the segmentation of the sclerotic hippocampus compared to that in healthy controls.

Segmentation of Gray and White Matter

Volumetric measurements of neocortical areas provide an indirect means of estimating regional neuronal number. Regional cortical GM and subcortical matter (hemispheric WM and subcortical nuclei volumes) has been assessed using block analysis (57). In this technique, the segmented images of each cerebral hemisphere are divided into a number of equal slices in an anterior–posterior axis, allowing measurement of interhemispheric volume ratios between blocks. In a study of patients with cortical dysgenesis, widespread changes were seen in apparently normal areas distant from the visually apparent areas of dysgenesis (57, 58).

It is noteworthy that segmentation methods applied so far to epilepsy have been semi-automatic because they involve, at least in some steps, the intervention of an operator. Moreover, automatic segmentations methods have provided only lobar volumes (29). In general, it remains to be seen whether the objectivity and increased reproducibility of an automated approach outweigh the decreased ability to delineate fine structure in the neocortex and the medial temporal lobe.

Completely automatic and accurate segmentation of individual brain structures is thus far an unsolved problem. However, automatic and efficient segmentation techniques open new possibilities for the processing of a large number of MRI data sets. With the refinement of segmentation techniques, future work should target separate analysis of GM and WM of individual brain regions (i.e. specific gyri), allowing comprehensive analysis of the whole brain instead of few target areas. It is, however, important to remember that a disadvantage of fully automatic processing concerns quality control, which is imperative for any type of quantitative analysis. Therefore, visual inspection of the results is still a necessity, particularly in difficult-to-segment areas such as the mesial temporal lobe.

ANALYSIS OF SHAPE

Shape analysis is emerging as an important area of medical image processing because it has the potential to improve both the accuracy of medical diagnosis and the pathophysiology of neurologic diseases. Analysis of shape enables evaluation of local details that are not evident in measurement of the total volume of a structure. In computational anatomy, statistical surface shape models have been shown to be more sensitive than volumetric MRI in detecting small losses of volume in the hippocampus, particularly in schizophrenia and Alzheimer's disease (59–63). Emerging techniques of deformation-based segmentation allowing the examination of the brain structures have been largely applied to the hippocampus, however other brain structures such as the corpus callosum have also been studied (43, 48–50, 52, 62–67).

Shape Analysis of the Hippocampus

Only a few reports in adults have demonstrated changes in hippocampal shape in patients with epilepsy (56, 68, 69). In a recent study, a previously validated technique of deformation-based hippocampal segmentations was applied in a small group of patients with documented unilateral mesial temporal sclerosis and TLE (68). Using composite images, shape differences between the epileptogenic, smaller hippocampus, and contralateral hippocampus were measured. Final shape differences were projected on the contralateral 'normal' side. Both patients with right and left hippocampal sclerosis showed similar regions of maximal inward deformation in the affected hippocampus, which were the medial and lateral aspect of the head, and posterior aspect of the tail. The authors reported that hippocampal shape abnormality in TLE patients was different from that in a previously described case of schizophrenia (59) and Alzheimer's disease (61). In the view of the authors, these results suggest

that specific 3D patterns of volume loss might occur in TLE. Similar findings were reported in a patient who developed status epilepticus in the context of acute encephalitis (69).

A new technique for shape analysis based on medial models is coming into view in the literature (66, 70). We used an algorithm developed by Bouix and Siddiqi at McGill University for analyzing anatomic structures from 3D MRI data using medial surfaces (64, 65). In this method, the medial surface of the hippocampus is defined as the locus of the centers of the interior spheres with maximal radius. The medial surface reflects the topologic and geometrical features of an object in a very compact form. Registering the medial surfaces describing different hippocampi in a common space allows statistical analysis of differences in shape between patients and normal control subjects (Fig. 8.3).

Our preliminary results of shape analysis using the radius function of the medial surfaces showed that in left TLE patients, deformation involves mostly the head–body transition area. In right TLE patients, there was a flattening of the head of the hippocampus and a bending of the hippocampal body (Fig. 8.4).

It is conceivable that, coupled with other methods in a proper statistical framework, results from shape analyses might increase the sensitivity of diagnosis of epilepsy and possible aid early detection of the disease. Future applications in TLE include analysis of newly diagnosed patients, patients with normal hippocampal volume, and those with familial forms.

Shape Analysis of the Sulci and Cortical Mantle

The problem of quantifying, as opposed to visualizing, the cortical surface and measuring its variability across subjects is difficult to express in mathematical terms because the boundaries of gyri and the extent of sulci are imprecise. Major sulci have variable branching patterns and many secondary gyri have a highly variable appearance or may be absent. However, mathematical models of structure and shape have the potential to be able to isolate cortical characteristics in a form that gives diagnostic information not easily available to the human observer.

Although disruption of normal gyral patterns and alteration of cortical ribbon are features of many structural abnormalities related to epilepsy, little work has been done in the analysis of neocortical shape for quantification of changes possibly related to neuronal damage or abnormal connectivity in this disorder. Most studies have relied upon visual inspection to identify gross abnormalities in gyration on the 3D surface-rendered MRI (71). However, similarly to volumetric MRI studies in the mesial temporal lobe, the identification of more subtle alterations may require quantitative analysis of hemispheric differences and comparison of individual gyral surface area or gyral/sulcal locations with previously established population norms. Measurements of GM and WM surface area and index of curvature of the gyri

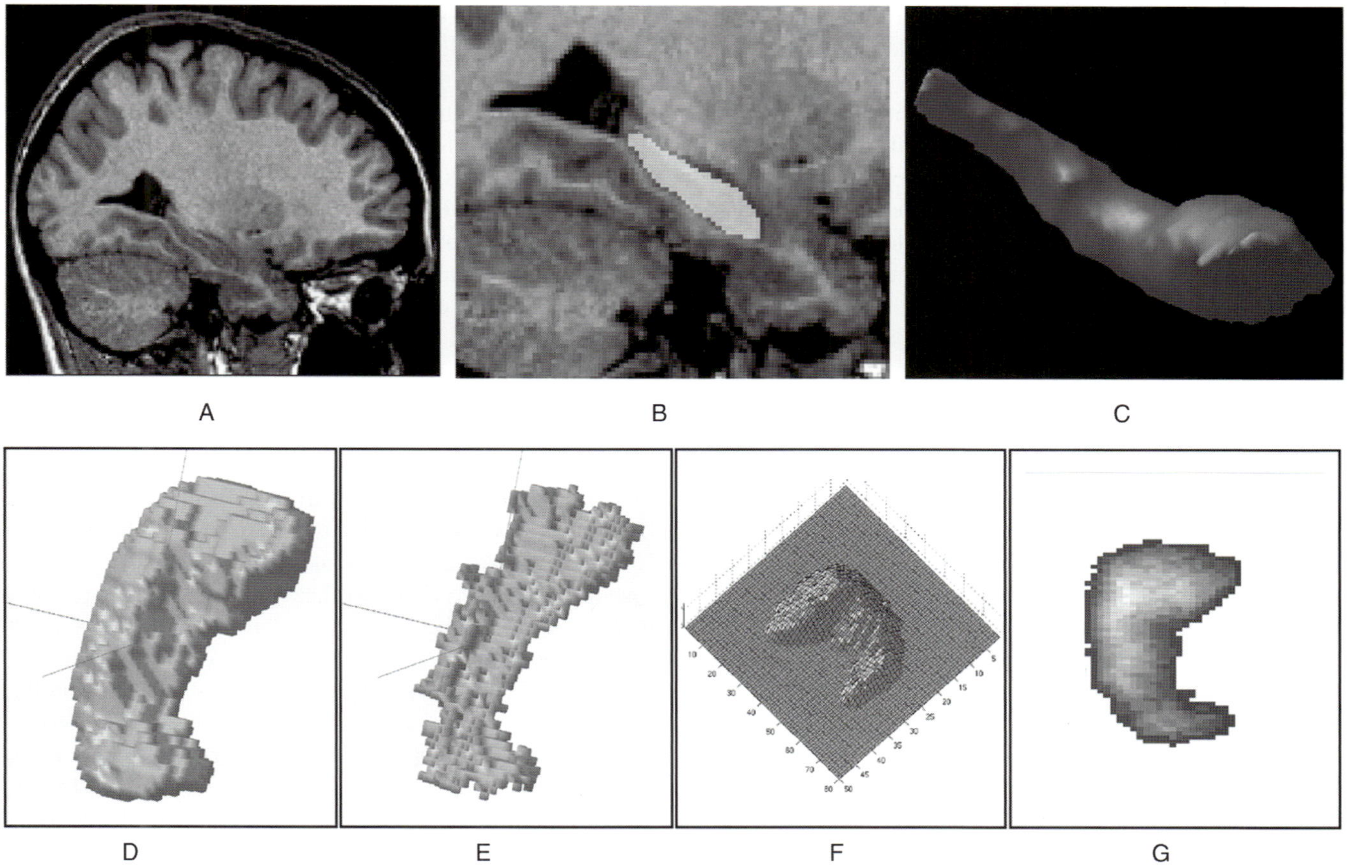

A   B   C

D   E   F   G

FIG. 8.3. Hippocampal shape analysis. **A.** Sagittal T1-weighted MRI. **B.** Hippocampal label. **C.** Three-dimensional view of the manually segmented hippocampus. **D.** Three-dimensionally rendered hippocampus. **E.** The most prominent sheet of the medial surface. **F.** The medial surface radius function as a surface plot. **G.** Two-dimensional intensity map, in which each point refers to the medial surface radius as a height function.

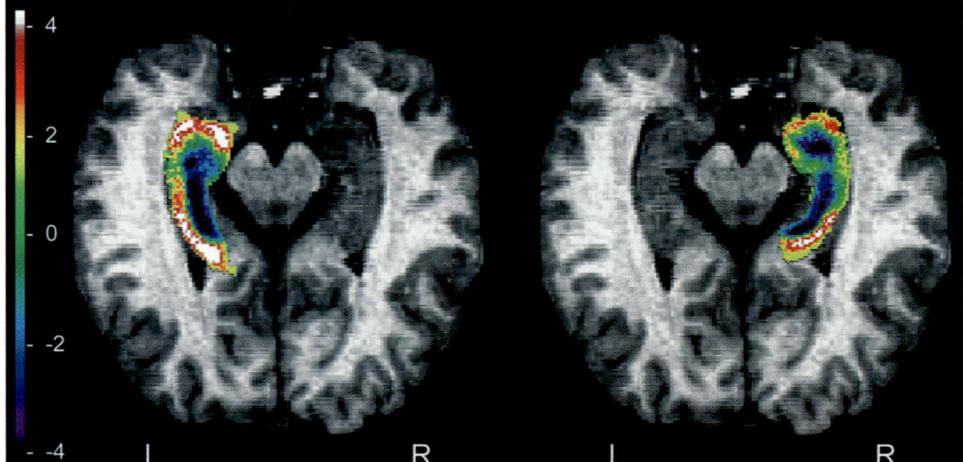

FIG. 8.4. Hippocampal shape analysis. Shape analysis showing the location of the deformation in the hippocampus ipsilateral to the seizure focus in patients with left (n = 20) and right (n = 20) temporal lobe epilepsy compared to controls (n = 40). The intensity of the image is directly proportional to the magnitude (and sign on the color bar) of the regression of the medial surface radius function and thus reveals information about the location of shape differences between patients and controls. Although changes in shape involve most of the hippocampus, in patients with left temporal lobe epilepsy the deformation (negative values) is located in the head-body transition area, whereas patients with right temporal lobe epilepsy present with a marked flattening of the hippocampal head.

have shown subtle abnormalities in neocortical structures in TLE (27) but their relationship to the epileptic foci and the occurrence of seizure remains unclear.

In an attempt to define subtle simplification of gyral patterns, some authors have applied fractal analysis to MRI images from patients with frontal lobe epilepsy (72) and cryptogenic epilepsy (73). Results indicated that, compared to a group of normal controls, abnormally low fractal dimension (an index of contour complexity) of the GM–WM interface and the WM surface was found in 10 of 16 patients with frontal lobe epilepsy and nine of 23 subjects with cryptogenic epilepsy. This method, which was implemented in two dimensions rather than 3D, provided a nonspecific index of complexity with low sensitivity that was unable to identify focal abnormalities. Nevertheless, it illustrates the potential of quantitative analysis for detecting anomalous cortical morphology, particularly if extended into 3D.

Recently, there has been a great interest within the brain imaging community in developing increasingly more advanced image analysis methods for characterizing sulcal shape. Automated or semi-automated methods for statistical models of sulci have relied on graphs constructed from 3D point sets (74, 75), on ribbons used to model the space between opposite sides of a sulcus (76, 77), or on curves located on the outer cortical surface (78). These methods allow intersubject sulcal shape comparisons of the major sulci (76) and can quantify a variety of characteristics, such as length, volume and indexes of curvature (79).

There is evidence that sulcal shapes might be linked to the underlying cytoarchitecture and related to connectivity of the brain, since they are influenced by forces exerted by connection fibers (80). Therefore, these methods seem an appropriate instrument to explore the hypothesis that abnormal neuronal connectivity produces abnormal cortical folding patterns. MR-based shape analysis could clarify which aspects of sulcal shape abnormalities are most relevant to brain pathology in epilepsy, particularly in malformations of cortical development.

CORTICAL THICKNESS MEASUREMENTS

While extensive manual segmentation of the cortical mantle on MRI is prohibitive, reliable automatic 3D segmentation and measurement of the cerebral cortex remains a challenging problem because of its convoluted nature. Measuring cortical thickness in an accurate yet fully automated fashion has the potential to provide maps of changes across the cortical ribbon with not only statistical significance as an output (such as produced by voxel based morphometry, see below) but also a meaningful metric of change, namely cortical thickness loss or gain measured in millimeters. This offers the potential to define clinical and statistical significance.

There have been only few studies attempting to measure cortical thickness from MRI data (81–87), most probably because of the inherent difficulty in executing the task correctly.

Two types of approach have been used: one attempting to replicate the jeweler's eyepiece measurement by measuring the distance from the brain surface to the white matter on a slice (85), the other trying to separate the two surfaces (GM–CSF and GM–WM), create object representation of these two surfaces, and then find the closest point on one surface given a point on the other (81–87).

The first approach faces the problem of selecting the correct slice angle along which to measure the thickness at any one point. That is a very difficult task, made even more difficult by the fact that MRI is discrete data rarely sampled higher than 1 mm spacing. The second approach, which uses a much more sophisticated series of data processing techniques, has to deal with three main issues: tissue classification, separation of the opposite banks of sulci that have been fused through the partial volume effect, and construction of the actual surfaces into some polygonal model or delineated boundaries.

Once the surfaces have been defined, the thickness at any one location has to be found. The most common approach is some variant of the straight-line measurement. The technique used involves picking a point on one of the surfaces (GM or WM surface) and finding the closest point on the other surface (81, 84, 88). In the method described by Jones et al. (82), cortical thickness is computed through by solving the Laplace's equation over the cortex with constant boundary values at the two interfaces. The solution of Laplace's equation describes a nested series of surfaces that make a smooth transition between the inner and outer surface. Field lines orthogonal to all intermediary surfaces between the two interfaces can then be computed, and the thickness at any point in the mantle can be found by integrating over these streamlines.

Very few studies have been dedicated to the measurement of cortical thickness in neurologic disorders. A recent study by Rosas et al. (86) showed that the cortical ribbon, compared to healthy controls, is thinner in Huntington's disease patients and that atrophy spreads to more anterior regions as the disease progresses.

To assess cortical thickness in TLE, we used deformable models described by McDonald at the Montreal Neurological Institute (84). The fully automated algorithm starts with the same spherical model for each subject, which is then deformed on to their respective Talairach registered and classified volumes to create a WM–GM surface and a GM–CSF surface (Fig. 8.5). The resulting nodes of each surface are thus guaranteed to both be in the cortical mantle as well as in comparable locations. This therefore allows for population analyses.

In the Montreal series, 32 patients with left TLE and left hippocampal atrophy on volumetric MRI, and 51 normal controls were studied. Decrease in cortical thickness occurred in the ipsilateral entorhinal cortex and hippocampus, and bilaterally in the frontal and central areas, suggesting a multilobar involvement (Fig. 8.6). The relationship between such measurements and the clinical parameters and disease progression remains to be determined.

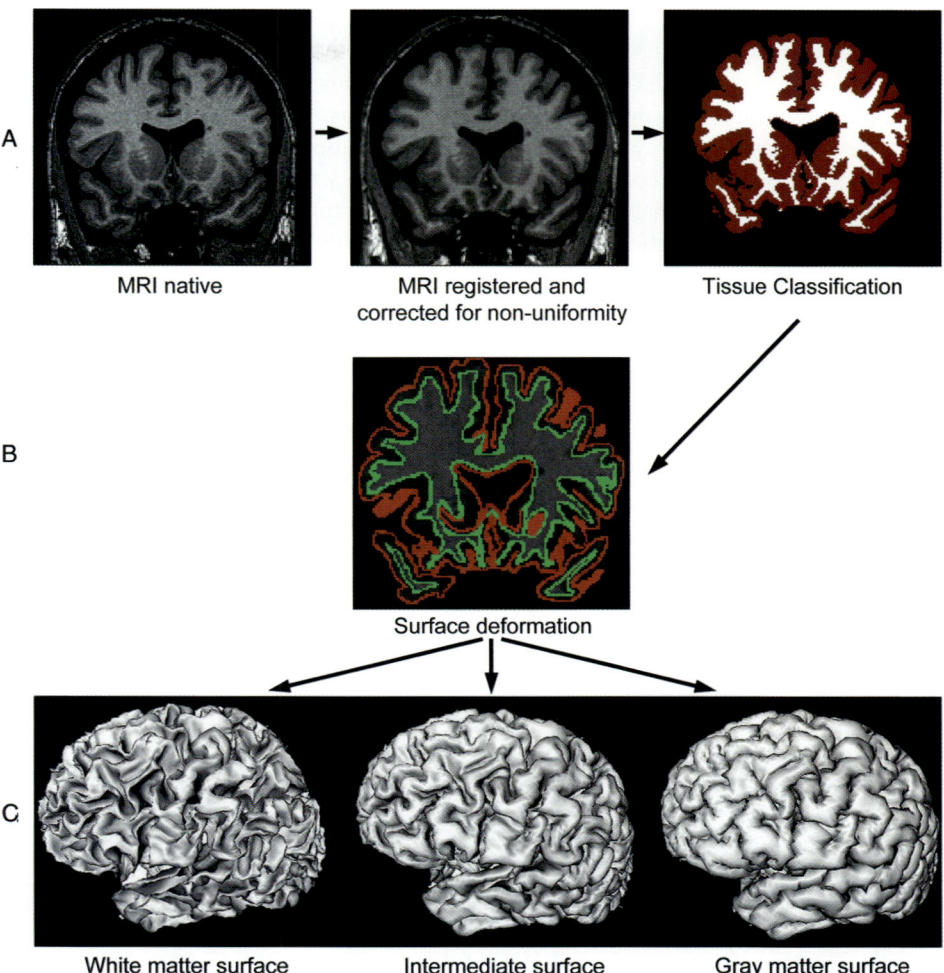

FIG. 8.5. Automated three-dimensional extraction of inner and outer surfaces of cerebral cortex from MRI for cortical thickness measurements. **A.** The native 3D T1-weighted MRI is registered in a standard stereotaxic space and corrected for non-uniformity, and classified into gray matter (GM), white matter (WM), and cerebrospinal fluid (CSF) using an artificial neural network classifier. Then a sphere is deformed to the WM–GM boundary as identified in the classification step. This will generate a WM surface. This surface is then expanded outwards towards the GM–CSF boundary to create a GM surface. **B.** Cross-section of the GM (red) and WM (green) surfaces superimposed on the classified volume. **C.** Left view of the inner, intermediate, and outer surfaces of a cerebral cortex. The intermediate surface is defined as the geometric mean between the GM and WM surfaces.

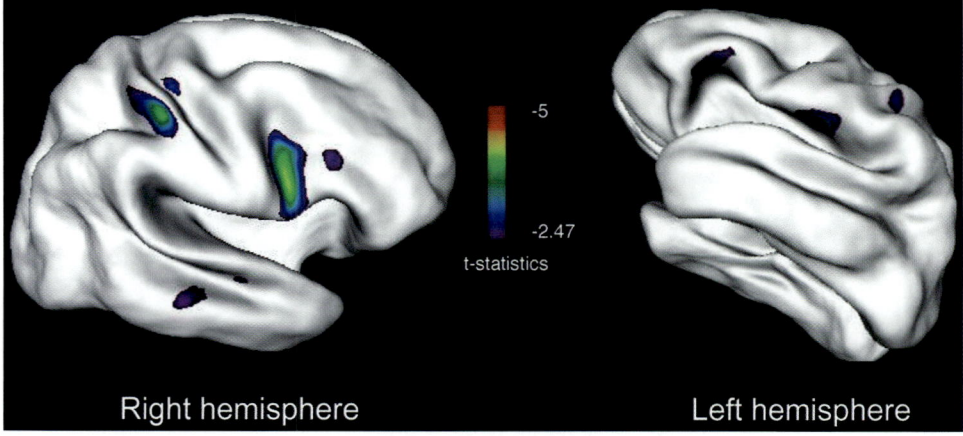

FIG. 8.6. Cortical thickness measurement in temporal lobe epilepsy. Bilateral frontal and central decrease in cortical thickness in patients with left temporal lobe epilepsy. Lateral views of the left and right hemisphere are shown.

VOXEL-BASED MORPHOMETRY

Volume and geometry are only a part of the information provided by MRI. Pathology also causes changes in water relaxation behavior that are manifested by gray-level variation. Voxel-based morphometry (VBM), a recent imaging technique that was originally developed for functional MRI analysis, is a powerful tool for analyzing subtle differences in signal intensity (89).

The context for VBM can be set by dividing medical image analysis techniques in two broad categories: structure-based and voxel-based methods. Structure-based methods add information to an image by conveying knowledge from human expertise. They imply clustering voxels together according to some meaningful representation to the user, allowing further statistical analysis of the structure. An example of structure-based methodology is manual segmentation of the hippocampus from MRI and subsequent volume estimation of the collection of voxels labeled by an expert observer. The goal of voxel-based methods (segmentation, registration, or morphometry) is to measure some properties at the voxel level and extract meaningful information, without relying on a subjective intermediary processing stage. Furthermore, VBM allows the investigation of brain tissue abnormalities with no *a priori* region of interest, enabling a comprehensive and unbiased analysis of global brain structure.

At its simplest, VBM involves a voxel-wise comparison of the local 'concentration' (see below) of some property between two groups of subjects. VBM relies heavily on an accurate co-registration process before comparing different MRI volumes at a voxel level. Typically, linear registration is used to conform all brains to the same orientation and size. Any differences due to misregistration will result in added noise to the statistical results. Nonlinear registration can be used to further conform all subjects to a common reference volume at a local level.

After tissue classification, images are smoothed by convolving with an isotropic gaussian kernel. Therefore, each voxel in the smoothed images contains the average concentration around the voxel. This is often referred as tissue 'density' or 'concentration' (89). Voxel-wise parametric statistical tests are used to compare the smoothed concentration maps

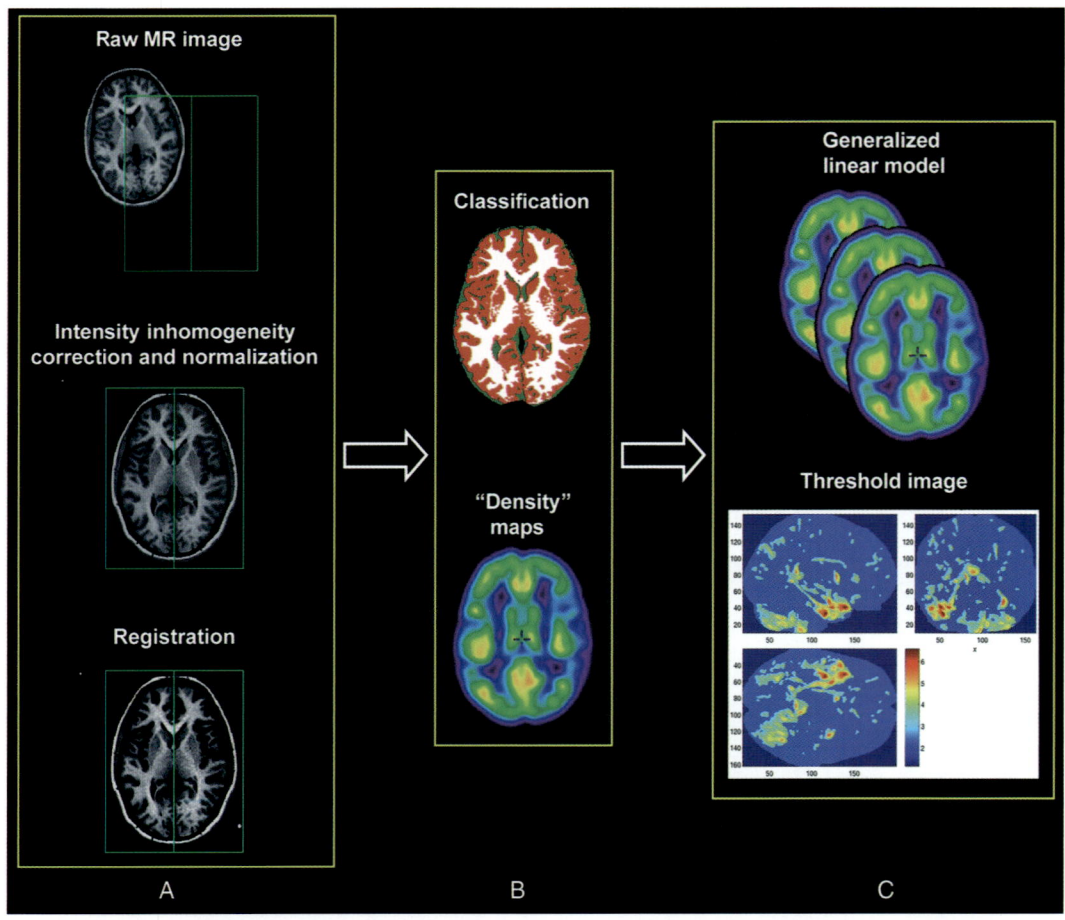

FIG. 8.7. Voxel-based morphology. **A.** Automated correction for intensity nonuniformity; normalization of gray-level intensities to a common scale across subjects; registration of images to a standardized stereotaxic space to adjust for differences in total brain volume and orientation. **B.** Classification of brain tissue into gray matter (GM), white matter (WM), and CSF; blurring of GM and WM binary masks with an isotropic gaussian kernel to generate 3D maps of GM and WM 'density'. **C.** Statistical maps of differences between patient and control densities obtained using a general linear model.

from the two groups. Corrections for multiple comparisons are made using the theory of gaussian random fields (90) (Fig. 8.7). Meaningful clinical results are usually found when large clusters of voxels are significant. Many neuroimaging laboratories in the world have the capability to perform VBM using the SPM package (89).

Voxel-based morphometry has been used to reveal pathologic changes in gray or white matter in neurologic conditions such as Alzheimer's disease (91) and schizophrenia (92).

As one of the MRI features of mesial temporal sclerosis is hypointense signal on T1-weighted images, VBM has potential for mapping the spatial distribution of abnormalities along the hippocampal axis and in extrahippocampal structures. VBM has previously been used to indicate region-specific grey matter abnormalities in patients with TLE and hippocampal atrophy (93, 94), juvenile myoclonic epilepsy (95), affective aggression and TLE (96), and malformations of cortical development (97, 98). In TLE, VBM has produced conflicting results showing significant clusters of decreased GM intensity in the epileptogenic hippocampus in some studies (93, 94) and no abnormalities in others (96, 98). However, VBM was able to show consistently across different studies neocortical GM reduction or excess, either lateralized or not to the epileptic focus, demonstrating abnormalities beyond the visualized lesions.

We studied 40 patients with right intractable TLE, 47 patients with left TLE, and 51 neurologically normal controls. Volumetric MRI showed hippocampal atrophy ipsilateral to the seizure focus in all patients. Blurring of GM and WM masks was done using an isotropic gaussian kernel with full-width half maximum of 5 mm to generate 3D maps of GM and WM 'density.' Patients with left and right TLE had a diffuse GM reduction in the hippocampus ipsilateral to the seizure focus and bilateral thalamic GM reduction. Left TLE patients also had ipsilateral GM reduction in temporopolar and superior temporal cortices, and bilateral frontal and parietal GM reduction. Compared to normal controls, patients with left and right TLE showed a diffuse reduction of temporal lobe WM (temporopolar area, temporal stem, parahippocampal, superior, middle, inferior, and fusiform gyri) ipsilateral to the seizure focus. We also found bilateral WM reduction in the cerebellum, and WM reduction in the body of corpus callosum. There was also bilateral WM reduction in parietal and parieto-occipital lobe in right-TLE patients (Fig. 8.8).

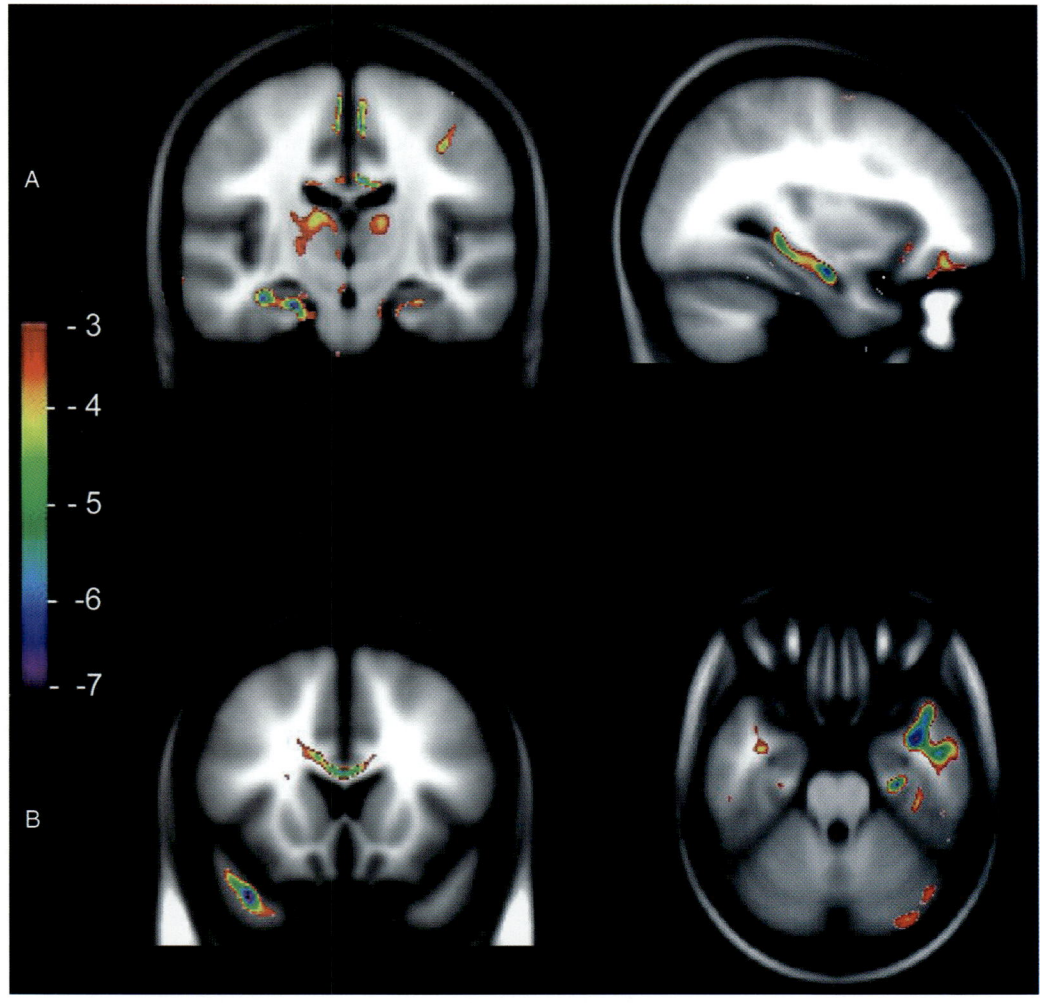

FIG. 8.8. Voxel-based morphometry. Selected areas of (**A**) decreased gray matter and (**B**) decreased white matter concentration in patients with left (left) and right (right) temporal lobe epilepsy.

These results show that limbic pathology extends beyond the hippocampus and involves the temporopolar cortex and the thalamus. Moreover, there are extensive WM changes throughout the temporal lobe with anterior predominance. GM and WM reduction is also present in frontal and parietal lobes. Reduction in GM concentration reported in previous studies and in our patients most probably corresponds to GM atrophy. The pathologic correlates of an increase in GM concentration found in previous studies are less clear (93, 98, 99). Our results showed that regions of increased GM density corresponded to reduction in WM density. Therefore, the increased GM density reported in previous studies might be simply explained by a decrease in the adjacent WM density, which was not analyzed.

In TLE, it has also been shown that extrahippocampal GM abnormalities may be correlated with duration of epilepsy, suggesting secondary brain damage (94).

Although VBM is a relatively straightforward technique, some technical aspects deserve further discussion. Results of VBM depend on the quality of image registration, segmentation, classification, and intensity nonuniformity correction. Modification of some steps in the analysis may be tested to further improve the technique, such as nonlinear registration to conform all brains to a template. The size of the kernel used for smoothing is also an important factor for interpreting results and should be comparable to the size of the expected regional differences between the groups of brains. In VBM studies in epilepsy the used kernel size (14–10 mm) was obviously larger than the expected dimension of abnormalities (e.g. atrophy) of brain structures, such as, for example, the hippocampus.

TEXTURE ANALYSIS

Morphology and texture are important features for visual assessment of an image. Morphology refers to the analysis of shape-related properties of structures within an image, including, for example, cortical thickness. The texture of an image can be described by the distribution of brightness and darkness within that image. Computer-based texture analysis of digital images provides statistical methods capable of identifying the relationship between neighboring pixels over the specific region of interest, often considering the probability that certain intensities are found in specific spatial locations with respect to each other. These techniques result in numerical feature descriptors about spatial gray level variations in pixel neighborhoods (100), which can be used for tissue characterization.

First-order texture methods measure intensity-based properties of an image, such as mean intensity, variance of intensity, or intensity gradient. These types of property can generally be appreciated through visual analysis. Second-order texture methods analyze the spatial distribution of intensity patterns within an image that are not easily perceived through visual analysis.

In medical imaging, texture analysis has been shown to increase the level of diagnostic information extracted from many modalities such as MRI and ultrasound, and to characterize differences in appearances unrecognizable by visual observation (101, 102). Reported applications include classification of pathologic tissue in liver, thyroid, breast, kidney, prostate, and the heart, and characterization of brain tumors. Texture analysis has been used to identify pathology in Alzheimer's disease (103) and multiple sclerosis (104). The usefulness of applying texture analysis to brain MRI in part arises from an intuitive parallel between changes in spatial distributions of gray-level intensity patterns and abnormal tissue organization (102, 105).

In epilepsy, texture analysis has been applied to improve lesion detection in focal cortical dysplasia (37, 106, 107) and TLE (108).

Malformations of cortical development are increasingly recognized as an important cause of focal epilepsy, particularly in younger patients (109). Indeed, focal cortical dysplasia (FCD) (110) is the most common form of developmental disorder in patients with pharmacologically intractable partial epilepsy referred for presurgical evaluation. In many patients with neuronal migration defects, the abnormality is possibly much more widespread across the hemisphere than the changes visible on MRI would lead one to expect. This may be part of the reason why seizures do not always stop entirely following surgical treatment, although the improvement following surgery in the great majority of these patients is well worthwhile.

The interpretation of MRI features of these malformations requires particular attention to the analysis of cortical GM, GM–WM boundary, WM, and periventricular region. On T1-weighted MRI, FCD is mainly characterized by variable degrees of cortical thickening and a poorly defined transition between GM and WM, but also by an hyperintense signal within the dysplastic lesion with respect to normal cortex (111). FCD lesions are mostly located in extratemporal areas. As discussed above, minor abnormalities may only be detected when the volumetric data is reformatted as a tangential slice or as a surface display of the 3D reconstruction (1) However, the inherent complexity of the brain's convolutional pattern makes the visual identification of FCD lesions difficult.

In our own research, by applying texture analysis to MRI, we sought to develop a computer-based method to assist in the detection of FCD in patients with pharmacologically intractable epilepsy. Our initial approach was to apply morphologic and first-order texture models of the MRI characteristics of FCD. The models were implemented in a voxel-wise fashion, such that a set of feature maps could be generated for each patient. These features were chosen to model in vivo the pathologic characteristics of FCD. We selected 16 patients in whom FCD had been histologically proven at operation. In eight patients, FCD had been recognized on conventional MRI prior to the surgery. In the remaining eight patients, preoperative MRI had been reported as normal. Details about modeling of the different characteristics of FCD were published elsewhere (107).

In brief, the following voxel-wise operators were applied to the 3D T1-weighted MRI for each patient:

- a gray-matter run-length operator to model GM thickness

- an absolute gradient operator to quantify the blurring of the GM/WM interface
- an operator to model hyperintense T1 signal within GM through intensity measurement of a voxel relative to the threshold intensity between GM and WM (termed 'relative intensity'; Fig. 8.9).

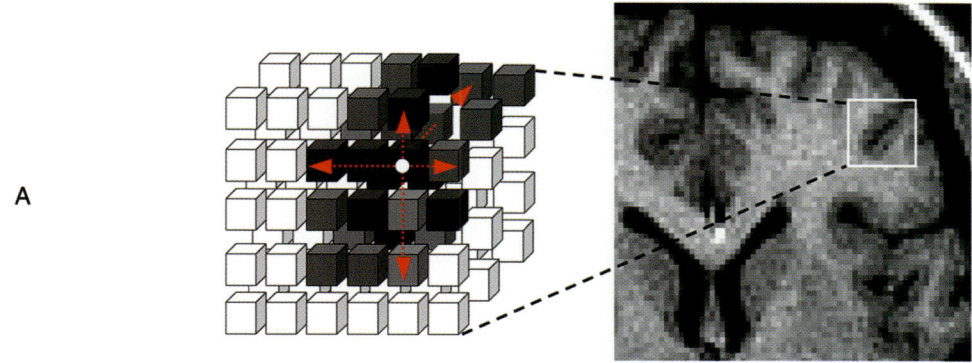

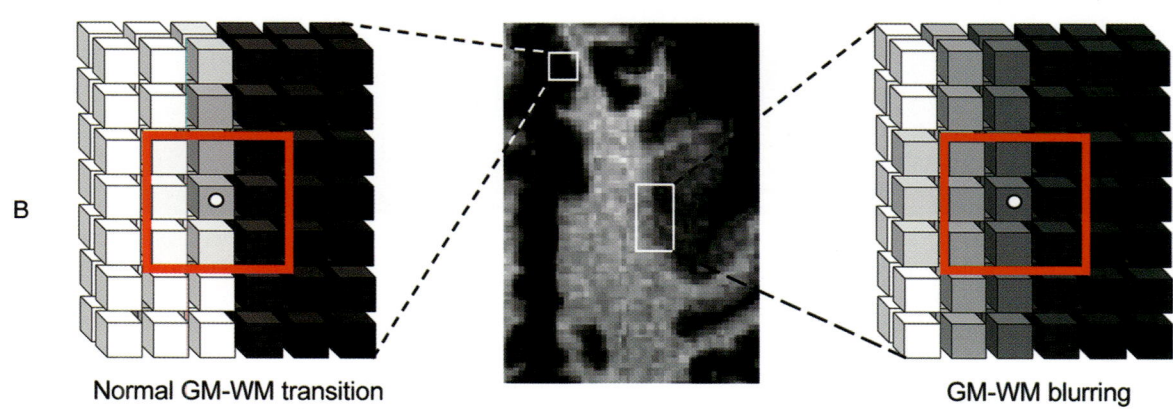

Normal GM-WM transition   GM-WM blurring

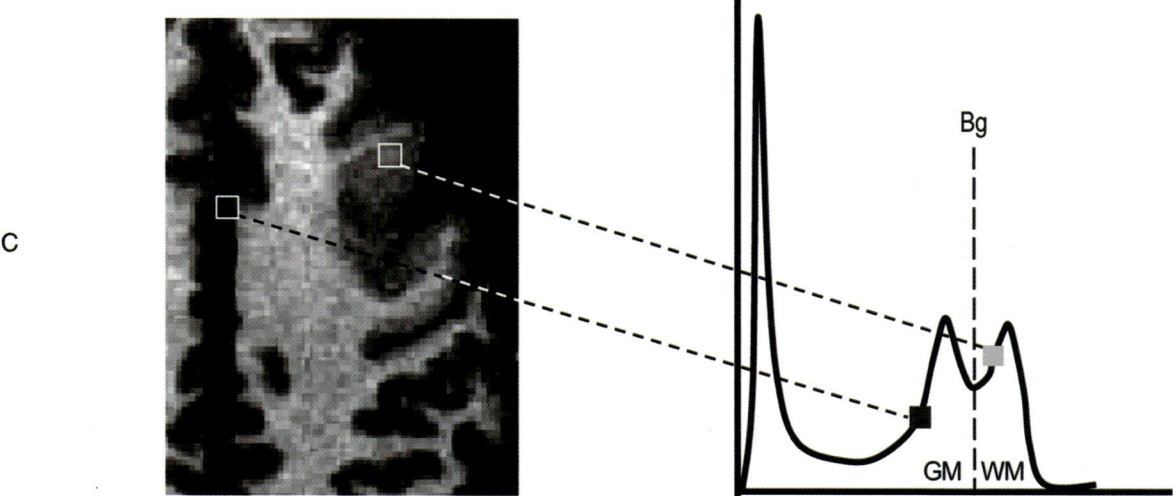

FIG. 8.9. Schematic representation of models of: (**A**) cortical thickness; (**B**) blurring of gray matter (GM) – white matter (WM) transition; and (**C**) relative intensity in focal cortical dysplasia. **A.** A small region of cortex and adjacent WM (box) is represented and magnified. To model cortical thickening, each voxel (dot) in the MRI volume was used as the starting point for GM counting performed in each discrete direction. **B.** To model GM–WM transition, the absolute gradient of gray level intensities was calculated in a cube centered on each voxel. Examples of regions of interest with normal GM–WM transition (left) with a steep gradient and blurred GM-WM transition (right) with progressive gradient are schematically represented. **C.** The gray level intensities signal within the FCD lesion was modeled by calculating the absolute difference between the intensity of a given voxel and the intensity at the GM–WM boundary Bg as defined by the image histogram. This allowed the relative position of each voxel to be calculated with respect to Bg.

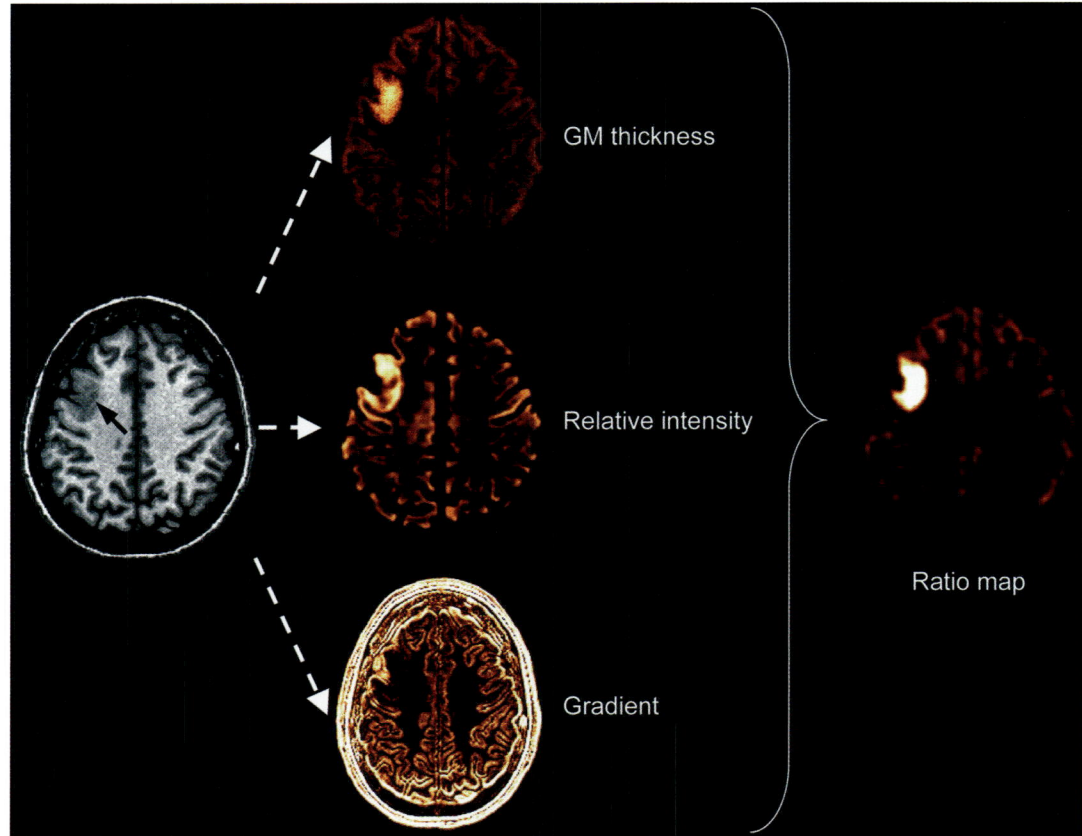

FIG. 8.10. A representative example of a lesion of focal cortical dysplasia in the frontal lobe (arrow). The maps show increased gray matter (GM) thickness and lesion intensity, and a reduction in the gradient. The ratio map (GM thickness × relative intensity/gray level intensity gradient) enhances the contrast and maximizes lesion visibility.

To maximize visibility of FCD lesions, the three feature maps were combined into a composite map (Fig. 8.10). Our results showed that the composite maps yielded a significantly increased sensitivity of lesion detection relative to conventional MRI (88% vs 50%) by maintaining high specificity (95% vs 100%). In this work we demonstrated for the first time in a controlled fashion that the application of computer-based models of the MRI characteristics of FCD pathology could significantly improve the sensitivity of lesion detection.

After demonstrating that our method could be improved by incorporating more sophisticated models of the MRI characteristics of FCD pathology (37) (Fig. 8.11), we sought to develop an automated approach for the detection of FCD (106). We developed a two-stage, computer-based classifier to identify FCD lesions using morphologic and first-order features presented above (see Fig. 8.9) and second-order texture analysis. Computational models of MRI characteristics of FCD provided visually discernible information, while second-order texture analysis was used to quantify less available information regarding tissue organization through the quantification of spatial relationships of gray-level intensity pairs (Figs 8.12, 8.13). We studied the preoperative MRI of 18 patients with histologically confirmed FCD. FCD was detected on conventional MRI during standard presurgical evaluation in 11 of the 18, resulting in a sensitivity of 61%. The classifier correctly identified FCD lesions in 15 of 18 patients (83%). Representative examples are shown in Figure 8.14.

In addition to the high sensitivity of lesion detection, another equally important result is that no lesional voxels were identified in any control subject. This finding is especially relevant in light of the fact that in five patients the classifier identified a lesional cluster that did not colocalize with a manual lesion label. Retrospective visual analysis of the individual feature maps input revealed that these lesional clusters exhibited a pattern of features similar to the known FCD lesions. However, no EEG abnormalities data were found in these regions and retrospective visual inspection of these regions did not show any FCD. Furthermore, we found no clinical or histopathologic characteristics that would differentiate these five patients from the others. Yet the absence of any false positives in control subjects, combined with reports of diffuse or nonfocal cortical involvement in FCD (110, 113, 114), suggests that these clusters may indeed indicate abnormal regions that are otherwise undetectable via conventional means.

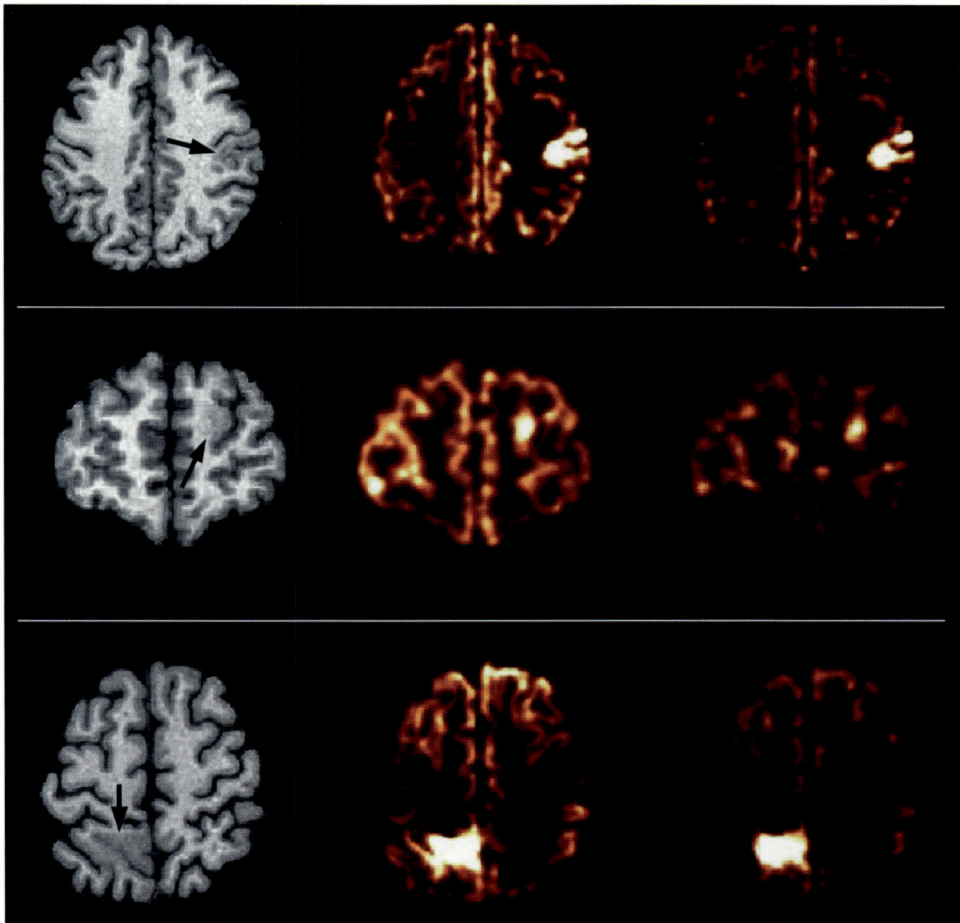

FIG. 8.11. Improved contrast in focal cortical dysplasia models. Within each panel, the conventional T1-weighted MRI is in the left-hand column, the original composite map set is in the middle column, and the improved composite map is in the right-hand column. Lesion locations are indicated on the conventional MRI by arrows. Intensity within nonlesional cortex is reduced in the improved composite map relative to the original composite map for all examples.

The classifier improved upon our previous techniques by providing an automated, objective approach to lesion detection. An advantage of 3D texture analysis, as well as the cortical thickness and gradient models among the first order features, is that they operate in three dimensions. This allows the simultaneous consideration of information from consecutive slices of the brain, whereas a human observer performing standard visual analysis examines the brain volume a slice at a time and therefore must mentally synthesize information from consecutive slices.

In a preliminary study of TLE patients with unilateral hippocampal atrophy texture analysis has been able to detect abnormalities in the contralateral hippocampus that were undetected by visual inspection of the MR images (108). In an attempt to lateralize the seizure focus in TLE patients with normal hippocampal and amygdalar volumetric MRI using texture analysis, we studied 26 TLE patients and 30 aged- and sex-matched control subjects. Leave-one-out linear discriminant analysis (with stepwise feature selection) trained on the MRI second-order texture data of the hippocampus

and the amygdala allowed correct lateralization of the seizure focus in all patients.

Our results indicate that texture analysis provides evidence for brain structural damage that is not evident through visual and volumetric analysis, and suggest that this technique could be a powerful tool for lesion identification in focal epilepsy related to malformations of cortical development and particularly in patients with no detectable structural lesion, so-called 'MRI-negative' or cryptogenic cases.

FUTURE DIRECTIONS

Widespread availability of powerful computing facilities and sophisticated image processing software, combined with the high spatial resolution and excellent tissue contrast provide by high-field MRI, will probably continue to expand the power of image processing. There is little doubt that this

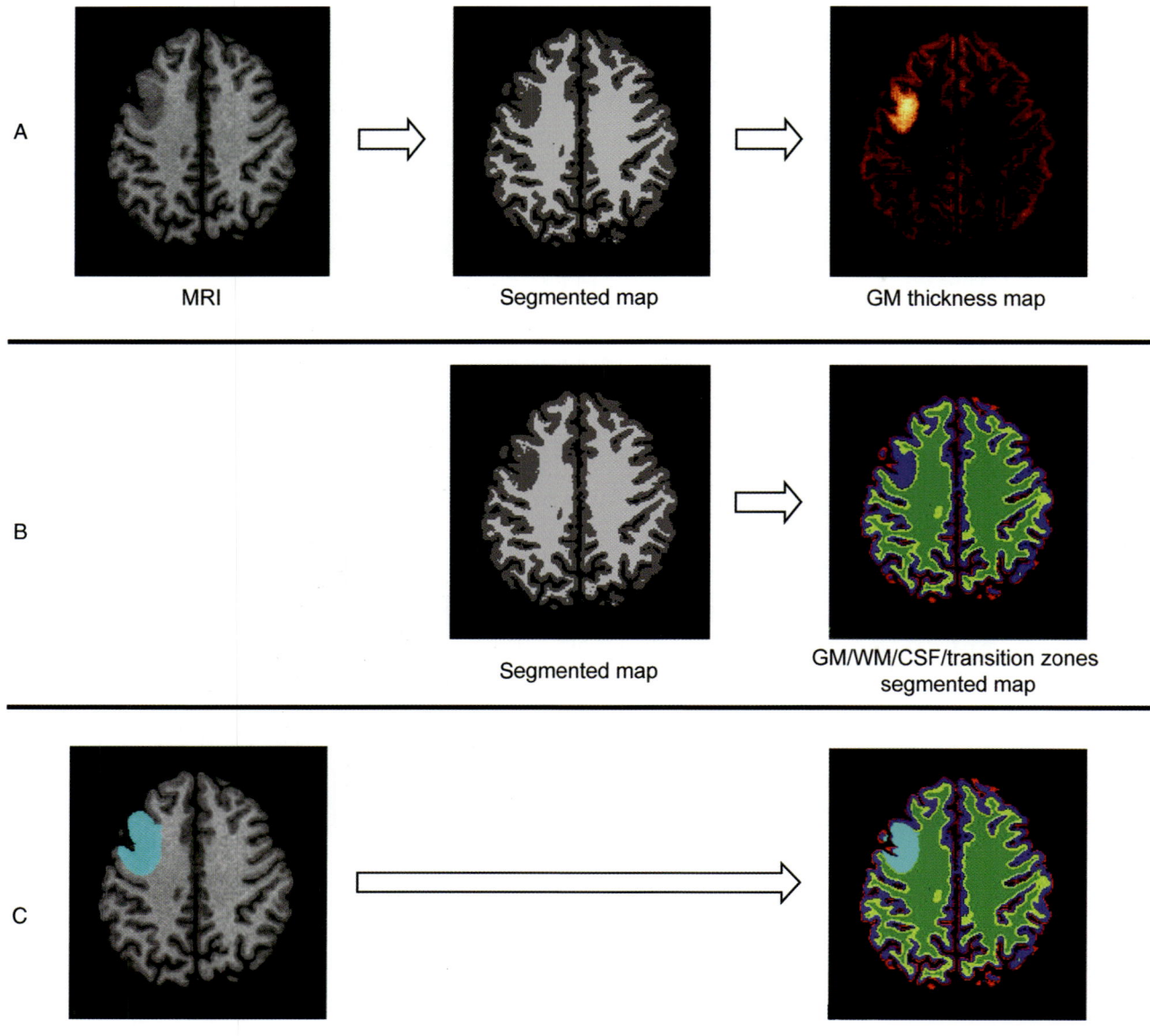

A MRI → Segmented map → GM thickness map

B Segmented map → GM/WM/CSF/transition zones segmented map

C Manual lesion label on MRI → 6-class segmented map

FIG. 8.12. Automatic classification of focal cortical dysplasia. **A.** T1-weighted MRI volumes are segmented into gray matter (GM), white matter (WM), and CSF, resulting in a GM/WM/CSF segmented map, which is used as a basis for measuring cortical thickness. **B.** The GM/WM/CSF segmented maps are further segmented into more classes for use in training the classifiers. GM/WM and GM/CSF transition classes are defined by analyzing a neighborhood of a fixed size surrounding each voxel within the segmented. A voxel is determined to belong to the GM/WM transition class (yellow) if at least 30% of neighboring voxels are GM and at least 30% of neighboring voxels are WM. A similar algorithm is used for the GM/CSF transition class. The result is a segmented map exhibiting the five following classes: GM, WM, CSF, GM/WM transition, and GM/CSF transition (GM/WM/CSF/transition zones segmented map). **C.** Lesions of focal cortical dysplasia are manually segmented on T1-weighted MRI (left). Adding the lesion labels to the GM/WM/CSF/transition zones segmented map results in a six-class segmented map (right).

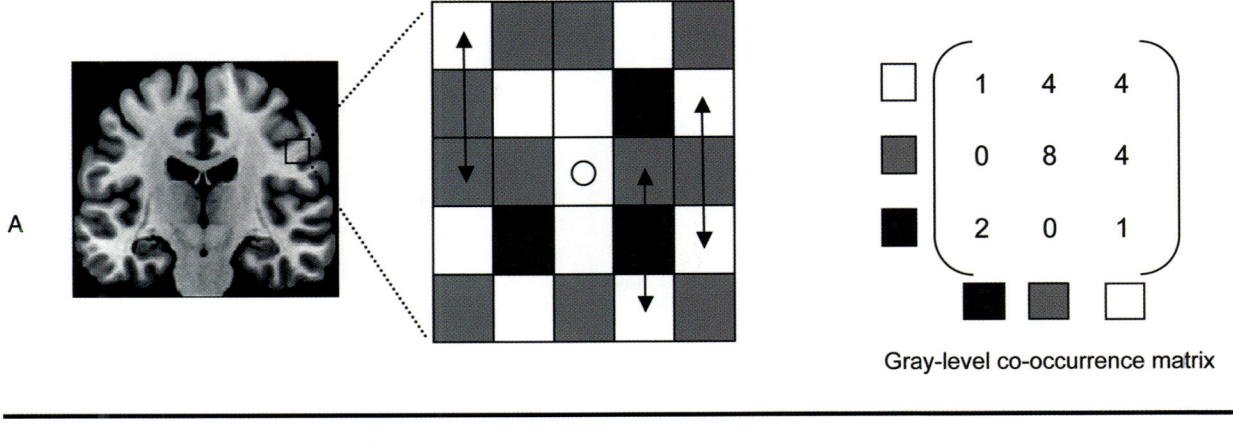

Gray-level co-occurrence matrix

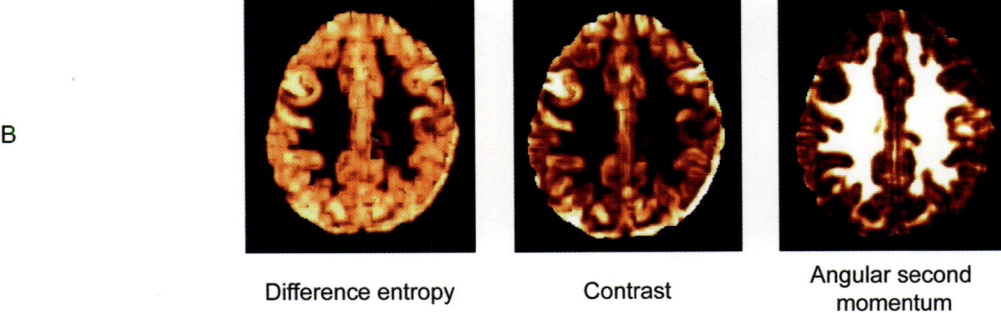

Difference entropy   Contrast   Angular second momentum

FIG. 8.13. Automatic classification of focal cortical dysplasia: construction of second-order texture maps. **A.** A region of predetermined size is constructed around each voxel (center circle in the schematic magnification). Within this region, the number of occurrences of the various pairs of voxel-intensities separated by a given distance in a given direction (sample pairs indicated by arrows) is counted to produce a co-occurrence matrix. Second-order texture feature operators are then calculated on the co-occurrence matrix. The entire MRI volume is examined using this procedure. **B.** Representative axial slices from second-order texture maps used to construct the automated classifier.

increasing sophistication will improve our understanding of the causes and consequences of epilepsy, possibly by combining different quantitative structural imaging methods described above. Structural imaging results will lay foundations for subsequent investigation of targeted electrophysiologic measurements, neurochemical and physiologic imaging assessments, including measures of synaptic markers (PET and SPECT imaging) or functional imaging (fMRI, MR spectroscopy, and PET).

Longitudinal studies using these novel and sensitive automatic MR-based methods may serve as a basis for modeling disease progression. The few longitudinal studies published so far have relied on operator-dependent methods (115–117). Improvements in the accuracy in data registration and the use of fully automated techniques are critical to this area of research. Ultimately, any MRI lesion has to be correlated with the other parameters ensuing from a comprehensive pre-surgical evaluation.

Some of the general problems related to imaging analysis methods such as reproducibility, low spatial resolution, long processing time, and availability of sufficient computer power are being increasingly overcome and will allow their widespread use. Therefore, as for volumetric MRI measurement of the hippocampus, it is conceivable that some of the

methods discussed above will be usable in routine clinical practice in the near future.

SUMMARY AND CONCLUSIONS

Acquisition techniques with gradient-echo techniques allow for an improved signal-to-noise ratio, whole brain coverage with thin slices in times compatible with clinical examinations, and minimal partial volume effects. The impact of this improved imaging data, when combined with new image processing techniques, is very promising.

The necessity for obtaining high reproducibility and the need to increase efficiency has motivated the development of computer-assisted automated procedures. These techniques are promising because, unlike visual assessment, they provide reliable, consistent, and reproducible data, and are easy to automate.

These techniques have the potential to reveal more clearly the nature, location, and extent of brain abnormalities and could eventually improve diagnostic yield, leading to further reduction in the requirement for invasive EEG recording and in the number of patients diagnosed with cryptogenic epilepsy. The abundance of techniques available

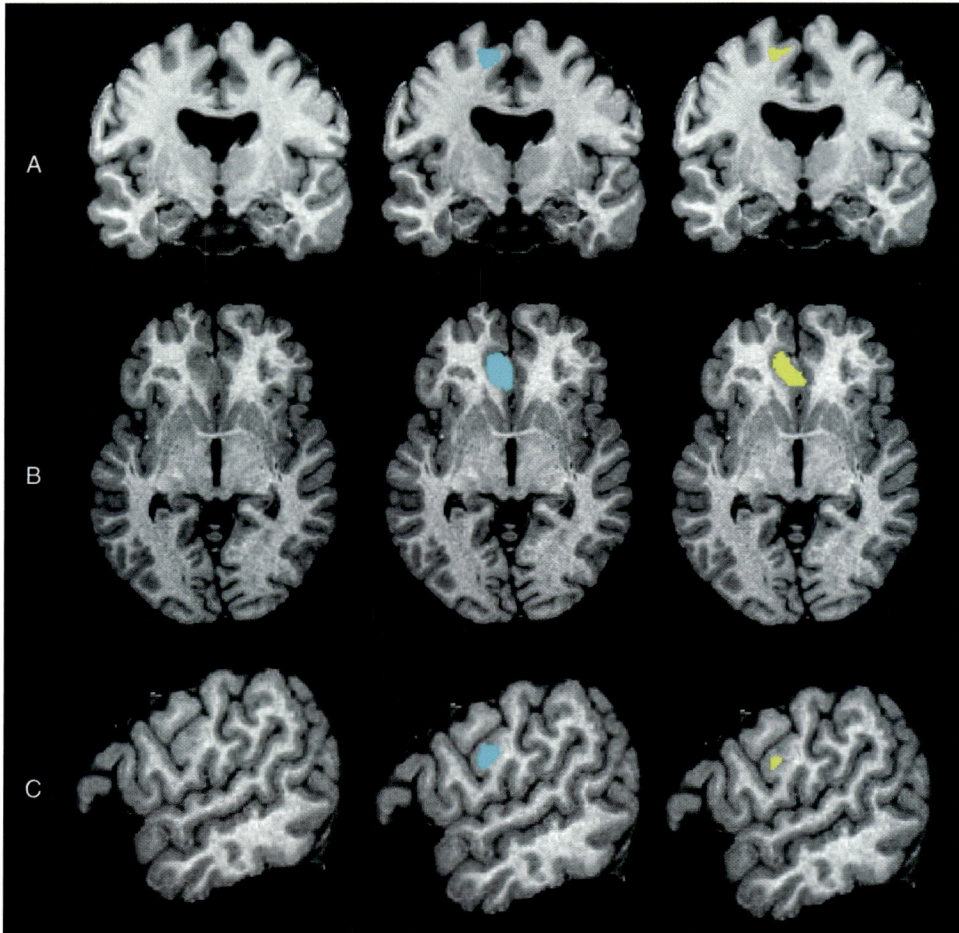

FIG. 8.14. Automatic classification of focal cortical dysplasia. Three examples (**A–C**) of automated focal cortical dysplasia lesion identification. Left: T1-weighted MRI. Center: MRI with manual lesion label shown in blue. Right: MRI with lesion identified automatically by the classifier shown in yellow.

to researchers makes it difficult to predict which image processing techniques will have an actual impact on the clinical practice. It is fundamental to bear in mind that the clinical input is determinant in deciding which features to investigate and which technique may be most useful.

By demonstrating diffuse abnormalities not identified by eye because of anatomic variability and the subtle nature of the changes, the information provided by novel image processing methods may prove to be useful to predict seizure outcome of surgical resection by demonstrating a more widespread abnormality of the brain. Even if the sensitivity of these techniques turns out not to be better but only equal to the manually segmented volumes, their application would represent a great improvement in procedures, since these methods are automated and objective. So far, many of these methods have been applied to population-based studies, allowing a better and more global understanding of the disease. In the future, these novel techniques should be tailored to provide information in individual patients, making their impact more relevant at a clinical level.

These quantitative methods will further enhance our ability to push the limits of the never-ending search for 'invisible' lesions and significantly improve the selection of patients for seizure surgery. Although some methods are relatively well established, others are in their infancy. It is hoped that these new techniques ultimately will become more widely available and permit lesion identification in many more patients being evaluated in specialized centers. Such studies could result in new predictors for the treatment of epilepsy by allowing studying the relationship between subtle anatomic changes and clinical symptoms, cognitive signs and response to treatment.

ACKNOWLEDGMENTS

Most of the work presented here is the result of collaborations with Neda Bernasconi, Samson Antel, Louis Collins, Alan Evans, Kelim Siddiqi, and Doug Arnold. We wish to thank Simon Duchesne, Jason Lerch, Najmeh Khalili, and

Roch Comeau for their invaluable help and useful suggestions. I am grateful to the Canadian Institute of Health Research (CIHR) for funding research in this area.

REFERENCES

1. Bastos AC, Comeau RM, Andermann F, et al. Diagnosis of subtle focal dysplastic lesions: curvilinear reformatting from three-dimensional magnetic resonance imaging. *Ann Neurol* 1999;46:88–94.

2. Schulze-Bonhage AH, Huppertz HJ, Comeau RM, et al. Visualization of subdural strip and grid electrodes using curvilinear reformatting of 3D MR imaging data sets. *Am J Neuroradiol* 2002;23:400–403.

3. Musse O, Armspach JP, Namer IJ, et al. Data-driven curvilinear reconstructions of 3D MR images: application to cryptogenic extratemporal epilepsy. *Magn Reson Imaging* 2002;16:1227–1235.

4. Collins DL, Neelin P, Peters TM, Evans AC. Automatic 3D inter-subject registration of MR volumetric data in standardized Talairach space. *J Comput Assist Tomogr* 1994;18 192–205.

5. Talairach J, Tournoux P. *Co-planar stereotaxic atlas of the human brain.* New York: Thieme Medical, 1988.

6. Zijdenbos AP, Forghani R, Evans AC. Automatic 'pipeline' analysis of 3-D MRI data for clinical trials: application to multiple sclerosis. *IEEE Trans Med Imaging* 2002;21:1280–1291.

7. Sled JG, Pike GB. Standing-wave and RF penetration artifacts caused by elliptic geometry: an electrodynamic analysis of MRI. *IEEE Trans Med Imaging* 1998;17 653–662.

8. Sled JG, Zijdenbos AP, Evans AC. A comparison of retrospective intensity non-uniformity correction methods for MRI. *Inform Proc Med Imag* 1997;459–464.

9. Kovacevic N, Lobaugh NJ, Bronskill MJ, et al. A robust method for extraction and automatic segmentation of brain images. *Neuroimage* 2002;17:1087–1100.

10. Shattuck DW, Sandor-Leahy SR, Schaper KA, et al. Magnetic resonance image tissue classification using a partial volume model. *Neuroimage* 2001;13:856–876.

11. Duncan JS. Imaging and epilepsy. *Brain* 1997;120:339–377.

12. Cook MJ, Fish DR, Shorvon SD, et al. Hippocampal volumetric and morphometric studies in frontal and temporal lobe epilepsy. *Brain* 1992;115:1001–1015.

13. Jack CR Jr, Bentley MD, Twomey CK, Zinsmeister AR. MR imaging-based volume measurements of the hippocampal formation and anterior temporal lobe: validation studies. *Radiology* 1990;176:205–209.

14. Watson C, Andermann F, Gloor P, et al. Anatomic basis of amygdaloid and hippocampal volume measurement by magnetic resonance imaging. *Neurology* 1992;42:1743–1750.

15. Bernasconi N, Bernasconi A, Andermann F, et al. Entorhinal cortex in temporal lobe epilepsy: a quantitative MRI study. *Neurology* 1999;52:1870–1876.

16. Pruessner JC, Li LM, Serles W, et al. Volumetry of hippocampus and amygdala with high-resolution MRI and three-dimensional analysis software: minimizing the discrepancies between laboratories. *Cereb Cortex* 2000;10:433–442.

17. Cascino GD, Jack CR Jr, Parisi JE, et al. Magnetic resonance imaging-based volume studies in temporal lobe epilepsy: pathological correlations. *Ann Neurol* 1991;30:31–36.

18. Kuznecky R, Cascino GD, Palmini A, et al. Structural neuroimaging. In: Engel J Jr, ed. *Surgical treatment of the epilepsies.* New York: Raven Press, 1993:197–209.

19. Kuznecky RI, Murro A, King D, et al. Magnetic resonance imaging in childhood intractable partial epilepsies: pathologic correlations. *Neurology* 1993;43:681–687.

20. Margerison JH, Corsellis JA. Epilepsy and the temporal lobes. A clinical, electroencephalographic and neuropathological study of the brain in epilepsy, with particular reference to the temporal lobes. *Brain* 1966;89:499–530.

21. Bernasconi N, Bernasconi A, Caramanos Z, et al. Mesial temporal damage in temporal lobe epilepsy: a volumetric MRI study of the hippocampus, amygdala and parahippocampal region. *Brain* 2003; 126:462–469.

22. Jutila L, Ylinen A, Partanen K, et al. MR volumetry of the entorhinal, perirhinal, and temporopolar cortices in drug-refractory temporal lobe epilepsy. *Am J Neuroradiol* 2001;22:1490–1501.

23. Salmenpera T, Kalviainen R, Partanen K, Pitkanen A. Quantitative MRI volumetry of the entorhinal cortex in temporal lobe epilepsy. *Seizure* 2000;9:208–215.

24. Bernasconi N, Bernasconi A, Caramanos Z, et al. Entorhinal cortex atrophy in epilepsy patients exhibiting normal hippocampal volumes. *Neurology* 2001;56:1335–1339.

25. Briellmann RS, Jackson GD, Kalnins R, Berkovic SF. Hemicranial volume deficits in patients with temporal lobe epilepsy with and without hippocampal sclerosis. *Epilepsia* 1998;39:1174–1181.

26. Coste S, Ryvlin P, Hermier M, et al. Temporopolar changes in temporal lobe epilepsy: a quantitative MRI-based study. *Neurology* 2002;59:855–861.

27. Lee JW, Andermann F, Dubeau F, et al. Morphometric analysis of the temporal lobe in temporal lobe epilepsy. *Epilepsia* 1998;39:727–736.

28. Mitchell LA, Jackson GD, Kalnins RM, et al. The anterior temporal lobe in TLE: quantitative MRI and histopathological assessment. *Soc Magn Reson Med* 1998:285.

29. Moran NF, Lemieux L, Kitchen ND, et al. Extrahippocampal temporal lobe atrophy in temporal lobe epilepsy and mesial temporal sclerosis. *Brain* 2001;124:167–175.

30. DeCarli C, Hatta J, Fazilat S, et al. Extratemporal atrophy in patients with complex partial seizures of left temporal origin. *Ann Neurol* 1998;43:41–45.

31. Dreifuss S, Vingerhoets FJ, Lazeyras F, et al. Volumetric measurements of subcortical nuclei in patients with temporal lobe epilepsy. *Neurology* 2001;57:1636–1641.

32. Natsume J, Bernasconi N, Andermann F, Bernasconi A. MRI volumetry of the thalamus in temporal, extratemporal, and idiopathic generalized epilepsy. *Neurology* 2003;60:1296–1300.

33. Haller JW, Christensen GE, Joshi SC, et al. Hippocampal MR imaging morphometry by means of general pattern matching. *Radiology* 1996; 199:787–791.

34. Barra V, Boire JY. Tissue segmentation on MR images of the brain by possibilistic clustering on a 3D wavelet representation. *J Magn Reson Imaging* 12000;1:267–278.

35. Niessen W, Vincken KL, Weickert J, Viergever M. Three-dimensional MR brain segmentation. In: Proceedings of the IEEE International Conference on Computer Vision, 1998: 53–57.

36. Aboutanos GB, Nikanne J, Watkins N, Dawant BM. Model creation and deformation for the automatic segmentation of the brain in MR images. *IEEE Trans Biomed Eng* 1999;46:1346–1356.

37. Antel SB, Bernasconi A, Bernasconi N, et al. Computational models of MRI characteristics of focal cortical dysplasia improve lesion detection. *Neuroimage* 2002;17:1755–1760.

38. Baillard C, Hellier P, Barillot C. Segmentation of brain 3D MR images using level sets and dense registration. *Med Image Anal* 2001; 5:185–194.

39. Christensen GE, Joshi SC, Miller MI. Volumetric transformation of brain anatomy. *IEEE Trans Med Imaging* 1997;16:864–877.

40. Collins DL, Holmes CJ, Peters TM, Evans AC. Automatic 3-D model-based neuroanatomical segmentation. *Hum Brain Map* 1995;3:190–208.

41. Collins DL, Zijdenbos AP, Baare WFC, Evans AC. ANIMAL+ INSECT: improved cortical structure segmentation. In: Kuba A, ed. Image processing in medical imaging. Heidelberg: Springer Verlag, 1999:210–223.

42. Dawant BM, Hartmann SL, Thirion JP, et al. Automatic 3-D segmentation of internal structures of the head in MR images using a combination of similarity and free-form transformations: Part I, Methodology and validation on normal subjects. *IEEE Trans Med Imaging* 1999;18:909–916.

43. Duchesne S, Pruessner J, Collins DL. Appearance-based segmentation of medial temporal lobe structures. *Neuroimage* 2002;17:515–531.

44. Duta N, Sonka M. Segmentation and interpretation of MR brain images: an improved active shape model. *IEEE Trans Med Imaging* 1998;17:1049–1062.

45. Ghanei A, Soltanian-Zadeh H, Windham JP. A 3D deformable surface model for segmentation of objects from volumetric data in medical images. *Comput Biol Med* 1998;28:239–253.

46. Hartmann SL, Parks MH, Martin PR, Dawant BM. Automatic 3-D segmentation of internal structures of the head in MR images using a combination of similarity and free-form transformations: Part II, validation on severely atrophied brains. *IEEE Trans Med Imaging* 1999;18:917–926.

47. Kelemen A, Szekely G, Gerig G. Elastic model-based segmentation of 3-D neuroradiological data sets. *IEEE Trans Med Imaging* 1999;18:828–839.

48. Pitiot A, Toga AW, Thompson PM. Adaptive elastic segmentation of brain MRI via shape-model-guided evolutionary programming. *IEEE Trans Med Imaging* 2002;21:910–923.

49. Shen D, Herskovits EH, Davatzikos C. An adaptive-focus statistical shape model for segmentation and shape modeling of 3-D brain structures. *IEEE Trans Med Imaging* 2001;20:257–270.

50. Shen D, Moffat S, Resnick SM, Davatzikos C. Measuring size and shape of the hippocampus in MR images using a deformable shape model. *Neuroimage* 2002;15:422–434.

51. Szekely G, Kelemen A, Brechbuhler C, Gerig G. Segmentation of 2-D and 3-D objects from MRI volume data using constrained elastic deformations of flexible Fourier contour and surface models. *Med Image Anal* 1996;1:19–34.

52. Van Ginneken B, Frangi AF, Staal JJ, et al. Active shape model segmentation with optimal features. *IEEE Trans Med Imaging* 2002;21:924–933.

53. Webb J, Guimond A, Eldridge P, et al. Automatic detection of hippocampal atrophy on magnetic resonance images. *Magn Reson Imaging* 1999;17:1149–1161.

54. Ashton EA, Parker KJ, Berg MJ, Chen CW. A novel volumetric feature extraction technique with applications to MR images. *IEEE Trans Med Imaging* 1997;16:365–371.

55. Hogan RE, Mark KE, Choudhuri I, et al. Magnetic resonance imaging deformation-based segmentation of the hippocampus in patients with mesial temporal sclerosis and temporal lobe epilepsy. *J Digit Imaging* 2000;13:217–218.

56. Hogan RE, Mark KE, Wang L, et al. Mesial temporal sclerosis and temporal lobe epilepsy: MR imaging deformation-based segmentation of the hippocampus in five patients. *Radiology* 2000;216:291–297.

57. Sisodiya SM, Free S, Stevens JM, et al. Widespread cerebral structural changes in patients with cortical dysgenesis and epilepsy. *Brain* 1995;118:1039–1050.

58. Sisodiya SM, Free SL. Disproportion of cerebral surface areas and volumes in cerebral dysgenesis. MRI-based evidence for connectional abnormalities. *Brain* 1997;120:271–281.

59. Csernansky JG, Joshi S, Wang L, et al. Hippocampal morphometry in schizophrenia by high dimensional brain mapping. *Proc Natl Acad Sci USA* 1998;95:11406–11411.

60. Csernansky JG, Wang L, Jones D, et al. Hippocampal deformities in schizophrenia characterized by high dimensional brain mapping. *Am J Psychiatry* 2002;159:2000–2006.

61. Csernansky JG, Wang L, Joshi S, et al. Early DAT is distinguished from aging by high-dimensional mapping of the hippocampus. Dementia of the Alzheimer type. *Neurology* 2000;55:1636–1643.

62. Posener JA, Wang L, Price JL, et al. High-dimensional mapping of the hippocampus in depression. *Am J Psychiatry* 2003;160:83–89.

63. Wang L, Joshi SC, Miller MI, Csernansky JG. Statistical analysis of hippocampal asymmetry in schizophrenia. *Neuroimage* 2001;14:531–545.

64. Bouix S, Siddiqi K. *Computing medial surfaces.* 2000;Vol 55.

65. Bouix, S. Siddiqi, K. *Divergence-based medial surfaces.* Dublin, 2000:613–618.

66. Joshi S, Pizer S, Fletcher PT, et al. Multiscale deformable model segmentation and statistical shape analysis using medial descriptions. *IEEE Trans Med Imaging* 2002;21:538–550.

67. Shenton ME, Gerig G, McCarley RW, et al. Amygdala-hippocampal shape differences in schizophrenia: the application of 3D shape models to volumetric MR data. *Psychiatry Res* 2002;115:15–35.

68. Hogan RE, Bucholz RD, Choudhuri I, et al. Shape analysis of hippocampal surface structure in patients with unilateral mesial temporal sclerosis. *J Digit Imaging* 2000;13:39–42.

69. Kaiboriboon K, Hogan RE. 2002 Hippocampal shape analysis in status epilepticus associated with acute encephalitis. *AJNR Am J Neuroradiol* 23:1003–1006.

70. Pizer SM, Fritsch DS, Yushkevich PA, et al. Segmentation, registration, and measurement of shape variation via image object shape. *IEEE Trans Med Imaging* 1999;18:851–865.

71. Sisodiya SM, Stevens JM, Fish DR, et al. The demonstration of gyral abnormalities in patients with cryptogenic partial epilepsy using three-dimensional MRI. *Arch Neurol* 1996;53:28–34.

72. Cook MJ, Free SL, Manford MR, et al. Fractal description of cerebral cortical patterns in frontal lobe epilepsy. *Eur Neurol* 1995;35:327–335.

73. Free S, Sisodiya SM, Cook MJ, et al. Three-dimensional fractal analysis of the white matter surface from magnetic resonance images of the human brain. *Cereb Cortex* 1996;6:830–836.

74. Mangin JF, Frouin V, Bloch I, et al. From 3D magnetic resonance images to structural representations of the cortex topography using topology preserving deformations. *J Math Imag Vision* 1995;5:297–318.

75. Tao X, Prince JL, Davatzikos C. Using a statistical shape model to extract sulcal curves on the outer cortex of the human brain. *IEEE Trans Med Imaging* 2002;21:513–524.

76. Le Goualher G, Argenti AM, Duyme M, et al. Statistical sulcal shape comparisons: application to the detection of genetic encoding of the central sulcus shape. *Neuroimage* 2000;11:564–574.

77. Le Goualher G, Procyk E, Collins DL, et al. Automated extraction and variability analysis of sulcal neuroanatomy. *IEEE Trans Med Imaging* 1999;18:206–217.

78. Vaillant M, Davatzikos C. Hierarchical matching of cortical features for deformable brain image registration. In: International Conference on Information Processing in Medical Imaging (IPMI), 1999: 182–195.

79. Batchelor PG, Castellano Smith AD, Hill DL, et al. Measures of folding applied to the development of the human fetal brain. *IEEE Trans Med Imaging* 2002;21:953–965.

80. Van Essen DC. A tension-based theory of morphogenesis and compact wiring in the central nervous system. *Nature* 1997;385:313–318.

81. Fischl B, Dale AM. Measuring the thickness of the human cerebral cortex from magnetic resonance images. *Proc Natl Acad Sci USA* 2000;97:11050–11055.

82. Jones SE, Buchbinder BR, Aharon I. Three-dimensional mapping of cortical thickness using Laplace's equation. *Hum Brain Map* 2000;11:12–32.

83. Kabani N, Le Goualher G, MacDonald D, Evans AC. Measurement of cortical thickness using an automated 3-D algorithm: a validation study. Neuroimage 2001;13:375–380.

84. MacDonald D, Kabani N, Avis D, Evans AC. Automated 3-D extraction of inner and outer surfaces of cerebral cortex from MRI. *Neuroimage* 2000;12:340–356.

85. Meyer JR, Roychowdhury S, Russell EJ, et al. Location of the central sulcus via cortical thickness of the precentral and postcentral gyri on MR. *Am J Neuroradiol* 1996;17:1699–1706.

86. Rosas HD, Liu AK, Hersch S, et al. Regional and progressive thinning of the cortical ribbon in Huntington's disease. *Neurology* 2002;58:695–701.

87. Zeng X, Staib LH, Schultz RT, Duncan JS. Segmentation and measurement of the cortex from 3-D MR images using coupled-surfaces propagation. *IEEE Trans Med Imaging* 1999;18:927–937.

88. Magnotta VA, Andreasen NC, Schultz SK, et al. Quantitative in vivo measurement of gyrification in the human brain: changes associated with aging. *Cereb Cortex* 1999;9:151–160.

89. Ashburner J, Friston KJ. Voxel-based morphometry–the methods. *Neuroimage* 2000;11:805–821.

90. Worsley KJ, Liao CH, Aston J, et al. A general statistical analysis for fMRI data. *Neuroimage* 2002;15:1–15.

91. Baron JC, Chetelat G, Desgranges B, et al. In vivo mapping of gray matter loss with voxel-based morphometry in mild Alzheimer's disease. *Neuroimage* 2001;14:298–309.

92. Wright IC, McGuire PK, Poline JB, et al. A voxel-based method for the statistical analysis of gray and white matter density applied to schizophrenia. *Neuroimage* 1995;2:244–252.

93. Keller SS, Mackay CE, Barrick TR, et al. Voxel-based morphometric comparison of hippocampal and extrahippocampal abnormalities in patients with left and right hippocampal atrophy. *Neuroimage* 2002;16:23–31.

94. Keller SS, Wieshmann UC, Mackay CE, et al. Voxel based morphometry of grey matter abnormalities in patients with medically intractable temporal lobe epilepsy: effects of side of seizure onset and epilepsy duration. *J Neurol Neurosurg Psychiatry* 2002;73:648–655.

95. Woermann FG, Free SL, Koepp MJ, et al. Abnormal cerebral structure in juvenile myoclonic epilepsy demonstrated with voxel-based analysis of MRI. *Brain* 1999;122:2101–2108.

96. Woermann FG, van Elst LT, Koepp MJ, et al. Reduction of frontal neocortical grey matter associated with affective aggression in patients with temporal lobe epilepsy: an objective voxel by voxel analysis of automatically segmented MRI. *J Neurol Neurosurg Psychiatry* 2000;68:162–169.

97. Richardson MP, Friston KJ, Sisodiya SM, et al. Cortical grey matter and benzodiazepine receptors in malformations of cortical development. A voxel-based comparison of structural and functional imaging data. *Brain* 1997;120:1961–1973.

98. Woermann FG, Free SL, Koepp MJ, et al. Voxel-by-voxel comparison of automatically segmented cerebral gray matter–A rater-independent comparison of structural MRI in patients with epilepsy. *Neuroimage* 1999;10:373–384.

99. Keller S, Mackay C, Webb J, et al. Voxel based morphometry of hippocampal and extra-hippocampal effects of unilateral temporal lobe epilepsy. *Neuroimage* 2001;13:803.

100. Haralick RM, Shanmugam K, Dinstein I. Textural features for image classification. *IEEE Trans Sys Man Cyber* 1973;SMC-3:610–621.

101. Garra BS, Krasner BH, Horii SC, et al. Improving the distinction between benign and malignant breast lesions: the value of sonographic texture analysis. *Ultrason Imaging* 1993;15:267–285.

102. Lerski RA, Straughan K, Schad LR, et al. MR image texture analysis–an approach to tissue characterization. *Magn Reson Imaging* 1993;11:873–887.

103. Freeborough PA, Fox NC. MR image texture analysis applied to the diagnosis and tracking of Alzheimer's disease. *IEEE Trans Med Imaging* 1998;17:475–479.

104. Mathias JM, Tofts PS, Losseff NA. Texture analysis of spinal cord pathology in multiple sclerosis. *Magn Reson Med* 1999;42:929–935.

105. Schad LR, Bluml S, Zuna I. MR tissue characterization of intracranial tumors by means of texture analysis. *Magn Reson Imaging* 1993;11:889–896.

106. Antel SB, Collins DL, Bernasconi N, et al. Automated detection of focal cortical dysplasia lesions using computational models of their MRI characteristics and texture analysis. *Neuroimage* 2003;19:1748–1759.

107. Bernasconi, A. Antel, SB. Collins, DL, et al. Texture analysis and morphological processing of magnetic resonance imaging assist detection of focal cortical dysplasia in extra-temporal partial epilepsy. *Ann Neurol* 2001;49:770–775.

108. Yu O, Mauss Y, Namer IJ, Chambron J. Existence of contralateral abnormalities revealed by texture analysis in unilateral intractable hippocampal epilepsy. *Magn Reson Imaging* 2001;19:1305–1310.

109. Barkovich AJ, Kuzniecky RI, Jackson GD, et al. Classification system for malformations of cortical development: update 2001. *Neurology* 2001;57:2168–2178.

110. Taylor DC, Falconer MA, Bruton CJ, Corsellis JAN. Focal dysplasia of the cerebral cortex in epilepsy. *J Neurol Neurosurg Psychiatry* 1971;34:369–387.

111. Barkovich AJ, Kuzniecky RI. Neuroimaging of focal malformations of cortical development. *J Clin Neurophysiol* 1996;13:481–494.

113. Prayson RA, Estes ML. Cortical dysplasia: a histopathologic study of 52 cases of partial lobectomy in patients with epilepsy. *Hum Pathol* 1995;26:493–500.

114. Prayson RA, Spreafico R, Vinters HV. Pathologic characteristics of the cortical dysplasias. *Neurosurg Clin North Am* 2002;13:17–25.

115. Crum WR, Scahill RI, Fox NC. Automated hippocampal segmentation by regional fluid registration of serial MRI: validation and application in Alzheimer's disease. *Neuroimage* 2001;13:847–855.

116. Liu RS, Lemieux L, Bell GS, et al. A longitudinal quantitative MRI study of community-based patients with chronic epilepsy and newly diagnosed seizures: methodology and preliminary findings. *Neuroimage* 2001;14:231–243.

117. Liu RS, Lemieux L, Bell GS, et al. Progressive neocortical damage in epilepsy. *Ann Neurol* 2003;53:312–324.

CHAPTER 9

Imaging and Neuropsychology

Michael M. Saling

NEUROPSYCHOLOGY IN EPILEPSY

In the modern neuroscientific era, a very close interplay between neuropsychological model building and neuroimaging is developing. It is the underlying thesis of this chapter that cognitive architecture has an impact on patterns of activation observed during functional neuroimaging and on patterns of correspondence between structural MR measures and task performance, or correlations between resting glucose metabolism on PET and out-of-scanner task performances. In order to contextualize the argument, this chapter provides a conceptual introduction to the neuropsychology of focal epilepsy, with an emphasis on memory and language function, and I then move on to consider the significance of functional neuroimaging on neurocognitive model building in this field. Finally, I present some views on preoperative evaluation and decision making from a neuropsychological perspective. In this respect, too, neuropsychology and neuroimaging are natural allies, and the interaction between them is central to the approach outlined here.

Neuropsychology, as it name suggests, is an interdisciplinary field with two major aims. The first is to understand how psychological domains such as perception, language, cognition, and action are represented in, and regulated by, the normal brain. Much use has been made of the time-honored lesion method for the purpose of 'fractionating' psychological processes into fundamental components, and then demonstrating a double dissociation between lesion location and component functions (1). A well-known example is the fractionation of memory into immediate (primary) and recent (secondary) components. Bilateral mesial temporal lesions produce recent memory disorders with preservation of immediate memory (2). Left temporoparietal lesions have the opposite effect (2, 3). Double dissociations of this

type disclose the architecture of neurocognitive systems, provide important insights into the cerebral representation of complex functions, and allow for the localization of damage on the basis of well characterized cognitive disorders. High-resolution structural neuroimaging makes it possible to define brain lesions and cognitive function contemporaneously, opening up a new era of structurofunctional correlation in neuropsychology. Functional neuroimaging has been recruited with enthusiasm to address the question of cerebral representation without the need for drawing inferences from lesioned to normal brain.

A second aim of neuropsychology is to describe neurologic diseases in terms of their impact on psychological function, for the specific purpose of expanding clinical knowledge in the form of a neuropsychological syndromology. Neuropsychology has played a major role in differentiating, *inter alia*, primary dementias or stroke syndromes, and these broad directions are also reflected in neuropsychological approaches to the focal epilepsies.

Systematic neuropsychological study of patients with cerebral disease or injury preceded the advent of neuroimaging by several decades. The principal methodology was the lesion method. It involved careful description (qualitative and quantitative) of cognitive and behavioral change that was then correlated with anatomic pathology. It soon became clear that neuropsychological methods were able to localize lesions in the major associative cortices, previously considered to be 'silent.' The earliest application of neuropsychology to the field of focal epilepsy was based on the localizing significance of neuropsychological findings, underpinned by the seminal work of Brenda Milner and her colleagues at the Montreal Neurologic Institute (4). The development of technology that allowed the substance of the brain to be imaged, or regional cerebral function to be disclosed with a high degree of anatomic resolution, had a large and fundamental impact on the clinical neurosciences, and neuropsychology was no exception. Neuropsychologists rapidly embraced functional neuroimaging, and cognitive science has magnified the scope of functional neuroimaging to include, among other things, the very real possibility of clinical applications for cognitive activation techniques.

One of the most robust findings in neuropsychology is that bilateral damage of the hippocampi causes profound memory impairment, that is, amnesia (2, 5). The key characteristic of amnesic states is a failure to encode personal events and therefore the passage of time itself. The seminal case in the field of epilepsy is the famous HM (6). Conversely, it is well accepted that unilateral hippocampal damage causes a more restricted form of memory loss (7). Here the individual retains the ability to lay down personal memories and it therefore retains an ongoing and temporally coherent autobiographical record. Against this background, however, the affected individual has trouble learning new information that is exclusively represented in one symbolic framework or another. In the case of left mesial temporal damage, verbal information is difficult to acquire. Written or spoken information is forgotten. Right mesial temporal damage diminishes the ability to remember information that is inherently spatial. These difficulties represent the material specific impairments, and are commonly encountered in the field of temporal lobe epilepsy. Importantly, material that can be represented in more than one way can ameliorate the effects of a material specific memory disorder. This means, in turn, that the proper assessment of material specific disorders depends on theoretically and empirically well-targeted probes.

UNDERSTANDING MEMORY FUNCTION: A MODEL FOR THE FOCAL EPILEPSIES

Cognitive Architecture of Memory

The domain that we refer to as 'memory' is made up of multiple cognitive processes, some of which function in a surprisingly autonomous fashion. Neuropsychological evaluation of temporal lobe epilepsy deals predominantly with the *declarative memory system* and the interplay between its various components (5). The property that sets the declarative memory system apart is that its contents are amenable to conscious access. We are able to think about them, talk about them, or manipulate them in the spotlight of full awareness. Two broad systems contribute to declarative memory, *primary* and *secondary*. Primary memories are processed by a capacity-limited mechanism that can only contain as much information as can be held simultaneously in conscious awareness (one or two sentences, a single arithmetic problem, or a short list of separate items). The contents of primary memory decay rapidly (within seconds) to make way for the next items in the continuous stream of information that enters awareness. Decay of specific primary memory content can be

suspended if that content is actively manipulated. Reciting a string of incoming digits in reverse order is a good example of this. Active manipulation of the contents of primary memory is referred to as *working memory*. Primary memory forms the basis of ongoing awareness, production and comprehension of language, and reasoning. It is an 'on-line' processing system, and is mediated by neocortex.

The retention of information for more than a few seconds (anything from minutes to years) depends on the *secondary memory system*. To all intents and purposes its capacity is unlimited. It consists of two components, *episodic* and *semantic* (8, 9). The episodic system forms memories that are unique to the individual, define individual life histories, and ultimately contribute to the sense of self. Personal memories are context-specific. In other words, personal memories are inextricably bound-up with a specific chronologic point in the individual's history, a specific place, and a specific emotional state. The event and its associated spatiotemporal and emotional context technically constitute a memory episode. Amnesia is a disturbance of episodic memory. From a neurologic point of view, episodic memory is fundamentally dependent on mesial structures that include the hippocampal system and its diencephalic and cingulate projections (2).

By contrast, the semantic memory system is impersonal. It is a permanent store of our knowledge of the natural, constructed, and sociocultural world, that is, our stock of facts and meanings. The content of semantic memory is not specific to the individual but to a greater or lesser extent is held in common by all human beings. No particular significance attaches to the contexts in which the information was acquired. Unlike the 'one-off' acquisition of episodic memories, semantic memories are acquired by repetition and slow accretion over multiple contexts (think for example of the acquisition of vocabulary). Accordingly, semantic memories are not stored together with contextual information and are therefore context-independent. The neurologic substrate of semantic memory is an extensive neocortical network (10). Semantic memory is fundamentally preserved in amnestic disorders caused by focal midline lesions, but the neurologic substrates of episodic and semantic memory might interface in the anteromesial temporal region (11).

By virtue of their sheer magnitude, the stored contents of episodic and semantic memory are maintained below the level of awareness until they are specifically retrieved and temporarily held in working memory. Consider the following examples:

- When a person is asked to recite the months of the year in reverse order, stored knowledge of the names of the months and their chronologic order is retrieved from semantic memory and held in primary memory where the operation of reversal is performed
- When asked to recall the guests who attended a wedding, the context-specific event is retrieved from episodic memory and surveyed in working memory until the question has been answered.

Interactions of this type are mediated by projections between posterior association cortex and dorsolateral prefrontal cortex (in the case of retrieval from semantic memory), and those between the hippocampal system and dorsolateral prefrontal cortex (in the case of retrieval from episodic memory).

Fundamental to our approach to the evaluation of memory in temporal lobe epilepsy is the notion that the episodic and semantic systems operate in an *associative* or *relational* fashion (12). An episode is formed when an event is associated with a spatiotemporal and emotional context. The event itself is a complex of individual components that must be associated with one another if the event is to be remembered as nonfragmented. Similarly, an item of vocabulary is an association between a symbol (word) and the object it signifies, to take a semantic example. It can be said that associative or relational processing is the building block of the declarative memory system (5).

Arbitrary Associative Learning: A Third Component

Thus far I have presented a fairly conventional dichotomous view of secondary memory. In the assessment setting, neuropsychologists elicit secondary memory function by asking to patient to learn and retain a body of new information, the quantity of which exceeds the capacity or *span* of primary memory. Practically, this involves the presentation of words lists, test, geometric configurations, faces, or pictures of objects that are to be learned and recalled. New learning paradigms are often regarded as tapping episodic memory. In my view, new learning of this type does not conform to the special nature of episodic memory. The use of new learning paradigms in neuroimaging research in an attempt to reveal the functional neuroanatomy of episodic memory has led to a confusing picture.

Further, new learning paradigms do not fit entirely with the notion of semantic memory. Some of the material that makes up new learning tasks has features in common with previously established semantic links. Consider the following word pair *bird–pelican*. Remembering this pair is greatly assisted if one knows that a pelican is a bird. Nevertheless, the pair could equally have been *bird–dove* or *bird–eagle*. In this sense the pairing *bird–pelican* is arbitrary. The successful acquisition of a list of category–exemplar word pairs therefore depends on prior semantic memories as well as the capacity to absorb the essentially arbitrary aspects of the list. The semantic component in a word pair can be reduced almost completely, as in a pair such as *desk–lake*. To learn a list of randomly conjoined pairs, the individual must now rely heavily on what amounts to a rote process, which I term *arbitrary associative learning*. I propose that the secondary memory system requires a third component, which is responsible for the rapid uptake of links or relations that have yet to be established in episodic or semantic memory, or which might conflict with pre-established knowledge.

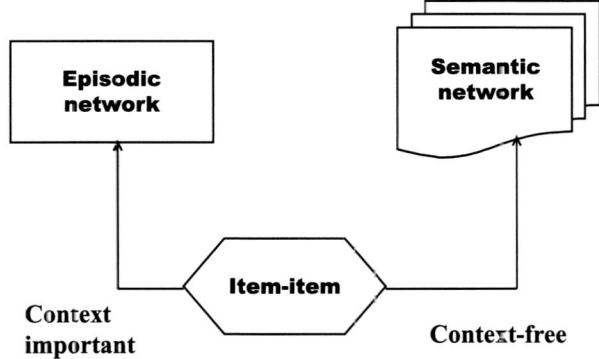

FIG. 9.1. An alternative view of the declarative memory system.

A further example may serve to show the generality of this idea. In anticipation of the imminent arrival of guests, the host hurriedly tidies the sitting room by hiding objects in the nearest and easiest-to-get-at location. In order to remember where those things are when the guests have left, the host must encode an association between object and temporary location. This association is novel in the sense that a pre-established basis for placing a particular object in a particular temporary place does not exist. Arbitrary associative learning provides basic relational input to the episodic and semantic systems (Fig. 9.1). This concept is fundamental to our view of the temporal lobe organization of memory and the application of our model to the neuropsychological evaluation of temporal lobe epilepsy.

FUNCTIONAL NEUROANATOMY OF DECLARATIVE MEMORY

Research in this area is expanding rapidly, and space does not permit an exhaustive treatment. I will simply tease out some fundamental trends that I consider important for the approach being elaborated here.

Primary Memory and its Intersection with Language

As mentioned previously, primary memory (including working memory) is a neocortical function. Cognitive models of working memory portray it as a complex hierarchical system or systems (1). Whether there is a single working memory system that subserves all cognitive domains (language, spatial cognition, and the like), or a separate working memory system for each domain (modular organization of cognition), is controversial. The essential point is that working memory in its entirety must be represented in the brain in a widely distributed fashion.

A great deal of the research effort in the functional neuroimaging of cognition has been devoted to working memory. Language paradigms are now being used with increasing frequency in the preoperative evaluation of surgical candidates with intractable focal epilepsies, possibly even rivaling the

Wada technique in the language lateralization (see Chapter 10). One commonly used paradigm, letter fluency, has a complex cognitive architecture, which includes a substantial working memory component. As words are generated, the patient has to hold these in a primary memory store and monitor this stock of responses for repetitions and other rule breaks (13). Letter fluency activates a number of specific cortical regions that reflect the linguistic components of the task. Like many other working memory paradigms, it also activates the left middle frontal gyrus, corresponding with Brodmann areas 9 and 46 (i.e. in dorsolateral prefrontal cortex; Fig. 9.2).

While it would be a mistake to assume that the working memory system is fully 'located' in the dorsolateral prefrontal cortex, it is not unreasonable to regard this region as a nodal coordinating locus of a widely represented working memory network (14). Left dorsolateral prefrontal activation in response to letter fluency tasks can be thought of as reflecting the working memory basis of language, and therefore has language lateralizing significance. Our group has shown

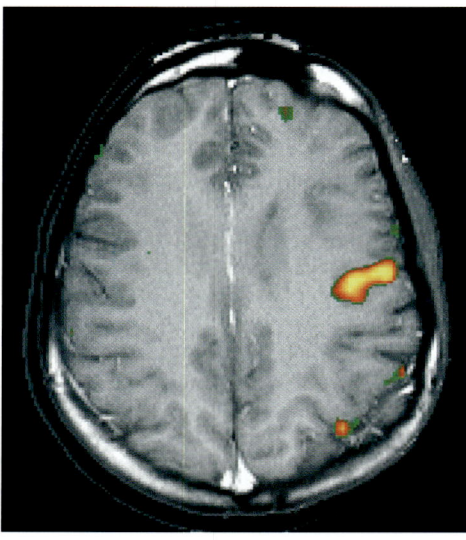

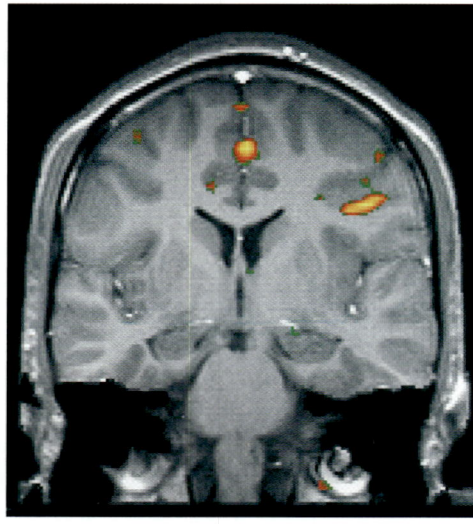

FIG. 9.2. Left dorsolateral prefrontal and anterior cingulate activation produced by a letter fluency task.

that there is a close correspondence between the pattern of activation produced by letter fluency tasks and that produced by noun–verb generation tasks.

Dorsolateral prefrontal cortex is likely to be the neural substrate, at least in part, of the so-called *executive* or *supervisory* component of working memory. Executive function, as the term implies, involves the control of lower level functions, and therefore deals with allocation of processing resources, as well as the planning and modulation of cognitive processes. It is important to note, in the present context, that executive function also underlies retrieval of information from the secondary memory system (see below). Retrieval processes are resource intensive, and proceed on the basis of an ongoing record of what information has or has not been accessed at any point in the process.

Secondary Memory

Functional neuroimaging research on memory has been colored by the assumption that new learning tasks are necessarily processed via the episodic system, and should, therefore, elicit hippocampal activation. A survey of this literature reveals that activation of the hippocampus proper is seldom observed, but parahippocampal or fusiform activation is more common (15). This, in turn, has spawned the view that the hippocampus is not critically involved in episodic memory, despite decades of lesion research that suggest the opposite. Recent work has shown, however, that paradigms tapping recall of truly personal memories in spatiotemporal and emotional context do activate hippocampus proper (16). New learning paradigms, such as verbal paired associate learning, activate structures in the parahippocampal region but not the hippocampus proper. In other words, there appears to be an intratemporal anatomic dissociation in normal studies that parallels the cognitive distinction I have drawn between 'episodic' and 'new learning' systems.

In a recent PET study (17) with [¹⁵O]H₂O to measure regional cerebral blood flow, we found that arbitrary paired associate learning activates a left hemisphere network involving parahippocampal region, fusiform gyrus, and dorsolateral prefrontal cortex. Amongst these regions the change in left parahippocampal regional cerebral blood flow was the most prominent, and extended along the rostrocaudal axis of the region to involve perirhinal cortex. The hippocampus proper did not activate. It seems likely, then, that structures within the parahippocampal region (entorhinal cortex, perirhinal cortex, and posterior parahippocampal cortex) constitute a processing node for arbitrary associative learning.

DISORDERS OF SECONDARY MEMORY IN TEMPORAL LOBE EPILEPSY

In most cases the neuropathology of temporal lobe epilepsy has a unilateral emphasis, and intractable seizures are often relieved by unilateral anterior temporal lobectomy. Largely on the basis of postresection findings, Brenda Milner and her colleagues demonstrated a double dissociation between material (i.e. whether the memory task is verbal or spatial in nature) and laterality of the resection (left versus right): right temporal resections produced impairments in nonverbal or visuospatial memory (with preservation of verbal memory) (18), and left temporal resections produced impairments in verbal memory (with preservation of nonverbal memory) (7). This came to be known as the *material-specificity* hypothesis (7). Importantly, verbal-specific and visuospatial-specific disorders are fundamentally impairments of new learning. Episodic memory remains intact. It is only when both mesial temporal regions are disrupted that episodic memory is profoundly impaired. In other words, bitemporal damage is necessary for the clinical phenomenon of amnesia, as the case of HM demonstrated so vividly.

The material-specificity model and the bitemporal model of amnesia formed the basis of neuropsychological practice in temporal lobe epileptology (19). While there have been no convincing exceptions to the bitemporal model of amnesia, the material-specificity model, at least in its strong form, has required some modification (20). Interpretation of postlobectomy findings in anatomocognitive terms is difficult because multiple structures are involved. En bloc anterior temporal lobe resection removes not only sclerotic hippocampal tissue but also amygdala, parahippocampal region, and lateral temporal cortex. Some early attempts to identify the anatomic basis of material-specific memory impairments were based on relationships between the extent of resection of hippocampal or neocortical tissue and memory performance. Ultimately this correlative approach was limited by the fact that the extent of resection was often dictated by the nature and extent of epileptogenic pathology, and that the extent of mesial and lateral resection is itself interrelated.

Reliable MR visualization of hippocampal sclerosis (21) provided a new opportunity to study the impact of well lateralized epileptogenic lesions on material-specific memory impairments at the preoperative stage when neuropsychological decision making is most needed. The following sections summarize some trends that have emerged from preoperative research.

Visuospatial-specific Impairments and Right Hippocampal Sclerosis

The association between right hippocampal sclerosis and visuospatial memory impairment is not as robust as the material-specificity hypothesis predicts (22). While some patients do perform poorly on tasks that involve the acquisition of topographic or figural information, these impairments are also seen in cases with left hippocampal sclerosis, making it difficult to discriminate between left and right hippocampal sclerosis groups on the basis of visuospatial memory impairments (23). Some visuospatial tasks do appear to discriminate

between left and right hippocampal sclerosis. There are preliminary indications that tasks involving navigation through simulated three-dimensional environments are more closely related to right hippocampal function (24) and might eventually form a valid basis for interrogating this region in TLE.

Verbal-specific Memory Impairments and Left Hippocampal Sclerosis

The link between verbal-specific memory impairments and left hippocampal sclerosis is considerably more reliable (25–30) but not as straightforward as was previously supposed (20, 25, 26, 30, 31). Like language, verbal memory is hierarchically organized. It extends from the encoding of single letters to the recall of complex narrative. Much of the previous (and some contemporary) research is predicated on the assumption that verbal memory is unitary; that is, there is no real distinction between learning a random string of words, for example, or recalling grammatically complex text. In terms of this view, a lesion that disrupts one aspect of verbal memory will disrupt all other aspects. Also in line with this unitary view, verbal memory is often quantified as a global index that summates performance over a number of different verbal memory tasks (e.g. word list learning, verbal paired associate learning, and recall of narrative). The origins of this procedure lie in a psychometric notion that correlation means identity. For some clinical purposes such as documentation of impairment in diffuse disorders (moderately advanced dementia or closed head injury) the summation of different memory tests might serve us quite well. In the detection of focal impairment, however, the unitary view has led to insensitivity at the diagnostic level, and has obscured what we now believe to be a high degree of specialization within the temporal lobe (30–33).

Comparison between groups of TLE patients with MR-documented and pathologically confirmed right or left hippocampal sclerosis has confirmed that verbal memory impairments are selectively related to left-sided damage. This association, however, does not apply to all forms of verbal memory. There is a marked and robust impairment of memory for arbitrary paired associates in left hippocampal sclerosis, and this paradigm reliably differentiates left from right hippocampal sclerosis (30). Memory for semantically related paired associates, text, or lists of single words, on the other hand, shows small left–right effects in some samples of patients but not in others. When an effect is present it is secondary to language factors (34, 35). The latter group of tasks are either explicitly semantically structured (related word pairs or text), or susceptible to the imposition of semantic structure in the course of learning (single word lists). In either case, pre-established semantic relations support learning. Semantically structured tasks, however, decline selectively after anterior temporal lobectomy, which imposes an additional neocortical lesion, and show prominent left-right effects postoperatively. Arbitrary associative learning shows no further change after temporal lobe resection (35).

The following general picture emerges from the lesion studies: arbitrary associative learning appears to be primarily dependent on mesial temporal structures as evidenced by its sensitivity to the effects of mesial temporal damage. Semantically structured tasks seem to be more dependent on neocortical structures, as suggested by a drop in performance after anterior temporal lobectomy. Thus, preoperative lateralization of verbal memory is *task-specific* (30) while lateralization of verbal memory after left en bloc anterior temporal lobectomy is not (35).

Computational modeling suggests that that the brain must represent semantically structured and newly acquired arbitrary information in nonoverlapping neural substrates to protect semantic networks from catastrophic interference (36). The convergence of this notion and the differential impairment of arbitrary and structured forms of verbal memory caused by left hippocampal sclerosis and lateral temporal damage are consistent with the hypothesis that there is intratemporal specialization in the regulation of verbal memory.

Left Temporal Specialization: The Contribution of Functional Neuroimaging

This hypothesis carries important implications for the preoperative evaluation of TLE and the prediction of postoperative changes in verbal memory. Nevertheless, it is difficult to demonstrate intratemporal specialization in a compeling fashion in the context of lesion methodology because naturally occurring epileptogenic pathology in the temporal lobe usually encompasses a number of regions.

In order to test the hypothesis we exploited the finding that mesial temporal foci are associated with variable patterns of resting glucose metabolism (37). Since cerebral glucose metabolism reflects neuronal function, variations in glucose uptake provide an ideal substrate for correlational mapping of cognitive processes. Our approach was to correlate measures of arbitrary or semantically related verbal paired associate learning with resting [18]fluorodeoxyglucose uptake in a PET environment in a sample of patients with left TLE and MR evidence of well lateralized ipsilateral hippocampal sclerosis.

The key finding was a dissociation between temporal region and task property (arbitrary versus semantically structured associates): arbitrary associative learning correlated with glucose uptake in the left perirhinal region (Fig. 9.3), while learning of semantically related paired associates correlated with uptake in the left anterior inferior temporal neocortex (Fig. 9.4). No peak correlations were found in the hippocampus proper.

Regression modeling revealed that arbitrary associative learning was predicted solely by glucose uptake in the left perirhinal region. Semantically structured associative learning was predicted primarily by uptake in left anterior inferior temporal neocortex and secondarily by uptake in the ipsilateral perirhinal region. This is encapsulated in the model depicted in Figure 9.5.

Mesial Temporal Pathology and Arbitrary Associative Learning

The role of the hippocampus in the regulation of new learning has been emphasized to the exclusion of other mesial temporal lobe structures. This parallels the emphasis on the hippocampus as the primary generator of epileptic activity in TLE. Greater attention is now being devoted to the study of cell loss in entorhinal, perirhinal, and parahippocampal cortex. Recent findings show that volume loss in TLE is not restricted to the hippocampus, but is also seen in entorhinal, and perirhinal cortex (38). As mentioned above, functional neuroimaging studies of memory show that new learning tasks typically activate sites in the parahippocampal region, and a number of lines of evidence now suggest that the anterior portion of the parahippocampal region (entorhinal and perirhinal cortices) are crucial substrates for associative learning (39–43).

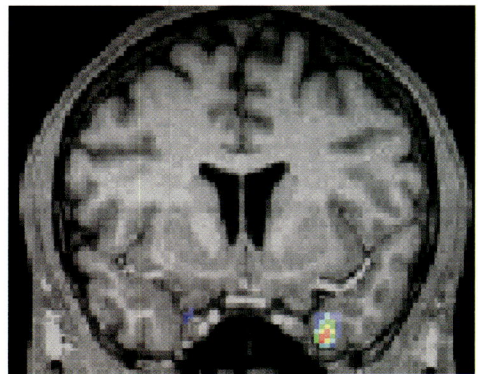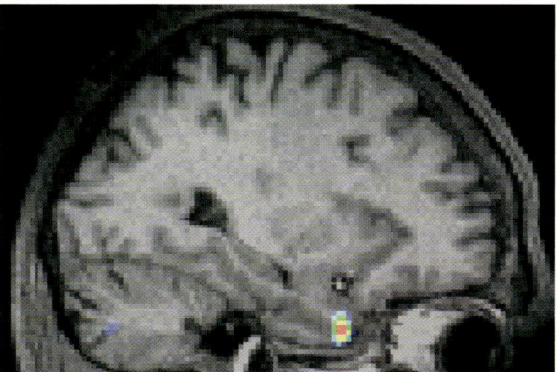

FIG. 9.3. Peak correlation between arbitrary paired associative learning and glucose uptake in the perirhinal region. (With permission from Weintrob et al. 2002 (32).)

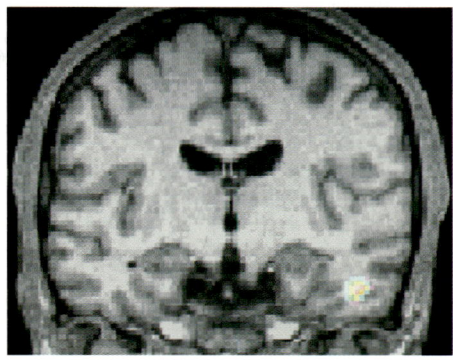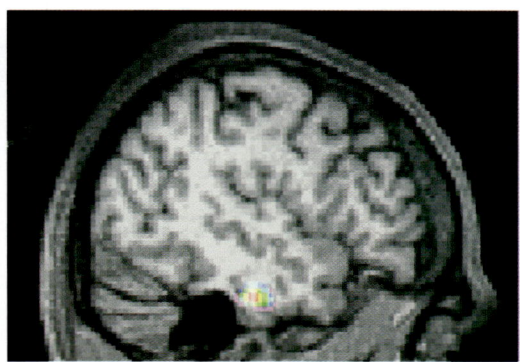

FIG. 9.4. Peak correlation between semantically related associative learning and glucose uptake in anterolateral temporal neocortex. (With permission from Weintrob et al. 2002 (32).)

A quantitative relationship exists between T2 relaxation times and measures of arbitrary new learning, such that increments in T2 signal are associated with worsening memory (33). This has been interpreted as a direct (and exclusive) effect of hippocampal cell loss. Given a positive relationship, however, between hippocampal and anterior parahippocampal cell loss, these findings might reflect broader mesial temporal involvement in arbitrary associative learning.

Mesial and Lateral Memory Patterns in Left Temporal Lobe Epilepsy

When memory disturbances in TLE are conceptualized in this way, it is possible to define reasonably distinctive patterns of memory impairment in patients with left temporal foci. The patterns described here are not purely theoretically derived, but are seen in the clinical setting.

Left Mesial Temporal Lobe Epilepsy

The underlying pathology is commonly mesial temporal sclerosis, often associated with characteristic anterior temporal lobe changes such as loss of differentiation at the gray–white junction, decreased T1 signal, and increased T2 signal on MRI. As far as we know at this stage, the mesial temporal cell loss and gliosis is the key cause of the neuropsychological features. Mild confrontation naming deficits are commonly seen, although these are seldom reflected at a conversational level: spontaneous language output is usually normal. The memory impairment is task-specific, with poor

acquisition of arbitrary verbal material. Memory tasks with a significant semantic component are performed at normal or near-normal levels. Recall of visuospatial material is variable, but generally normal.

From a functional point of view these patients have preserved episodic memory, and are therefore well oriented and able to recall personal details. As far as daily information is concerned, they are able to recall broad outlines (such as the overall gist of a news item, conversation, or text) but have trouble in recalling specific details. These features are summarized in Table 9.1. It is worth noting that the disturbances are less pronounced in the case of nonsclerotic and circumscribed epileptogenic lesions (some dysplastic lesions, cavernomas, or neoplastic changes), or generally in adult-onset seizures.

Left Lateral Temporal Lobe Epilepsy

Seizures of left temporal origin arise from a variety of pathologies. Developmental anomalies are frequently seen, and can be quite subtle. Neuropsychological impairments in this group are difficult to document preoperatively, but when present tend to show up as mild inefficiencies in language-based cognition, including inefficient recall of text and other forms of semantically structured information. Mesial temporal memory function is normal.

Memory Patterns in Right and Bilateral Temporal Lobe Epilepsy

Right Temporal Lobe Epilepsy

Depending on the locus and nature of the underlying pathology, these patients exhibit a variety of impairments in visuospatial function, including poor learning and recall of topographic, figural, or facial information. Verbal memory is generally normal. Confrontation naming impairments are sometimes seen in patients with right mesial temporal sclerosis.

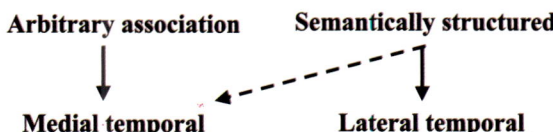

FIG. 9.5. A neuropsychological model of verbal learning.

TABLE 9.1. *Neuropsychological Features of Left Mesial Temporal Lobe Epilepsy*

Neurocognitive Domain	Clinical Features
Language	
Impaired confrontation naming	Fluent conversational language with minimal or no word-finding difficulties
Memory	
Intact episodic memory	Able to recall contextualized personal events
Poor uptake of arbitrary associations	
Normal or near normal semantic memory; able to utilize previously established semantic knowledge to support new learning	Able to recall general ideas, themes or gist: difficulty with recall of specific details
Variable but predominantly normal spatial memory	Normal route-finding, topographical orientation, facial recognition, constructional skills

Bilateral Temporal Lobe Epilepsy

Bilateral mesial temporal sclerosis and independent bitemporal seizure foci are associated with material nonspecific or *general* memory impairments; that is, verbal and spatial memory is impaired. Functionally, these patients are unreliable in the recall of personal events and should be regarded as partially amnesic. General memory impairments are also seen in cases with long-standing unilateral temporal foci with prominent spread of seizure activity to the contralateral temporal lobe.

PREOPERATIVE DECISION MAKING

Neuropsychological investigation has been an important component of the presurgical work-up of patients with intractable TLE. The rationale for this type of investigation stems from the fact that temporal lobe structures involved in the genesis of epileptiform discharges are also crucial and nodal components of the memory network. Classically, the objective of neuropsychological assessment was twofold:

- to assist in localizing seizure foci by demonstrating material-specific impairments
- to anticipate dysfunction, and possibly significant structural damage affecting temporal lobe structures contralateral to the putative seizure focus, with the ultimate aim of avoiding a postoperative amnesic state.

Advances in imaging technology have added to electroencephalography the confirmatory power of characterizing epileptogenic tissue in terms of a number of neurobiologic dimensions such as changes in volume, cellular reactivity, interictal metabolism, and local hyperperfusion during the ictus. As a result, the risk of performing a temporal lobe resection in the presence of an abnormal contralateral temporal lobe has been minimized. In the light of precise imaging one might even be tempted to consider whether temporal lobe resection in the presence of biologically minor contralateral

abnormalities is as undesirable as was previously thought. Nevertheless, the measurement of structural, metabolic, blood flow, or electrophysiologic changes cannot substitute for the direct characterization of memory or other cognitive functions.

As much of this chapter has illustrated, neuroanatomic concepts of memory are still evolving. It is unlikely that the structural basis of memory in the temporal lobe has been fully explored and conceptualized. The relationship of neurobiologic markers to cognitive function is complex, particularly with respect to the issue of reorganization of function in the face of neurologic disease. The contribution of partially damaged tissue, whether sclerotic or dysplastic, to the integrated operation of memory is not well understood. Finally, the specifics of neuropsychological outcome after surgery cannot be predicted on the basis of neuropathologic factors alone. The combination of neurocognitive evaluation with structural or functional imaging (including cognitive activation studies), forms the basis of our approach, and has led to reduced reliance on amobarbital for studies of language and memory lateralization.

The Problem of 'Incongruous' Memory

For a number of decades preoperative evaluation has been heavily driven by the strong form of the material-specificity hypothesis. In terms of this model, right temporal foci should be associated with impaired visuospatial memory and intact verbal memory, while the reverse should be true in left temporal foci. Deviations from this pattern are regarded as incongruous, and are often thought of as preoperative complications, perhaps raising the question of bitemporal involvement. It is becoming clear that lateralization of memory function is more complex than the double dissociation predicted by the strong form of the material-specificity hypothesis. Incongruity in the pattern of memory breakdown is not necessarily of concern, but the issue should be approached with caution on a case-by-case basis. Decision making is often blurred when theoretically unfocused and poorly targeted measures are used.

It is now well accepted that cases with early-onset seizures, definite unilateral mesial temporal sclerosis, extra-hippocampal atrophy of the ipsilateral temporal lobe, and a moderate to severe material-specific impairment of memory function (congruent with the affected side) are at least risk for postoperative memory impairments after a standard anterior temporal lobectomy. Conversely, cases with very mild unilateral mesial temporal sclerosis and very mild or no material-specific memory impairment are highly likely to experience a postoperative drop in memory. This principle applies equally to left- or right-sided foci. There are, however, some considerations that are specific to the side of the focus.

Right-sided Foci

In cases with a right-sided focus and well defined ipsilateral hippocampal sclerosis, the presence of impaired arbitrary verbal associative learning raises the question of bitemporal involvement. The base-rate of this pattern in purely right mesial temporal sclerosis is low. On the other hand, impairments in semantically structured forms of verbal memory are not as suggestive because impairment of this type do occur in right-sided cases. When mesial temporal sclerosis is mild and visuospatial memory is entirely normal, the possibility of postoperative difficulties in remembering new faces, learning new routes, or recalling diagrammatic or architectural information should be considered.

Left-sided Foci

Most cases with a left-sided focus and definite ipsilateral mesial temporal sclerosis will exhibit impaired verbal memory, the key feature of which is abnormal arbitrary associative learning. Some of these cases also exhibit impairments in one or more aspects of nonverbal memory. Because the base-rate of the latter finding on standard testing is reasonably high in the presence of a normal right hippocampus, it does not necessarily constitute evidence of a general memory impairment and is not an automatic contraindication to a left anterior temporal resection. We occasionally encounter a rather different pattern in cases with severe left hippocampal sclerosis: arbitrary verbal associative learning is normal but visuospatial memory is severely impaired. One interpretation is reorganization of verbal memory function, possibly to the contralateral hemisphere, with 'crowding out' of the resident function (namely, visuospatial memory). Alternatively, it might suggest that the parahippocampal region is unaffected, and that verbal memory is being supported at an entorhinal or perirhinal level. At this stage of our knowledge, a pattern of this type should prompt careful study of the parahippocampal region. If this is abnormal, then reorganization, or even interhemispheric transfer, might be a viable hypothesis.

FUTURE DIRECTIONS

The work discussed here suggests that there is an essential complementarity between functional neuroimaging approaches to cognition in focal epilepsy and the lesion method that has long formed the basis of neuropsychology: both are capable of fractionating or dissociating neurocognitive systems. The use of neuroimaging in this way is predicated on two assumptions:

- tasks with differing cognitive architectures are capable of producing reliably different patterns of activation
- there is an invariant relationship between the various cognitive subcomponents of a task, and their neural substrates.

The first assumption has been seriously challenged by the well-known fact that a bewildering array of tasks activate certain common regions such as dorsolateral prefrontal cortex and the anterior cingulate region. This could serve to suggest, however, that all these tasks rest on common cognitive fundamentals such as working memory and selective attention. The differential patterns of correlation between arbitrary and semantic forms of verbal memory and resting glucose uptake in patients with left hippocampal sclerosis reinforces the notion that high-level differences in cognitive architecture are represented in different regions of the temporal lobe and should therefore produce differential patterns of activation. In other words, functional neuroimaging could and should be used to test the predictions of neurocognitive models, with the advantage that the technique is not limited by the anatomic proclivities of naturally occurring pathologies.

Null findings in functional neuroimaging do pose a problem: when a task gives rise to a reliable cerebral change it can be concluded that there is some sort of relationship between the task and the activated region, but the opposite interpretation is not unequivocal when no cerebral change is observed (44). This is particularly pertinent in the silence of the hippocampus proper when challenged by new learning paradigms. The model I have proposed here is predicated on the interpretation that the hippocampus is not particularly 'interested' in low-level associative processes but is recruited specifically in response to the complex associative process that underlies truly episodic memories. Binder and Detre (Chapter 10) raise the possibility that the nonresponsiveness of the hippocampus to learning tasks might be the result of a technical issue. Hopefully, future work will help to resolve this. A central aim of this chapter was to show that the imaging fractionation of verbal memory function corresponds with the different patterns of verbal memory impairment seen in mesial and lateral TLE. This is a powerful justification for continuing efforts to take a cognitive model-testing approach to functional neuroimaging research in the focal epilepsies. Further, patterns of cerebral activation are capable of reflecting individual differences (13), and could be used to advantage in preoperative evaluation. This theme is taken up further in Chapter 10 .

REFERENCES

1. Shallice T. From neuropsychology to mental structure. Cambridge: Cambridge University Press, 1988.
2. Bauer RM, Grande L, Valenstein E. Amnesic disorders. In: Valenstein E, ed. Clinical neuropsychology, 4th ed. New York: Oxford University Press, 2003:495–573.
3. Vallar G, Shallice T. Neuropsychological impairments of short-term memory. New York: Cambridge University Press, 1990.
4. Milner B. Psychological aspects of focal epilepsy and its neurosurgical management. In: Walter R, ed. Neurosurgical management of the epilepsies. New York: Raven Press, 1975:299–332.
5. Cohen NJ, Eichenbaum H. Memory, amnesia, and the hippocampal system. Cambridge, MA: MIT Press, 1994.
6. Milner B, Corkin S, Teuber HL. Further analysis of the hippocampal amnesic syndrome: 14 year followup study of H. M. Neuropsychologia 1968;6:215–234.
7. Milner B. Memory and the medial temporal regions of the brain. In: Broadbent DE, ed. Biology of memory. New York: Academic Press, 1970:29–50.
8. Tulving E. Episodic and semantic memory. In: Donaldson W, ed. Organization of memory. New York: Academic Press, 1972:382–403.
9. Tulving E. Episodic memory: from mind to brain. Annu Rev Psychol 2002;53:1–25.
10. Saffran EM, Sholl A. Clues to the functional and neural architecture of word meaning. In: Hagoort P, ed. The neurocognition of language. New York: Oxford University Press, 2000:241–272.
11. Kensinger EA, Siri S, Cappa SF, Corkin S. Role of the anterior temporal lobe in repetition and semantic priming: evidence from a patient with a category-specific deficit. Neuropsychologia 2003;41:71–84.
12. Savage GR, Saling MM, Davis CW, Berkovic SF. Direct and indirect measures of verbal relational memory following anterior temporal lobectomy. Neuropsychologia 2002;40:302–316.
13. Wood AG, Saling MM, Abbott DF, Jackson GD. A neurocognitive account of frontal lobe involvement in orthographic lexical retrieval: an fMRI study. Neuroimage 2001;14:162–169.
14. Nyberg L, Marklund P, Persson J, et al. Common prefrontal activations during working memory, episodic memory, and semantic memory. Neuropsychologia 2003;41:371–377.
15. Nyberg L, McIntosh AR, Houle S, et al. Activation of medial temporal structures during episodic memory retrieval. Nature 1996;380:715–717.
16. Maguire EA, Mummery CJ. Differential modulation of a common memory retrieval network revealed by positron emission tomography. Hippocampus 1999;9:54–61.
17. Weintrob DL, Saling MM, Reutens DCE, et al. Verbal memory in TLE: differing consequences of functional and structural changes in the left temporal lobe. Epilepsia 2000;41:S80.
18. Milner B. Visual recognition and recall after right temporal-lobe excisions in man. Neuropsychologia 1968;6:191–210.
19. Jones-Gotman M, Smith ML, Zatorre RJ. Neuropsychological testing for localizing and lateralizing the epileptogenic region. In: Engel J, ed. Surgical treatment of the epilepsies, 2nd ed. New York: Raven Press, 1993:245–261.
20. Dobbins IG, Kroll NEA, Tulving E, et al. Unilateral medial temporal lobe memory impairment: type deficit, function deficit, or both? Neuropsychologia 1998;36:115–127.
21. Jackson GD, Berkovic SF, Tress BM, et al. Hippocampal sclerosis can be reliably detected by magnetic resonance imaging. Neurology 1990;40:1869–1875.
22. Piguet O, Saling MM, O'Shea MF, et al. Rey figure distortions discriminate right and left foci in temporal lobe epilepsy. Arch Clin Neuropsychol 1994;9:451–460.
23. Saling MM, O'Shea MF, Desmond P, Berkovic SF. Topographical memory in temporal lobe epilepsy: Laterality effects depend on surgery. Epilepsia 1995;36:S120.
24. Maguire E. Hippocampal and parietal involvement in human topographical memory: evidence from functional neuroimaging. In: O'Keefe J, ed. The hippocampal and parietal foundations of spatial cognition. Oxford: Oxford University Press, 1999:405–415.
25. Baxendale SA. The hippocampus: functional and structural correlations. Seizure 1995;4:105–117.
26. Bell BD, Davies KG. Anterior temporal lobectomy, hippocampal sclerosis, and memory: recent neuropsychological findings. Neuropsychol Rev 1998;8:25–41.
27. Hermann BP, Wyler AR, Bush AJ, Tabatabai FR. Differential effects of left and right anterior temporal lobectomy on verbal learning and memory performance. Epilepsia 1992;33:289–297.
28. Oxbury JM, Oxbury SM. Memory and the human temporal lobes. In: Milner AD, ed. Comparative neuropsychology. New York: Oxford University Press, 1998:95–108.
29. Rausch R. Differences in cognitive function with left and right temporal lobe dysfunction. In: Zaidel E, ed. The dual brain: hemispheric specialization in humans. New York: Guilford Press, 1985:247–261.
30. Saling MM, Berkovic SF, O'Shea MF, et al. Lateralization of verbal memory and unilateral hippocampal sclerosis: evidence of task-specific effects. J Clin Exp Neuropsychol 1993;15:608–618.
31. Rausch R, Babb TL. Evidence for memory specialization within the mesial temporal lobe in man. In: Engel J, ed. Fundamental mechanisms of human brain function. New York: Raven Press, 1987.
32. Weintrob DL, Saling MM, Berkovic SF, et al. Verbal memory in left temporal lobe epilepsy: Evidence for task-related localization. Ann Neurol 2002;51:442–447.
33. Wood AG, Saling MM, O'Shea MF, et al. Reorganization of verbal memory and language: a case of dissociation. J Int Neuropsychol Soc 1999;5:69–74.
34. Hermann BP, Seidenberg M, Haltiner A, Wyler AR. Adequacy of language function and verbal memory performance in unilateral temporal lobe epilepsy. Cortex 1992;28:423–433.
35. Saling MM, O'Shea MF, Weintrob DL, et al. Medial and lateral contributions to verbal memory: evidence from temporal lobe epilepsy. In: Suzuki K, ed. Frontiers of human memory. Sendai: Tohoku University Press, 2002:151–158.
36. McClelland JL, McNaughton BL, O'Reilly RC. Why there are complementary learning systems in the hippocampus and neocortex: insights from the successes and failures of connectionist models of learning and memory. Psychol Rev 1995;102:419–457.
37. Savic I, Altshuler L, Baxter L, Engel J Jr. Pattern of interictal hypometabolism in PET scans with fludeoxyglucose F-18 reflects prior seizure types in patients with mesial temporal lobe seizures. Arch Neurol 1997;54:129–136.
38. Bernasconi N, Bernasconi A, Caramanos Z, et al. Mesial temporal damage in temporal lobe epilepsy: a volumetric MRI study of the hippocampus, amygdala and parahippocampal region. Brain 2003;126:462–469.
39. Bilkey DK. Long-term potentiation in the in vitro perirhinal cortex displays associative properties. Brain Res 1996;733:297–300.
40. Buckley MJ, Gaffan D. Perirhinal cortex ablation impairs configural learning and paired-associate learning equally. Neuropsychologia 1998;36:535–546.
41. Bunsey M, Eichenbaum H. Critical role of the parahippocampal region for paired-associate learning in rats. Behav Neurosci 1993;107:740–747.
42. Miyashita Y, Okuno H, Tokuyama W, et al. Feedback signal from medial temporal lobe mediates visual associative mnemonic codes of inferotemporal neurons. Brain Res Cogn Brain Res 1996;5:81–86.
43. Pihlajamaki M, Tanila H, Hanninen T, et al. Encoding of novel picture pairs activates the perirhinal cortex: an fMRI study. Hippocampus 2003;13:67–80.
44. Rugg M. Functional neuroimaging in cognitive neuroscience. In: Hagoort P, ed. The neurocognition of language. New York: Oxford University Press, 2000:14–36.

CHAPTER 10

Functional MRI in Epilepsy

Jeffrey R. Binder and John A. Detre

INTRODUCTION

The goal of functional neuroimaging is to map the activity of the living brain in space and time. Electrophysiologic methods such as magnetoencephalography and electroencephalography offer direct measurements of neural activity with high temporal resolution but are limited by difficulties in defining the spatial location and extent of activation. Neuroimaging methods based on metabolic and vascular parameters, while offering limited temporal resolution, provide excellent spatial resolution and localization of brain function. One such method, functional magnetic resonance imaging (fMRI), enables completely noninvasive imaging of changes in blood oxygenation and perfusion. In recent years fMRI has become the most widely used modality for visualizing regional brain activation and is beginning to find widespread application in clinical neuroscience.

Unlike positron emission tomography (PET), fMRI does not require exposure to ionizing radiation. fMRI can thus be performed many times in the same subject without additional health risks, providing improved statistical power, measures of test–retest reliability, the ability to monitor changes in activation serially over time, and the potential for exploring a wide range of activation tasks. Compared to PET, fMRI provides superior temporal and spatial resolution and increased sensitivity for detecting task activation in individual subjects through signal averaging. On the other hand, PET provides a greater repertoire of image contrast sources. Whereas fMRI is primarily sensitive to hemodynamic changes, PET images can reflect blood flow, glucose utilization, oxygen consumption, and receptor binding. The latter occurs at concentrations well below the sensitivity of MRI, and can only be measured in vivo with radioactive tracers, although fMRI can be used to visualize pharmacological

effects indirectly (1–3). PET also provides a silent environment that is not affected by electromagnetic interference or the presence of ferrous objects. However, PET scanning is less widely available and significantly more costly than fMRI because of the need for on-line tracer synthesis.

In this review, we discuss the physiologic bases and contrast mechanisms underlying susceptibility-based and perfusion-based fMRI signals, and review the potential applications of fMRI in the management of epilepsy.

PHYSIOLOGY OF FUNCTIONAL NEUROIMAGING

Nearly all studies of task-specific activation using functional neuroimaging rely on the fact that regional changes in brain metabolism produce regional changes in cerebral blood flow (CBF), herein referred to as activation–flow coupling. Regional CBF changes are used as a surrogate marker for changes in regional brain function; thus uncoupling of blood flow and metabolism or neural function may result in false-negative or false-positive neuroimaging signals. Changes in blood flow and metabolism occur with excitatory or inhibitory neurotransmission, both of which are energy consuming processes (4).

Studies in both animal models and human subjects using a variety of modalities have shown that, in normal brain, blood flow changes occur following a latency of 0.5–1.5 seconds and build to a peak in approximately 4–8 seconds, even for stimuli of much shorter duration (5). The activation–flow coupling response is so stereotyped in normal subjects that it may be taken as a constant in statistical models used to analyze fMRI data. However, there are likely to be pathologic alterations in activation–flow coupling in certain disease states, as well as both regional variations and individual variations in activation–flow coupling in normals (6). For example, in patients with severe stenosis of arteries supplying a given brain region, delayed vascular transit times may be observed, along with an attenuation of functionally induced hemodynamic changes (7, 8).

Surprisingly little is known about the physiology underlying activation–flow coupling. The phenomenon was originally described in 1890 by Roy and Sherrington (9). Studies since that time have failed to identify a specific hormonal or metabolic factor that mediates activation–flow coupling (5). The recent identification of nitric oxide gas as a highly vasoactive and rapidly diffusible substance suggested the possibility of this chemical serving as a mediator, but a variety of other metabolites and even direct synaptic connections have also been proposed. Even the purpose of activation–flow coupling remains undetermined. While it is often assumed that a regional CBF increase is required to supply oxygen and nutrients, studies of brain energy metabolism in response to functional activation have not conclusively supported this idea (10), and more recent data confirm that cerebral blood flow changes are not regulated by glycolytic demands (11). Additionally, blood flow effects can be pharmacologically decoupled from brain activation without loss of electrophysiologic responses (12). An alternative possibility is that regional blood flow increases to remove toxic waste products of metabolism. The extent to which non-neuronal constituents of brain parenchyma contribute to the overall metabolic rate is also uncertain and might be variable. Nonetheless, at least in normal subjects, regional blood flow changes have typically colocalized with known functional specialization.

BIOPHYSICAL BASIS OF FUNCTIONAL MAGNETIC RESONANCE IMAGING

The term fMRI typically refers to MRI scanning in which some or all tissue contrast arises from nonstructural factors such as changes in blood flow and/or metabolism. Such changes are typically on the order of only a few percent or less of the overall signal intensity, but modern MRI scanners are stable enough to measure such small changes reliably. Further, signal averaging across multiple acquisitions or trials is carried out to strengthen the activation-related signal relative to background noise. The primary contrast phenomena exploited for fMRI are blood-oxygenation-level-dependent (BOLD) contrast and perfusion contrast obtained using arterial spin labeling (ASL), which uses electromagnetically labeled arterial blood water as a flow tracer. Because BOLD contrast is easier to obtain and generally provides higher signal-to-noise for task specific activation, it has been widely adopted as the method of choice for most fMRI applications.

BOLD Functional Magnetic Resonance Imaging

BOLD contrast reflects a complex interaction between blood flow, blood volume, and hemoglobin oxygenation (13–15). Functional contrast is obtained because the iron present in hemoglobin becomes paramagnetic only when it is deoxygenated (16, 17), producing a local susceptibility increase manifested as a change in T2*, among other effects (Fig. 10.1A). This change in hemoglobin oxygenation can be observed using a variety of pulse sequences, including routine gradient-echo sequences and gradient-echo echoplanar sequences, which particularly emphasize T2* effects. With regional brain activation, a reduction in T2* is observed, reflecting a decrease in regional deoxyhemoglobin. This has been attributed to increases in CBF that exceed increases in oxygen metabolism (10), although the precise basis for this mismatch is uncertain. Some modeling studies based on the physiology of blood flow changes and oxygen diffusion suggest that large changes in flow may be required to increase oxygen delivery even to a small extent (18).

Task-specific BOLD signal changes are not directly quantifiable in physiologic units and instead are expressed as a percentage signal change or as a statistical significance level based on a particular statistical model. Absolute or resting function cannot be easily assessed, and for clinical studies it may be difficult to know whether any observed abnormalities are due to baseline or task-specific effects. A typical BOLD response consists of a 0.5–5% change in regional image intensity that develops over 2–8 seconds following task initiation, typically with an initial peak or overshoot, a somewhat lower plateau for sustained tasks, and often an undershoot of the baseline following task completion. The peak latency of several seconds represents a major limiting factor in the temporal resolution of functional imaging methods that rely on activation–flow coupling. There is some evidence that prior to the increase in regional CBF, there is a more localized decrease in hemoglobin oxygenation, presumably due to a more rapid increase in oxygen utilization than in blood flow. This has been best visualized in calcarine cortex using optical methods in animal models (19) and more recently in fMRI studies in animals and humans (20, 21). If reliably obtainable, this signal could provide a means of improving both the spatial and temporal resolution of fMRI.

Activation-induced CBF changes vary in size depending on the nature of the contrast between baseline and activation states. There are also probably variations due to task performance, effort, age, gender, medications, presence of vascular disease, and other factors. Sensitivity to T2* changes increases at higher magnetic field strengths, such that BOLD signal changes at 4.0 T may approach 25% when comparing simple sensorimotor tasks with a resting baseline.

Perfusion Functional Magnetic Resonance Imaging

Cerebral perfusion can also be measured directly using endogenous contrast with ASL (22–24). This class of technique uses magnetically labeled arterial blood water as a diffusible tracer for blood flow measurements (Fig. 10.1B),

BOLD

ASL

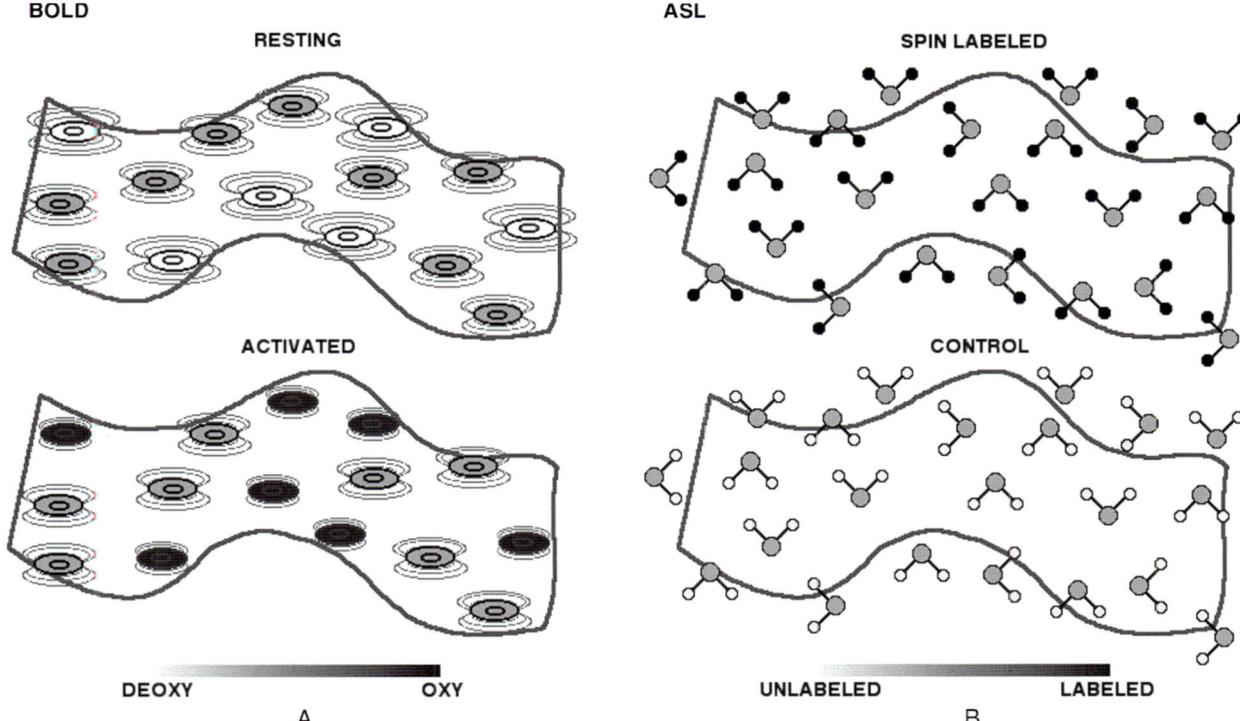

FIG. 10.1. Mechanisms for noninvasively obtaining functional contrast using MRI. Physiologic effects in a microvessel are illustrated. **A.** Blood-oxygenation-level-dependent (BOLD) contrast is attributed to paramagnetic properties of deoxyhemoglobin in red blood cells, which produces distortions in the local magnetic field, manifested as signal loss on T2*-weighted images. With task activation there are regional increases in CBF that exceed increases in oxygen utilization, resulting in deoxyhemoglobin dilution and therefore a regional signal increase. BOLD effects are largely intravascular. **B.** Arterial spin labeling (ASL) uses electromagnetic labeling of arterial blood water protons as a tracer for flow quantification. The effects of ASL are measured by comparison with a control image acquired without ASL; the difference between these images reflects the distribution of the spin label. Because water is diffusible, the tracer can leave the microvasculature and enter the tissue.

in a manner analogous to that used for oxygen-15 PET scanning (25). The 'magnetic' tracer has a decay rate of T1, which is sufficiently long to allow perfusion of the microvasculature and tissue to be detected. ASL techniques are capable of quantifying cerebral blood flow in well characterized physiologic units of ml/100 g/min, or may be used in a qualitative fashion similar to BOLD fMRI (24, 26, 27). Use of ASL for functional imaging has been less widespread because it is more difficult to implement and produces a smaller signal-to-noise ratio (SNR). A number of groups have reported successful detection of focal activation using perfusion contrast obtained with pulsed (24, 26, 27) or continuous ASL (28, 29). The recent development of multislice ASL (30) has considerably enhanced its utility.

Studies of resting CBF using ASL methods are likely to have clinical utility in diagnosing and managing many central nervous system disorders. For example, specific patterns of blood flow reduction are found in chronic epilepsy, cerebrovascular disease, and degenerative disorders such as Alzheimer's disease. Because flow can be quantified directly, comparison of resting cerebral blood flow across patient groups or before and after pharmacologic interventions can be readily carried out. ASL perfusion fMRI was recently shown to be sensitive to interictal hypometabolism in TLE (31).

There is also growing evidence that ASL methods have advantages over BOLD contrast for imaging task-specific activation. The ASL effect is not dependent on T2* and therefore CBF changes can be detected in regions of high static susceptibility with ASL methods (32). Because CBF is measured using pairwise subtraction between ASL and control labeling, low-frequency drift effects are eliminated. This renders ASL images equally sensitive to gradual versus rapid changes in brain function (33), and broadens the range of statistical procedures that can be used for data analysis (34). Finally, because CBF measurements made using ASL are in physiologic units that are insensitive to scanner effects, there seems to be less variability in task activation across subjects in group analyses (33, 34).

Hemodynamic parameters such as cerebral blood volume and mean transit time can also be measured by imaging the passage and distribution of exogenous MRI contrast agents such as gadolinium-DPTA. This approach was used to generate the first report of fMRI in humans during photic stimulation (35). However, because contrast administration is required for each measurement, its use for task activation studies has waned, although modifications of this approach are used for functional blood volume imaging in animal models (36). Contrast bolus tracking methods remain in wide use for detecting resting hemodynamic abnormalities in a variety of clinical settings (37).

Spatial Resolution and Image Distortion

While MRI is capable of imaging structures in the micron range (38), SNR varies directly with voxel size, and signal averaging time for extremely small voxels would probably be prohibitive for most human applications. In addition, degradation by motion becomes a very significant problem with high-resolution imaging, particularly since even normal physiologic motion such as that induced by arterial pulsatility can be in the order of millimeters. This can be mitigated to some extent by cardiac gating, which has allowed visualization of activation in small brain regions not otherwise achievable (39). The spatial precision of activation–flow coupling is also unknown, but current thinking is that flow effects are considerably less localized than metabolic effects. However, at least in some brain regions, the vascular supply is organized in a very functionally precise manner. This has been demonstrated for rat whisker barrel cortex where the cortical regions subserving each whisker appear to have a dedicated microvascular supply (40). Although these regions are less than 1 mm, it was possible to visualize them in the rat brain using high-field fMRI (41). It has also been possible to visualize similarly sized ocular dominance columns in calcarine cortex in cats (20) and in humans (42).

Because T2*-weighted BOLD images are based on susceptibility contrast, they are also very sensitive to bulk static susceptibility effects, leading to signal loss or distortion at tissue–air and tissue–bone interfaces such as the orbital frontal cortex and inferior temporal lobe (43). This susceptibility-induced BOLD signal dropout, if primarily arising from through-plane field gradients, can be largely recovered by Z-shimming techniques, which require multiple image acquisitions with different amplitudes of slice refocusing gradient (44, 45) or additional k-space coverage (46). A single-shot Z-shimming approach was recently described that does not require sacrificing temporal resolution (47). Because it is based on spin labeling rather than susceptibility contrasts, ASL imaging is not affected by bulk static susceptibility.

Data Acquisition

Many data acquisition variables are under investigator control, while others reflect limitations of the scanner hardware. One obvious decision involves the size of the image voxels, which partly determines the spatial resolution of the activation image. Small voxels are desirable but MR signal decreases with decreasing voxel volume and susceptibility to noise from small head movements increases, resulting in limits on SNR with small voxels. Scanning at higher magnetic field strengths (i.e. 3 T or higher) provides stronger signals, partially offsetting the SNR problem, so smaller

voxels are generally more practical at high field. As the voxel size is made smaller, however, more time is needed to image the same volume of brain, resulting in trade-offs between image resolution and either the extent of brain imaged or the temporal resolution. Factors such as gradient strength, slew rate, and gradient switching speed vary across hardware platforms and determine how rapidly a volume of voxels can be acquired, although there are also safety factors that ultimately limit acquisition speed.

Susceptibility-induced BOLD signal dropout generally increases at higher field because intravoxel gradients tend to be stronger and spin dephasing faster. These effects can be countered to a large extent by shortening the echo time and using smaller voxels, and by more sophisticated high-order shimming. Another relative difficulty encountered at high fields is the shortening of T1, which leads to loss of gray–white contrast in standard T1-weighted anatomic images.

The very rapid image acquisition that makes high temporal resolution fMRI possible is based on single-shot k-space sampling techniques such as echoplanar imaging (EPI) (48), which allows an entire two-dimensional image to be acquired in less than 100 ms. Single-shot EPI is the most popular acquisition method, but spiral k-space sampling (49), partial k-space EPI (50), multishot EPI (45, 49), and other techniques are also used and have a variety of advantages and disadvantages. In addition to the choice of k-space acquisition method, T2*-weighted contrast can be based on either gradient-echo or spin-echo pulse sequences. Spin-echo sequences, while less sensitive overall, are considerably less sensitive to BOLD signals arising from large draining veins and so may provide more precise localization of neural responses (51).

Images are typically acquired continuously during fMRI, with acquisition of one volume followed immediately by acquisition of the next volume, but an alternative for studies using auditory stimuli is 'clustered (or 'sparse') acquisition' (52, 53). In this approach, there is a period of silence (typically 5–10 s) following each volume acquisition. The purpose of the silence is (1) to allow the brain regions responding to the scanner noise to return to baseline levels of activation prior to the next volume acquisition, and (2) to allow presentation of the auditory stimuli without interference by the scanner noise. This method appears to improve detection of activation in primary auditory areas. Drawbacks include the longer time needed to obtain an adequate number of images and the fact that the restricted sampling in time of the hemodynamic response does not allow its time course to be determined.

In addition to image acquisition, most fMRI experiments involve acquisition of behavioral data. Typically, subjects are presented with either visual or auditory stimuli and asked to perform tasks that require a response to the stimuli. Increasingly, investigators using fMRI are concerned with acquiring a detailed record of the task performance so that the resulting brain activation data can be accurately interpreted. For motor tasks, this may include measurement of initiation time and movement rate (54). For perceptual and cognitive tasks, key presses are often used to monitor accuracy and response time.

FUNCTIONAL MAGNETIC RESONANCE IMAGING EXPERIMENTAL DESIGN AND DATA ANALYSIS

In a typical fMRI study, images through the brain are acquired every few seconds for several minutes. Early fMRI studies exclusively used blocked-trial designs with alternating epochs of task and control conditions, each consisting of multiple trials. This approach maximizes sensitivity, since large signal changes are sustained, and also minimizes dependence on an accurate estimate of the hemodynamic response. The power spectrum of BOLD fMRI data collected from human subjects in the absence of any experimental task or time-varying stimuli demonstrate greater power at low frequencies, which can be well characterized by a 1/frequency $(1/f)$ function (55), or by more complicated modeling with special smoothing techniques (56). This temporal autocorrelation causes relative reductions in sensitivity for block designs with fundamental frequencies below 0.01 Hz (57).

More recently, many investigators have explored techniques that allow fMRI responses to individual task stimuli to be segregated (58). These 'event-related' approaches allow different classes of stimuli to be randomized, reducing habituation effects, and also permit analysis of fMRI data based on subject performance on individual trials (59, 60). One application of this approach is to conduct separate analyses of trials that are performed correctly and incorrectly. This is potentially very useful in clinical studies that compare task activation between control and patient groups that differ in task performance, or across different patients. If patients fail to perform well on a task, decreased activation of the appropriate brain region might be expected. On the other hand, if, despite decreased performance an increased effort is required, regional activation might be expected to increase (61). Similarly, enhanced performance in some patients could be associated with either an increase or a decrease in activation in a given brain region (62). Using an event-related approach, regional brain activation following only correctly or incorrectly performed trials can be retrospectively compared across subjects or across control and patient groups, independent of overall performance on the task.

A very different approach to functional brain imaging in clinical populations that circumvents the issue of task performance is to correlate neurocognitive deficits with alterations in resting brain function using quantitative functional imaging such as CBF measurements using ASL techniques. Since only resting perfusion is measured, the interpretation of the imaging data is not confounded by task performance.

Comparison of functional localization across subjects presents additional challenges in the interpretation of clinical functional neuroimaging studies. Many such comparisons have been accomplished through the use of transformation into standard neuroanatomic spaces such as Talairach space (63), although more complicated algorithms are available, including those that attempt to unfold cerebral gyri (64, 65). These algorithms rely on characteristic signal intensities of gray matter, white matter, and cerebral spinal fluid, which can be altered in the presence of lesions such as tumors, strokes, or focal atrophy. When lesions are large, they may distort the brain sufficiently to make automated or semi-automatic morphing into a standard space impossible.

The standard approach to detecting task-specific functional activation begins with a model of what the hemodynamic response, and thus the BOLD signal, should look like. These approaches are illustrated in Figure 10.2 for blocked and event-related designs. Activation is then identified by statistical analysis of the time series data in each voxel of the image volume with respect to the modeled response. This was first accomplished using a simple correlation analysis (66), although multiple linear regression methods including a variety of confounds (such as linear drift and head movement) are now more common, and nonparametric approaches as well as task-independent approaches are being developed. A linearity between neural activity and hemodynamic responses is often assumed in these models, especially for event-related analyses, though deviations from linearity clearly occur. For both resting and activation studies, time series data must be examined and corrected for motion effects, and task-correlated motion (movement of the head induced by performance of the task) may be particularly difficult to distinguish from functional activation. A thresholded statistical map is ultimately superimposed on high resolution anatomic images or other representations of the brain. Thresholding for significance is complicated, and requires consideration of spatial and temporal autocorrelation in the data as well as false positive activation that may

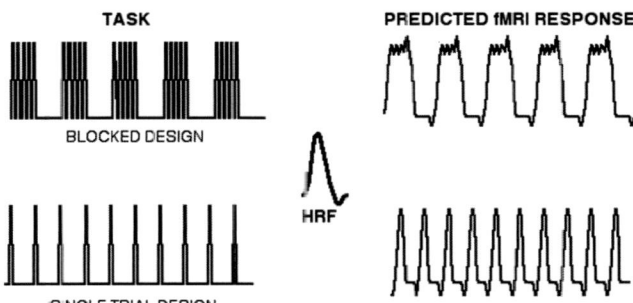

FIG. 10.2. Experimental designs for task activation studies. Stimuli may be blocked or presented individually. The predicted fMRI response is obtained by convolving the administered task with the hemodynamic response function, which may be assumed or measured. Because the hemodynamic response is prolonged and delayed, blocks of sequential stimuli produce a response with a sustained peak, whereas the responses to widely spaced individual stimuli can still be segregated. Data analysis procedures typically use pixel-by-pixel regression analyses to identify pixels in which signal changes correlate significantly with the predicted responses.

result from multiple comparisons, since three-dimensional images typically contain thousands of voxels.

Thorough reviews of fMRI task design, data analysis, and available software packages have been published previously (57, 67–72).

PREOPERATIVE MAPPING OF SENSORIMOTOR CORTEX

Motor Activation

A large number of fMRI studies have demonstrated primary sensorimotor cortex activation along the central sulcus during movement (73–77), including demonstration of the somatotopic organization of this region (78–80). Movement not only engages motor cortex but also provides tactile and proprioceptive sensory input, so activation is not confined to the motor cortex (anterior bank of the central sulcus) but rather involves primary motor and sensory areas. Finger movements are used most commonly, since face or proximal limb movements increase the likelihood of unacceptable movement artifacts. The magnitude of activation in primary motor cortex is directly dependent on the rate of finger movement (81, 82). Complex, sequential movements of individual digits produce additional activation in associated regions such as premotor cortex, supplementary motor area, and postcentral sulcus bilaterally (54, 76). Thus, the expected activation pattern is largely determined by the particular movement parameters selected for the activation task. A simple and commonly used procedure is to have the patient oppose the fingers sequentially to the thumb as quickly as possible. Many studies have used repetitive opening and closing of the fist.

Such tasks appear to reliably activate sensorimotor cortex in the central sulcus, and have been used in a number of patient studies (83–95). The clinical utility of such maps is in functional localization prior to surgery in this region for tumor or seizure focus resection. When the lesion is in close proximity to primary sensorimotor cortex along the central sulcus, precise localization of the activated region relative to the lesion could potentially help predict whether a sensorimotor deficit is likely to occur from lesion resection. It might also be possible to minimize any resulting deficit by purposefully sparing activated and immediately surrounding regions, although no quantitative studies have verified the effectiveness of such an approach. fMRI information is perhaps particularly useful when anatomic structures are distorted by mass effects making it difficult to ascertain the location of the central sulcus with certainty. Motor cortex localization with fMRI has generally been highly concordant with intraoperative electrocortical stimulation mapping (83, 85, 86, 89–91, 94, 95).

As with all fMRI studies, the activation pattern observed in motor studies is determined not solely by the activation task but rather by the contrast between activation and 'baseline' states. Pujol et al. favor an activation paradigm in which finger movements of one hand are compared directly to finger movements of the other hand rather than to a resting baseline (91). In addition to activating contralateral primary sensorimotor cortex, both these conditions activate the premotor, postcentral, and supplementary motor areas bilaterally. When the conditions are contrasted, these bilateral activations are thus subtracted away, leaving only activation in the contralateral central sulcus. This protocol successfully identified the central sulcus in 82% of 50 patients with brain tumors. Failure to activate the central sulcus was associated with pre-existing paresis of the contralateral hand, older age, and head motion. Correct localization by fMRI was confirmed in all of the 22 patients studied with intraoperative cortical stimulation.

Activation of motor cortex in patients with severe contralateral paresis is an important problem, since these patients are likely to have lesions in or near the motor strip and so have the greatest need for preoperative mapping. One potential solution to this problem is to activate the premotor area by movement of the ipsilesional (unimpaired) hand (96), from which the location of the central sulcus can be estimated. The success of this approach obviously depends on whether the lesion also impairs activation of the precentral sulcus. Another problem encountered in motor studies is that performance of a motor task may cause the patient to move the body and head slightly, resulting in false-positive signals in the fMRI data referred to as task-correlated motion artifacts (97). Careful instruction and training of the patient, measures to comfortably restrict head motion, use of small rather than large movements for the activation task, and proximal fixation of the limb to be moved should minimize such artifacts (98).

Somatosensory Activation

Many fMRI studies have focused on activation of the somatosensory system (99–114). Stimuli have included light touch with air puffs or other tactile stimuli (106, 110, 112, 113), scratching of the palm (98), vibration (104–106), electrical stimulation (100, 101, 107–109, 114) noxious stimuli (99, 111), and proprioception induced by passive joint movement (112). Activated areas usually include primary somatosensory cortex (SI) along the central sulcus and postcentral gyrus, secondary cortex (SII) in the parietal operculum, insula, and more posterior ventral parietal areas (PV). Many studies have demonstrated somatotopic organization in primary somatosensory cortex, whereas association areas are not clearly somatotopic (102, 104, 106, 108, 109, 113). As with the motor system, unilateral stimulation activates primary cortex only in the contralateral hemisphere but secondary areas bilaterally (101, 103, 107).

It is still uncertain what stimulus is the most effective, although indications are that pain stimuli are somewhat less reliable for evoking SI activation than more dynamic stimuli (111). Activation magnitude in SI depends on the intensity of stimulation (100, 108), the size of the stimulated body surface (99, 111), and the rate of stimulation (114). Responses in secondary areas seem to be less influenced by these variables but are probably more dependent on level of attention paid to the stimulus (101) and on whether stimulation is delivered unilaterally or bilaterally (103).

Somatosensory activation can be used to localize the central sulcus preoperatively and is applicable even in patients with severe hemiparesis, unless the patient also has severe hemianesthesia. Sensory activation also has the advantage of not requiring movement that could cause artifacts. One study of 94 brain tumor patients found a lower incidence of severe movement artifacts with a somatosensory paradigm (repetitive brushing of the palm) compared to a motor paradigm, but significantly higher percentage signal increases with the motor paradigm (98). The authors concluded that somatosensory paradigms were less sensitive than motor paradigms, but it is unclear whether repetitive brushing of the palm represents an optimal sensory stimulus.

PREOPERATIVE MAPPING OF LANGUAGE SYSTEMS

The aim of localizing language functions preoperatively is to minimize postoperative language deficits, such as anomia, that can result from epilepsy surgery (115). Functional brain mapping techniques can contribute to this process in several ways. By determining the location of important language functions, mapping techniques might help predict the risk of postoperative language deficits. During the surgical procedure itself, functional maps might be used to minimize such deficits by avoiding important functional areas.

Language Activation Protocols

Although fMRI and PET have been used extensively to study normal language processing, the areas identified in different studies have varied markedly, probably owing to use of different language activation tasks, control tasks, imaging techniques, and data-processing methods (116).

Language is not a single process but rather involves specialized sensory systems for speech, text, and object recognition; access to whole-word information; access to word meaning; processing of syntax; and multiple mechanisms for written and spoken language production. Neuropsychological studies suggest some degree of modularity of organization of these language subsystems (117) and it is unlikely that any single activation procedure could identify all of them. Some commonly used task combinations and the brain regions they typically 'activate' are shown in Table 10.1.

A few examples may be illustrative of some main issues in task design. Numerous studies over the past decade have shown that hearing words – whether the task involves passive listening, repeating, or categorizing – activates the superior temporal gyrus bilaterally when compared to a resting state (Fig. 10.3A) (118–121). The symmetry of this activation may be surprising but a consideration of the task contrast (complex sounds compared to no sounds) reveals that the 'rest' baseline contains no controls for primary or secondary auditory processes that engage auditory cortex in both superior temporal gyri (123). Thus, much of the activation produced by contrasting word-listening versus no sound could be due to prelinguistic auditory processing. These activation patterns bear almost no relationship to language dominance measured by Wada testing (124). Another problem in using such a paradigm for language mapping is that left-lateralized brain areas associated with semantic processing are probably active during the 'rest' state (125). Thus any activity in these regions during the word-listening task would be difficult to detect when compared to 'rest'.

Similar problems occur in designs that contrast reading or naming tasks with a resting or visual fixation baseline. The resting condition contains little in the way of controls for prelinguistic visual form recognition processes in ventral occipitotemporal regions, which thus dominate the activation map. Benson et al. found that such procedures do not reliably produce lateralized activation and do not correlate with language dominance measured by Wada testing (126).

More widely used than listening, repeating reading, and object naming tasks are 'word generation' tasks (also called

TABLE 10.1. *Some Task Contrasts Used for Language Mapping and the Regions in which Robust Activations are Typically Observed*

	Ventrolateral Prefrontal	Dorsal Prefrontal	Superior Temporal	Ventrolateral Temporal	Ventral Occipital	Angular Gyrus
Hearing words vs rest			B			
Hearing words vs nonspeech sounds			L > R			
Word generation vs rest	L > R			L > R	B	
Word generation vs reading	L					
Object naming vs rest	B			L > R	B	
Semantic decision vs sensory discrimination	L	L	L > R	L		L
Semantic decision vs phonological decision		L		L		L
Reading sentences vs letterstrings	L > R		L > R	L > R		

L, left hemisphere; R, right hemisphere; B, bilateral.

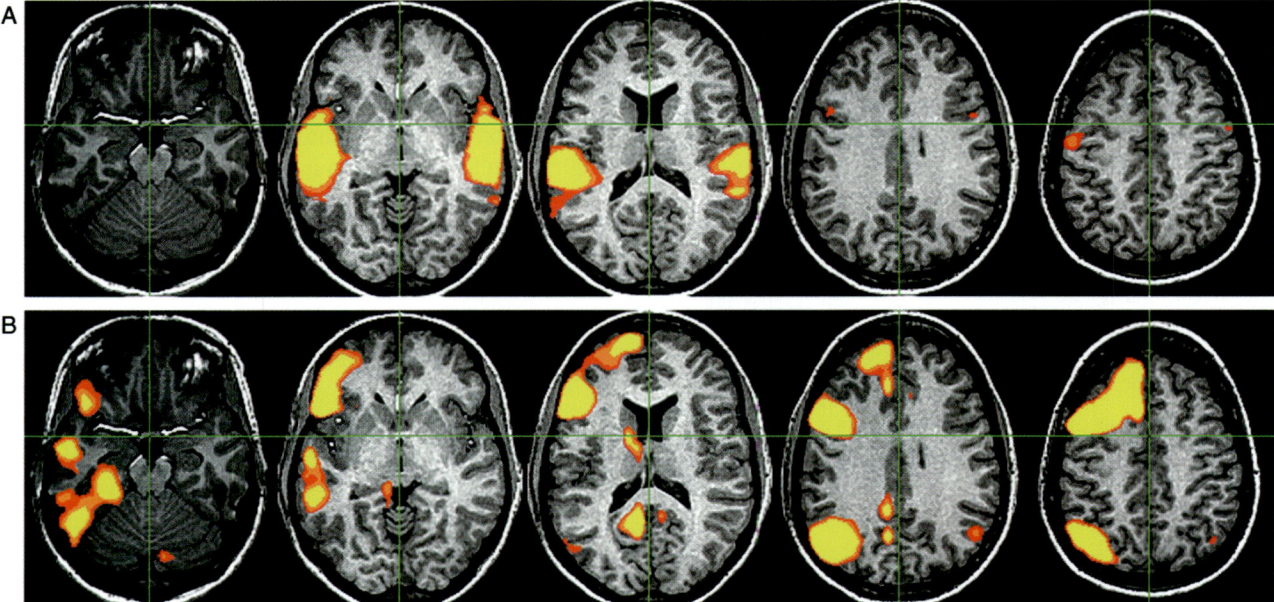

FIG. 10.3. Group average fMRI activation patterns in neurologically normal, right-handed volunteers during two language paradigms. **A.** Listening to spoken words contrasted with resting (28 subjects) Superior temporal activation occurs bilaterally. **B.** Semantic decision on auditory words contrasted with a tone decision control task (30 subjects). Activation is strongly left-lateralized in multiple prefrontal and sensory association cortices. The images are serial axial sections spaced at 15 mm intervals through stereotaxic space, starting at z = −15. The left hemisphere is on the reader's left. Green lines indicate stereotaxic *x* and *y* axes. (Reprinted with permission from Binder et al. 2002 (122).)

fluency tasks) that require word retrieval in response to a verbal cue. Subjects are given a beginning letter, a semantic category, or a word, and must retrieve a phonologically or semantically associated word. This task strongly activates the dominant inferior and dorsolateral frontal lobe, including prefrontal and premotor areas (121, 127–129). Posterior language areas such as middle and inferior temporal gyri, fusiform gyrus, and angular gyrus are only weakly activated by the word generation task compared to a resting state or a word reading control (121, 127–129).

Another approach involves pairing a word comprehension task with a nonlinguistic sensory discrimination task (130–136). These tasks can be given in either the visual or auditory modality. The sensory discrimination task controls for primary sensory, attentional, working memory, and motor aspects of the language task. The resulting activation pattern is strongly left-lateralized and involves both prefrontal and posterior association areas (Fig. 10.3B). An attractive feature of these paradigms is that measured behavioral responses, consisting of simple button presses for stimuli that meet response criteria, permit task performance to be quantified.

Normative Studies

Several language mapping protocols have been carried out in relatively large samples of normal subjects (137–142). All these protocols produced left-lateralized activation patterns in right-handed subjects. Lateralization has often been quantified using some type of left–right difference score. One commonly used version is based on the left–right difference in the number of activated voxels (activation volume),

normalized by the total number of activated voxels (i.e. $[L-R]/[L+R]$). This index varies from −1 (all activated voxels in the right hemisphere) to +1 (all activated voxels in the left hemisphere). This type of index depends on the statistical threshold used to identify voxels as 'active' and tends to increase with increasingly stringent thresholds because of the elimination of false-positive voxels in both hemispheres (143, 144). Others have advocated measures based on magnitude rather than volume of activation (126, 145). Lateralization indexes (LI) can be computed for the entire hemisphere or for homologous regions of interest (ROIs). Focusing on language-related ROIs avoids the problem of nonspecific or nonlanguage activation in bilateral sensory, motor, and executive systems that is characteristic of some task contrasts (144).

Language lateralization as measured by fMRI in several large samples of normal right-handed adults ranges from strong left dominance (LI near +1) to roughly symmetrical representation (LI near 0) (139, 140). As a group, left-handed and ambidextrous subjects show a relative rightward shift of language functions compared to right-handed subjects (139, 141, 146). This difference reflects a group tendency only, due to the fact that a larger minority (20–25%) are symmetrical or right dominant; most left-handed and ambidextrous subjects are, like right-handers, left-dominant for language. These estimates of language dominance and handedness effects in normal subjects agree very well with earlier Wada language studies in patients with late-onset seizures (140, 147, 148).

Sex differences in language lateralization were reported in a few fMRI studies (138, 149). Other PET (150, 151), fMRI (139, 141, 152), and functional transcranial Doppler (153) studies, together involving over 600 normal subjects, have failed to find differences between men and women in lateralization of language functions. Two studies reported age effects on language dominance in adults, manifested as a decline in the LI (greater symmetry of language processing) with increasing age (140, 141). Similar declines in hemispheric specialization have been observed for other cognitive domains (154, 155), and may reflect recruitment of homologous functional regions as compensation for age-related declines in neural functional capacity. Level of education had no effect on LI in the one study in which it was assessed (140).

Two fMRI studies directly compared LIs from a sample of normal adults with LIs from patients with epilepsy (140, 143). Both studies included only right-handed individuals to avoid confounding effects of handedness. Patients with epilepsy had a higher incidence of atypical (symmetric or right-lateralized) language dominance; this was particularly true for patients with left sided seizure foci (143). In one study there was a clear relationship between LI and age of onset of seizures ($r = 0.50$, $p < 0.001$), with language tending to shift more toward the right hemisphere with earlier onset (140). These effects are in agreement with Wada studies showing effects of side of seizure focus and age at onset on language lateralization (147, 148, 156, 157).

Wada Test Comparisons

Preliminary results suggest a high level of agreement between fMRI and Wada tests on measures of language lateralization (Table 10.2) (124, 126, 131, 135, 143, 158–165). Most of these studies, however, involved relatively small sample sizes (7–20 patients) and relatively few crossed-dominant individuals. A variety of task contrasts have been employed, including semantic decision versus sensory discrimination (131, 135, 160), semantic decision versus orthographic decision (161), word generation versus rest (124, 126, 143, 159, 162–165), rhyme decision (158), object naming (126, 163), and word or sentence reading (126, 163). In the largest of these early studies, an fMRI language laterality index based on a semantic decision versus sensory discrimination contrast was compared to an analogous index based on the Wada test in 22 epilepsy patients (160). The two indices were highly correlated ($r = 0.96$) and there were no disagreements in dominance classification. In a subsequent analysis using the same methods, dominance classification by Wada and fMRI was concordant in 48 of 49 (98%) consecutive patients with valid examinations (166).

While semantic decision and word generation paradigms generally produce high (90–100%) concordance rates (although see Worthington et al. 1997 (167)), results obtained with sentence listening versus rest (124), object naming versus rest (126), and object naming versus sensory discrimination (163) protocols were not correlated with Wada results. This lack of concordance probably stems from the fact that these contrasts produce strong activation in auditory and visual sensory systems that are not strongly lateralized, and only weak activation in prefrontal language areas. Word generation tasks, on the other hand, produce strong frontal activation but relatively weak temporal and parietal activation. The most concordant results obtained with these tasks are thus based on activation in a frontal ROI.

TABLE 10.2 Wada–fMRI Language Lateralization Comparisons

Lead Author, year	n	Language Task	Control Task	Result
Desmond, 1995	7	Semantic decision (vis words)	Orthographic decision	100% concordance
Binder, 1996	22	Semantic decision (aud words)	Tone Monitoring	100% concordance $r = 0.96$
Bahn, 1997	7	Covert phonological word gen	Rest	100% concordance
Hertz-Pannier, 1997	6	Covert or overt word gen	Rest	100% concordance
Worthington, 1997	12	Covert phonological word gen	Rest	56% concordance
Yetkin, 1998	13	Covert phonological word gen	Rest	100% concordance $r = 0.91$
Benson, 1999	12	Covert verb gen	Fixation	100% concordance
		Covert object naming	Fixation	n.s. lateralization
		Covert word reading	Fixation	n.s. lateralization
Lehéricy, 2000	10	Covert semantic word gen	Rest	$r = 0.88$ for a frontal ROI
		Covert sentence repetition	Rest	n.s. correlation
		Passive story listening	Nonword listening	n.s. correlation
Baciu, 2001	8	Rhyme detection (vis words)	Shape decision	100% concordance
Binder, 2001	49	Semantic decision (aud words)	Tone Monitoring	98% concordance
Carpentier, 2001	10	Semantic/syntactic decision	Sensory discrimination	90% concordance
Spreer, 2002	13	Semantic matching (vis words)	Color matching	100% concordance frontal ROI
Rutten, 2003	18	Covert verb gen	Shape decision	72% concordance verb gen
		Covert semantic word gen	Rest	83% combining all tasks
		Covert object naming	Shape decision	n.s. concordance for others
		Covert sentence reading	Shape decision	
Adcock, 2003	19	Covert phonological word gen	Rest	100% concordance
Sabbah, 2003	20	Covert semantic word gen	Rest	95% concordance

ROI, region of interest.

This characteristic of the word generation tasks is potentially problematic for clinical applications in patients with temporal lobe pathology, for several reasons. First, it is possible that language lateralization in such cases could differ for the frontal and temporal lobes, and it would be preferable to know the dominance pattern in the region in which surgery is to be undertaken. Second, if the goal is not simply to determine language dominance but rather to detect language-related cortex with optimal sensitivity for surgical planning, then lack of dominant temporal or parietal lobe activation represents a clear failure of the task paradigm.

Another major limitation of the word generation task is that it requires spoken responses, which are somewhat problematic for fMRI studies. As a result, all the cited studies used 'covert' responding, in which subjects are asked simply to 'think of' words. The absence of behavioral confirmation of task performance is not a problem if the goal is simply to calculate a lateralization index in the setting of at least some measurable activation. If, on the other hand, there is little or no activation, or the goal is to localize activation with optimal sensitivity, it can never be known whether lack of activation implies lack of cortical function or is simply an artifact of poor task compliance.

Comparisons with Cortical Stimulation Mapping

A number of studies have compared fMRI language maps with language maps obtained using cortical stimulation mapping (126, 131, 168–175). These studies are of great potential interest because they permit a test of whether fMRI activation foci represent 'critical' language areas. Some regions activated during language tasks may play a minor, supportive role rather than a critical role, and resection of these active foci may not necessarily produce clinically relevant deficits. It is thus vital to distinguish these noncritical areas from those that are critical to normal function. The assumption underlying the cortical stimulation technique is that the temporary deactivation induced by electrical interference will identify any such critical areas.

The published studies comparing fMRI and cortical stimulation report encouraging results. These reports involved relatively small samples (<15 patients). Methods for comparing the activation maps have tended to be qualitative and subjective rather than quantitative and objective, with a few exceptions (168, 172). Fitzgerald et al. reported, in 11 patients, an average sensitivity of 81% and specificity of 53% when using fMRI to predict 'critical' language sites on intraoperative cortical stimulation mapping, employing a criterion that the fMRI focus in question spatially overlap the stimulation site (168). When the criterion was loosened to include instances in which the fMRI focus was within 2 cm of the stimulation site, sensitivity improved to 92% but specificity was 0%. Sensitivity and specificity were highly variable across subjects. Rutten et al. found an average sensitivity of 92% and specificity of 61%, but this analysis was

performed after removing three patients (out of 11) in whom cortical stimulation mapping showed no language sites (172). Moreover, the fMRI data appear to have been used during surgery to select the sites for cortical stimulation, so the measurements being compared were not made independently.

Several factors make these comparisons particularly difficult to carry out. One problem is in matching the task characteristics across the two modalities. fMRI studies usually employ controls for nonlinguistic aspects of task performance, whereas this is typically not true of stimulation mapping studies. For example, stimulation studies often focus on speech arrest, which can result from disruption of motor or attentional systems as well as language systems (176). A second difficulty is the fact that many fMRI activation foci lie buried in the depths of sulci, which are not available for stimulation mapping. Thus, it reasonable to expect that many foci of activation observed by fMRI simply will not be tested adequately during cortical stimulation mapping.

Finally, the assumptions forming the basis for the cortical stimulation technique have yet to be adequately tested. There is, for example, very little evidence that resection of 'critical' areas detected by cortical stimulation necessarily leads to postoperative language deficits. One study, in fact, showed that the likelihood of finding 'critical' foci in the left anterior temporal lobe was higher among patients with poor language function, even though these patients are less likely to show language decline after left anterior temporal lobectomy (177, 178). Moreover, there is very little evidence that cortical stimulation mapping has any effect on preventing language decline (115), suggesting that there are critical language areas that may not be detected by focal electrical interference. This lack of sensitivity might occur, for example, if language functions were redundantly distributed across a number of nearby zones, several of which fell within the resection area but none of which produced a language deficit when deactivated in isolation.

Prediction of Language Outcome

It could be argued that neither the Wada test nor cortical stimulation mapping constitute an ideal 'gold standard' against which to judge fMRI language maps. Both these tests have recognized limitations, and both differ sufficiently from fMRI in terms of methodology and level of spatial detail that it is probably unreasonable to expect strong concordance with fMRI maps. A more meaningful measure of the validity of fMRI language maps is how well they predict postoperative language deficits. The purpose of preoperative language mapping, after all, is to assess the risk of such deficits and (in the case of cortical stimulation mapping) to minimize their severity. If fMRI can predict postoperative language deficits as well as, or better than, the Wada test, then what need is there to compare fMRI directly with the Wada?

Sabsevitz et al. (179) assessed the ability of preoperative fMRI to predict naming decline in 24 consecutively encountered patients undergoing left anterior temporal lobectomy (ATL). fMRI employed a semantic decision versus sensory discrimination protocol. All left ATL patients also underwent Wada testing and intraoperative cortical stimulation mapping, and surgeries were performed blind to the fMRI data. Compared to a control group of 32 right ATL patients, the left ATL group declined postoperatively on the 60-item Boston Naming Test ($p < 0.001$). Within the left ATL group, however, there was considerable variability, with 13 patients (54%) showing significant declines relative to the control group and the remainder no decline. A laterality index based on fMRI activation in a temporal lobe region of interest was strongly correlated with outcome ($r = -0.64$, $p < 0.001$), such that the degree of language lateralization toward the surgical (left) hemisphere was related to poorer naming outcome, whereas language lateralization toward the nonsurgical (right) hemisphere was associated with less or no decline (Fig. 10.4). Of note, an LI based on a frontal lobe ROI was considerably less predictive ($r = -0.47$, $p < 0.05$), suggesting that an optimal LI is one that indexes lateralization near the surgical resection area. The fMRI temporal lobe LI showed 100% sensitivity, 73% specificity, and a positive predictive value of 81% for predicting significant decline. By comparison, the Wada language LI showed a somewhat weaker correlation with decline ($r = -0.50$, $p < 0.05$), 92% sensitivity, 43% specificity, and a positive predictive value of 67%.

These results suggest that preoperative fMRI could be used to stratify patients in terms of risk for language decline, allowing patients and physicians to more accurately weigh the risks and benefits of brain surgery. It is crucial to note, however, that these results hold only for the particular methods used in the study and may not generalize to other fMRI protocols, analysis methods, patient populations, or surgical procedures. Future studies should not only confirm these results using larger patient samples but also test their generalizability to other protocols.

'Tailoring' Resections

It remains to be established how useful fMRI language activation maps will be for more precise planning of surgical resections. At least three significant problems complicate progress:

- inconsistencies in language maps produced by different activation protocols
- the failure to date to find an activation protocol that reliably activates the anterior temporal lobe, where the majority of epilepsy surgeries are performed
- an inadequate understanding of the specificity of fMRI activations.

As indicated earlier, different fMRI language activation protocols in current clinical use produce markedly different patterns of activation (116, 180, 181). While it is plausible to anticipate minor variation in activation profiles due to differential demands on separate subcomponents of language functions by different activation tasks, it is unlikely that this accounts for the full range of variance in these studies. Rather, these findings suggest that activation maps are strongly dependent on the specific contrast made between language and control tasks used in the activation protocol (see discussion above). Of note, none of the language activation protocols currently in common use are associated with robust anterior temporal lobe activation. Because the dominant anterior temporal lobe is known to contribute to language processes (119, 132–186), and left anterior temporal lobectomy not infrequently results in language decline (187–190), it follows that these protocols are not detecting crucial language areas. Clearly, further language activation task development is necessary. It may also be necessary, as some have suggested (163, 181), to incorporate multiple activation protocols before a complete picture of language zones in an individual can be discerned.

In addition to these issues concerning sensitivity of the activation protocol, it is conceivable that some regions activated during language tasks may play a minor or nonspecific role rather than a critical role in language. Resection of these 'active' foci may not necessarily produce clinically relevant or persisting deficits. Thus, those who would use fMRI activation maps to decide which brain regions can be resected in an individual patient run two risks:

- resection of critical language zones that are 'not activated' because of insensitivity of the particular language activation protocol employed resulting in postoperative language decline

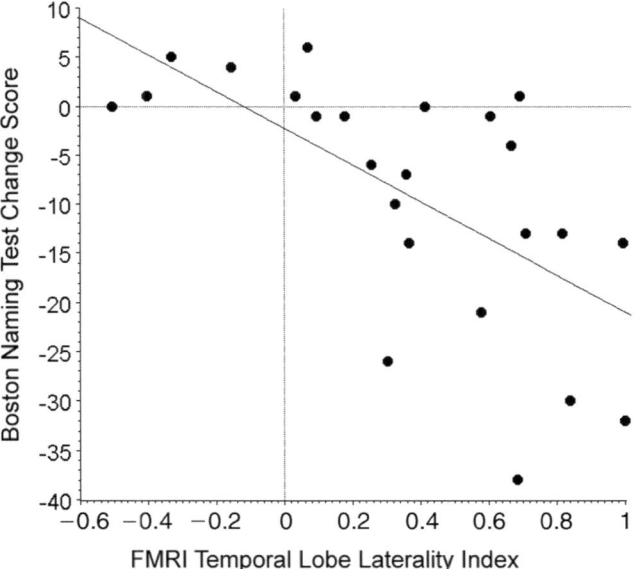

FIG. 10.4. Scatterplot depicting the relationship between preoperative lateralization of language-related brain activation in a temporal lobe region of interest and postoperative decline in confrontation-naming performance. (Reprinted with permission from Sabsevitz et al. 2003 (179).)

• sparing of 'activated' regions that are actually not critical for language, resulting in suboptimal seizure control.

Only through very carefully designed studies – in which resections are performed blind to the fMRI data, standardized procedures are used for assessing outcome, and quantitative measures are made of the anatomic and functional lesion – will the usefulness of fMRI language maps for 'tailoring' surgical resections be determined.

PREOPERATIVE MAPPING OF MEDIAL TEMPORAL LOBE MEMORY SYSTEMS

The hippocampus and associated medial temporal lobe structures subserve episodic memory function, and amnestic syndromes are accordingly the most significant cognitive deficits resulting from temporal lobectomy. The selective intracarotid amobarbital, or Wada, test was initially developed to determine lateralization of speech dominance (191) and was subsequently extended to evaluate lateralized asymmetries in memory function in an effort to additionally predict the occurrence of amnestic syndromes following resections (192). While the Wada test has been the gold standard for preoperative lateralization of language and memory function, it is invasive and provides only a limited period of time for testing. Other problems associated with Wada testing include known injection-side order effects (193, 194), variable cross-flow of amobarbital to the contralateral hemisphere, and the fact that the hippocampus is not actually supplied by the anterior circulation and is therefore deafferented rather than directly anesthetized during Wada testing.

For the reasons noted above, presurgical mapping of memory function in temporal lobe epilepsy (TLE) is an obvious application for clinical fMRI. The primary goal would be to determine the extent to which the affected versus unaffected temporal lobes are engaged during memory processes. This information would presumably be of use in determining the risks of amnestic complications from temporal lobectomy. Further, if prospective studies clearly demonstrate that resection in a region of fMRI activation results in a decrement in memory performance, fMRI data might further be used in planning specific resections in individual cases to avoid postsurgical amnesia. Because memory function is subserved by the same brain regions that typically harbor the seizure focus itself, memory activation patterns observed with fMRI may also contribute to seizure lateralization in TLE and to prediction of seizure-free outcome from temporal lobectomy, as has been demonstrated for the memory portion of the Wada test (195, 196) and interictal metabolic imaging (197, 198).

However, applications of fMRI to memory lateralization have thus far been much less studied than language lateralization, and are also more challenging for a variety of reasons. The hippocampus has been notoriously difficult to activate reliably. This may be at least partly attributable to difficulties in disengaging memory function for a control condition, as well as identifying a good active task. The hippocampus is also in a region of comparatively high static susceptibility, resulting in decreased sensitivity for BOLD fMRI. Efforts to overcome these obstacles include the use of Z-shimming (199) or ultrathin slices (200) to minimize susceptibility artifacts, or the use of ASL contrast with susceptibility-independent imaging sequences. Finally, as compared to language functions, which are subserved by large cortical regions through the hemisphere, the hippocampal formation has a much smaller volume of tissue and therefore SNR for detecting hippocampal activation is greatly reduced. Future studies will move to higher magnetic field strengths to increase sensitivity of fMRI in the medial temporal region. Multicoil arrays may also improve sensitivity, though the medial temporal cortex is actually rather far from the surface.

Episodic memory is typically engaged during fMRI by explicit or incidental encoding tasks, with subsequent recognition testing to verify encoding success. A variety of stimulus materials have been used for this purpose, though encoding of complex visual scenes, as originally described by Stern et al. (201) has been the most widely used task. This task produces bilateral activation. Encoding of material-specific stimuli has also been used in an attempt to selectively engage right or left hemispheric memory systems (202, 203). Several groups have also examined both novel and familiar stimuli (204–206), finding that contrasting novel versus familiar stimuli yields robust activation in the hippocampal formation.

While the hippocampus proper is the brain region most commonly associated with episodic memory function,[207] fMRI studies have often demonstrated that much of the activation is located more posteriorly in the parahippocampal formation, at least for visual stimuli (200, 201, 208). The hippocampal system comprises two cytoarchitectonically distinct regions. The hippocampal formation, which includes the horn of Ammon, dentate gyrus, and subiculum, consists of three-layered allocortex, whereas the parahippocampus, which includes the entorhinal and posterior medial parahippocampal cortices, consists of six-layered mesocortex. The parahippocampus receives convergent input from the various cortical sensory association areas. In turn, the parahippocampus provides the majority of cortical input to the hippocampal formation, with which it is reciprocally connected. A majority of the afferent and efferent signals between the cerebral cortex and the hippocampal formation are relayed via the parahippocampus. Afferent signals of cortical origin follow the transhippocampal loop. Signals enter the entorhinal cortex and pass through the dentate gyrus, sectors CA1, CA2, and CA3 of the hippocampus proper, and the subiculum, before returning to the entorhinal cortex, whence they are re-projected back to the areas from which they originated. Because extrahippocampal lesions that interrupt the transhippocampal loop impair the formation of long-term declarative memory, it appears that the back-projection of signals from the hippocampus to the cerebral cortex via the parahippocampus may be essential for declarative memory encoding (209).

In most fMRI studies, activation within the entire medial temporal lobe has been considered. Sperling et al (206). found that encoding of novel versus familiar stimuli yielded activation more anteriorly in the medial temporal region. The use of a blocked design maximizes sensitivity and minimizes the need for accurate models of when encoding actually takes place during stimulus processing and of the hemodynamic response. In contrast, event-related designs allow segregation of successfully and unsuccessfully encoded trials (60), which may be useful in matching patients and controls for task performance.

Encoding of complex visual scenes resulted in asymmetrical activation in a small series of patients with primarily right-sided unilateral TLE (210) (Fig. 10.5). In this study, a simple asymmetry index was calculated based on right and left sided regions of interest. Golby et al (211). subsequently used novel versus familiar stimuli of various modalities, and also found decreased activation ipsilateral to the seizure focus in another small series of patients with unilateral TLE. The use of material-specific stimuli may more closely approximate the Wada memory test, although if normal activation is unilateral, an asymmetry index cannot be calculated and some internal reference will be required to calibrate the observed activation in patients.

These studies also compared fMRI memory lateralization with that obtained by Wada testing, demonstrating that memory lateralization by these two modalities agreed to a large extent. However, because fMRI examines endogenous function while the Wada test is fundamentally a lesion study, it is also reasonable to expect that these modalities may differ, and that the findings obtained with each modality may be complementary rather than entirely duplicative (212). Reductions in fMRI memory activation also appear to correctly lateralize seizure foci in the majority of cases (213, 214), and very preliminary results also suggest that postsurgical amnesia correlates with fMRI activation ipsilateral to the resection.[215] Binder et al (213). found that anterior hippocampal activation during memory encoding correlated better with seizure lateralization than activation in other medial temporal regions.

Complex cognitive functions such as memory typically activate a distributed network of brain regions, not all of which are critical for task performance. Conversely, some critical regions may not be activated due to limitations in sensitivity or task design. fMRI studies of memory in TLE represent an ideal clinical application for this new modality and provide an excellent model for validating fMRI more generally. TLE is a relatively stereotyped disorder that is confined to a small brain region; therefore, only a limited number of activation paradigms must be developed to assess its function. Furthermore, since temporal lobectomy is currently clinically indicated in many patients with TLE regardless of fMRI findings, it provides an opportunity to determine the consequences of resection in or near a region of focal activation. The use of fMRI before and after temporal lobectomy also provides a model for studying neuroplastic responses in human brain.

As with any new diagnostic or therapeutic modality, fMRI memory localization should be carefully validated in a prospective fashion before use in routine clinical management. In addition to the technical improvements in fMRI acquisition described above, more robust data analysis procedures are also required to reliably detect activation in the relatively small hippocampal formation. Machulda et al (216). observed that fMRI localization within the hippocampal formation varied with thresholding parameters, although laterality did not. Activation also varies with memory performance (60). The test–retest reliability of memory activation paradigms is uncertain and needs to be more firmly established. Existing data suggest substantial variability in activation volume from scan to scan (217), although the location of this activation was relatively constant. These shortcomings will hopefully be addressed through a more thorough understanding of the sources of variability between subjects and scans, the development of more sensitive fMRI methods, and

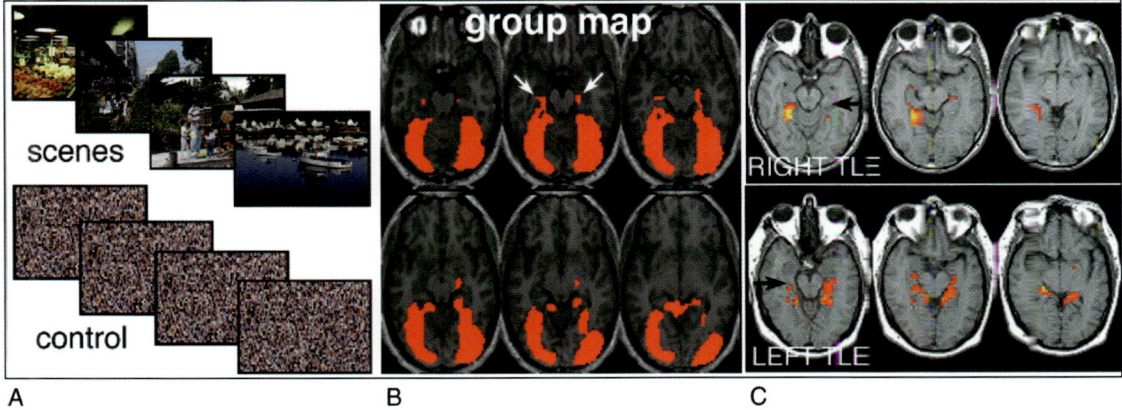

FIG. 10.5. Functional MRI of episodic memory in TLE. **A.** Examples of complex visual scenes and control images used during a scene encoding task. The control is a single randomly retiled image. Subjects are asked to remember the scenes for subsequent testing. **B.** Group activation map (*n* = 17) using a random effects model showing activation in visual association cortex and extending into the medial temporal lobe and hippocampus (arrows). **C.** Suprathreshold activation in a medial temporal region of interest in patients with right (top) and left (bottom) TLE. Decreased activation is observed in the region ipsilateral to the seizure focus (arrows).

optimization of activation tasks and analysis procedures. It is likely that fMRI localization and lateralization of memory function will ultimately contribute to the presurgical management of TLE and other medial temporal lobe lesions.

REFERENCES

1. Nguyen TV, Brownell AL, Iris Chen YC, et al. Detection of the effects of dopamine receptor supersensitivity using pharmacological MRI and correlations with PET. *Synapse* 2000;36:57–65.
2. Stein EA. fMRI: a new tool for the in vivo localization of drug actions in the brain. *J Anal Toxicol* 2001;25:419–424.
3. Zhang Z, Andersen A, Grondin R, et al. Pharmacological MRI mapping of age-associated changes in basal ganglia circuitry of awake rhesus monkeys. *Neuroimage* 2001;14:1159–1167.
4. Nudo RJ, Masterson RB. Stimulation-induced [^{14}C]2-deoxyglucose labeling of the synaptic activity in the central auditory system. *J Comp Neurol* 1986;245:553–565.
5. Villringer A, Dirnagl U. Coupling of brain activity and cerebral blood flow: basis of functional neuroimaging. *Cereb Brain Metab Rev* 1995; 7:240–276.
6. Aguirre GK, Zarahn E, D'Esposito M. The variability of human, BOLD hemodynamic responses. *Neuroimage* 1998;8:360–369.
7. Powers WJ, Fox PT, Raichle ME. The effect of carotid artery disease on the cerebrovascular response to physiologic stimulation. *Neurology* 1988;38:1475–1478.
8. Stoll M, Seidel A, Schimrigk K, Hamann GF. Hand gripping and acetazolamide effect in normal persons and patients with carotid artery disease. *J Neuroimaging* 1998;8:27–31.
9. Roy CS, Sherrington CS. On the regulation of the blood-supply of the brain. *J Physiol* (Lond) 1890;11:85–108.
10. Fox PT, Raichle ME. Focal physiological uncoupling of cerebral blood flow and oxidative metabolism during somatosensory stimulation in human subjects. *Proc Natl Acad Sci USA* 1986;83:1140–1144.
11. Powers WJ, Hirsch IB, Cryer PE. Effect of stepped hypoglycemia on regional cerebral blood flow response to physiological brain activation. *Am J Physiol* 1996;270:H554–H559.
12. Lindauer U, Megow D, Schultze J, et al. Nitric oxide synthase inhibition does not affect somatosensory evoked potentials in the rat. *Neurosci Lett* 1996;216:207–210.
13. Kwong KK, Belliveau JW, Chesler DA, et al. Dynamic magnetic resonance imaging of human brain activity during primary sensory stimulation. *Proc Natl Acad Sci USA* 1992;89:5675–5679.
14. Mandeville JB, Marota JJA, Ayata C, et al. MRI measurement of the temporal evolution of relative CMRO2 during rat forepaw stimulation. *Magn Reson Med* 1999;42:944–951.
15. Ogawa S, Menon RS, Tank DW, et al. Functional brain mapping by blood oxygenation level-dependent contrast magnetic resonance imaging. A comparison of signal characteristics with a biophysical model. *Biophysics J* 1993;64:803–812.
16. Ogawa S, Lee TM, Kay AR, Tank DW. Brain magnetic resonance imaging with contrast dependent on blood oxygenation. *Proc Natl Acad Sci USA* 1990;87:9868–9872.
17. Thulborn KR, Waterton JC, Matthews PM, Radda GK. Oxygenation dependence of the transverse relaxation time of water protons in whole blood at high field. *Biochim Biophys Acta* 1982;714:263–270.
18. Buxton RB, Frank LR. A model for the coupling between cerebral blood flow and oxygen metabolism during neural stimulation. *J Cereb Blood Flow Metab* 1997;17:64–72.
19. Malonek D, Grinvald A. Interactions between electrical activity and cortical microcirculation revealed by imaging spectroscopy: implications for functional brain mapping. *Science* 1996;272:551–554.
20. Kim D-S, Duong TQ, Kim S-G. Magnetic resonance imaging of iso-orientation domains in cat visual cortex using early negative BOLD signals. *Soc Neurosci Abstr* 1999;25:783.

21. Yacoub E, Le TH, Ugurbil K, Hu X. Further evaluation of the initial negative response in functional magnetic resonance imaging. *Magn Reson Med* 1999;41:436–441.
22. Alsop DC, Detre JA. Reduced transit-time sensitivity in noninvasive magnetic resonance imaging of human cerebral blood flow. *J Cereb Blood Flow Metab* 1996;16:1236–1249.
23. Detre JA, Leigh JS, Williams DS, Koretsky AP. Perfusion imaging. *Magn Reson Med* 1992;23:37–45.
24. Edelman RR, Siewert B, Darby DG, et al. Qualitative mapping of cerebral blood flow and functional localization with echo-planar MR imaging and signal targeting with alternating radio frequency. *Radiology* 1994;192:513–520.
25. Detre JA, Zhang W, Roberts DA, et al. Tissue specific perfusion imaging using arterial spin labeling. *Nucl Magn Reson Biomed* 1994; 7:75–82.
26. Kim SG. Quantification of relative cerebral blood flow change by flow-sensitive alternating inversion recovery (FAIR) technique: application to functional mapping. *Magn Reson Med* 1995, 34:293–301.
27. Kwong KK, Chesler DA, Weisskoff RM, et al. MR perfusion studies with T1-weighted echo planar imaging. *Magn Reson Med* 1995;34: 878–887.
28. Talagala SL, Noll DC. Functional MRI using steady state arterial water labeling. *Magn Reson Med* 1998;39:179–183.
29. Ye F, Smith A, Yang Y, et al. Quantitation of regional cerebral blood flow increases during motor activation: a steady-state arterial spin tagging study. *Neuroimage* 1997;6:104–112.
30. Alsop DC, Detre JA. Multisection cerebral blood flow MR imaging with continuous arterial spin labeling. *Radiology* 1998;208:410–416.
31. Wolf RL, Alsop DC, French JA, et al. Detection of mesial temporal lobe hypoperfusion in patients with temporal lobe epilepsy using arterial spin labeled perfusion MRI. *Am J Neuroradiol* 2001;22: 1334–1341.
32. Wang J, Li L, Roc AC, et al. Reduced susceptibility effects in perfusion fMRI with single-shot spin-echo EPI acquisitions at 1.5 Tesla. *Magn Reson Imaging* 2004;22:1–7.
33. Wang J, Aguirre GK, Kimberg DY, et al. Arterial spin labeling perfusion fMRI with very low task frequency. *Magn Reson Med* 2003;49:796–802.
34. Aguirre GK, Detre JA, Alsop DC. Experimental design and the relative sensitivity of BOLD and perfusion fMRI. *Neuroimage* 2002;15: 488–500.
35. Belliveau JW, Kennedy DN, McKinstry RC, et al. Functional mapping of the human visual cortex by magnetic resonance imaging. *Science* 1991;254:716–719.
36. Mandeville JB, Marota JJ, Kosofsky BE, et al. Dynamic functional imaging of relative cerebral blood volume during rat forepaw stimulation. *Magn Reson Med* 1998;39:15–24.
37. Lev MH, Rosen BR. Clinical applications of intracranial perfusion MR imaging. Neuroimaging Clin North Am 1999;9:309–331.
38. Johnson GA, Thompson MB, Drayer BP. Three-dimensional MRI microscopy of the normal rat brain. *Magn Reson Med* 1987;4:351–365.
39. Guimaraes AR, Melcher JR, Talavage TM, et al. Imaging subcortical auditory activity in humans. *Hum Brain Mapp* 1998;6:33–41.
40. Woolsey TA, Rovainen CM, Cox SB, et al. Neuronal units linked to microvascular modules in cerebral cortex: response elements for imaging the brain. *Cereb Cortex* 1996;6:647–660.
41. Yang X, Hyder F, Shulman RG. Activation of single whisker barrel in rat localized by functional magnetic resonance imaging. *Proc Natl Acad Sci USA* 1996;93:475–478.
42. Menon RS, Ogawa S, Strupp J, Ugurbil K. Ocular dominance columns in human V1 demonstrated by functional magnetic resonance imaging. *J Neurophysiol* 1997;77:2780–2787.
43. Ojemann JG, Akbudak E, Snyder AZ, et al. Anatomic localization and quantitative analysis of gradient refocused echo-planar fMRI susceptibility artifacts. *Neuroimage* 1997;6:156–167.
44. Constable RT, Spencer DD. Composite image formation in z-shimmed functional MRI. *Magn Reson Med* 1999;42:110–117.

45. Yang QX, Dardzinski BJ, Li S, Smith MB. Multi-gradient echo with susceptibility in homogeneity compensation (MGESIC): demonstration of fMRI in the olfactory cortex at 3.0T. *Magn Reson Med* 1997; 37:331–335.

46. Glover G. 3D z-shim method for reduction of susceptibility effects in BOLD fMRI. *Magn Reson Med* 1999;42:290–299.

47. Song AW. Single-shot EPI with signal recovery from the susceptibility-induced losses. *Magn Reson Med* 2001;46:407–411.

48. Mansfield P. Multi-planar image formation using NMR spin echoes. *J Physics* 1977;C10:L55–L58.

49. Noll DC, Stenger VA, Vazquez AL, Peltier SJ. Spiral scanning in fMRI. In: Moonen CTW, Bandettini PA, eds. Functional MRI. Berlin: Springer, 1999:149–160.

50. Hyde JS, Biswal BB, Jesmanowicz A. High-resolution fMRI using multislice partial k-space GR-EPI with cubic voxels. *Magn Reson Med* 2001;46:114–125.

51. Kennan RP. Gradient echo and spin echo methods for functional MRI. In: Moonen CTW, Bandettini PA, eds. Functional MRI. Berlin: Springer, 1999:127–136.

52. Edmister WB, Talavage TM, Ledden PJ, Weisskoff RM. Improved auditory cortex imaging using clustered volume acquisition. *Hum Brain Mapp* 1999;7:89–97.

53. Hall DA, Haggard MP, Akeroyd MA, et al. Sparse temporal sampling in auditory fMRI. *Hum Brain Mapp* 1999;7:213–223.

54. Harrington DL, Rao SM, Haaland KY, et al. Specialized neural systems underlying representations of sequential movements. *J Cogn Neurosci* 2000;12:56–77.

55. Zarahn E, Aguirre GK, D'Esposito M. Empirical analyses of BOLD fMRI statistics. I. Spatially unsmoothed data collected under null-hypothesis conditions. *Neuroimage* 1997;5:179–197.

56. Woolrich MW, Ripley BD, Brady M, Smith SM. Temporal autocorrelation in univariate linear modeling of FMRI data. *Neuroimage* 2001;14:1370–1386.

57. Aguirre GK, D'Esposito M. Experimental design for brain fMRI. In: Moonen CTW, Bandettini PA, eds. Functional MRI. Berlin: Springer, 1999:369–380.

58. Buckner RL, Bandettini PA, O'Craven KM, et al. Detection of cortical activation during averaged single trials of a cognitive task using functional magnetic resonance imaging. *Proc Natl Acad Sci USA* 1996;93:14878–14883.

59. Brewer JB, Zhao Z, Desmond JE, et al. Making memories: Brain activity that predicts how well visual experience will be remembered. *Science* 1998;281:1185–1188.

60. Wagner AD, Schacter DL, Rotte M, et al. Building memories: remembering and forgetting of verbal experiences as predicted by brain activity. *Science* 1998;281:1188–1191.

61. Tagaris GA, Kim SG, Strupp JP, et al. Quantitative relations between parietal activation and performance in mental rotation. *Neuroreport* 1996;7:773–776.

62. Furey ML, Pietrini P, Haxby JV, et al. Cholinergic stimulation alters performance and task-specific regional cerebral blood flow during working memory. *Proc Natl Acad Sci USA* 1997;94:6512–6516.

63. Talairach J, Tournoux P. Co-planar stereotaxic atlas of the human brain. New York: Thieme, 1988.

64. Dale AM, Fischl B, Sereno MI. Cortical surface-based analysis. I. Segmentation and surface reconstruction. *Neuroimage* 1999;9:179–194.

65. Fischl B, Sereno MI, Dale AM. Cortical surface-based analysis. II: Inflation, flattening, and a surface-based coordinate system. *Neuroimage* 1999;9:195–207.

66. Bandettini PA, Jesmanowicz A, Wong EC, Hyde JS. Processing strategies for time-course data sets in functional MRI of the human brain. *Magn Reson Med* 1993;30:161–173.

67. Bullmore E, Brammer M, Williams SCR, et al. Statistical methods of estimation and inference for functional MR image analysis. *Magn Reson Med* 1996;35:261–277.

68. Frank LR, Buxton RB, Wong EC. Probabilistic analysis of functional magnetic resonance imaging data. *Magn Reson Med* 1998;39:132–148.

69. Friston KJ, Jezzard P, Turner R. Analysis of functional MRI time-series. *Hum Brain Mapp* 1994;1:153–171.

70. Friston KJ, Holmes A, Poline JB, et al. Detecting activations in PET and fMRI: levels of inference and power. *Neuroimage* 1996;4:223–235.

71. Gold S, Christian B, Arndt S, et al. Functional MRI statistical software packages: A comparative analysis. *Hum Brain Mapp* 1998;6:73–84.

72. Rosen BR, Buckner RL, Dale AM. Event-related functional MRI: past, present, and future. *Proc Natl Acad Sci USA* 1998;95:773–780

73. Bandettini PA, Wong EC, Hinks RS, et al. Time course EPI of human brain function during task activation. *Magn Reson Med* 1992;25:390–397.

74. Kim S-G, Ashe J, Hendrich K, et al. Functional magnetic resonance imaging of motor cortex: hemispheric asymmetry and handedness. *Science* 1993;261:615–617.

75. Ramsay NF, Kirkby BS, Van Gelderen P, et al. Functional mapping of human sensorimotor cortex with 3D BOLD fMRI correlates highly with H2(15)O PET rCBF. *J Cereb Blood Flow Metab* 1996;17:670–679.

76. Rao SM, Binder JR, Bandettini PA, et al. Functional magnetic resonance imaging of complex human movements. *Neurology* 1993; 43:2311–2318.

77. Wildgruber D, Erb M, Klose U, Grodd W. Sequential activation of supplementary motor area and primary motor cortex during self-paced finger movement in human evaluated by functional MRI. *Neurosci Lett* 1997;227:161–164.

78. Lotze M, Erb M, Flor H, et al. FMRI evaluation of somatotopic representation in human primary motor cortex. *Neuroimage* 2000;11: 473–481.

79. Maldjian JA, Gottschalk A, Patel RS, et al. The sensory somatotopic map of the human hand demonstrated at 4 Tesla. *Neuroimage* 1999;11:473–481.

80. Rao SM, Binder JR, Hammeke TA, et al. Somatotopic mapping of the human primary motor cortex with functional magnetic resonance imaging. *Neurology* 1995;45:919–924.

81. Jäncke L, Specht L, Mirzazade S, et al. A parametric analysis of the 'rate effect' in the sensorimotor cortex: a functional magnetic resonance imaging analysis in human subjects. *Neurosci Lett* 1998;252:37–40.

82. Rao SM, Bandettini PA, Binder JR, et al. Relationship between movement rate and functional magnetic resonance signal change in human primary motor cortex. *J Cereb Blood Flow Metab* 1996;16: 1250–1254.

83. Achten E, Jackson GD, Cameron JA, et al. Presurgical evaluation of the motor hand area with fMRI in patients with tumors and dysplastic lesions. *Radiology* 1999;210:529–538.

84. Atlas SW, Howard RS, Maldjian J, et al. Functional magnetic resonance imaging of regional brain activity in patients with intracerebral gliomas: findings and implications for clinical management. *Neurosurgery* 1996;38:329–338.

85. Chapman PH, Buchbinder BR, Cosgrove GR, Jiang HJ. Functional magnetic resonance imaging for cortical mapping in pediatric neurosurgery. *Ped Neurosurg* 1996;23:122–125.

86. Jack CR, Thompson RM, Butts RK, et al. Sensory motor cortex: correlation of presurgical mapping with functional MR imaging and invasive cortical mapping. *Radiology* 1994;190:85–92.

87. Kahn T, Schwabe B, Bettag M, et al. Mapping of the cortical motor hand area with functional MR imaging and MR imaging-guided laser-induced interstitial thermotherapy of brain tumors. Work in progress. *Radiology* 1996;200:149–157.

88. Maldjian J, Atlas SW, Howard RS, et al. Functional magnetic resonance imaging of regional brain activity in patients with intracerebral arteriovenous malformations before surgical or endovascular therapy. *J Neurosurg* 1996;84:477–483.

89. Mueller WM, Yetkin FZ, Hammeke TA, et al. Functional magnetic resonance imaging mapping of the motor cortex in patients with cerebral tumors. *Neurosurgery* 1996;39:515–520.

90. Puce A, Constable RT, Luby ML, et al. Functional magnetic resonance imaging of sensory and motor cortex: comparison with electrophysiological localization. *J Neurosurg* 1995;83:262–270.

91. Pujol J, Conesa G, Deus J, et al. Clinical application of functional magnetic resonance imaging in presurgical identification of the central sulcus. *J Neurosurg* 1998;88:863–869.

92. Righini A, de Divitiis O, Prinster A, et al. Functional MRI: primary motor cortex localization in patients with brain tumors. *J Comput Assist Tomogr* 1996;20:702–708.

93. Schad LR, Bock M, Baudendistel K, et al. Improved target volume definition in radiosurgery of arteriovenous malformations by stereotactic correlation of MRA, MRI, blood bolus tagging, and functional MRI. *Eur Radiol* 1996;6:38–45.

94. Schlosser MJ, McCarthy G, Fulbright RK, et al. Cerebral vascular malformations adjacent to sensorimotor and visual cortex. Functional magnetic resonance imaging studies before and after therapeutic intervention. *Stroke* 1997;28:1130–1137.

95. Yousry TA, Schmid UD, Jassoy AG, et al. Topography of the cortical motor hand area: prospective study with functional MR imaging and direct motor mapping at surgery. *Radiology* 1995;195:23–29.

96. Stippich C, Kapfer D, Hempel E, et al. Robust localization of the contralateral precentral gyrus in hemiparetic patients using the unimpaired ipsilateral hand: a clinical functional magnetic resonance imaging protocol. *Neurosci Lett* 2000;285:155–159.

97. Hajnal JV, Myers R, Oatridge A, et al. Artifacts due to stimulus correlated motion in functional imaging of the brain. *Magn Reson Med* 1994;31:283–291.

98. Hoeller M, Krings T, Reinges MH, et al. Movement artefacts and MR BOLD signal increase during different paradigms for mapping the sensorimotor cortex. *Acta Neurochir* (Wien) 2002;144:279–284.

99. Apkarian AV, Gelnar PA, Krauss BR, Szeverenyi NM. Cortical responses to thermal pain depend on stimulus size: a functional MRI study. *J Neurophysiol* 2000;83:3113–3122.

100. Arthurs OJ, Williams EJ, Carpenter TA, et al. Linear coupling between functional magnetic resonance imaging and evoked potential amplitude in human somatosensory cortex. *Neuroscience* 2000;101:803–806.

101. Backes WH, Mess WH, van Kranen-Mastenbroek V, Reulen JP. Somatosensory cortex responses to median nerve stimulation: fMRI effects of current amplitude and selective attention. *Clin Neurophysiol* 2000;111:1738–1744.

102. Disbrow E, Roberts T, Krubitzer L. Somatotopic organization of cortical fields in the lateral sulcus of *Homo sapiens*: evidence for SII and PV. *J Comp Neurol* 2000;418:1–21.

103. Disbrow E, Roberts T, Poeppel D, Krubitzer L. Evidence for interhemispheric processing of inputs from the hands in human S2 and PV. *J Neurophysiol* 2001;85:2236–2244.

104. Gelnar PA, Krauss BR, Szeverenyi NM, Apkarian AV. Fingertip representation in the human somatosensory cortex: an fMRI study. *Neuroimage* 1998;7:261–283.

105. Golaszewski SM, Siedentopf CM, Baldauf E, et al. Functional magnetic resonance imaging of the human sensorimotor cortex using a novel vibrotactile stimulator. *Neuroimage* 2002;17:421–430.

106. Hodge CJJ, Huckins SC, Szeverenyi NM, et al. Patterns of lateral sensory cortical activation determined using functional magnetic resonance imaging. *J Neurosurg* 1998;89:769–779.

107. Korvenoja A, Huttunen J, Salli E, et al. Activation of multiple cortical areas in response to somatosensory stimulation: combined magnetoencephalographic and functional magnetic resonance imaging. *Hum Brain Mapp* 1999;8:13–27.

108. Krause T, Kurth R, Ruben J, et al. Representational overlap of adjacent fingers in multiple areas of human primary somatosensory cortex depends on electrical stimulus intensity: an fMRI study. *Brain Res* 2001;899:36–46.

109. Kurth R, Villringer K, Mackert BM, et al. fMRI assessment of soma-totopy in human Brodmann area 3b by electrical finger stimulation. *Neuroreport* 1998;9:207–212.

110. Moore CI, Stern CE, Corkin S, et al. Segregation of somatosensory activation in the human rolandic cortex using fMRI. *J Neurophysiol* 2000;84:558–569.

111. Peyron R, Laurent B, Garcia-Larrea L. Functional imaging of brain responses to pain. A review and meta-analysis. *Neurophysiol Clin* 2000;30:263–288.

112. Rausch M, Spengler F, Eysel UT. Proprioception acts as the main source of input in human S-I activation experiments: a functional MRI study. *Neuroreport* 1998;9:2865–2868.

113. Servos P, Zacks J, Rumelhart DE, Glover GH. Somatotopy of the human arm using fMRI. *Neuroreport* 1998;9:605–609.

114. Takanashi M, Abe K, Yanagihara T, et al. Effects of stimulus presentation rate on the activity of primary somatosensory cortex: a functional magnetic resonance imaging study in humans. *Brain Res Bull* 2001;54:125–129.

115. Hermann BP, Perrine K, Chelune GJ, et al. Visual confrontation naming following left anterior temporal lobectomy: a comparison of surgical approaches. *Neuropsychology* 1999;13:3–9.

116. Binder JR, Price CJ. Functional imaging of language. In: Cabeza R, Kingstone A, eds. Handbook of functional neuroimaging of cognition. Cambridge, MA: MIT Press, 2001:187–251.

117. Shallice T. From neuropsychology to mental structure. Cambridge: Cambridge University Press, 1989.

118. Binder JR, Frost JA, Hammeke TA, et al. Human temporal lobe activation by speech and nonspeech sounds. *Cereb Cortex* 2000;10:512–528.

119. Mazoyer BM, Tzourio N, Frak V, et al. The cortical representation of speech. *J Cogn Neurosci* 1993;5:467–479.

120. Price CJ, Wise RJS, Warburton EA, et al. Hearing and saying. The functional neuro-anatomy of auditory word processing. *Brain* 1996;119:919–931.

121. Wise R, Chollet F, Hadar U, et al. Distribution of cortical neural networks involved in word comprehension and word retrieval. *Brain* 1991;114:1803–1817.

122. Binder JR, Achten E, Constable RT, et al. Functional MRI in epilepsy. *Epilepsia* 2002;43(Suppl 1):51–63.

123. Henschen SE. On the hearing sphere. Acta Otolaryngol (Stockh) 1918–1919;1:423–486.

124. Lehéricy S, Cohen L, Bazin B, et al. Functional MR evaluation of temporal and frontal language dominance compared with the Wada test. *Neurology* 2000;54:1625–1633.

125. Binder JR, Frost JA, Hammeke TA, et al. Conceptual processing during the conscious resting state: a functional MRI study. *J Cogn Neurosci* 1999;11:80–93.

126. Benson RR, FitzGerald DB, LeSeuer LL, et al. Language dominance determined by whole brain functional MRI in patients with brain lesions. *Neurology* 1999;52:798–809.

127. Petersen SE, Fox PT, Posner MI, et al. Positron emission tomographic studies of the cortical anatomy of single-word processing. *Nature* 1988;331:585–589.

128. Raichle ME, Fiez JA, Videen TO, et al. Practice-related changes in human brain functional anatomy during nonmotor learning. *Cereb Cortex* 1994;4:8–26.

129. Warburton E, Wise RJS, Price CJ, et al. Noun and verb retrieval by normal subjects. Studies with PET. *Brain* 1996;119:159–179.

130. Binder JR, Frost JA, Hammeke TA, et al. Human brain language areas identified by functional MRI. *J Neurosci* 1997;17:353–362.

131. Carpentier A, Pugh KR, Westerveld M, et al. Functional MRI of language processing: dependence on input modality and temporal lobe epilepsy. *Epilepsia* 2001;42:1241–1254.

132. Demb JB, Desmond JE, Wagner AD, et al. Semantic encoding and retrieval in the left inferior prefrontal cortex: a functional MRI study of task difficulty and process specificity. *J Neurosci* 1995;15:5870–5878.

133. Démonet J-F, Chollet F, Ramsay S, et al. The anatomy of phonological and semantic processing in normal subjects. *Brain* 1992;115:1753–1768.

134. Müller R-A, Kleinhans N, Courchesne E. Linguistic theory and neuroimaging evidence: an fMRI study of Broca's area in lexical semantics. *Neuropsychologia* 2003;41:1199–1207.

135. Spreer J, Arnold S, Quiske A, et al. Determination of hemisphere dominance for language: comparison of frontal and temporal fMRI activation with intracarotid amytal testing. *Neuroradiology* 2002;44: 467–474.

136. Vandenberghe R, Price C, Wise R, et al. Functional anatomy of a common semantic system for words and pictures. *Nature* 1996;383: 254–256.

137. Hund-Georgiadis M, Lex U, Friederici AD, von Cramon DY. Non-invasive regime for language lateralization in right- and left-handers by means of functional MRI and dichotic listening. *Exp Brain Res* 2002;145:166–176.

138. Pugh KR, Shaywitz BA, Shaywitz SE, et al. Cerebral organization of component processes in reading. *Brain* 1996;119:1221–1238.

139. Pujol J, Deus J, Losilla JM, Capdevila A. Cerebral lateralization of language in normal left-handed people studied by functional MRI. *Neurology* 1999;52:1038–1043.

140. Springer JA, Binder JR, Hammeke TA, et al. Language dominance in neurologically normal and epilepsy subjects: a functional MRI study. *Brain* 1999;122:2033–2045.

141. Szaflarski JP, Binder JR, Possing ET, et al. Language lateralization in left-handed and ambidextrous people: fMRI data. *Neurology* 2002; 59:238–244.

142. Vikingstad EM, George KP, Johnson AF, Cao Y. Cortical language lateralization in right handed normal subjects using functional magnetic resonance imaging. *J Neurol Sc* 2000i;175:17–27.

143. Adcock JE, Wise RG, Oxbury JM, et al. Quantitative fMRI assessment of the differences in lateralization of language-related brain activation in patients with temporal lobe epilepsy. *Neuroimage* 2003;18:423–438.

144. Rutten GJ, Ramsey N, van Rijen P, van Veelen C. Reproducibility of fMRI-determined language lateralization in individual subjects. *Brain Lang* 2002;80:421–437.

145. Liégois F, Connelly A, Salmond CH, et al. A direct test for lateralization of language activation using fMRI: Comparison with invasive assessments in children with epilepsy. *Neuroimage* 2002; 17:1861–1867.

146. Knecht S, Dräger B, Deppe M, et al. Handedness and hemispheric language dominance in healthy humans. *Brain* 2000;123: 2512–2518.

147. Loring DW, Meador KJ, Lee GP, et al. Cerebral language lateralization: Evidence from intracarotid amobarbital testing. *Neuropsychologia* 1990;28:831–838.

148. Rasmussen T, Milner B. The role of early left-brain injury in determining lateralization of cerebral speech functions. *Ann NY Acad Sci* 1977;299:355–369.

149. Shaywitz BA, Shaywitz SE, Pugh KR, et al. Sex differences in the functional organization of the brain for language. *Nature* 1995;373: 607–609.

150. Buckner RL, Raichle ME, Petersen SE. Dissociation of human prefrontal cortical areas across different speech production tasks and gender groups. *J Neurosci* 1995;74:2163–2173.

151. Price CJ, Moore CJ, Friston KJ. Getting sex into perspective. *Neuroimage* 1996;3:S586.

152. Frost JA, Binder JR, Springer JA, et al. Language processing is strongly left lateralized in both sexes: evidence from FMRI. *Brain* 1999;122:199–208.

153. Knecht S, Deppe M, Dräger B, et al. Language lateralization in healthy right-handers. *Brain* 2000;123:74–81.

154. Grady CL, Maisog JM, Horwitz B, et al. Age-related changes in cortical blood flow activation during visual processing of faces and location. *J Neurosci* 1994;14:1450–1462.

155. Grady CL, McIntosh AR, Bookstein F, et al. Age-related changes in regional cerebral blood flow during working memory for faces. *Neuroimage* 1998;8:409–425.

156. Risse GL, Gates JR, Fangman MC. A reconsideration of bilateral language representation based on the intracarotid amobarbital procedure. *Brain Lang* 1997;33:118–132.

157. Woods RP, Dodrill CB, Ojemann GA. Brain injury, handedness, and speech lateralization in a series of amobarbital studies. *Ann Neurol* 1988;23:510–518.

158. Baciu M, Kahane P, Minotti L, et al. Functional MRI assessment of the hemispheric predominance for language in epileptic patients using a simple rhyme detection task. *Epileptic Disorders* 2001;3:117–124.

159. Bahn MM, Lin W, Silbergeld DL, et al. Localization of language cortices by functional MR imaging compared with intracarotid amobarbital hemispheric sedation. *Am J Radiol* 1997;169:575–579.

160. Binder JR, Swanson SJ, Hammeke TA, et al. Determination of language dominance using functional MRI: a comparison with the Wada test. *Neurology* 1996;46:978–984.

161. Desmond JE, Sum JM, Wagner AD, et al. Functional MRI measurement of language lateralization in Wada-tested patients. *Brain* 1995;118:1411–1419.

162. Hertz-Pannier L, Gaillard WD, Mott S, et al. Noninvasive assessment of language dominance in children and adolescents with functional MRI: a preliminary study. *Neurology* 1997;48:1003–1012.

163. Rutten G-J, Ramsey N, van Rijen P, et al. fMRI-determined language lateralization in patients with unilateral or mixed language dominance according to the Wada test. *Neuroimage* 2004;in press.

164. Sabbah P, Chassoux F, Leveque C, et al. Functional MR imaging in assessment of language dominance in epileptic patients. *Neuroimage* 2003;18:460–467.

165. Yetkin FZ, Swanson S, Fischer M, et al. Functional MR of frontal lobe activation: Comparison with Wada language results. *Am J Neuroradiol* 1998;19:1095–1098.

166. Binder JR, Hammeke TA, Possing ET, et al. Reliability and validity of language dominance assessment with functional MRI. *Neurology* 2001;56(Suppl 3):A158.

167. Worthington C, Vincent DJ, Bryant AE, et al. Comparison of functional magnetic resonance imaging for language localization and intracarotid speech amytal testing in presurgical evaluation for intractable epilepsy. *Stereotactic Functional Neurosurg* 1997;69:197–201.

168. Fitzgerald DB, Cosgrove GR, Ronner S, et al. Location of language in the cortex: a comparison between functional MR imaging and electrocortical stimulation. *Am J Neuroradiol* 1997;18:1529–1539.

169. Lurito JT, Lowe MJ, Sartorius C, Mathews VP. 1997 Comparison of fMRI and intraoperative direct cortical stimulation in localization of receptive language areas. *J Comput Assist Tomogr* 1997;24:99–105.

170. Ruge MI, Victor JD, Hosain S, et al. Concordance between functional magnetic resonance imaging and intraoperative language mapping. *Stereotactic Functional Neurosurg* 1999;72:95–102.

171. Rutten GJM, van Rijen PC, van Veelen CWM, Ramsey NF. Language area localization with three-dimensional functional magnetic resonance imaging matches intrasulcal electrostimulation in Broca's area. *Ann Neurol* 1999;46:405–408.

172. Rutten GJM, Ramsey NF, van Rijen PC, et al. Development of a functional magnetic resonance imaging protocol for intraoperative localization of critical temporoparietal language areas. *Ann Neurol* 2002;51:350–360.

173. Schlosser MJ, Luby M, Spencer DD, et al. Comparative localization of auditory comprehension by using functional magnetic resonance imaging and cortical stimulation. *J Neurosurg* 1999;91:626–635.

174. Stapleton SR, Kiriakipoulos E, Mikulis D, et al. Combined utility of functional MRI, cortical mapping, and frameless stereotaxy in the resection of lesions in eloquent areas of brain in children. *Ped Neurosurg* 1997;26:68–82.

175. Yetkin FZ, Mueller WM, Morris GL, et al. Functional MR activation correlated with intraoperative cortical mapping. *Am J Neuroradiol* 1997;18:1311–1315.

176. Benbadis SR, Binder JR, Swanson SJ, et al. Is speech arrest during Wada testing a valid method for determining hemispheric representation of language? *Brain Lang* 1998;65:441–446.

177. Chelune GJ. Using neuropsychological data to forecast postsurgical cognitive outcome. In: Lüders H, ed. *Epilepsy surgery*. New York: Raven Press, 1991:477–485.

178. Schwartz TH, Devinsky O, Doyle W, Perrine K. Preoperative predictors of anterior temporal language areas. *J Neurosurg* 1998;89: 962–970.

179. Sabsevitz DS, Swanson SJ, Hammeke TA, et al. Use of preoperative functional neuroimaging to predict language deficits from epilepsy surgery. *Neurology* 2003;60:1788–1792.

180. Detre JA, Floyd TF. Functional MRI and its applications to the clinical neurosciences. *Neuroscientist* 2001;7:64–79.

181. Gaillard WD, Theodore WH. Mapping language in epilepsy with functional neuroimaging. *Neuroscientist* 2000;6:391–401.

182. Damasio H, Grabowski TJ, Tranel D, et al. A neural basis for lexical retrieval. *Nature* 1996;380:499–505.

183. Grabowski TJ, Damasio H, Tranel D, et al. A role for left temporal pole in the retrieval of words for unique entities. *Hum Brain Mapp* 2001;13:199–212.

184. Hamberger MJ, Goodman RR, Perrine K, Tamny TR. Anatomic dissociation of auditory and visual naming in the lateral temporal cortex. *Neurology* 2001;56:56–61.

185. Price CJ, Moore CJ, Humphreys GW, Wise RJS. Segregating semantic from phonological processes during reading. *J Cogn Neurosci* 1997;9:727–733.

186. Scott SK, Blank C, Rosen S, Wise RJS. Identification of a pathway for intelligible speech in the left temporal lobe. *Brain* 2000; 123:2400–2406.

187. Bell BD, Davies KG, Hermann BP, Walters G. Confrontation naming after anterior temporal lobectomy is related to age of acquisition of the object names. *Neuropsychologia* 2000;38:83–92.

188. Davies KG, Bell BD, Bush AJ, et al. Naming decline after left anterior temporal lobectomy correlates with pathological status of resected hippocampus. *Epilepsia* 1998;39:407–419.

189. Hermann BP, Wyler AR, Somes G, Clement L Dysnomia after left anterior temporal lobectomy without functional mapping: frequency and correlates. *Neurosurgery*. 1994;35:52–57.

190. Langfit JT, Rausch R. Word-finding deficits persist after left anterotemporal lobectomy. Arch Neurol 1996;53:72–76.

191. Wada J, Rasmussen T. Intracarotid injection of sodium amytal for the lateralization of cerebral speech dominance. *J Neurosurg* 1960;17: 266–282.

192. Milner B, Branch C, Rasmussen T. Study of short-term memory after intracarotid injection of sodium amytal. *Trans Am Neurol Assoc* 1962;87:224–226.

193. Glosser G, Cole L, French J, et al. Is there a reason to inject the side of presumed epileptic focus first in the Intracarotid Amobarbital Test? Presented at the 1997 Meeting of the American Epilepsy Society, April 1997: Boston, MA.

194. Glosser G, Cole LC, Deutsch GK, et al. Hemispheric symmetries in arousal affect outcome of the intracarotid amobarbital test. *Neurology* 1999;52:1583–1590.

195. Loring DW, Meador KJ, Lee GP, et al. Wada memory performance predicts seizure outcome following anterior temporal lobectomy. *Neurology* 1994;44:2322–2324.

196. Sperling MR, Saykin AJ, Glosser G, et al. Predictors of outcome after anterior temporal lobectomy: the intracarotid amobarbital test. *Neurology* 1994;44:2325–2330.

197. Manno EM, Sperling MR, Ding X, et al. Predictors of outcome after anterior temporal lobectomy: positron emission tomography. *Neurology* 1994;44:2331–2336.

198. Weinand ME, Carter LP. Surface cortical cerebral blood flow monitoring and single photon emission computed tomography: prognostic factors for selecting temporal lobectomy candidates. *Seizure* 1994;3: 55–59.

199. Constable RT, Carpentier A, Pugh K, et al. Investigation of the hippocampal formation using a randomized event-related paradigm and z-shimmed functional MRI. *Neuroimage* 2000;12:55–62.

200. Fransson P, Merboldt KD, Ingvar M, et al. Functional MRI with reduced susceptibility artifact: high-resolution mapping of episodic memory encoding. *Neuroreport* 2001;12:1415–1420.

201. Stern CE, Corkin S, González RG, et al. The hippocampal formation participates in novel picture encoding: Evidence from functional magnetic resonance imaging. *Proc Natl Acad Sci USA* 1996;93: 8660–8665.

202. Golby AJ, Poldrack RA, Brewer JB, et al. Material-specific lateralization in the medial temporal lobe and prefrontal cortex during memory encoding. *Brain* 2001;124:1841–1854.

203. Reber PJ, Wong EC, Buxton RB. Encoding activity in the medial temporal lobe examined with anatomically constrained fMRI analysis. *Hippocampus* 2002;12:363–376.

204. Hunkin NM, Mayes AR, Gregory LJ, et al. Novelty-related activation within the medial temporal lobes. *Neuropsychologia* 2002;40: 1456–1464.

205. Kirchhoff BA, Wagner AD, Maril A, Stern CE. Prefrontal-temporal circuitry for episodic encoding and subsequent memory. *J Neurosci* 2000;20:6173–6180.

206. Sperling RA, Bates JF, Cocchiarella AJ, et al. Encoding novel face-name associations: a functional MRI study. *Hum Brain Mapp* 2001;14:129–139.

207. Squire LR. Memory and the hippocampus: a synthesis from findings with rats, monkeys, and humans. *Psychol Rev* 1992;99:195–231.

208. Rombouts SA, Machielsen WC, Witter MP, et al. Visual association encoding activates the medial temporal lobe: a functional magnetic resonance imaging study. *Hippocampus* 1997;7:594–601.

209. Gloor P. The temporal lobe and limbic system. New York: Oxford University Press, 1997.

210. Detre JA, Maccotta L, King D, et al. Functional MRI lateralization of memory in temporal lobe epilepsy. *Neurology* 1998;50:926–932.

211. Golby AJ, Poldrack RA, Illes J, et al. Memory lateralization in medial temporal lobe epilepsy assessed by functional MRI. *Epilepsia* 2002;43:855–863.

212. Killgore WDS, Glosser G, Casasanto D, et al. Functional MRI and the Wada test provide complementary information for predicting post-operative seizure control. *Seizure* 2000;8:450–455.

213. Binder JR, Bellgowan PSF, Swanson SJ, et al. FMRI activation asymmetry predicts side of seizure focus in temporal lobe epilepsy. *Neuroimage* 2000;11:S155.

214. Jokeit H, Okujava M, Woermann FG. Memory fMRI lateralizes temporal lobe epilepsy. *Neurology* 2001;57:1786–1793.

215. Casasanto DJ, Glosser G, Killgore WDS, et al. Presurgical fMRI predicts memory outcome following anterior temporal lobectomy. *J Int Neuropsychol Soc* 2001;7:183.

216. Machulda MM, Ward HA, Cha R, et al. Functional inferences vary with the method of analysis in fMRI. *Neuroimage* 2001;14:1122–1127.

217. Machielsen WC, Rombouts SA, Barkhof F, et al. FMRI of visual encoding: reproducibility of activation. *Hum Brain Mapp* 2000;9: 156–164.

CHAPTER 11

Magnetic Resonance Neurophysiology: Simultaneous EEG and fMRI

Anthony B. Waites, David F. Abbott, Steven W. Fleming and Graeme D. Jackson

INTRODUCTION

This chapter describes techniques that combine the spatial resolution of MRI with the temporal resolution of the electro-encephalogram (EEG) by concurrently acquiring EEG and functional MRI (fMRI). This is one of the most exciting new advances in epileptology and we believe that it will form the basis of major new insights into mechanisms of seizure generation and epilepsy concepts. Like fMRI when it was first developed, it has become possible because of technology advances. In this case it is the ability to measure the few millivolts of the EEG scalp signal in the hostile environment of the MR scanner where up to several volts of artifact have to be dealt with.

Electroencephalography has been a mainstay of the clinical diagnosis of epilepsy for decades, and a vast array of abnormal interictal and ictal cerebral electrical activity has been identified with the epilepsy syndromes. While its utility is unquestioned, EEG is only capable of revealing part of the information required to understand epileptic phenomena. The temporal resolution of EEG is high but its spatial resolution is relatively low, a problem that until recently could only be partially solved by the use of invasive methods such as intracranial recordings including surface or depth electrodes. The behavior of the cerebral vasculature during particular electrical events is also poorly understood, although it has been known for some time that dramatic blood flow changes, often large, occur during seizures (1).

Functional MRI allows one to explore the local vascular response, and indirectly the coupled neural response to particular stimuli. As described in Chapter 10, fMRI has found clinical use in the mapping of areas of eloquent cortex by localizing cerebral blood-oxygen-dependent (BOLD) signal changes while subjects perform certain tasks.

BOLD changes also occur during seizures, and these can be measured with fMRI (2–4). It is extremely difficult to perform such measurements, however, for it requires the subject to have a seizure in the scanner during fMRI acquisition, while remaining very still so that the study is not ruined by motion artifact. It is much more feasible to scan a subject while abnormal subclinical interictal events are occurring, such as spike and slow wave activity. It is clear that BOLD changes also occur around the time of these events, either as a result of the abnormal electrical activity or perhaps even leading up to it. Unfortunately, BOLD signal fluctuations alone are generally too small to delineate regions of abnormality if the timing of the related electrical activity is not known. EEG can give us that timing information if it can be performed within the MR scanner.

In this chapter we describe the technological advances that have led to the ability to concurrently acquire EEG and fMRI data. We review the results of the few studies to date that have made use of this technology, including figures primarily from our own work as examples of applications of the method. We conclude that simultaneous EEG and fMRI is a powerful technique that is certain to further our understanding of the mechanisms of epilepsy, and is likely to revolutionize clinical diagnosis and management through greater understanding of this and other diseases.

THE EVOLVING AND EXPANDING ROLE OF MAGNETIC RESONANCE IMAGING

In addition to providing unsurpassed anatomic detail, MR can provide images that reflect a number of physiologic processes. fMRI shows increased signal-intensity in areas of high blood flow as a result of a fall in deoxyhemoglobin, as detected by BOLD contrast techniques (5–8). fMRI has been used to localize brain areas associated with many motor, sensory, and cognitive tasks. Oxygenated hemoglobin (oxyHb) has magnetic properties similar to surrounding brain tissue, while deoxyHb does not. The T2*-weighted MR imaging technique used is very sensitive to changes in local magnetic properties. Sequential images can be rapidly obtained giving fMRI the unique ability to provide excellent temporal as well as spatial information. MR spectroscopy can detect metabolites important in neuronal function such as N-acetyl aspartate, creatine, choline and phosphocholine, glutamine and glutamate, and lactate (see Chapter 13). Diffusion-weighted MRI detects cell swelling (see Chapter 12) and, like MR spectroscopy, may show persisting changes some time after the event.

Successful surgical treatment of epilepsy is dependent upon accurate localization of the seizure focus. While standard MRI imaging will frequently reveal a causative anatomic abnormality in temporal lobe epilepsy, this is often not the case in extratemporal epilepsy.

WHERE DOES fMRI/EEG FIT IN EPILEPSY INVESTIGATIONS?

To define the epilepsy process it is conceptually necessary to define three parameters that provide information in different domains (dimensional quality or axis). These are:

- the clinical context of the seizure
- the fixed or structural focal abnormality in the brain
- the functional site of origin of ictal activity (see Chapter 1).

Of these we have a long epileptologic tradition to define the first, many imaging methods to define the second, and few methods to define the third. The importance of simultaneous fMRI/EEG is that it provides additional and new tools to help define the intermittent functional events at the core of epileptic seizures.

There is considerable evidence that partial epileptic seizures cause intense cerebral activation and regional increases in blood flow. Increased blood flow, often large in magnitude and extent, has been demonstrated with ictal single-photon-emission computed tomography (SPECT; Chapter 14). Focal increases in metabolism have been demonstrated with ictal positron-emission tomography (PET) in some patients with partial onset seizures (Chapter 15). Ictal PET studies in patients with generalized epilepsies have produced variable results but tend to argue against regional or general increases in cerebral metabolism. Compared to these techniques, ictal fMRI has the advantage both of high spatial resolution and the ability to sample brain function with relatively good temporal resolution compared to these other imaging techniques (but still poor compared to EEG and magnetoencephalography, MEG). fMRI/EEG therefore

has the potential to demonstrate important aspects of the generation of seizures, the vizualization of which has not previously been possible. As will be seen in later parts of this chapter, much of this potential is starting to be realized.

Whereas EEG delivers excellent information on the timing of the spikes, it is poor in precisely locating the source of the discharges. Sophisticated EEG analysis techniques, such as dipole modeling, can improve the localization qualities of scalp EEG (9). Intracerebral EEG allows recording directly from the seizure focus, or from a brain area in close proximity to the seizure focus. Whereas intracerebral EEG gives very precise temporal and spatial information, it is invasive and expensive, and thus limited to a small proportion of subjects. Furthermore, it is restricted to the implanted brain area. Therefore, there is a clear need for a noninvasive, whole brain investigation tool to localize the seizure focus.

Another problem is that only about 70% of patients with refractory focal epilepsy show a lesion on MR imaging, which in many instances reflects the seizure onset zone (see Chapter 2). Advances in neuroimaging techniques have greatly improved detection of structural abnormalities associated with the seizure focus. However, in some patients no abnormality can be detected, or in the presence of a larger lesion it may not be clear which parts of the lesion are responsible for seizure generation. The application of fMRI/EEG techniques to this problem uses the spatial localization qualities of fMRI combined with the temporal precision of discharges on EEG recording.

In 1994, we first demonstrated that functional MRI is a potential tool for seizure focus localization in a 4-year-old child who had frequent focal motor seizures (2). Such early studies used clinical signs for seizure detection, as EEG recording during scanning was not possible at that stage. Now, 10 years later, many of the technical problems are solved, and several centers worldwide now report successful studies with a combination of EEG recording and MR imaging with the aim of seizure focus localization.

TECHNICAL CONSIDERATIONS

As we have argued above, combined fMRI/EEG is a very promising methodology that combines knowledge about neuronal activity and its metabolic response. The human EEG, recorded on the scalp for clinical purposes, is in the range of 10–200 μV. Clinical MRI systems operate with magnetic fields up to 3 T. Technical problems associated with the technique include EEG artifacts caused by the high-intensity magnetic field and rapidly changing field gradients.

Any movement of a conductor in the static magnetic field can induce a voltage in the lead, which, as well as degrading image quality, can be potentially dangerous for the patient, unless safety precautions are taken (10). Movement can be due to patient head movement, cardiac-induced scalp/head movements, and vibration of the leads due to scanner noise.

One way to overcome artifacts associated with the gradient switching of MR image acquisition is to record EEG only during times when the patient is in the magnet but there is no MR imaging. The MR images are acquired after visual identification of a spike (spike image) and after periods of normal EEG background (control image). The time lag of several seconds between the spike event and the acquisition allows acquisition of the image during the peak of the hemodynamic response (11). This method is relatively simple; however, it has the disadvantage that only a small time window after a discharge can be assessed, and no EEG information can be obtained during scanning. Successful spike-triggered fMRI has been reported by several groups (12–21).

Truly concurrent fMRI/EEG recording is technically more challenging but has great potential for clinical and scientific neurologic applications. In contrast to spike-triggered fMRI the entire hemodynamic response after a discharge can be assessed, and the continuous imaging and EEG recording allows investigation of changes prior, during, and after interictal and ictal discharges. Several methods have been developed to reduce the ballistocardiogram (22, 23) and the artifact caused by currents induced by rapidly changing magnetic gradients (24–27). In contrast to the averaging of many interictal epileptiform discharges (IEDs), performed with spike-triggered fMRI, continuous fMRI/EEG assesses each discharge as a single event. In order to assess whether single spikes are associated with sufficient fMRI activation to be useful, one study assessed the BOLD response after each spike in a patient with focal epilepsy (21). About one-third of the 43 assessed spikes were associated with a significant BOLD signal change, suggesting that this method is feasible. Further demonstrations of the feasibility of continuous EEG during fMRI can be found in recent publications (28–32).

WHAT IS MEASURED BY FMRI/EEG?

Logothetis et al. co-registered intracranial recordings of neuronal signal and functional MRI in monkeys. They found that the focal BOLD signal change primarily measured the input and processing of neuronal information within that focal region, detected as measured changes in local field potentials (7, 33). This indicates that BOLD signal reflects neuronal activity in a focal brain area. Interictal discharges reflect spontaneous neuronal activity, and therefore it seems reasonable that fMRI/EEG might be able to identify the anatomic area from which interictal discharges arise. It has been shown that interictal spiking produces focal increases in cerebral blood flow and glucose metabolism (34). The area of blood flow increase corresponded to the site of maximal ictal EEG abnormality recorded with implanted electrodes (34). As part of the BOLD response can be explained by blood flow increase, this is a further indication that the area identified by fMRI/EEG represents the seizure focus.

The BOLD response to single IEDs can vary (35). However, the shape of the hemodynamic response after interictal discharges is often similar to other fMRI experiments (29). The areas identified by fMRI/EEG seem to be reproducible, at least in one study, which assessed a single patient on four separate occasions (20).

PRACTICAL ISSUES FOR PERFORMING ENCEPHALOGRAPHY INSIDE THE MAGNETIC RESONANCE IMAGING SCANNER

Many obstacles need to be overcome to achieve successful EEG recording in MRI scanners. The MR environment is a hostile one for recording EEG. High-field (3 T) recordings are even more difficult than with 1.5 T systems. Nonetheless, it can be done, and a number of centers have developed solutions. We describe here some of the more significant issues that one must consider if these studies are to be successfully undertaken.

Patient Safety

The most important consideration while recording EEG in a scanning MRI is patient safety. To record EEG in an MRI, electrodes are placed on the patient's scalp. These are connected via EEG leads to the EEG amplifier, which in turn is connected to a recording device. Apart from the normal safety considerations observed while recording EEG, a number of new safety concerns need to be addressed before recording in a scanning MRI can be performed safely.

Magnetic Field Attractive Force

Ferrous materials becoming projectiles in the magnetic field can injure patients. All ferrous material will be attracted to the magnet, the force of attraction depending on the type, shape, and mass of the material. For the safety of the patients, all materials used for the EEG system should be nonferrous.

Radiofrequency Burning

Without careful preparation, patients can be burnt when connected to conductors in a scanning MRI. Radiofrequency energy generated while scanning induces high voltages in loops formed by EEG leads – up to 8000 V/m^2 at 1.5 T (36). If current flow through the patient due to this voltage is not restricted the patient can be burned. Low-impedance paths for current flow could be due to:

- low input impedance of a faulty EEG amplifier channel
- low impedance through low-pass radiofrequency filter on the input to EEG channels

- low impedance caused by capacitive coupling between the EEG leads
- low impedance caused by bad insulation on cables shorting together or to the patient
- multiple ground electrodes (36).

Although avoiding all the above should remove the risk of burning, using high-impedance leads or current-limiting resistors can reduce the risk further. It has been shown at 1.5 T with a circularly polarized coil (36) that including more than 13k series resistors as close to the EEG electrodes as possible will limit current flow to safe levels. The current flow can also be reduced by minimizing the loop areas formed by the EEG leads, as the voltage induced is directly proportional to the loop area.

Magnetic Resonance Imaging Artifacts – Degradation of Image Quality

The main obstacles to the acquisition of good-quality MRI images during a simultaneous fMRI/EEG experiment are susceptibility artifact induced by the leads and electrodes, and radiofrequency interference induced by the EEG electronics equipment degrading acquired fMRI images. The former can be minimized by use of nonmetallic electrodes and the latter by placing the EEG recording equipment outside the scanner room. One can use a shielded headbox located in the magnet room to convert and transmit via optical fiber the signals from the EEG leads, with a reciprocal converter located outside of the magnet room.

Limitations of Electroencephalography in the Scanner

The acquisition of EEG within the MRI scanner is difficult. Movement of a conductor in a magnetic field generates a voltage or electromotive force (EMF). Power generation utilities use magnets of less than 1 T in strength to generate voltages in excess of 300 000 V. The human EEG, recorded on the scalp for clinical purposes, is in the range of 10–300 μV. Clinical MRI systems typically operate with magnetic fields of up to 3 T. In order to record the very low EEG signal reliably in an MR system, these induced artifactual signals must be isolated from the EEG and removed. A typical EEG recorded in a 3 T scanner is shown in Figure 11.1. When the scanner is off, pulse artifact can be seen. The gradient artifact hides all EEG signal during the periods of scanning.

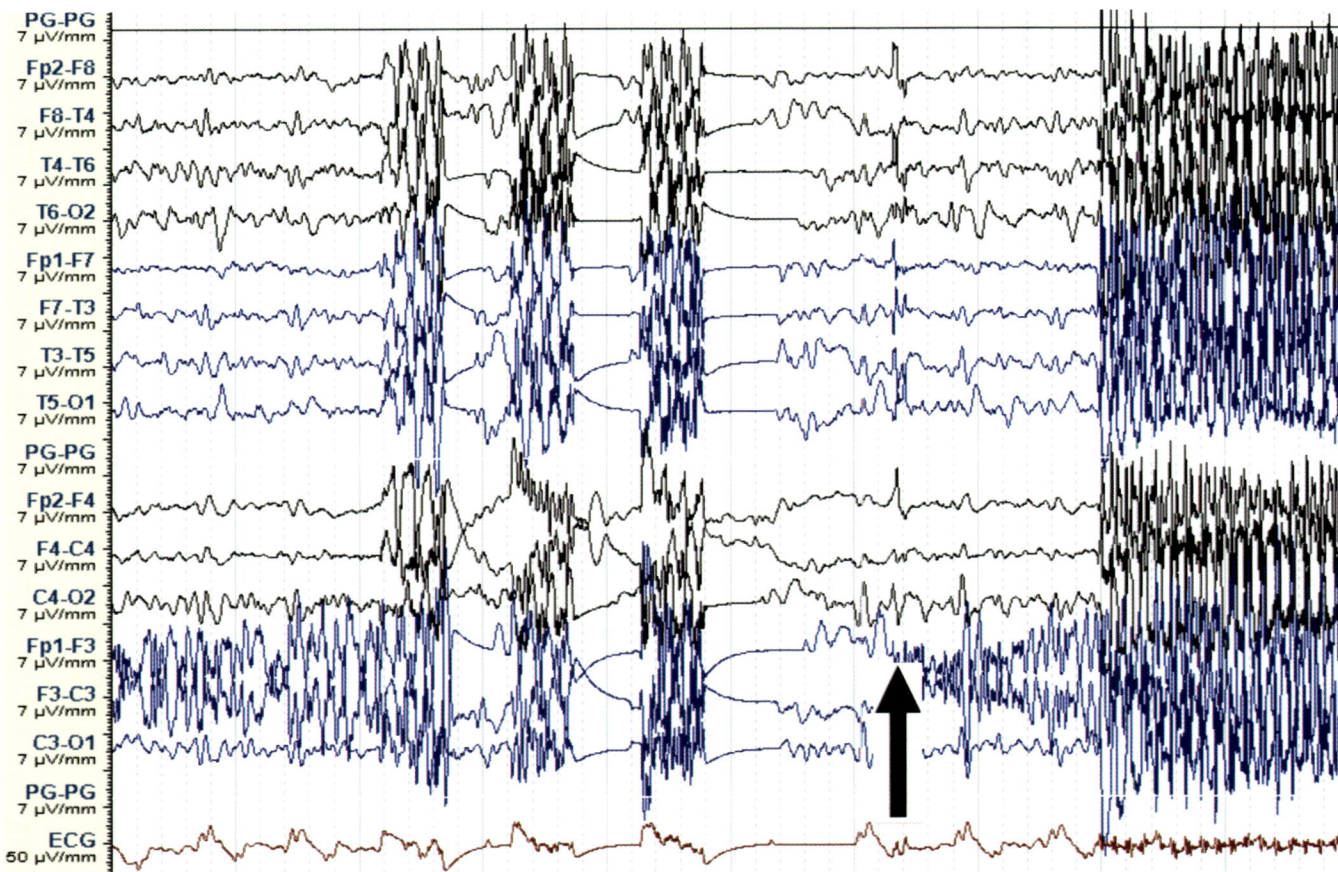

FIG. 11.1. Raw (uncorrected) EEG signal acquired within a 3 T MR scanner. The displayed panel shows EEG and ECG signals before scanning (left), during prescan (middle) and after commencement of the EPI scan (right). Gradient artifact obscures all other EEG signals during scanning. The pulse artifact is present throughout the EEG (seen by aligning the ECG with the peak in the QRS complex). At least one possible candidate spike is seen in the trace (arrow).

Gradient-induced Artifacts

In order to record the very low level EEG in an MR system we must deal with the large EMF induced in the EEG leads during scanning. These gradient induced artifacts are caused by conductive loops formed by the EEG leads and scalp being exposed to the changing gradient fields.

The Scale of the Gradient Induced Artifacts

Knowing the gradient slew rate (the rate of change of the gradient field) and the size and position of the conductive loop, we can calculate the approximate EMF induced using Faraday's law:

$$EMF = -d\Phi/dt.$$

It must be noted that the actual voltage induced in EEG leads depends on the area of the loops and their position relative to the gradient fields, which in turn depends on the EEG montage and patient positioning.

In this case the rate of change of flux ($d\Phi/dt$) is the result of slewing (rapidly changing) the X, Y, Z gradients. The rate of change of magnetic flux is a function of

- gradient slew rate
- the area of a closed path normal to, and enclosing the flux, and
- the distance between the normal surface and the magnetic center of the gradients (iso-center).

Pulsing one gradient, on a system capable of 150 T/m/s, assuming a loop area of 0.1 m × 0.1 m @ 0.1 m from iso-center:

$$
\begin{aligned}
EMF &= -d\Phi/dt \quad &(1)\\
&= -A \times dB/dt\\
&= -(0.1 \times 0.1 \times 0.1) \times 150\\
&= 0.15\,V \text{ peak or } 0.3\,V \text{ p–p for both positive- and}\\
&\quad \text{negative-going gradient changes.}
\end{aligned}
$$

This is at least three orders of magnitude larger than the EEG signal, so without counter-measures gradient-induced artifacts will completely obscure the EEG data (22, 36).

Dealing with Gradient-induced Artifacts

From Equation (1) it is evident that the gradient-induced EMF is directly proportional to the loop area and slew rate (dB/dt). Although the slew rate is fixed, twisting the EEG leads together as close to the head as possible can reduce the area (37).

Spike-triggered Acquisition

The most obvious solution to gradient artifact is only to operate the EEG equipment while the scanner is not acquiring images. One such approach is spike-triggered fMRI, where the EEG is observed by an expert electroencephalographer in real-time until an event of interest occurs (such as a spike and slow wave event), at which point the radiographer is instructed to acquire a single MR imaging volume and the EEG equipment is switched off. If enough events are captured and compared to baseline images (acquired after periods of normal EEG activity), areas of activation or deactivation (where signal increase or decrease is present only immediately after a spike) can be inferred (13, 38).

The main problems with this approach are practical. The acquisition is time-consuming, since scans are acquired only infrequently. Further, the shape of the hemodynamic response cannot be measured, since to avoid changing intensity and contrast in the images due to T1 effects, only a single image is acquired following each spike or rest event. In order to avoid possible spikes occurring during MR scanning when the EEG is unmonitored, a pause of at least 15 seconds is inserted following an MR acquisition (Fig. 11.2). This creates a further limitation, as some patients have very frequent interictal discharges (every few seconds), so it would be impossible to unambiguously interpret BOLD changes in a spike-triggered study of these subjects.

Interleaved Techniques

In order to increase the signal to noise of a study, it would be advantageous to increase the number of images acquired per unit time. This has been achieved using interleaved fMRI and EEG. In its simplest form, EEG is acquired for a period of time, then the EEG equipment is switched off while some MR images are acquired, and then image acquisition is

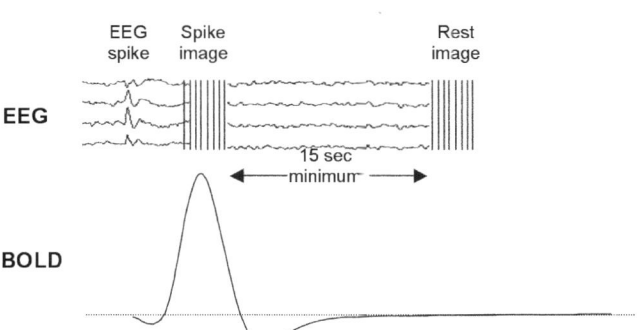

FIG. 11.2. Spike-triggered fMRI-EEG BOLD response to the spike is sampled by waiting 3 seconds following the spike, which aligns the single MR image volume with the maximum of the hemodynamic response. A series of single rest scans are acquired after a period of EEG inactivity. The 15-second minimum delay assures no BOLD response to a missed EEG spike during MR acquisition, as well as allowing full T1 relaxation.

stopped so that more EEG can be acquired, and so on. (28, 39). The problem here is that there is a variable time between acquisitions, since some are preceded by an EEG period. The nonequilibrium of spin effects result in different T1 image contrast between the first few images acquired when MR scanning commences after a period without scanning. In conventional fMRI these first few images are usually discarded, but here the first image acquired is likely to be the most important, as the BOLD signal change related to the spike will have substantially decayed by the time the spins have reached equilibrium.

A logical extension of the interleaved EEG/fMRI acquisition is a 'near simultaneous' method where the timing of each EEG and fMRI acquisition is short. Rather than acquiring a block of fMRI followed by a block of EEG, a single fMRI acquisition is performed with an effective repetition time sufficiently long to allow a short period of EEG acquisition before the next fMRI acquisition. The EPI fMRI sequence used must allow all slices to be acquired very quickly followed by a 'silent' period where a few seconds of EEG can be acquired (28, 39). This method mitigates many of the problems of slow interleaved EEG and fMRI blocks, however as there is still a time period of half a second or more where EEG must be switched off while the fMRI acquisition occurs. Thus there is the possibility that some spikes could be missed, thus creating problems of interpretation and possibly leading to decreased power in a study.

SIMULTANEOUS AND CONTINUOUS EEG AND FMRI

The ideal is to obtain simultaneous and continuous high quality fMRI and EEG data without gradient artifact and in real time.

In most published examples, near real time can be achieved using some sort of post-processing of the EEG. There have been various strategies for the removal of the gradient artifact during simultaneous and continuous EEG.

The first strategy uses a hard-wired montage of electrodes. By a careful positioning of electrode leads, the loop area and therefore the artifact can be reduced dramatically. In combination with low-pass filtering, to remove the high-frequency gradient switching component of the artifact, the residual signal is a combination of the EEG signal and frequency components related to the scanning rate (images per second). Unfortunately, filtering cannot be used to remove these components as they are in the same range as the EEG signal.

The second strategy is to attempt to eliminate the gradient artifact using a post-processing filter. This approach requires a wide-bandwidth, high dynamic range EEG acquisition system, in order to adequately sample both the large artifactual signal and the EEG signal of interest. The artifact is removed by applying narrow rejection filters targeted at the frequencies of the imaging gradients (26). These frequencies are known

from the imaging protocol, and are verifiable by looking at the Fourier transform of the EEG signal, where the gradient switching frequency and its harmonics can be seen as spikes in the frequency distribution.

Another approach is to sparsely sample the EEG in a manner that avoids measurement during the gradient switching (40). By repositioning the gradients in relation to the EEG sampling frequency, it is possible to sample only when the imaging gradients are constant. This method leads to a compromise in measurement performance with regard to the achievable TR, imaging volume, and EEG sampling frequency.

Movement-induced Artifacts

As stated earlier, movement of the electrodes or leads in the magnetic field can generate a further artifact. This movement can be periodic, due to pulsatile blood flow effects in the scalp, or random, due to random patient head motion. These movements cause slight changes in the position of the EEG leads near the scalp (41, 42). If these movements change the amount of magnetic flux enclosed in the loop then they will induce an EMF in the EEG leads.

The Scale of Movement Induced Artifacts

In this case the rate of change of flux ($d\Phi/dt$) is the result of the loop area exposed to the main field changing. The rate of change of flux is a function of the rate of change in area of a closed path normal to, and enclosing the flux of the main MR field, and the field strength of the magnet. Assuming a field of 3 T, a loop area of $0.1\,m \times 0.1\,m$, $0.1\,mm$ movement of one side of the loop over $40\,mSec$ (cardiac QR segment) then

$$
\begin{aligned}
EMF &= -d\Phi/dt & (2)\\
&= -B \times dA/dt\\
&= -3 \times (0.1 \times (0.1 - 0.0999))/0.04\\
&= 750\,\mu V.
\end{aligned}
$$

This is more than double the size of a large EEG signal.

Movement artifacts may be reduced by restricting patient and cable movement and by reducing the area of loops formed by the head and EEG leads. The periodic component of the cardioballistic movement artifact has been successfully removed by post-processing (24, 41). The combined effects of correction for gradient artifact and cardioballistic artifact leads to an EEG signal that approaches the quality of EEG outside the magnet (Fig. 11.3).

The performance of the algorithm for correcting cardioballistic artifact is largely dependent on the accurate identification of the timing of the peak of the QRS complex in the ECG, which depends on the quality of the ECG. In the MR scanner, especially at high field, the ECG becomes broad, making accurate timing difficult to obtain.

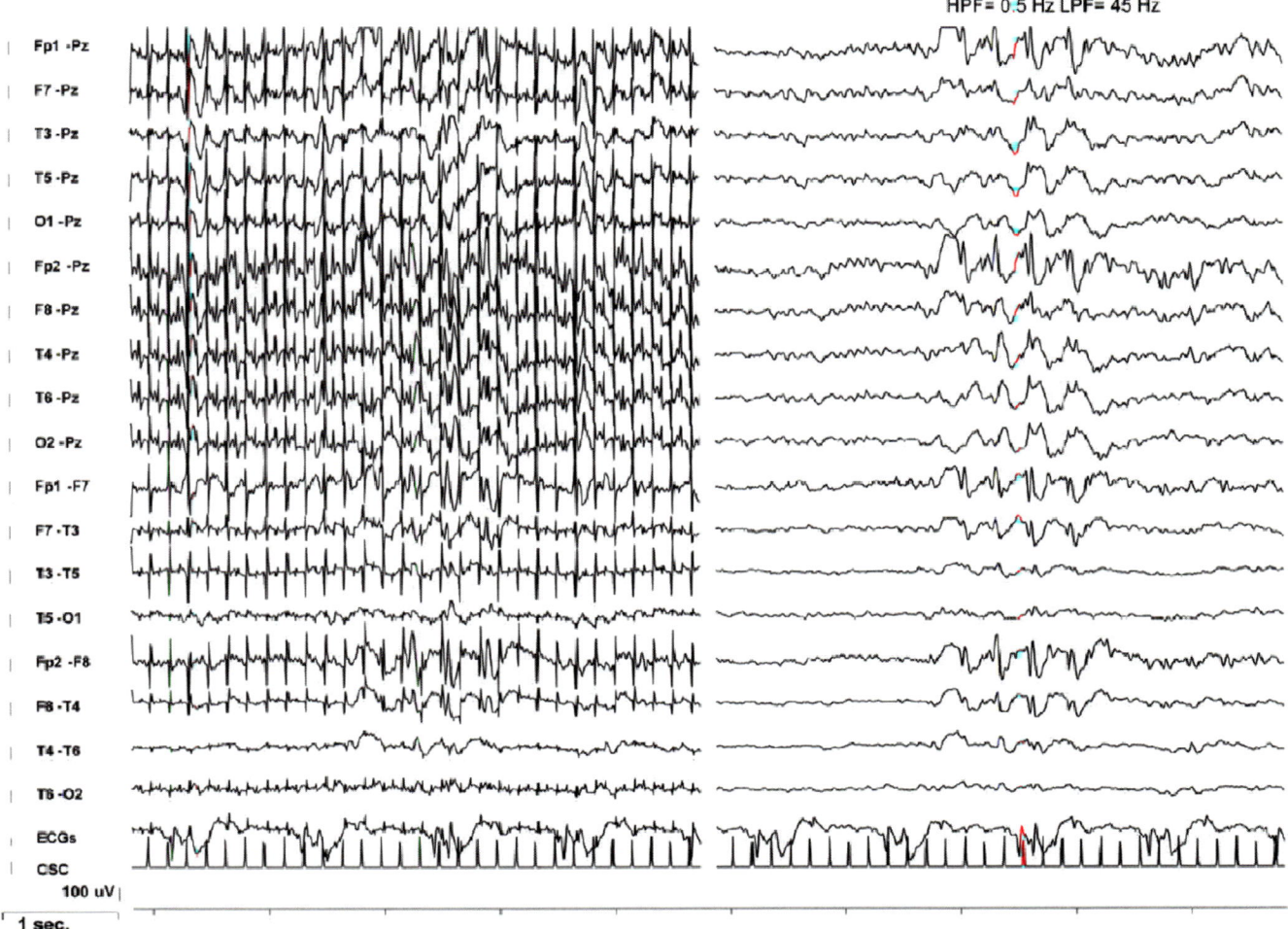

FIG. 11.3. Typical in-scanner (1.5 T) EEG before (left) and after (right) removal of pulse artifact and gradient artifact. (With permission from Salek-Haddadi et al. 2003 (44).)

This makes the quality of artifact removal variable and subject-specific.

A further problem, not so easy to deal with, is random patient motion. This can lead to a random and isolated EEG artifact, which cannot be easily corrected. In some cases these artifacts can look disturbingly like the epileptogenic transients that we are trying to identify. Motion detection may be essential to identify these as artifacts. This also makes it absolutely critical to have an experienced epileptologist present who can identify true EEG events of interest based on their spatial and temporal characteristics.

Image Analysis

Spike-triggered analysis is simple to perform. Since only a single image is acquired following each spike or rest event, there are no requirements to model the hemodynamic response. One may simply group scans into rest and spike categories and perform a Student's *t*-test to judge significance.

Most recent studies from major centers have focused on continuous, simultaneously acquired fMRI and EEG.

Analysis of these data uses a method known as spike-related fMRI-EEG (29, 35, 43). This approach follows simultaneous acquisition of fMRI and EEG with post-scan EEG analysis. The EEG is first processed to minimize the pulse and gradient artifacts mentioned above, then read by an epileptologist to classify all EEG changes. Those considered to be IEDs are then treated as events of interest in an event-related analysis of the fMRI data. This involves creating a model timecourse that is switched on during the IED and convolving this function with an appropriate hemodynamic response function (HRF) to model the delay caused by the vascular origin of the BOLD contrast in fMRI. This basis function is included in the analysis, and variance correlated to this model is compared to residual variance. Voxels are considered to be activated during the IEDs when the modeled variance is significant compared to the residual variance. The main benefit of the spike-related approach is the increased amount of data acquired, so that shorter studies can lead to a significant result. Further, continuous acquisition of data allows the measurement of the actual HRF of a region.

As summarized by Salek-Haddadi et al (44), studies vary in their analysis approach, including acquisition method

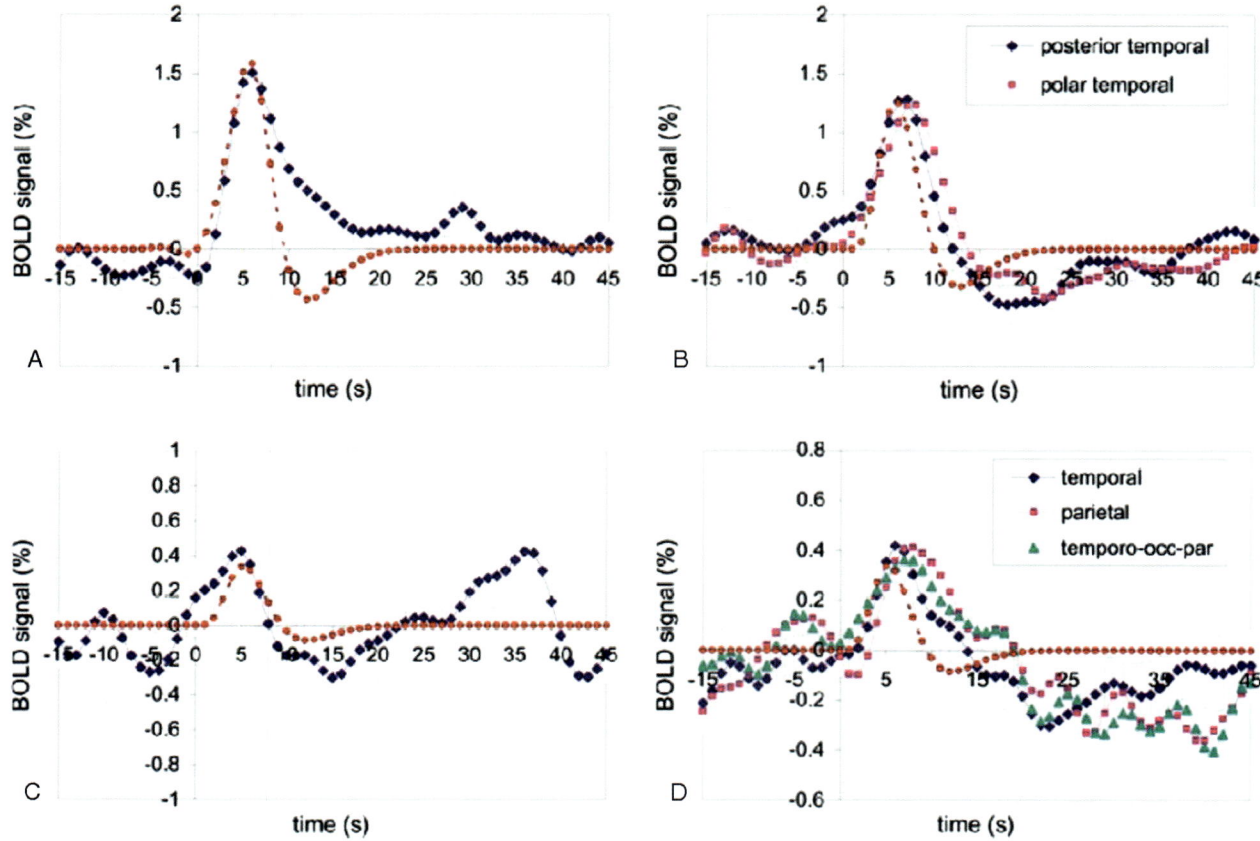

FIG. 11.4. Timecourse of measured BOLD response to IEDs for four subjects. The *red* dashed line represents the fitted canonical hemodynamic response to spikes. The four subject's responses (**A–D**) show significant variation from the standard response, but interregional differences (shown in **B, D**) appear to be small. (With permission from Benar et al. 2002 (35).)

(spike-triggered or continuous, spike-related), HRF model (canonical HRF, or a set of cosine or Gaussian basis functions), as well as the statistical threshold reported as significant. The standard SPM approach is to fit a canonical HRF derived from cognitive studies to the data (45, 46). It is simple to implement but inflexible, since it expects the BOLD response to follow the form of the canonical HRF, which may not be valid for IEDs. Fitting the BOLD response is also possible using a set of basis functions such as cosine or gamma functions. This approach is more flexible, and can model many different forms of the HRF. The advantage of this approach is that it will detect nonstandard BOLD responses, but it is also more likely to detect false positives, such as non-BOLD-related variance possibly due to artifacts.

The basis function approach has been applied to epilepsy (29). That study found that the detected HRF had a somewhat similar form to the canonical HRF but reached its peak at a later time for that subject (10 s compared to 5 s for the canonical model).

Another strategy is to try to directly measure the (average) BOLD timecourse following an IED (35, 47). The problem with this approach is that a timecourse must be measured from a specific region. The choice of this region has been based on the position of activations using an initial standard

SPM analysis, which selects for regions that have a response similar in form to the canonical HRF, and is thus preselecting for similar responses. Despite this limitation, distinct differences were seen between subjects in the observed BOLD timecourse (Fig. 11.4).

All these approaches are likely to be statistically valid but may detect different aspects of the BOLD response, both with regard to spatial distribution and timecourse.

APPLICATION OF THESE TECHNIQUES TO EPILEPSY

Ictal fMRI

As we commented above and in Chapter 2, in order to understand the epilepsy process it is necessary to determine the clinical context of the seizure, a structural focal abnormality of the brain, and the functional site of origin of ictal activity. Often the clinical context is known from the clinical history and presenting features. Many tests give access to the anatomic area that is abnormal and unchanging with time (e.g. PET, MRI, neuropsychological tests, and others). To date only the clinical observation of the seizure with video monitoring, the EEG, and ictal SPECT provide specific information about the ictal onset. Surface EEG provides limited spatial information and, while intracranial EEG may more precisely localize the origin of seizures, it is highly invasive and is therefore restricted to selected patients. Dynamic imaging that aims to detect changes at the time of the seizure has been limited by the inability to predict when seizures will occur. To date only injecting at the time of a seizure followed by SPECT imaging at a subsequent time have been routinely used (ictal SPECT). PET, while having the capacity to reveal blood flow and metabolic changes, is limited in its temporal resolution and has poor spatial resolution compared to MRI (see also Chapter 14).

Early fMRI studies of epilepsy focused on the ictal state, since, in the absence of EEG information, this state was easiest to identify, typically using prior anatomic information and searching for focal variance changes (2–4, 48).

We first reported ictal fMRI activity in 1994 (2). The patient was a 4-year-old boy with Rasmussen's encephalitis. Single-slice fMRI was taken though the area of maximal anatomic abnormality, with one slice being taken every 10 seconds for 10 minutes. The child had recurrent simple partial seizures involving the right face. The images were then analyzed by subtracting baseline images from those obtained during clinical seizures. This study demonstrated that seizures were associated with a regional increase in BOLD contrast in specific gyri in the left hemisphere, and also that the rise in BOLD signal commenced at least 60 seconds prior to clinical seizure onset (Fig. 11.5). This same area occasionally showed a similar intensity increase at a time when there was no clinical seizure. This suggested to us that the seizure focus might display a spectrum of activity, ranging from subclinical seizure activity associated with minor EEG activations

(interictal spikes) to full clinical seizures, and that both exhibit a similar pattern of fMRI activation.

Other similar observations have followed that support the concept that subclinical epileptiform activity occurs at the seizure focus and is detectable by fMRI.

Detre et al. (3) reported a case study that suggested fMRI could localize the epileptiform focus during subclinical seizure activity. The subject was a 25-year-old with multiple daily simple partial seizures of the right face. Analysis was based on subtraction of the mean pixel intensity over the 11 minutes epoch from each slice. There were marked fluctuations in signal intensity from the presumed epileptogenic zone despite there being no clinical seizures. Confirmation that this was the epileptogenic zone was later provided by placement of intracranial electrodes prior to resective surgery. This fMRI study defined the area of final electrocorticography-guided surgical resection more precisely than did ictal SPECT, PET, and EEG. This study was limited by the absence of EEG monitoring during the fMRI study, prohibiting correlation between electrical discharges and blood flow changes. However, it is interesting to note that the rise in blood flow from the epileptogenic zone occurred gradually over 30 seconds, suggesting a gradual build up of activity over this time.

To date the most satisfying approach to analyzing fMRI data of the ictal state was that presented by Salek-Haddadi et al. (32), performed using continuous fMRI/EEG. They studied a 47-year-old man with a 2-year history of generalized tonic–clonic seizures, as well as frequent partial seizures with inactivity but without auras. The fMRI/EEG study investigated a single focal unilateral subclinical seizure that occurred during a 35-minute scanning session. They detected the onset and duration of the seizure using the EEG

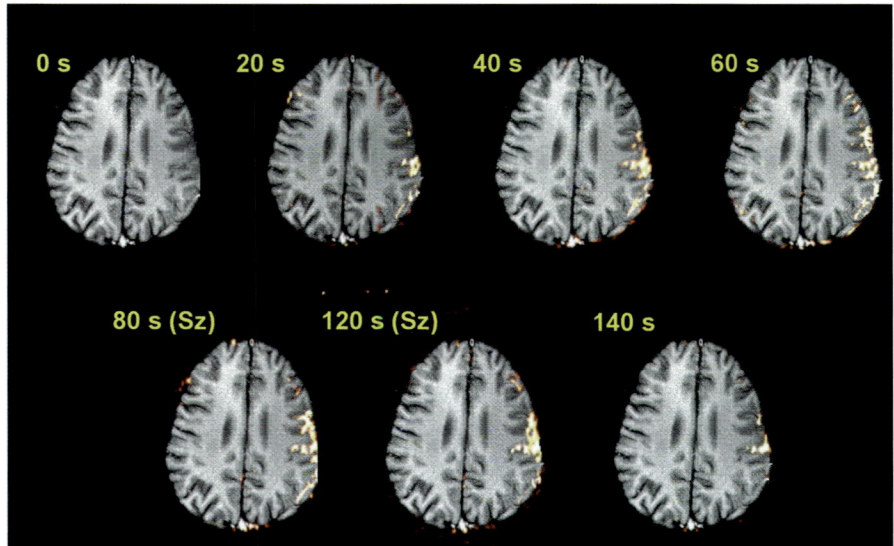

FIG. 11.5. First demonstrated in-scanner ictal event recorded with fMRI. Standard anatomic images are shown with a superimposed fMRI image that was obtained during a focal seizure. The timing of each scan is presented. At $T = 80\,s$, the clinical seizure began, and persisted to $T = 120\,s$. (From Jackson 1994 (69), reprinted by permission of the journal *Epilepsia*.)

signal, then fitted a flexible model to the variance in a window of 45 seconds duration around the seizure. This approach makes no assumption about the response during any specific part of the seizure. The study found that the seizure response in a cluster of 917 voxels approximately followed a sine wave with a period of 102 seconds. This cluster was centered over the left temporal and insular cortices, and was concordant with the EEG localization (F7/T3).

Development of Continuous EEG fMRI for Clinical Use

The development of spike-triggered and latterly continuous and simultaneous fMRI/EEG has been undertaken with considerable focus by the Queen Square group in London. They have demonstrated the practicality of this technology (22, 36, 41) and have shown that it can localize the seizure focus in partial epilepsy (20, 49). In one recent case, thalamic activation was seen during partial seizures that occurred in the MR imaging system (32). All of this work has been at 1.5 T, where many interictal epileptiform events are needed to obtain a successful study. At 3 T, successful studies can be seen with as few as two spikes in some cases. An example of such a subject with only two EEG events, but that reached significance ($p < 0.05$, corrected for multiple comparisons) is shown in Figure 11.6.

In the past few years a number of studies have been published attempting to understand the origin of interictal spikes associated with different clinical epilepsies. In these studies, the fMRI/EEG technology has been used primarily as a means of understanding basic phenomena associated with the type of epilepsy under study. This is likely to be an area where these techniques will have major impact.

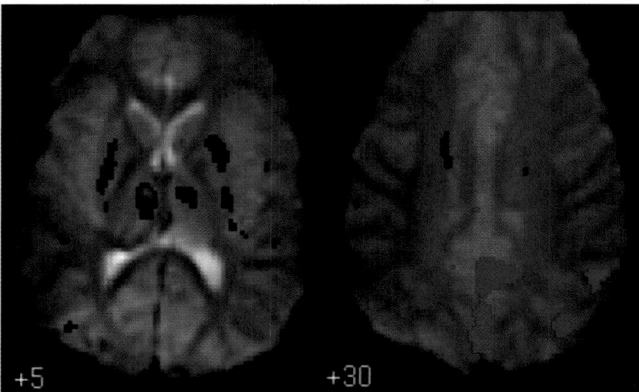

FIG. 11.6. Significant fMRI/EEG activation *(red)* and deactivation *(blue)* detected in a patient with idiopathic generalized epilepsy in a case where only two spike and wave events were detected in the EEG during a 30-minute study. The threshold for display is *p* <0.05, corrected for multiple comparisons. Deactivation in the posterior cingulate region agrees with published data (62), as does activation bilaterally in the thalamus (70).

Benign Epilepsy with Centrotemporal Spikes

Benign epilepsy with centrotemporal spikes (BECTS, rolandic epilepsy) is a common childhood epilepsy disorder (50–52). Age of onset is from 3 to 13 years, with an excellent prognosis for remission in adolescence (53). Seizures typically begin with numbness or paresthesias on one side of the mouth or cheek, followed by hemifacial twitching, difficulty speaking, and at times clonic movements of the ipsilateral arm. Some attacks evolve into a secondarily generalized convulsion (54). Although seizures are infrequent, the interictal EEG reveals frequent high-amplitude epileptiform discharges with a characteristic electrical field, of negativity over the central and temporal regions, and positivity over frontal regions (55, 56).

In individuals with BECTS spikes, we have shown spike-related BOLD signal increases in the pre- and postcentral gyrus (57). In the group of subjects with electroclinically typical BECTS, spikes were associated with significant BOLD increases in the precentral gyrus and decreases in the medial frontal region (Fig. 11.7). Activity in this area is consistent with the facial sensorimotor involvement in BECTS seizures. It appears that these regions are involved in spike discharges and therefore the pathophysiology of this epilepsy disorder. Spike-triggered fMRI is a useful tool for exploring mechanisms of spike and seizure generation underlying specific epilepsy syndromes. Newer techniques such as continuous EEG-fMRI with event related analysis may allow exploration of the temporal association between the activated and deactivated regions we observe.

Reading Epilepsy

Reading epilepsy is an unusual syndrome, in which seizures can be precipitated by reading either silently or out-loud (58). The syndrome typically has its onset in the mid-teens, is nonprogressive and rarely spontaneously remits (59, 60). Most subjects describe 'jerks ' or 'clicks' of the jaw, commencing shortly after beginning reading and building in frequency as reading continues.

We recorded EEG inside our 3 T MRI scanner and acquired spike-triggered fMRI in a patient with reading epilepsy (61). Spike-related fMRI BOLD activity is seen bilaterally in the precentral gyrus, central sulcus, and globus pallidus, suggesting that the spikes of reading epilepsy involve cortical and subcortical structures. We also performed a block design fMRI study of reading in two subjects with reading epilepsy to demonstrate those brain regions recruited by the reading task. Comparison of fMRI activations seen during spiking with those during reading showed overlap of activation in the posterior extent of the dorsolateral prefrontal cortex (Fig. 11.8). In this patient with reading epilepsy, epileptiform activity may involve local spread of cortical activity from brain regions recruited by the working memory component of the reading task into the adjacent

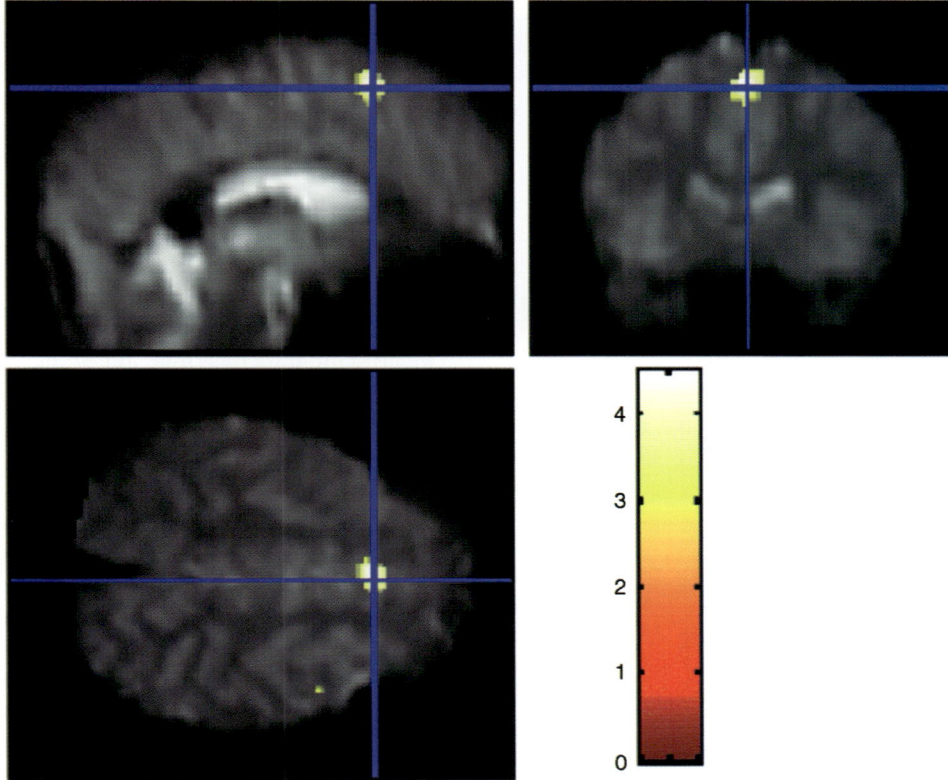

FIG. 11.7. Results of group analysis showing spike-related signal decreases for four subjects with electroclinical features consistent with typical BECTS. Medial frontal deactivation is seen ($T = 4.72$) although the peak voxel is just under the threshold for significance after correction for multiple comparisons ($p = 0.055$). On the coronal and sagittal views it can be seen that this is in the medial part of the superior frontal gyrus, superior to the cingulate sulcus, in the region of the supplementary motor area.

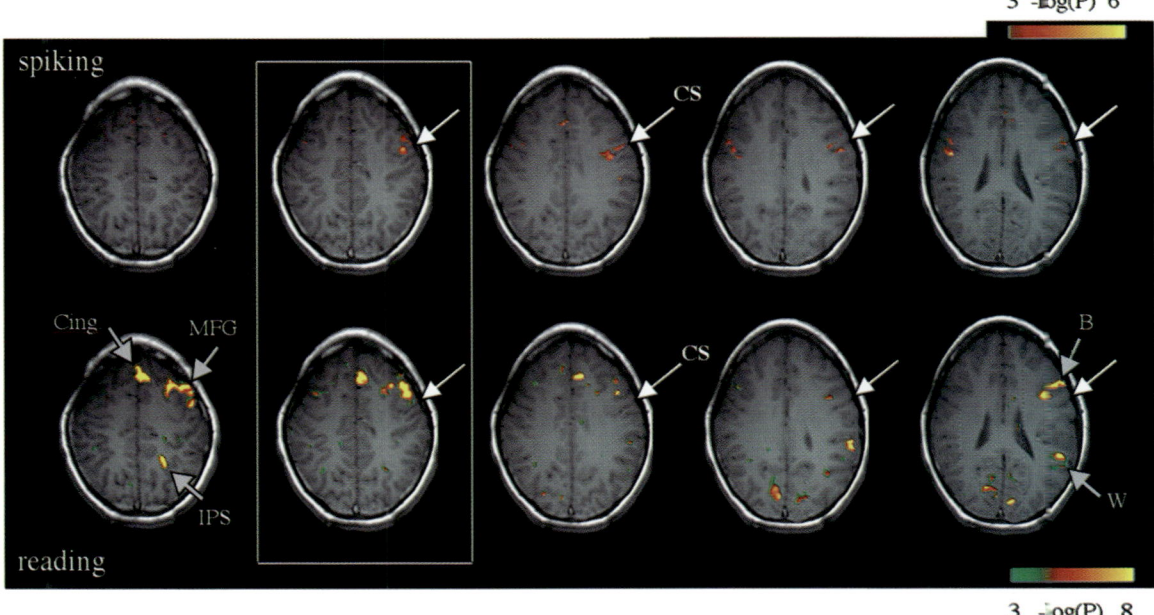

FIG. 11.8. Cortical fMRI activity seen with spiking (top row) compared to reading (not spiking – 30 s reading, 30 s rest for four cycles, bottom row). T-statistic maps have been overlaid on to T1-weighted images to allow better anatomic definition. The location of the central sulcus (CS) is indicated by the white arrows. The boxed slice shows spike-related activity overlapping with reading related activity in the posterior middle frontal gyrus (working memory area) but also extending into the precentral gyrus. Lower slices show the more extensive and bilateral involvement of the precentral gyrus and central sulcus. Spike related activity is separate from reading related activity in Broca's and Wernicke's areas. (With permission from Archer et al. 2003 (71).)

areas of motor cortex, and subsequent activity in a cortical subcortical circuit.

Idiopathic Generalized Epilepsy

Idiopathic generalized epilepsy (IGE) is a common disorder, accounting for 40% of individuals with epilepsy, in which epileptiform activity appears synchronously over both hemispheres. Generalized spike and slow wave discharges (S&W) recorded on scalp EEG are pathognomonic of IGE. These discharges show bursts of bilateral, symmetrical spike and wave or poly-spike and wave at a rate of 2.5–5 Hz. S&W discharges are seen over the whole head but often have a bifrontal predominance. Single or brief runs of discharges occur interictally, with more prolonged runs associated with absence attacks.

In a recent fMRI study of spontaneous S&W discharges in idiopathic generalized epilepsy, some S&W-related fMRI activations were seen bilaterally in the precentral gyrus, while no significant change in BOLD signal was observed in the thalamus (62). In contrast, we found significant deactivation of the posterior cingulate and the cuneus/precuneus, as well as left greater than right angular gyrus (Fig. 11.9A). This was a robust finding, being present in all the individuals with more than four spikes and significant on group analysis. These regions may have a special role in the electroclinical phenomenon of S&W and 'absence.' This role

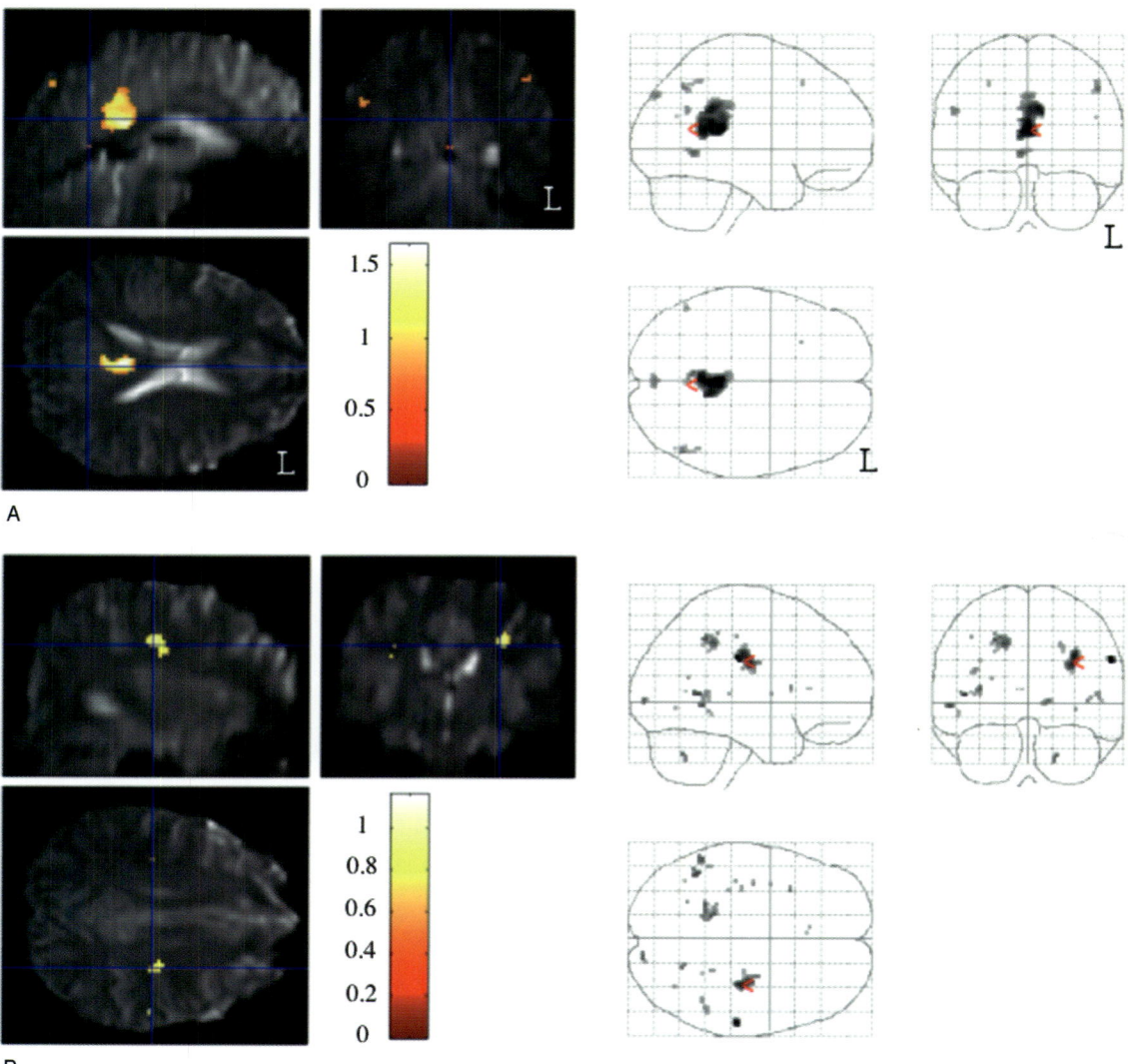

FIG. 11.9. Group analysis (conjunction) of five patients with IGE, showing spike-related 'deactivation' (**A**) and activation (**B**). On the left, results have been overlaid on to averaged, normalized EPI of subject D, and thresholded at $p < 0.001$ uncorrected. *Blue* lines represent slice plane of the orthogonal images, with *t*-scores indicated in the color scale. On the right, results are displayed as a 'glass brain' projection. (With permission from Archer et al. 2003 (62).)

might be causative, with reduced activity in the cingulate facilitating the onset of S&W. Alternatively, reduced activity in the posterior cingulate may be the consequence of S&W activity. Decreased posterior cingulate activity may be a marker of altered thalamocortical activity and might be important in the pathogenesis of S&W.

Spike and wave related increases in BOLD signal were observed bilaterally in the depths of the precentral sulcus in some individuals and on group analysis (Fig. 11.9B). Activations were in a similar posterior frontal location across subjects but only partially overlapped. Spike-triggered fMRI, by its nature, does not provide information about the time course of the changes in BOLD signal observed. Thus the changes we observe may precede the S&W or follow it. Activity bilaterally in the precentral sulcus might be relevant to the frontal predominance of S&W discharges seen in these and many other patients with IGE, suggesting a preferential activation of these regions. Alternatively, given that some authors have suggested that it is a burst of cortical activity that initiates S&W epileptiform activity (63), this region may be involved in the initiation of S&W in these subjects.

Focal Epilepsy

Focal epilepsy includes a variety of disorders, including hippocampal sclerosis and malformations of cortical development. The spikes of focal epilepsies are often harder to detect in the MR environment, primarily they are detected only in one or a few EEG channels, making them harder to distinguish from artifact. Despite this difficulty, a number of studies have attempted to study focal epilepsy with fMRI/EEG.

One recent study considered the feasibility of imaging focal epilepsies using fMRI/EEG (49). They considered a series of 10 patients and found that in six of these patients, reproducible BOLD activation was detected that was concurrent with EEG localization. In a similar study, Lazeyras et al. (13) studied 11 patients, and found that seven showed fMRI/EEG results that confirmed the clinical diagnosis. In six subjects, intracranial electrodes were implanted, and in five of these patients, the fMRI focus was confirmed by the intracranial recordings.

Use of Simultaneous fMRI/EEG in Animal Models

We have applied the technology of simultaneous fMRI/EEG to a penicillin-induced sheep model of epilepsy (64). This model allows close monitoring of parameters such as the EEG, ECG, breathing, oxygen saturation, temperature, and blood pressure. During unilateral electrographic seizures, focal BOLD signal changes occurred at the seizure focus and ipsilateral amygdala, suggesting the presence of a cortico–subcortical loop (Fig. 11.10). This observation illustrates the potential of the model for understanding seizure generation, spread, and possibly the consequences of repeated seizures on the brain.

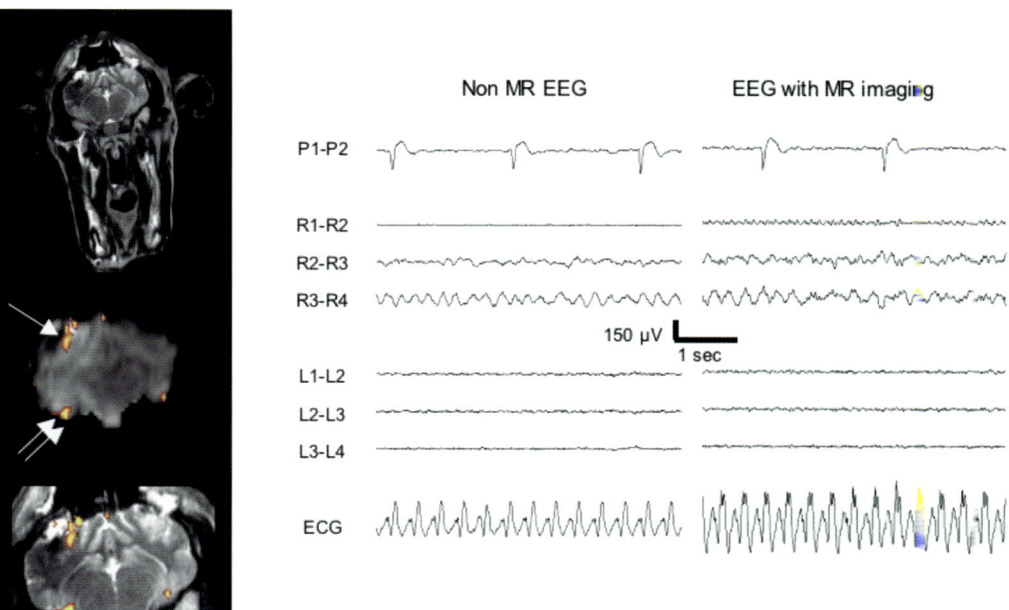

FIG. 11.10. Animal model of epilepsy studied with fMRI/EEG. The left panel shows amygdala activation (double arrows) due to seizure activity induced by cortical injection of penicillin in a sheep (single arrow). The right panel shows simultaneously acquired EEG. In this case the EEG tells us when the neural events are occurring, and the MR shows us the spatial location and extent of the neural network. Measuring the neural response with this temporal and spatial resolution gives us insights into the subcortical brain response not obtainable in any other way.

Novel fMRI Approaches to Epilepsy Imaging

One limitation of the fMRI/EEG analysis philosophy is that it uses, as inputs, events detected using EEG, and may thus suffer from the bias of EEG, which is most sensitive to radial sources that are close to the brain surface and less so to tangential sources such as in the sulcal walls, where opposing dipoles may cancel out (65). In order to overcome this possible limitation, and maintain sensitivity to possible deep sources of IEDs, other methods have been suggested to detect IED-related BOLD changes.

One option to avoiding the bias of EEG is to use other indicators of epileptiform activity. In a recent study, we imaged a patient with myoclonic jerks of the right foot. The patient, a 26-year-old woman, showed an abnormal gyrus extending anteriorly off the left central sulcus approximately 2 cm lateral to the interhemispheric fissure. This gyrus had thickened gray matter at its depth and blurring of the gray–white junction, features suggestive of dysplasia. In this subject we were interested in localizing the focus of origin of the jerks, so the timing of these jerks were obtained from concurrent video monitoring and included in the fMRI analysis as events of interest. Activation was seen in the dysplastic cortex, in the foot area of motor cortex, and the left supplementary motor area (Fig. 11.11A). Extracting the timecourse of the hemodynamic response for these regions, it was observed that the dysplastic cortex and SMA showed activation which lead the foot area by around 2 seconds (Fig. 11.11B). This temporal shift may in future yield information regarding the evolution of interictal activity into a seizure.

Temporal Clustering Analysis

Another approach is to use an exploratory, data-driven method to detect focal changes. One possible candidate in this regard is temporal clustering analysis. This technique has been applied to epilepsy in a recent study (66), and involves identifying time points when many voxels are at their maximum intensity, presumably because of seizure-based changes. No simultaneous EEG was recorded but, by looking for a particular subset of the variance, specifically changes of between 2% and 10% from the resting BOLD intensity level, they were able to detect focal regions in six patients with temporal lobe epilepsy. In all subjects, the maximum t score was in the hemisphere ipsilateral to subsequent surgical resection. In four subjects, activation was found in the ipsilateral temporal lobe. This approach has been shown to be sensitive to seizure-related BOLD changes – the only remaining issue is whether it is also sensitive to artifactual changes, such as motion.

Functional Connectivity

Another candidate method for further exploring fMRI data of the interictal state is functional connectivity (67, 68). By performing an initial spike-related analysis using spikes identified using EEG, one can identify a focal region involved in the seizure generation network, and probably associated with generation of those spikes detectable by scalp electrodes (Fig. 11.12A). These regions are presumably a subset of all regions involved in the epileptogenic circuit that is sought after. By using the signal timecourse of

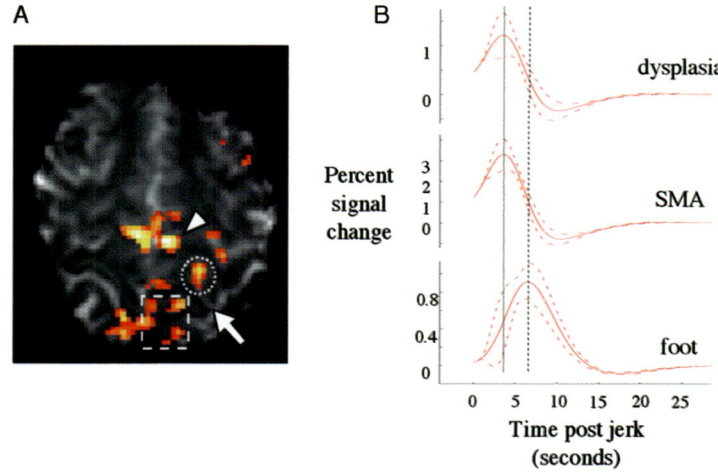

FIG. 11.11. Event-related fMRI study of myoclonic jerks of the right foot. **A.** Activation map overlaid on the EPI of the subject. The arrow indicates the dysplastic 'drumstick'-shaped gyrus at its junction with the central sulcus. The arrowhead indicates the possibly abnormal gyrus in the region of the supplementary motor area (SMA). The dashed square indicates activation associated with the foot motor area. **B.** Fitted response and standard errors of the hemodynamic response to foot jerks from the data seen in **A**. The fitted hemodynamic response peaks earlier in the dysplastic cortex and SMA regions than in the foot area.

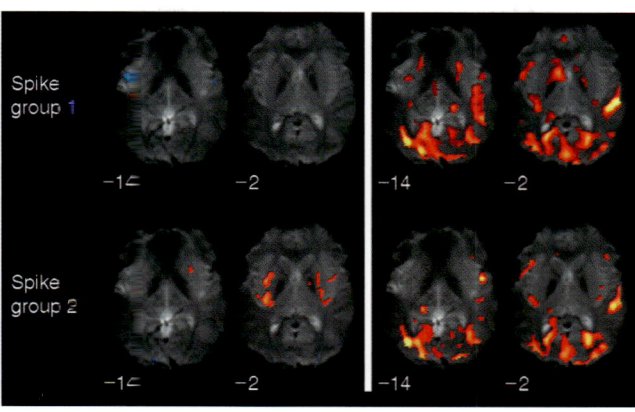

A   B

FIG. 11.12. Combined fMRI/EEG and functional connectivity (FC) analysis of a patient with IGE. **A.** Event-related analysis of spikes with two morphologies (group 1: 12 spikes, upper panels; group 2: 2 spikes, lower panels) show different patterns of activation *(red)* and deactivation *(blue)*. **B.** Connectivity analysis shows greater sensitivity, yielding a widespread network that is consistent for the two spike groups, indicating that FC is more sensitive to the underlying seizure network.

this region, a wider network is identified including subcortical regions (Fig. 11.12B).

REFERENCES

1. Penfield W. The evidence for a cerebral vascular mechanism in epilepsy. *Ann Intern Med* 1933;7:303–310.
2. Jackson GD, Connelly A, Cross JH, et al. Functional magnetic resonance imaging of focal seizures. *Neurology* 1994;44:850–856.
3. Detre JA, Sirven JI, Alsop DC, et al. Localisation of subclinical ictal activity by functional magnetic resonance imaging: correlation with invasive monitoring. *Ann Neurol* 1995;38:618–624.
4. Detre J, Alsop D, Aguirre G, Sperling M. Coupling of cortical and thalamic ictal activity in human partial epilepsy: demonstration by functional magnetic resonance imaging. *Epilepsia* 1996;37:657–661.
5. Ogawa, S, Lee TM Kay AR, Tank DW. Brain magnetic resonance imaging with contrast dependent on blood oxygenation. *Proc Natl Acad Sci* 1990;87:9868–9872.
6. Logothetis N, Pauls J, Augath M, et al. Neurophysiological investigation of the basis of the fMRI signal. *Nature* 2001;412:150–157.
7. Logothetis NK. The neural basis of the blood-oxygen-level-dependent functional magnetic resonance imaging signal. *Philos Trans R Soc Lond B Biol Sci* 2002;357:1003–1037.
8. Logothetis NK. The underpinnings of the BOLD functional magnetic resonance imaging signal. *J Neurosci* 2003;23:3963–71.
9. Merlet I, Gotman J. Dipole modeling of scalp electroencephalogram epileptic discharges: correlation with intracerebral fields. *Clin Neurophysiol* 2001;112:414–430.
10. Lemieux L, Allen PJ, Franconi F, et al. Recording of EEG during fMRI experiment: patient safety. *Magn Reson Med* 1997;38:943–952.
11. Liao CH, Worsley KJ, Poline J-B, et al. Estimating the delay of the fMRI response. *Neuroimage* 2002;16:593–606.
12. Krakow K, Woermann FG, Symms MR, et al. EEG-triggered functional MRI of interictal epileptiform activity in patients with partial seizures. *Brain* 1999;122:1679–1688.
13. Lazeyras F, Blanke O, Perrig S, et al. EEG-triggered functional MRI in patients with pharmacoresistant epilepsy. *J Magn Reson Imaging* 2000;12:177–185.
14. Krakow K, Lemieux L, Messina D, et al. Spatio-temporal imaging of focal interictal epileptiform activity using EEG-triggered functional MRI. *Epileptic Disord* 2001;3:67–74.
15. Jager L, Werhahn KJ, Hoffmann A, et al. Focal epileptiform activity in the brain: detection with spike-related functional MR imaging – preliminary results *Radiology* 2002;223:860–869.
16. Archer JS, Abbott DF, Waites AB, Jackson G. fMRI deactivation of the posterior cingulate during generalised spike and wave. *Neuroimage* 2003;20:1915–1922.
17. Archer JS, Briellmann RS, Abbott DF, et al. Benign epilepsy with centro-temporal spikes: spike triggered fMRI shows somato-sensory cortex activity. *Epilepsia* 2003;44:200–204.
18. Archer JS, Briellmann RS, Syngeniotis A, et al. Spike triggered fMRI in reading epilepsy: involvement of left frontal cortex working memory areas. *Neurology* 2003;60:415–421.
19. Seeck M, Lazeyras F, Michel CM, et al. Non-invasive epileptic focus localization using EEG-triggered functional MRI and electromagnetic tomography. *Electroencephalogr Clin Neurophysiol* 1998;106 508–512.
20. Symms MR, Allen PJ, Woermann FG, et al. Reproducible localization of interictal epileptiform discharges using EEG-triggered fMRI. *Phys Med Biol* 1999;44:N161–N168.
21. Krakow K, Messina D, Lemieux L, et al. Functional MRI activation of individual interictal epileptiform spikes. *Neuroimage* 2001;13 502–505.
22. Allen PJ, Josephs O, Turner R. A method for removing imaging artifact from continuous EEG recorded during functional MRI. *Neuroimage* 2000;12:230–239.
23. Bonmassar G, Purdon PL, Jaaskelainen IP, et al. Motion and ballistocardiogram artifact removal for interleaved recording of EEG and EPs during fMRI. *Neuroimage* 2002;16:1127–1141.
24. Benar C, Aghakhani Y, Wang Y, et al. Quality of EEG in simultaneous EEG-fMRI for epilepsy. *Clin Neurophysiol* 2003;114:569–580.
25. Anami K, Mori T, Tanaka F, et al. Stepping stone sampling for retrieving artifact-free electroencephalogram during functional magnetic resonance imaging. *Neuroimage* 2003;19:281–295
26. Hoffmann A, Jager L, Werhahn KJ, et al. Electroencephalography during functional echo-planar imaging: detection of epileptic spikes using post-processing methods. *Magn Reson Med* 2000;44:791–798.
27. Goldman RI, Stern JM, Engel J Jr, Cohen MS. Acquiring simultaneous EEG and functional MRI. *Clin Neurophysiol* 2000;111:1974–1980.
28. Baudewig J, Bittermann HJ, Paulus W, Frahm J. Simultaneous EEG and functional MRI of epileptic activity a case report. *Clin Neurophysiol* 2001 112:1196–1200.
29. Lemieux L, Salek-Haddadi A, Josephs O, et al. Event-related fMRI with simultaneous and continuous EEG: description of the method and initial case report. *Neuroimage* 2001;14:780–787.
30. Al-Asmi A, Benar CG, Gross DW, et al. fMRI activation in continuous and spike-triggered EEG-fMRI studies of epileptic spikes. *Epilepsia* 2003;44:1328–1339.
31. Salek-Haddadi A, Lemieux L, Merschhemke M, et al. Functional magnetic resonance imaging of human absence seizures. *Ann Neurol* 2003;53:663–667.
32. Salek-Haddadi A, Merschhemke M, Lemieux L, Fish DR. Simultaneous EEG-correlated ictal fMRI. *Neuroimage* 2002;16:32–40.
33. Logothetis NK, Pauls J, Augath M, et al. Neurophysiological investigation of the basis of the fMRI signal. *Nature* 2001;412:150–157.
34. Bittar RG, Andermann F, Olivier A, et al. Interictal spikes increase cerebral glucose metabolism and blood flow: a PET study. *Epilepsia* 1999;40:170–178.
35. Benar CG, Gross DW, Wang Y, et al. The BOLD response to interictal epileptiform discharges. *Neuroimage* 2002;17:1182–1192.
36. Lemieux L, Allen P, Franconi F, et al. Recording of EEG during fMRI experiments: patient safety. *Magn Reson Med* 1997;38:943–952.

37. Goldman R, Stern J, Engel J, Cohen M. Acquiring simultaneous EEG and functional MRI. *Clin Neurophysiol* 2000;111:1974–1980.

38. Archer J, Briellmann R, Abbott D, et al. Spike triggered fMRI: a technique for understanding the aetiology if epileptiform activity. *Neuroimage* 2001;13:S768.

39. Bonmassar G, Schwartz D, Liu A, et al. Spatiotemporal brain imaging of visual-evoked activity using interleaved EEG and fMRI recordings. *Neuroimage* 2001;13:1035–1043.

40. Anami K, Mori T, Tanaka F, et al. Stepping stone sampling for retrieving artifact-free electroencephalogram during functional magnetic resonance imaging. *Neuroimage* 2003;19:281–295.

41. Allen PJ, Polizzi G, Krakow K, et al. Identification of EEG events in the MR scanner: the problem of pulse artifact and a method for its subtraction. *Neuroimage* 1998;8:229–239.

42. Muri R, Felbinger J, Rosler K, et al. Recording of electrical brain activity in a magnetic resonance environment: distorting effects of the static magnetic field. *Magn Reson Med* 1998;39:18–22.

43. Iannetti GD, Di Bonaventura C, Pantano P, et al. fMRI/EEG in paroxysmal activity elicited by elimination of central vision and fixation. *Neurology* 2002;58:976–979.

44. Salek-Haddadi A, Friston KJ, Lemieux L, Fish DR. Studying spontaneous EEG activity with fMRI. *Brain Res Rev* 2003;43:110–133.

45. Friston K, Holmes A, Worsley K, et al. Statistical parametric maps in functional imaging: a general linear approach. *Hum Brain Mapp* 1995;2:189–210.

46. Josephs O, Henson RN. Event-related functional magnetic resonance imaging: modelling, inference and optimization. *Philos Trans R Soc Lond B Biol Sci* 1999;354:1215–1228.

47. Kang JK, Benar C, Al-Asmi A, et al. Using patient-specific hemodynamic response functions in combined EEG-fMRI studies in epilepsy. *Neuroimage* 2003;20:1162–1170.

48. Krings T, Topper R, Foltys H, et al. Cortical activation patterns during complex motor tasks in piano players and control subjects. A functional imaging study. *Neurosci Lett* 2000;278:189–193.

49. Krakow K, Woermann F, Symms M, et al. EEG-triggered functional MRI of interictal epileptiform activity in patients with partial seizures. *Brain* 1999;122:1679–1688.

50. Cavazzutti G. Epidemiology of different types of epilepsy in school age children of Modena, Italy. *Epilepsia* 1980;21:57–62.

51. Pazzaglia P, D'Alessandro R, Lozito A, Lugaresi E. Classification of the epilepsies according to the symptomatology of the seizures: practical value and prognostic implications. *Epilepsia* 1982;23:343–350.

52. Nayrac P, Beaussart M. Les pointes-ondes prerolandiques: expression EEG tres particuliere. *Rev Neurol* 1958;99:201–206.

53. Blom S, Heijbel J. Benign epilepsy of childhood with centro-temporal EEG foci: a follow-up study in adulthood of patients initially studied as children. *Epilepsia* 1982;23:629–631.

54. Loiseau P, Beaussart M. The seizures of benign childhood epilepsy with rolandic paroxysmal discharges. *Epilepsia* 1973;14:381–389.

55. Gastaut Y. Un element deroutant de la symptomatologie electroen-cephalographique: les pointes prerolandiques sans signification focale. *Rev Neurol* 1952;87:488–490.

56. Lerman P. Benign partial epilepsy with centro-temporal spikes. In: Roger J, et al, eds. Epileptic syndromes in infancy, childhood and adolescence. London: John Libbey, 1992:150–158.

57. Archer J, Briellmann R, Abbott D, et al. Benign epilepsy with centro-temporal spikes: spike triggered fMRI shows somato-sensory cortex activity. *Epilepsia* 2003;44:200–204.

58. Bickford R, Whelan J, Klass D, Corbin K. Reading epilepsy: clinical and electroencephalographic studies of a new syndrome. *Trans Am Neurol Assoc* 1956;81:100–102.

59. Radhakrishnan K, Silbert P, Klass D. Reading epilepsy: an appraisal of 20 patients diagnosed at the Mayo Clinic, Rochester, Minnesota, between 1949 and 1989, and delineation of the epileptic syndrome. *Brain* 1995;118:75–89.

60. Koutroumanidis M, Koepp M, Richardson M, et al. The variants of reading epilepsy: a clinical and video-EEG study of 17 patients with reading induced seizures. *Brain* 1998;121:1409–1427.

61. Archer J, Briellmann R, Syngeniotis A, et al. Spike triggered fMRI in reading epilepsy: involvement of left frontal cortex working memory area. *Neurology* 2003;60:415–421.

62. Archer JS, Abbott DF, Waites AB, Jackson GD. fMRI 'deactivation' of the posterior cingulate during generalized spike and wave. *Neuroimage* 2003;20:1915–1922.

63. McCormick D, Contreras D. On the cellular and network bases of epileptic seizures. *Annu Rev Physiol* 2001;63:815–846.

64. Opdam H, Federico P, Jackson G, et al. A sheep model for the study of focal epilepsy with concurrent intracranial EEG and functional MRI. *Epilepsia* 2002;43:779–787.

65. Gloor P. Neuronal generators and the problem of localization in electroencephalography: application of volume conductor theory to electroencephalography. *J Clin Neurophysiol* 1985;2:327–354.

66. Morgan VL, Price RR, Arain A, et al. Resting functional MRI with temporal clustering analysis for localization of epileptic activity without EEG. *Neuroimage* 2004;21:473–481.

67. Friston KJ, Frith CD, Liddle PF, Frackowiak RS. Functional connectivity: the principal-component analysis of large (PET) data sets. *J Cereb Blood Flow Metab* 1993;13:5–14.

68. Biswal B, Yetkin FZ, Haughton VM, Hyde JS. Functional connectivity in the motor cortex of resting human brain using echo-planar MRI. *Magn Reson Med* 1995;34:537–541.

69. Jackson GD. New techniques in magnetic resonance and epilepsy. *Epilepsia* 1994;35(Suppl 6):S2–S13.

70. Salek-Haddadi A, Lemieux L, Merschhemeke M, et al. Functional magnetic resonance imaging of human absence seizures. *Ann Neurol* 2003;53:663–667.

71. Archer JS, Briellmann RS, Syngeniotis A, et al. Spike-triggered fMRI in reading epilepsy: involvement of left frontal cortex working memory area. *Neurology* 2003;60:415–421.

CHAPTER 12

MR Diffusion and Perfusion Imaging in Epilepsy

Alan Connelly

Magnetic resonance imaging has an important role to play in the investigation of patients with epilepsy, not only with respect to providing exquisite anatomic detail but increasingly by means of information from images based on physiologic and functional parameters. This chapter outlines the present and potential contributions to the field from MR diffusion and perfusion images of the brain. It is not intended to constitute an exhaustive literature review but rather to give an overview of the underlying principles of the methods, to outline some of the technical constraints involved, and to discuss potential applications of both the existing methods and developments that might reasonably be expected in the near future. To this end, the initial section describes some of the basic theory of diffusion and perfusion MRI, and includes some discussion of methods of analysis and their implications. Subsequent sections describe the application of these methods to patients with epilepsy, followed by a discussion of potential future developments.

BACKGROUND

Magnetic Resonance Diffusion Imaging

Diffusion

The term 'diffusion' is used to describe the random microscopic translational motion of molecules (brownian motion), in which the overall mean displacement of a population of molecules remains zero. This is in contrast to flow, in which there is coherent motion in a particular direction. In a large population of freely diffusing molecules, such as in a mobile

liquid, the 'diffusion volume' would be expected to be spherical, with the radius of the sphere increasing as the square root of the time that diffusion is allowed to evolve. (Such behavior might be observed, for example, in a droplet of dye in a container of water, where the color would spread equally in all directions.) Diffusion behavior in an in vivo environment, however, is more complex, since molecules are not in such a homogeneous, unhindered environment; the movement of molecules observed in practice is therefore dependent on the nature of any barriers to diffusion.

Diffusion-weighted Imaging

The signal intensity on an MR image can be made dependent on the rate of water diffusion in the brain by the presence of additional magnetic field gradients (in its most common form, this would consist of two identical gradients, one either side of a refocusing pulse in a spin-echo sequence). Diffusion of water in the presence of these gradients introduces signal loss in an image. The resulting MR image intensity would be weighted according to the rate of water diffusion, with high-diffusivity regions giving relatively low signal intensity, while regions of low diffusivity would give a relatively high signal intensity. However, diffusion-weighted (DW) images, by being sensitized to the microscopic movement of water, are highly sensitive to the effects of brain motion, such that conventional multi-shot images suffer severe degradation when diffusion weighted gradients are added. Although there are several potential solutions to this problem, single-shot DW echo-planar imaging (EPI) (1) is by far the most common method in use at present; concomitant

315

limitations of this solution include image distortions in regions of high magnetic susceptibility gradients (e.g. in the region of the inferior temporal lobes or the frontal sinuses), and reduced spatial resolution (typically of the order of 2 mm).

The degree of diffusion weighting in an MR image is dependent on a combination of the strength of the diffusion gradient, the length of time the diffusion gradient is on, and the time between the pair of diffusion gradients (2). These contributions to diffusion weighting are collectively described by a 'b-value'; the higher the value of b, the greater the degree of diffusion weighting. The value of b can be increased by increasing any or all of the listed contributions. However, exactly analogously to T1-weighted or T2-weighted imaging, the image intensity on diffusion-weighted imaging (DWI) is dependent on a number of factors in addition to diffusion. In DWI, the image intensity is weighted not only by water diffusivity but also by proton density and the relaxation times, T1 and T2. The contribution of diffusion can be isolated by quantification; i.e. by calculation of what is usually referred to as the apparent diffusion coefficient (ADC), the contributions from overall water content and from relaxation times can be eliminated, leaving only diffusion information. (The term *apparent* diffusion coefficient is used since the measured diffusion in vivo is dependent not only on water diffusivity, but also on factors such as barrier permeability and diffusion time.)

Diffusion Tensor Imaging

Diffusion that is the same in all directions (*isotropic diffusion*) can be described simply by a directionless number, namely the diffusion coefficient D (in vivo, this would be the ADC), since the direction of measurement of this number is unimportant. D can be determined in an isotropic system by making two measurements at different b values, with the diffusion weighting in any arbitrary direction. However, this is not the case for *anisotropic diffusion*, where the water diffusivity is different in different directions; this can potentially confound data reproducibility but may also provide further important information, as discussed below. Diffusion in an anisotropic system cannot be described by a simple number, but is characterized by a diffusion tensor (again, in vivo this would be an apparent diffusion tensor), in the form of the matrix D:

$$\mathbf{D} = \begin{pmatrix} D_{xx} & D_{xy} & D_{xz} \\ D_{yx} & D_{yy} & D_{yz} \\ D_{zx} & D_{zy} & D_{zz} \end{pmatrix}$$

where the diagonal elements indicate the molecular mobility in orthogonal directions, and the off-diagonal elements express how diffusion in one direction is correlated with that in a perpendicular direction.

In effect, rather than diffusivity being characterized by a sphere (as in the isotropic case), anisotropic diffusion is characterized by the size, shape, and orientation of a diffusion ellipsoid, with three potentially non-equal axes representing different diffusivities in three orthogonal directions. Characterization of this ellipsoid requires at least six DW images to be acquired, each with diffusion weighting in a different, independent direction, resulting in a minimum of seven measurements in total (six diffusion directions, plus one measurement with low diffusion weighting, typically $b = 0$) (3). It is increasingly common, however, to acquire many more diffusion directions than this minimum (e.g. 20 directions + three averages of the $b = 0$ image), since this both increases the signal-to-noise ratio and minimizes directional bias in the diffusion measures obtained.

Biological Applications of Diffusion Tensor Imaging

In tissues with microstructure that is randomly oriented on the scale of an image voxel, water diffusivity appears to be the same in all directions; e.g. the extensive dendritic arborization in gray matter results in apparent isotropic diffusion on the macroscopic scale of an MR image. However, in tissues with highly organized microstructure, such as in white matter, water diffuses more rapidly along the direction of the fiber tracts than perpendicular to this direction (anisotropic diffusion); in the latter direction, the cell membranes and myelin layers present greater obstacles to the free movement of water than are present parallel to the long axis of the axons. Therefore, to obtain a reproducible measure of diffusion in the brain, it is not meaningful to calculate the ADC in a single direction. The axes of the cells (or their diffusion ellipsoids) will be arbitrarily oriented with respect to the fixed x, y, and z axes of the magnet, resulting in a misleadingly inhomogeneous (and orientation dependent) DW signal intensity. Diffusion tensor MRI (DTI) provides all the information required to calculate an appropriate diffusion ellipsoid for each voxel of an imaging volume (4). (Specifically, it provides a measurement of the effective diffusion tensor, D, in each voxel of an imaging volume.)

Orientation-independent Parameters

In order for any parameter that is used to characterize diffusion in vivo to be biologically meaningful, it must be indicative of some aspect of cellular status, and not an artifact of the relative orientation of the brain to the fixed x, y, and z axes of the MR scanner's gradient system. This potential problem arises due to the inherent anisotropy of diffusion within the brain, such that a measurement made in a single direction on two occasions, for example, would give different results if the head orientation were different on each occasion, even if there was no change in diffusivity.

Fortunately, it is possible to obtain a measure of the orientationally averaged diffusivity (i.e. one that reflects the average of diffusion coefficients measured in all spatial directions) that is robust to head orientation, by calculating the average of the ADCs measured in three orthogonal directions. However, such a measure does contain some directional bias, since only three directions have been sampled, yet inferences are drawn assuming averaging over all spatial directions. Also, it should be noted that it is not possible to calculate a robust indicator of the degree of diffusion anisotropy from the limited information available from such sampling of diffusion in only three directions.

If enough data are acquired to characterize the diffusion tensor D (see above for a discussion of the minimum required), it is possible to calculate new quantitative scalar parameters that relate to specific features of the diffusion process (a scalar quantity being one that has only magnitude, i.e. a simple number). As already indicated, the most useful scalar quantities are those designed to be rotationally invariant, i.e. independent of the coordinate system in which the MR measurement is made and of the orientation of the brain with respect to the magnet. The most commonly used rotationally invariant scalar measure that characterizes the bulk diffusion properties of the tissue, independent of the orientation of the fibers, is the *Trace* of the diffusion tensor (*Trace(D)*) (4), which provides a measure of the orientationally averaged diffusivity. (The trace of a matrix is the sum of the diagonal elements; i.e. *Trace(D)* = $D_{xx} + D_{yy} + D_{zz}$; note that the ADC_{av} described above is generally a good approximation to *Trace(D)*.)

The most fundamental rotationally invariant quantities are the three principal diffusivities (known as eigenvalues) of D, which are the principal diffusion coefficients along the three coordinate directions that constitute the local 'fiber frame of reference' in each voxel (Fig. 12.1). Each eigenvalue is associated with a direction (or eigenvector) that is intrinsic to the tissue. The three eigenvectors of D are mutually perpendicular and define a local fiber frame of reference (effectively, the orientation of the diffusion ellipsoid at any given location; see Fig. 12.1). In each voxel, the eigenvalues (conventionally labeled λ_1 to λ_3) can be sorted in order of decreasing magnitude (λ_1 = highest diffusivity, λ_2 = intermediate diffusivity, and λ_3 = lowest diffusivity). In anisotropic tissues consisting of ordered parallel bundles, the largest eigenvalue, λ_1, represents the diffusion coefficient along the direction parallel to the fiber, while λ_2 and λ_3 represent the diffusion coefficients in the transverse directions (4).

Widely used rotationally invariant scalar measures that are applicable in anisotropic systems include indices of the relative anisotropy and fractional anisotropy (FA) (5). These provide measures of the degree to which diffusion is different in different directions; in other words, how much the diffusion ellipsoid's shape deviates from being spherical, indicating that the diffusivity in different directions is

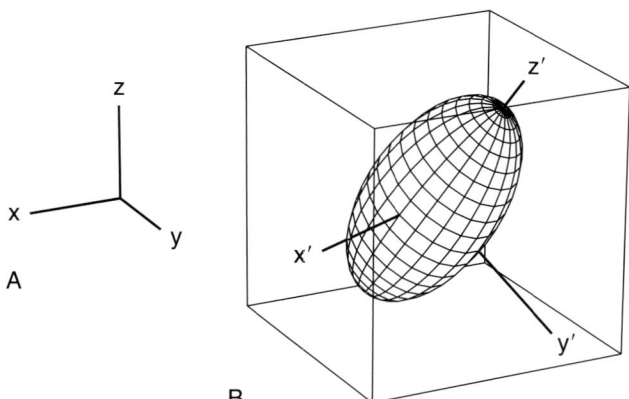

FIG. 12.1. A. An *x*, *y*, *z* coordinate system representing the spatial frame of reference of the laboratory (i.e. within the magnet). **B.** A typical diffusion ellipsoid within a voxel; such an ellipsoid can have any arbitrary orientation with respect to the reference frame. The appropriate coordinate system for this ellipsoid (i.e. *x'*, *y'*, and *z'*) can be calculated from the principal directions of the diffusion tensor; i.e. the eigenvectors of the tensor (see text) are aligned along the *x'*,*y'*, and *z'* axes. The three principal diffusivities of the diffusion tensor (known as eigenvalues; see text) are the principal diffusion coefficients along the three coordinate directions that constitute the local 'fiber frame of reference' in each voxel.

unequal, such as is typically found in white matter regions with parallel arrangement of fibers. For example, FA is particularly high in the corpus callosum, which has a highly ordered arrangement of white matter fibers. Figure 12.2 shows examples of both *Trace(D)* and FA maps, together with information corresponding to the direction of highest diffusivity.

Fiber-tracking

The eigenvectors of the diffusion tensor provide unique directional information that can be used to infer interesting features of tissue in vivo. In particular, measurements of the eigenvector associated with the largest eigenvalue (λ_1) in each voxel (i.e. the direction of the longest axis of the diffusion ellipsoid) can be used to construct maps of white matter fiber direction within an imaging volume, on the assumption that the largest diffusivity is oriented along the direction of the fiber tract (Fig. 12.2). This information has been demonstrated to provide the potential for noninvasive fiber tractography in the brain, and this is currently a very active area of research (see, for example, references 6–10). Nevertheless, no present tracking algorithm has yet been shown to be sufficiently robust for clinical applications, and many technical issues remain to be addressed.

Also, in addition to the limitations of any particular tracking algorithm, a more fundamental problem is that the diffusion tensor does not provide sufficient information to determine the correct fiber orientation in voxels that contain significant partial volume effects, such as crossing or 'kissing' fibers, which unfortunately are not uncommon at the spatial

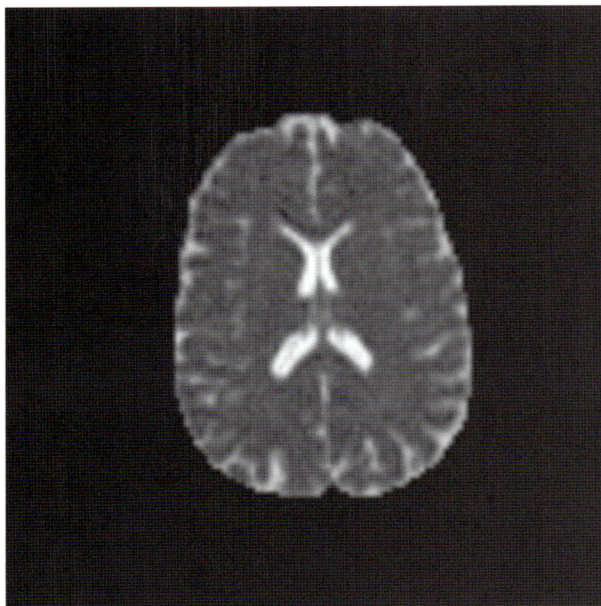

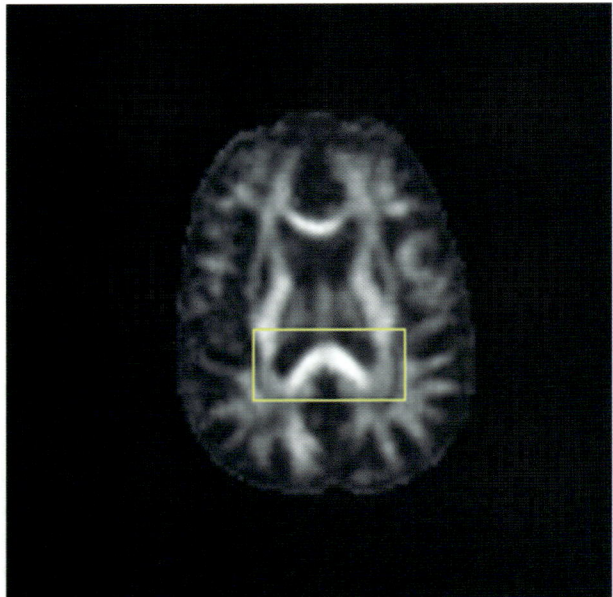

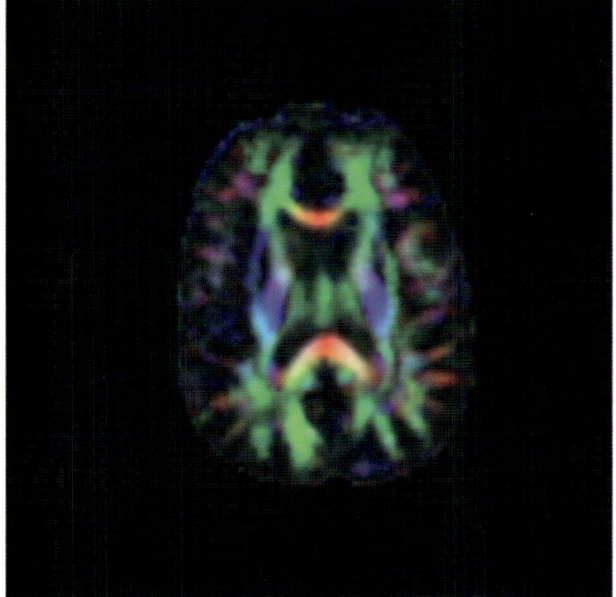

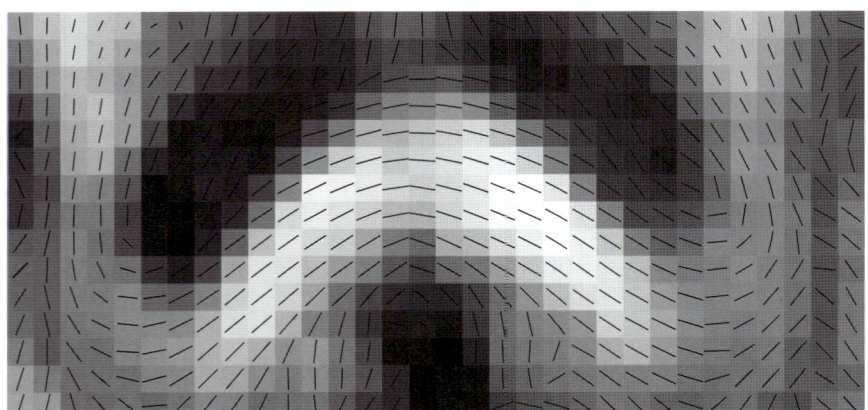

FIG. 12.2. Examples of maps that can be generated from the diffusion tensor. **A.** A map of the mean diffusivity, generated from calculating *Trace* (***D***). **B.** A map of the fractional anisotropy (FA). **C.** A *color-coded* map of the major eigenvector of the diffusion tensor weighted by the corresponding FA map. The major eigenvector is that associated with the largest eigenvalue (λ_1), and indicates the direction of the highest diffusivity (see text). *Red* = left–right, *green* = anterior–posterior, and *blue* = through-plane. It can be seen from a combination of all three maps that *gray* matter and *white* matter have similar average diffusivity values but low FA and high FA values respectively. **D.** An indication of the direction of the major eigenvector overlaid on the section of the FA map highlighted in **B**. It is apparent that there is high coherence of the eigenvectors between voxels in the corpus callosum and the internal capsule but less orientational coherence in the voxels located in gray-matter regions.

resolution that is possible for DTI. A number of other approaches have been proposed, such as diffusion spectroscopic imaging (DSI; a technique based on q-space imaging) (11) and high angular resolution imaging (12), each of which requires particular data acquisition conditions to be fulfilled. The former in particular suffers from a totally impractical imaging time (of the order of 4 hours), while it remains unclear in the latter how the ADC profile relates to the underlying fiber architecture. Further work is required, therefore, before robust inferences can be made concerning fiber orientations in regions containing crossing fibers.

Mechanisms of Diffusion-weighted Imaging Signal Changes

Much of the work to date to investigate the basis for signal abnormalities observed in DWI has been carried out in the context of cerebral ischemia. Nevertheless, the underlying biophysical mechanisms are likely to be relevant in the interpretation of the findings in patients with epilepsy. The DWI evidence of an early reduction of ADC in cerebral ischemia has been attributed to a shift of extracellular water to intracellular compartments as a result of a disruption of ion homeostasis (13). This is believed to occur as a result of the following chain of events: a decreased blood supply following an initial insult reduces the amount of oxygen and glucose delivered to the tissue, and this is accompanied by a decrease in the available adenosine triphosphate (ATP). ATP normally provides energy to pump Na^+ out of and K^+ into the cell to maintain ionic homeostasis. When the supply of ATP ceases, there is an accumulation of intracellular Na^+, causing an influx of water into the cell by osmosis, which leads to cell swelling (cytotoxic edema) and, in time, cell death. Later work (14, 15) supported Moseley's early hypothesis, and it is now generally accepted that a drop in the tissue water ADC in ischemic tissue is associated with the development of cytotoxic edema.

Despite this demonstrated association between cytotoxic edema and ADC, the exact biophysical mechanisms of water ADC reduction remain uncertain. Several hypotheses have been suggested, including: a reduction in extracellular diffusion due to an increase in the tortuosity of the extracellular space that occurs after cell swelling (16, 17); a reduction in cell membrane permeability (18); and a decrease in intracellular diffusivity (as evidenced by reduction in the diffusivity of intracellular metabolites (19) or intracellular ^{133}Cs (20)), either by a decrease in the intracellular circulation or an increase in viscosity. It is possible that more than one of these mechanisms contributes to the observed reduction in ADC, since there is some evidence for each.

In epilepsy, reduced ADC has been observed in a number of different animal models of status epilepticus and has been attributed to disruption in ion homeostasis resulting in movement of water from the extra- to the intracellular space, or to cytoplasmic dysfunction. The epilepsy models have

important differences from ischemia models, in that the former showed no reduction in ATP, and no hypoperfusion, while in the latter these appeared to be contributory factors. However, a common feature to both models is the presence of cell swelling, suggesting that the mechanisms for a reduction in diffusion may have similarities in both cases, despite the different nature of the cellular insult. The subsequent increase above control values in the ADC of tissue water that is generally observed in ischemia after around 1 week is believed to be associated with cell lysis, the loss of cellular barriers, and vasogenic edema. However, any process that results in an expansion of extracellular space, such as the significant cell loss often associated with epilepsy, would be expected also to result in an increased ADC.

Magnetic Resonance Perfusion Imaging

The terms *perfusion* and *cerebral blood flow* (CBF) are often used indistinguishably to refer to the volume of blood delivered to the capillary bed of a block of tissue in a given period of time, with units therefore of ml/100g/min. It is important to distinguish between perfusion, which takes place at the capillary level (and is visualized on perfusion MRI), and bulk flow through major vessels (such as is visualized on MR angiography). Perfusion MRI offers some advantages when compared to the widely used perfusion techniques of single-photon-emission computed tomography (SPECT) or positron-emission tomography (PET), not least in terms of the absence of ionizing radiation in MRI. In addition, since MRI can also provide structural information, a combined structural/functional MRI examination becomes possible, at least interictally, in the evaluation of patients with epilepsy. However, because all currently available MRI perfusion methods employ short-lived tracers, imaging of *ictal* events requires the patient to already be in the MRI scanner at the time of the seizures. As a result, *ictal* studies using MR perfusion imaging will be particularly difficult in most cases.

There are two general MR approaches to the assessment of perfusion, which differ with regard to their respective use of an exogenous and endogenous MR-visible tracer. The first MRI approach, *dynamic susceptibility contrast* (DSC) MRI, or 'bolus tracking,' relies on the injection of a bolus of paramagnetic contrast agent. The second approach involves magnetic labeling of inflowing water protons in blood using MR techniques that are known collectively as *arterial spin labeling* (ASL). The majority of the work published to date on perfusion MRI has been related to the investigation of cerebral ischemia, although there is increasing interest within the field of epilepsy, with a number of promising applications reported in recent years. Across a range of applications, bolus tracking has been the most widely used technique for MR perfusion imaging, and is in clinical use in many institutions. Although ASL has several advantages compared to bolus tracking, a number of drawbacks to the approach have resulted in a relatively limited clinical implementation to date.

Since the theory underlying both the bolus tracking and ASL methods is extensive (see Calamante et al. 1999 (21) for a detailed review), only a brief summary of some important aspects is given below.

Bolus Tracking Magnetic Resonance Imaging

Clinically approved MR contrast agents do not cross the intact blood–brain barrier, and therefore can be considered as intravascular contrast agents in the absence of breakdown of the blood–brain barrier. If a bolus of paramagnetic contrast agent (e.g. gadolinium-DTPA) is injected intravenously, its passage through the brain produces a transient decrease in signal intensity on a series of spin-echo or gradient-echo images (22), due respectively to a reduction in the relaxation times T2 or T2* induced by the gadolinium. In the capillary phase, this signal loss is primarily in the tissue (despite the intravascular nature of the contrast agent), since the effects on the T2 relaxation rate extend through space, and the capillaries themselves occupy typically only 3–5% of tissue volume.

Assuming a linear relationship between the change in relaxation rate and the concentration of contrast agent ($C(t)$), the latter can be calculated on a pixel-by-pixel basis. The concentration in a region of interest (ROI) in the tissue can be related to CBF by the following expression (21):

$$C(t) = k \, \text{CBF} \, (\text{AIF} \otimes R(t)) \tag{1}$$

where k is a proportionality constant, AIF is the arterial input function (i.e. the concentration of tracer entering the ROI at time t), and $R(t)$ is the residue function, which describes the fraction of contrast agent remaining in the ROI at time t, following the injection of an ideal, infinitely narrow, bolus at time zero. The symbol $\otimes$ indicates the mathematical operation known as a convolution; the convolution of the AIF with the residue function accounts for the fact that, for the nonideal bolus used in practice, part of the spread in the concentration–time curve is due to the finite length of the actual bolus as it arrives in the brain. If unaccounted for, this dispersion would be interpreted by the model as occurring within the ROI itself, leading to a considerable underestimation of CBF.

Although it is not appropriate here to go into detail about the assumptions and implications of Equation (1), it is important to note that the concentration of contrast agent (and therefore the signal intensity time curve) depends not only on CBF but also on the AIF and the residue function. Therefore, the actual concentration–time curve measured for any given ROI can be influenced not only by the perfusion of the ROI but also by the injection conditions and the vascular structure.

Deconvolution Analysis

There are two commonly used approaches to the analysis and quantification of bolus tracking data. The first of these requires measurement of the AIF in order to solve Equation (1) using a technique known as deconvolution (21, 23). This method is time-consuming and computationally intensive but can provide direct physiologic information about CBF, cerebral blood volume (CBV), and mean transit time (MTT; the average time for the tracer to pass through the vasculature after the injection of an ideal bolus).

There are two main concerns with this approach. First, it is generally believed to produce only relative measurements of perfusion (24, 25), primarily because of uncertainty with respect to the two proportionality constants involved. The first of these constants relates the measured signal intensity changes to the concentration of contrast agent (assuming a linear relationship), while the second constant (k in Equation (1)) reflects the influence of brain density and hematocrit concentration on the relationship between the concentration–time curve and CBF. Neither of these constants can be determined easily in vivo, and fixed values are normally assumed throughout the brain. However, the validity of such assumed conversion factors under varied physiologic conditions remains to be determined.

Some studies have attempted to obtain absolute measurements by reference to other techniques such as PET (see, for example, Ostergaard et al. 1998 (26)) and, although the values in healthy volunteers are consistent with expected CBF, again a full validation under various physiologic conditions is still required. Until then, absolute values of perfusion should be interpreted with caution.

The second concern with the deconvolution approach is related to the measurement of the AIF. This is generally estimated from the concentration–time curve from pixels within a major artery (e.g. the middle cerebral artery). Therefore, the measured bolus can be further delayed and dispersed on its transit from that artery to the ROI. This is sometimes observed in cases of abnormal vasculature, such as in occlusion, stenosis, or in the presence of collateral flow. This extra delay and dispersion is interpreted by the model as occurring within the ROI, which leads to an underestimation of CBF, overestimation of MTT, and possible underestimation of CBV (27). Therefore, although this problem is less severe in the context of epilepsy than in that of stroke, special care still must be taken when interpreting perfusion data in the presence of delays and dispersion.

Summary Parameters

The second approach to the analysis of bolus tracking data is to use so-called 'summary parameters' calculated directly from the profile of the concentration–time curve as indirect perfusion measures. There are several different parameters, such as bolus arrival time (BAT), time to peak (TTP; i.e. time until the maximum of $C(t)$), maximum peak concentration (MPC; i.e. maximum value of $C(t)$), full width at half maximum (FWHM) of the curve, area under the peak, etc. The use of this approach is common since the analysis of data is fast and straightforward and does not require measurement of the AIF.

It has become common to use particular summary parameters as approximations to specific physiological measures; for example, MPC as 'CBF,' FWHM as 'MTT,' the first moment of $C(t)$ as 'MTT' (a better approximation than FWHM), and CBV divided by 'MTT' as 'CBF index' (or CBF_i). However, it is important to note that these are only approximations, and in some circumstances not good approximations, to the desired parameters. Except for the area under the peak (which is proportional to CBV), all other summary parameters can provide only indirect physiological measures, since they can be affected by changes in any of CBF, CBV, and MTT (28). Furthermore, as mentioned above, they also can be influenced by injection conditions (volume injected, injection rate, cannula size, etc.) and the vascular structure, as well as by the cardiac output of the patient.

As a result, changes in the summary parameters could represent not only changes in perfusion but also changes in any of these conditions. Therefore, although they can be effective in the identification of abnormal regions (e.g. a region with prolonged TTP will represent a region that is 'hemodynamically abnormal'), the interpretation of such abnormality in terms of cerebral perfusion is not straight forward (28, 29) In particular, differences in AIF between patients, or between studies in an individual patient, can produce variability in the summary parameters larger than that due to the abnormality under investigation (29). Therefore, if they are used for setting thresholds, for comparison between patients, or in follow-up studies, misleading results can be obtained that should be interpreted with caution.

It should be noted that, since the transit time of the bolus through the tissue is only a few seconds, a fast imaging technique is required to properly characterize the peak. The most commonly used technique is EPI, which allows several slices to be acquired with a time resolution of 1–2 seconds. However, EPI suffers from several drawbacks, such as low resolution and image distortions. Therefore, image quality is commonly sacrificed to achieve the necessary time resolution for the analysis of bolus tracking data.

Arterial Spin Labeling

Arterial spin labeling (ASL) is a totally noninvasive MR method that uses water protons as a freely diffusible tracer and has the potential for measuring perfusion quantitatively. An MR image can be sensitized to the effect of inflowing blood if the blood is in a different magnetic state from that of the static tissue. ASL techniques use this principle by magnetically labeling blood flowing into the slices of interest (30, 31). The inflowing blood water exchanges with tissue water, causing a change in the local tissue magnetization that is directly related to perfusion. A perfusion-weighted image can be generated by the subtraction of an image in which inflowing spins have been labeled from an image in which spin labeling has not been performed. Absolute quantification of perfusion can be obtained if other parameters (such as tissue T_1, the T_1 of blood, the blood–brain partition coefficient (λ) of water, the efficiency of spin labeling (α), and the transit time from the labeling site to the tissue) are also measured (see Calamante et al. 1999 (21) for a review).

It should be noted that some of these values, in particular T_1(blood), λ, and α, are difficult to measure, with the result that standard values are often assumed. However, it has been shown that there is the potential for considerable variability in these parameters, and the assumption of generic values constitutes a potential source of error in CBF determination.

Under the general heading of ASL, two distinct subgroups exist: continuous ASL (CASL) and pulsed ASL (PASL). In the first subgroup, CASL, the arterial spins can be magnetically labeled either by continuous inversion using a long off-resonance radiofrequency pulse (31) or by repeated slice selective saturation pulses (30) (saturation produces a smaller signal change but deposits significantly less radiofrequency power). The labeling is realized by the application of the labeling pulse to a plane through the blood vessels in the neck, which have the required flow direction (perpendicular to the labeling plane) and velocity for CASL. A steady state develops where the regional magnetization in the brain is directly related to CBF (21) and the acquisition of a control image in which the blood is not labeled allows the formation of a perfusion-weighted image by subtraction.

One consequence of the labeling method in CASL is that there is a high radiofrequency power deposition. This may limit the utility of this approach in some patients and might present a particular problem in pediatric studies (because of low body weight) or in patients with compromised blood flow.

In the other ASL subgroup, PASL, the arterial labeling is achieved by using a short (typically ≈ 10 ms) radiofrequency pulse (32–34), and CBF can be obtained from the time-dependent signal change created by the exchange of the labeled blood and brain tissue water. As an example, Figure 12.3 shows a schematic representation of a particular PASL method, flow-sensitive alternating inversion recovery (FAIR) (33, 34); a perfusion-weighted image is generated from the difference between label and control images. A detailed description of the different ASL techniques and the mathematical models used for quantification is not appropriate to this text and the reader is referred to recent reviews (21, 35), for a more extensive description than that given here.

Two of the main limitations of ASL (which have contributed to its slow incorporation in the clinical setting relative to bolus tracking) are low signal-to-noise and possible long (and unknown) transit times from the labeling site to the tissue, and these are discussed briefly below:

Low Signal-to-Noise

The signal-to-noise ratio of subtraction images is inherently poor since measured signal intensity changes due to

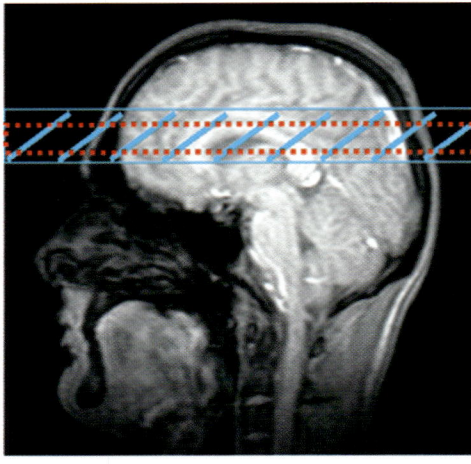 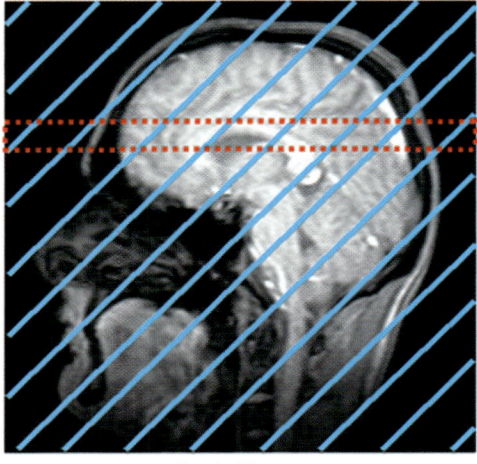

Label image   Control image

FIG. 12.3. Schematic diagram illustrating the image pairs acquired using the FAIR PASL technique (see text). The dotted *red lines* indicate the position of the axial slice from which a perfusion image will be obtained, and regions of inverted magnetization are indicated by the *blue* diagonal lines. An image is acquired at time TI after the inversion pulse in each case, and the difference between label and control images results in a perfusion-weighted image.

perfusion are small (the relative signal difference in the perfusion-weighted image is only of the order of 1% at 1.5 Tesla), and many averages (typically 40–60) are required to generate high quality images, leading to long scan times. Since a T_1 map is also required for perfusion quantification, the typical ASL scan time is 5–10 time longer than for bolus tracking MRI.

Long Transit Times

The transit time (δ) from the labeling site to the tissue can be very long, particularly in the presence of hemodynamic abnormalities, and the magnetic labeling of the blood is diminished, reducing even further the sensitivity of the technique. Also, transit times within an imaging slice have been demonstrated to be heterogeneous, resulting in a potential source of error in CBF calculation.

It is perhaps more obvious why transit time might be a problem in CASL, in that the labeling plane is some distance away from the slices in which perfusion is measured. However, because of slice profile imperfections, transit time is also commonly problematic in PASL. For example, the most commonly used PASL method is FAIR (33, 34) (see Fig. 12.3). Interactions between inversion and excitation slice profiles mean that the inversion (labeling) slice in FAIR-type sequences is commonly ≈3 times the width of the imaging slice (ideal = 1:1) to avoid subtraction errors between the two images. Thus the flow of labeled blood into the image slice is delayed, resulting in the problems described above.

The measurement of δ is not straightforward, requiring characterization of the bi-exponential relationship between the ASL signal and inversion time (TI), which is too time-consuming for practical clinical use. Furthermore, fitting for δ on a pixel-by-pixel basis is very unstable because of signal-to-noise ratio issues.

An alternative approach is to minimize the effect of δ. Wong et al (36). have described a modification (QUIPPS) that can be applied to PASL sequences, which renders them relatively insensitive to transit time, but the required sequence parameters can become impractical if δ is very long. In the case of CASL, Alsop and Detre[37] have also introduced a sequence modification, consisting of the insertion of a postlabeling delay prior to image acquisition. If this delay is longer than the longest transit time, and the quantification equations are modified accordingly, then the resulting perfusion maps are insensitive to variations in transit time.

The inherently low signal-to-noise ratio of ASL, combined with extended transit times, results in particularly poor perfusion sensitivity in pathologic low-flow states. Therefore, although ASL techniques are in theory able to calculate CBF in absolute units, clinical applications to date have been limited.

APPLICATIONS OF MAGNETIC RESONANCE DIFFUSION AND PERFUSION IN EPILEPSY

As stated in the introduction to this chapter, the aim of this section is not to present a comprehensive review of the literature but rather to describe and discuss examples of work that is believed to demonstrate the role of diffusion imaging in the study of patients with epilepsy. A similar approach will be taken in the following section with respect to the role of MR perfusion in epilepsy.

Diffusion Imaging in Epilepsy

Diffusion imaging has been applied both to the specific examination of the hippocampus in patients with temporal lobe epilepsy (TLE), and to the investigation of the brain as a whole in non-TLE patients. Examples of reports that are illustrative of each are discussed below.

Ictal Diffusion Imaging

As mentioned above, a number of animal models, in which seizures were induced by a range of methods with different underlying mechanisms, have established that seizure activity can produce a short-term reduction in diffusivity in the vicinity of the seizure origin. Methods of seizure induction have included the administration of bicuculline (a $GABA_A$ antagonist) (38), kainic acid (a glutaminergic agent) (39), or cortical electroshocks (40).

The reduction in diffusion following seizures is very short-lived, with the result that few *ictal* studies have been carried out in patients. Those that have been performed, however, indicate that the detected ADC reduction may provide information related to seizure localization. For example, in a case report of a patient with nonconvulsive status epilepticus, Flacke et al (41). showed that there was an 18% reduction in ADC in the left temporoparietal region that was confined to a focal section of the cortical ribbon. The ADC in this region was normal on follow-up imaging 1 month later, at a time when the patient had recovered and had a normal EEG. Calistri et al (42). showed similar findings in a patient with epilepsia partialis continua. In this patient, a 35% ADC reduction was observed in the right frontoparietal region (ipsilateral to the seizures), and in the contralateral cerebellum. Both of these regions also showed hyperperfusion in similar locations, and both had normal ADC and perfusion in follow-up studies over 2–15 days.

It seems likely that what was observed in these studies is evidence of reversible cytotoxic edema associated with focal seizure activity, analogous to that observed in the animal models. The focal nature of the observed changes in conjunction with their transient nature suggest that they may be associated with epileptogenic tissue (and in the latter case, additional areas remote from but functionally connected to the epileptogenic cortex), and may therefore provide important localizing information regarding recent seizure activity.

Interictal Diffusion Imaging

Hippocampal

Perhaps reflecting the logistical difficulties in performing the above work, the majority of studies that have used DTI to investigate patients with epilepsy have been carried out *interictally*. In a study of eight patients with mesial temporal lobe epilepsy and five control subjects, Hugg et al (43). reported increased ADC_{av} in hippocampi ipsilateral to the seizure focus compared both to contralateral and to control hippocampi (Fig. 12.4). Quantitative hippocampal T2 relaxation and volumetric measurements were also performed on

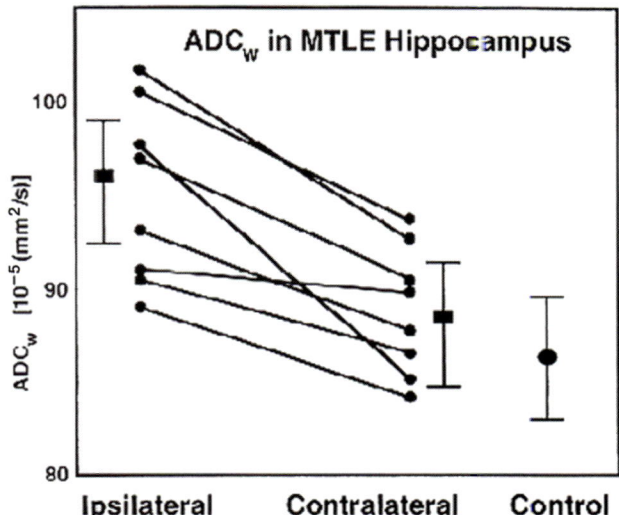

FIG. 12.4. Apparent diffusion coefficient values from the hippocampal epileptic focus and contralateral hippocampus. Normal control values are also shown as mean from right and left hippocampus. (Courtesy of R. Kuzniecky, M.D. and J. Hugg, Ph.D)

these patients, and the ADC_{av} findings were reported to be correlated with these measures (although data were not presented). An anisotropy index (AI) was also calculated, but was not found to be different between groups. It should be noted, however, that the diffusion data in this study were acquired in only three diffusion-sensitized directions, and as a result the AI calculated is not a robust parameter since it is head-orientation-dependent (see section on diffusion tensor imaging, above).

In a further study of hippocampal diffusion measures in 14 patients with partial seizures, Wieshmann et al (44). showed significantly elevated ADC_{av} values in sclerotic hippocampi compared to nonsclerotic hippocampi in patients or controls. Hippocampal sclerosis (HS) was determined by the MR criteria of elevated T2 relaxation time and small hippocampal volume. Quantitative measures of each of these were obtained in both patients and controls, and good correlations were found between ADC and both T2 and hippocampal volume. It is interesting to note that there were two outliers in the ADC values from the non-HS patient hippocampi, which were not different from the ADC values found in HS; these two hippocampi had significantly elevated T2 relaxation times, but could not be classified as HS since the volumes were normal.

As in the study described above, the AI values calculated in this study were also based on data from only three directions and are therefore orientation-dependent. As a result, a very high variance was found in the AI measures (in control subjects, 46% vs 4% for ADC_{av}). Although a reduction in AI was observed in the group data when comparing HS with non-HS, only a very weak correlation was observed between AI and T2 or volume measures.

Both the above studies show similar principal findings, namely that there is a significant increase in ADC_{av} in HS, indicating an increase in water mobility in such hippocampi.

One possible explanation for this observation is an increase in membrane permeability as a result of cellular insult. However, such changes have been demonstrated only in more severe and acute circumstances than those present in HS, and it seems more likely that the observed changes in ADC_{av} result from an increase in extracellular space due to neuronal loss in affected hippocampi.

The study by Hugg et al (43). found no relationship between AI and hippocampal abnormality, whereas Wieshmann et al (44). reported a significant difference between HS and non-HS AI results, although in the absence of a meaningful correlation with T2 or volume data. It is worth noting in this context that anisotropy measures would be expected to be an insensitive indicator of abnormalities of hippocampal diffusivity, since, in such a gray matter structure, diffusion would be almost isotropic in normal hippocampi, making detection of a decrease in AI very difficult. With this in mind, it is perhaps not surprising that no significant changes were observed in the study by Hugg et al (43)., since in addition the patient numbers were small and the AI measure used was orientation-dependent. A similar explanation could be used with respect to the lack of correlation between the AI and T2 or volume findings in the study by Wieshmann et al. (44). However, the latter did report a significant decrease in AI in HS, despite also using an orientation-dependent measure of anisotropy.

These data suggest a decrease in the degree of orientational organization of the cells in HS with respect to a normal hippocampus, which may result simply from the same increase in extracellular space that underlies the observed increase in ADC_{av}. However, the suggestion by the authors that this may be related to the reduction in dendritic branching that is known to be associated with epileptogenesis raises an interesting question. It has been shown that, in embryonic or early postnatal mouse brain, the cortical gray matter has a relatively high diffusion anisotropy, which diminishes over time to the near-zero adult value (45). These findings suggest the existence of ordered, oriented microstructure in the gray matter of the developing brain, which becomes less ordered with time. This has been explained by a largely parallel orientation of migrating neuronal cells initially, with the subsequent proliferation of dendritic branching rendering diffusion pseudoisotropic on the MR spatial scale. Therefore, in the context of HS, loss of dendritic branching and increase in extracellular space may in fact have conflicting effects on the measured AI.

Thus it appears, both from first principles and from empirical data, that ADV_{av} is the diffusion measure that would be expected to provide greatest sensitivity in detecting hippocampal abnormality in HS.

Extrahippocampal

In addition to the above investigations directed specifically to the hippocampus, a number of studies have examined the relationship between DTI and epileptogenic structural abnormalities on an ROI basis. For example, in a study of 18 patients with structural lesions, including infarcts, injuries, malformations of cortical development (MCDs), and tumors, anisotropy was reported to be reduced in all lesions and ADC_{av} to be increased in approximately 70% (46). This suggests a loss of directional organization in many lesions, irrespective of etiology.

However, in many circumstances, there are significant limitations to using only an ROI approach in the investigation of DTI abnormalities. This is of particular relevance when investigating patients with localization-related epilepsy in conjunction with normal conventional MRI (MRI-negative patients), since in many cases no prior investigation site can be identified. The identification of focal abnormalities in such patients may be of particular importance because surgical treatment without an abnormality on preoperative imaging is often associated with a poor outcome. Also, even in patients who have identifiable lesions on conventional structural imaging, other methodologies have demonstrated previously that there may be more extensive abnormalities that do not have a macroscopic structural correlate, which could have an influence on surgical decision making.

The alternative approach of voxel-by-voxel image analysis is not only more objective, it also enables the evaluation of the whole brain rather than just specific regions. It has been demonstrated that DTI analyzed on a voxel-by-voxel basis can identify areas of abnormality in both mean diffusivity and FA. In particular, two large studies from the same group, using identical protocols, reported the findings in 22 patients with MCD (47) and in 10 patients with acquired epileptogenic lesions, together with 30 MRI-negative patients (48). Both studies included the same 30 healthy control subjects.

Diffusion weighting was applied in each of seven independent directions, enabling the calculation of rotationally invariant maps of both mean diffusivity and FA for each subject, with data acquired from 26 slices. Normalization to a template and statistical analysis of the maps were performed using the program SPM (SPM96; Wellcome Department of Imaging Neuroscience, London, UK). The maps from each subject were statistically compared on a voxel-by-voxel basis to 30 control subjects and significant increases or decreases were detected at an individual voxel level. Since such analyses give only the location and statistical significance of any differences, additional ROI analysis was performed in selected regions of abnormality to determine the magnitude of the changes underlying the detected differences.

Areas of reduced anisotropy were found in 17/22 patients with MCDs, in 15 of whom the changes corresponded to all or part of the MCD (47). None of the four patients with band heterotopia had FA changes in the region of the MCD itself. In six patients, reduced FA was detected in regions outside the MCD that appeared normal on conventional MRI. In two of the 22 patients, an increase in FA was detected in white matter adjacent to MCD. In 10 patients, an increase in the mean diffusivity was observed, in eight of whom the changes included the MCD, but in nine there were mean diffusivity changes that included normal appearing gray and white matter. In seven patients, the regions of increased mean diffusivity were more extensive than those observed on the FA maps.

These findings are interesting for a number of reasons. The FA maps were more sensitive in detecting the MCD, presumably because the difference between gray matter and white matter is relatively large in FA maps and almost negligible on mean diffusivity maps. The reduction in FA detected in the MCDs is presumably due in large part to the comparison of abnormally located gray matter to regions that are white matter in controls. However, it is potentially of greater interest that abnormalities were detected beyond the regions of visible MCD in many cases. These findings suggest that either the MCD is more extensive than is detectable on conventional imaging or the normal appearing white matter is in fact abnormal, with perhaps reduced cell density. The latter suggestion would be corroborated by the observation in some cases of more extensive increases in mean diffusivity, possibly indicating increased extracellular space due to failure of neurogenesis or subsequent cell loss.

The increased FA detected in two patients could be due to the presence of white matter that has been displaced by the MCD being compared to gray matter in the normal control subjects, or to white matter fibers that are more densely packed. From the results obtained from ROI analysis of the increased FA region in the normal-appearing occipital lobe in one of the patients, it appears that the latter explanation is the more likely in this case – the measured FA is very high for this region, giving a value more typical of structures such as the corpus callosum and therefore suggestive of unusually highly ordered occipital white matter.

Rugg-Gunn et al (48). demonstrated that DTI analyzed using SPM is sensitive in patients with acquired cerebral damage (five head injury, three infarction, one focal leukoencephalitis, one perinatal injury), identifying significant increases in mean diffusivity and significant reductions of anisotropy in all patients (41). In three of these 10 patients, FA was decreased in additional normal appearing regions while, in three further patients, mean diffusivity was increased in areas that were also normal on conventional MRI.

Individual analyses of the 30 patients with partial seizures and normal conventional MRI identified areas of significantly abnormal diffusion in nine patients. In only two of these nine was the abnormality found to be in FA, and in one of these there was good agreement with electroclinical seizure onset. Eight of the nine patients with abnormal diffusion showed increased mean diffusivity, with six of these in locations consistent with electroclinical seizure localization (Fig. 12.5 shows example images from one of the latter patients). Group analysis of nine MRI-negative patients with electroclinical seizure onset localizing to the left temporal region revealed a significant increase of diffusivity and a significant reduction in anisotropy within the white matter of the left temporal lobe (Fig. 12.6). A similar analysis in six patients with right temporal lobe seizures showed no significant diffusion abnormality (although there was a trend to indicate reduced FA).

The findings in patients with acquired lesions in the above study indicate that the mean diffusivity and FA are equally sensitive to the detection of such lesions, in contrast to the reported findings in MCD, where FA was significantly more sensitive in detecting abnormality in the MCD itself. This perhaps emphasizes the likelihood that the detection of MCD using a voxel-by-voxel comparison of normalized FA maps (by SPM, in this case) is strongly influenced by the comparison of heterotopic gray matter (low FA) with white matter (high FA) in the equivalent location in controls.

With respect to the acquired lesion findings more generally, it is perhaps of less significance that abnormalities of diffusion were detected in all acquired lesions (since these were already clearly discernible on conventional MR imaging) than that a significant number of abnormalities were detected in otherwise normal appearing regions. These were observed both as additional abnormalities in the patients

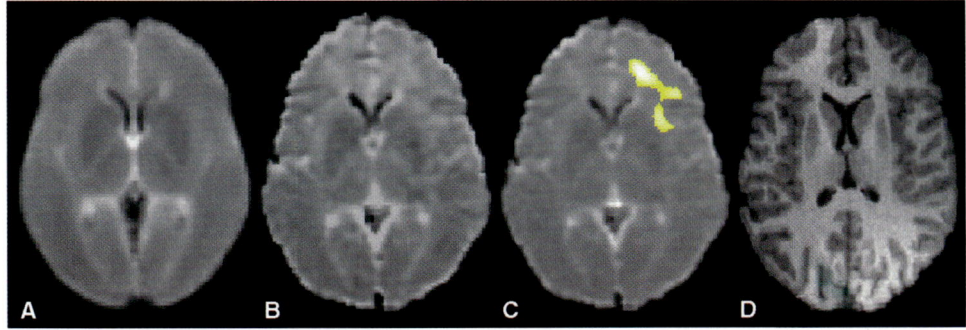

FIG. 12.5. Images from a patient with right frontal lobe epilepsy who had normal conventional MRI. Normalized axial average diffusivity maps at the same slice position for the averaged 30 control subjects (**A**), and the patient (**B**). (**C**) The region of significantly increased diffusivity is superimposed on the map shown in (**B**). (**D**) An equivalent slice from the patient's T1-weighted images, for anatomic reference. Note that right on the image is the patient's right. (From Rugg-Gunn FJ, Eriksson SH, Symms MR, et al. Diffusion tensor imaging of cryptogenic and acquired partial epilepsies. Brain 2001;124:627–636, by permission of Oxford University Press; figure courtesy of Dr F. Rugg-Gunn, National Society for Epilepsy and Epilepsy Research Group, Chalfont St Peter, UK.)

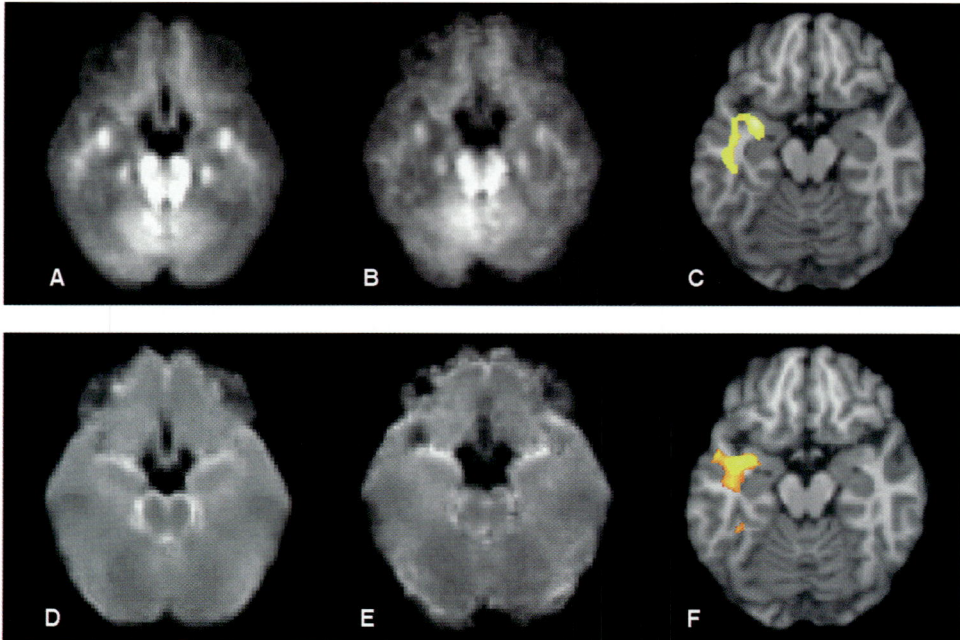

FIG. 12.6. Averaged images from a group of nine patients with left temporal lobe epilepsy and normal conventional MRI. (**A**) and (**B**); normalized axial *anisotropy maps* at the same slice position for the averaged 30 control subjects (**A**) and for the 9 TLE patients (**B**). (**D**) and (**E**); normalized axial *average diffusivity maps* at the same slice position for the averaged 30 control subjects (**D**) and for the nine TLE patients (**E**). The regions of decreased anisotropy and increased diffusivity (c and d respectively) are superimposed on normalized T1-weighted SPM templates at the same slice position. These regions are localized to the left temporal lobe. Note that right on the image is the patient's right. (From Rugg-Gunn FJ, Eriksson SH, Symms MR, *et al.* Diffusion tensor imaging of cryptogenic and acquired partial epilepsies. Brain 2001;124:627–636, by permission of Oxford University Press; figure courtesy of Dr F. Rugg-Gunn, National Society for Epilepsy and Epilepsy Research Group, Chalfont St Peter, UK.)

with visible lesions, and in nine of the 30 patients with no detectable structural abnormality. In the latter, the mean diffusivity measures showed significantly greater sensitivity to the detection of diffusion abnormality than was observed using FA data.

These significant differences in the diffusion indices in individual MRI-negative patients suggest that minor structural disorganization may exist in occult epileptogenic cerebral lesions. This could be due to a number of factors, including for example undetected neuronal dysgenesis, or atrophy, gliosis, and expansion of the extracellular space as a result of chronic seizures. The group effect observed in patients with left temporal lobe epilepsy indicates that there may be similar subtle abnormalities throughout the temporal lobe in such patients that are below the sensitivity of detection in individual patients. This may explain the failure to observe significant changes in the patients with right temporal lobe epilepsy, since there were fewer of these patients than left-affected patients.

It is of obvious importance in investigating patients with partial epilepsy that the identification of focal abnormality can be done on an individual basis. However, such group data can be viewed as establishing that abnormalities of diffusion do exist in normal appearing regions. It may be hoped, therefore, that, with improvements in DTI and analysis methods, further occult epileptogenic regions may be identified in individual patients, potentially leading to more invasive diagnostic procedures and possible epilepsy surgery in otherwise nonlesional patients.

Discussion: Diffusion in Epilepsy

The applicability of diffusion imaging to the investigation of patients with epilepsy will be dependent on a number of factors. The MR pulse sequences and hardware capable of performing these are becoming more widely available, such that on state-of-the-art scanners, DTI data acquisition will soon become relatively routine. The generation of rotationally invariant parameter maps should in principle also become straightforward.

However, what might remain more difficult is the analysis required to identify abnormalities that have no detectable structural correlate. Such investigations will not usually be possible by means of user-defined ROIs but are likely to require some form of statistical analysis on a voxel-by-voxel basis, such as the SPM-based studies described above. This will inherently require comparison with normative data, and will therefore necessitate some form of spatial normalization prior to analysis. Although there is no reason in principle why the spatial normalization step cannot be incorporated into the manufacturer-based software of many MR systems, it is likely that the control data will be locally generated and may therefore entail significant offline processing. While these restrictions may have only a small influence on practice within centers with research personnel who have the appropriate image-processing skills, they may pose at least a short-term constraint on these techniques becoming widespread.

The properties of water diffusion in tissues, as measured by DTI, are affected by tissue constituents such as macromolecules, membranes, and organelles, as well as by tissue microstructure and organization. A DTI study therefore potentially provides information that cannot be obtained using conventional, tissue-compositional-based or relaxometry-based MRI methods.

However, when considering the role of DTI in epilepsy, it is of interest to consider the nature of the information that results. In many cases, the abnormalities detected are related to changes in either the average diffusivity or the anisotropy of diffusion in white matter regions. Since epilepsy is essentially a disease of gray matter, or rather the seizures themselves will originate in gray matter regions, it remains to be seen what contribution will be made to patient diagnosis and treatment from the detection of exclusively white matter abnormalities. It is of course arguable that such abnormalities may be related to adjacent and as yet undetected gray matter abnormalities, and that what is required is improvement in the sensitivity of detection of the latter. This is similar to the argument presented above that group studies showing otherwise undetected abnormality can establish, in principle, that there are pathologic alterations in diffusion that merit further efforts to visualize in individuals.

A potential barrier to achieving further understanding of the role of DTI in epilepsy investigations is the somewhat circular difficulty in determining the clinical significance of the findings. It would not be ethical at present to perform surgery on any patient in whom the sole evidence of a focal lesion is a diffusion abnormality, even if this were consistent with electroclinical seizure localization. As a result, it is difficult to envisage rapid progress taking place in determining how important such lesions may be. Epilepsy surgery may well take place in those patients who have focal hippocampal abnormalities or focal acquired lesions, but these patients will in general have other evidence as to lesion type and location. The additional information from DTI would not contribute significantly to the decision to operate, nor would our understanding of the usefulness of DTI information be enhanced. It is highly unlikely that either the MCD patients or the MRI-negative patients will proceed to surgery, since the former are recognized generally to have poor outcome, while there will be insufficient evidence of a focal lesion in the latter. Given that it is in the latter group that the DTI findings are potentially most useful, it may be a considerable time before enough corroborating information is available to enable full advantage to be taken of this additional information.

Perfusion Magnetic Resonance Imaging in Epilepsy

As discussed earlier, MR perfusion imaging has some important advantages when compared to alternative methods

such as SPECT and PET. However, a major limitation with respect to the study of epilepsy is that ictal imaging is usually highly impractical. To undertake any form of MR perfusion imaging, it is necessary first that the subject is lying within the magnet when the contrast agent is injected or the magnetic labeling is applied, and second that no subject movement occurs during data collection, which takes place typically over a period of minutes. The first condition requires that the patient has sufficiently frequent seizures that they can be expected to occur during the MR examination, while the second condition excludes patients in whom seizures are associated with movement.

Ictal Perfusion Magnetic Resonance Imaging

Despite these practical difficulties, a few such *ictal* studies have taken place, usually in individual patients with focal status epilepticus (SE). Warach et al (49). performed both *ictal* SPECT and *ictal* MR bolus tracking investigations in a patient who presented with focal SE following treatment for a medulloblastoma. The *ictal* SPECT imaging showed hyperperfusion throughout the temporal/parietal/occipital regions, while repeat examination 2 weeks later when there was no longer epileptic activity showed symmetric perfusion of the left and right hemispheres. The MR investigations were analyzed only in terms of cerebral blood volume, with no CBF calculation; nevertheless, the *ictal* scan showed changes associated with seizure activity, with increased CBV in the right parietal region, which had resolved at the time of the later investigation. During the *ictal* MR investigation, the patient's seizures took the form of left visual field hallucinations, which did not preclude acquiring movement-free data.

Flacke et al (41). used a combination of DTI and bolus tracking perfusion MRI to investigate a patient with nonconvulsive SE both during a period of seizure activity, and 1 month later when his EEG had returned to normal. The mean diffusivity findings (see previous section) showed a focal reduction in ADC_{av} in the left temporoparietal area during the *ictal* scan, which had resolved 1 month later. The perfusion data were analyzed in terms of CBV and a surrogate for MTT (not defined), which were used to calculate a CBF index (where $CBF_i = CBV/'MTT'$). CBF_i was demonstrated to be elevated in the left temporoparietal region, and, consistent with the EEG and DTI findings, had returned to normal at follow-up.

Calistri et al (42). also reported both DTI and bolus tracking perfusion findings in a patient with epilepsia partialis continua. The patient underwent MR examination on admission, then subsequently at 15 days afterwards, by which time all abnormal electrical activity had disappeared from the EEG. The initial MR investigation revealed reduced average diffusivity and increased perfusion in the right frontoparietal cortex (ipsilateral to seizures), and in the contralateral cerebellum. Both the diffusion and perfusion findings had returned to normal at the later time point.

Together, these reports indicate that MR diffusion and perfusion studies provide noninvasive information regarding the evolution of focal SE. The abnormal electrical activity in SE is accompanied by a focal increase in CBF and has also been shown to be associated with perturbation of membrane ion homeostasis, with elevation of the extracellular potassium concentration and an influx of sodium, calcium, and water following the osmotic gradient, resulting in cell swelling. The latter has been demonstrated in the context of cerebral ischemia to be accompanied by a decrease in the average diffusivity, as was also manifest *ictally* in the above SE investigations. However, unlike in ischemia, the observed increase in perfusion in SE suggests that the cell energy state is maintained, with the ADC returning to within the normal range in the absence of seizures.

Other circumstances in which ADC reduction has been shown to be reversible include transient ischemic attacks and hyperacute stroke (50). In these cases, the normalization of ADC is most probably due to the restoration of CBF before irreversible cellular damage has occurred. In SE, the observed return to normal of the diffusivity on seizure cessation presumably reflects a different mechanism of disruption of ion homeostasis in the context of elevated perfusion, namely that it results from abnormal electrical activity rather than compromised energy status. It is possible, however, that the acute cytotoxic edema implied by the reduced ADC during SE may be associated with longer-term neuronal loss if the seizures are prolonged, despite the observed recovery of the ADC and normalization of the CBF. The combination of MR diffusion and perfusion imaging appears to provide evidence for cellular compromise associated with seizure activity, and therefore could contribute to the identification of the site of recent seizures.

Interictal Perfusion Magnetic Resonance Imaging

For the practical reasons already outlined, the application of *ictal* perfusion MRI will be restricted to a minority of patients with epilepsy. Nevertheless, since *interictal* hypoperfusion (in association with hypometabolism) has been shown to have lateralizing value, there remains a potential wider role for perfusion MRI in the investigation of focal seizures. As might be expected, studies of this type have involved larger groups of patients than typically reported for *ictal* studies.

Continuous Arterial Spin Labeling

Wolf et al (51). performed continuous ASL (CASL) perfusion studies *interictally* in 12 patients with temporal lobe epilepsy (TLE), and also in 12 normal controls. Continuous labeling (or control labeling; see background) was applied at the level of the cervicomedullary junction, and CBF was measured in eight axial slices. A postlabeling delay of 1.2 s was used to minimize the effects of transit time from the labeling plane to the imaged plane. In addition, ^{18}F-fluorodeoxyglucose (FDG) PET studies were also performed in 11 of the patients as part of their clinical evaluation, enabling comparison between metabolic and perfusion lateralization indices.

Electroclinical assessment indicated that seven patients had right TLE and five had left TLE. Because of the presence of both left and right TLE patients, an absolute index of asymmetry was used for comparison with controls. It was found that, although there was asymmetry present in the patient perfusion data, it was not significantly different from control asymmetry, which showed a systematically higher CBF in the left temporal lobe. Nevertheless, the CASL perfusion asymmetry index in patients showed good correlations both with the clinical lateralization and with the FDG-PET hypometabolism laterality.

Global CBF values were greatly reduced in many of the epilepsy patients, which may be explained by the fact that the patients were being treated with anticonvulsive medications. For comparison of CBF between patients and controls, therefore, it was necessary to normalize the CBF values obtained from the mesial temporal lobes to the global CBF values. After normalization, it was found that only the left TLE patients showed a significant decrease in CBF in the ipsilateral hemisphere compared to control values. In the right TLE patients, no significant decrease in normalized CBF was observed with respect to controls, although there was a significant difference between ipsilateral and contralateral mesial temporal lobe CBF in both right and left TLE patients, with the ipsilateral value significantly lower.

This study indicates that it is feasible to perform CASL perfusion imaging in patients with epilepsy and that additional lateralization information may be obtained. The latter appears to be substantiated by the good correlation between CBF lateralization and both clinical and FDG-PET lateralization. It has been suggested that FDG metabolic data are more useful for seizure localization than blood-flow-based PET studies, because of the uncoupling of CBF and metabolism interictally. Therefore, the apparent correspondence between FDG-PET and MR perfusion laterality findings in this study is encouraging.

A number of important considerations were also made apparent, however. The difference in global CBF between patients and controls indicates the need for caution in interpreting CBF measures, particularly when ROI analysis is used. If an ROI alone were to be sampled, an apparent focal difference in CBF between patients and controls could result from what is in reality a global CBF change. Normalization could be performed using the global value (as in this study), or by reference to another region of the brain, although at the expense of an increase in variance in both cases. Another important factor to be considered is the influence of the control group. In the particular population included in the above work, there was a systemic difference between left and right mesial temporal lobe CBF. If this is a general phenomenon, the implications are, first, that it may be difficult to detect a reduction in CBF in the right TLE group (although relative asymmetry should be maintained), and second, that without control data an asymmetry in right TLE patients could be interpreted as significant when it is in fact within a normal trend.

Pulsed Arterial Spin Labeling

Liu et al (52). also performed an ASL perfusion study, but in this case they used a pulsed ASL (PASL) technique known as FAIR-HASTE. FAIR describes the particular PASL protocol used (see Fig. 12.3), while HASTE (half-Fourier single shot turbo spin-echo) is used for data acquisition. The latter was chosen due to its relative insensitivity to image distortions in regions of high magnetic susceptibility gradients, such as the temporal lobes.

The work describes the investigation of eight patients with TLE using both PASL and $H_2^{15}O$-PET. The PET data were acquired prior to the MR studies, and the results were used to select an optimal slice position for the single-slice PASL data collection; namely, an axial slice through the temporal lobes corresponding to that with the most significant asymmetry on $H_2^{15}O$-PET. Both the MR and PET data were analyzed in terms of an asymmetry index, and correlation between the findings was investigated.

Although a reasonably good correlation was observed between the PET and ASL data, it was also apparent that there was considerable scatter in the data, and that the slope of the linear fit was significantly different from 1. This suggests that, although the two measures of perfusion are related, they are by no means identical, which may be due to differences in sensitivity to particular vessel dimension or variability in anatomic location of ROI sampling. No information is given in this work as to how the perfusion asymmetries relate to seizure localization, with the result that it is not possible to conclude which of the techniques performed better with respect to seizure location. However, it is particularly restrictive that the ASL data required prior location information from the PET data in order to sample a suitable single slice.

Nevertheless, the similarity of the FDG/ASL findings in the study discussed above, and the correlation described between $H_2^{15}O$-PET and ASL in this work suggest that, in principle, ASL may be able to provide useful additional lateralizing information, particularly given the restricted availability of PET imaging, although further work is needed to provide a robust basis for such a conclusion.

Bolus Tracking Magnetic Resonance Imaging

In a bolus tracking study, Wu et al (53). acquired MR blood volume data from nine TLE patients interictally and one SE patient ictally. FDG-PET data were also acquired in eight of the 10 patients (seven interictal, one ictal). In all cases, the

MR perfusion data were used to construct only CBV maps. For the interictal TLE studies, bolus tracking perfusion data were acquired from a single coronal slice, in each case using a T2*-weighted fast low-angle shot (FLASH) sequence. ROIs were outlined in both hippocampi in each case, and the CBV was measured. Because of the presence of multiple lesions in the patient with SE, bolus tracking was performed using EPI, enabling five axial slices to be acquired with a time resolution of 1.5 seconds. In addition, in both ictal and interictal investigations, CBV measurements were made in a ROI of normal frontal white matter.

Ratios of CBV (hippocampus) or CBV (lesion) to the frontal white matter CBV were calculated for the interictal or ictal studies respectively. In seven of the nine interictal patients, the hippocampus/white matter CBV ratio was lower in the left hippocampus. In six of these cases, the left hippocampus was atrophic, while no atrophy was observed in the other. In the six patients with left-sided lower CBV in whom FDG-PET was performed, left temporal hypometabolism was identified in all cases. The remaining two from the nine interictal patients had lower CBV ratio in the right hippocampus, which was again concordant with the hippocampal atrophy findings, and with the hypometabolism observed in the one patient who had FDG-PET.

The ictal data from this study are somewhat less convincing than the interictal data, with the former suffering from a less well-delineated means of determining a suitable ROI. Although increased CBV is suggested to be present in the vicinity of the observed lesions, this is not exclusive to these regions and is therefore of limited localizing value.

The interictal data from the above study are perhaps surprisingly well correlated with the structural and metabolic findings, given that only CBV measures were used. An argument is advanced that information about CBF can be inferred from the CBV data 'under certain conditions,' but this is not the case, as can be seen from the information given in the background section of this chapter. In order to calculate CBF, a measure of MTT would be required; the assumption made in this work would render CBV and CBF as always the same, which is clearly not a reasonable conclusion. Nevertheless, the CBV data themselves appear to enable the inference of meaningful lateralization assignments, thereby suggesting that bolus tracking MR data may be able to make a contribution to seizure lateralization in such patients. It might reasonably be argued that the additional information available from CBF measures in such studies would strengthen this conclusion.

Discussion: Perfusion in Epilepsy

Information regarding cerebral perfusion has long been recognized as important in the investigation of partial epilepsy. MR perfusion imaging therefore appears to offer the attractive prospect of obtaining such information non-invasively, including the avoidance of ionizing radiation.

The benign nature of the investigation also lends itself to the performance of serial studies, which could enable an understanding of the evolution or progression of a condition. However, it should be acknowledged that there are a number of disadvantages to obtaining perfusion data by means of MRI.

The most obvious drawback is the probable difficulty in the majority of patients of obtaining *ictal* information. It has become well established that SPECT is far more successful in correctly identifying an epileptogenic region when both *interictal* and *ictal* studies are combined, while *interictal* SPECT in particular does not have a high success rate when used independently. Therefore, the information that perfusion MRI will be able to provide will be limited in many cases, although it remains to be seen whether the potential improvement in image quality of MRI compared to SPECT will produce more robust interictal findings.

It is also worth noting that, in terms of data processing, the procedure involved in obtaining perfusion MRI measures is unlikely to be as robust in the near future as for the equivalent DTI parameters. The acquisition of the images required for bolus tracking perfusion imaging will be relatively trivial on any scanner equipped to perform EPI, which should include virtually every recent scanner. EPI (or some equivalent very rapid acquisition method) is frequently used to collect the data, since a time resolution of less than 2 seconds is required to delineate the concentration-time curve adequately. As a result, to enable the acquisition of multiple slices within this time frame, each image must be acquired extremely quickly. Although not used in the epilepsy work discussed above, there are many reports related to ischemia (the major application of bolus tracking to date) showing multislice acquisition of such EPI data, indicating that this acquisition software is widely available.

The required data analysis, however, presents a far more difficult problem than that for DTI. Full analysis of bolus tracking data requires the deconvolution of Equation (1) (see above) to enable maps of CBF, CBV, and MTT to be calculated. However, this is not a trivial procedure to carry out reliably in an automated way. Currently, those research groups that use this technique extensively generally perform the data processing offline from the scanner, using some form of in-house software. It is perhaps significant in this respect that, in the reports discussed above, no such calculations were performed, with the consequence that none of the bolus tracking studies reported true CBF values.

Among a number of problems with automating such a process is the difficulty in identifying suitable image voxels in which to measure the arterial input function (AIF), which is required to perform the deconvolution. It is essential that such voxels are placed within a region that samples the arterial concentration of contrast agent, which usually requires careful manual placement of the sampled regions within a large artery (e.g. the middle cerebral artery) while minimizing partial volume with surrounding tissue. (Note: it is also essential if deconvolution analysis is planned that one of the multislice images acquired is positioned to contain such an artery with minimal through-slice partial volume.) Significant partial volume error will result in significant underestimation of the AIF, with corresponding overestimation of the CBF. Recent work by Alsop et al (54). suggests a potential method for the measurement of a 'local' AIF, which may improve current approaches, although this work is at an early stage at present.

A further requirement in bolus tracking is that the data analysis is confined to the first passage of the bolus of contrast and that the effects of recirculated contrast are in some way removed or ignored. This can be done by fitting the early part of the concentration-time curve to a model function (usually a gamma-variate function), and extending the resulting function to longer times. Such a fitting routine is difficult to perform robustly on a pixel-by-pixel basis, because of low signal-to-noise. The alternative to fitting the curve is to analyze only that part of the curve that precedes the recirculation peak; this not only requires information regarding the optimal time point at which to stop the analysis but also results in an underestimation of the CBV, since CBV is obtained from the area under the curve and the whole curve is no longer sampled.

The problems associated with automated analysis have delayed the implementation by scanner manufacturers of software capable of performing a full analysis of bolus tracking data. It is probable that this situation will change in the future, although care should be taken in using data that have been generated on a 'black-box' basis, since there is great potential for error in converting the raw MR images into perfusion parameter maps.

The alternative approach to MR perfusion imaging, namely ASL, has a greater potential than bolus tracking to be able to produce absolute values of CBF but does not provide information on CBV. The issue of absolute quantification is arguably not so important in epilepsy applications because of the potentially confounding effect of anticonvulsant medication on global CBF (see above), which may necessitate normalization to a reference CBF in order to identify focal abnormalities robustly.

The practical difficulties that might be encountered in producing reliable ASL parameter maps are somewhat different from those described for bolus tracking. Unlike the case of bolus tracking, the acquisition of the required images is much more demanding in ASL. Since essentially the data are produced by taking the difference between control images and perfusion-labeled images (with the difference expected to be of the order of 1% at a field strength of 1.5 T), careful setting up of the MR acquisition sequence on a particular scanner is required, in combination with very good scanner stability. In addition, the suggested solutions to transit time problems (discussed in the background section) for both continuous ASL and pulsed ASL each result in a reduction of the magnetic label applied to the flowing blood, with the consequence of a further reduction in the subtraction signal, particularly when blood flow is very low.

It remains to be seen whether the problems relating to transit time will prove significant in the low flow situations encountered *interictally*. In the interim, although current studies have suggested that it is feasible to obtain laterality information by means of ASL measurements, further data are required to establish the reliability of the method in the study of patients with epilepsy.

SUMMARY

Diffusion tensor imaging can provide measures of both average diffusivity and FA, and appears to provide further information in patients with epilepsy than that available from conventional MRI, with the identification of additional abnormalities both in patients with structural lesions and in those with partial seizures who have unremarkable conventional MRI scans. The clinical utility of these methods remains to be established. It is to be hoped that, with the increasingly wide availability of MR scanners capable of acquiring such data, in combination with the provision of software to calculate meaningful parameters, the clinical utility may gradually become established.

Although it is a desirable end that DTI tractography may be used to identify the connectivity of epileptogenic areas and epileptic networks, it is uncertain at present whether it will be feasible to obtain adequate information to identify the functionally relevant tracts with sufficient reliability. There are a number of technical problems that make this difficult, in particular related to signal-to-noise ratio, spatial resolution, and partial volume issues. However, perhaps the most difficult problem is to resolve crossing fibers, for which there is to date no practically feasible yet robust solution. This is a very active area of research, however, and it is possible that, in the coming years, a viable method will be found to extract fiber directionality from water diffusivity information that is sufficiently robust to the above problems for clinical use.

Perfusion imaging provides the promise of being able to make acute and serial studies of cerebral blood delivery, which may make a useful contribution to seizure lateralization and localization in the evaluation of patients with partial seizures. This is to some extent already feasible for interictal studies and it is likely that the availability and reliability of the perfusion information will improve. However, it is well known that the efficacy of interictal information in identifying epileptogenic regions is limited. A significant practical limitation, therefore, will continue to be the difficulty in obtaining *ictal* MR perfusion information, for which patient confusion and movement associated with seizures will frequently present a considerable difficulty.

REFERENCES

1. Turner R, Le Bihan D. Single shot diffusion imaging at 2 Tesla. *J Magn Reson* 1990;86:445–452.
2. Tanner JE, Stejskal EO. Restricted self-diffusion of protons in colloidal systems by the pulsed-gradient, spin-echo method. *J Chem Phys* 1968;49:1768–1778.
3. Basser PJ, Pierpaoli C. A simplified method to measure the diffusion tensor from seven MR images. *Magn Reson Med* 1998;39:928–934.
4. Basser PJ, Mattiello J, LeBihan D. Estimation of the effective self-diffusion tensor from the NMR spin echo. *J Magn Reson B* 1994;103:247–254.
5. Pierpaoli C, Basser PJ. Towards a quantitative assessment of diffusion anisotropy. *Magn Reson Med* 1996;36:893–906.
6. Mori S, Crain BJ, Chacko VP, van Zijl PCM. Three-dimensional tracking of axonal projections in the brain by magnetic resonance imaging. *Ann Neurol* 1999;45:255–269.
7. Jones DK, Simmons A, Williams SCR, Horsfield MA. Non-invasive assessment of axonal fiber connectivity in the human brain via diffusion tensor MRI. *Magn Reson Med* 1999;42:37–41.
8. Conturo TE, Lori NF, Cull TS, et al. Tracking neuronal fiber pathways in the living human brain. *Proc Natl Acad Sci USA* 1999;96:10422–10427.
9. Basser PJ, Pajevic S, Pierpaoli C, et al. In vivo fiber tractography using DT-MRI data. *Magn Reson Med* 2000;44:625–632.
10. Tournier J-D, Calamante F, Gadian DG, Connelly A. Diffusion-weighted magnetic resonance imaging fibre-tracking using a front evolution algorithm. *Neuroimage* 2003;20:276–288.
11. Wedeen VJ, Reese TG, Tuch DS, et al. Mapping fibre orientation spectra in cerebral white matter with Fourier-transform diffusion MRI. In: Proceedings of the International Society for Magnetic Resonance in Medicine, 2000.
12. Tuch DS, Reese TG, Wiegell MR, et al. High angular resolution diffusion imaging reveals intravoxel white matter fiber heterogeneity. *Magn Reson Med* 2002;48:577–582.
13. Moseley ME, Cohen Y, Mintorovitch J, et al. Early detection of regional cerebral ischemia in cats: comparison of diffusion- and T2-weighted MRI and spectroscopy. *Magn Reson Med* 1990;14:330–460.
14. Benveniste H, Hedlund LW, Johnson GA. Mechanism of the detection of acute cerebral ischaemia in rats by diffusion-weighted magnetic resonance microscopy. *Stroke* 1992;23:746–754.
15. Busza AL, Allen L, King MD, et al. Diffusion-weighted imaging studies of cerebral ischemia in gerbils. Potential relevance to energy failure. *Stroke* 1992;23:1602–1612.
16. Latour LL, Svoboda K, Mitra PP, Sotak CH. Time-dependent diffusion of water in a biological model system. *Proc Natl Acad Sci USA* 1994;91:1229–1233.
17. Norris DG, Niendorf T, Leibfritz D. Healthy and infarcted brain tissues studied at short diffusion times: the origins of apparent restriction and the reduction in apparent diffusion coefficient. *NMR Biomed* 1994;7:304–310.
18. Helpern JA, Ordridge RJ, Knight RA. The effect of cell membrane water permeability on the apparent diffusion coefficient of water. In: Proceedings of the Society for Magnetic Resonance in Medicine 1992:1201.
19. Wick M, Nagatomo Y, Prielmeier F, Frahm J. Alteration of intracellular metabolite diffusion in rat brain in vivo during ischemia and reperfusion. *Stroke* 1995;26:1930–1933.
20. Neil JJ, Duong TQ, Ackerman JJH. Evaluation of intracellular diffusion in normal and globally-ischemic rat brain via 133Cs NMR. *Magn Reson Med* 1996;35:329–335.
21. Calamante F, Thomas DL, Pell GS, et al. Measuring cerebral blood flow using magnetic resonance techniques. *J Cereb Blood Flow Metab* 1999;19:701–735.
22. Rosen BR, Belliveau JW, Vevea JM, Brady TJ. Perfusion imaging with NMR contrast agents. *Magn Reson Med* 1990;14:249–265.
23. Ostergaard L, Weisskoff RM, Chesler DA, et al. High resolution measurement of cerebral blood flow using intravascular tracer bolus passages. Part I. Mathematical approach and statistical analysis. *Magn Reson Med* 1996;36:715–725.
24. Sorensen AG. What is the meaning of quantitative CBF? *Am J Neuroradiol* 2001;22:235–236.
25. Calamante F, Gadian DG, Connelly A. Quantification of perfusion using bolus tracking MRI in stroke. Assumptions, limitations, and potential implications for clinical use. *Stroke* 2002;33:1146–1151.

26. Ostergaard L, Johannsen P, Poulsen PH, et al. Cerebral blood flow measurements by magnetic resonance imaging bolus tracking: comparison with [O-15] H₂O positron emission tomography in humans. *J Cereb Blood Flow Metab* 1998;18:935–940.

27. Calamante F, Gadian DG, Connelly A. Delay and dispersion effects in dynamic susceptibility contrast MRI: simulations using Singular Value Decomposition. *Magn Reson Med* 2000;44:466–473.

28. Weisskoff RM, Chesler DA, Boxerman JL, Rosen BR. Pitfalls in MR measurement of tissue blood flow with intravascular tracers: Which mean transit-time? *Magn Reson Med* 1993;29:553–559.

29. Perthen JE, Calamante F, Gadian DG, Connelly A. Is quantification of bolus tracking MRI reliable without deconvolution? *Magn Reson Med* 2002;47:61–67.

30. Detre JA, Leigh JS, Williams DS, Koretsky AP. Perfusion imaging. *Magn Reson Med* 1992;23:37–45.

31. Williams DS, Detre JA, Leigh JS, Koretsky AP. Magnetic resonance imaging of perfusion using spin inversion of arterial water. *Proc Natl Acad Sci USA* 1992;89:212–216.

32. Edelman RR, Siewart B, Darby DG, et al. Qualitative mapping of cerebral blood-flow and functional localization with echo-planar MR-imaging and signal targeting with alternating radio-frequency. *Radiology* 1994;192:513–520.

33. Kwong KK, Chesler DA, Weisskoff RM, et al. MR perfusion studies with T1-weighted echo-planar imaging. *Magn Reson Med* 1995;34: 878–887.

34. Kim SG. Quantification of relative cerebral blood flow change by flow-sensitive alternating inversion recovery (FAIR) technique – application to functional mapping. *Magn Reson Med* 1995;34:293–301.

35. Barbier EL, Lamalle L, Decorps M. Methodology of brain perfusion imaging. *J Magn Reson Imaging* 2001;13:496–520.

36. Wong EC, Buxton RB, Frank LR. Quantitative imaging of perfusion using a single subtraction (QUIPSS and QUIPSS II). *Magn Reson Med* 1998;39:702–708.

37. Alsop DC, Detre JA. Reduced transit time sensitivity in non-invasive magnetic resonance imaging of human cerebral blood-flow. *J Cereb Blood Flow Metab* 1996;16:1236–1249.

38. Zhong J, Petroff OAC, Prichard JW, Gore JC. Changes in water diffusion and relaxation properties of rat cerebrum during status epilepticus. *Magn Reson Med* 1993;30:241–246.

39. Nakasu Y, Nakasu S, Morikawa S, et al. Diffusion-weighted MR in experimental sustained seizures elicited with kainic acid. *Am J Neuroradiol* 1995;16:1185–1192.

40. Zhong J, Petroff OAC, Pleban LA, et al. Reversible reproducible reduction of brain water apparent diffusion coefficient by cortical electroshocks. *Magn Reson Med* 1997;37:1–6.

41. Flacke S, Wullner U, Keller E, et al. Reversible changes in echo planar perfusion- and diffusion-weighted MRI in status epilepticus. *Neuroradiology* 2000;42:92–95.

42. Calistri V, Caramia F, Bianco F, et al. Visualization of evolving status epilepticus with diffusion and perfusion MR imaging. *Am J Neuroradiol* 2003;24:671–673.

43. Hugg JW, Butterworth EJ, Kuzniecky RI. Diffusion mapping applied to mesial temporal lobe epilepsy: Preliminary observations. *Neurology* 1999;53:173–176.

44. Wieshmann UC, Clark CA, Symms MR, et al. Water diffusion in the human hippocampus in epilepsy. *Magn Reson Imaging* 1999;17:29–36.

45. Mori S, Itoh R, Zhang J, et al. Diffusion tensor imaging of the developing mouse brain. *Magn Reson Med* 2001;46:18–23.

46. Wieshmann UC, Clark CA, Symms MR, et al. Reduced anisotropy of water diffusion in structural cerebral abnormalities demonstrated with diffusion tensor imaging. *Magn Reson Imaging* 1999b;17:1269–1274.

47. Eriksson SH, Rugg-Gunn FJ, Symms MR, et al. Diffusion tensor imaging in patients with epilepsy and malformations of cortical development. *Brain* 2001;124:617–626.

48. Rugg-Gunn FJ, Eriksson SH, Symms MR, et al. Diffusion tensor imaging of cryptogenic and acquired partial epilepsies. *Brain* 2001; 124:627–636.

49. Warach S, Levin JM, Schomer DL, et al. Hyperperfusion of ictal seizure focus demonstrated by MR perfusion imaging. *Am J Neuroradiol* 1994;15:965–968.

50. Grant PE, He J, Halpern EF, et al. Frequency and clinical context of decreased apparent diffusion coefficient reversal in the human brain. *Radiology* 2001;221:43–50.

51. Wolf RL, Alsop DC, Levy-Reis I, et al. Detection of mesial temporal lobe hypoperfusion in patients with temporal lobe epilepsy by use of arterial spin labeled perfusion MR imaging. *Am J Neuroradiol* 2001;22:1334–1341.

52. Liu H-L, Kochunov P, Hou J, et al. Perfusion-weighted imaging of interictal hypoperfusion in temporal lobe epilepsy using FAIR-HASTE: Comparison with H₂¹⁵O PET measurements. *Magn Reson Med* 2001;45:431–435.

53. Wu RH, Bruening R, Noachter S, et al. MR measurement of regional relative cerebral blood volume in epilepsy. *J Magn Reson Imaging* 1999;9:435–440.

54. Alsop DC, Wedmid A, Schlaug G. Defining a local input function for perfusion quantification with bolus contrast MRI. In: Proceedings of the International Society for Magnetic Resonance in Medicine 2002:659.

CHAPTER 13

Magnetic Resonance Spectroscopy

Hoby Hetherington, Ognen Petroff, Graeme D. Jackson, Ruben I. Kuzniecky,
Regula S. Briellmann and R. Mark Wellard

For many clinicians and radiologists, magnetic resonance spectroscopy (MRS) has long held great promise of being able to noninvasively measure the biochemistry of the living brain. Available for measurement are many important chemical properties such as metabolite and neurotransmitter concentrations, lactate, pH, energy metabolism, and even metabolic rate constants that are fundamental to brain function and of importance in disease. It is fair to say that, in typical practice, MRS has become a routine and important test in only a few situations, in a few centers, with a limited range of applied techniques and for a limited range of diseases. The future importance of this technology is only vaguely recognized, if at all.

While the acquisition of MR spectra is possible on many MR systems, only a small amount of the potential of MRS is currently used. As this field matures, a range of measurements of clinical importance will become available. Clarifying the potential as well as the issues involved in achieving this is the aim of this chapter.

The chapter is divided into three sections, which deal with issues that we believe are essential information for a proper understanding of MRS. The first two sections review the basics of MR physics and brain biochemical systems. The third section reviews the clinical applications of MRS.

The first section, by Hoby Hetherington, deals primarily with determining what MRS can measure and the underlying MR physics of how this can be achieved. This is fundamental to understanding what is possible with MRS and what the limitations of these measurements are.

The second section, by Ognen Petroff, provides a detailed discussion of the biochemistry of the systems that determine the concentrations of substances that are measured by MRS. As well as highlighting the important window to brain biochemistry that MRS provides, this information is essential for understanding and interpreting changes in brain chemistry that are measured by MRS.

The third section, by Graeme Jackson, Ruben Kuzniecky, Regula Briellmann and Mark Wellard, reviews the current state of the literature in MRS of epilepsy. This section emphasizes clinical applications and how information from MRS can inform clinical decisions.

Magnetic Resonance Spectroscopy: Principles and Techniques

Hoby Hetherington

OVERVIEW

In-vivo MRS offers the unique ability to noninvasively measure the chemical composition of living tissue. Although there are a large number of NMR visible nuclei, the most commonly used in the in vivo human brain are ^{1}H, ^{31}P, and ^{13}C. In the next three sections, the information content and major methods used for spectroscopic studies in the brain will be discussed. Unlike other forms of spectroscopy, the physics underlying MR spectroscopy offers the unique ability to 'engineer' acquisition methods to optimize the measurement of different compounds. Therefore we will also discuss the rationale, advantages, and limitations behind the major acquisition methods used. The text does not try to provide an exhaustive theoretical background for the development of new sequences but rather focuses on the primary technical and biologic issues that govern the selection of different methods.

^{1}H SPECTROSCOPY

^{1}H Information Content

Because of its high sensitivity and it wealth of information content, ^{1}H spectroscopy has become the most widely used nucleus for the investigation of in-vivo metabolism in the human brain. ^{1}H spectroscopy offers the unique ability to monitor a variety of metabolites and processes ranging from markers of neuronal injury and loss (N-acetyl aspartate) through the product of anaerobic metabolism (lactate) to direct measures of the primary inhibitory and excitatory neurotransmitters (gamma-amino butyric acid – GABA – and glutamate). However this wealth of information, when combined with the relatively small range of frequencies over which these resonances occur, results in substantial spectral overlap, making quantification of the resonances difficult. Therefore a variety of acquisition methods specific for individual resonances or groups of resonances have been developed. In general, no single method is capable of delivering optimal sensitivity and specificity for all major resonances of interest simultaneously. The investigator must therefore often tailor the particular study to the compound or class of compounds most relevant to the investigatory goals.

In the following sections we will discuss the major methods available and their biologic information content. As a whole, there are three broad groups of resonances of interest for neuroscientists:

- non-J-coupled high-concentration singlet resonances, which can be measured using relatively simple and widely available methods
- J-coupled resonances of high concentration that require either high-performance hardware or specially optimized sequences and sophisticated postacquisition analysis routines
- J-modulating resonances of low concentration that require more sophisticated acquisition methods.

High-concentration Singlets

The most widely used resonances, because of their relatively large brain concentration (11–30 mmol/l in proton intensity), biologic significance, and ease of acquisition, are N-acetyl aspartate (NAA), creatine (Cr), and choline (Ch). For neurologic studies, NAA, which is synthesized only in neuronal mitochondria (1), has proved to be a valuable marker for assessing neuronal loss and damage (2–4). Because of its greater content in astrocytes in comparison to neurons (1), elevations in the creatine resonance, reflecting the summation of phosphocreatine and creatine, have been interpreted as reflecting gliosis (5–7). Choline has largely been used as a marker for elevated membrane turnover (6, 7). Epileptogenic regions are typically characterized by a combination of neuronal loss and damage with or without reactive gliosis. As such, NAA is typically decreased while creatine and choline may remain unchanged or become elevated (8,9). Thus, either measures of NAA content or ratios of NAA:Cr, NAA:Ch, and NAA:(Cr+Ch) have been used to identify regions of metabolic abnormalities (8, 9).

Although these compounds contain a number of different ^{1}H resonances, the most commonly used are 2.02 ppm resonance of NAA, the 3.02 ppm resonance of creatine and the 3.17 ppm resonance of choline (Fig. 13.1). All three of these resonances are not J-coupled. Thus these ^{1}H nuclei appear as single, narrow resonances, reflecting the summed intensity of all ^{1}H nuclei in the group (three for NAA and creatinine; nine for choline). In addition to their narrow resonance structures and high multiplicity, the concentrations of NAA, creatine and choline are amongst the highest in human brain.

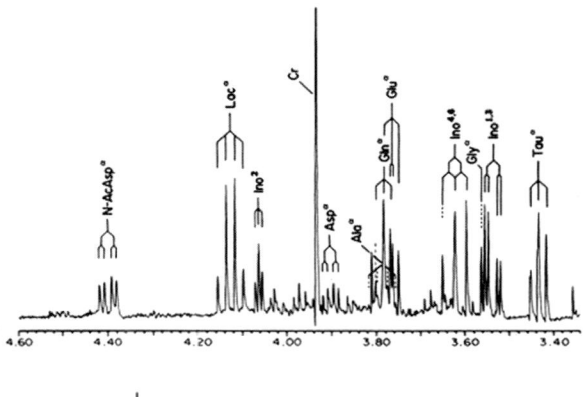

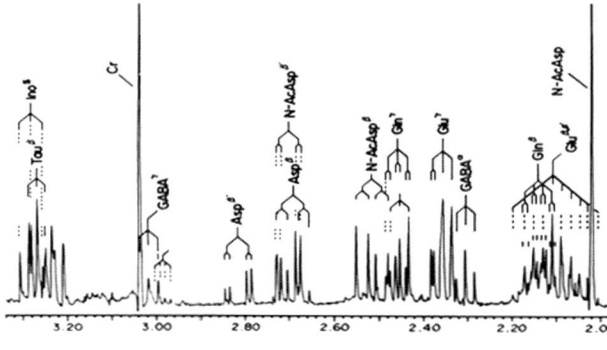

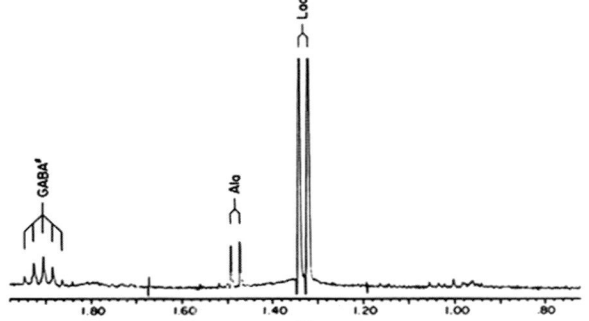

FIG. 13.1. High-resolution spectrum from a perchloric acid extract of rat brain showing the major ^{1}H resonances. (Courtesy of KL Behar; with permission from Behar and Ogino 1991 (10).)

Quantitative studies of NAA, creatinine and choline have reported in-vivo cerebral levels of approximately 10 mmol/l for NAA, 6–9 mmol/l for creatine, and 1.2–1.8 mmol/l for choline, depending upon tissue type (gray vs white matter) and cerebral location (cerebrum vs cerebellum) (11, 12). Thus, combining the tissue contents with the multiplicity of the resonance (three for NAA and Cr) and (nine for Ch), the in-vivo resonances of these three compounds reflect ^{1}H intensities of 11–30 mmol/l.

High-concentration Multiplets

Amongst the next highest molecules in concentration in the human brain are glutamate and glutamine. Glutamate is the primary excitatory neurotransmitter in mammalian brain. Additionally, glutamate occupies a key role in linking

neurotransmission and energetics via its role in the glutamate–glutamine cycle in neurons and astrocytes and its interconvertability with α-ketoglutarate, a key intermediate in the tricarboxylic acid (TCA) cycle. Glutamine occupies a crucial role in returning carbon equivalents of neurotransmitter glutamate taken up by astrocytes back to neurons and detoxification of excess ammonia loads. Thus measurements of glutamate and glutamine can provide insight into imbalances in glutamate metabolism and hyperexcitability in patients with epilepsy.

Glutamate demonstrates three non-exchangeable ^{1}H resonances, which appear as triplets or higher-order multiplets depending upon the field strength. The most commonly used resonance for quantification is the 2.35 ppm resonance that appears at high field as a triplet with resonance intensities of approximately 1:2:1 (see Fig. 13.1). Given its multiplicity of 2, and concentration of 5–10 mmol/l depending upon location and tissue type, a total intensity of 10–20 mmol/l is distributed across the three lines. Thus the central line glutamate is smaller than that of NAA by a factor of 3–6. The structure of glutamine is similar to that of glutamate; its upfield resonances are also seen as triplets and higher order multiplets. Because of the lower concentration of glutamine in the brain (3–6 mmol/l), the center line of its 2.48 ppm resonance is a factor of 5–10 smaller than that of NAA.

As described, J-coupling splits these resonances into multiple lines, which reduces the overall sensitivity and broadens the spectral range, making overlap with other molecules and each other problematic. Typically this overlap can be accounted for only through sophisticated postacquisition modeling programs using extensive *a priori* assumptions, very high signal-to-noise ratio (SNR) spectra and system/acquisition-dependent variables (13). Additionally, the J-coupling also results in phase modulation of the individual resonance lines, such that, depending upon the echo time used, the resonance lines may be either positive, negative, or near zero (Fig. 13.2). To overcome this effect, most investigators have typically used sequences with very short echo times so as to acquire the data before significant J-modulation occurs. This both limits the type of sequence that can be used to acquire the data and places greater demands on the MR system hardware.

Low-concentration Multiplets

In addition to the compounds already described, other significant metabolites of interest for epileptologists include GABA, lactate and beta-hydroxybutyrate (BHB). GABA, the primary inhibitory neurotransmitter, is known to be globally decreased in a variety of epilepsies. Lactate, the end product of anaerobic glycolysis, is known to accumulate during seizures in animal models and has been observed to remain elevated in the immediate postictal period in humans (14). BHB is the primary alternate fuel for the brain when glucose levels are depressed and the metabolic target of the ketogenic diet, a treatment used for childhood epilepsies.

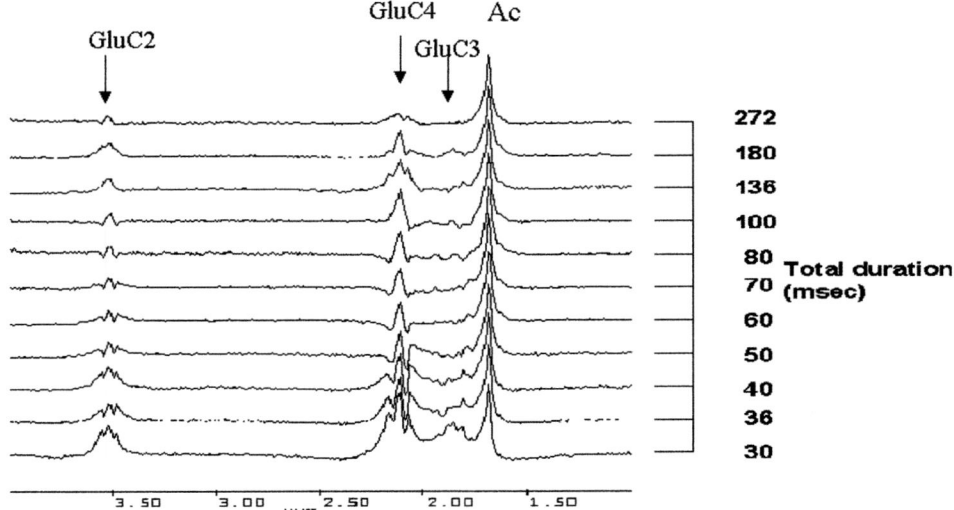

FIG. 13.2. Spectra acquired with varying echo times from a sample of glutamate and acetate at 4.1 T, showing the J-modulation characteristics of glutamate as a function of echo time.

Like glutamate and glutamine, GABA, lactate, and BHB are also J-coupled. Specifically, GABA features three upfield resonances (two triplets and a higher-order multiplet). Lactate has two resonances, a doublet and a quartet, while BHB has three resonances, a doublet, a quartet, and a higher-order multiplet. However, unlike glutamate and glutamine, their concentrations in the human brain are typically at or below 1 mmol/l. Brain GABA levels have been estimated to be 1–1.2 mmol/l, while cerebral lactate levels are typically of the order of 0.5–0.7 mmol/l. BHB is typically well below 100 μmol/l, except during ketosis, when brain levels may reach 0.5–1.0 mmol/l. Given the range in multiplicities, three for the 1.33 ppm lactate and 1.20 ppm BHB doublets and two for the 3.00 ppm GABA triplet, the resonance intensities are a factor of 20–40 smaller than those of NAA (see Fig. 13.1).

Because of the low concentration of these compounds and their overlap with other resonances such as creatine and macromolecules, their detection using standard sequences is prone to large uncertainties. To overcome this limitation, advanced MR methods known as spectral editing sequences have been developed (15–18). These sequences make use of the unique J-coupling properties of the individual resonances and are not available on most clinical systems. Additionally, because of the low concentration, SNR limitations restrict the minimum volume resolution achievable. Thus to date most of the studies measuring GABA, lactate, and BHB in the in-vivo human brain have been performed using surface coils, which sample peripheral regions of the brain.

Water Suppression and Lipid Suppression

As described, the ^{1}H spectrum contains a wealth of metabolic information. However the metabolites of interest

vary in effective concentrations ranging from 1 to 30 mmol/l in ^{1}H intensity. Overshadowing these resonances are the tissue water signal, representing 70–110 mol/l ^{1}H intensity, and the molar signals arising from lipids. Fortunately, the lipid signals arising from brain tissue under normal conditions are immobile, such that they are extremely broad, decay rapidly, and are generally not detectable. However, the tissue water and extracerebral lipids arising from muscle and fat are detectable, and represent large potentially interfering resonances. Independent of which resonances are to be observed, the tissue water and the extracerebral lipid resonances must always be suppressed.

Water Suppression

To date the most widely used methods for water suppression rely on frequency difference between the tissue water signal at 4.67 ppm and the most commonly observed metabolites (0.9–4.1 ppm). The most common method for water suppression (CHESS) uses a frequency-selective excitation pulse followed by a large gradient pulse (19). This has two effects. First the radiofrequency (RF) pulse reduces the amount of longitudinal water magnetization that can be excited and detected by the remainder of the pulse sequence. Second, the gradient pulse disperses the water magnetization in the transverse plane over all available angles, such that its vector sum is zero. The extent to which the water resonance is suppressed is directly determined by the extent to which a perfect 90 pulse is achieved. Inhomogeneities in the transmit system or errors in calibration can dramatically reduce the efficiency of water suppression. To overcome this limitation for moderate calibration errors or moderate inhomogeneities in the RF coils, a variety of multi-pulse

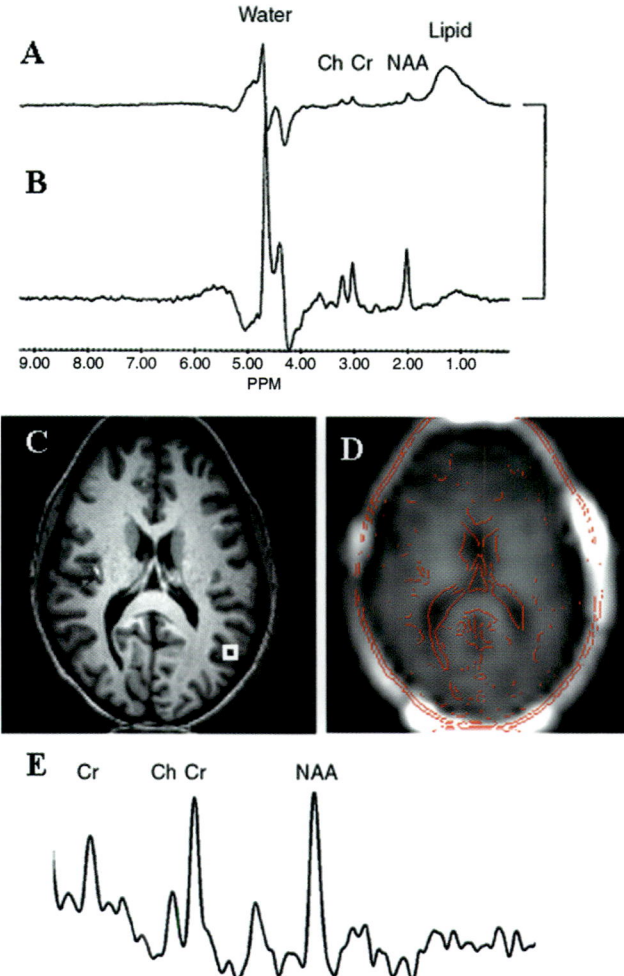

FIG. 13.3. A, B. Single-scan spectra from a 10 mm thick slice in human brain. The spectra in **A** were acquired without an initial non-selective inversion pulse, while **B** was acquired with an inversion pulse and 265 ms delay. The dominant extracranial lipid resonance seen in **A** is dramatically suppressed (>50-fold) in **B**. **C, D.** A scout image and the corresponding NAA image acquired using the single plane selection method. **E.** A spectrum (0.5 ml) from the cortical periphery; its location is designated in C by the white square. (With permission from Hetherington et al. 1994 (279).)

suppression schemes using varying flip angle have been developed (20).

An alternative approach uses specially crafted excitation or refocusing pulses to excite only the metabolites and avoid the water resonance. These pulses are simple to apply (simple block shapes and fixed delays) and because of their symmetry provide near complete water suppression independent of the applied RF field or any heterogeneities in it (Fig. 13.3A). The primary limitation to these pulses is that the spectral profile delivered is not rectangular, and small variations (<5–10%) in efficiency occur across the excitation band (21). Additionally, for resonances that are extremely close to the water resonance (<0.5 ppm away) the required pulse trains become too long in duration.

Lipid Suppression

Although brain lipids are largely invisible using conventional pulse sequences, extracerebral lipids arising from muscle and scalp are visible and can dominate the ¹H spectrum. To exclude these resonances, three primary methods have been employed. The most common method uses volume localization sequences to limit the acquired data to a three-dimensional (3D) volume entirely within the brain (see Clinical applications, below). By restricting the spectral data to brain tissue only, the extracerebral lipid resonances are eliminated.

However, in circumstances where peripheral cortical regions might be of interest, as in neocortical epilepsies, restriction of the volume of interest to a rectangle may preclude sampling of the desired region. For studies where the entire brain within a slice, or a peripheral cortical location, is to be evaluated, use of an alternative method can be more effective. Because of the short T1 and T2 relaxation times of the lipids relative to metabolites, sequences using either T1 or T2 weighting can be used to suppress lipid resonances. Early measurements using low field (1.5 T) systems often used long-echo (T_E 136 or 272 ms) sequences to suppress the lipid resonances. Unfortunately, because of the dramatic reduction of metabolite T2s with increasing field strength, this approach at higher fields (>3.0 T) results in substantial SNR loses, offsetting the gain in SNR afforded by higher-field magnets (21). Alternately, use of an initial inversion recovery pulse followed by an optimized delay can reduce the lipid signal by a factor of 40–100, while the metabolites are only reduced by a factor of 2 (Fig. 13.3A,B). This sequence when combined with spectroscopic imaging methods (see Clinical applications, below) can then be used to map metabolic abnormalities from peripheral cortical locations (Fig. 13.C–E).

Spectroscopic Localization

Unlike measurements of excised tissue, in-vivo measurements require some form of volume localization to provide interpretable data. Specifically, the region or regions of the brain giving rise to the acquired spectrum must be well defined. To date there are two primary schemes for providing localized spectra: single-voxel methods and spectroscopic imaging methods. For single-voxel methods a single moderately sized region of the brain (typically 2–8 ml) is acquired. Spectroscopic imaging methods simultaneously acquire many smaller voxels (0.5–2 ml) spanning a larger 2D or 3D region of the brain. By acquiring the data in spectroscopic imaging mode, each acquisition step contributes full SNR to every reconstructed location. To a first approximation, the minimum time required to achieve sufficient SNR for every voxel in the SI data set is equivalent to the amount of time required for the identical SNR from a similar-sized single-voxel acquisition. Acquisition of additional spectra from other locations using a single-voxel method would then require additional scans, thereby substantially lengthening the duration of the study.

Although the efficiency of collection and information content of spectroscopic imaging methods is substantially higher than single-voxel methods, the acquisition, analysis, and interpretation are also significantly more complex. Although most early MR studies of epilepsy utilized single-voxel methods (3), the desire to map the extent of the metabolic alterations has made spectroscopic imaging the method of choice for most recent studies of nonmodulating multiplets. Because of the complexities of pulse sequence design for measuring J-modulating resonances, to date most studies of glutamate and glutamine have used single-volume acquisitions. However, recently advanced methods for spectroscopic imaging studies of glutamate and glutamine have been reported, offering the advantages of regional mapping. Finally, because of the low concentrations of GABA, lactate and BHB, and the requirement for spectral editing sequences, virtually all these measurements have been performed using single-volume methods.

Single-volume Localization Methods

As described, the first attempts to acquire localized spectra from the human brain used acquisition methods that selected a single well-localized volume. Although a variety of methods and combination methods have been reported, the most common methods are stimulated echo acquisition mode (STEAM; Fig. 13.4A) and point resolved spectroscopy (PRESS; Fig. 13.4B) (19). These sequences are similar in that volume localization is achieved using three spatially selective pulses to define a cubic volume in three-dimensional space. Specifically, each pulse serves to excite or refocus a slice, such that at the conclusion of the sequence the three-dimensional rectangular volume reflecting the intersection or overlap of the three pulses yields detectable signal. However the methods differ in that STEAM acquires a stimulated echo using three slice-selective 90 pulses, whereas PRESS acquires a double spin echo using a slice-selective 90 pulse and two-slice selective 180 refocusing pulses. This difference allows STEAM sequences to be acquired with very short T_{ES} (<20 ms) but at a cost of a factor of 2 in SNR, whereas PRESS typically uses longer echo times (>40 ms) because of the requirement to form two spin echoes, but retains full SNR.

For STEAM, the 50% reduction in sensitivity is a significant limitation with regards to minimum volume sizes. Thus STEAM data are typically acquired using volumes of 2–8 ml. However the ability to acquire data with short T_{ES} (<20 ms) minimizes J-modulation losses in compounds such as glutamate and glutamine (22, 23). For PRESS-based acquisitions, the retention of full SNR makes it an ideal

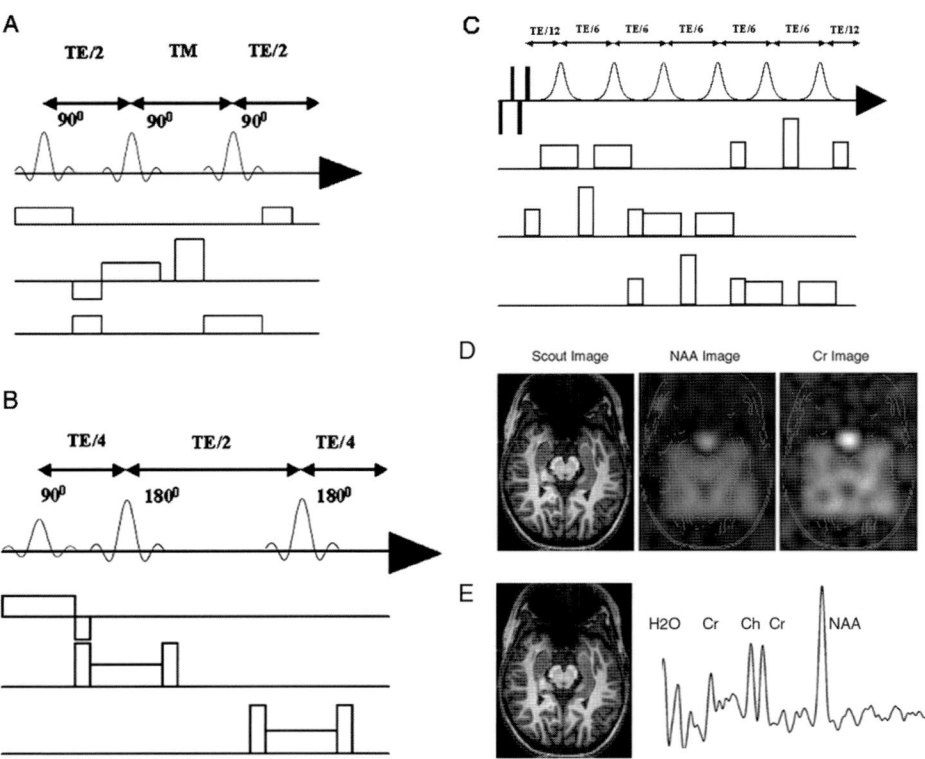

FIG. 13.4. Pulse sequence diagrams for (**A**) STEAM; (**B**) PRESS; and (**C**) Adiabatic LASER sequence, **D, E.** Data acquired using the sequence displayed in **C** from the human hippocampus, including NAA and creatinine images, and a representative spectrum from the hippocampus. The data were acquired at 4.0 T in the human hippocampus.

method when the total echo time is not a limitation and SNR is limiting (e.g. measurements of NAA, creatinine, and choline). Thus PRESS-based localization sequences are commonly used in conjunction with spectroscopic imaging when peripheral regions are not of interest. In this case the localization provided by the PRESS sequence is used to exclude unwanted regions such as near the sinuses and auditory canals, where significant susceptibility induced static field inhomogeneity artifacts occur.

At higher B_0 field strengths (>3 T) the electrical and geometric properties of the human head begin to dominate the achieved homogeneity of the RF coils used for transmission and detection (24). This inhomogeneity manifests itself by making the efficiency of pulse sequence spatially dependent. For PRESS acquisitions the B_1 dependence induces a $\sin^5(\theta)$ weighting where θ is the applied pulse angle. Thus, for inhomogeneities of 20%, a 27% reduction in signal amplitude can occur independent of any change in metabolite concentration. To overcome this effect, the PRESS sequence can be modified to utilize adiabatic refocusing pulses (25). These pulses achieve perfect refocusing over a wide range of RF values (θ), such that there is no degradation in signal creation efficiency. Figure 13.4C shows an example of an adiabatic version of the PRESS sequence, the LASER sequence, in which all three dimensions of localization are achieved using adiabatic refocusing pulses. When used with an adiabatic excitation pulse, the pulse angle dependence of this sequence is zero. This minimizes errors and uncertainties in quantification of the acquired spectra.

Spectroscopic Imaging

By simultaneously acquiring data from multiple volumes, spectroscopic imaging methods have become the method of choice for mapping metabolic alterations in the lateralization and localization of seizure foci using ^{1}H spectroscopy. To provide regional information, phase encoding gradients in one, two, or three dimensions are applied after the initial excitation pulse. The gradient strength is then linearly incremented such that the signal from each location varies in a sinusoidal fashion. The frequency of the sinusoidal variation varies linearly with distance from the center of the magnet. Fourier transformation of the data with respect to the gradient step in each of the acquired directions (one, two, or three dimensions), resolves the signals into their discrete sinusoidal frequencies, and thus their respective distances from the magnet center. For a 2D encoding sequence, where 32 encodes are acquired in each direction ($32 \times 32 = 1024$ encodes total) a 32×32 map is generated with a spectrum associated with each location in the map. The resonance intensity for a single species (e.g. NAA) can then be determined for each location and a metabolic image of NAA can be constructed. Typically, the data is then interpreted by super-imposing an anatomic image over the spectroscopic imaging map.

As described, spectroscopic imaging studies can be carried out in one, two, or three dimensions. However because of the requirement to obtain good water suppression over the entire acquired volume, and the strong B_0 inhomogeneities associated with locations adjacent to the oral cavity, 3D spectroscopic imaging of the entire brain is not generally possible. Additionally, even for 2D studies of a single plane, the susceptibility effects from the sinuses and ear canals limit homogeneity from slices taken along the temporal pole to the more medial locations, including the hippocampus and mid brain. Thus, single-voxel localization schemes such as PRESS and LASER are often used to select and extend 2D volume within a slice (eg $10 \times 8 \times 1$ cm) and spectroscopic imaging is then performed over that volume. Figure 13.4C–E show an example using the LASER sequence and a semiselective excitation pulse.

Measurements of *N*-Acetyl Aspartate, Creatine and Choline

As described, because of their high concentration, multiplicity, singlet structure, and absence of J-coupling, NAA, creatine and choline can be easily measured by routine spectroscopic imaging methods. Because of the ability to acquire more than a single location at a time and the variations in metabolite content as a function of tissue content, the accurate analysis of spectroscopic imaging data presents significant hurdles. At the resolutions typically attainable (0.5–2 ml) with volume head coils, significant mixing of gray matter, white matter, and cerebrospinal fluid (CSF) occurs, such that typically individual voxels span the gamut from pure gray matter to pure white matter.

Additionally, variations due to brain region, cerebrum versus cerebellum, can also have profound effects on the measured spectra. Although NAA has been reported to be relatively constant across gray and white matter (Table 13.1, Fig. 13.5), creatine is known to be 30–50% higher in gray matter as opposed to white matter. Thus, the common practice of reporting ratios of NAA or choline relative creatine, results in substantial variability on a voxel-by-voxel basis in normal controls. If this heterogeneity is not accounted for, false positives for the detection of neuronal loss/damage (higher than average gray matter, higher than average Cr/NAA) or false negatives (higher than average white matter, lower than average Cr/NAA) can occur when using the Cr/NAA ratio to identify epileptogenic regions (26).

To overcome this limitation and identify true differences in metabolic content it is necessary to compare each voxel to its anticipated control value, corrected for tissue content heterogeneity. This can be done by:

- determining the metabolite content of 'pure' gray and white matter voxels using a regression analysis
- determining the amount of gray matter, white matter and CSF in the voxel, and

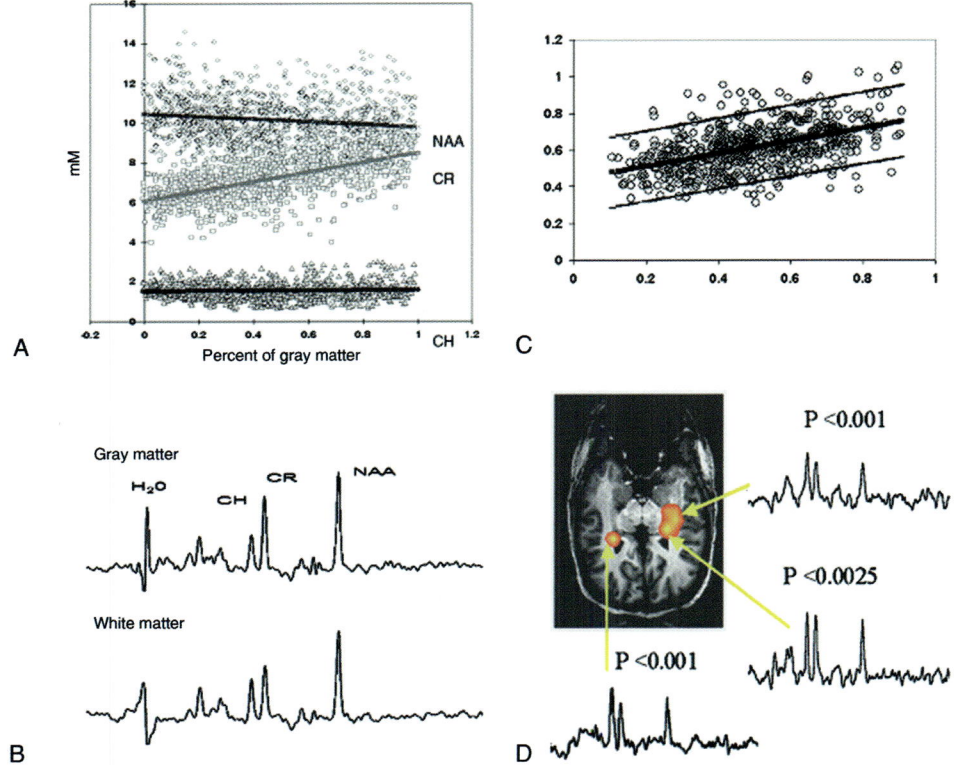

FIG. 13.5. A. Plot of the quantitative values of NAA, CR and CH as function of gray matter content. **B.** Representative spectra from gray and white matter, highlighting the higher levels of creatine in human gray matter. **C.** A regression analysis of CR/NAA as a function of gray matter content from the in-vivo human temporal lobe at the level of the hippocampus. **D.** The regression analysis was used to identify regions of metabolic abnormality (color overlays) in a patient with temporal lobe epilepsy. (With permission from Chu et al. 2000 (26).)

- combining these values to calculate a predicted metabolite content or ratio.

If this data is further combined with the statistical variation seen in normal controls, the significance of the differences from control for any given voxel in a patient study can then be assessed. This data can then be presented in terms of color-coded maps overlaid on the anatomic images for easy interpretation (Fig. 13.5).

Measurements of Glutamate and Glutamine

Because of their J-coupling, significant losses in intensity occur in glutamate and glutamine if sequences using even moderate echo times (T_E >20 ms) are used (Fig. 13.6A). Thus, most studies designed to measure these compounds have used STEAM sequences to acquire the data (Fig. 13.6B). However, because of the short echo, the STEAM spectra contain substantial contributions from macromolecular resonances (Fig. 13.6C) that distort the baseline under these resonances.

To overcome this limitation, three primary approaches have been employed. In one approach a 'metabolite suppressed' spectra, a spectrum containing only macromolecule components, can be acquired using a long inversion-recovery sequence. Subtraction of the resulting spectra provides a macromolecule-'free' spectrum simplifying spectral interpretation (Fig. 13.6D). However, subtraction of the 'metabolite suppressed spectra' reduces the overall SNR and lengthens the study time through requirement of a second scan. Alternately, other investigators have used reference spectra from normal controls to serve as a model for subtraction from subsequent data sets (27). However this assumes that the macromolecular components are invariant to disease process, which is not true in stroke (28) and unknown in epilepsy.

A third approach is to refocus or eliminate the effects of J-modulation, so as to allow longer echo evolution periods that reduce macromolecule components through T2 losses. Recently, two approaches for acquiring spectroscopic images of glutamate in the in-vivo human brain have been reported. The first method uses a novel pulse sequence in which the J-modulation of glutamate and glutamine is refocused by use of a polarization transfer or multiple-quantum transfer step (29). Although highly effective, the phase of the transverse magnetization at the time of the transfer pulse must be carefully adjusted, otherwise substantial SNR losses occur. More recently, an optimally timed LASER sequence has been used to acquire spectroscopic images of

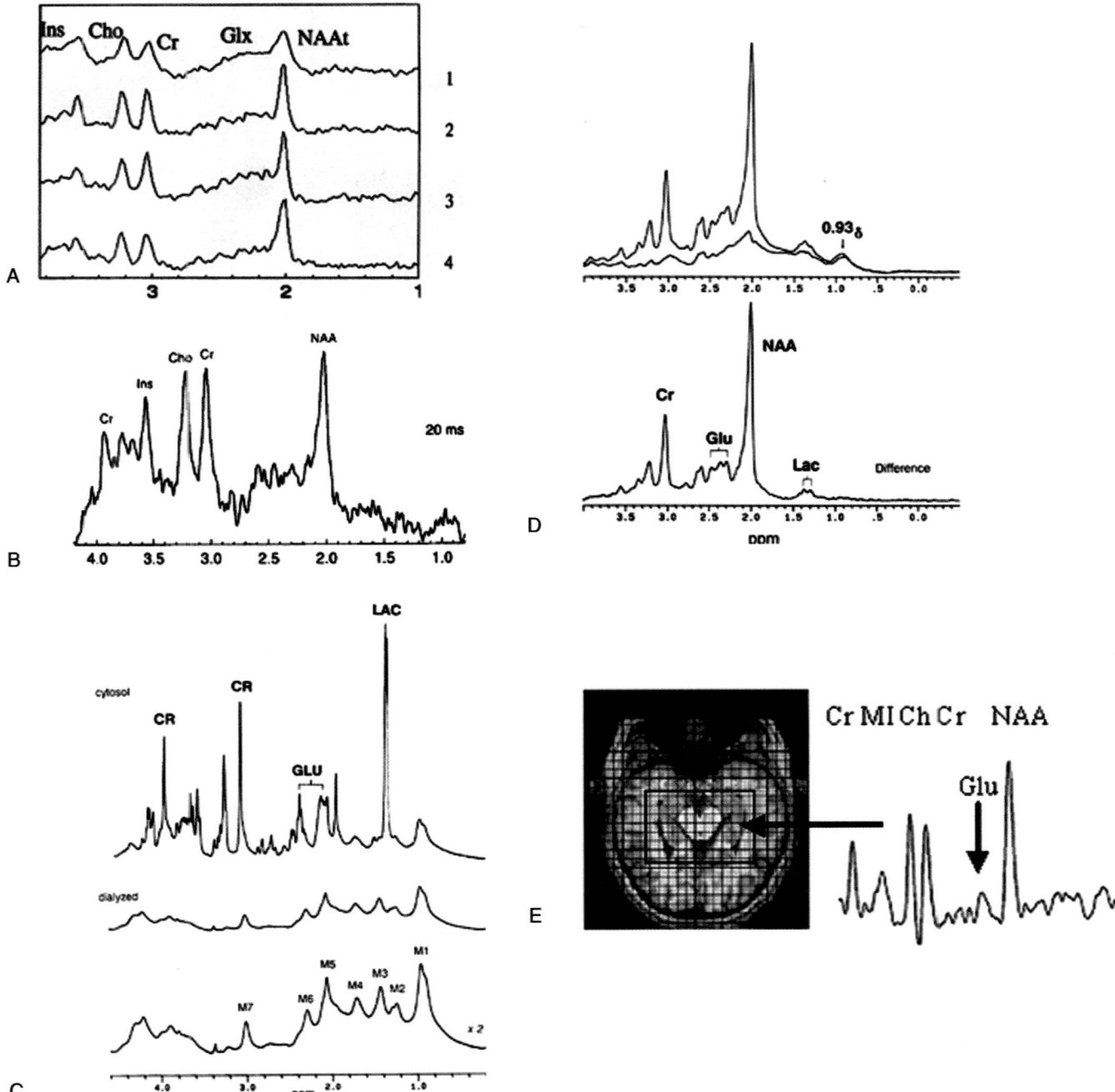

FIG. 13.6. A, B. Volume-localized spectra of glutamate from the human hippocampus acquired using PRESS and STEAM methods. **C.** High-resolution spectra acquired from an ex-vivo rat brain, demonstrating the presence of macromolecular resonances that appear in the high-molecular-weight dialyzed fraction of the brain. **D.** These resonances are suppressed in the in-vivo human brain. Specifically, the top spectrum represents both low-molecular-weight metabolites and high-molecular-weight macromolecular resonances, while the middle spectrum is acquired with an initial inversion pulse to suppress low-molecular-weight metabolite resonances. Differencing of these spectra yields the third spectrum, containing only the low-molecular-weight metabolites. Note the improvement in spectral resolution in the region about glutamate (2.35 ppm). **E.** A 1 ml spectrum acquired from the human hippocampus using a modified LASER method. (**A.** with permission from Simister et al. 2002; (23) **B.** with permission from Choi et al. 1999; (22) **C.** and **D.** with permission from Behar et al. 1994 (272).)

glutamate from the adult hippocampus (Fig. 13.6E). Because of the special characteristics of the adiabatic selection pulses, they serve not only to localize the signal but also to suppress homonuclear J-modulation through time averaging of the coupling Hamiltonian. By increasing

the echo time to 40–50 ms, these sequences suppress the macromolecular resonances beneath glutamate and glutamine, providing for flat baselines and removing the requirement for fitting or subtracting macromolecular contributions.

Independent of the acquisition or localization method used, at 1.5 T extensive overlap between the glutamate and glutamine resonances occurs, such that advanced fitting algorithms using *a priori* knowledge are required to interpret the data. Additionally, at 1.5 T the simple triplet systems seen for the C-4 resonances of glutamate and glutamine degenerate into strongly coupled systems, making fitting and analysis highly dependent on the acquisition parameters used. At higher field strengths (4 T and above), the glutamate and glutamine spin systems simplify, and approach a weak-coupling limit, displaying more classical coupling patterns. Even at 4 T, the most downfield line of the 2.35 glutamate resonance overlaps the most upfield line of the 2.48 ppm glutamine resonance. Thus high B_0 homogeneity is a requisite for accurate fitting of the acquired data.

Measurements of Gamma-amino Butyric Acid, Lactate, and Beta-hydroxybutyrate

Unlike glutamate and glutamine, the typically low concentrations of GABA, lactate, and BHB ($\approx$1 mmol/l or less) makes their observation challenging both for SNR and spectral overlap reasons. As described previously, the multiplet structure and low concentration results in a 20–40-fold reduction in peak intensity in comparison to NAA. To compensate for this increase, a similar 20–40 volume increase is required, e.g. 20–40 ml volumes or alternatively the use of a more sensitive detector, such as a surface coil. Surface coils of 7–10 cm diameter typically provide increases in SNR ranging from 3–5 over that of volume coils, bringing the require volumes sizes down to approximately 5–10 ml for the accurate measurement of submillimolar concentrations of GABA, lactate, and BHB. However the increased SNR comes at that sacrifice of limited penetration into the brain (typically $\approx$5 cm) from the brain surface. Thus to date most MR studies of GABA, lactate, and BHB have been performed using surface coils focusing on the occipital lobe.

Even when adequate SNR can be obtained, the GABA, lactate, and BHB resonances are overlapped by other resonances of much higher concentration, such as creatine, glutamate, glutamine, and macromolecule resonances. To overcome this limitation, specialized spectral editing sequences have been developed. These sequences utilize the unique J-coupling properties of the molecules to selective induce/inhibit J-modulation in the spectrum (Fig. 13.7A). For GABA, the 3.00 ppm C-4 resonance is typically the target for observation. On alternate scans a selective 180 pulse is applied to its J-coupled partner at 1.9 ppm. When the 180 pulse is applied with the correct timing interval, (one-quarter J or approximately 34 ms) the J-modulation is reversed, and the C-4 resonance appears as an in-phase triplet (Fig. 13.7B). When the pulse is not applied, the outer lines of the triplet undergo J-modulation and their phase inverts. Resonances such as creatine that are not J-coupled do not experience J-modulation and thus are not affected by the selective 180 pulse applied to the 1.9 ppm position.

When the spectra are subtracted only the outer lines of the GABA triplet remain, and the creatine resonance is eliminated.

Despite the elimination of the creatine resonance, a macromolecule resonance also overlaps the GABA position. Unfortunately the macromolecule resonance is also J-coupled with a similar coupling constant. To further complicate the problem, the macromolecule resonance's coupled partner is located at 1.7 ppm, only 0.2 ppm away from the GABA resonance. Thus the selective inversion pulse must be highly selective to avoid inverting the macromolecule resonance and thus also causing 'co-editing' of the macromolecule resonance.

At field strengths of 3 T and lower, because of the small frequency differences (less than 24 Hz) it is not possible to selectively edit only the GABA resonance. To overcome this approach, three methods have been reported. The first uses a 'metabolite suppressed' spectrum to subtract out the macromolecule component (30). However this method requires additional measurements and a spectral subtraction. A second approach uses a 'macromolecule-optimized' measurement and a mathematical correction to the GABA-edited spectrum based on the efficiencies and selectivity of the two inversion pulses (17) (Fig. 13.7C).

The third approach, and perhaps the simplest and most efficient, has been recently described by Henry (31). In this approach, the two spectra to be subtracted are acquired with the inversion pulse centered at 1.9 ppm, and 1.5 ppm. It is assumed that the 1.5 ppm centered inversion pulse does not affect the GABA 1.9 ppm resonance; therefore the 3.0 ppm GABA resonance should J-modulate normally. However the macromolecule resonance at 3.0 ppm should see the same degree of J-modulation in both acquisitions, since both inversion pulses are centered 0.2 ppm (1.9 and 1.5 ppm) away from its 1.7 ppm coupled partner. Thus automatically the macromolecule contributions to the final edited spectrum are canceled.

As a final note, the selectivity of the inversion pulse is critical in these approaches. Specifically, if the inversion pulse applied at 1.5 ppm also affects the 1.9 ppm resonance of GABA, the final edited GABA intensity will be reduced and, in the limit that the pulse selectivity is poor, the GABA resonance may be completely eliminated.

Unlike GABA, lactate and BHB have methyl resonances that are split by a single J-coupled ^1H partner, giving rise to two up-field doublet resonances at 1.33 and 1.21 ppm respectively. Although they are not obscured by other major cerebral metabolites, their position is overlapped by a number of macromolecule resonances and may be obscured by residual lipid resonances. When lactate levels are elevated by more than 200% (concentrations greater than 2 mmol/l), the resonance is usually detectable in standard localized PRESS and spectra as an inverted doublet at $h = 136$ ms and an upright doublet at 272 ms. To confirm the identity, typically both the $T_E = 136$ and $T_E = 272$ ms spectra are collected and the phase modulation of the resonance at 1.33 ppm is used to confirmation the resonance as lactate.

For more subtle changes in lactate or BHB, less than 1 mmol/l, spectral editing sequences offer the highest

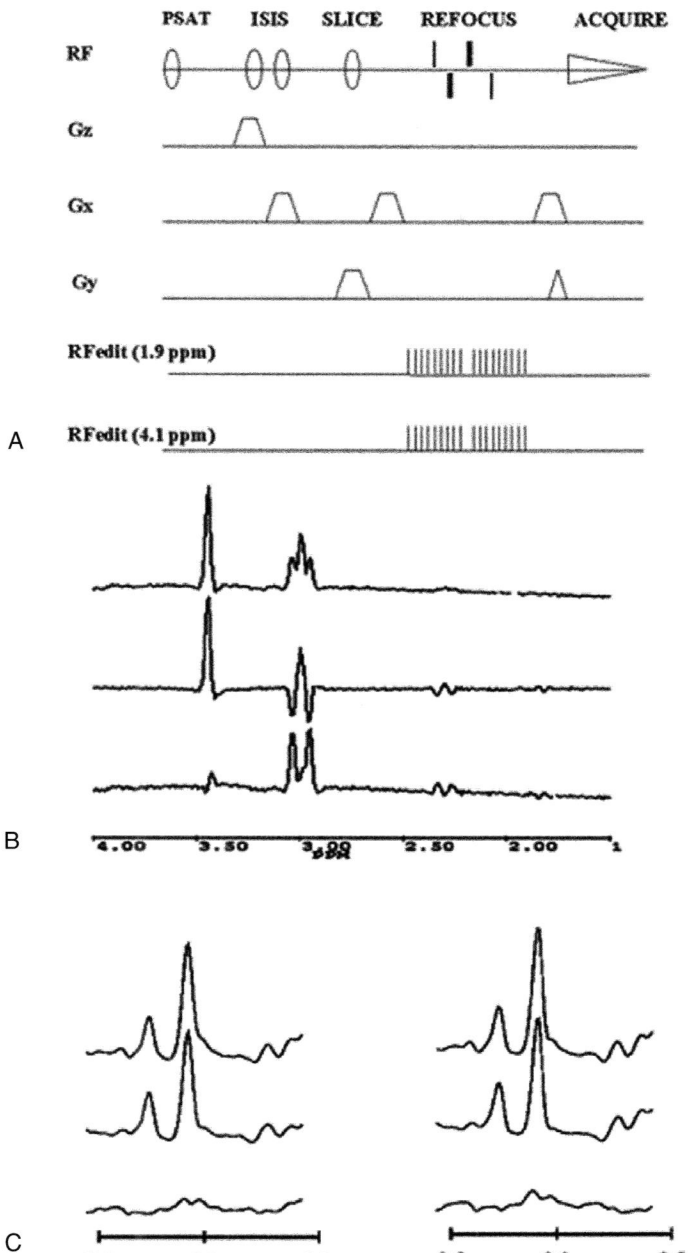

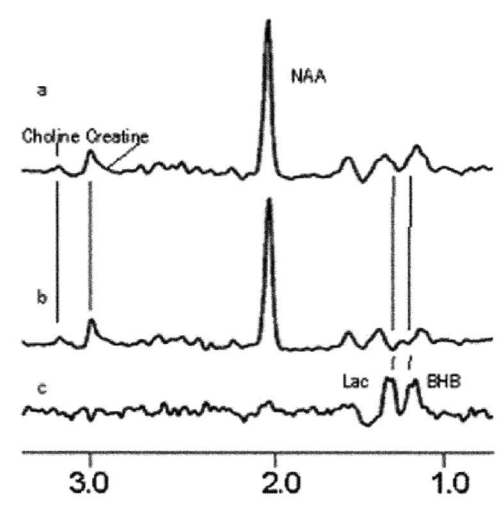

FIG. 13.7. A. A GABA spectral editing sequence. **B.** The corresponding spectra, from a solution of GABA and glycine. **C.** In-vivo data in the human brain. In **B** the top spectrum is acquired without an inversion pulse to the GABA C-3 resonance, such that GABA C-4 triplet resonance has not J-modulated, whereas the second spectrum was acquired with the inversion pulse, resulting in J-modulation of the GABA C-4 resonance. Application of the inversion pulse at either the GABA C-3 (1.9 ppm) resonance or the macromolecule (MM) resonance (1.7 ppm) yield the corresponding predominantly GABA or MM edited spectra. **D.** The use of the analogous spectral editing method for measuring lactate and beta-hydroxy butyrate (BHB) in the human brain. (With permission from Hetherington et al. 1998 (280).)

sensitivity and specificity. Unlike GABA, where 50% of the intensity is lost in the editing study, full sensitivity can be obtained for the lactate and BHB up-field doublets. For these resonances a selective 180 pulse is applied to the coupled partner (4.11 ppm for lactate, 4.2 ppm for BHB) at $T_E = 68$ ms. The spectra can then be subtracted to obtain the edited methyl resonances. Fortunately, the overlying macromolecular resonances do not have coupled partners in the vicinity of 4 ppm, such that editing of these resonances is dramatically simplified. Figure 13.7D shows an example of the measurement of lactate and BHB from a child being treated with the ketogenic diet. Of note, the BHB resonance in the normal, not ketotic, brain is less than 100 μm, whereas in this child the brain concentration is in excess of 1 mmol/l, indicating its availability for oxidative use.

^{31}P SPECTROSCOPY

Information content

Unlike ^{1}H spectra, where the ubiquity of the ^{1}H resonance provides a vast array of resonances to observe, the ^{31}P spectrum is limited in its content, reflecting five primary groups of resonances: phosphocreatine (PCr), inorganic phosphate (Pi), adenosine triphosphate (ATP), and phosphomonoester (PME) and -diester (PDE) (Fig. 13.8). Therefore, although limited in the types of resonance that can be measured, the ^{31}P spectrum provides great detail with regard to the bioenergetic status of the tissue (PCr, ATP, and Pi). This has proved quite useful in studies of temporal lobe epilepsy (TLE), where marked energetic impairment, decreased PCr/Pi

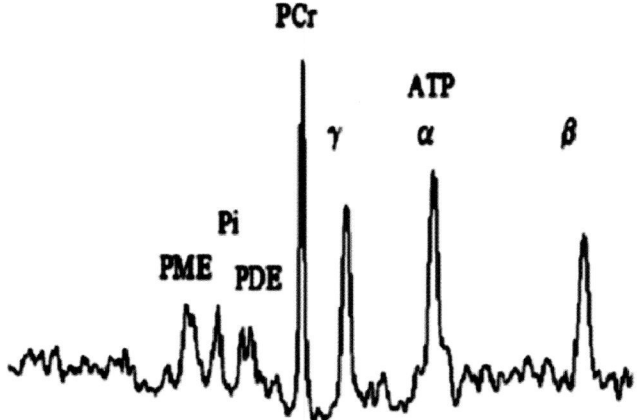

FIG. 13.8. A ³¹P spectrum of human brain acquired at 4 T from a 12 ml volume. The spectrum displays resonances from phosphomonoesters (PME), inorganic phosphate (Pi), phosphodiesters (PDE), phosphocreatine (PCr), and adenosine triphosphate (α,β,γ resonances).

and PCr/ATP, is present in both the ipsilateral and contralateral hippocampi. Additionally, because of the chemical exchange characteristics of the Pi resonance, pH can be determined from its chemical shift. Similarly, although less used, the free magnesium content pMg can be determined from the chemical shift of the β-ATP resonance. The PDE and PME resonances give information about lipid head-groups.

Because of the relatively large chemical shift range and the relatively low number of major resonances, the ³¹P spectrum is relatively free of spectral overlap, such that advanced spectral editing methods are not required. Similarly, with the exception of broad resonances arising from calcium phosphate in the skull and immobilized lipid head groups, which are exceptionally broad, the ³¹P spectrum is free of overlapping dominant resonances that must be suppressed. Thus, methodologically, ³¹P spectra are relatively easy to acquire and analyze. However, because of its decreased gyromagnetic ratio, 40% of the ¹H nucleus, the lack of multiplicity (one ³¹P nucleus per resonance as opposed to three ¹H nuclei for methyl groups), and the relatively low brain concentrations <4 mmol/l, the available SNR in the ³¹P spectrum is limited. Additionally both heteronuclear ¹H–³¹P and homonuclear ³¹P–³¹P J-coupling act to broaden the ATP, PME, and PDE resonances, further reducing resonance intensity. Therefore the primary challenges for ³¹P spectroscopy in the brain are to achieve adequate SNR in localized spectra and to compensate for the effects of tissue heterogeneity.

Localization of ³¹P Spectra

Unlike ¹H resonances, the T2s of many ³¹P species are relatively short (<50 ms) and the homonuclear coupling constants are large (≈15 Hz). Together these factors limit the use of single-shot localization methods, such as STEAM and PRESS, that use relatively lengthy echo periods. Therefore initial single-voxel ³¹P studies of human brain used an

alternate method, image-selected in-vivo spectroscopy, ISIS, which is based on an addition/subtraction scheme combined with spatially selective inversion pulses (32). Because of the low SNR of the ³¹P spectrum and the resultant necessity for prolonged acquisition periods to achieve adequate SNR, spectroscopic imaging approaches are also widely used in the acquisition of ³¹P data (33, 34).

Single-voxel Localization: ISIS

The ISIS sequence provides one-, two- and three-dimensional localized volumes by concatenating spatially selective inversion pulses applied in orthogonal directions. For example, a 1D ISIS sequence is depicted in Figure 13.9. In this method, the slice of interest is inverted on alternate scans prior to excitation and acquisition. For the two scans, the slice of interest contributes spectra that are opposite in phase, while the nonselected region retains the same phase. Subtraction of the two spectra results in cancellation of data from outside the selected slice (Fig. 13.9A). Extension of this method to two dimensions results in a requirement of four scans (Fig. 13.9B). The rectangle selected is then defined by the four possible combinations of the two spatially selective inversion pulses. To attain full 3D localization a minimum of eight scans are required consisting of all possible combinations (on/off) for application of the three spatially selective inversion pulses (Fig. 13.9C). Figure 13.9D shows an example of a 3D localized ³¹P spectrum from the human brain at 1.5 T.

Because of the low gyromagnetic ratio of the ³¹P nucleus, the strength of the RF field is substantially (2.5 times) weaker than that of the ¹H nucleus for similar peak powers. This results in a 2.5-fold reduction in maximum bandwidth for spatially selective pulses. The reduced bandwidth results in the use of proportionately weaker gradients for slice selection. Since the gradient strengths (in Hz/mm) are weaker, the natural frequency difference between different resonance lines (in Hz) now mimics a difference in spatial position. This in turn causes signals arising from different resonances to originate from different volumes. When this is combined with the relatively large bandwidth of the ³¹P spectrum, twice that of ¹Hs, substantial misregistrations occur because of these chemical shift displacement errors. Fortunately, spectroscopic imaging methods do not suffer from this type of error and are therefore ideal for ³¹P spectroscopy.

Spectroscopic Imaging

Since spectroscopic imaging methods do not result in CSDE errors, they have become the method of choice for ³¹P spectroscopy in the human brain. At 4 T and higher, nominal volume sizes of 12 ml or smaller are possible with volume head coils with acquisition times of less than 1 hour. Figure 13.10 shows an example of a ³¹P spectrum acquired from the human brain using a 3.4 ml nominal voxel. In this

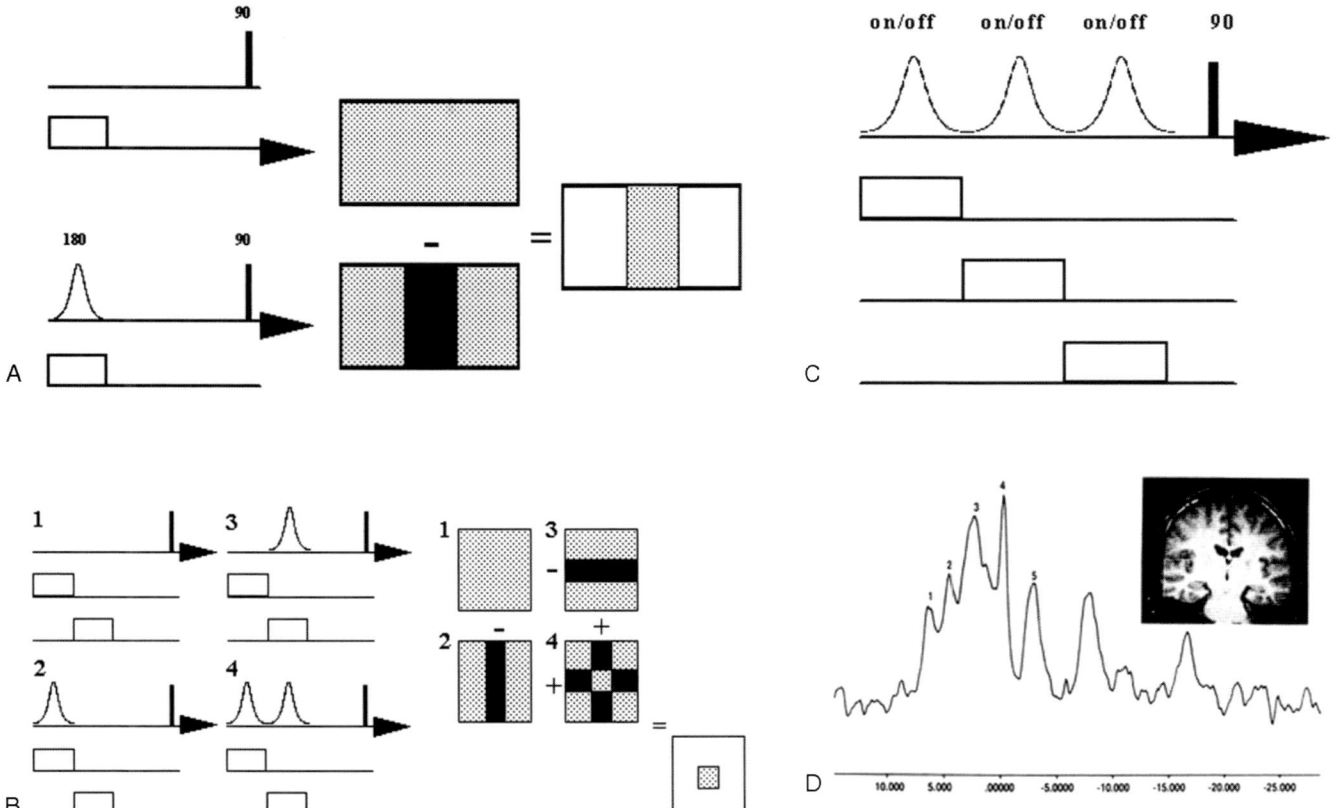

FIG. 13.9. The ISIS localization sequences for (**A**) 1D; (**B**) 2D; and (**C**) 3D. The subtraction scheme providing 1D and 2D localization is depicted in **A** and **B**. **D**. ISIS localizes spectrum from the human temporal lobe acquired at 1.5 T. (With permission from Kuzniecky et al. 1992 (262).)

spectrum the resonances of PCr, ATP, Pi, and PDE and PME are all well resolved and easily quantifiable. Despite the spectral quality, three additional factors can limit the interpretability of the ^{31}P data:

- the spatial distribution of tissue contributing to the acquired voxel
- natural tissue heterogeneity in the ^{31}P spectrum
- the coarseness of the spectroscopic imaging grid.

Unlike single-voxel acquisition methods, where the spatial extent of the selected volume resembles a cube with steeply inclined sides, spectroscopic imaging voxels can have a more extended profile with substantial contributions from distant locations in the brain. Specifically, the spatial extent of the sampled volume for each voxel is governed by its point spread function, which includes effects from both the phase encoding scheme used (e.g. rectangular vs spherical) and any postacquisition filtering.

Figure 13.11 shows four examples of different sampling and processing schemes. The first scheme (Fig. 13.11A) uses a simple rectangular sampling (256 linearly stepped values, 16 in each direction) without any postacquisition filtering. As can be seen, there are substantial ripples that result in both positive and negative signal contributions from

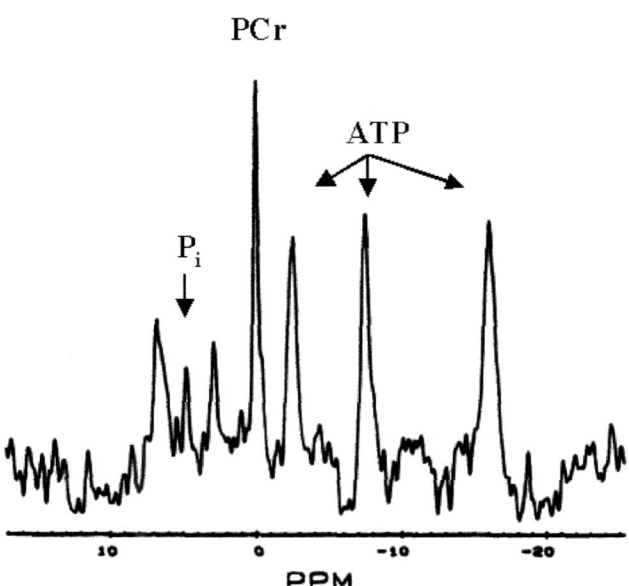

FIG. 13.10. A ^{31}P spectrum acquired from the human brain at 4.1 T using a 3.4 ml volume.

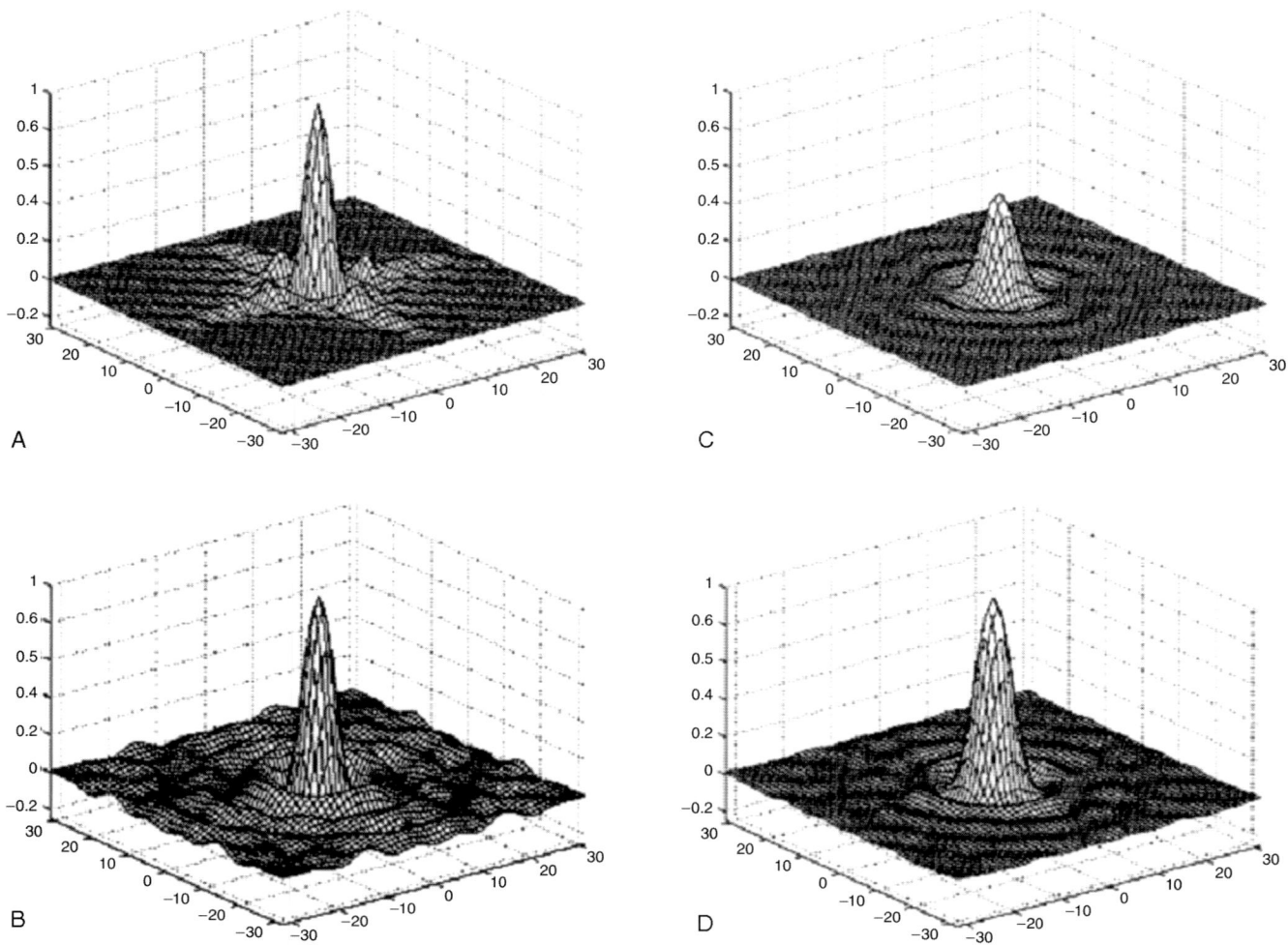

FIG. 13.11. The point-spread functions (PSF) for different encoding and postprocessing schemes. **A.** Rectangular sampling. **B.** Circular sampling. **C.** Circular sampling and postacquisition apodization with a cosine filter. **D.** A cosine-weighted acquisition without postacquisition apodization.

different brain regions. In scheme B, the analogous sampling scheme is used, with the exception that only samples within a circle tangential to the edges of the rectangle are acquired (193 samples in total). In this case the ripples are not as prominent along the major axes but rather appear as concentric circles, and the width of the selected volume is also increased.

Scheme C uses the same sampling scheme as B, with the exception that postacquisition filtering with a cosine function (multiplication with a cosine function) has been applied before spatial transformation. As can be seen the ripples have been reduced. The reduction in the ripples comes at the cost of increased width, and decreased maximum SNR at the center of the object. The decreased SNR is reflected by the central peak being less than 1.0 on the vertical axis. Finally, Figure 13.11D displays the analogous acquisition-weighted scheme without any postacquisition filtering. In this scheme the number of acquisitions for each encoding step varies according to a cosine distribution. The result is nearly identical to Figure 13.11C but there is no loss in SNR.

However, it should be noted that the minimum number of acquisitions has been increased by a factor of 8 to 1576 samples. Thus extensive acquisition-based weighting may not be possible in 3D localized measurements because of the excessive minimum acquisition times required.

Metabolite Heterogeneity

Just as ^{1}H metabolite content varies between gray and white matter, so does the content of various ^{31}P metabolites. Specifically, ATP ranges from 3.41 ± 0.33 mmol/l in cerebral white matter to 2.19 ± 0.33 in gray matter to 1.75 ± 0.58 mmol/l in mixed cerebellar volumes (35). Even larger differences are seen in skeletal muscle surrounding the brain, where ATP content approaches 8.5 ± 1.9 mmol/l. For PCr the variation between cerebral gray matter, cerebral white matter, and mixed cerebellar volumes is substantially less (3.53 ± 0.33, 3.33 ± 0.33, 3.75 ± 0.66 mmol/l respectively). However PCr content in the skeletal muscle is even higher, approaching 25.4 ± 2.3 mmol/l. Thus for arbitrary volumes, dramatic differences can be seen on a voxel-by-voxel basis as the tissue content changes.

Figure 13.12A, B shows examples of this variation for a row spanning both temporal lobes and a rectangle spanning the posterior aspect of the hippocampi and cerebellum. As can be seen (Fig. 13.12A), the ratio of PCr/ATP is highest near the skull, arising from skeletal muscle contributions and lowest from regions high in white matter content. Similarly, the ATP content in the spectra drops dramatically, despite relatively constant PCr levels when cerebellar contributions increase.

To overcome this limitation, the analogous method used to compensate for tissue heterogeneity in the ^{1}H spectrum can be applied. Specifically, using the calculated 'pure' tissue values for PCr and ATP from the different tissue types, and the tissue content of the voxel (including its point-spread function), an expected metabolite concentration can be calculated. Figure 13.12C shows plots of the measured and predicted PCr and ATP content for the volumes displayed in Figure 13.12A, B. Despite the twofold variation in measured content, virtually all the variation is explainable in terms of differences in tissue content. Figure 13.12D shows an example from a patient with TLE, quantifying the decrement in PCR/ATP from the ipsilateral lobe in comparison to the control value from an equivalent tissue mixture.

Voxel Positioning

Although the tissue composition can be corrected for, the relatively coarse spatial resolution of the ^{31}P spectroscopic images, and the arbitrary relationship between the location of anatomic structures within the brain and the magnet center, can present significant difficulties. Specifically, if a volume of interest, such as the ipsilateral hippocampus, falls at the intersection of the sampling limits of 8 pixels, its contribution to any single pixel will be so small (12.5%) that any metabolic alteration present may not be detectable against the background of what may be normal tissue. To overcome this problem postacquisition voxel-shifting methods are commonly

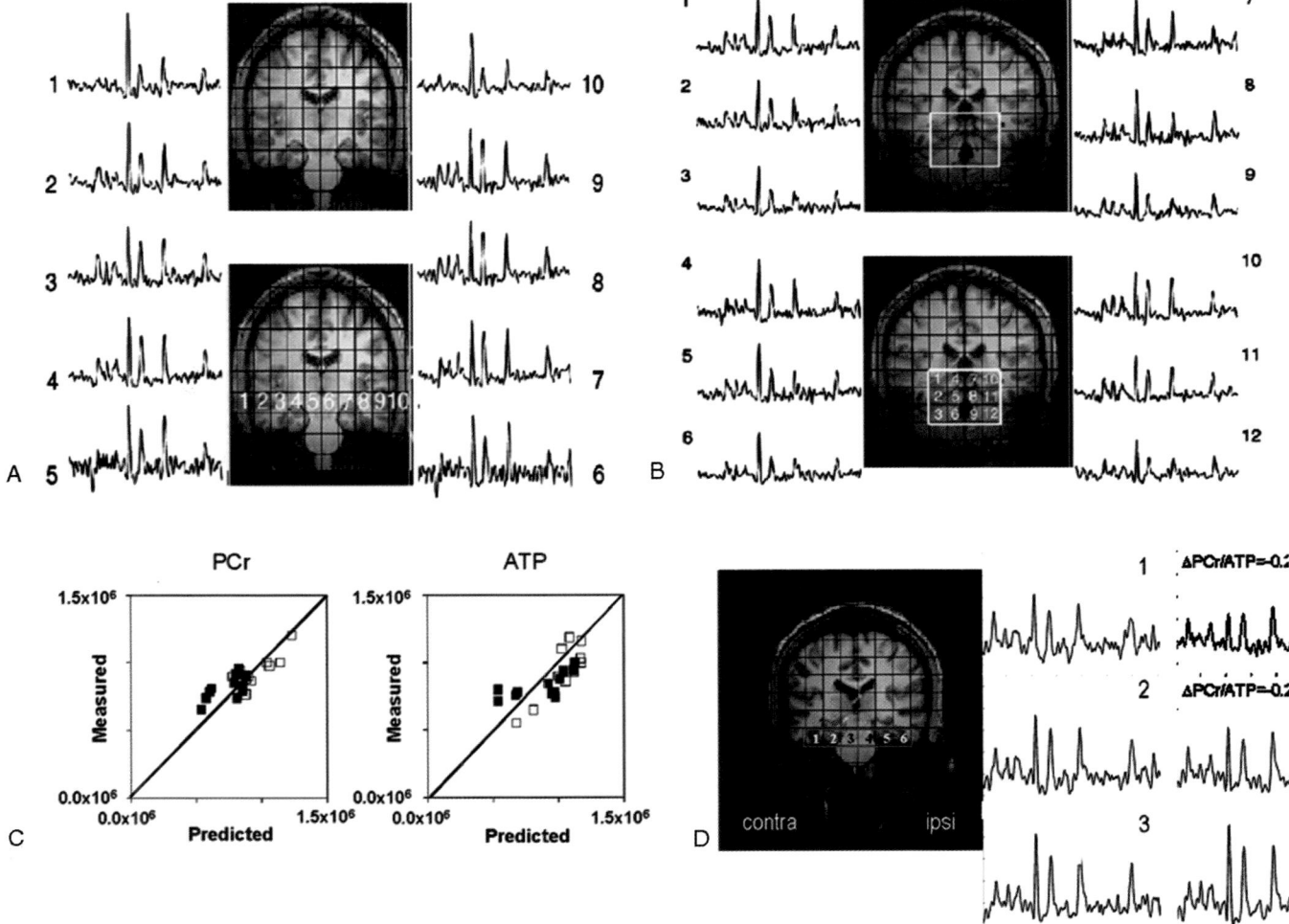

FIG. 13.12. ^{31}P spectra acquired from a row spanning the hippocampi bilaterally and a rectangle encompassing both the hippocampus and cerebellum. Plots of the expected PCr and ATP content (based on tissue composition) and the measured values for the spectra presented are displayed. (With permission from Hetherington et al. 2001 (35).)

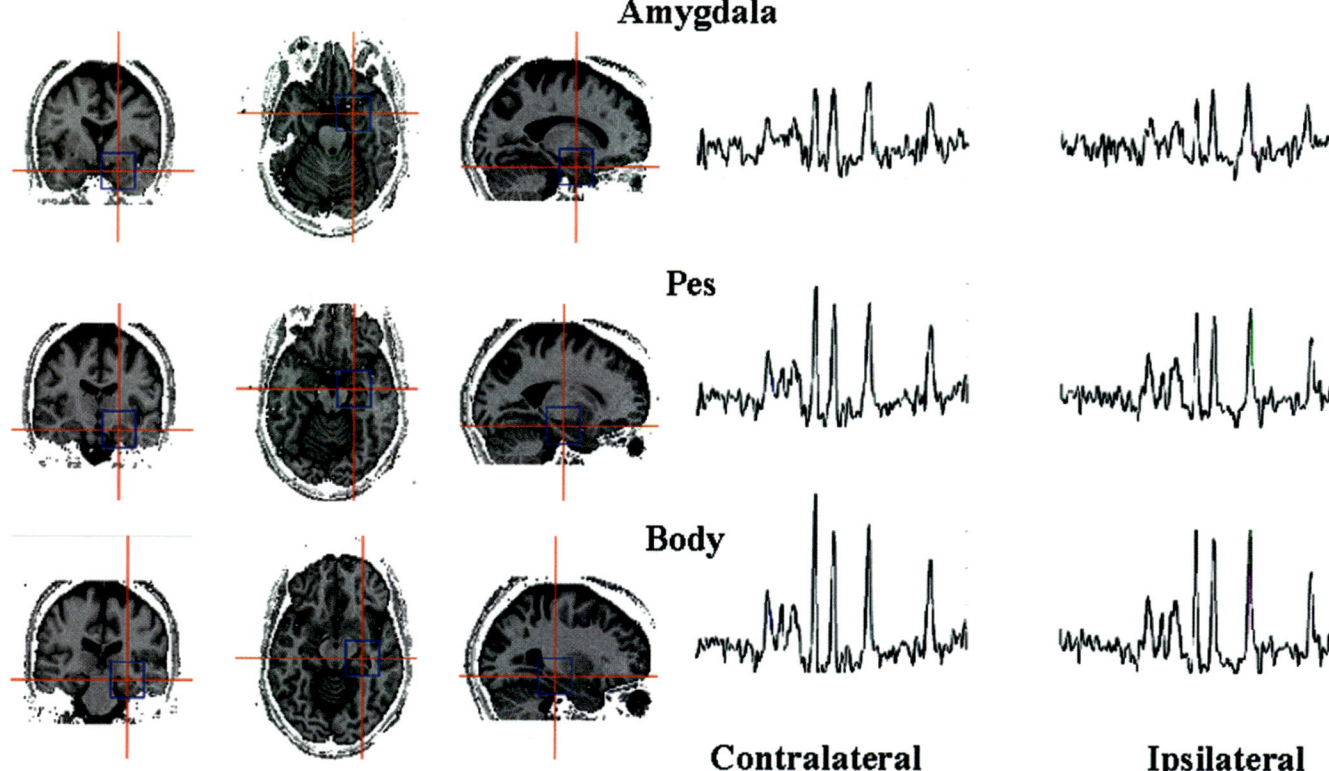

Amygdala

Pes

Body

Contralateral   **Ipsilateral**

FIG. 13.13. Spectra acquired from the amygdala, pes, and hippocampal body from a patient with temporal lobe epilepsy. The locations of the spectra are displayed in the images. The PCr/ATP ratio is decreased more substantially in the ipsilateral lobe in comparison to the contralateral lobe and anteriorly.

employed. In this method, the central coordinates of specific regions to be analyzed are identified on anatomic images. These coordinates are then used to shift the spectroscopic imaging voxels so that they are centered over the region of interest. If the data is collected as a 3D set, the resulting spectroscopic imaging voxels can be placed with an accuracy limited only by the resolution in the anatomic images (typically 1.5 mm or less). Although the spectroscopic imaging voxel's point-spread function is not altered, the voxel is guaranteed to maximally contain the region of interest.

Figure 13.13 shows an example of this method. Spectra spanning the hippocampal formations of a patient with TLE have been reconstructed from the amygdala, pes, and hippocampus. As can be seen, there is greater energetic impairment (decreased PCr/ATP) in the ipsilateral lobe as compared to the contralateral lobe and greater impairment bilaterally from more anterior locations.

^{13}C SPECTROSCOPY

Information Content

Like ^{31}P spectroscopy, ^{13}C spectroscopy suffers from low sensitivity (gyromagnetic ratio one-quarter of ^{1}H) and low multiplicity (one nucleus per resonance group). However, unlike ^{1}H and ^{31}P spectroscopy, the ^{13}C nucleus is only 1.1% naturally abundant, making detection of in-vivo levels of major metabolites in the absence of external enrichment especially difficult. Typically large volumes (>100 ml) with acquisition times of 30 minutes or more are employed.

Despite this limitation, the 1.1% natural abundance enables dynamic metabolic rate studies to be performed. For brain, after administration of ^{13}C-labeled glucose, the glucose label enters the carbon backbones of major metabolites, including glutamate, glutamine, GABA, aspartate, and lactate. When specifically labeled substrates are used (C1-labeled vs C2-labeled glucose), the pattern of labeling gives crucial information regarding the relative ratio of different pathways. Most recently, alternative sources of ^{13}C label such as acetate and BHB, which are favored by glial and neuronal cells respectively, have been used to provide cell-specific turnover information. Using this methodology, the rates of glutamate–glutamine cycling between neurons and astrocytes have been measured. Thus, despite the limitations of SNR, ^{13}C spectroscopy provides unique information not available by other means.

To overcome these limitations a variety of specialized pulse sequences have been developed to enhance the sensitivity of the measurements. The first method, polarization transfer (36) transfers magnetization from the ^{1}H nuclei to their covalently bound ^{13}C partners, using their J-coupling properties. Once transferred, the magnetization is then detectable as increased signal in the ^{13}C spectrum. The second method, heteronuclear editing or proton observe carbon edit (POCE) (37), uses the ^{1}H–^{13}C coupling to selectively observe only those ^{1}H signals bound to ^{13}C nuclei in the ^{1}H spectrum.

Polarization Transfer Methods

As described, polarization transfer methods move magnetization from ^{1}H nuclei to their respective J-coupled ^{13}C nuclei. Since the ^{1}H magnetization is a factor of 4 greater than that of the ^{13}C nucleus, the typical increase in ^{13}C signal

can be as high as a factor of 4. Despite this increase, the ^{13}C magnetization is still detected with the intrinsic sensitivity of ^{13}C, so that the method is inherently less sensitive than directly detecting the ^{1}H signal. Thus brain studies to date acquired from the occipital lobe have typically used surface coils and 70–140 ml volumes (36, 38).

Since the ^{13}C spectrum is much broader than the ^{1}H spectrum, 200 ppm versus 10 ppm, many resonances that are poorly resolved in the ^{1}H spectrum, e.g. the C3 and C4 resonances of glutamate and glutamine, are well resolved. This advantage makes the method ideal for measurements of neurotransmitter cycling rate, when labeling in the C-3 and C-4 positions of glutamate and glutamine must be resolved. Figure 13.14 shows a polarization transfer sequence and representative data from a human brain.

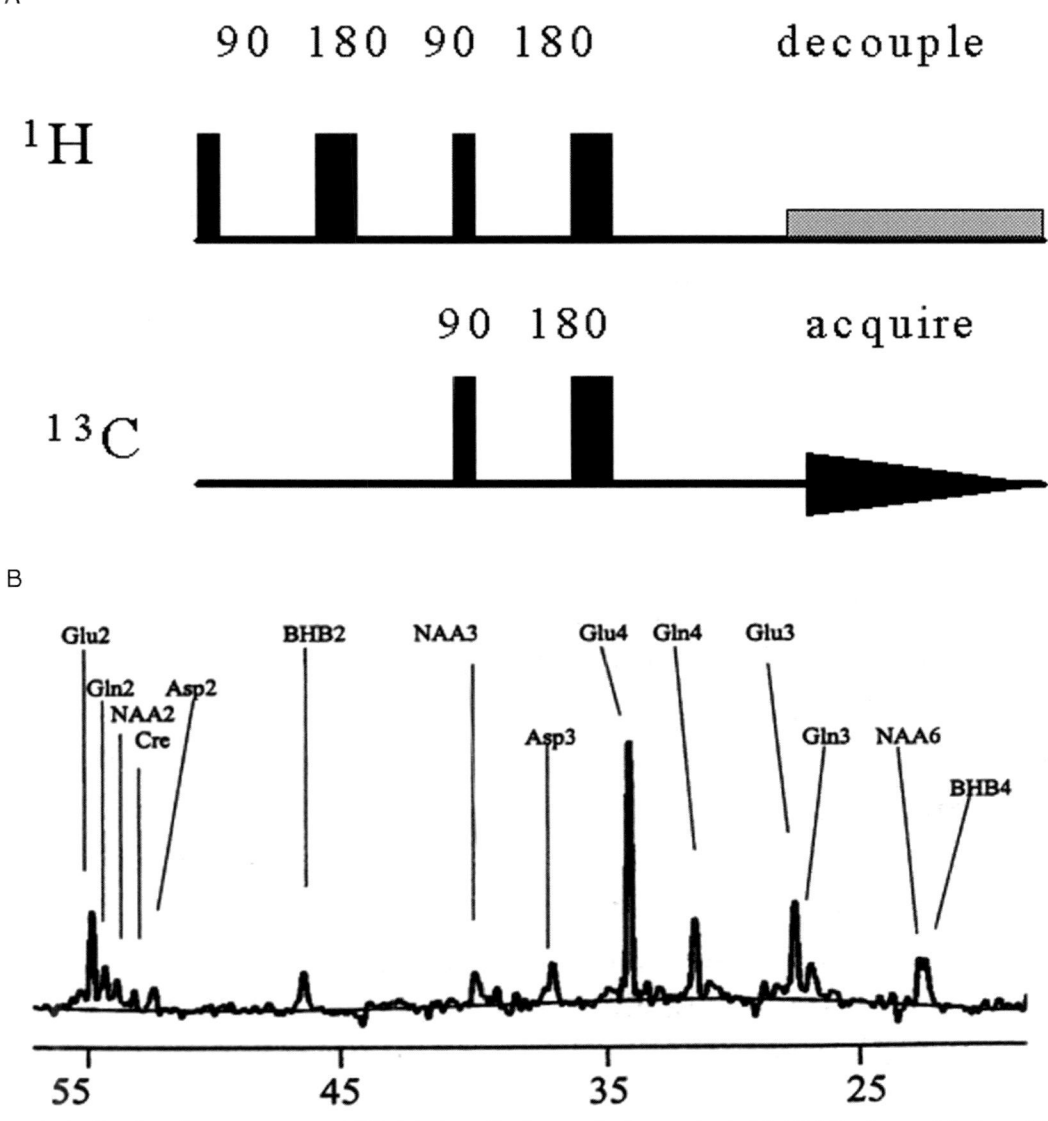

FIG. 13.14. The polarization transfer sequence and ^{13}C data from the human brain acquired at 2.1 T following an infusion of ^{13}C-labeled beta-hydroxy butyrate (BHB). The labeled resonances are aspartate (asp), BHB, creatine (cre), glutamate (glu), glutamine (gln), and *N*-acetyl aspartate (NAA). (With permission from Pan et al. 2002 (71).)

Proton Observe Carbon Edit

Unlike the polarization transfer methods, POCE excites and acquires ^{1}H signals. Similar to the homonuclear editing methods used for measuring GABA, lactate, and BHB, the POCE method utilizes the ^{1}H–^{13}C heteronuclear J-coupling to selectively resolve only those ^{1}H nuclei bonded to ^{13}C nuclei. In this case, the editing is performed using alternate applications of a ^{13}C inversion pulse applied with $T_E = \frac{1}{2}J$ or 3.8 ms. Similar to the polarization transfer method, decoupling during the acquisition, in this case ^{13}C decoupling, is required to maximize sensitivity. Because of the stringent timing requirements and relatively short echo times required, volume localization is typically achieved using one or two dimensions of ISIS, in combination with slice selective refocusing or excitation (Fig. 13.15).

Although the spectral resolution of the POCE sequence is limited by the intrinsic characteristics of the ^{1}H spectrum, and therefore worse than that achievable with polarization transfer, the enhanced sensitivity allows for much smaller volumes, 6 ml for surface coils and 20 ml for volume coils, with more rapid sampling rates (4–5 min acquisitions). In measurements of the TCA cycle rate, the rapid detection of the labeling of the C-4 resonance of glutamate is the most critical factor. As such, POCE methods provide better performance for TCA cycle turnover measurements (smaller volumes, shorter acquisition periods) in comparison to polarization transfer.

As in ^{1}H and ^{31}P spectroscopy, tissue heterogeneity can have significant effects on the calculated rates. Specifically, the absolute rate calculated, V_{TCA}, is directly proportional to the amount of glutamate in the volume. Further, significant differences between gray and white matter TCA cycle rates (white matter is a factor of 3–4 slower) distorts the shape of turnover curves, resulting in large errors in rate constants (up to 30%) when the tissue content is not factored in (39). Thus, careful attention to the tissue composition of the volumes being measured is critical to the biologic interpretation of the data.

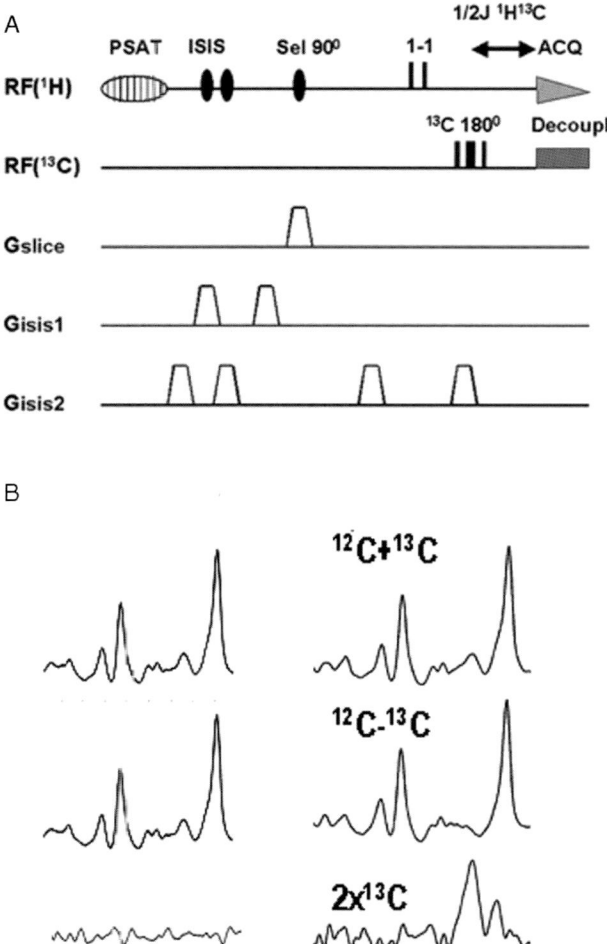

FIG. 13.15. From a 6 ml volume in the human brain at 4 T. The in-vivo data was acquired (left) prior to (before label incorporation into glutamate) and (right) after infusion of ^{13}C glucose (high level of ^{13}C incorporation into glutamate). (With permission from Pan et al. 2000 (39).)

Biochemistry for Magnetic Resonance Spectroscopy

Ognen Petroff

GLUTAMATE METABOLISM

In the normal adult brain, the glutamate concentration of gray matter primarily reflects the glutamate concentration in glutamatergic neurons, the glutamate content of which is far greater than that of nonglutamatergic neurons or glia (40). Neuronal glutamate is lost during glutamate transmitter release and is taken up by glia, where it is recycled by glutamine synthetase (GS) (41). With increased excitatory activity, the rate of neuronal glutamate loss would be greater. Glutamate lost from the neuron is replaced through phosphate-activated glutaminase (PAG) acting upon glutamine synthesized in the glia (42, 43).

The glutamate–glutamine cycle is the main pathway of astroglial glutamate uptake and may be measured by MRS. Astroglia replace neuronal glutamate through the glutamate–glutamine cycle, supplemented in certain situations by the glial release of TCA cycle intermediates, including alpha-ketoglutarate (2-oxoglutarate), citrate, and succinate. Neurons lack the enzymes required for de novo synthesis of glutamate and therefore depend on astroglia to provide substrates for the synthesis of glutamate lost during neurotransmission (44). The complete pathway is called the glutamate–glutamine cycle.

Although the pathways of astroglial glutamate uptake and cycling were well established from cellular studies, their physiologic importance was controversial prior to recent invivo studies using MRS (45). Because the neurotransmitter glutamate is packaged in vesicles (46, 47), the concept arose of a small, nonmetabolic 'transmitter' pool, which did not interact with the large 'metabolic' glutamate pool. The initial studies that brought this concept into question were,

it was found, using carbon MRS ([^{13}C]-MRS), a high rate of glutamine labeling from 1-^{13}C-glucose (36) in the human occipital parietal lobe. To test whether this rapid labeling was due to the glutamate–glutamine cycle, a series of MRS studies in healthy rat models were undertaken to determine whether glutamine was synthesized primarily from the glutamate–glutamine cycle or from ammonia detoxification, as was previously believed (48). Labeling from ammonia detoxification, which involves net anaplerosis, was measured using 2-^{13}C glucose and ^{15}N ammonia as label precursors, both of which require anaplerosis to label glutamine at specific carbon positions (49, 50).

Magnetic resonance spectroscopy studies in the rat cerebral cortex have shown that the rate of the glutamate–glutamine cycle is coupled in a close to 1:1 ratio to neuronal (primarily glutamatergic) glucose oxidation above the rate measured with an isoelectric electroencephalogram (EEG) (51). There is a highly significant association between electrical activity measured using EEG, the rate of glucose consumption, the TCA cycle (oxygen consumption), and glutamate–glutamine cycling (Fig. 13.16). Changes in rate of glutamate turnover and thus the glutamate–glutamine cycle are proportional to EEG power and changes in the neuronal spiking frequency (52–54). Measuring the rate of glutamate–glutamine cycle reflects the rate of glutamatergic neurotransmission through a wide range of conditions from pentobarbital coma with an isoelectric EEG through sensory stimulation with evoked potentials.

The rate of metabolism of the TCA cycle and the glutamate–glutamine cycle varies with the species studied. Basal rates of glucose uptake, glycolysis, TCA cycle (oxygen consumption), and the glutamate–glutamine cycle are twofold faster

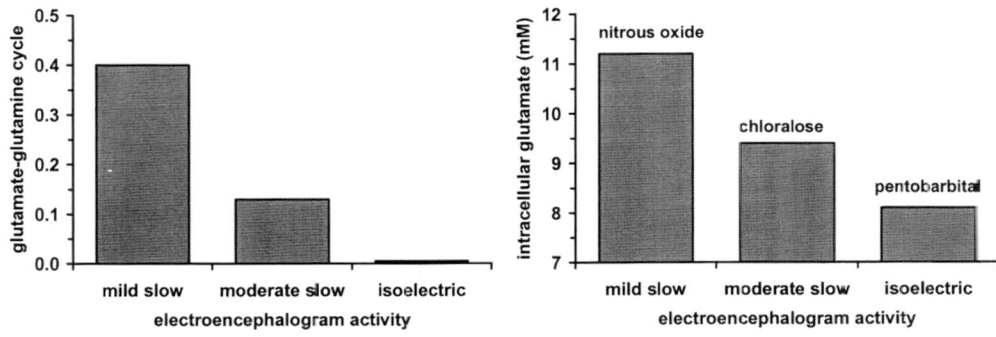

FIG. 13.16. The rate of the glutamate–glutamine cycle decreases in proportion to the decrease in neural activity as measured using scalp electroencephalography. Brain glutamate content also decreases in parallel to the change in neural activity as the depth of anesthesia increases. (From data in Sibson et al. 1998 (51).)

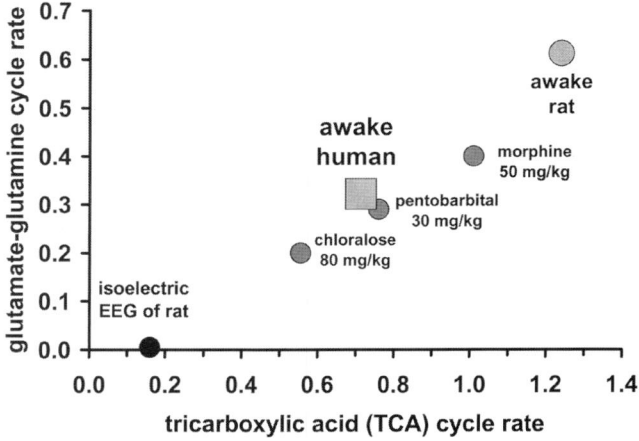

FIG. 13.17. The glutamate–glutamine cycle rate changes in proportion to the rate of the tricarboxylic acid (TCA) cycle under a variety of levels of brain activity, e.g. depth of anesthesia. Data derived from Sibson et al. 1998 (51), Hyder et al. 2001 (52), Shen et al. 1999 (55), and Kanamatsu & Tsukada 1999 (56).

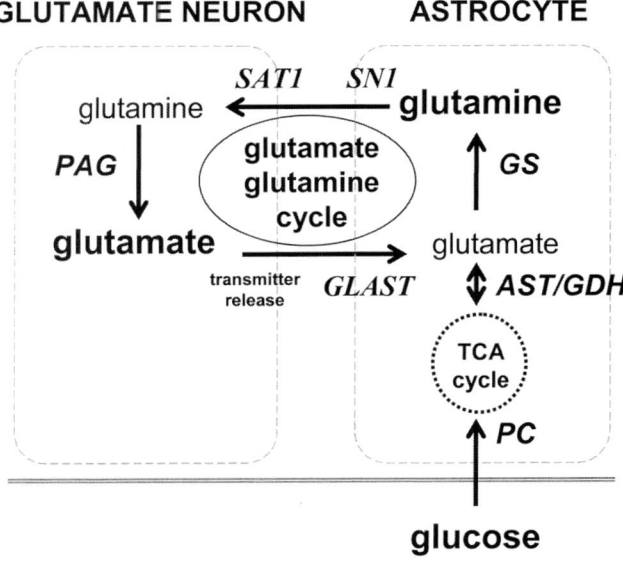

FIG. 13.18. The glutamate–glutamine cycle and the anaplerotic pathway used by the brain for the de-novo synthesis of glutamate from glucose. AST, aspartate transaminase; GDH, glutamate dehydrogenase; GLAST, glutamate aspartate transporter; GS, glutamine synthetase; PAG, phosphate activate glutaminase; PC, pyruvate carboxylase; SAT1, system-A transporter; SN1, system-N transporter.

in rats than in humans (Fig. 13.17). Using the glutamate–glutamine cycle/TCA cycle ratio compensates for the nearly twofold difference in cerebral metabolic rates. The ratio is similar in both rat (0.49, SE 0.05) and human brain (0.46, SE 0.04) (55, 56). Although the glutamate–glutamine cycle/TCA cycle ratio is clearly decreased by surgical-grade anesthesia with chloralose, the effects are minor compared with the major decrease seen during pentobarbital coma with an isoelectric EEG. Intracellular glutamate concentrations of the rat forebrain also decrease in parallel with the decrease in electrical activity. Glutamatergic neurotransmission and cellular glutamate content appear to decrease in parallel.

In many animal models of epilepsy, extracellular and intracellular glutamate concentrations increase markedly with the onset of seizures (57, 58). Intracellular glutamate content is increased interictally in the epileptogenic zone. Basal extracellular glutamate concentrations, measured by microdialysis or supraperfusion of the pial cortex, also are increased interictally.

GLUTAMATE–GLUTAMINE CYCLE

The components of the glutamate–glutamine cycle (Fig. 13.18) include the following steps.

1. Vesicular or nonvesicular release of glutamate takes place from the glutamatergic neuron into the synaptic cleft/extracellular space.
2. Astroglial uptake of glutamate plays a key role in maintaining the low extracellular levels needed for proper receptor-mediated functions. Studies of glutamatergic synapses have shown them to be closely surrounded by glial end processes possessing high densities of glutamate transporters. Glutamate transporters are sodium-dependent

and electrogenic and have an affinity, K_m, of 1–3 μmol/l, which is in the range of normal estimated extracellular glutamate concentration (59, 60). Reuptake of glutamate from the extracellular space is accomplished primarily by glia using the sodium-dependent, electrogenic glutamate transporters EAAT1 (GLAST) and EAAT2 (GLT-1) (41). Under normal conditions, GLAST and GLT-1 are located on astrocytic membranes and terminate excitatory neurotransmission by first binding glutamate (buffering) then transporting glutamate into the astrocytic cytosol in an energy (ATP)-consuming step. The physiologic importance of astroglial glutamate transport was demonstrated in studies in which antisense oligonuclectides directed against the astrocytic glutamate and aspartate transporters GLT1 or GLAST in vivo resulted in elevated extracellular glutamate in vivo and excitotoxicity (61). The large majority of cortical glutamate uptake after release is astroglial and tightly coupled to the glial sodium–potassium ATPase and therefore glial energy metabolism. Under severely depolarizing conditions of elevated extracellular potassium and glutamate, which can occur during a seizure, glutamate transporters reverse catastrophically releasing glutamate and aspartate (62).

3. Rising glial cytosolic glutamate stimulates GS, which consumes one glutamate, one ATP (complexed with magnesium), and one ammonia (NH_3) molecule to synthesize one glutamine, one ADP, one Pi, one free magnesium and releases acid, lowering cytosolic pH (63). In the brain, GS is an enzyme of primary neurochemical importance, since it converts neurotoxic ammonia and the

neurotransmitter glutamate into glutamine. Nonbrain GS responds to end-product (glutamine and its derivatives) feedback inhibition, whereas brain GS does not.

4. Glial release of glutamine is tightly controlled (64–66). The system-N (SN1) transporter is coupled to the hydrogen and sodium ion gradients and thus tightly coupled to the sodium–potassium ATPase, which consumes ATP and generates Pi, hydrogen ion, ADP, and free magnesium under physiologic conditions. Intracellular acidification promotes the uptake of glutamine and down the sodium gradient into the cell and releases hydrogen ion into the extracellular fluid. Glial alkalosis (pH ≈7.4) slows the release of glutamine. When the SN1 transporter is blocked, intracellular pH drops toward 6.5. Because of its electroneutral character, glutamine transport readily reverses under physiologic conditions and during a seizure. The SN1 transporter system is primarily localized to glia near synaptic terminals.

5. Conversely, the system-A transporter (SAT1 and SAT2) is expressed almost exclusively by neurons rather than glia (66). It exhibits particularly high levels of expression by inhibitory neurons with the location of SAT1 at the nerve terminal. SAT1 and SAT2 proteins all mediate electrogenic transport due to the uptake of sodium ion and neutral amino acid, i.e. glutamine, unopposed although modulated by hydrogen ion. Because it is electrogenic, SAT1 is more resistant to reversal under physiologic conditions, but can fail with collapse of the sodium gradient and intracellular acidosis; the changes that occur during a seizure.

6. Glutamine is converted to glutamate and ammonia by PAG (67–69). This enzyme is usually bound to the mitochondrial membrane (inner or outer) and can translocate from one to the other surface. PAG bound to the inner mitochondrial membrane appears to be largely inactive. PAG activity is activated by Pi and, therefore, is intimately coupled to energy-state and cytosolic pH. Fatty acids, valproate, NMDA receptor antagonists, and free calcium stimulate PAG activity. The primary inhibitors of PAG include glutamate, ammonia, and hydrogen ions. Other potent inhibitors of PAG activity include NAA, leucine, homocysteine, histidine, glycine, and taurine.

7. Cytosolic glutamate is repackaged into vesicles by a specific energy-dependent vesicular glutamate transporter (VGLUT1) (41). Vesicular uptake of glutamate is driven by membrane potential and the hydrogen ion gradient. VGLUT1 appears to be a vesicular membrane-bound ATPase that pumps hydrogen ions and glutamate into the vesicle. It also appears to be a Pi transporter.

Magnetic Resonance Spectroscopy Methods used to Measure the Glutamate–Glutamine Cycle

Several strategies were developed to measure glutamate–glutamine cycling and the TCA cycle using glucose, acetate,

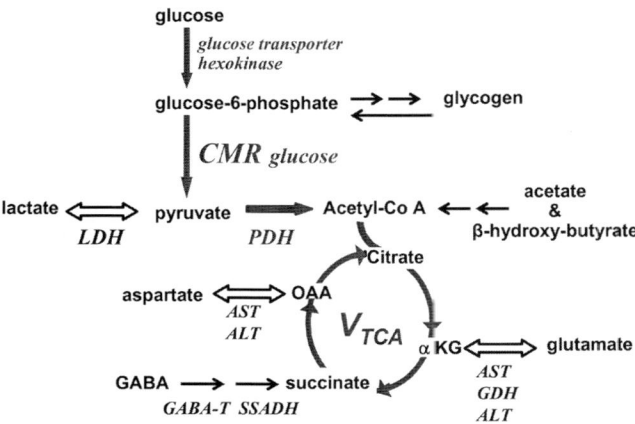

FIG. 13.19. The primary route of glucose metabolism in brain. Acetyl-CoA, acetyl coenzyme A; ALT, alanine transaminase; AST, aspartate transaminase; CMR, cerebral metabolic rate; GABA-T, GABA transaminase; GDH, glutamate dehydrogenase; α-KG, alpha-ketoglutarate; LDH; lactate dehydrogenase; CAA, oxaloacetic acid; PDH, pyruvate dehydrogenase; SSADH, succinic semi-aldehyde dehydrogenase.

and BHB labeled with ^{13}C, a nonradioactive isotope of carbon and in-vivo MRS (38, 50, 70, 71). Dynamic measurements of the rate of incorporation of ^{13}C into brain glutamate and glutamine may be used to measure the rate of glucose uptake, glycolysis, the TCA cycle, glycogen, and the synthesis of glutamate, glutamine, and aspartate (Fig. 13.19). Several enzymes catalyze the fast chemical exchange between alpha-ketoglutarate and glutamate, including aspartate transaminase, alanine transaminase, glutamate dehydrogenase, and GABA transaminase (GABA-T).

Measuring the Glutamate–Glutamine Cycle at Steady-state using 2-^{13}C Glucose

Several strategies were developed for determining the ratio of the glutamate–glutamine cycle to TCA cycle from steady state ^{13}C-labeling patterns of glutamate and glutamine at steady-state. One strategy takes advantage of the label from 2-^{13}C-glucose being incorporated into the internal positions of glutamate and glutamine only through the glia (50, 72). Label from 2-^{13}C-glucose, which enters the TCA cycle through pyruvate dehydrogenase, is incorporated into (5–13) C-glutamate and 1-^{13}C-glutamate. It does not label the internal positions of glutamate or glutamine. In contrast, ^{13}C-label entering the TCA cycle from the anaplerotic pathway through pyruvate carboxylase will label glial glutamine C2 and C3 initially because both pyruvate carboxylase and GS are found exclusively in glia. Subsequently, labeled glutamine will be taken up by the neurons to replenish released glutamate by the glutamate–glutamine cycle. The labeling in neuronal C3-glutamate is diluted relative to the precursor C3 glutamine as a result of unlabeled carbons entering through the neuronal TCA cycle ($V_{unlabeled}$). From the ratio of

C3-glutamine to C3-glutamate labeling at isotopic steady state, the ratio of the rate of glutamate–glutamine cycle to TCA cycle (V_{cycle}/V_{TCA}) may be calculated. Because steady-state labeling analysis is used, the results are to a first order independent of whether label exchange between the mitochondrial and cytosolic glutamate pools is rapid relative to the TCA cycle, in contrast to the analysis of ^{13}C time course data (dynamic measurements). The main assumptions in the analysis of labeling results are that pyruvate carboxylase is localized to the astrocyte and that the majority of glutamate is in the neuron.

Measuring the Glutamate–Glutamine using 2-^{13}C Acetate

Acetate is an ideal tracer for studying glial metabolism and neurotransmitter cycling (Fig. 13.20). A complication for studying neuronal/glial neurotransmitter cycles in vivo is that most isotope-labeled precursors will be incorporated by both cell types. This limitation is overcome by ^{13}C-labeled acetate, which is almost exclusively metabolized in glia, as has been validated by in-vivo studies in animals and humans (70, 73, 74).

Recently, 2-^{13}C-acetate was used to selectively measure the contribution of astroglial oxidative metabolism to total substrate oxidation and the rate of total neuronal-glial glutamate cycling in human brain by ^{13}C MRS (70, 73). The strategy is similar to the use of 2-^{13}C-glucose in that the stable-isotope tracer enters the glutamate–glutamine cycle through glia. The glial specificity of 2-^{13}C-glucose requires that pyruvate carboxylase is expressed almost exclusively in glia. The glial specificity of 2-^{13}C-acetate requires that the glial monocarboxylic acid transporter is highly selective for acetate compared to the neuronal one, which prefers lactate (75, 76).

Dynamic and steady-state in-vivo C13-MRS measurements of the glutamate–glutamine cycle/TCA cycle ratio made concurrently in the occipital lobe of healthy humans are identical. Both values are in good agreement with those made using $_{-}$-^{13}C-glucose in the same group of subjects on a separate experimental day. This strategy has been used in ^{13}C-MRS studies of a rat model of TLE, 1 and 14 days after kainic acid injection (77).

Extensive studies in animals have shown that changes in glutamate release and metabolism may play an important role in the origin and spread of seizure activity. Glutamate metabolism is coupled closely to mitochondrial respiration and ATP synthesis. Glia efficiently remove glutamate released by neurons and help to terminate the action of released glutamate. In-vitro and in-vivo studies indicate that a major portion of glutamate transported into glia is converted to glutamine (neutral metabolite) and returned to neurons for the resynthesis of glutamate. Disturbances of the glutamate–glutamine cycle, reflected by increased intracellular glutamate levels and impaired glutamate clearance, could be an important metabolic change associated with epileptogenesis.

Intracellular glutamate concentrations are elevated in the epileptogenic human hippocampus (78). Compared with autopsy samples, mean hippocampal intracellular glutamate is elevated in mesial TLE patients with normal-appearing hippocampi on the presurgical, clinical MRI and minimal neuron loss by histopathologic examination. Mean cellular glutamate levels of the epileptogenic hippocampus with pathologically verified hippocampal sclerosis fall within the normal range (autopsy-based).

The elevation is even more striking when cellular glutamate levels are corrected for neuron loss. Above-normal glutamate levels are present in almost half the hippocampi with the greatest neuron loss. Intracellular glutamate concentrations must be exceedingly high in the remaining glutamatergic neurons, or above-normal, intracellular, glutamate concentrations must be present in the remaining nonglutamatergic neurons or glia. Cellular glutamate decreases in proportion to neuronal loss or simplification (loss of neuronal volume

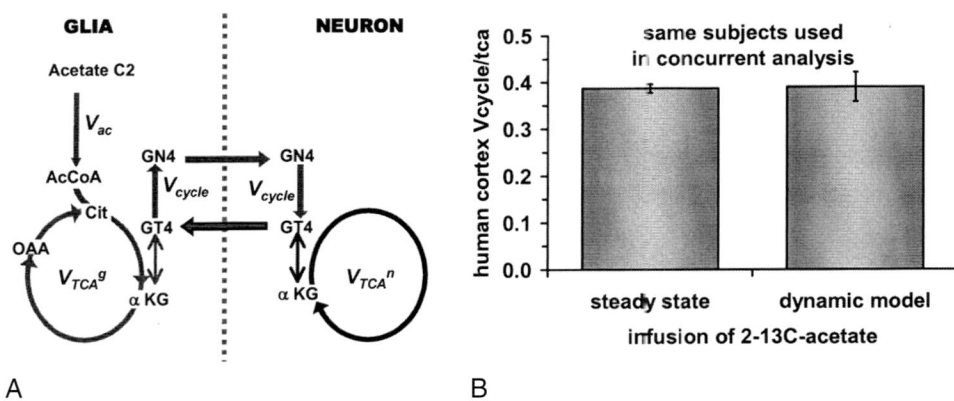

A   B

FIG. 13.20. A. 2-^{13}C-acetate metabolism in human brain. AcCoA, acetyl coenzyme A; α-KG, alpha-ketoglutarate; Cit, citrate; GN4, 4–^{13}C-glutamaine; GT4, 2-^{13}C-glutamate; OAA, oxaloacetic acid. **B.** The ratio of the glutamate–glutamine cycle to TCA cycle rates, measured using serial spectra, are the same as those measured in single spectrum, collected after steady-state is achieved. Serial spectra collected during the dynamic phase of the experiment and the steady-state spectrum at the end are obtained from the same volunteer. From data published by Lebon et al. 2002 (70).

through shrinkage of dendrite, synapses, and other processes). The neuron loss, particularly of large glutamatergic neurons, and glial proliferation should decrease glutamate concentrations in the sclerotic hippocampus. The findings suggest that there appears to be a relative increase in cellular glutamate content in the epileptogenic human hippocampus. Whether this increase in glutamate is localized in the remaining neurons or proliferating glia remains to be determined. There are no significant associations seen between tissue glutamate concentrations and neuron loss or glial density.

The findings raise two possibilities. Either the remaining neurons, mainly 'GABAergic', have extremely high intracellular glutamate content, or a subpopulation of glial cells must have high glutamate content. Cell culture studies suggest that glial precursor cells have high intracellular glutamate content (79, 80). Above-normal intracellular glutamate concentrations could contribute to the above-normal release of glutamate measured in the epileptogenic human hippocampus during spontaneous seizures. The high glutamate content would be expected to contribute to the epileptic state by increasing network excitability and promoting excitotoxicity.

Measuring the Glutamate–Glutamine Cycle in the Epileptic Human Hippocampus

The glutamate–glutamine cycle/TCA cycle ratio (Fig. 13.21) is severely compromised in almost all patients with hippocampal sclerosis (72). Using glutamate–glutamine cycle/TCA cycle ratios automatically corrects for the decreased glucose and TCA cycle (oxygen) metabolism that characterizes the epileptogenic hippocampus during the interictal state. Paradoxically, widespread hypometabolism centered on the epileptogenic region appears to characterize the interictal state in ≈80% of patients with mesial TLE (81). The decrease in glucose uptake has been attributed to hippocampal neuron loss and the widespread involvement to diaschisis.

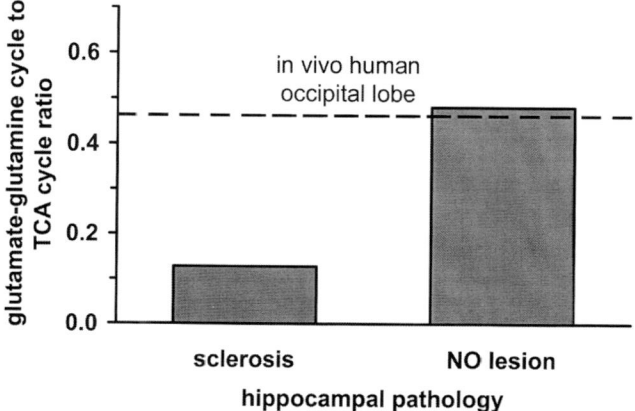

FIG. 13.21. The ratio of the glutamate–glutamine cycle rate normalized to the tricarboxylic acid cycle rate is very low in hippocampal sclerosis. (From data in Petroff et al. 2002 (82).)

Overall, there is only a weak association between brain volume and cerebral metabolism measured using positron emission tomography (PET) with about 13% of the variance attributable to atrophy (82). This relationship breaks down even further in the epileptogenic regions, suggesting that the hypometabolism is not mainly due to neuron loss. Quantitative pathologic studies show that hippocampal neuron loss does not account for the severity of the hypometabolism. Hypometabolism measured using fluorodeoxyglucose (FDG-PET) improves after successful surgery, which suggests that the epileptic state rather than neuron loss is the dominant factor (83).

Unexpectedly, normal glutamate–glutamine cycle/TCA cycle ratios are seen in patients with mesial TLE and normal-appearing hippocampi on the presurgical, clinical MRI and minimal neuron loss by histopathologic examination (see Fig. 13.21). This suggests that interictal, glutamatergic neurotransmission remains in the normal range for patients with normal-appearing hippocampi by MRI, despite the elevated intracellular glutamate.

No associations with antiepileptic drugs in use at the time of surgery, duration of the epilepsy, gender, or age were seen that did not reflect the pathology. There were no significant associations between glutamate–glutamine cycle/TCA cycle ratio and hippocampal glutamate or glutamine content seen that did not reflect the pathology. Measurements of the glutamate–glutamine cycle/neuronal TCA cycle ratio in the normal human hippocampus are not available. The closest comparisons to these results are recent measurements using in-vivo ^{13}C-MRS in the human occipital-parietal lobe and the awake and lightly anesthetized rat forebrain (84, 85). Under low light, unstimulated conditions, values range between 0.4 and 0.5.

The relative rate of the glutamate–glutamine cycle to glutamate synthesis is decreased in epileptic hippocampi that show sclerosis. The association with histopathology is striking. Neuron–glia cycling is not low in all epileptic hippocampi; it is lowest in those with significant loss of neurons and glial proliferation. Because this ratio is calculated from the relative labeling of the glutamate (primarily neuronal) and glutamine (synthesized in glia) pools, as opposed to absolute flux rates, the low glutamate–glutamine cycle/neuronal TCA cycle ratio is not simply due to reduced cellular density or generalized hypometabolism. If the remaining neurons and glia were functioning normally the ratio of the glutamate–glutamine cycle to the neuronal TCA cycle would be independent of neuronal loss.

Glutamate Concentrations in Epilepsy

Extensive studies in animals have shown that changes in glutamate release and metabolism may play an important role in the origin and spread of seizure activity. Glutamate metabolism is coupled closely to mitochondrial respiration and ATP synthesis. Glia efficiently remove glutamate released by neurons and help to terminate the action of released glutamate. In-vitro and in-vivo studies indicate that a major portion of the glutamate transported into glia is converted to glutamine (neutral metabolite) and returned to neurons for the resynthesis of glutamate. Disturbances of the glutamate–glutamine cycle, reflected by increased intracellular glutamate levels and impaired glutamate clearance, could be an important metabolic change associated with epileptogenesis.

In many animal models of epilepsy, extracellular and intracellular glutamate concentrations increase markedly with the onset of seizures (72, 86, 87). Intracellular glutamate content is increased interictally in the epileptogenic zone. Basal extracellular glutamate concentrations, measured by microdialysis or supraperfusion of the pial cortex, also are increased interictally.

Intracellular Glutamate in the Epileptogenic Human Hippocampus

Intracellular glutamate concentrations are elevated in the epileptogenic human hippocampus (Fig. 13.22) (88). Compared with the autopsy series mean, mean hippocampal intracellular glutamate is elevated in mesial TLE patients with normal-appearing hippocampi on the presurgical, clinical MRI and minimal neuron loss by histopathologic examination. Mean cellular glutamate levels of the epileptogenic hippocampus with pathologically verified hippocampal sclerosis fall within the normal range (autopsy-based).

The elevation is even more striking when cellular glutamate levels are corrected for neuron loss. Above-normal glutamate levels are present in almost half the hippocampi with the greatest neuron loss. Intracellular glutamate concentrations must be exceedingly high in the remaining glutamatergic neurons or above-normal, intracellular, glutamate concentrations must be present in the remaining nonglutamatergic neurons or glia. Cellular glutamate decreases in proportion to neuronal loss or simplification (loss of neuronal volume through shrinkage of dendrite, synapses, and other processes). The neuron loss, particularly of large glutamatergic neurons, and glial proliferation should decrease glutamate concentrations in the sclerotic hippocampus. The findings suggest that there appears to be a relative increase in cellular glutamate content in the epileptogenic human hippocampus. Whether this increase glutamate is localized in the remaining neurons or proliferating glia remains to be determined. There are no significant associations seen between tissue glutamate concentrations and neuron loss or glial density. The findings raise two possibilities. Either the remaining neurons, mainly 'GABAergic', have extremely high intracellular glutamate content or a subpopulation of glial cells must have high glutamate content. Cell culture studies suggest that glial precursor cells have high intracellular glutamate content (79, 80). Above-normal intracellular glutamate concentrations could contribute to the above-normal release of glutamate measured in the epileptogenic human hippocampus during spontaneous seizures. The high glutamate content would be expected to contribute to the epileptic state by increasing network excitability and promoting excitotoxicity.

Neocortical Glutamate Content in Human Epilepsies

Neocortical intracellular glutamate levels are increased in the epileptic human brain (Fig. 13.23) (86, 89, 90). Biopsies of human temporal lobe cortex ipsilateral to the epileptogenic hippocampus show that glutamate is elevated by 2.3 µmol/g in spiking cortex compared with adjacent non-spiking cortex.

Cellular Glutamate Content and Antiepileptic Drugs

Magnetic resonance spectroscopy measurements show that cellular glutamate levels (Fig. 13.24), measured in visual cortex remote from the presumed seizure focus in the

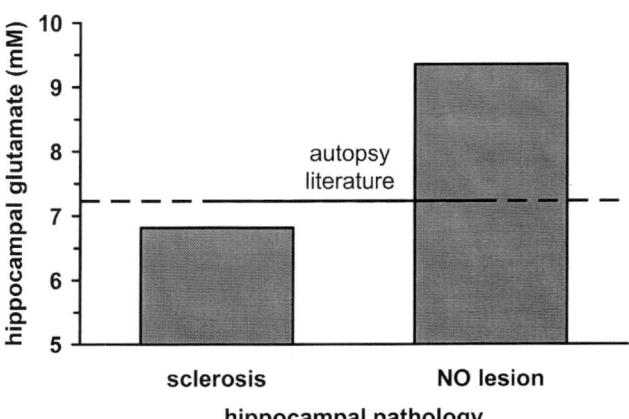

FIG. 13.22. Intracellular glutamate content is above normal in the epileptogenic hippocampus. The increase becomes marked when correct. (From data in Petroff et al. 2002 (82).)

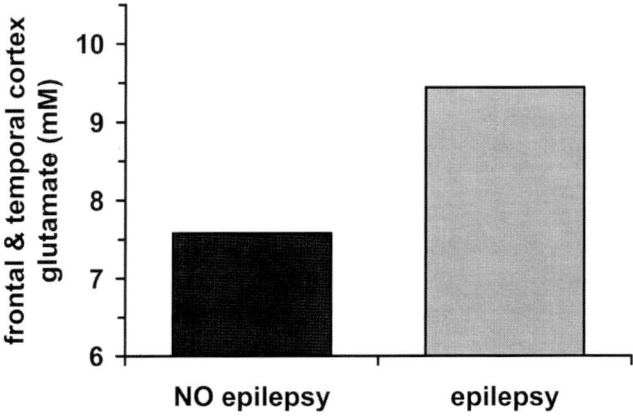

FIG. 13.23. Cortical glutamate content is increased in biopsies of patients with epilepsy compared to those without epilepsy. (From data in Perry 1982.)

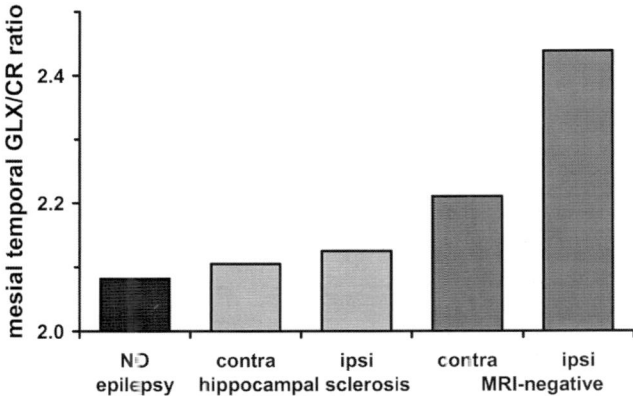

FIG. 13.24. Occipital lobe glutamate content is above normal in patients with refractory localization-related epilepsy treated with carbamazepine or phenytoin. (From data in Petroff et al. 1999, 2000 (86, 90).)

temporal or frontal lobes, are increased in patients with refractory complex partial seizures (86, 89, 90). Occipital lobe glutamate levels were below normal in 44% of patients treated with carbamazepine or phenytoin, 40% on valproate, 29% on gabapentin, and none on vigabatrin. Mean brain glutamate levels were lower on vigabatrin than on carbamazepine or phenytoin. Patients taking phenobarbital or primidone appeared to have the lowest levels on cortical glutamate. Whether a decrease in brain glutamate is associated with improved seizure control requires serial measurements in a larger sample of patients.

Cellular Glutamate is Highest Ipsilateral to the Epileptogenic Human Hippocampus

The glutamate plus glutamine levels (GLX) appear to be increased in the temporal lobe ipsilateral to the seizure onset (Fig. 13.25) (91, 92). The level appears to be even higher

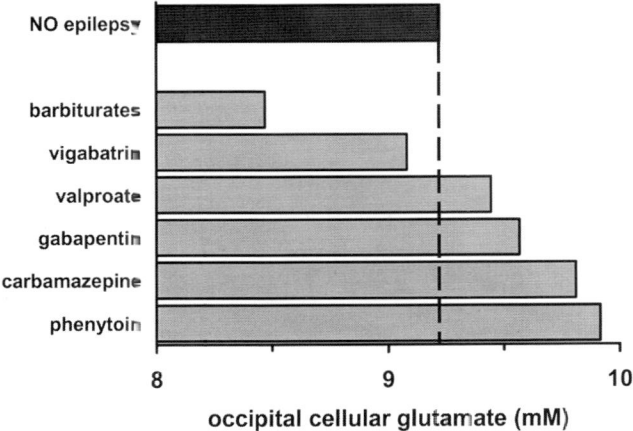

FIG. 13.25. The glutamate plus glutamine to total creatine ratio (GLX/Cr) is above normal in the mesial temporal lobes of patients with temporal lobe epilepsy (TLE) without lesions seen by MRI. The GLX/Cr ratio is increased ipsilateral to the seizure focus in TLE. (From data in Woermann et al. 1999 (91).)

ipsilateral to the seizure focus in patient without abnormalities on MRI (MR-negative). Neurotransmitter glutamate release from synaptosomes is drastically reduced if either ATP or cytosolic glutamate concentrations are depleted, which is consistent with a critical role for cytosolic glutamate metabolism for maintaining the vesicular pool. As a result of the relationship between cytosolic and vesicular glutamate concentrations, an increase in cytosolic glutamate may enhance both vesicular and nonvesicular glutamate release. Serial in-vivo MRS studies measuring the relationship between cellular glutamate levels and cortical excitability have not been reported. The increased neocortical glutamate levels ipsilateral to the epileptogenic temporal lobe suggest that increased intracellular glutamate content could contribute to the hyperexcitability of the epileptic network, facilitating spread of seizure activity to brain regions outside of the ictal onset zone. Spectroscopic imaging of brain glutamate should improve our understanding of both focal and generalized epilepsies and may become very useful in mapping epileptic networks (39).

In MRI-negative patients, the GLX levels appear to be increased in the temporal lobe ipsilateral to the seizure onset (92, 91). Neurotransmitter glutamate release from synaptosomes is drastically reduced if either ATP or cytosolic glutamate concentrations are depleted, which is consistent with a critical role for cytosolic glutamate metabolism for maintaining the vesicular pool. As a result of the relationship between cytosolic and vesicular glutamate concentrations, an increase in cytosolic glutamate may enhance both vesicular and nonvesicular glutamate release. Although it is attractive to speculate that increased cellular glutamate levels may contribute to widespread cortical excitability thus facilitating the spread of the seizure from the epileptogenic zone to become generalized, serial in-vivo MRS studies measuring the relationship between cellular glutamate levels and cortical excitability have not been reported. Spectroscopic imaging of brain glutamate should improve our understanding of both focal and generalized epilepsies (29).

GAMMA-AMINO BUTYRIC ACID METABOLISM

Gamma-amino butyric acid has had a central role in neural control theory since it was first discovered in 1950 (93). It is the major inhibitory neurotransmitter in human cortex. GABA serves as the primary inhibitory neurotransmitter at 20–44% of cortical neurons (94). MRS has been in clinical use for a number of years and permits serial, noninvasive measurements of certain cerebral metabolites without discomfort or known hazards. Continuing MRS development has resulted in techniques for the measurement of intracellular GABA and its major metabolites noninvasively, and safely in the brain of healthy human subjects (17, 95–98). Recently, MR methods to image GABA have been developed (55).

Several lines of evidence support a major role for GABA levels affecting GABA release and by this mechanism having a key role in the regulation of cortical excitability. Studies in cell culture and brain slice have shown directly that increasing cellular GABA levels increases tonic GABA release and in response to physiologic activation (99, 100). Primate models of photosensitive epilepsy have low GABA levels and seizures improve with GABAergic drugs (101, 102). Similarly, antiepileptic drugs that increase GABA or enhance GABAergic inhibition block the photoparoxysmal response in photosensitivity epilepsies (103, 104). Drug-induced enhancement of GABAergic inhibition reduces abnormal flash-evoked potentials in parallel with an improvement in the associated myoclonus (105).

Myoclonus without loss of consciousness, characteristic of juvenile myoclonic epilepsy (JME) and other myoclonic epilepsy syndromes, is attributed to a defect in GABAergic inhibition (106). Spontaneous and photosensitive seizures are seen in alcohol and other drug withdrawal states characterized by downregulation of the GABA-A receptors or low occipital GABA levels (107). MRS-based measurements show low GABA levels in the visual cortex of patients, consistent with the enhanced cortical excitability observed in JME (108). In primates, light deprivation results in decreased glutamic acid decarboxylase (GAD) content within several days and decreased genetic transcription (GAD mRNA) within several weeks (94, 109). Long-term deprivation of visual input leads to marked changes in the excitability and function of the visual cortex. Recent studies show an association between increasing excitability in the visual cortex and decreasing GABA concentrations, induced by 1–2 hours of light-deprivation in healthy human subjects (110).

Two-thirds of patients with refractory, localization-related epilepsy treated with traditional antiepileptic drugs have below-normal occipital lobe GABA levels (86). Below-normal GABA levels in the visual cortex are associated with poor seizure control, not with being seizure-free (111). GABAergic neurons are decreased in the human epileptogenic neocortex associated with TLE, low-grade tumors, and cortical malformations (94, 112–114). Loss of GABAergic processes is seen in some cases. Circulating autoantibodies against GAD occur in some patients with refractory epilepsy (115). Below-normal cellular GABA levels in the visual cortex contribute to enhanced cortical excitability and therefore to the potential for seizures. What is unknown is whether the low cellular GABA is caused by frequent seizures or is an epiphenomenon.

Some studies have shown that patients with epileptiform abnormalities on interictal EEG recorded shortly after a seizure are more likely to have another seizure within 2 years than those with normal EEGs (116). These interictal epileptiform abnormalities probably reflect increased cortical excitability and serve as a biomarker of epileptogenicity. Similarly, localization of the site of termination of seizures of focal origin to cortical regions other than the onset is associated with a poorer surgical prognosis (117). This observation raises the possibility of additional abnormal epileptogenic cortical regions with impaired seizure-terminating capabilities, i.e. increased cortical excitability.

The presence of interictal epileptiform discharges extending beyond the area of resection correlates with poor surgical outcome in patients with extrahippocampal epilepsy (118). In contrast, patients with focal interictal epileptiform discharges included in surgical resection have good surgical outcomes. This observation suggests that increased cortical excitability outside the epileptogenic region predicts failure to become seizure-free after surgery. The observations are consistent with the hypothesis that increased cortical excitability beyond the epileptogenic region appears to contribute to continued seizure activity.

Intracellular GABA plus homocarnosine levels measured in the visual cortex, remote from the presumed seizure focus in the temporal or frontal lobes, are lowest in those patients with epileptiform abnormalities on interictal EEG (111). The associations between the interictal EEG and cellular GABA plus homocarnosine are similar to the associations between the EEG and the likelihood that seizures will recur. Low cortical cellular GABA levels could contribute to increased cortical excitability, which allows the focal seizure to spread and become generalized. Below-normal cellular GABA plus homocarnosine, measured by in-vivo MRS, could become a useful marker for epileptogenicity.

Combined with other EEG and other neuroimaging methods, MRS-based imaging of GABA, homocarnosine, and glutamate may become useful modalities in the evaluation of patients presenting with possible seizures.

GABA is formed from the alpha-decarboxylation of glutamate by GAD and is metabolized to succinate by the sequential actions of GABA-T and succinic semi-aldehyde dehydrogenase (SSADH). The activity of GAD is believed to be primarily responsible for regulating the steady-state concentration of GABA in vivo through the pyridoxal-5′-phosphate-dependent interconversion of active (holo-GAD) and inactive forms (apo-GAD) (93). Apo-GAD accounts for at least 50% of total GAD present in the brain. The activation of GAD is stimulated by Pi and inhibited by ATP, GABA, and aspartate. ATP promotes the formation of apo-GAD and stabilizes it. The activation of apo-GAD to holo-GAD by pyridoxal phosphate is a two-step process. The reversible association of apo-GAD with activated pyridoxine is rapid (ATP inhibits binding of apo-GAD with pyridoxal phosphate). Pi antagonizes the inhibitory effects of ATP and, through allosteric mechanisms, accelerates the formation of holo-GAD from the apo-GAD/pyridoxyl-phosphate intermediate. GAD is activated by changes in energy state – depolarization, acidosis, increased carbon dioxide, low bicarbonate, low phosphocreatine, increased magnesium, increased ADP, and decreased ATP.

GAD consists of two major isoforms, GAD65 and GAD67, that are the products of two different genes located in humans on chromosomes 2 and 10 (119). The two isoforms have different distributions and functions (120). GAD65 appears to comprise the bulk of GAD protein in the brain but most of it is in the inactive, apoenzyme, form. This isoform is localized primarily in synapses, perhaps associated with vesicles, and usually operates at a small fraction of its maximal catalytic capacity. Because the equilibria under physiologic conditions strongly favor the apoenzyme form, GAD65 activity is very sensitive to changes in energy state (Pi, phosphocreatine, pH, magnesium, ADP, ATP) and the availability of pyridoxal phosphate (activated vitamin B6).

GAD65 may control GABAergic function in phasic inhibitory neurons (acting as a point-to-point, fast neurotransmitter) by maintaining vesicular GABA concentrations. Holo-GAD (active enzyme) levels remain unchanged in mice deficient in GAD65, but apo-GAD (inactive) levels are greatly reduced. Not unexpectedly, GABA levels are about the same in wild-type and homozygous GAD65-deficient mice. Mild stress induces spontaneous seizures affecting limbic structures in these mice and they are very sensitive to convulsants.

The GABA concentration of neocortex primarily reflects the fractional volume of GABAergic neurons weighted by the GABA content of those neurons. Under normal conditions, the GABA content of GABAergic neurons (50–100 mmol/l in nerve terminals) is far greater than that of non-GABAergic neurons or glia (42). GAD67 has a wider distribution in the neuronal cytosol, being expressed in cell bodies, axons, dendrites, and synapses. The vesicular pool of GABA, thought to be synthesized under normal condition primarily by GAD65, comprises ≈30% of the GABA content, whereas GAD67 appears to synthesize ≈70% of brain GABA (93). GAD67 has a wider distribution in the neuronal cytosol, being expressed in cell bodies, axons, dendrites, and synapses.

In individual neurons, the ratio of GAD65 to GAD67 mRNA varies with cell type. Higher levels of GAD67 mRNA are seen usually in neurons known to be tonically firing. GAD67 mRNA is more abundant than GAD65 mRNA in most regions of the brain. In the adult primate visual cortex 18% of neurons express GAD67 mRNA, whereas 13% express GAD65 mRNA (121). Most of GAD67 is in the holo-GAD form, actively synthesizing GABA. In individual neurons, the ratio of GAD65 to GAD67 mRNA varies with cell type. Experiments with GAD67 'knock-out' mice lend further support to the hypothesis that changes in brain GABA concentration are more affected by changes in GAD67 expression and activity than by changes in GAD65 (122–124).

Changes in cytosolic GABA concentrations alter cellular physiology in a variety of ways. The distribution of GAD67 appears to coincide with the distribution of the neuronal GABA transporter (GAT1), suggesting that cytosolic GABA synthesized by this GAD isoform may have a significant paracrine function, perhaps through transporter reversal (100, 125). Release of GABA through transporter reversal has been demonstrated with physiologic stimuli. Tonic release of GABA increases with increasing cytosolic GABA, resulting in increased basal extracellular levels. Dynamic insertion of GABA transporters into the plasma membrane occurs in response to increased extracellular GABA. Increased transporter availability interacting with higher cytosolic GABA would act in a synergistic fashion to magnify GABAergic effects.

In patients evaluated for epilepsy surgery, microdialysis-based GABA measurements show a decrease in the seizure-induced release of GABA in the epileptogenic hippocampus, where the seizure started, compared to the contralateral one (126). The deficiency of GABA release is attributed in part to a dysfunction of the GABA transporter system (GAT1) (127). Low cytosolic GABA levels could contribute to the deficiency of GABA release. In some patients, the epileptogenic hippocampus is gliotic (hippocampal sclerosis); in others, patients with mesial TLE histology show no significant gliosis. What is unknown is whether genetic polymorphisms or acquired injuries, e.g. anti-GAD or anti-GAT1 antibodies, contribute to the deficient release of GABA through low GABA levels, deficient GAT1 expression, or GAT1 dysfunction.

Both glutamate and glutamine are immediate amino acid precursors of GABA. The glial specific enzyme, GS, and the neuronal enzymes, PAG and GAD, are important regulatory enzymes of GABA homeostasis (93, 128) (Fig. 13.26). In the GABA–glutamine cycle, GABA released from cells (by either vesicular release or transporter reversal), taken up by surrounding glia, converted to glutamine, released by glia, taken up by neurons, is converted back to glutamate, which serves a substrate for GABA synthesis, thus completing the cycle. Only glia contain the enzymes needed to synthesize glutamine and new TCA cycle intermediates.

The GABA–glutamine cycle parallels the glutamate–glutamine cycle. GABA, released from neurons by vesicular

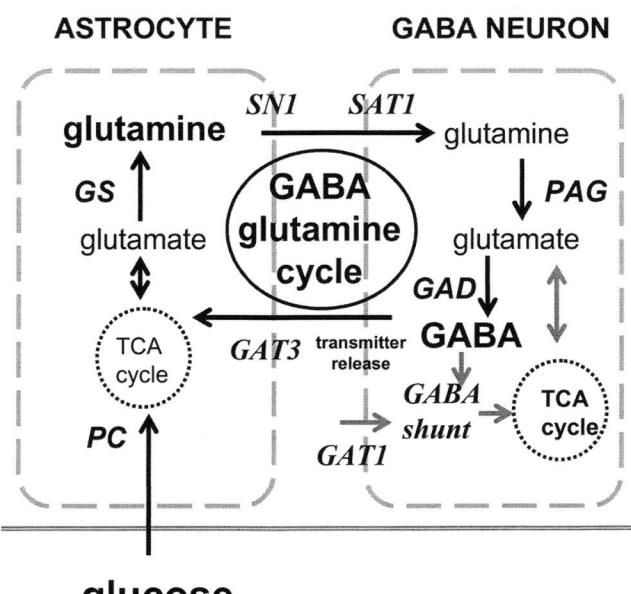

FIG. 13.26. Schematic of the GABA–glutamine cycle and the anaplerotic pathway used by the brain for the de-novo synthesis of GABA from glucose. GAD, glutamic acid decarboxylase; GAT1, neuronal GABA transporter; GAT3, glial GABA transporter; GS, glutamine synthetase; PAG, phosphate activate glutaminase; PC, pyruvate carboxylase; SAT1, system-A transporter; SN1, system-N transporter.

or nonvesicular routes, is taken up by glia through the sodium-dependent GABA transporter (GAT3). In the mitochondria, it is converted by the sequential actions of GABA-T and SSADH into succinate, a critical TCA cycle intermediate. The GABA-T plus SSADH complex is referred to as the 'GABA shunt'. Glutamate is synthesized from alpha-ketoglutarate, another key TCA intermediate, through the action of GABA-T. Rising glial cytosolic glutamate stimulates glutamate synthesis by GS. Glial release of glutamine is tightly controlled by the SN1 transporter. The system-A transporter (SAT1 and SAT2), which actively takes up extracellular glutamine, exhibits particularly high levels of expression by GABAergic neurons with the location of SAT1 at the nerve terminal. Glutamine is converted to glutamate and ammonia by PAG. The GABA–glutamine cycle is completed by the GAD, which synthesizes GABA from glutamate. A portion of the GABA released into the synaptic cleft is taken up by the neuronal sodium-dependent GABA transporter (GAT1). In glutamatergic and GABAergic neurons, GABA enters the GABA shunt to be recycled to the TCA cycle as succinate.

Both glutamine and GABA are critical anaplerotic substrates, maintaining neuronal mitochondrial synthetic function. GABAergic neurons appear to be unable to synthesize GABA de novo from glucose or lactate. Glutamine produced from exogenous glutamate is readily released in cultured astrocytes and GABA synthesis is stimulated by glutamine in synaptosomes, cell cultures, and brain slices, where it serves as a major precursor of the releasable pool of glutamate and GABA (75, 129–131). This suggests that GAD activity, and hence GABA synthesis, is limited by the availability of intracellular glutamate in GABAergic neurons.

The GABA–Glutamate Cycle

Another cycle, the glutamate-GABA cycle, potentially exists (Fig. 13.27). Glutamatergic neurons appear to express GABA transporters (GAT1) and GABA-T/SSADH. GABA released by GABA-containing cells can be taken up by glutamatergic cells and recycled to form glutamate. Conversely, GABAergic neurons can take up extracellular glutamate. Glutamate transporters are localized primarily on glia and on certain GABAergic neurons, not glutamatergic ones. Glutamate, taken up by GABAergic neurons, stimulates GAD and thus GABA synthesis, thereby increasing GABA levels. GAD67 transcription and expression is upregulated in response to injury (93). Enhanced activity of the glutamate-GABA cycle could be an adaptive metabolic response to excess glutamate release, helping to mitigate excitotoxicity.

Epileptogenesis and GABA

Clearly, many factors affect seizure generation. The traditional view on epileptogenesis is centered on changes

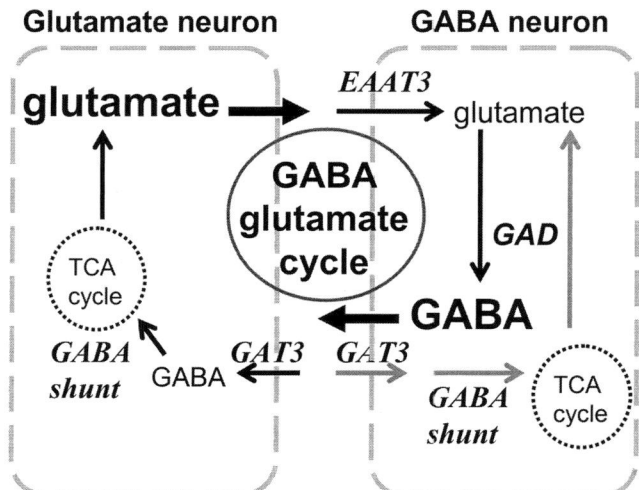

FIG. 13.27. The GABA–glutamate cycle. EAAT3, neuronal glutamate transporter; GAD, glutamic acid decarboxylase; GAT1, neuronal GABA transporter; GAT3, glial GABA transporter.

in the intrinsic properties of populations of neurons and neuron-to-neuron interactions within the seizure-onset zone. A population of excitatory neurons begins to generate barrages of action potentials (intrinsic bursts). Glutamatergic synaptic transmission increases by way of recurrent neuronal connections, which develop in response to the epileptogenic injury. There is a decrease in the efficiency of inhibitory connections (GABA-mediated) (132, 133). In the appropriate setting, GABAergic neurotransmission can become excitatory. GABA acts as an excitatory neurotransmitter during fetal development and astrocytes express GAD in the fetal central nervous system (134, 135). Low expression of the neuron-specific potassium chloride co-transporter (KCC2) in pyramidal neurons in the epileptic hippocampus has been suggested as a possible mechanism for the excitatory actions of GABA.

GABA plays an important role in mammalian epilepsy (136, 137). GABA is the major inhibitory neurotransmitter in the brain of mammals, including humans. Reviews by several investigators have stressed the role of GABA in epilepsy and emphasized the developmental aspects of GABA physiology, with implications for childhood epilepsy. Animal models using advanced molecular genetic techniques such as knockout mutations have identified the role of genes affecting ion channels, the synapse (including release and uptake of neurotransmitters), synaptic receptors and the neural network that result in epilepsy (138). Many of these mutations result in alterations of GABA and glutamate physiology. A recently described mutation of a nonspecific alkaline phosphatase results in markedly reduced brain GABA and intractable seizures (139).

In addition, rare genetic disorders of GABA metabolism have been identified in a few hundred children (140). These disorders include pyridoxine-dependent epilepsies, GABA-T deficiency and succinic-semialdehyde-dehydrogenase deficiency (141–143). Subjects with pyridoxine-dependent epilepsies have been observed to have extremely low CSF GABA levels, elevated glutamate, and low levels of brain GABA. Recent reports have suggested that similar changes in CSF GABA occur in children with infantile spasms (144). Despite the known role of pyridoxine (vitamin B6) as an important co-factor for GAD, a key regulatory enzyme of GABA metabolism, characterization of the molecular defect in pyridoxine-dependent epilepsies has yet to be discovered. However, mutations in the γ_2 subunit of the GABA-A receptor were recently reported to cause familial epilepsy with febrile seizures or absence (145, 146).

Measurements of cerebral GABA levels will provide a more efficient procedure for identifying families carrying genes affecting GABA metabolism, and will facilitate the identification of the specific mutated genes. MRS-based GABA and homocarnosine imaging may become useful in extending the phenotype to detect presymptomatic family members of patients with inherited causes of low brain GABA and epilepsy.

Studies using MRS have found reduced cellular GABA levels in the human visual cortex in localization-related epilepsies. Below-normal GABA levels in the visual cortex are associated with poor seizure control in refractory localization-related epilepsy syndromes (108, 111, 147–149). Whether low GABA levels are the cause or the result of frequent seizures is unknown.

It is surprising that intracellular GABA levels are below normal in many patients with poor seizure control, particularly in regions presumably remote from the epileptogenic areas (most often temporal and frontal lobes in our series). Both GABA concentrations and synthesis rates increase in most seizure models (57). Serial MRS measurements, made in the occipital lobe cortex before and after a series of bilateral electroconvulsive therapy treatments with documented electrographic seizures, show GABA increases in most morbidly depressed patients (150). One plausible hypothesis is that below-normal cellular GABA levels in the visual cortex contribute to enhanced cortical excitability and therefore to the potential for seizures. Low cellular GABA levels reflect an intrinsic alteration in GABA metabolism and are not sufficient in themselves to cause epilepsy in most patients. Low neocortical GABA levels contribute to the expression of seizure disorders in the localization-related epilepsies by increasing cortical excitability in a global fashion, thereby facilitating the spread of seizure to regions remote from the epileptogenic zone.

Cortical Excitability and GABA Content

Some studies have shown that patients with epileptiform abnormalities on interictal EEG recorded shortly after a seizure are more likely to have another seizure within 2 years than those with normal EEGs (116). These interictal epileptiform abnormalities probably reflect increased cortical excitability and serve as a biomarker of epileptogenicity. Similarly, localization of the site of termination of seizures of focal origin to cortical regions other than the onset is associated with a poorer surgical prognosis (117). This observation raises the possibility of additional abnormal epileptogenic cortical regions with impaired seizure-terminating capabilities, i.e. increased cortical excitability.

The presence of interictal epileptiform discharges extending beyond the area of resection correlates with poor surgical outcome in patients with extrahippocampal epilepsy (118). In contrast, patients with focal interictal epileptiform discharges included in surgical resection have good surgical outcomes. This observation suggests that increased cortical excitability outside the epileptogenic region predicts failure to become seizure-free after surgery. The observations are consistent with the hypothesis that increased cortical excitability beyond the epileptogenic region appears to contribute continued seizure activity.

Intracellular GABA plus homocarnosine levels measured in the visual cortex, remote from the presumed seizure focus in the temporal or frontal lobes, are lowest in those patients with epileptiform abnormalities on interictal EEG (Fig. 13.28) (111). The associations between the interictal EEG and cellular GABA plus homocarnosine are similar to the associations between the EEG and the likelihood that seizures will recur. Low cortical cellular GABA levels could contribute to increased cortical excitability, which allows the focal seizure to spread and become generalized. Below-normal cellular GABA plus homocarnosine, measured by in-vivo MRS, could become a useful marker for epileptogenicity. Combined with other EEG and other neuro-imaging methods, MRS-based imaging of GABA, homocarnosine, and

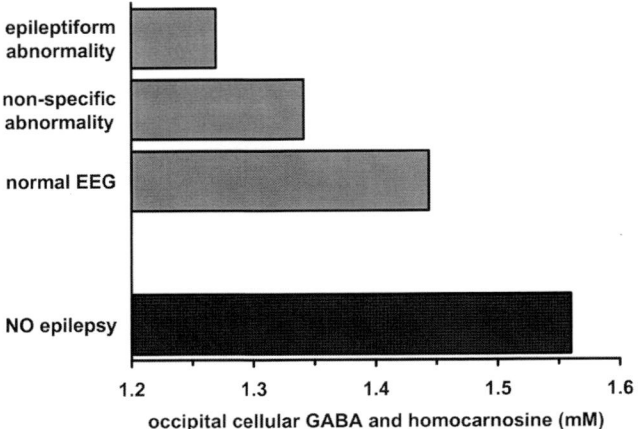

FIG. 13.28. The occipital GABA plus homocarnosine content of the occipital lobe, remote from the seizure focus, is below normal in patients with refractory, complex partial seizures. Those patients with epileptiform discharges on interictal EEG have the lowest levels. (From data in Petroff et al. 1996 (111).)

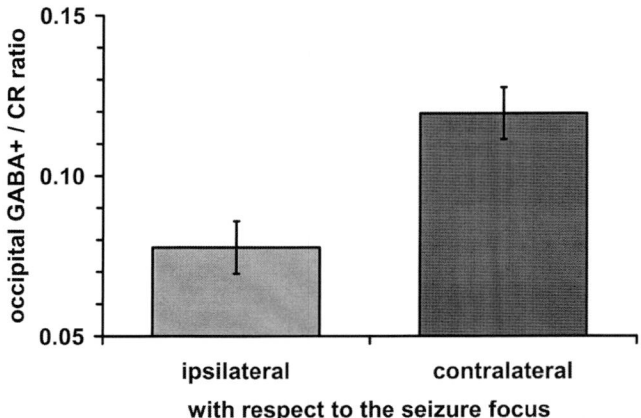

FIG. 13.29. Proton-MRS measurements of the GABA+ to creatine (GABA+/Cr) ratio of the occipital lobe ipsilateral and contralateral to the seizure focus in patients with temporal lobe epilepsy show that the ratio is significantly less on the ipsilateral side. Low GABA may define the epileptic network in localization-related epilepsies. (From data in Mueller et al. 2001 (151).)

glutamate may become useful modalities in the evaluation of patients presenting with possible seizures.

Occipital GABA Levels are Reduced Ipsilateral to Epileptic Focus

Occipital-posterior-temporal lobe GABA+/Cr ratios are reported to be 30% lower ipsilateral to the seizure focus (Fig. 13.29) (151). The ratios are lowest ipsilateral to the seizure focus in those patients who achieved good seizure control after GABA levels are increased with vigabatrin. Vigabatrin is a GABA-T inhibitor that increases intracellular and extracellular GABA and homocarnosine (147, 148). This suggests that increased GABA may contribute to the reduction in symptoms. A recent review proposes that human epilepsy is a disorder of large neural networks (152). The electrical hyperexcitability associated with seizure activity reverberates within the neural structures of the network to culminate in the eventual expression of seizures. The low neocortical GABA levels ipsilateral to the epileptogenic temporal lobe suggest that low cellular GABA could contribute to the hyperexcitability of the epileptic network.

Imaging GABA may become very useful in mapping epileptic networks. MRS-based GABA, homocarnosine, and glutamate imaging may become a key part of the presurgical evaluation of patients with refractory localization-related epilepsies. GABA and glutamate imaging may be useful for the localization of the epileptogenic network. Bilateral below-normal GABA or homocarnosine may herald the recurrence of seizures after epilepsy surgery.

Effects of Antiepileptic Drugs on Cortical GABA Content

The use of the traditional antiepileptic drugs do not appear to have a major effect on intracellular GABA and homocarnosine levels measured in the visual cortex using MRS (86, 90, 149). In patients with refractory localization-related epilepsies treated with carbamazepine, phenytoin, phenobarbital, primidone, valproate, or combinations of these drugs, cortical GABA and homocarnosine levels are low. In animal models, valproate is reported to increase intracellular GABA by inhibiting SSADH and possibly stimulating GABA synthesis.

Daily use of vigabatrin, topiramate, gabapentin, or zonisamide appears to be associated with increased cellular GABA plus homocarnosine (Fig. 13.30). Vigabatrin is a potent, irreversible inhibitor of GABA-T that is known to increase the cytosolic and vesicular GABA content of neurons, the cytosolic GABA content of glia, and extracellular and serum GABA concentration (147). Topiramate and gabapentin clearly raise GABA and homocarnosine in human brain but have no clear-cut effect in rodent models (153–156).

In drug-free volunteers without epilepsy, topiramate, gabapentin, and lamotrigine increased intracellular brain

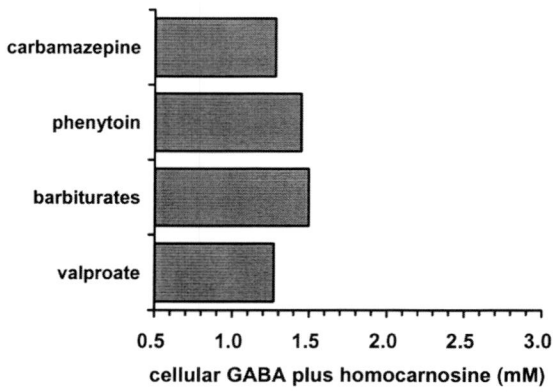

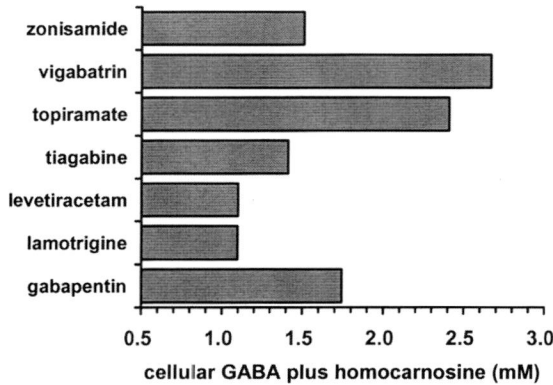

FIG. 13.30. Treatment with vigabatrin, topiramate, gabapentin, or zonisamide appears to be associated with increased cellular GABA plus homocarnosine, measured in the occipital lobe using proton-MRS. (From data in Petroff et al. 1999, 2000 (86, 90).)

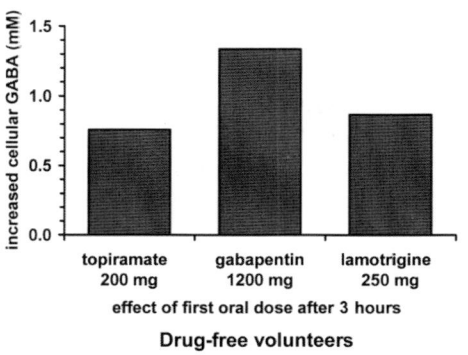
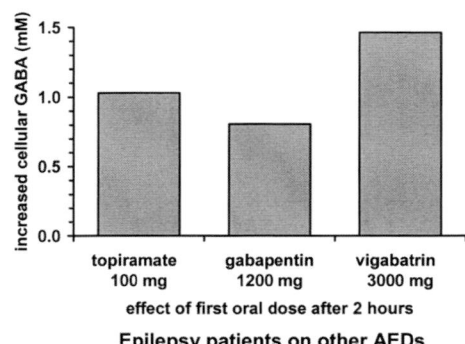

FIG. 13.31. A. Serial proton-MRS measurements show that topiramate, gabapentin, and lamotrigine increase intracellular brain GABA within 3 hours of the first oral dose. **B.** Similarly, topiramate, or vigabatrin increase intracellular GABA levels in the visual cortex within 1–2 hours in patients with epilepsy. (From data in Kuzniecky et al. 2002 (155) and Petroff et al. 1999, 2000, 2001(86, 90, 148).)

GABA with 3 hours of the first oral dose (155, 157) (Fig. 13.31). Increased levels are maintained for at least 4 weeks on daily doses of topiramate 400 mg, gabapentin 2400 mg, and lamotrigine 500 mg.

In patients with refractory localization-related epilepsies, the first oral doses of gabapentin, topiramate, or vigabatrin increase intracellular GABA levels in the visual cortex within 1–2 hours of the first oral dose (Fig. 13.31) (153, 154, 158). In-vivo MRS-based studies of GABA metabolism have shown that human and rodent GABA metabolism are clearly different. Whether GABA metabolism is different in young children remains to be further evaluated (159). Using GABA, homocarnosine, and glutamate imaging may help tailor the selection of anti-epileptic drugs to individualize therapy for the neurotransmitter/neurometabolic condition of the patient. An epilepsy patient with low GABA or homocarnosine may benefit from a drug that increases cellular GABA or homocarnosine or perhaps lowers cellular glutamate. Vigabatrin and phenobarbital, drugs that are thought to exert their anticonvulsant effects through the GABAergic system, appear to lower cellular glutamate too.

HOMOCARNOSINE: A UNIQUE ASPECT OF PRIMATE GAMMA-AMINO BUTYRIC ACID METABOLISM

Homocarnosine, a dipeptide of GABA and histidine unique to brain, is present in human brain in greater amounts (0.3–1.6 mmol/l) than in other mammals (<0.07 mmol/l). Homocarnosine is an inhibitory neuromodulator synthesized in the neuron from GABA and histidine (160–162). Immunohistology studies for homocarnosine suggest a cytosolic localization in human brain, most probably in subclasses of GABAergic neurons. In the human neocortex and white matter tracts, homocarnosine immunoreactivity is seen along projecting fibers rather than in GABAergic interneurons. Autopsy-based studies show that regional homocarnosine and GABA levels vary independently (163).

Homocarnosine concentrations are three- to sixfold higher in adults than in infants.

Human CSF GABA consists of micromolar concentrations of homocarnosine and pyrrolidinone (the internal lactam of GABA), small amounts of other GABA containing peptides, and nanomolar quantities of free GABA (164). It comprises approximately 40% of the GABA measured in human CSF after acid extraction of human CSF. The histidyl portion of the homocarnosine molecule is sensitive to pH with a pK in the physiologic range (6.86) (165). The chemical shift of the homocarnosine resonances can be used to measure the pH of the human brain (7.06) in the homocarnosine-specific (neuronal cytosol) compartment. It has been proposed that homocarnosine contributes to intracellular buffering.

Although homocarnosine may serve as an important inhibitory neuromodulator in the human brain, little is known about the regulation of its synthesis (166). Homocarnosine is synthesized in the cytosol of a subclass of GABAergic neurons by the enzyme homocarnosine synthetase (161) (Fig. 13.32). Human homocarnosine synthetase activity is

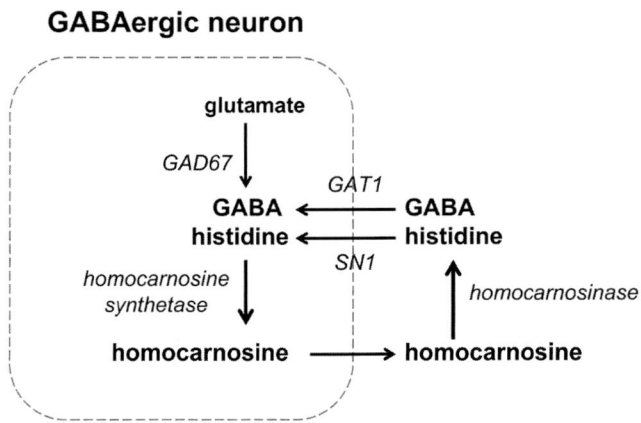

FIG. 13.32. Homocarnosine synthesis. GAD67, glutamic acid decarboxylase isoform 67 kDa; GAT1, neuronal GABA transporter; SN1, system-N transporter.

highest in the occipital cortex, basal ganglia, and cervical cord and lowest in the cerebellar cortex. Immunoreactivity is seen in neuronal cell bodies, axons, and synapses, correlating well with the cytosolic distribution of homocarnosine itself (162). The distribution of homocarnosine synthetase appears to correlate better with the reported distribution of GAD67 than for GAD65. Not unexpectedly, regional homocarnosine and GABA levels do not correlate (163). The substrates for the enzyme are histidine and GABA and ATP. The products include homocarnosine, ADP, free magnesium, and a hydrogen ion.

In vitro, human homocarnosine synthetase has a V_{max} of 18 nmol/g/h and a Km for GABA of 8.8 mmol/l. The Km for histidine is approximately 1 mmol/l based upon studies of the rat enzyme (carnosine-homocarnosine synthetase) (167). Substrate availability, based on estimated cytosolic concentrations of GABA (5–10 mmol/l) and histidine (0.1–0.2 mmol/l), may limit homocarnosine synthetase activity. Consistent with substrate limitation, in-vivo MRS-based studies have shown that homocarnosine concentrations increase following administration of drugs that elevate GABA, but only after a delay of at least 24 hours (153, 154, 158).

Whether homocarnosine is packaged in vesicles and co-released with GABA remains unresolved. GABAergic neurons often co-release a variety of short peptides with GABA. Alternatively, homocarnosine may be released through GABA-transporter (GAT1) reversal. This possibility is less likely because homocarnosine is a significantly larger molecule than GABA and positively charged.

A specific enzyme, homocarnosinase (human serum carnosinase), rapidly hydrolyzes homocarnosine. It has an extracellular location associated with a subtype of GABAergic synapses. Homocarnosine is hydrolyzed in the extracellular space into GABA and histidine. Neurons are unable to synthesize histidine and utilize the SN1 transporter, which has a greater affinity for histidine than glutamine. SN1 is coupled to the hydrogen and sodium ion gradients. Intracellular acidification promotes the uptake of histidine as it stimulates GAD67 to synthesize GABA. Homocarnosinase immunoreactivity is associated with synapses of projecting fibers, localization suggesting that homocarnosine may act as an important modulator of excitability in the human neocortex.

Homocarnosinosis, secondary to the inherited absence of homocarnosinase, has been reported (140, 160, 166). The phenotype is unclear. Some patients are neurologically normal, others have cognitive and developmental problems, spinal muscular atrophy, or seizures. Diagnosis requires CSF or MRS analysis because homocarnosine that enters the blood is rapidly hydrolyzed by carnosinase, a serum enzyme that is present in normal amounts in patients with homocarnosinosis.

The regulation of homocarnosine concentrations is poorly understood. Restriction of histidine lowers the abnormally elevated homocarnosine levels associated with a dysfunctional degradative enzyme, homocarnosinase (168). CSF homocarnosine levels are elevated 6–24 hours after the first dose of vigabatrin, the GABA-T inhibitor that raises GABA levels in the CSF, cytosol, and vesicles (169). CSF studies in patients suggest that above-normal levels of homocarnosine may contribute to improved seizure control (170).

Homocarnosine Content and Seizure Control

The primary effect of vigabatrin at low daily doses (1–2 g/d) appears to be an increase in intracellular GABA. At standard doses (3–4 g/d), homocarnosine continues to increase with minimal change in cortical GABA. Greater than 50% improvement in seizure frequency was reported with higher homocarnosine levels in most patients treated with vigabatrin (Fig. 13.33) (148). Patients whose seizure control more than doubled had higher homocarnosine concentrations than patients who did not benefit ($p < 0.05$). Mean GABA levels were the same in patients who improved and those who did not improve. Increased homocarnosine failed to benefit some patients. The increase in homocarnosine contributed to improved seizure control.

Patients with refractory localization-related epilepsies often have below-normal intracellular GABA and homocarnosine measured by in-vivo MRS in the visual cortex. Low cellular GABA and poor seizure control are associated in such patients treated with valproate or lamotrigine (Fig. 13.34). Surprisingly, patients with JME, even those with excellent seizure control (no convulsions in years), often have cellular GABA levels lower than patients with poorly controlled complex partial seizures (108). Over half (69%) of patients with JME treated with valproate or lamotrigine had GABA levels more than 2 SD below-normal. The discordant finding of low GABA and excellent seizure control in JME may be explained by the normal homocarnosine levels. Patients with refractory complex partial seizures have below-normal mean GABA and homocarnosine levels; patients with JME had the lowest mean GABA levels, yet had normal homocarnosine levels.

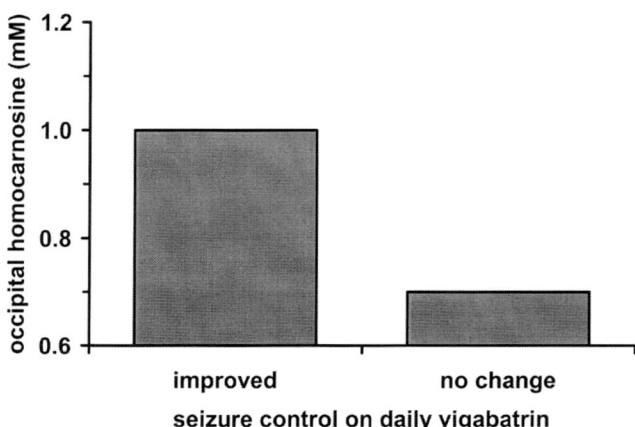

FIG. 13.33. Improved seizure control is associated with increased homocarnosine concentrations in epilepsy patients treated with vigabatrin. (From data in Petroff et al. 1998 (148).)

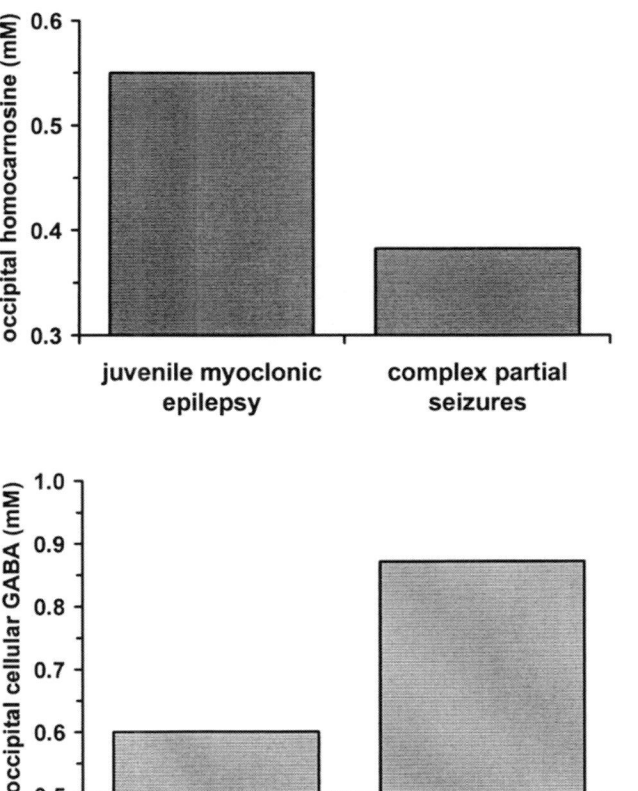

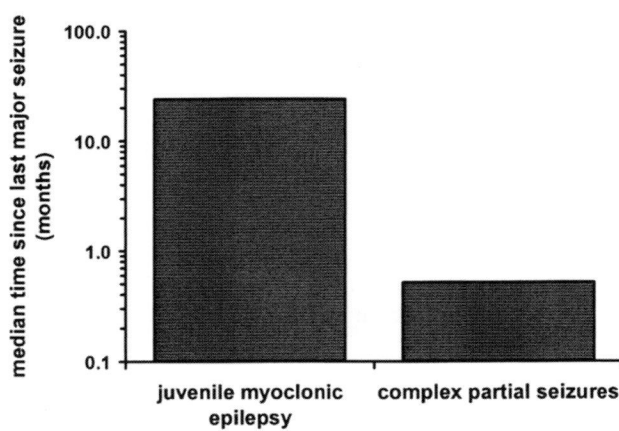

FIG. 13.34. Excellent seizure control is associated with increased homocarnosine concentrations in patients with juvenile myoclonic epilepsy. (From data in Petroff et al. 2001 (154).)

Higher levels of homocarnosine were associated with better seizure control in all patients, irrespective of seizure type. All patients with below-normal homocarnosine had poor seizure control – several seizures with loss of contact per month. All patients with JME had normal homocarnosine levels; those with the lowest homocarnosine levels had had at least one seizure with loss of contact within the past year. Log-linear regression revealed a significant association between homocarnosine levels and seizure control. These results indicate that higher brain homocarnosine levels strongly correlate with better seizure control in human epilepsy. However, while this correlation implies a causal linkage, it does not prove that homocarnosine directly decreases cortical excitability and by this mechanism improves seizure control.

Hydrolysis of homocarnosine has been proposed as an alternate metabolic pathway to rapidly increase GABAergic activity and thus serve as an important inhibitory neuromodulator in human neocortex. Intraventricular injections show that homocarnosine has anticonvulsant properties. It may interact directly with GABA receptors or after hydrolysis to GABA and histidine (162).

The mechanisms of homocarnosine release, possible synaptic co-release with GABA or, more likely, nonsynaptic routes, are obscure. Paracrine models appear to be favored, with homocarnosine serving as an inhibitory modulator rather than a point-to-point synaptic signaling. Release of homocarnosine could contribute to glutamate–GABA cycling and reflect an adaptive response to excess extracellular glutamate. Homocarnosine may modulate synaptic transmission directly by altering the availability of zinc (171). Because homocarnosine is an excellent chelator of zinc and copper with relatively little affinity for calcium or magnesium, it can buffer zinc and copper levels with little impact on calcium. Alternatively, histidine, another excellent chelator of zinc, may be the primary effector. Having a strong zinc chelator at the GABA receptor should enhance the inhibitory action of GABA, particularly at those GABA receptors expressing the gamma-subunit (172, 173). Zinc also synchronizes release of GABA and modulates glutamatergic receptors (174). Thus homocarnosine can modulate neuronal excitability through a number of mechanisms. Low homocarnosine could reflect decreased fractional volumes of homocarnosine-containing neurons, expression of homocarnosine synthetase, or downregulation of homocarnosine synthetase activity.

A number of the new antiepileptic drugs—topiramate, lamotrigine, levetiracetam, gabapentin—increase cellular homocarnosine. Daily use of vigabatrin, gabapentin, and topiramate increases intracellular concentrations of GABA and homocarnosine (Fig. 13.35) (88, 153, 154, 158). Surprisingly, daily use of levetiracetam appears to increase intracellular homocarnosine without appreciably increasing intracellular GABA.

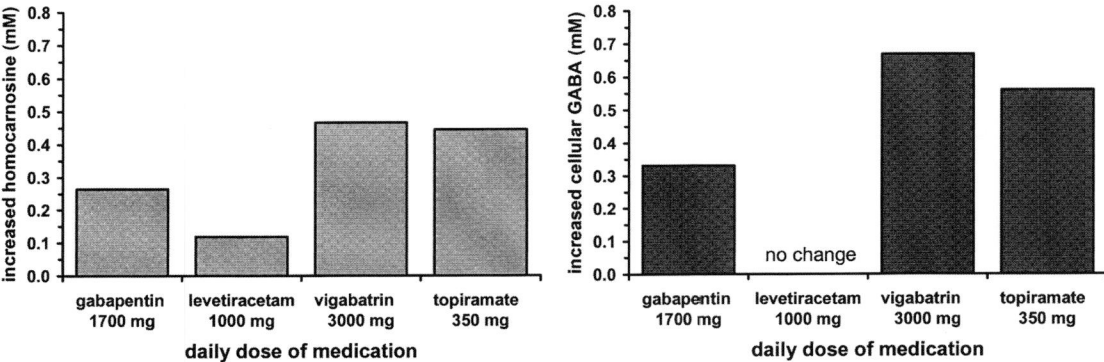

FIG. 13.35. Treatment with topiramate, vigabatrin, gabapentin, and levetiracetam increases cortical homocarnosine content. (From data in Petroff et al. 1999, 2000, 2001 (86, 90, 148).)

N-ACETYL ASPARTATE METABOLISM

N-acetyl aspartate is the most concentrated organic metabolite unique to the central nervous system. The singlet resonance from the three hydrogen atoms of the terminal methyl group of the N-acetyl portion of NAA serves as a useful marker of normal adult nervous tissue. NAA levels and the NAA-to-creatine (NAA/Cr) ratio are decreased in a wide variety of neurologic problems. Mitochondrial dysfunction or loss of neurons and axons are a common feature. Following a stroke, NAA levels decline over a period of several days. The loss of NAA after a stroke reflects the loss of neurons (175). Pathology studies of the dementias clearly demonstrate a significant association between neuron loss and low NAA levels (176). Studies of chronic plaques in multiple sclerosis show a significant correlation between axon loss and low NAA levels (177, 178). Studies of wallerian degeneration in rat optic nerve support this relationship— less NAA correlates with the degree of axon loss. (179)

Studies of human inborn errors of metabolism cast doubt on the tight association between low NAA levels and neuron loss. Martin and colleagues report brain spectra that appear to show no NAA, which were obtained from a disable child with neurodevelopmental retardation and moderately delayed myelination (180). Naturally, the report generated a lively discussion (181). Yet, the primary observations remain valid—little or no NAA is present in MR spectra obtained from voxels from multiple regions of brain using routine clinical MRS methodology. NAA levels are extremely low in a transgenic mouse model of Huntington's disease (182). Low NAA levels occurred in the absence of neuronal death as measured by postmortem Nissl staining and neuronal counting, but in the presence of nuclear inclusion bodies.

Reversible decreases in NAA are seen following traumatic brain injury (183). Serial measurements of NAA in acute multiple sclerosis plaques show a pattern of decline and recovery. The observations suggest that a metabolic component contributes to the reversible decrease of NAA (184, 185). In the mitochondrial cytopathies, below-normal NAA, low phosphocreatine, and elevated lactate levels are seen in all patients, including those without signs and symptoms of brain involvement and with normal MRIs (186–189). These changes are most prominent in patients with myoclonic epilepsy or stroke. Some of the MRS-based findings appear to be partially reversible with therapy. In-vitro studies using isolated neuronal mitochondria, neuron cultures, and perfused slice systems show that a variety of mitochondrial toxins may be used to inhibit NAA synthesis with only a modest impairment of ATP synthesis (190, 191). The findings in the mitochondrial disease are similar to those seen in the localization-related epilepsies. Mitochondrial dysfunction is one of the characteristics of the epileptogenic human hippocampus (192).

The NAA content of brain is controlled by the rate of synthesis in mitochondria, less the rate of neuronal release or oxidation (191, 193). When NAA is released there is an obligate loss of TCA cycle metabolites, i.e. alpha-ketoglutarate or oxaloacetic acid (Fig. 13.36). Glia exclusively contain the anaplerotic enzymes necessary for the *de novo* synthesis of TCA cycle intermediates. The glutamate–glutamine cycle between neurons and glia is the dominant mechanism used to replenish neuronal TCA cycle intermediates (44). In the adult nervous system, NAA is synthesized from acetyl co-enzyme A (acetyl CoA) and aspartate by NAA synthetase by the mitochondrial enzyme NAA synthetase (L-aspartate N-acetyl-transferase).

The mechanism by which NAA enters the cytosol is unclear. One possibility is through a dicarboxylate transporter, e.g. malate or succinate. It accumulates in the cytosol on many but not all neurons, especially in large axons. NAA does not participate in neuronal metabolism except in a subset of glutamatergic neurons (196). Another neuron-specific enzyme, NAAG synthase (NAA-L-glutamate ligase), synthesizes a dipeptide, NAA-glutamate (NAAG) (195). The mechanism by which NAA is released from the neuronal cytosol is unknown. One attractive possibility is reversal of the sodium-dependent, electrogenic, dicarboxylate transporter (NaDC3) during neuronal or axonal depolarization (196).

NAA is hydrolyzed by myelin-associated aspartoacylase (N-acyl-L-aspartate amido-II-hydrolase) to aspartate and

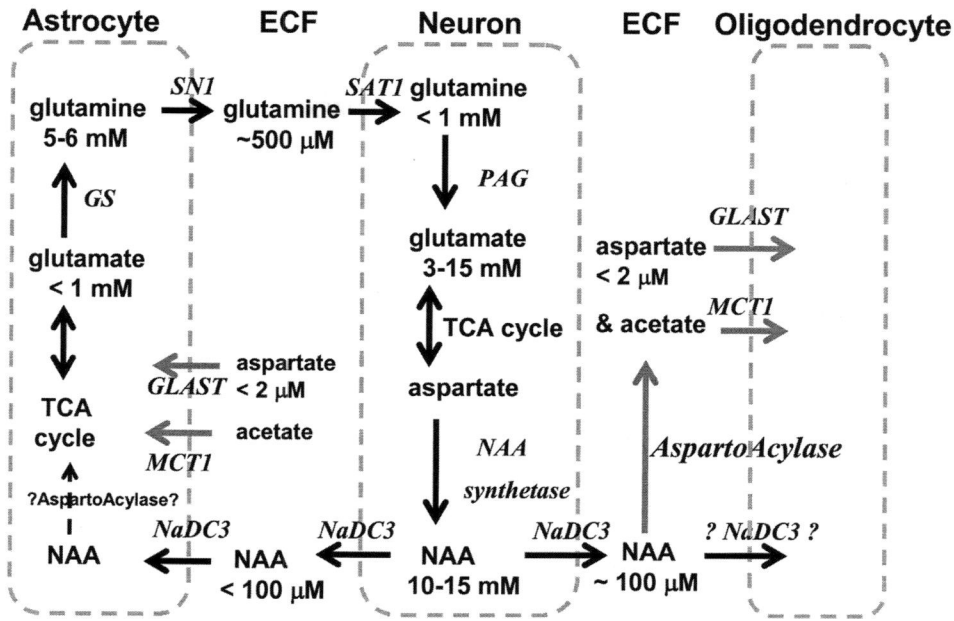

FIG. 13.36. *N*-acetyl aspartate metabolism. ECF, extracellular fluid; GLAST, glutamate aspartate transporter; GS, glutamine synthetase; MCT1, glial monocarboxylic acid transporter; NaDC3, dicarboxylic acid transporter; PAG, phosphate activated glutaminase; SAT1, system-A transporter; SN1, system-N transporter.

acetate (197). Aspartate and acetate are taken-up primarily by glial transporters (GLAST and MCAT1) (41, 76). Astrocytes take up NAA directly using NaDC3, which is functionally very active in glia (198). Dicarboxylic acids and NAA do not readily cross the intact blood–brain barrier and are therefore 'trapped' in the central nervous system. Labeling studies suggest that NAA is primarily hydrolyzed in oligodendrocytes that are myelinating. However, type-2 astrocytes express large amounts of aspartoacylase, suggesting that they too can metabolize NAA.

Mutation of aspartoacylase leads to Canavan's disease, which is an autosomal recessive leukodystrophy resulting in spongy degeneration of white matter tracts of the brain with a 50% increase in brain NAA and the NAA aciduria (193, 199). In-vivo MRS studies using ^{13}C-labeled glucose have shown that NAA turnover is coupled to glutamate turnover. NAA synthesis rates are reduced in patients with Canavan's disease in proportion to the slow rate of catabolism. The slow rate of NAA turnover indicates that elevated NAA levels inhibit NAA synthesis (product inhibition). The NAA aciduria indicates that the NAA leaks across the blood–brain barrier and is not metabolized to a significant extent by the liver or kidney.

What is the Role of NAA in the Central Nervous System?

The exact function of NAA in the nervous system has eluded definition (194, 195, 197, 200). One role is to serve as a substrate for NAAG, an excitatory neuromodulator. Another is that NAA itself appears to be an excitatory neuromodulator. Intraventricular injection of NAA produced epileptiform discharges. Hippocampal slice preparations perfused with NAA brain produces repetitive firing of hippocampal CA3 neurons. Genomic deletion within a region in which the aspartoacylase gene is located result in the tremor rat with absence-like seizures and spongiform degeneration. NAA has been proposed as a neuron–glia signaling system, perhaps critical for the formation of nodes of Ranvier.

A third, more intriguing hypothesis is that NAA serves as an osmolite controlling volume regulation as a putative component of a molecular water pump (aquaporin) (200). This proposal suggests that NAA synthesis and transport is used to remove the water generated by mitochondrial oxidative metabolism, thus minimizing the potential edema that would be the functional consequence of rapid oxidation metabolism. Oxidation of 1 mol of glucose yields 6 mol of water and carbon dioxide. Oxidation of 1 mol of BHB ('ketone body') yields 4 mol of water and carbon dioxide. A consequence of this hypothesis would be a metabolic coupling between the rates of the TCA cycle and NAA synthesis.

Other less likely hypotheses include a role in shuttling acetyl groups from neuronal mitochondria to myelin. In the fetal brain, taurine content is high. As taurine levels decrease, NAA levels rise in a reciprocal fashion. The apparent diffusion coefficients of ATP and phosphocreatine (PCr) lengthen in parallel. NAA may facilitate diffusion of ATP and PCr in dendrites, axons, myelinating oligodendrocytes, and other regions where the distances (diffusion path length) between mitochondria producing ATP and the transporters and enzymes consuming ATP are long. The apparent diffusion coefficients of the high-energy phosphates (ATP and PCr) are faster in NAA solutions compared to other major osmolites, e.g. taurine or myoinositol (mI) (201).

NAA Content is Decreased Ipsilateral to the Seizure Focus

In the localization-related human epilepsies, NAA and NAA/Cr ratios are decreased in the epileptogenic temporal lobe (9, 202, 203). In human TLE, low NAA levels are often widespread and can affect the temporal lobe contralateral to the epileptogenic hippocampus (Fig. 13.37) and correlate with interictal hypometabolism measured using PET (204). The widespread changes seen using PET and MRS are attributed to diaschisis. Neuron loss or dysfunction has been shown to decrease NAA. Below-normal NAA can provide evidence of temporal lobe or hippocampal abnormalities in epilepsy patients who show no abnormality on extensive MRI investigation (205). Lesser decreases in NAA are seen in the temporal lobe contralateral to the epileptogenic one. Below-normal NAA levels in the temporal lobe, contralateral to the epileptogenic one removed by surgery, often herald a poor outcome (206). Very low NAA levels in the temporal lobe contralateral to the one removed by surgery suggest bilateral dysfunction of the temporal lobes. The surgical outcome may be less than expected because of cognitive problems or recurrent epilepsy. A recent study reports significant negative associations between epilepsy duration and mesial temporal lobe NAA/CR ratios, both ipsilateral and contralateral to the epileptogenic temporal lobe (207). In regions with low levels prior to surgery, NAA can recover to nearly normal values following successful temporal lobectomy (9, 208). Most of the recovery occurs within 6 months and 95% by 2 years (209).

In patients with a frontal or parietal-central epileptogenic focus (neocortical epilepsy), spectroscopic imaging of NAA is useful in localizing the epileptogenic zone (210, 211).

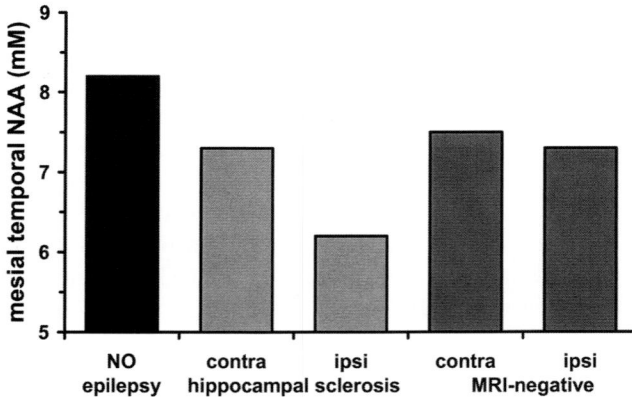

FIG. 13.37. Mean NAA content is below normal in the mesial temporal lobes of patients with temporal lobe epilepsy (TLE). NAA is lowest ipsilateral to the seizure focus in TLE with hippocampal sclerosis. (From data published by Woermann et al. 1999 (91).)

Seizure frequency correlates with the magnitude of the decrease in NAA in the seizure focus (212). In epilepsia partialis continua, cortical NAA levels are lowest in the seizure focus. Partial recovery occurs when seizures remit (213). Extremely low NAA levels are seen in the epileptic focus associated with developmental malformation with normal or increased neuron densities (214). This suggests that the NAA content of neurons in the epileptogenic zone must be decreased, probably because of impaired mitochondrial synthesis rather than enhanced neuronal release and catabolism by glial.

Whether decreased NAA levels of the mesial temporal lobe reflect hippocampal neuron loss remain unclear. A prior study of the epileptogenic human hippocampus resected at surgery reports that NAA content is significantly lower in 'sclerotic gliotic' specimens than those that are 'histologically unremarkable' (215). Another semiquantitative study involving eight patients suggests that there is an association between low NAA levels by in-vivo MRS and severity of hippocampal sclerosis (216). A larger study reports no association between the hippocampal Cr/NAA ratios measured in vivo by MRS and neuron/glia ratios of portion of the resected hippocampi (217).

A recent surgical series showed that there are no significant associations between hippocampal neuron loss and the cellular content of NAA despite a more than a threefold difference in neuron loss and a twofold increase in glial density (Fig. 13.38) (78). A highly significant association between hippocampal NAA and glutamate content is seen, with weak associations between NAA and aspartate and glutamate and aspartate. The association between NAA and glutamate content suggests that NAA and glutamate metabolism are linked closely in the epileptogenic hippocampus. Aspartate is the precursor of NAA and a weak association is not unexpected. Both aspartate and glutamate are in rapid chemical exchange with TCA cycle intermediates (malate and alpha-ketoglutarate) and an association is expected.

The modest decreases in glutamate and NAA in the hippocampi with more than 70% neuron loss and a doubling of glial density are unexpected. In the adult nervous system, NAA appears to be localized to neuronal cytosol (195, 219). It would appear unlikely that the intracellular NAA and glutamate content is increased two- to threefold in the remaining neurons of the most gliotic hippocampi. A more probable explanation is that proliferating glial cells contain significant amounts of NAA and glutamate. In cell cultures, the NAA and total creatine content of O2A-oligodendrocyte precursor cells are higher than in cerebellar neurons (79). A recent study shows that 'mature oligodendrocytes' grown in cell culture with ciliary neurotrophic factor contain high levels of intracellular total creatine and NAA, comparable to levels reported in a variety of neuronal cultures (80).

The NAA content measured in hippocampal sclerosis with TLE is too high for the degree of neuron loss. One hypothesis is that NAA is synthesized by glial precursor cells and reactive glia. Enzyme and transporter expression,

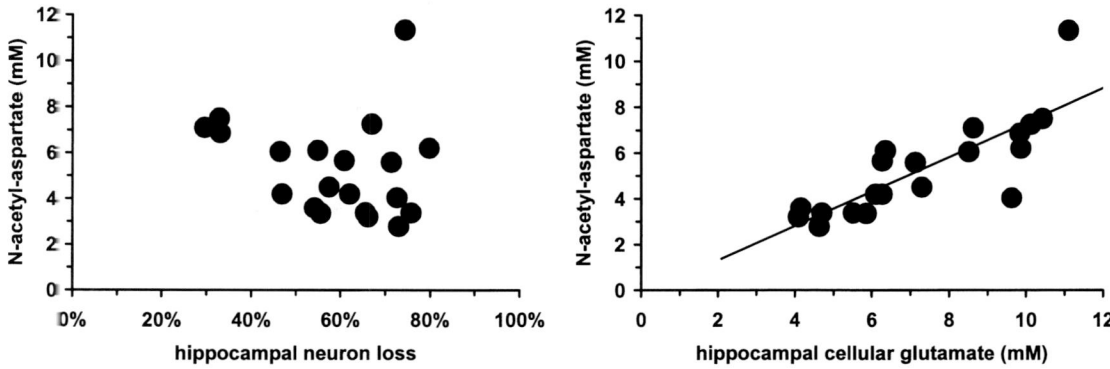

FIG. 13.38. There is no significant association between hippocampal neuron loss and the cellular content of NAA in the epileptogenic human hippocampus. There is a strong linear correlation between intracellular glutamate and NAA.

function, and localization are altered in the epileptogenic human hippocampus with sclerosis. An alternative hypothesis would invoke a pool of NAA 'trapped' in astrocytes, which may have a very slow metabolic turnover rate. MR spectra of a cellular fraction of rat and human brain enriched in glial cells show significant amounts of NAA (221). Histopathologic studies identifying subpopulations of glial cells and the co-localization of enzymes and transporters critical for NAA synthesis will resolve these issues.

ACKNOWLEDGMENT

Funding was provided by NIH-NINDS grants NS39092, NS6208 and NS32518. I would like to thank my colleagues in the research including Kevin L. Behar, Leonardo G. Cohen, Laura D. Errante, Fahmeed Hyder, Richard H. Mattson, James W. Prichard, Douglas L. Rothman, Robert G. Shulman, Nicole R. Sibson, Dennis D. Spencer, and Anne Williamson.

Clinical Applications of Magnetic Resonance Spectroscopy in Epilepsy

Graeme D. Jackson, Ruben I. Kuzniecky, Regula S. Briellmann and Mark R. Wellard

As a noninvasive technique for investigating brain metabolites, MRS enables the study of metabolic abnormalities in patients with epilepsy. The information available from MRS complements the detailed structural information that is provided by conventional MR. The value of MRS lies in its role as a means for the diagnosis of the epileptogenic lesion, where it may help to define the extent of a surgical resection or to predict postoperative outcome (7, 220). MRS may give important insights into the mechanisms of seizure generation and termination, and into the pharmacodynamics of antiepileptic drugs, and may thus help in deciding which patients may tolerate particular drugs. With its broad application, MRS has been used in the clinical context to solve the riddle of seizure focus localization in patients without obvious MR abnormalities ('MR-negative' epilepsy). Over more than two decades, MRS has developed a prominent role in research applications where the basic seizure disorder process is investigated.

Early studies using ^{31}P MR spectroscopy to study a rabbit model of status epilepticus were carried out in the 1980s by Prichard and colleagues at Yale (221, 222), showing changes in energy stores and pH. Later it was shown that lactate was elevated for a prolonged time following brief seizures (223, 224), and ^{13}C MRS documented that this elevation was the result of continuing turnover of the lactate pool (225).

Brain lactate is elevated by seizure activity, as demonstrated by conventional biochemical studies of excised tissue. In vivo animal studies using proton MRS allowed more dynamic studies and a better appreciation of how persistent lactate elevation is after even brief convulsive seizure (20–22). Selective neuronal injury by kainate-induced status epilepticus in rats was associated with focal reduction of NAA determined by proton MRS imaging, even before T2-weighted MRI changes were observed (23).

Najm et al. (24) used proton MRS to identify specific in-situ metabolic markers for seizures and seizure-induced neuronal damage in rat brains. They pretreated rats with placebo or cycloheximide 1 hour before kainic acid injection and then scanned rat brains at the level of the hippocampus before, during, and 24 hours after seizures. They found a significant increase in lactate ratios in kainic-acid-treated rats during and 24 hours after seizure onset; however, this increase was prevented by cycloheximide pretreatment. They suggest that in-situ lactate increase is a marker of seizure-induced neuronal damage and that there is no significant increase of in-situ lactate during seizures that do not lead to neuronal damage (234).

In 1986, a ^{31}P MR spectroscopy study of infants (226) showed that the phosphocreatine (PCr)/Pi ratio was decreased during seizures in the seizure focus, and returned to normal after the seizure ended. Elevated lactate in a region of chronic encephalitis in a patient with Rasmussen's encephalitis was reported using proton MR spectroscopy. (227) The first large study with proton MR spectroscopy in TLE was reported by Connelly and co-workers in 1994 (3). Figure 13.39 shows an MRS investigation in a patient who had a seizure of temporal lobe origin hours before the scan. Lactate increase is observed in the right temporal lobe. Many subsequent studies have demonstrated metabolic changes associated with epilepsy; both associated with the seizure focus and in other areas, possibly related to seizure spread. These include studies of proton, phosphorus and carbon nuclei.

PROTON MAGNETIC RESONANCE SPECTROSCOPY IN EPILEPSY

Proton (^{1}H) MRS provides information on about 30 brain metabolites. Of major interest for the investigation of

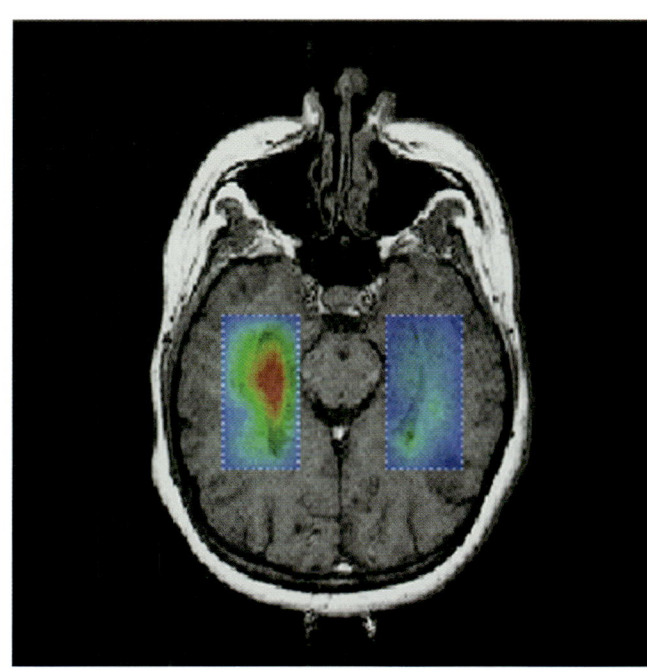

FIG. 13.39. Spectra from both temporal lobes in a patient following a temporal lobe seizure. Note the elevation of lactate in correspondence to the epileptogenic temporal lobe. (Courtesy of Dr T. Ng, UAB, Birmingham, USA.)

epilepsy patients are: NAA, choline-containing metabolites (Cho), creatine/phosphocreatine (Cr), lactate, all of which are measurable using short- or long-echo acquisitions. Spectra acquired with short-echo times provide information about these metabolites as well as mI, GLX, aspartate, and alanine, in addition to several other metabolites (228), some of which require spectral editing techniques for detection (e.g. GABA). A reduction in the NAA signal, or in its ratio to other metabolite signals, is commonly interpreted as indicative of neuronal loss or impaired neuronal function. It has been suggested that Cr and Cho are concentrated in glial cells (79). Increased Cho suggests gliosis and elevated membrane turnover (228). mI is a putative marker of gliosis and an organic osmolyte (229) involved in cellular volume control (230). Studies in animals have identified rapid reduction of mI as a mechanism of brain volume regulation following hyponatremia, with levels being slow to return to normal on normalization of the osmotic environment (231).

Proton MRS is of particular importance in epilepsy patients with brain tumors. The characteristic elevation of choline makes MRS a valuable tool for the diagnosis of tumors and their differentiation from other lesions (232). There is also good evidence that the metabolite profile can differentiate between tumor types (233). For example, lesions with normal Cho levels may strongly argue against the presence of a fast growing tumor.

Temporal Lobe Epilepsy and Proton Magnetic Resonance Spectroscopy

Lateralizing MRS abnormalities have been described in TLE patients, beginning in 1994 (3). They have been

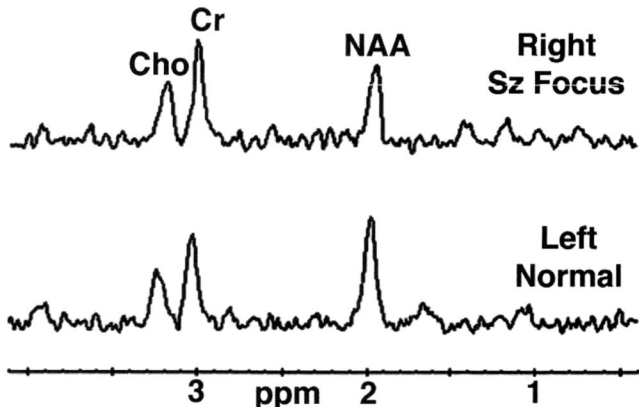

FIG. 13.40. Proton spectrum obtained from 1 ml voxels in the temporal lobe of a patient with temporal lobe epilepsy. Spectrum shows reduction in NAA in the epileptogenic temporal lobe.

replicated in adults (5, 9, 234, 235) and children (236, 237). The abnormalities typically consist of reduced NAA signal and increased choline and mI signals, suggestive of gliosis (234). A typical spectrum and the acquisition plane obtained from the temporal lobes of a patient with TLE are shown in Figures 13.40 and 13.41. These MRS findings are consistent with the histopathologic characteristics of reduced neuron cell counts and increased glial cell numbers. More recently, increased mI has been reported as a consequence of induction of Na+/mI cotransporter (SMIT) following seizure activity (229) associated with glial proliferation in the seizure focus.

Proton MRS studies have shown focal reductions of NAA signal in patients with nonlesional TLE (25, 26, 28–42), with good correlation with EEG abnormalities and severity of

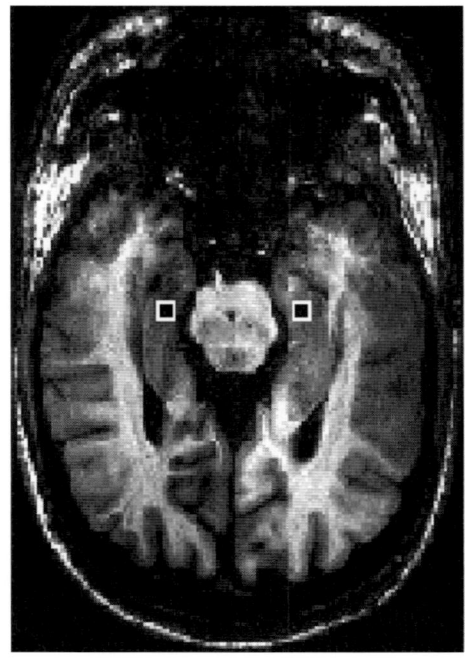
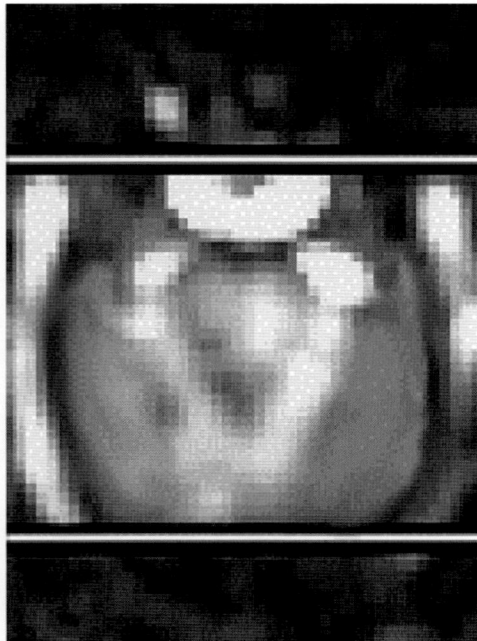

FIG. 13.41. Spectroscopic plane and scout image for acquisition of MRS imaging.

cell loss. The results of published MRS studies suggest that, in patients with partial epilepsy, there is a metabolic abnormality throughout the brain, with patterns of asymmetry and focal accentuation that are useful for noninvasive localization of epileptogenic foci (25–39, 43–46). The MRS findings may have prognostic value for seizure outcome as well (39, 47, 48).

Clinical correlative studies suggest that proton MRS may be extremely sensitive in detecting metabolic changes in dysfunctional epileptogenic regions. In a series of 100 consecutive patients with TLE, Cendes et al. (31) reported abnormal NAA/Cr values in at least one temporal lobe in all but one patient; they were low bilaterally in 54%. The asymmetry between right and left sides of NAA/Cr lateralized 86/93 (92.5%) of patients who had lateralization by ictal EEG. There were seven patients with no clear lateralization by EEG. The MRS imaging lateralization was ipsilateral to the EEG in all but two patients who had bilateral TLE and bilateral AM-HF atrophy greater on the same side as the MRS imaging. Twelve of 13 patients with normal MRIVol had a significant decrease of NAA/Cr within the mesial temporal lobe ipsilateral to the ictal EEG focus (Fig. 13.42). Seven of these underwent surgery and the histopathology showed mild mesial temporal sclerosis.

The above mentioned study (31) showed a direct correlation between the measure of NAA/Cr and MRI volumes of the hippocampus. However, another study by Kuzniecky et al. showed no correlation between the measure of hippocampal specific Cr/NAA and MRI volumes in 34 patients (238). Methodologic and statistical regional analysis differences may account for the discrepancy between studies. Some degree of dissociation between severity of NAA abnormality and hippocampal volume or cell loss is not unexpected. This includes the finding of abnormal NAA measures in normal volume hippocampi (both ipsilateral and contralateral to site of seizure onset) and the reversibility or correction of NAA abnormalities in patients who become seizure free after surgery (14, 15).

Significance of Reduced NAA in Temporal Lobe Epilepsy: Histopathologic Correlations

One of the major questions regarding MRS imaging in TLE is whether the observed NAA changes correlate directly with a reduction in neuronal populations. The only quantitative study to date that addresses this question was carried out in our laboratory. A total of 40 patients undergoing TLE surgery were studied with MRI volumes of the hippocampus and quantitative neuronal/glial cell counts of the resected hippocampus. Autopsy controls were used for the neuropathologic studies.

Correlations of hippocampal volumes with the hippocampal neuronal/glial (N/G) ratios revealed a significant interdependence ($r = 0.465$, $p < 0.01$). Analysis of the Cr/NAA ratios from the patient's resected hippocampus with the CA N/G ratio of hippocampal samples independently or as a group showed no significant correlations ($r = -0.04$, $p < 0.8$).

These findings indicate that hippocampal atrophy computed by MRI volumetry correlates with hippocampal N/G ratios in the resected hippocampus of patients with TLE. However, the metabolic measurements obtained with MRS imaging do not correlate with the same hippocampal N/G ratios. These findings suggest that the MRS metabolic measures reflect neuronal and glial dysfunction rather than absolute neuronal cell loss as previously assumed.

To our knowledge, this is the first study correlating quantitative hippocampal histopathology and MRS imaging in

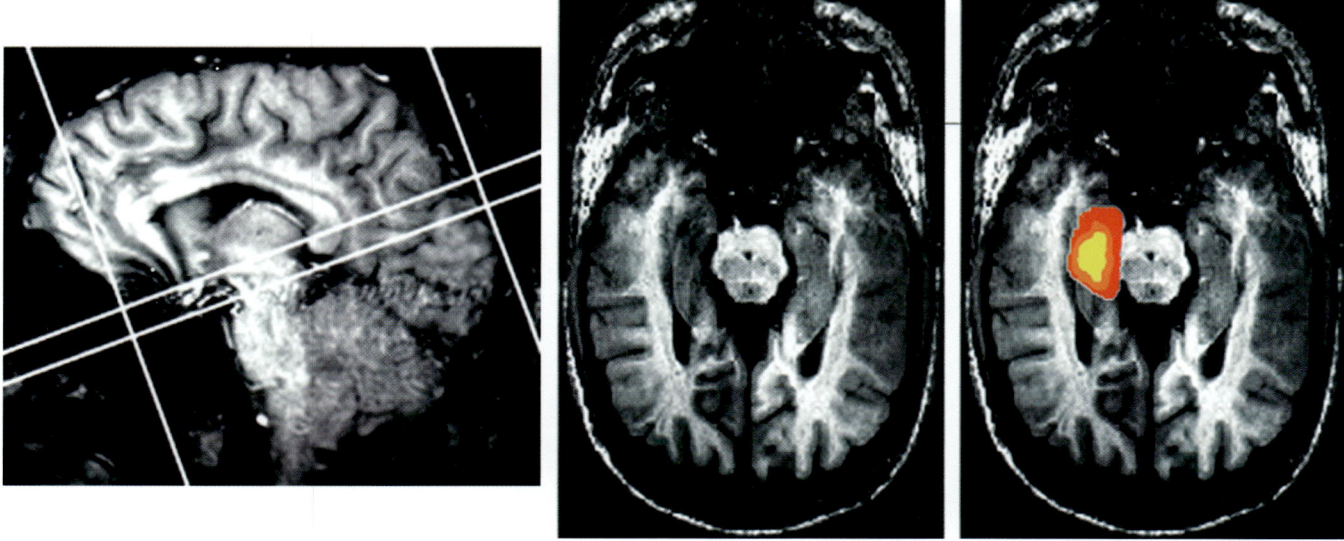

FIG. 13.42. Spectroscopic imaging demonstrating abnormal CR/NAA in both temporal lobes in a patient with bilateral temporal lobe epilepsy.

temporal lobe patients. Our results are in disagreement with the findings of Duc et al. (216) who reported a linear correlation between NAA concentrations and hippocampal sclerosis. The above study however, included a small number of patients ($n = 8$) and it is likely that the data was influenced by restriction of range. More important, however, is the expected inaccuracy of the qualitative determination of hippocampal sclerosis that may have resulted in an apparent correlation (216).

Several animal and human studies support our findings that the metabolic ratios measured by MRS imaging do not directly reflect neuronal cell loss in epileptic tissue. First, data derived from volumetric-MRS imaging correlations have concluded that both techniques are lateralizing and concordant but the degree of metabolic change does not directly correlate with hippocampal volume loss (238). Second, PET studies suggest that the decreases in glucose metabolism do not correlate with CA1 neuronal cell loss (81). This could be secondary to the fact that hypometabolism in PET reflects synaptic density changes leading to hypometabolism rather than cell loss. Third, recent correlative studies suggest that PET hypometabolism and MRS changes do not directly correlate (207).

Even more relevant to the results presented here, however, is MRS data suggesting that the metabolic abnormalities may reflect neuronal–glial dysfunction rather than neuronal cell loss. A study reported metabolic abnormalities in regions that showed no significant neuronal cell density or N/G ratio differences when compared to control brain samples in patients with epileptogenic developmental malformations (214). Furthermore, a number of studies have indicated that, after cessation of seizures, MRS imaging metabolism normalizes in the peri-ictal region or in contralateral regions such as the hippocampus (9, 208). Finally, animal experiments suggest that NAA changes are detected prior to neuronal cell loss and reflect metabolic changes that can be reversible (208). Taken together, the lack of a direct relationship between the histopathologic findings and MRS imaging values and the results of previous studies strongly support the functional nature of the proton MRS metabolic changes in epilepsy.

These findings support the concept that the metabolic dysfunction measured by MRS and the hippocampal volume loss detected by MRI volumetry do not have the same neuropathologic basis. These observations support the use of proton MRS imaging not only as a functional imaging technique that provides lateralization in epilepsy but also as a tool that provides further information about the status of brain function.

The spatial relationship between the NAA decrease and the underlying mechanisms causing neuronal damage is unclear. We often observe that spectra are abnormal in regions close to the epileptogenic temporal lobes. The results of MRS studies need to be carefully evaluated since reproducibility is important, especially in the context of minor metabolic differences (Fig. 13.43). It has been observed that the neuronal damage as measured by NAA can extend to areas at a distance from the lesion, and that the timing of the insult may contribute to the widespread neuronal damage (54). It remains to be seen if this is relevant for the severity of epilepsy. However, if we use the NAA signal as a parameter of neuronal function we may be able to understand how these variables inter-relate to each other. The side of maximum NAA reduction often coincides with the side of EEG abnormality.

The relationship between interictal spiking and underlying neuronal function and epileptogenic state is unclear. Serles et al. (55) showed a trend toward higher interictal spike frequencies on surface EEG in regions of pronounced neuronal metabolic damage or dysfunction. This suggests that both variables parallel an underlying pathologic substrate, although the pathophysiologic processes may be distinct. On the other hand, Maton et al. (57) found that bilateral Cr/NAA abnormalities were three times as frequent as the detection of bitemporal interictal spikes. Figure 13.44 shows bilateral temporal lobe abnormalities in a patient with asymmetric disease. Thus, as with PET and MRI Vol, measures of interictal NAA disturbances do not appear to be completely linked with the EEG measure of neurophysiologic epileptiform disturbance.

Magnetic resonance spectroscopy may be helpful in the identification of the seizure focus in refractory focal epilepsy patients without obvious MR abnormalities. Some studies reported MRS metabolite abnormalities in patients with focal epilepsy, without obvious structural MR abnormalities (91, 205, 239). They consisted of decreased NAA and increased Cho, lateralized to the seizure focus, similar to the patients with hippocampal sclerosis. However, the specificity of these abnormalities has been questioned. Metabolic abnormalities have been found not only in seizure foci (234) but also in areas distant from the seizure focus (234), such as the contralateral temporal lobe (209). Figure 13.45 shows the contralateral involvement with contralateral NAA deficit in a girl with unilateral lesion on the MR.

Contralateral MRS Abnormalities

Bilateral temporal lobe MRS abnormalities have been found in up to 50% of TLE patients (205, 240). The significance of bilateral abnormalities is poorly understood, partly because pathologic specimens are rarely available from the temporal lobe contralateral to the seizure focus. However, autopsy studies suggest a high prevalence of bilateral hippocampal abnormalities in TLE patients (241, 242). This is consistent with quantitative MRI studies reporting the frequent occurrence of bilateral abnormalities (243, 244). It has been shown that contralateral NAA abnormalities measured by MRS are reversible with time, suggesting transient neuronal dysfunction (209). The presence of bilateral metabolic changes has been associated with poor postoperative seizure outcome (220, 245), in particular when the metabolic dysfunction is worse in the contralateral areas of resection.

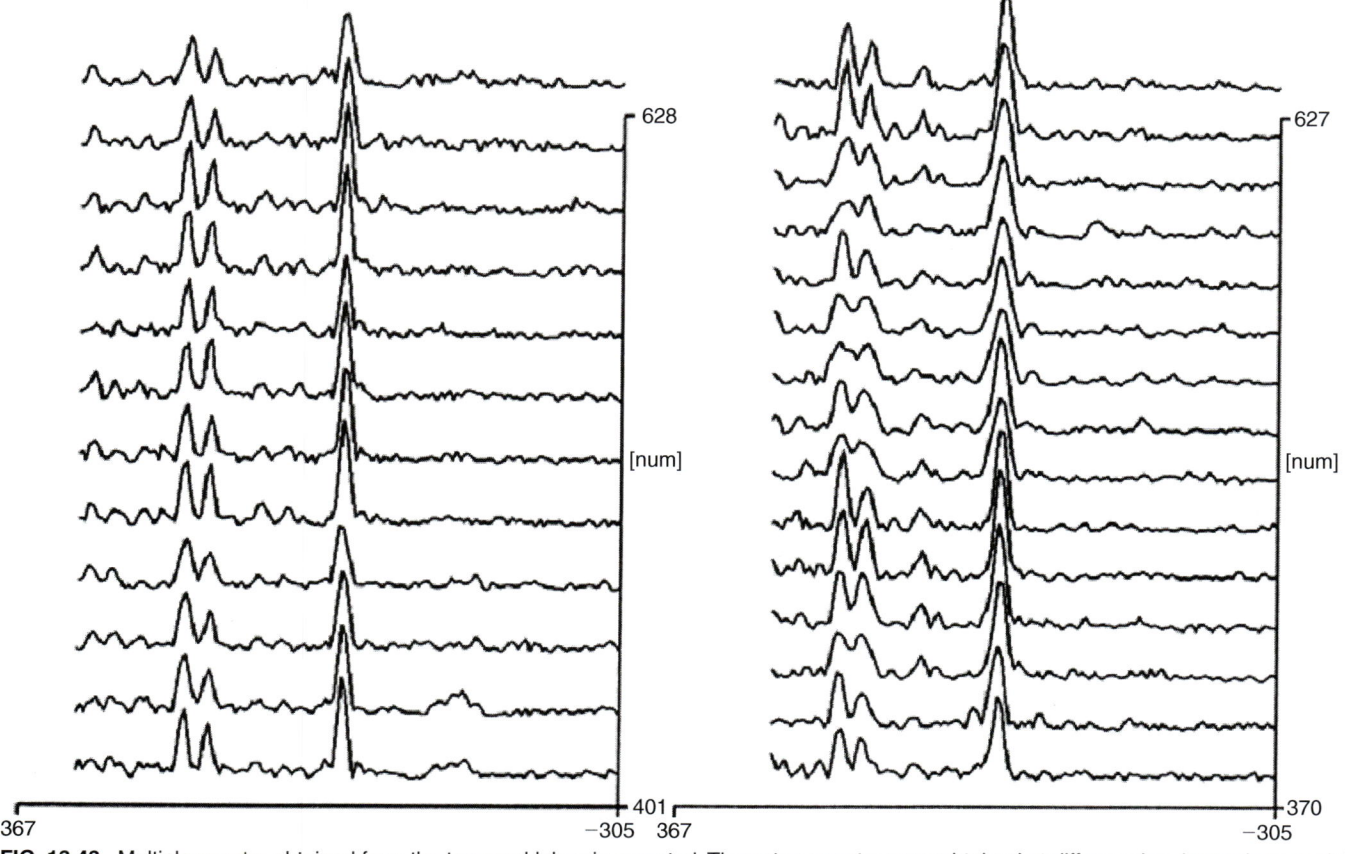

FIG. 13.43. Multiple spectra obtained from the temporal lobes in a control. These two spectra were obtained at different time intervals to study reproducibility effects.

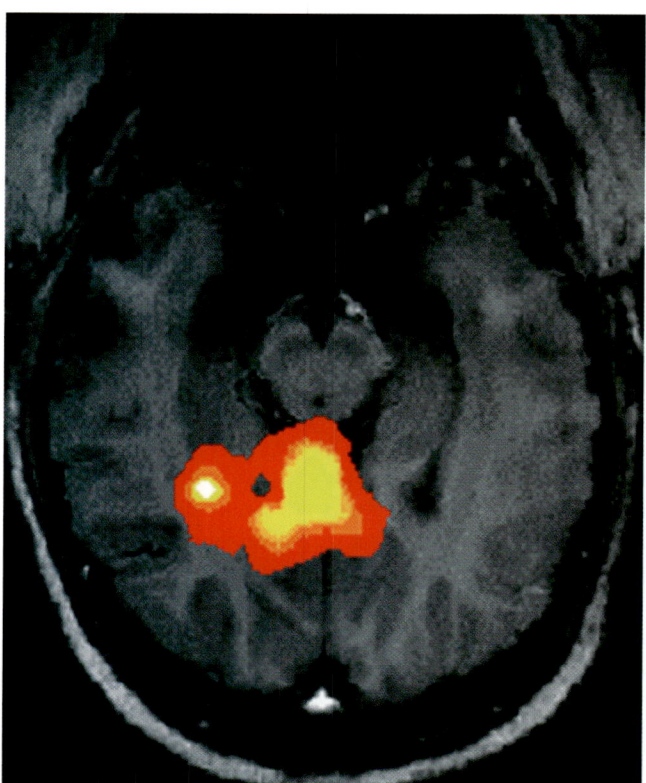

FIG. 13.44. Spectroscopic plane and image demonstrating unilateral metabolic abnormalities in a patient with unilateral temporal lobe epilepsy. Localization was obtained through these procedures.

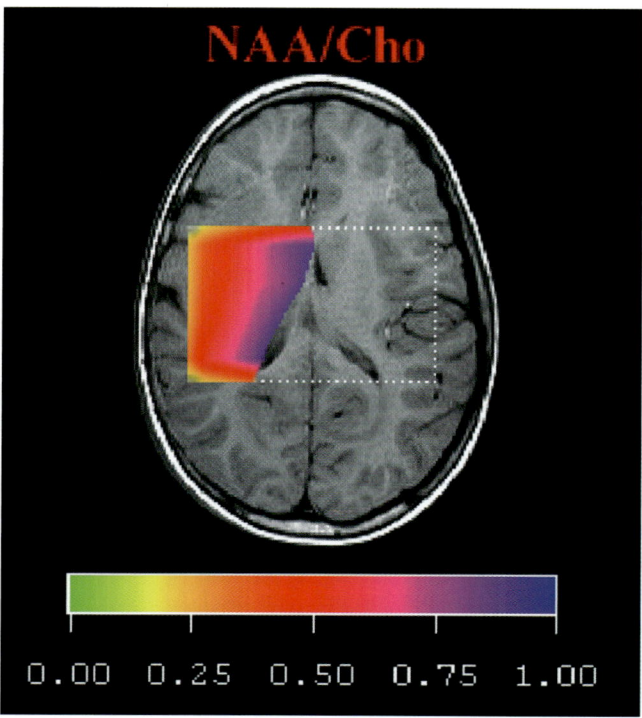

FIG. 13.45. Metabolite map of NAA/Cho ratios reveals an area larger than the MRI abnormal area, suggesting diffused pathology. (Courtesy of Dr T. Ng, UAB, Birmingham, USA.)

Widespread Proton Magnetic Resonance Spectroscopy Abnormalities

Whereas the presence of bilateral temporal lobe abnormalities may be consistent with the presence of independent bilateral foci, there is also the possibility that the contralateral changes may reflect abnormalities due to seizure spread. In severe TLE, functional abnormalities beyond the seizure focus have been documented by PET (246) and SPECT (247). Metabolite changes in brain lobes other than that harboring the seizure focus suggest that seizure spread may cause changes detectable by MRS. Widespread MRS abnormalities have been found in several studies (9, 235, 238, 248–250).

Our experience suggests that frontal lobe reduction of mI concentrations is observed in both TLE with hippocampal sclerosis and in mild TLE (250) and may be due to either a short-term change following recent seizure activity or a cumulative effect of chronic seizures. A recent report has shown reduced frontal lobe NAA in severe refractory TLE (7). When compared to volumetric changes, also known to occur in brain lobes distant to the seizure focus, MRS abnormalities were not associated with volumetric deficits in the frontal grey and white matter (249). This suggests that the widespread MRS abnormalities in TLE may have a different origin from the widespread volumetric changes or that the metabolite changes may precede the structural changes.

Proton MRS has proved to be a sensitive measure to detect metabolic pathologies in patients with TLE; however, it remains to be clarified whether this additional information adds to the overall management of the patient. With its high sensitivity, metabolite abnormalities in brain regions, distinct from the seizure focus, can be detected and it remains difficult to disentangle which abnormalities are due to causes or consequences of seizures. Some indication can be taken from a large study performed on 82 patients with refractory TLE, which found in both the ipsilateral and contralateral temporal lobe an NAA/Cr ratio that was negatively correlated with the duration of epilepsy (207). Patients with frequent generalized tonic-clonic seizures had lower NAA/Cr than patients with no or rare generalized tonic–clonic seizures. This suggests that ongoing seizures may induce additional neuronal damage, which will progress in parallel to the duration of the epilepsy.

Extratemporal Lobe Epilepsy and Proton Magnetic Resonance Spectroscopy

In contrast to the numerous proton MRS studies of TLE patients, there are only few reports in other types of partial epilepsy (211, 251, 252). Support for frontal lobe involvement in 15 JME patients, in the form of reduced NAA, has been presented (252). These studies suggest that the potential of correct seizure focus lateralization is less than in TLE.

In one study comparing the coincidence rate between the seizure focus and the reduction of the NAA/Cr ratio, correct lateralization was present in 19 of the 21 TLE patients but only in four of the seven frontal lobe epilepsy patients (251). Widespread NA reduction was observed to be greatest at the seizure focus in a study of 20 patients with epilepsy of frontal or central/postcentral origin, suggesting that the MRS abnormalities in extratemporal epilepsy might therefore not be localized enough to readily specify the seizure focus (211). Figure 13.45 shows bilateral frontal lobe spectra in a patient with focal cortical dysplasia, in which the direction of the MRS abnormalities suggested a pathology on the left side.

In extratemporal lobe epilepsy, the seizure focus is usually neocortical. In contrast, in patients with hypothalamic hamartoma, seizure onset is in the subcortical lesion (253, 254). Patients with hypothalamic hamartoma usually have frequent gelastic seizures starting early in life and may show cognitive impairment and behavioral disturbances.

Preliminary data suggests that MRS may be useful for the evaluation of other forms of partial epilepsies (40, 43, 44, 54), including those associated with cortical developmental malformations (214). Li et al. (239) and Kuzniecky et al. (214) demonstrated that different types of cortical developmental malformation show different degrees of decrease of NAA. In cortical dysplasia, the relative NAA signal is very low. This disorder appears to result from abnormal neuronal and glial cell differentiation and proliferation, and the lesion contains structurally abnormal neurons with abnormal synaptic activity and connectivity, thus explaining the reduced NAA values. In polymicrogyria, where the NAA values were normal or slightly abnormal, the malformation is due to an abnormal cortical organization caused by a postmigrational insult and the neurons are mature. Heterotopia consist of a large number of neurons that failed to initiate or complete the migration process. In heterotopia, because of the high number of neurons, one would expect a relative increase of the NAA signal. This assumption is based on histopathologic studies showing normal-appearing neurons and on early fluorodeoxyglucose PET studies showing patterns of glucose uptake similar to normal cortex. However, proton MRS have shown NAA signal intensity to be variably normal or abnormal in patients with heterotopia. This suggests that at least some of these apparently normal neurons are, in fact, dysfunctional.

Our laboratory has also found (214) that patients with focal cortical dysplasia have a significant correlation between the metabolic abnormalities and the frequency of seizures but not with the degree of interictal EEG discharges. Quantitative neuronal and glial cell counts revealed no statistically significant correlation between cell loss and the abnormal metabolic ratios in those who underwent surgery. These findings suggest that MRS imaging-based metabolic abnormalities in patients with cortical developmental malformation are complex and influenced by a number of factors.

Phosphorus Magnetic Resonance Spectroscopy in Epilepsy

Phosphorus-31 magnetic resonance spectroscopy allows evaluation of the energetic state of the brain, by providing a measure of nucleoside triphosphates (predominantly ATP), PCr, PMEs, PDEs and Pi in brain tissue (255). Figure 13.46 shows phosphorus spectra in controls at 1.5 T versus 4.1 T. The information about the levels of high-energy phosphate metabolites is derived from ATP and PCr. Typically the PCr/ATP ratio is quoted as an indicator of the tissue energy status. While cerebral ATP is depleted only under severe metabolic conditions, changes in PCr have been observed with ^{31}P MRS following neuronal activity (256). The PME peak predominantly comprises phosphatidylethanolamine and phosphatidylcholine (precursors of cell membranes (257)). The PDE resonance includes glycerophosphatidylcholine (GPCh), glycerophosphatidylethanolamine (GPEth) and mobile phospholipids. The GPCh and GPEth represent membrane breakdown products (257) but the majority of the signal (>80%) probably originates from intracellular mobile phospholipids. Additionally, the chemical shift of the Pi resonance provides an excellent measure of intracellular pHi (258). Changes in the relative PME and PDE concentrations have been associated with membrane turnover (259). Figure 13.10 shows phosphorus spectra obtained at very high field strength of 4.1T.

Phosphoesters are of considerable interest because they represent precursors of membrane synthesis and breakdown products. However, these metabolites contain both protons and phosphorus in close proximity. The components absorb energy from each other, making their MR detection, differentiation, and quantification difficult. It is possible to increase the sensitivity and improve the differentiation of phosphoesters by simultaneously transmitting two radio frequency signals, one of which is tuned to the proton nuclei to disrupt the interaction between proton and phosphorus nuclei (known as decoupling). The increase in signal is more than 50%, which is sufficient to allow quantification of the different phosphoester components in the tissue. An added advantage of this technique is the reduction in time taken for data acquisition, reducing potential patient discomfort.

In ^{31}P MRS studies of epilepsy patients, changes in PCr can be expected following neuronal activity (256). During and shortly after a seizure, changes in pHi and high-energy phosphates may be found (222). Interestingly, these metabolites have been reported to be abnormal in relatively seizure-free patients (34). ^{31}P MRS also provides information on mobile PME and PDE associated with membranes (260). ^{31}P MRS has shown potential for lateralizing metabolic dysfunction (34). Decreased PCr/Pi was observed in 65–75% of patients with TLE (261). This may relate to the timing of measurements relative to recent seizure activity. Altered ^{31}P metabolites and pHi have been reported in the postictal period. An important feature of the findings reported to date is that abnormalities are present in regions that are normal to a range of other measurements, including MRI. They may therefore be unique markers for an early stage of the processes by which normal neurons are recruited into the permanently epileptogenic neuronal population.

TEMPORAL LOBE EPILEPSY AND PHOSPHORUS MAGNETIC RESONANCE SPECTROSCOPY

Several groups have investigated a potential reduction in pH in patients with TLE (261, 262–264). In one study (262) there were significant differences between patients and controls with respect to the PCr/Pi ratio. However, no significant differences were found between patients and controls with respect to pH. In contrast, others have found an elevation of pH, along with increased Pi and reduced PME in the ipsilateral temporal lobe (263, 264). Reduced ATP/Pi and PCr/Pi ratios in the temporal lobe were predictive for the side of the seizure focus in more than 70% of patients studied (34). Overall, the results of these studies are controversial, although it appears that some phosphorus metabolite abnormalities are indeed present in the epileptogenic temporal lobe. Variations between the reports may originate from a difference in timing of the MRS study, relative to seizures. However, high field studies (4.1 T) with excellent spectral resolution have indicated that pH is indeed normal in the interictal state (Fig. 13.47).

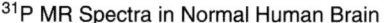

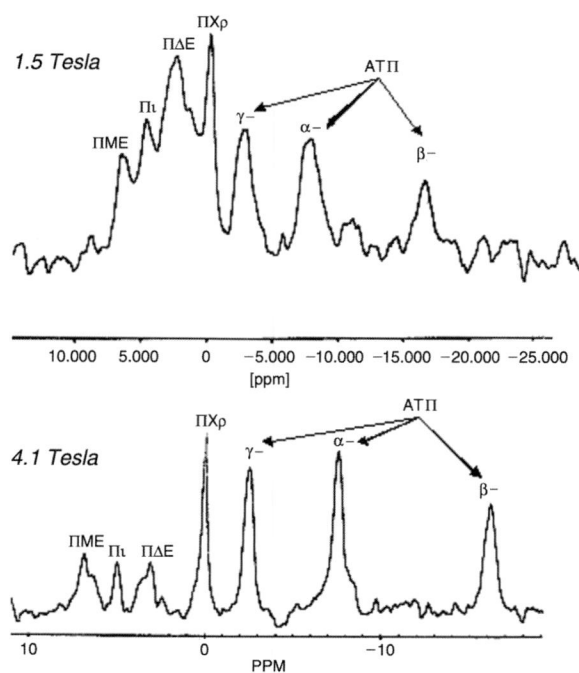

FIG. 13.46. Phosphorus spectra obtained from a normal volunteer at 1.5 T and 4.1 T. Note spectrum baseline improvement and enhanced spectral resolution at high field.

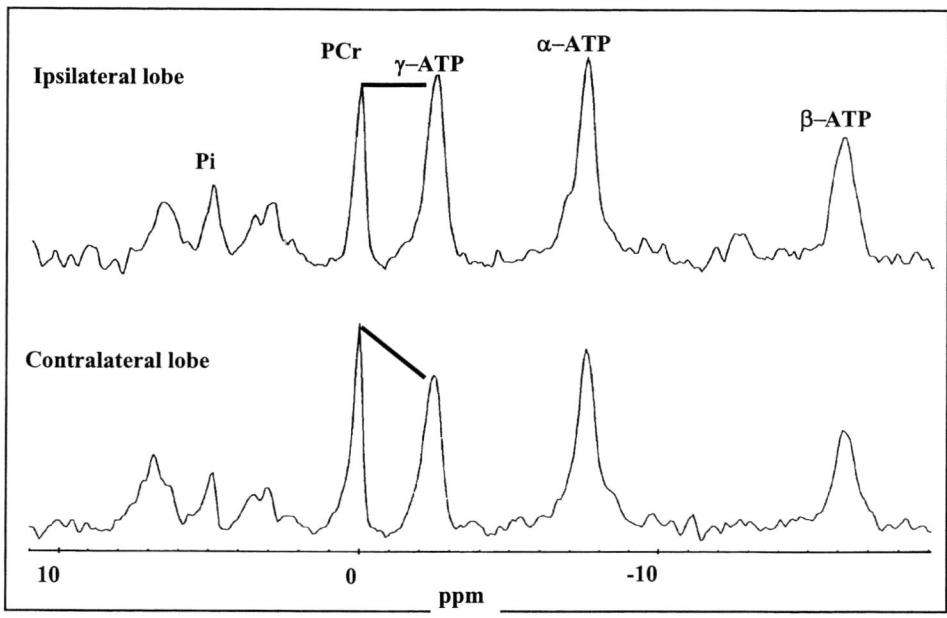

FIG. 13.47. Phosphorus spectra from a patient with temporal lobe epilepsy. Note the abnormality in ATP/PCr and increased Pi in the affected temporal lobe.

OTHER NUCLEI FOR MAGNETIC RESONANCE SPECTROSCOPY IN EPILEPSY

The increased SNR available with a high magnetic field allows the detection of less sensitive nuclei. MR spectroscopy performed at a magnetic field strength of 3 T or above facilitates the use of other nuclei than protons and phosphorus. These nuclei include carbon (13C), sodium (23Na) and fluorine (19F). The low natural abundance of 13C can be used to advantage if enriched in exogenous metabolites. The metabolic fate of 13C-labeled substrates can be followed to determine flux through metabolic pathways with the appearance of newly labeled metabolites in sequential spectra. For example, administration of 13C-labeled glucose and acetate can be used to study the TCA cycle and glutamine–glutamate cycling (265). Metabolite flux in such studies can also be used to determine the kinetics of the metabolic pathways (38). In-vitro 13C MRS has already been used to show reduced glutamate–glutamine cycling in surgically resected tissue from epileptogenic hippocampus (72). This technique has also been used to examine other metabolite pathways in animals (130) and it is likely that such studies eventually will be extended to humans.

Studies including other nuclei are rare. There is only one 23Na study of epilepsy reported (266). This is an area yet to be examined with current high-field facilities. The nucleus 19F is not naturally present in vivo and has yet to be used for the study of epilepsy in humans. However, there are studies using MRS of this nucleus in animal models of epilepsy (267) and other diseases to examine the fate of 19F-labeled compounds (268).

HIGH-FIELD MAGNETIC RESONANCE SPECTROSCOPY AND FUTURE DIRECTION

Magnetic resonance spectroscopy, as an imaging technique based on relatively low signal levels, benefits substantially by moving to a higher magnetic field strength scanner. High magnetic field strength scanners achieve a higher SNR, which is the ratio of the amplitude of the desired signal to the amplitude of the noise that contaminates that signal when it is measured. The improvement in SNR from doubling the operational frequency is dependent on the imaging sequence and the parameters used but is approximately a factor of 1.7 for a fixed scan time (269). In practice, an increase in SNR allows shorter acquisition times for a given resolution, higher resolution for a given imaging time, or a combination of both. The dispersion of individual peaks contributing to a spectrum increases with magnetic field strength. Therefore, MRS gains in quality as the spectral dispersion and SNR increase with higher field magnetic strength, allowing separation of metabolite peaks that would otherwise not be distinguishable. In addition to improving the robustness of measured signal, one can also consider scanning with smaller voxel sizes. Figure 13.46 demonstrates the gain in quality of MR spectra from 1.5 T and 3 T. Overall, the increased SNR allows more precise quantification of common metabolites, and assessment of a broader range of metabolites, particularly for short echo time studies.

The future lies in the development of new, faster MRS acquisition protocols (270, 271) as well as in the refinement of existing techniques. This should allow the use of techniques that would otherwise require acquisition times greater than are practicable for human studies. This includes techniques such as spectral editing of *J*-coupled resonances measured with subtraction techniques such as those used for GABA (272, 273) and sequences that inherently detect only weak signals, such as those detected by multiple quantum techniques. An example of such a multiple quantum measurement is the measurement of intracellular sodium, rather than the total sodium signal obtained with a standard ^{23}Na MRS acquisition. These and related issues are discussed by Hetherington and Petroff in the previous sections of this chapter.

Future developments in MRS may enable the technique to benefit the investigation of seizure generation by correlating metabolism with interictal discharges (274, 275). MRS may also be of use in monitoring the progression of neuronal damage due to ongoing seizure activity (207). There is also the possibility that MRS will help to evaluate anticonvulsant therapy in vivo (276).

CONCLUSION

There is no doubt that ^{1}H and ^{31}P spectroscopy detects relevant metabolite changes in patients with TLE. Numerous studies confirm reduction in NAA and in the ratio of phosphocreatine/Pi (277). In his 1999 review, Kuzniecky concluded that proton MRS, using single-voxel or chemical shift imaging, lateralized TLE in 65–96% of cases, with bilateral changes seen in 35–45% of cases, while phosphorus MRS showed a lateralizing PCr/Pi ratio in 65–75% of the TLE patients (278). There are indications that these changes are reversible with seizure treatment. Improvements in MRS technology, such as the ability to calculate absolute concentrations, to account for differences between gray and white matter, and to achieve better spectral resolution by use of a higher magnetic field strength, will now allow more extensive use of this 'old' MR technique for patients with epilepsy (279, 280).

REFERENCES

1. Urenjak J, et al. Specific expression of *N*-acetylaspartate in neurons, oligodendrocyte-type-2 astrocyte progenitors and immature oligodendrocytes in vitro. *J Neurochem* 1992;59:55–61.
2. Hugg JW, et al. Proton MR spectroscopic imaging detects neuron loss more sensitively than MRI in focal epilepsy. In: Book of Abstracts, Society of Magnetic Resonance in Medicine. Berlin: Society of Magnetic Resonance in Medicine, 1992.
3. Connelly A, Jackson GD, Duncan JS, et al. Magnetic resonance spectroscopy on temporal lobe epilepsy. Neurology 1994;44:1411–1417.
4. Cendes, F, et al. Lateralization of temporal lobe epilepsy based on regional metabolic abnormalities in proton MRS. Ann Neurol 1994; 35:211–216.
5. Hetherington, H, et al. Proton nuclear magnetic resonance spectroscopic imaging of human temporal lobe epilepsy at 4.1 T. Ann Neurol 1995;38:396–404.
6. Pan, J, et al. Metabolic differences between multiple sclerosis subtypes measured by quantitative MR spectroscopy. Mult Scler 2002;8:200–206.
7. Suhy J, et al. ^{1}H MRSI predicts surgical outcome in MRI-negative temporal lobe epilepsy. *Neurology* 2002;58:821–823.
8. Hugg JW, et al. Neuron loss localizes human temporal lobe epilepsy by in vivo proton magnetic resonance spectroscopic imaging. *Ann Neurol* 1993;34:788–794.
9. Cendes F, Caramanos Z, Andermann F, et al. Proton magnetic resonance spectroscopic imaging and magnetic resonance imaging volumetry in the lateralization of temporal lobe epilepsy: a series of 100 patients. *Ann Neurol* 1997;42:737–746.
10. Behar KL, Ogino T. Assignment of resonances in the ^{1}H spectrum of rat brain by two dimensional shift correlated and J-resolved NMR spectroscopy. *Magn Reson Med* 1991;17:285–303.
11. Kreis R, Ernest T, Ross B. Absolute quantitation of water and metabolites in human brain: metabolite concentrations. *J Magn Reson* 1993;102:9–19.
12. Hetherington, H, et al. Evaluation of cerebral gray and white matter metabolite differences by SI at 4.1T. *Magn Reson Med* 1994; 32:565–571.
13. Provencher S. Automatic quantitation of localized in vivo ^{1}H spectra with LCModel. *NMR Biomed* 2001;14:260–264.
14. Ng T, et al. Temporal lobe epilepsy: presurgical localization with proton chemical shift imaging. *Radiology* 1994;193:465–471.
15. Hetherington H, Pohost G. Numerical optimization of semi-selective pulses as applied to human skeletal muscle at 4.1T. In: Book of Abstracts, Society of Magnetic Resonance in Medicine. Berlin: Society of Magnetic Resonance in Medicine, 1992.
16. Hetherington HP, et al. Application of high field spectroscopic imaging in the evaluation of temporal lobe epilepsy. Magn Reson Imaging 1995;13:1175–1180.
17. Rothman DL, Petroff OA, Behar KL, Mattson RH. Localized ^{1}H NMR measurements of gamma-aminobutyric acid in human brain in vivo. *Proc Natl Acad Sci* 1993;90(12):5662–5666.
18. Rothman DL, et al. Homonuclear ^{1}H-double resonance difference spectroscopy of the rat brain in vivo. *Proc Natl Acad Sci USA* 1984;81:6330–6334.
19. Frahm J, Merboldt K, Hanicke J. Localized proton spectroscopy using localized echos. *J Magn Reson* 1987;72:502.
20. Ogg R, Kingsley P, Taylor JS. WET: a T1 and B1 insensitive water suppression method for in vivo localized ^{1}H NMR spectroscopy. *J Magn Reson* 1994;104:1–10.
21. Hetherington H, et al. Quantitative proton SI of human brain at 4.1 T using image segmentation. *Magn Reson Med* 1996;36:21–29.
22. Choi CG, Frahm J. Localized proton MRS of the human hippocampus: metabolite concentrations and relaxation times. *Magn Reson Med* 1999;41:204–207.
23. Simister RJ, Woermann FG, McLean MA, et al. A short-echo-time proton magnetic resonance spectroscopic imaging study of temporal lobe epilepsy. *Epilepsia* 2002;43:1021–1031.
24. Vaughan JT, et al. High frequency volume coils for clinical NMR imaging and spectroscopy. *Magn Reson Med* 1994;32:206–218.
25. Bartha R, et al. In vivo ^{1}H$_2$O T2 measurements in the human occipital lobe at 4T and 7T by Carr–Purcell MRI. *Magn Reson Imaging* 2002;47:742–750.
26. Chu WJ, Kuzniecky RI, Hugg JW, et al. Statistically driven identification of focal metabolic abnormalities in temporal lobe epilepsy with corrections for tissue heterogeneity using ^{1}H spectroscopic imaging. *Magn Reson Med* 2000;43:359–367.
27. Pfeuffer J, et al. Toward an in vivo neurochemical profile in the rat brain. *Magn Reson Imaging* 1999;141:104–120.
28. Graham G, et al. Spectroscopic assessment of alterations in macromolecule and small molecule metabolites in human brain after stroke. *Stroke* 2001;32:2797–2802.
29. Pan JW, et al. Evaluation of multiple sclerosis by ^{1}H spectroscopic imaging at 4.1 T. *Magn Reson Med* 1996;36:72–77.
30. Behar K, et al. Detection of metabolites in rabbit brain by ^{13}C NMR spectroscopy following administration of 1-^{13}C glucose. *Magn Reson Med* 1986;3:911–922.
31. Henry P, et al. GABA editing without macromolecule contamination. *Magn Reson Imaging* 2001;45:517–520.

32. Ordidge R, Connely A, Lohman J. Image selected in vivo spectroscopy; a new technique for spatially selective NMR spectroscopy. *J Magn Reson* 1986;66:283.

33. Hugg JW, et al. Lateralization of human focal epilepsy by ^{31}P magnetic resonance spectroscopic imaging. *Neurology* 1992;42:2011–2018.

34. Chu WJ, Hetherington HP, Kuzniecky RI. Lateralization of human temporal lobe epilepsy by ^{31}P NMR spectroscopic imaging at 4.1 T. *Neurology* 1998;51(2):472–479.

35. Hetherington HP, Spencer DD, Vaughan JT, Pan JW. Quantitative (31)P Spectroscopic Imaging of Human Brain at 4 Tesla: assessment of gray and white matter differences of phosphocreatine and ATP. *Magn Reson Med* 2001;45:46–52.

36. Gruetter R, et al. Localized ^{13}C NMR spectroscopy in the human brain of amino acid labeling from D-[1-^{13}C]glucose. *J Neurochem* 1994;63:1377–1385.

37. Fitzpatrick S, et al. The flux from glucose to glutamate in the rat brain in vivo as determined by ^{1}H observed ^{13}C edited NMR Spectroscopy. *J. Cereb Blood Flow Metab* 1989;10:170.

38. Shen J, Petersen KF, Behar KL. Determination of the rate of the glutamate/glutamine cycle in the human brain by in vivo ^{13}C NMR. *Proc Natl Acad Sci USA* 1999;96:8235–8240.

39. Pan JW, Stein DT, Telang F, et al. Spectroscopic imaging of glutamate C-4 turnover in human brain. *Magn Reson Med* 2000;44: 673–679.

40. Ottersen OP, Zhang N, Walberg F. Metabolic compartmentation of glutamate and glutamine: morphological evidence obtained by quantitative immunocytochemistry in rat cerebellum. *Neuroscience* 1992;46:519–534.

41. Danbolt NC. Glutamate uptake. *Prog Neurobiol* 2001;65:1–105.

42. Fonnum F. Regulation of the synthesis of the transmitter glutamate pool. *Prog Biophys Mol Biol* 1993;60:47–57.

43. Conti F, Minelli A. Glutamate immunoreactivity in rat cerebral cortex is reversibly abolished by 6-diazo-5-oxo-L-norleucine (DON), an inhibitor of phosphate-activated glutaminase. *J Histochem Cytochem* 1994;42:717–726.

44. Hertz L, et al. Astrocytes: glutamate producers for neurons. *J Neurosci Res* 1999;57:417–428.

45. Erecinska M, Silver IA. Metabolism and role of glutamate in mammalian brain. *Prog Neurobiol* 1990;35:245–296.

46. Maycox P, Hell JW, Jahn R. Amino acid neurotransmission: spotlight on synaptic vesicles. *Trends Neurosci* 1990;13:83–87.

47. Nicholls D, Attwell D. The release and uptake of excitatory amino acids. *Trends Pharmacol Sci* 1990;11:462–468.

48. Cooper AJ, Plum F. Biochemistry and physiology of brain ammonia. *Physiol Rev* 1987;67:440–519.

49. Shen J, et al. ^{15}N-NMR spectroscopy studies of ammonia transport and glutamine synthesis in the hyperammonemic rat brain. *Dev Neurosci* 1998;20:434–443.

50. Sibson NR, et al. In vivo (13)C NMR measurement of neurotransmitter glutamate cycling, anaplerosis and TCA cycle flux in rat brain during. *J Neurochem* 2001;76:975–989.

51. Sibson NR, et al. Stoichiometric coupling of brain glucose metabolism and glutamatergic neuronal activity. *Proc Natl Acad Sci USA* 1998;95:316–321.

52. Hyder F, et al. Quantitative functional imaging of the brain: towards mapping neuronal activity by BOLD fMRI. *NMR Biomed* 2001;14:413–431.

53. Smith AJ, et al. Cerebral energetics and spiking frequency: the neurophysiological basis of fMRI. *Proc Natl Acad Sci USA* 2002; 99:10765–10770.

54. Shulman RG, Hyder F, Rothman DL. Biophysical basis of brain activity: implications for neuroimaging. *Q Rev Biophys* 2002;35:287–325.

55. Shen J, Shungu DC, Rothman DL. In vivo chemical shift imaging of gamma-aminobutyric acid in the human brain. *Magn Reson Med* 1999;41:35–42.

56. Kanamatsu T, Tsukada Y. Effects of ammonia on the anaplerotic pathway and amino acid metabolism in the brain: an ex vivo ^{13}C NMR

57. spectroscopic study of rats after administering [2-^{13}C]] glucose with or without ammonium acetate. *Brain Res* 1999;841:11–19.

57. Bradford HF. Glutamate, GABA and epilepsy. *Prog Neurobiol* 1995;47:477–511.

58. Sherwin AL, van Gelder NM. Amino acid and catecholamine markers of metabolic abnormalities in human focal epilepsy. *Adv Neurol* 1986;44:1011–1032.

59. Bergles DE, Diamond JS, Jahr CE. Clearance of glutamate inside the synapse and beyond. *Curr Opin Neurobiol* 1999;9:293–298.

60. Dzubay JA, Jahr CE. The concentration of synaptically released glutamate outside of the climbing fiber-Purkinje cell synaptic cleft. *J Neurosci* 1999;19:5265–5274.

61. Rothstein JD, et al. Knockout of glutamate transporters reveals a major role for astroglial transport in excitotoxicity and clearance of glutamate. *Neuron* 1996;16:675–686.

62. Rossi DJ, Oshima T, Attwell D. Glutamate release in severe brain ischaemia is mainly by reversed uptake. *Nature* 2000;403:316–321.

63. Eisenberg D, et al. Structure-function relationships of glutamine synthetases. *Biochim Biophys Acta* 2000;1477:122–145.

64. Chaudhry FA, et al. Molecular analysis of system N suggests novel physiological roles in nitrogen metabolism and synaptic transmission. *Cell* 1999;99:769–780.

65. Chaudhry FA, et al. Glutamine uptake by neurons: interaction of protons with system A transporters. *J Neurosci* 2002;22:62–72.

66. Chaudhry FA, Reimer RJ, Edwards RH. The glutamine commute: take the N line and transfer to the A. *J Cell Biol* 2002;157:349–355.

67. Kvamme E, Roberg B, Torgner IA. Phosphate-activated glutaminase and mitochondrial glutamine transport in the brain. *Neurochem Res* 2000;25:1407–1419.

68. Albrecht J, et al. Modulation of glutamine uptake and phosphate-activated glutaminase activity in rat brain mitochondria by amino acids and their synthetic analogues. *Neurochem Int* 2000;36:341–347.

69. Kvamme E, Torgner IA, Roberg B. Kinetics and localization of brain phosphate activated glutaminase. *J Neurosci Res* 2001;66: 951–958.

70. Lebon V, et al. Astroglial contribution to brain energy metabolism in humans revealed by ^{13}C nuclear magnetic resonance spectroscopy: elucidation of the dominant pathway for neurotransmitter glutamate repletion and measurement of astrocytic oxidative metabolism. *J Neurosci* 2002;22:1523–1531.

71. Pan JW, de Graaf RA, Petersen KF, et al. [2,4-13C2]-β-hydroxybutyrate metabolism in human brain. *J Cereb Blood Flow Metab* 2002;22: 890–898.

72. Petroff, OA, Errante LD, Rothman DL. Glutamate–glutamine cycling in the epileptic human hippocampus. *Epilepsia* 2002;43:703–710.

73. Bluml S, et al. Tricarboxylic acid cycle of glia in the in vivo human brain. *NMR Biomed* 2002;15:1–5.

74. Cruz F, Cerdan S. Quantitative ^{13}C NMR studies of metabolic compartmentation in the adult mammalian brain. *NMR Biomed* 1999;12:451–462.

75. Waniewski RA, Martin DL. Preferential utilization of acetate by astrocytes is attributable to transport. *J Neurosci* 1998;18:5225–5233.

76. Hanu R, et al. Monocarboxylic acid transporters, MCT1 and MCT2, in cortical astrocytes in vitro and in vivo. *Am J Physiol Cell Physiol* 2000;278:C921–C230.

77. Qu H, et al. Glial-neuronal interactions following kainate injection in rats. *Neurochem Int* 2003;42:101–106.

78. Petroff OA, et al. Neuronal and glial metabolite content of the epileptogenic human hippocampus. *Ann Neurol* 2002;52:635–642.

79. Urenjak J, et al. Proton nuclear magnetic resonance spectroscopy unambiguously identifies different neural cell types. *J Neurosci* 1993;13:981–989.

80. Bhakoo KK, Pearce D. In vitro expression of N-acetyl aspartate by oligodendrocytes: implications for proton magnetic resonance spectroscopy signal in vivo. *J Neurochem* 2000;74:254–262.

81. Henry TR. PET: cerebral blood flow and glucose metabolism–presurgical localization. *Adv Neurol* 2000;83:105–120.

82. Theodore WH, et al. Hippocampal volume and glucose metabolism in temporal lobe epileptic foci. *Epilepsia* 2001;42:130–132.

83. Spanaki MV, et al. Postoperative changes in cerebral metabolism in temporal lobe epilepsy. *Arch Neurol* 2000;57:1447–1452.

84. Shen J, Rothman DL. Magnetic resonance spectroscopic approaches to studying neuronal: glial interactions. *Biol Psychiatry* 2002;52:694–700.

85. Rothman DL, et al. In vivo NMR studies of the glutamate neurotransmitter flux and neuroenergetics: implications for brain function. *Annu Rev Physiol* 2003;65:401–427.

86. Petroff OA, Mattson RH, Rothman DL. Proton MRS: GABA and glutamate. *Adv Neurol* 2000;83:261–271.

87. Sherwin AL. Neuroactive amino acids in focally epileptic human brain: a review. *Neurochem Res* 1999;24:1387–1395.

88. Petroff OA. GABA and glutamate in the human brain. *Neuroscientist* 2002;8:562–573.

89. Petroff OA, et al. Initial observations on effect of vigabatrin on in vivo ^{1}H spectroscopic measurements of gamma-aminobutyric acid, glutamate, and glutamine in human brain. *Epilepsia* 1995;36:457–464.

90. Petroff OA, et al. Effects of valproate and other antiepileptic drugs on brain glutamate, glutamine, and GABA in patients with refractory complex partial seizures. *Seizure* 1999;8:120–127.

91. Woermann FG, et al. Short echo time single-voxel ^{1}H magnetic resonance spectroscopy in magnetic resonance imaging-negative temporal lobe epilepsy: different biochemical profile compared with hippocampal sclerosis. *Ann Neurol* 1999;45:369–376.

92. Savic I, et al. In vivo measurements of glutamine + glutamate (Glx) and N-acetyl aspartate (NAA) levels in human partial epilepsy. *Acta Neurol Scand* 2000;102:179–188.

93. Martin & Tobin 2000.

94. Ribak & Yan 2000.

95. Hyder F, et al. Localized ^{1}H NMR measurements of 2-pyrrolidinone in human brain in vivo. *Magn Reson Med* 1999;41:889–96.

96. Shen J, Rothman DL, Brown P. In vivo GABA editing using a novel doubly selective multiple quantum filter. *Magn Reson Med* 2002;47:447–454.

97. Hanstock CC, Coupland NJ, Allen PS. GABA X2 multiplet measured pre- and post-administration of vigabatrin in human brain. *Magn Reson Med* 2002;48:617–623.

98. Terpstra M, Ugurbil K, Gruetter R. Direct in vivo measurement of human cerebral GABA concentration using MEGA-editing at 7 Tesla. *Magn Reson Med* 2002;47:1009–1012.

99. Gaspary HL, Wang W, Richerson GB. Carrier-mediated GABA release activates GABA receptors on hippocampal neurons. *J Neurophysiol* 1998;80:270–281.

100. Wu Y, Wang W, Richerson GB. GABA transaminase inhibition induces spontaneous and enhances depolarization-evoked GABA efflux via reversal of the GABA transporter. *J Neurosci* 2001; 21:2630–1639.

101. Menini C, Silva-Barrat C. The photosensitive epilepsy of the baboon. A model of generalized reflex epilepsy. *Adv Neurol* 1998;75:29–47.

102. Lloyd KG, et al. Cerebrospinal fluid amino acid and monoamine metabolite levels of *Papio papio*: correlation with photosensitivity. *Brain Res* 1986;363:390–394.

103. Kasteleijn-Nolst Trenite DG. Reflex seizures induced by intermittent light stimulation. *Adv Neurol* 1998;75:99–121.

104. Rimmer EM, Milligan NM, Richens A. A comparison of the acute effect of single doses of vigabatrin and sodium valproate on photosensitivity in epileptic patients. *Epilepsy Res* 1987;1:339–346.

105. Cracco JB, Rossini PM. Evoked responses and transcranial brain stimulation. Application to reflex epilepsy. *Adv Neurol* 1998;75:49–67.

106. Werhahn KJ, et al. Differential effects on motorcortical inhibition induced by blockade of GABA uptake in humans. *J Physiol* 1999;517:591–597.

107. Behar KL, et al. Preliminary evidence of low cortical GABA levels in localized ^{1}H-MR spectra of alcohol-dependent and hepatic encephalopathy patients. *Am J Psychiatry* 1999;156:952–954.

108. Petroff OA, et al. Homocarnosine and seizure control in juvenile myoclonic epilepsy and complex partial seizures. *Neurology* 2001;56:709–715.

109. Benson DL, Huntsman MM, Jones EG. Activity-dependent changes in GAD and preprotachykinin mRNAs in visual cortex of adult monkeys. *Cereb Cortex* 1994;4:40–51.

110. Boroojerdi, B, Bushara KO, Corwell B, et al. Enhanced excitability of the human visual cortex induced by short-term light deprivation. *Cereb Cortex* 2000;10:529–534.

111. Petroff OA, et al. Low brain GABA level is associated with poor seizure control. *Ann Neurol* 1996;40:908–911.

112. Haglund MM, et al. Changes in gamma-aminobutyric acid and somatostatin in epileptic cortex associated with low-grade gliomas. *J Neurosurg* 1992;77:209–216.

113. Marco P, et al. Inhibitory neurons in the human epileptogenic temporal neocortex. An immunocytochemical study. *Brain* 1996;119:1327–1347.

114. Spreafico R, et al. Cortical dysplasia: an immunocytochemical study of three patients. *Neurology* 1998;50:27–36.

115. Peltola J, et al. Autoantibodies to glutamic acid decarboxylase in patients with therapy-resistant epilepsy. *Neurology* 2000;55:46–50.

116. Van Donselaar CA, et al. Value of the electroencephalogram in adult patients with untreated idiopathic first seizures. *Arch Neurol* 1992;49:231–237.

117. Spencer SS, Spencer DD. Implications of seizure termination location in temporal lobe epilepsy. *Epilepsia* 1996;37:455–458.

118. Bautista RE, et al. Prediction of surgical outcome by interictal epileptiform abnormalities during intracranial EEG monitoring in patients with extrahippocampal seizures. *Epilepsia* 1999;40:880–890.

119. Bu DF, et al. Two human glutamate decarboxylases, 65-kDa GAD and 67-kDa GAD, are each encoded by a single gene. *Proc Natl Acad Sci USA* 1992;89:2115–2119.

120. Soghomonian JJ, Martin DL. Two isoforms of glutamate decarboxylase: why? *Trends Pharmacol Sci* 1998;19:500–505.

121. Hendrickson AE, et al. Differential localization of two glutamic acid decarboxylases (GAD65 and GAD67) in adult monkey visual cortex. *J Comp Neurol* 1994;343:566–581.

122. Kash SF, et al. Epilepsy in mice deficient in the 65-kDa isoform of glutamic acid decarboxylase. *Proc Natl Acad Sci USA* 1997;94:14060–14065.

123. Asada H, et al. Mice lacking the 65 kDa isoform of glutamic acid decarboxylase (GAD65) maintain normal levels of GAD67 and GABA in their brains but are susceptible to seizures. *Biochem Biophys Res Commun* 1996;229:891–895.

124. Ji F, Kanbara N, Obata K. GABA and histogenesis in fetal and neonatal mouse brain lacking both the isoforms of glutamic acid decarboxylase. *Neurosci Res* 1999;33:187–194.

125. Yasumi M, et al. Regional distribution of GABA transporter 1 (GAT1) mRNA in the rat brain: comparison with glutamic acid decarboxylase67 (GAD67) mRNA localization. *Brain Res Mol Brain Res* 1997;44:205–218.

126. During MJ, Ryder KM, Spencer DD. Hippocampal GABA transporter function in temporal-lobe epilepsy. *Nature* 1995;376:174–177.

127. Patrylo PR, Spencer DD, Williamson A. GABA uptake and heterotransport are impaired in the dentate gyrus of epileptic rats and humans with temporal lobe sclerosis. *J Neurophysiol* 2001; 85:1533–1542.

128. Martin DL, Rimvall K. Regulation of gamma-aminobutyric acid synthesis in the brain. *J Neurochem* 1993;60:395–407.

129. Kapetanovic IM, Yonekawa WD, Kupferberg HJ. Time-related loss of glutamine from hippocampal slices and concomitant changes in neurotransmitter amino acids. *J Neurochem* 1993;61:865–872.

130. Patel AB, Rothman DL, Cline GW. Glutamine is the major precursor for GABA synthesis in rat neocortex in vivo following acute GABA-transaminase inhibition. *Brain Res* 2001;919:207–220.

131. Behar KL, Rothman DL. In vivo nuclear magnetic resonance studies of glutamate-gamma-aminobutyric acid-glutamine cycling in rodent and human cortex: the central role of glutamine. *J Nutr* 2001; 131(Suppl):2498S–2504S.

132. Traub RD, et al. On the structure of ictal events in vitro. *Epilepsia* 1996;37:879–891.

133. Kohling R. Neuroscience. GABA becomes exciting. *Science* 2002;298:1350–1351.

134. Van den Pol AN, et al. Glutamate inhibits GABA excitatory activity in developing neurons. *J Neurosci* 1998;18:10749–10761.

135. Ochi S, et al. Transient presence of GABA in astrocytes of the developing optic nerve. Glia 1993;9:188–198.

136. Berkovic SF, Scheffer IE. Genetics of the epilepsies. Curr Opin Neurol 1999;12:177–182.

137. Berkovic SF, et al. Epilepsies in twins: genetics of the major epilepsy syndromes. *Ann Neurol* 1998;43:435–445.

138. Prasad AN, Prasad C, Stafstrom CE. Recent advances in the genetics of epilepsy: insights from human and animal studies. *Epilepsia* 1999;40:1329–1352.

139. Waymire KG, et al. Mice lacking tissue non-specific alkaline phosphatase die from seizures due to defective metabolism of vitamin B-6. *Nat Genet* 1995;11:45–51.

140. Jakobs C, Jaeken J, Gibson KM. Inherited disorders of GABA metabolism. *J Inherit Metab Dis* 1993;16:704–715.

141. Battaglioli G, et al. Glutamate decarboxylase is not genetically linked to pyridoxine-dependent seizures. *Neurology* 2000;55:309–311.

142. Gibson KM, et al. 4-Hydroxybutyric acid and the clinical phenotype of succinic semialdehyde dehydrogenase deficiency, an inborn error of GABA metabolism. *Neuropediatrics* 1998;29:14–22.

143. Medina-Kauwe LK, et al. 4-Aminobutyrate aminotransferase (GABA-transaminase) deficiency. *J Inherit Metab Dis* 1999; 22:414–427.

144. Ohtsuka Y, et al. Long-term follow-up of vitamin B_6-responsive West syndrome. *Pediatr Neurol* 2000;23:202–206.

145. Baulac S, et al. First genetic evidence of GABA(A) receptor dysfunction in epilepsy: a mutation in the gamma2-subunit gene. *Nat Genet* 2001;28:46–48.

146. Wallace RH, et al. Mutant GABA(A) receptor gamma2-subunit in childhood absence epilepsy and febrile seizures. *Nat Genet* 2001;28:49–52.

147. Petroff OA, Rothman DL. Measuring human brain GABA in vivo: effects of GABA-transaminase inhibition with vigabatrin. *Mol Neurobiol* 1998;16:97–121.

148. Petroff OA, et al. Vigabatrin increases human brain homocarnosine and improves seizure control. *Ann Neurol* 1998;44:948–952.

149. Petroff OA, Behar KL, Rothman DL. New NMR measurements in epilepsy. Measuring brain GABA in patients with complex partial seizures. *Adv Neurol* 1999;79:939–945.

150. Sanacora G, et al. Increased cortical GABA concentrations in depressed patients receiving ECT. *Am J Psychiatry* 2003;160:577–579.

151. Mueller SG, et al. Effects of vigabatrin on brain GABA+/CR signals in patients with epilepsy monitored by ^{1}H-NMR-spectroscopy: responder characteristics. *Epilepsia* 2001;42:29–40.

152. Spencer SS. Neural networks in human epilepsy: evidence of and implications for treatment. *Epilepsia* 2002;43:219–227.

153. Petroff OA, et al. Effects of gabapentin on brain GABA, homocarnosine, and pyrrolidinone in epilepsy patients. *Epilepsia* 2000;41:675–680.

154. Petroff OA, et al. Topiramate rapidly raises brain GABA in epilepsy patients. *Epilepsia* 2001;42:543–548.

155. Kuzniecky R, et al. Modulation of cerebral GABA by topiramate, lamotrigine, and gabapentin in healthy adults. *Neurology* 2002; 58:368–372.

156. Errante LD, et al. Gabapentin and vigabatrin increase GABA in the human neocortical slice. *Epilepsy Res* 2002;49:203–210.

157. Kuzniecky R, et al. Topiramate increases cerebral GABA in healthy humans. *Neurology* 1998;51:627–629.

158. Petroff OA, et al. Acute effects of vigabatrin on brain GABA and homocarnosine in patients with complex partial seizures. *Epilepsia* 1999;40:958–964.

159. Novotny EJ Jr, et al. GABA changes with vigabatrin in the developing human brain. Epilepsia 1999;40:462–466.

160. Perry TL, et al. Homocarnosinosis: increased content of homocarnosine and deficiency of homocarnosinase in brain. *J Neurochem* 1979;32:1637–1640.

161. Kish SJ, Perry TL, Hansen S. Regional distribution of homocarnosine, homocarnosine-carnosine synthetase and homocarnosinase in human brain. *J Neurochem* 1979;32:1629–1636.

162. Jackson MC, et al. Localization of a novel pathway for the liberation of GABA in the human CNS. *Brain Res Bull* 1994;33: 379–385.

163. Perry TL, et al. Regional distribution of amino acids in human brain obtained at autopsy. *J Neurochem* 1971;18:513–519.

164. Grove J, et al. Artifactual increases in the concentration of free GABA in samples of human cerebrospinal fluid are due to degradation of homocarnosine. *J Neurochem* 1982;39:1061–1065.

165. Rothman DL, et al. Homocarnosine and the measurement of neuronal pH in patients with epilepsy. *Magn Reson Med* 1997;38: 924–929.

166. Gjessing LR, et al. Inborn errors of carnosine and homocarnosine metabolism. *J Neural Transm Suppl* 1990;29:91–106.

167. Skaper SD, Das S, Marshall FD. Some properties of a homocarnosine-carnosine synthetase isolated from rat brain. *J Neurochem* 1973;21:1429–1445.

168. Lunde HA, Gjessing LR, Sjaastad O. Homocarnosinosis: influence of dietary restriction of histidine. Neurochem Res 1986;11:825–838.

169. Ben-Menachem E, et al. The effect of different vigabatrin treatment regimens on CSF biochemistry and seizure control in epileptic patients. *Br J Clin Pharmacol* 1989;27(Suppl 1):79S–85S.

170. Riekkinen PJ, et al. Cerebrospinal fluid GABA and seizure control with vigabatrin. *Br J Clin Pharmacol* 1989;27(Suppl 1):87S–94S.

171. Trombley PQ, Horning MS, Blakemore LJ. Carnosine modulates zinc and copper effects on amino acid receptors and synaptic transmission. *Neuroreport* 1998;9:3503–3507.

172. Smart TG, Xie X, Krishek BJ. Modulation of inhibitory and excitatory amino acid receptor ion channels by zinc. *Prog Neurobiol* 1994;42:393–341.

173. Buhl EH, Otis TS, Mody I. Zinc-induced collapse of augmented inhibition by GABA in a temporal lobe epilepsy model. *Science* 1996;271:369–373.

174. Williamson A, Patrylo PR. Neuroscientist 1999;5:362–370.

175. Petroff OA, et al. Spectroscopic imaging of stroke in humans: histopathology correlates of spectral changes. *Neurology* 1992;42:1349–1354.

176. Cheng LL, et al. Quantitative neuropathology by high resolution magic angle spinning proton magnetic resonance spectroscopy. *Proc Natl Acad Sci USA* 1997;94:6408–6413.

177. Bitsch A, et al. Inflammatory CNS demyelination: histopathologic correlation with in vivo quantitative proton MR spectroscopy. *Am J Neuroradiol* 1999;20:1619–1627.

178. Bjartmar C, Trapp BD. Axonal and neuronal degeneration in multiple sclerosis: mechanisms and functional consequences. *Curr Opin Neurol* 2001;14:271–258.

179. Bjartmar C, et al. *N*-acetylaspartate is an axon-specific marker of mature white matter in vivo: a biochemical and immunohistochemical study on the rat optic nerve. *Ann Neurol* 2002;51:51–58.

180. Martin E, et al. Absence of *N*-acetylaspartate in the human brain: impact on neurospectroscopy? *Ann Neurol* 2001;49:518–521.

181. Sullivan EV, et al. N-acetylaspartate–a marker of neuronal integrity. *Ann Neurol* 2001;50:823.

182. Jenkins BG, et al. Nonlinear decrease over time in *N*-acetyl aspartate levels in the absence of neuronal loss and increases in glutamine and glucose in transgenic Huntington's disease mice. *J Neurochem* 2000;74:2108–2119.

183. Signoretti S, et al. N-Acetylaspartate reduction as a measure of injury severity and mitochondrial dysfunction following diffuse traumatic brain injury. *J Neurotrauma* 2001;18:977–991.

184. De Stefano N, et al. Diffuse axonal and tissue injury in patients with multiple sclerosis with low cerebral lesion load and no disability. *Arch Neurol* 2002;59:1565–1571.

185. Matthews PM, Arnold DL. Magnetic resonance imaging of multiple sclerosis: new insights linking pathology to clinical evolution. *Curr Opin Neurol* 2001;14:279–287.

186. Argov Z, Arnold DL. MR spectroscopy and imaging in metabolic myopathies. *Neurol Clin* 2000;18:35–52.

187. Rango M, et al. Brain activation in normal subjects and in patients affected by mitochondrial disease without clinical central nervous system involvement: a phosphorus magnetic resonance spectroscopy study. *J Cereb Blood Flow Metab* 2001;21:85–91.

188. Barbiroli B, Iotti S, Lodi R. Improved brain and muscle mitochondrial respiration with CoQ. An in vivo study by ^{31}P-MR spectroscopy in patients with mitochondrial cytopathies. *Biofactors* 1999;9:253–260.

189. Kuwabara T, et al. Mitochondrial encephalomyopathy: elevated visual cortex lactate unresponsive to photic stimulation – a localized ^{1}H-MRS study. *Neurology* 1994;44:557–559.

190. Bates TE, et al. Inhibition of *N*-acetylaspartate production: implications for ^{1}H MRS studies in vivo. *Neuroreport* 1996;7:1397–1400.

191. Clark JB. *N*-acetyl aspartate: a marker for neuronal loss or mitochondrial dysfunction. *Dev Neurosci* 1998;20:271–276.

192. Brines ML, et al. Regional distributions of hippocampal Na$^+$,K$^+$-ATPase, cytochrome oxidase, and total protein in temporal lobe epilepsy. *Epilepsia* 1995;36:371–383.

193. Moreno A, Ross BD, Bluml S. Direct determination of the *N*-acetyl-L-aspartate synthesis rate in the human brain by ^{13}C MRS and [1-^{13}C]glucose infusion. *J Neurochem* 2001;77:347–350.

194. Neale, JH, Bzdega T, Wroblewska B. *N*-Acetylaspartylglutamate: the most abundant peptide neurotransmitter in the mammalian central nervous system. *J Neurochem* 2000;75:443–452.

195. Baslow MH. Functions of *N*-acetyl-L-aspartate and *N*-acetyl-L-aspartylglutamate in the vertebrate brain: role in glial cell-specific signaling. *J Neurochem* 2000;75:453–459.

196. Huang W, et al. Transport of *N*-acetylaspartate by the Na$^+$-dependent high-affinity dicarboxylate transporter NaDC3 and its relevance to the expression of the transporter in the brain. *J Pharmacol Exp Ther* 2000;295:392–403.

197. Bhakoo KK, Craig TJ, Styles P. Developmental and regional distribution of aspartoacylase in rat brain tissue. *J Neurochem* 2001;79:211–220.

198. Hassel B, Brathe A, Petersen D. Cerebral dicarboxylate transport and metabolism studied with isotopically labelled fumarate, malate and malonate. *J Neurochem* 2002;82:410–419.

199. Matalon R, Michals-Matalon K. Biochemistry and molecular biology of Canavan disease. *Neurochem Res* 1999;24:507–513.

200. Baslow MH. Evidence supporting a role for *N*-acetyl-L-aspartate as a molecular water pump in myelinated neurons in the central nervous system. An analytical review. *Neurochem Int* 2002;40:295–300.

201. Nakada T, Kwee IL. Maturational changes in intracellular high energy phosphate transport in rat brain. *Neuroreport* 1991;2:777–780.

202. Gadian DG, et al. ^{1}H magnetic resonance spectroscopy in the investigation of intractable epilepsy. *Acta Neurol Scand Suppl* 1994;152:116–121.

203. Maton BM, Kuzniecky RI. Proton MRS: *N*-acetyl aspartate, creatine, and choline. *Adv Neurol* 2000;83:253–259.

204. Knowlton RC, et al. Presurgical multimodality neuroimaging in electroencephalographic lateralized temporal lobe epilepsy. *Ann Neurol* 1997;42:829–837.

205. Connelly A, et al. Proton magnetic resonance spectroscopy in MRI-negative temporal lobe epilepsy. *Neurology* 1998;51:61–6.

206. Gadian DG, et al. Lateralization of brain function in childhood revealed by magnetic resonance spectroscopy. *Neurology* 1996;46:974–977.

207. Bernasconi A, et al. Proton magnetic resonance spectroscopic imaging suggests progressive neuronal damage in human temporal lobe epilepsy. *Prog Brain Res* 2002;135:297–304.

208. Hugg JW, et al. Normalization of contralateral metabolic function following temporal lobectomy demonstrated by ^{1}H magnetic resonance spectroscopic imaging. *Ann Neurol* 1996;40:236–239.

209. Serles W, et al. Time course of postoperative recovery of *N*-acetyl-aspartate in temporal lobe epilepsy. *Epilepsia* 2001;42:190–197.

210. Garcia PA, et al. Proton magnetic resonance spectroscopic imaging in patients with frontal lobe epilepsy. *Ann Neurol* 1995;37:279–281.

211. Stanley JA, et al. Proton magnetic resonance spectroscopic imaging in patients with extratemporal epilepsy. *Epilepsia* 1998;39:267–273.

212. Garcia PA, et al. Correlation of seizure frequency with *N*-acetyl-aspartate levels determined by ^{1}H magnetic resonance spectroscopic imaging. *Magn Reson Imaging* 1997;15:475–478.

213. Mueller SG, et al. Proton magnetic resonance spectroscopy characteristics of a focal cortical dysgenesis during status epilepticus and in the interictal state. *Seizure* 2001;10:518–524.

214. Kuzniecky R, Hetherington H, Pan J. Proton spectroscopic imaging at 4.1 tesla in patients with malformations of cortical development and epilepsy. *Neurology* 1997;48:1018–1024.

215. Peeling J, Sutherland G. ^{1}H magnetic resonance spectroscopy of extracts of human epileptic neocortex and hippocampus. *Neurology* 1993;43:589–594.

216. Duc CO, et al. Quantitative ^{1}H MRS in the evaluation of mesial temporal lobe epilepsy in vivo. *Magn Reson Imaging* 1998;16:969–979.

217. Kuzniecky R, et al. Magnetic resonance spectroscopic imaging in temporal lobe epilepsy: neuronal dysfunction or cell loss? *Arch Neurol* 2001;58:2048–2053.

218. Tsai G, Coyle JT. *N*-acetylaspartate in neuropsychiatric disorders. *Prog Neurobiol* 1995;46:531–540.

219. Petroff OA, Pleban LA, Spencer DD. Symbiosis between in vivo and in vitro NMR spectroscopy: the creatine, *N*-acetylaspartate, glutamate, and GABA content of the epileptic human brain. *Magn Reson Imaging* 1995;13:1197–1211.

220. Eberhardt KE, et al. The significance of bilateral CSI changes for the postoperative outcome in temporal lobe epilepsy. *J Comput Assist Tomogr* 2000;24:919–926.

221. Prichard JW, et al. Cerebral metabolic studies in vivo by ^{31}P NMR. *Proc Natl Acad Sci* USA 1983;80:2748–2751.

222. Petroff OA, Prichard JW, Behar KL. In vivo phosphorus nuclear magnetic resonance spectroscopy in status epilepticus. *Ann Neurol* 1984;16:169–177.

223. Prichard JW, et al. Cerebral lactate elevation by electroshock: a ^{1}H magnetic resonance. *Ann NY Acad Sci* 1987;508:54–63.

224. Young RS, et al. The effect of diazepam on neonatal seizure: in vivo ^{31}P and ^{1}H NMR study. *Pediatr Res* 1989;25:27–31.

225. Petroff OA, et al. Cerebral lactate turnover after electroshock: in vivo measurements by ^{1}H/^{13}C magnetic resonance spectroscopy. *J Cereb Blood Flow Metab* 1992;12:1022–1029.

226. Younkin DP, et al. Cerebral metabolic effects of neonatal seizures measured with in vivo ^{31}P NMR spectroscopy. *Ann Neurol* 1986;20:513–519.

227. Matthews PM, Andermann F, Arnold DL. A proton magnetic resonance spectroscopy study of focal epilepsy in humans. *Neurology* 1990;40:985–989.

228. Danielsen ER, Ross B. The clinical significance of metabolites. In: Ross B, ed. Magnetic resonance spectroscopy of neurological diseases. New York: Marcel Dekker, 1999:23–42.

229. Nonaka M, Kohmura E, Yamashita T. Kainic acid-induced seizure upregulates Na$^+$/myo-inositol cotransporter mRNA in rat brain. *Brain Res Mol Brain Res* 1999;70:179–186.

230. Gullans SR, Verbalis JG. Control of brain volume during hyperosmolar and hypoosmolar conditions. *Annu Rev Med* 1993;44:289–301.

231. Brand A, Leibfritz D, Richter-Landsberg C. Oxidative stress-induced metabolic alterations in rat brain astrocytes studied by multinuclear NMR spectroscopy. *J Neurosci Res* 1999;58:576–585.

232. Burtscher IM, Holtas S. Proton magnetic resonance spectroscopy in brain tumours: clinical applications. *Neuroradiology* 2001;43:345–352.

233. Moller-Hartmann W, Herminghaus S, Krings T. Clinical application of proton magnetic resonance spectroscopy in the diagnosis of intracranial mass lesions. *Neuroradiology* 2002;44:371–381.

234. Najm IM, et al. MRS metabolic markers of seizures and seizure-induced neuronal damage. Epilepsia 1998;39:244–250.

235. Meiners LC, et al. Proton magnetic resonance spectroscopy of temporal lobe white matter in patients with histologically proven hippocampal sclerosis. *J Magn Res Imag* 2000;11:25–31.

236. Cross JH, Connelly A, Jackson GD. Proton magnetic resonance spectroscopy in children with temporal lobe epilepsy. *Ann Neurol* 1996;39:107–113.

237. Holopainen IE, et al. Proton spectroscopy in children with epilepsy and febrile convulsions. Pediatr Neurol 1998;19:93–99.

238. Kuzniecky R, Hugg JW, Hetherington H. Relative utility of ^{1}H spectroscopic imaging and hippocampal volumetry in the lateralization of mesial temporal lobe epilepsy. Neurology 1998;51:66–71.

239. Li LM, et al. Proton magnetic resonance spectroscopic imaging studies in patients with newly diagnosed partial epilepsy. *Epilepsia* 2000;41:825–831.

240. Ende GR, Laxer KD, Knowlton RC. Radiology 1997;202:809–817.

241. Babb TL. Bilateral pathological damage in temporal lobe epilepsy. *Can J Neurol Sci* 1991;18:645–648.

242. Margerison JH, Corsellis JAN. Epilepsy and the temporal lobes. *Brain* 1966;89:499–530.

243. Barr WB, Ashtari M, Schaul N. Bilateral reductions in hippocampal volume in adults with epilepsy and a history of febrile seizures. *J Neurol Neurosurg Psychiatry* 1997;63:461–467.

244. Quigg M, et al. Volumetric magnetic resonance imaging evidence of bilateral hippocampal atrophy in mesial temporal lobe epilepsy. *Epilepsia* 1997;38:588–594.

245. Kuzniecky R, et al. Predictive value of ^{1}H MRSI for outcome in temporal lobectomy. *Neurology* 1999;53:694–698.

246. Arnold S, et al. Topography of interictal glucose hypometabolism in unilateral mesiotemporal epilepsy. *Neurology* 1996;46:1422–1430.

247. Rabinowicz AL, et al. Changes in regional cerebral blood flow beyond the temporal lobe in unilateral temporal lobe epilepsy. *Epilepsy* 1997;38:1011–1014.

248. Miller SP, et al. Medial temporal lobe neuronal damage in temporal and extratemporal lesional epilepsy. *Neurology* 2000;54:1465–1470.

249. Mueller SG, et al. Reduced extrahippocampal NAA in mesial temporal lobe epilepsy. Epilepsia 2002;43:1210–1216.

250. Wellard RM, Briellmann RS, Prichard JW, et al. Myoinositol abnormalities in temporal lobe epilepsy. *Epilepsia* 2003;44:815–821.

251. Kikuchi S, et al. A study of the relationship between the seizure focus and ^{1}H-MRS in temporal lobe epilepsy and frontal lobe epilepsy. *Psychiatry Clin Neurosci* 2000;54:455–459.

252. Savic I, et al. MR spectroscopy shows reduced frontal lobe concentrations of N-acetyl aspartate in patients with juvenile myoclonic epilepsy. *Epilepsia* 2000;41:290–296.

253. Cascino GD, et al. Gelastic seizures and hypothalamic hamartomas: evaluation of patients undergoing chronic intracranial EEG monitoring and outcome of surgical treatment. *Neurology* 1993;43:747–750.

254. Berkovic SF, et al. Hypothalamic hamartomas and ictal laughter: evaluation of a characteristic epileptic syndrome and diagnostic value of magnetic resonance imaging. *Ann Neurol* 1988;23:429–439.

255. Buchli R, Duc CO, Martin E. Assessment of absolute metabolite concentrations in human tissue by ^{31}P MRS in vivo. Part I: Cerebrum, cerebellum, cerebral gray and white matter. *Magn Reson Med* 1994;32:447–452.

256. Sappey-Marinier D, Calabrese G, Fein G, et al. Effect of photic stimulation on human visual cortex lactate and phosphates using ^{1}H and ^{31}P magnetic resonance spectroscopy. *J Cereb Blood Flow Metab* 1992;12:584–592.

257. Bretscher MS. Asymmetrical lipid bilayer structure for biological membranes. *Nature New Biol* 1972;236:11–12.

258. Gadian DG, Radda GK, Dawson MJ. pH measurements of cardiac and skeletal muscle using ^{31}P NMR. New York: Liss, 1982.

259. Bluml S, Tan J, Harris K, et al. Quantitative proton-decoupled ^{31}P MRS of the schizophrenic brain in vivo. *J Comput Assist Tomogr* 1999;23:272–275.

260. Gadian DG. NMR and its application to living systems, 2nd ed. New York: Oxford University Press, 1995.

261. Laxer KD, Hubesch B, Sappey-Marinier D. Increased pH and inorganic phosphate in temporal seizure foci demonstrated by [^{31}P]MRS. *Epilepsia* 1992;33:618–623.

262. Kuzniecky R, Elgavish GA, Hetherington HP, et al. In vivo ^{31}P nuclear magnetic resonance spectroscopy of human temporal lobe epilepsy. *Neurology* 1992;42:1586–1590.

263. Hugg JW, et al. Phosphorus-31 MR spectroscopic imaging (MRSI) of normal and pathological human brains. *Magn Reson Imag* 1992;10:227–243.

264. Van der Grond J, et al. Regional distribution of interictal ^{31}P metabolic changes in patients with temporal lobe epilepsy. *Epilepsia* 1998;39:527–536.

265. Bluml S, A. Moreno, and J.H. Hwang, 1-(13)C glucose magnetic resonance spectroscopy of pediatric and adult brain disorders. *NMR Biomed* 2001;14:19–32.

266. Schnall MD, et al. Triple nuclear NMR studies of cerebral metabolism during generalized seizure. *Magn Reson Med* 1988;6:15–23.

267. Eleff SM, et al. Concurrent measurements of cerebral blood flow, sodium, lactate, and high-energy phosphate metabolism using ^{19}F, ^{23}Na, ^{1}H, and ^{31}P nuclear magnetic resonance spectroscopy. *Magn Reson Med* 1988;7:412–424.

268. Strauss WL, et al. 19F magnetic resonance spectroscopy investigation in vivo of acute and steady-state brain fluvoxamine levels in obsessive-compulsive disorder. *Am J Psychiatry* 1997;154:516–22.

269. Vlaardingerbroek MT, Den Boer JA. Magnetic resonance imaging: theory and practice. New York: Springer, 1999.

270. Dreher W, Leibfritz D. Fast proton spectroscopic imaging with high signal-to-noise ratio: spectroscopic RARE. *Magn Reson Med* 2002;47:523–528.

271. Li, BS, Regal J, Gonen O. SNR versus resolution in 3D ^{1}H MRS of the human brain at high magnetic fields. *Magn Reson Med* 2001;46:1049–1053.

272. Behar KL, Rothman DL, Spencer DD, Petroff OA. Analysis of macromolecule resonances in ^{1}H NMR spectra of human brain, *Magn Reson Med* 1994;32:294–302.

273. Weber OM, et al. Effects of vigabatrin intake on brain GABA activity as monitored by spectrally edited magnetic resonance spectroscopy and positron emission tomography. *Magn Reson Imag* 1999;17:417–425.

274. Park SA, et al. Interictal epileptiform discharges relate to ^{1}H-MRS-detected metabolic abnormalities in mesial temporal lobe epilepsy. *Epilepsia* 2002;43:1385–1389.

275. Maton B, et al. Correlation of scalp EEG and ^{1}H-MRS metabolic abnormalities in temporal lobe epilepsy. *Epilepsia* 2001;42:417–422.

276. Braun J, et al. Volume-selective proton MR spectroscopy for in-vitro quantification of anticonvulsants. *Neuroradiology* 2001; 43:211–217.

277. Hetherington HP, Pan JW, Spencer DD. ^{1}H and ^{31}P spectroscopy and bioenergetics in the lateralization of seizures in temporal lobe epilepsy. *J Magn Reson Imaging* 2002;16:477–483.

278. Kuzniecky R. Magnetic resonance spectroscopy in focal epilepsy: ^{31}P and ^{1}H spectroscopy. *Rev Neurol (Paris)* 1999;155:495–498.

279. Hetherington HP, Pan JW, Mason GF, et al. 2D spectroscopic imaging of the human brain at 4 T. *Magn Reson Med* 1994;32:530–534.

280. Hetherington HP, Newcomer BR, Pan JW. Measurements of human cerebral GABA at 4.1T using numerically optimized pulses. *Magn Reson Med* 1998;39:6–10.

CHAPTER 14

Single-photon-emission Computed Tomography in Epilepsy

Christopher C. Rowe

INTRODUCTION

Ictal single-photon-emission computed tomography (SPECT) and positron-emission tomography (PET) are valuable clinical tools in the management of patients with medically resistant partial epilepsy who are under evaluation for surgical treatment. Both techniques provide useful and complementary data for localization of the seizure focus and are regularly employed in most epilepsy surgery centers. The sensitivity for detection of the seizure focus is higher than that of structural imaging (1) but, unlike MRI, these modalities give little indication of the underlying pathology. The clinical value of PET and SPECT is greater when co-registration with MRI is performed, not infrequently pointing to an area of subtle structural abnormality overlooked on the initial MR reading.

BLOOD FLOW AND METABOLISM IN PARTIAL SEIZURES

Interictal

Between seizures, the *interictal* period, cerebral blood flow (CBF) and metabolism may be normal or reduced. A reduction in these indices in the epileptogenic temporal lobe is frequently present in patients with temporal lobe epilepsy (TLE), while *interictal* regional abnormalities are less common in other forms of epilepsy in the absence of a structural abnormality. The mechanism for reduced blood flow and metabolism is unexplained and its relationship to neuronal loss is unclear. The area of hypometabolism is often more extensive than that of demonstrable abnormality in resected specimens (2).

The most common histologic abnormality in patients with mesial TLE is mesial temporal sclerosis, with loss of neurons and gliosis in the hippocampus and amygdala (3). In contrast to this localized abnormality, *interictal* hypoperfusion and hypometabolism may extend well into lateral temporal, frontal and parietal cortex (2).

Ictal Blood Flow and Metabolism

Regional cerebral blood flow (rCBF) in the epileptic focus increases by up to 300% during a seizure (4, 5). This phenomenon was first observed by Horsley in 1892 and has subsequently been documented in both humans and animal seizure models by a variety of techniques (6). The intra-arterial ^{133}Xe clearance technique was the first noninvasive method that allowed observation of these changes in humans, but this approach was not suitable for routine *ictal* imaging (4, 7).

More stable tracers such as HMPAO permit the study of *ictal* and *postictal* changes with more accuracy. In the immediate *postictal* period regional cerebral blood flow and metabolism are reduced to a greater extent than in the *interictal* period (Fig. 14.1). The exact onset and duration of the *postictal* period is not strictly defined as the electrical, behavioral, metabolic, and blood flow features of this phase vary greatly in duration between individuals (8).

PREOPERATIVE LOCALIZATION WITH SPECT

Electroencephalography (EEG) remains the 'gold standard' laboratory investigation for seizure localization.

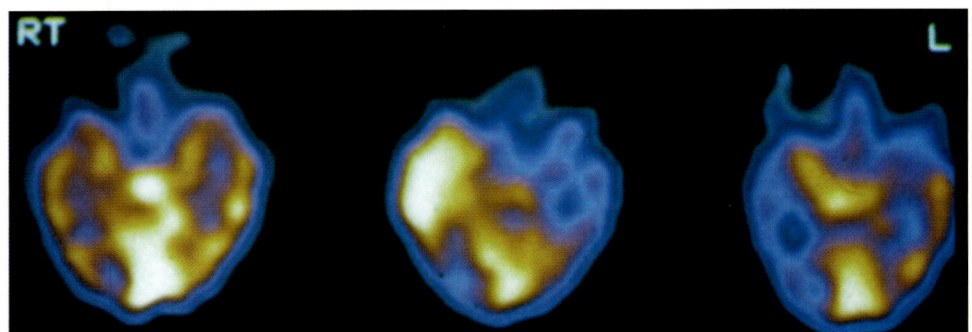

FIG. 14.1. SPECT demonstrating mild *interictal* right temporal lobe hypoperfusion (left panel), intense *ictal* hyperperfusion in the right temporal lobe with reduced perfusion in the left (middle panel), and marked *postictal* right lateral temporal hypoperfusion with residual anteromedial right temporal hyperperfusion (right panel). All studies are from the same patient with proven right TLE using Ceretec® (HMPAO). The *postictal* injection was given 3 minutes after completion of the seizure.

Ictal EEG from scalp electrodes does not permit confident localization in 40% of patients with TLE if used in isolation. However, in most patients confident localization can be achieved when *ictal* scalp EEG is supported by *ictal* clinical features and ancillary investigations such as MRI, *ictal* SPECT, and PET. In patients in whom investigations are contradictory, intracranial *ictal* EEG studies are performed. Serious complications including intracerebral hemorrhage and infection, although rare, have occurred following insertion of intracranial electrodes so noninvasive localization should always be attempted first.

SPECT IN TEMPORAL LOBE EPILEPSY

Optimal Image Presentation

The complete three-dimensional data set provided by SPECT enables selection of optimal image planes. The temporal lobes are best viewed by reconstructing transaxial slices parallel to the temporal lobe with coronal slices perpendicular to this plane (9–11). The temporal lobes run forward at a downward angle of approximately 35° from the anterior–posterior commissure (AC–PC) line. The AC–PC line can be approximated by joining the bottom of the frontal lobe and the occipital lobe on a midline sagittal slice and the temporal lobe plane is then derived from this line.

Asymmetry can be readily quantified in this plane using symmetrical regions of interest placed over the anterior temporal lobes. Asymmetry is normally less than 5%, while more than 10% is definitely abnormal. Region of interest quantification does not improve the sensitivity of seizure focus detection and is therefore usually only performed for research purposes (11, 12). Background subtraction and color scales are useful to enhance the mild degrees of temporal lobe asymmetry typically seen with SPECT in TLE.

Co-registration of SPECT with MRI is useful particularly for the interpretation of subtraction (*ictal* minus *interictal*) images.

Interictal SPECT

Interictal hypoperfusion was first demonstrated with SPECT in 1982 using ^{123}I iodoamphetamine and a dedicated single-slice SPECT device. *Ictal* hyperperfusion was also reported in the same study in several patients injected during seizures (13, 14). Since then many reports from seizure surgery centers have compared the results of *interictal* SPECT to *ictal* EEG localization or surgical outcome in patients with refractory temporal lobe epilepsy. A meta-analysis of these reports found that SPECT showed temporal lobe hypoperfusion on the side of the seizure focus in 55% and contralateral hypoperfusion leading to incorrect lateralization was present in 10% (15). SPECT studies in pediatric populations suggest similar clinical utility to adult studies.

Interictal SPECT does not have the sensitivity or accuracy of FDG-PET, as *interictal* blood flow changes are less marked than metabolic changes (16–18). Several studies have found better results imaging glucose metabolism than blood flow in the same patients with the same PET camera (19–21).

Interictal Variability

An alternative explanation for the lower sensitivity of SPECT compared with FDG-PET is that *interictal* blood flow and metabolism may be quite labile. Up to 10% of patients demonstrate *interictal* hyperperfusion but *interictal* hypermetabolism has not been described (22, 23). In most patients, *interictal* CBF findings are reproducible but examples of *interictal* temporal lobe hyperperfusion on the first study and hypoperfusion in the same area on a subsequent SPECT study have been documented, suggesting that temporal lobe perfusion may be labile in some individuals (12, 22, 24). The brain uptake of PET and SPECT blood flow tracers is principally a first-pass extraction process while FDG accumulates over 20–40 min. A transient increase in temporal lobe blood flow and metabolism may not be detected by FDG studies and so may give a better indication of the hypometabolic steady state. Improved localization can be obtained by repeating a SPECT study when the first result is negative or unexpected, further suggesting that *interictal* temporal lobe activity is variable (25).

Patterns of Hypoperfusion

The degree and extent of hypoperfusion, like that of hypometabolism, varies greatly from one individual to another. It most commonly involves the anterior pole of the temporal lobe and medial temporal region but involvement of lateral temporal cortex and ipsilateral frontal and parietal cortex is not uncommon. On occasion, hyperperfusion is observed. The degree of unilateral temporal lobe hypoperfusion correlates with the age at onset of seizures but not seizure frequency, patient age, or the likelihood of secondary generalization (12). The presence of left temporal lobe hypoperfusion reduces the risk of a postoperative decline in verbal short-term memory function after a left temporal lobectomy (26).

The Clinical Role of *Interictal* SPECT

Interictal SPECT has limited clinical value relative to other imaging procedures that have greater sensitivity and specificity, such as PET and MRI. There is less contrast between normal and abnormal areas with SPECT compared with PET and aggressive reading to improve sensitivity increases false localization. The main role for *interictal* SPECT is to aid interpretation of *ictal* SPECT studies by providing a baseline for visual comparison or image subtraction (Fig. 14.2).

ICTAL AND *POSTICTAL* SPECT

Ictal studies are obtained with injection during the electrical or clinical manifestation of a seizure. *Postictal* studies are obtained by injection after completion of a seizure. Some authors use the term 'peri-*ictal*' to refer to the *ictal* and early *postictal* phase given the variability of this period. The high first-pass extraction of ^{99m}Tc-exametazine (Ceretec®) and ^{99m}Tc-ECD (Neurolite®) with prolonged retention makes imaging of *ictal* cerebral blood flow feasible with these agents. [123]I iodoamphetamine (IMP) and ^{123}I-HIPDM are also suitable radiopharmaceuticals for *ictal* SPECT imaging but are more costly and less readily available. IMP, ECD, and stabilized Ceretec® do not require bedside reconstitution immediately prior to injection, permitting faster injections and less staff training. However, cost may be an issue due to

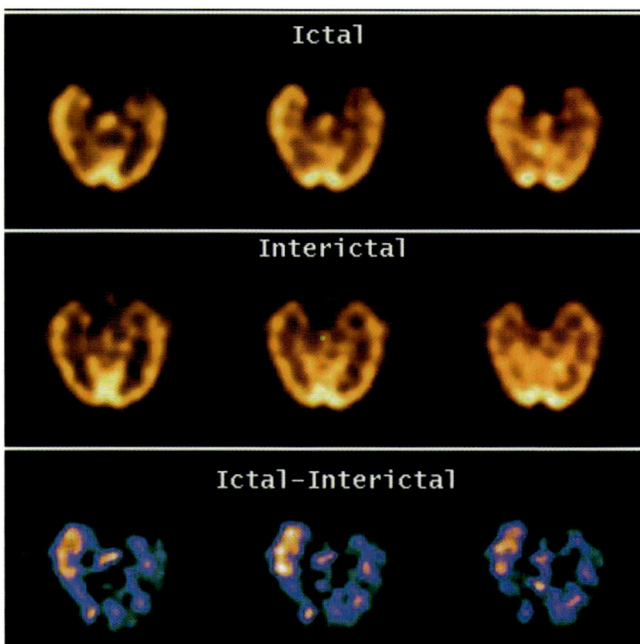

FIG. 14.2. Right temporal lobe epilepsy. Neurolite® (ECD) was injected during a seizure. Top row: *Ictal* SPECT. Middle row: *Interictal* SPECT. Bottom row. Subtraction of *interictal* from *ictal* SPECT images.

wastage on days when seizures do not occur, so some centers continue to use standard Ceretec® unless the seizures are suspected to be of extratemporal lobe origin or short duration. Those centers that have the shortest delay between seizure onset and injection of tracer have constant close observation of the patient by an EEG technologist or a nurse who gives the injection of tracer. Average injection delays of 10–30 seconds from seizure onset to injection are now achieved in many centers.

Sensitivity

Over 500 patients with unilateral temporal lobe epilepsy proven by *ictal* EEG, MRI, and other ancillary investigations or by seizure-free surgical outcome have been studied with *ictal* SPECT and the results published (10, 11, 25, 27–34). Correct identification of the seizure focus was achieved in over 90%, with incorrect lateralization in fewer than 5%. In a *postictal* series, with injection given on average 4 minutes after seizure onset, correct localization was achieved in 70%, with incorrect localization in fewer than 5% (8).

Patterns of *Ictal* Cerebral Blood Flow

Temporal lobe hyperperfusion will be seen with injection given during the seizure or up to 30 seconds after seizure completion (35). The area of hyperperfusion is variable but typically involves the anterior pole and medial temporal

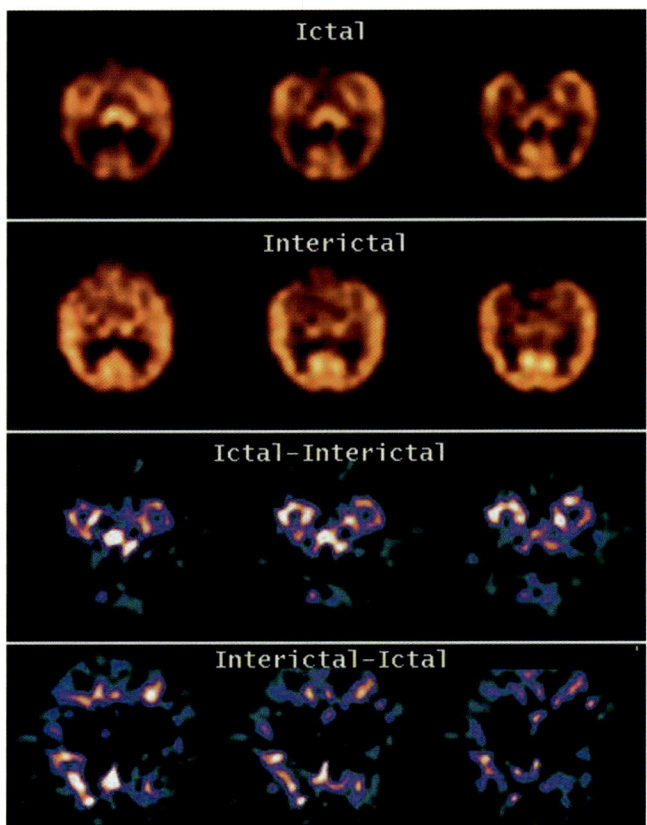

Ictal

Interictal

Ictal-Interictal

Interictal-Ictal

FIG. 14.3. Right temporal lobe seizure focus with *ictal* SPECT demonstrating bilateral changes. Interpretation of *ictal* SPECT may be difficult even in otherwise straightforward cases. This patient had right hippocampal sclerosis on MRI. *Ictal* SPECT showed hyperperfusion in the anterior part of both temporal lobes and widespread ictal hypoperfusion in the frontal lobes and parietotemporal areas. In this case both features were more apparent on the right and therefore consistent with right TLE.

lobe with a variable degree of lateral temporal cortex. Often, it is extensive and involves the anterior half of the temporal lobe. Hyperperfusion of the ipsilateral basal ganglia is common and correlates well with dystonic posturing of the contralateral arm during the seizure (36). Hyperperfusion of lesser extent may also be seen in the ipsilateral thalamus.

Propagation of the seizure also frequently leads to a variable degree of hyperperfusion in the contralateral medial temporal lobe (37). This is usually less extensive and of less intensity than in the temporal lobe from which the seizure originates (Fig. 14.3). Involvement of the ipsilateral insula cortex and basal frontal lobe is not infrequent. Secondarily generalized complex partial seizures will show unilateral blood flow increase if injection is given before generalization or if the seizure remains predominantly lateralized to one hemisphere. In such circumstances, hyperperfusion may be seen in the temporal lobe, ipsilateral motor cortex, basal ganglia and thalamus, and contralateral cerebellar cortex.

Ictal hyperperfusion is seen both with mesial temporal sclerosis and seizures as a result of structural lesions such as low-grade temporal lobe tumors, although the distribution is

sometimes unusual with the latter. One study found that foreign tissue lesions in the lateral temporal lobe were likely to show bilateral temporal lobe hyperperfusion, although greater on the side of the lesion (38). It is postulated that spread from the lateral cortex to the contralateral amygdala occurs through the anterior commissure. Posterolateral temporal lobe foci are also said to show more extensive hyperperfusion in the lateral cortex compared to medial temporal lobe foci (39). Involvement of the temporoparieto-occipital junction should raise the possibility of a posterior temporal focus.

Patterns of *Postictal* Cerebral Blood Flow

The area of *ictal* hyperperfusion is usually surrounded by hypoperfusion. The latter becomes the predominant feature in the *postictal* period and may extend widely to involve the entire ipsilateral hemisphere and the contralateral temporal lobe. *Postictal* hyperperfusion, if present, is usually restricted to the anteromedial temporal lobe and is rarely seen more than 5 minutes after seizure completion (8, 11, 35). The timing of the switch from an *ictal* to a *postictal* pattern of perfusion varies between individuals, as does the duration of the *postictal* change (8, 35). *Postictal* changes are more frequently bilateral and this, plus rapid resolution in some individuals, accounts for the reduced sensitivity of *postictal* imaging compared with *ictal* injection (8). The earlier the injection, the greater the chance of detecting useful blood flow changes. Injection more than 5 minutes from seizure completion will substantially reduce sensitivity.

Unilateral hyperperfusion has been reported in patients with independent bilateral temporal lobe foci. Bilateral temporal lobe *ictal* hyperperfusion in a patient with a unilateral focus is occasionally seen but less often than would be expected given the frequent spread of seizure activity to the contralateral temporal lobe on depth electrode recordings. In such cases, the side of greatest hyperperfusion usually correlates with the seizure focus.

SPECT IN EXTRATEMPORAL LOBE EPILEPSY

Intractable partial seizures may arise from a focus outside the temporal lobes. In most cases, there are clinical, MRI or EEG features that differentiate these seizures from TLE. In the absence of a causative structural lesion on MRI, such as a tumor or focal area of cortical dysplasia, localization of the focus is difficult. Such patients require extensive intracranial monitoring with subdural electrode grids and intracerebral depth electrodes. Despite these investigations, the focus may not be found and the results of surgery are not as good as those achieved with temporal lobe surgery.

It is in this challenging environment that FDG PET and *ictal* SPECT may have their greatest value. Accurate co-registration with MRI may permit detection of subtle structural abnormalities such as an area of cortical dysplasia and subtraction of *interictal* from *ictal* SPECT images is often useful.

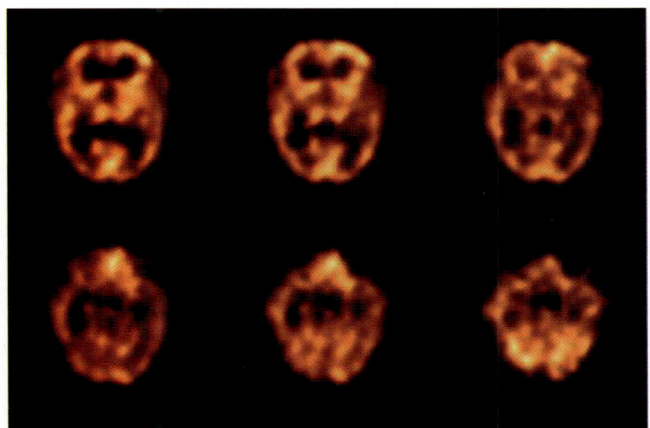

FIG. 14.4. *Ictal* SPECT in left frontal lobe epilepsy. In this patient both MRI and FDG PET were unable to localize the seizure focus.

Very early *ictal* injection is vital to minimize the confounding effects of seizure propagation.

Ictal SPECT studies may show focal hyperperfusion and are useful to differentiate temporal from extratemporal epilepsy, confirm the epileptogenicity of a structural lesion, and guide intracranial electrode placement in nonlesional cases (11, 33, 40–43). In a report of 41 nonlesional neocortical epilepsy cases, PET identified the focus

in 43% and *ictal* SPECT in 33% (44). In another report of 117 neocortical epilepsy cases, MRI found a relevant abnormality in 60%, PET in 78%, and *ictal* SPECT in 70% (45).

In frontal lobe epilepsy, *ictal* hyperperfusion has been demonstrated in various parts of the frontal lobes and is frequently accompanied by ipsilateral basal ganglia and contralateral cerebellar hyperfusion (41) (Figs 14.4, 14.5). A correlation between the site of frontal lobe hyperperfusion and different *ictal* clinical features has been shown (42). In parietal lobe epilepsy, *ictal* SPECT may show anterior parietal hyperperfusion when the *ictal* clinical features are characterized by sensorimotor manifestations and posterior parietal hyperperfusion when the seizures are psychoparetic in type (46).

In occipital lobe epilepsy, propagation of the seizure to one or both temporal lobes usually occurs. Very early *ictal* injection is required to find a focus in occipital lobe epilepsy and to avoid incorrect localization to the temporal lobe (Fig. 14.6). A study of 17 occipital lobe cases found PET identified the focus in 60% but *ictal* SPECT showed focal occipital hyperperfusion in only 29% but ipsilateral hyperperfusion in 76% predominantly in the temporal lobe (47).

Focal tonic seizures are thought to arise from the supplementary motor area. They are often of short duration so that true *ictal* SPECT is difficult to obtain. In one study of 15 patients with focal tonic seizures, *ictal* SPECT confirmed the location of the seizure focus in only 40% despite injection within 30 seconds of onset (48).

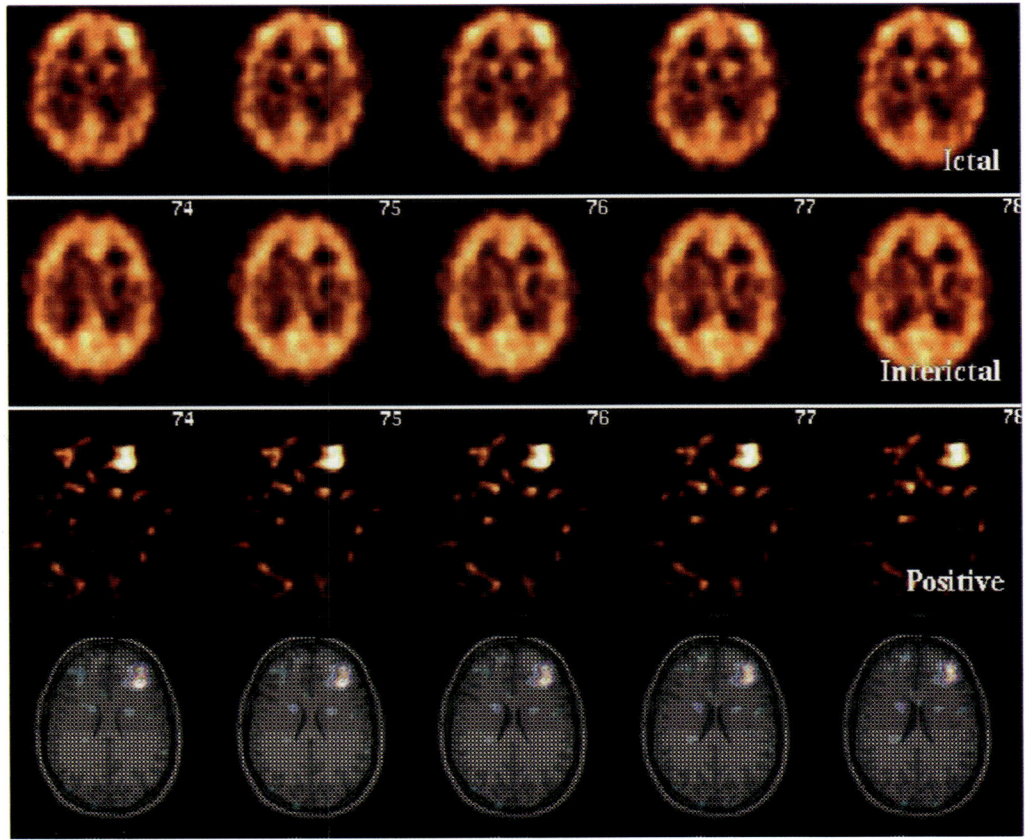

FIG. 14.5. Left frontal lobe seizure focus with co-registration of subtraction image and MRI.

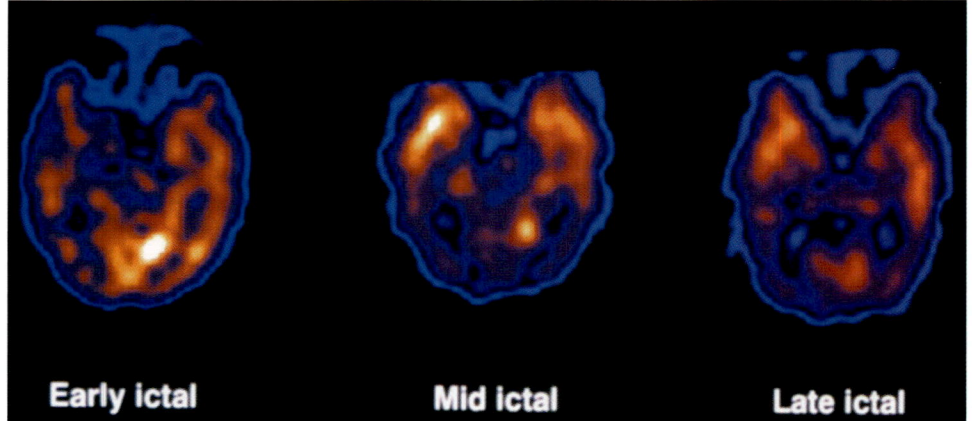

FIG. 14.6. Early, mid, and late *ictal* SPECT in a patient with a left occipital lobe seizure focus. Note the extensive temporal lobe hyperperfusion and the decline in occipital lobe uptake as the seizure progresses and recruits the temporal lobes.

Subtraction of *interictal* from *ictal* SPECT images with the difference image co-registered to the patient's MRI is important for detection of the seizure focus in extratemporal lobe seizures. Many centers have reported improved sensitivity using this technique compared to visual side-by-side comparison of *interictal* and *ictal* images (49–51). This technique has also been reported to identify cortical dysplasia associated with dysembryoplastic neuroepithelial tumors (DNET) (52).

FDG PET and *Ictal* SPECT Compared

Several reports have directly compared the performance of PET and *ictal* SPECT for seizure focus lateralization. In a study of 35 patients with TLE, *ictal* SPECT was marginally more sensitive than FDG PET for the lateralization of the focus, 89% versus 83% (53). In another report, FDG PET was marginally more sensitive than either *ictal* SPECT or MRI in 117 cases of neocortical epilepsy, with sensitivities of 78%, 70%, and 60% respectively (45). In one study of 41 nonlesional neocortical epilepsy patients, FDG PET and *ictal* SPECT had the same sensitivity of 56% but were described as complementary (44). Similar sensitivity was reported for both modalities in another report of 36 patients, although it defined the *ictal* SPECT seizure focus by focal hypoperfusion as well as hyperperfusion (30).

It therefore appears that *interictal* FDG PET and *ictal* SPECT have similar accuracy in seizure focus localization but may be complementary as one modality may be positive in a particular patient when the other is not.

Ictal SPECT and Surgical Outcome

In contrast to PET there is little data on the predictive value of *ictal* SPECT for seizure-free surgical outcome. A report of surgical outcome in 36 patients with extratemporal epilepsy found that concordance of SISCOM SPECT

(subtraction of MRI co-registered *interictal* from *ictal* images) with the site of surgery had independent predictive value over MRI and scalp *ictal* EEG for excellent seizure control (54).

OTHER SEIZURE DISORDERS

Intractable Neonatal and Early Infantile Seizures

Intractable seizures in this age group are associated with a poor prognosis and the seizures may contribute to the progressive neurologic deficit often seen in these children. *Ictal* SPECT has been used to investigate infants with infantile spasms (West's syndrome). While most showed diffuse changes, one-third showed focal cortical hyperperfusion (55). Hemispherectomy is employed in some patients with catastrophic seizures and contralateral hemiparesis. A favorable outcome is strongly predicted by abnormal blood flow or metabolic findings restricted to the side of surgery (56).

Lennox–Gastaut Syndrome

Lennox–Gastaut syndrome is a secondary generalized epileptic encephalopathy of childhood characterized by a variety of refractory seizure types including tonic, atonic, atypical absence and secondarily generalized tonic–clonic seizures, episodic slow spike and wave on EEG, and intellectual and behavioral difficulties. PET and SPECT studies of these patients have found a variety of abnormalities, both unifocal and multifocal, generalized reductions in metabolism and perfusion, and normal scans (57, 58). In the absence of a structural abnormality, the most common finding is diffuse hypometabolism. In some centers, surgical treatment is guided by PET and EEG findings with focal resection employed in those with a clearly defined focal abnormality. However, most centers do not use SPECT or PET in these patients since the yield for localization is very low.

Rasmussen's Syndrome

Rasmussen's syndrome, also known as smoldering encephalitis, is a rare form of childhood epilepsy characterized by intractable partial seizures and progressive hemiparesis. The only effective treatment is hemispherectomy although some patients have responded to antiviral therapy. SPECT shows focal or regional hypoperfusion or hyperperfusion (Fig. 14.7), which may be useful in defining a site for biopsy to confirm the diagnosis (59).

Gelastic Epilepsy and Hypothalamic Hamartoma

Laughing seizures (gelastic epilepsy) is classically due to hypothalamic hamartoma. Removal of the hamartoma is surgically challenging but if resection is complete the seizures are usually cured. *Ictal* SPECT demonstrates hyperperfusion of the hamartoma, confirming the etiology of the seizures (60), although, in some cases, propagation to cortical areas may be misleading, particularly if very early *ictal* injection is not obtained.

OTHER APPLICATIONS

Pseudoseizures

A common cause of apparently intractable epilepsy is pseudoseizure – seizure-like episodes that have a psychological basis. Up to 20% of patients admitted to seizure monitoring units for seizure characterization are found to have this problem. In the majority of cases distinction from genuine epilepsy can be readily made from observation of the episodes and surface EEG. In some cases diagnosis can be difficult and *ictal* SPECT imaging is useful. Vigorous voluntary motor activity does not induce rCBF increases of the same magnitude as seen with genuine partial seizures (61). Subtraction images appear to be more specific when using SPECT to support the diagnosis (62).

Unilateral Amytal Hemispheric Anesthesia (Wada Test)

The Wada test is employed in many patients prior to surgery for refractory epilepsy. Sodium amytal is injected into

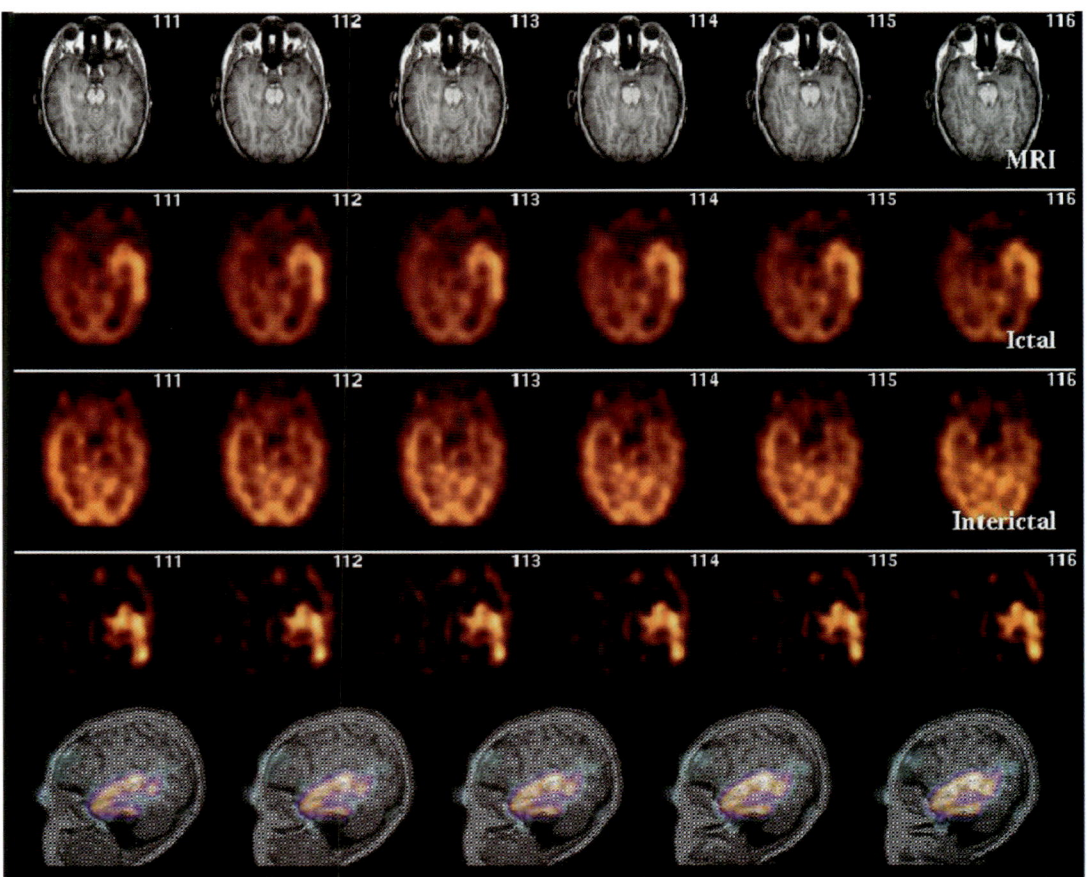

FIG. 14.7. *Ictal* and *interictal* SPECT in Rasmussen's encephalitis.

the internal carotid artery to induce a temporary state of hemianesthesia during which language and memory function of the unaffected hemisphere are tested. The memory function of the temporal lobe to be removed can be tested during contralateral hemianesthesia. Memory impairment then indicates temporal lobe dysfunction and provides indirect support for it being the seizure focus.

Much of the hippocampus is supplied by the posterior cerebral circulation and it is unclear if medial temporal structures are adequately anesthetized by intracarotid injection. Crossflow into the contralateral hemisphere may also complicate interpretation. Exametazime (HMPAO) injected through the arterial catheter clearly defines the distribution of amytal and has revealed crossflow not seen on angiography (63). Alternatively, it can be given intravenously shortly after the amytal to define the extent of cerebral suppression. Intravenous injection should be delayed for 30 seconds after the clinical effects of the amytal become apparent (64). A 25% or more reduction of regional brain activity is then seen and test results can be interpreted with knowledge of the location and extent of the amytal effect (64, 65).

NEURORECEPTOR IMAGING IN EPILEPSY

Benzodiazepine Receptor Studies

The benzodiazepine receptor and the gamma-aminobutyric acid (GABA) receptor form different parts of the same ionophore complex and both benzodiazepine and GABA-agonists inhibit brain activity. Several anticonvulsant drugs act through this mechanism.

A focal reduction in benzodiazepine receptors in temporal and extratemporal lobe foci has been demonstrated with PET and SPECT using the benzodiazepine receptor antagonist flumazenil labeled with ^{11}C or the iodinated derivative ^{123}I iomazenil (66). ^{11}C flumazenil PET can detect the benzodiazepine receptor density changes of hippocampal sclerosis and may be more sensitive than FDG-PET and MRI in detecting this pathology (67). In a study of postsurgical outcome after resection of neocortical seizure foci, the initial extent of reduced flumazenil binding and the amount of residual flumazenil abnormal cortex after resection were inversely correlated with success. The same was not true for FDG PET (68).

Iodine-123 iomazenil allows imaging of these receptors with SPECT. A multicenter European study found a reduction in benzodiazepine receptor binding with this agent at the presumed seizure focus in 72% of 92 patients with a variety of seizure types (69). However, in a study comparing ^{11}C flumazenil PET, FDG PET and ^{123}I iomazenil SPECT, the latter performed poorly (70). Like ^{11}C flumazenil PET studies, ^{123}I iomazenil SPECT may be a useful way to distinguish lateral from medial temporal lobe foci (71).

Cholinergic Receptor Studies

A reduction in binding of the muscarinic cholinergic receptor antagonist ^{123}I-iododexetimide has also been reported in TLE, usually localized to the area of hippocampal sclerosis (72, 73).

The Clinical Role of Neuroreceptor Studies

Neuroreceptor imaging with SPECT and PET is providing new insights into the biology of focal seizures. To date, available data suggest a complementary role for metabolic and receptor imaging in seizure focus localization in selected patients, particularly in those with extratemporal lobe seizures.

IMAGE ANALYSIS IN SPECT

SISCOM

Subtraction *ictal* SPECT with co-registration on MRI (SISCOM) is an elegant way to display *ictal* SPECT data. It has the advantage of anatomic correlation and may highlight an area of relative hyperperfusion or hypoperfusion not readily apparent on visual inspection. The SISCOM method as introduced by the Mayo Clinic group requires image smoothing with a third-order Metz filter on a 64 by 64 grid, normalizing the *ictal* and *interictal* SPECT scans to mean cerebral pixel counts, applying a user-chosen threshold to isolate cerebral cortex voxels, filling the ventricles using math morphology, and subtracting only the nonzero pixels. The scans are aligned with Wood's automated image registration (AIR) algorithm (49). The Mayo group have found that AIR and mutual information alignment both work well and are superior to surface matching (74).

However, small degrees of edge misalignment will result in large signals at gray–white matter junctions and the outer cortical edge. Experience and comparison back to the nonsubtracted images are needed to sort the noise from the areas of true *ictal* hyperperfusion and *ictal/postictal* hypoperfusion. Attempts have been made to reduce the noise in the subtraction images by compensating for the variation seen with paired *interictal* studies. The methods employed have used nonlinear intersubject registration to combine a group of subtraction images into standard anatomic space. The patient subtraction image was also nonlinearly registered to standard anatomic space and a voxel by voxel statistical comparison using statistical parametric mapping (SPM) or a similar method was performed. Although this has been reported to improve subtraction image quality, there are no data indicating that it improves the accuracy of seizure localization (75, 76).

Some authors claim a dramatic improvement in accuracy of localization compared to side-by-side visual comparison of *interictal* and *ictal* SPECT images (49, 77). However, in these papers the localization rates with side-by-side visual comparison were less than 50% even in the unilateral TLE patients. Furthermore, there was very poor correlation between the readers. These results are not consistent with the vast majority of papers on *ictal* SPECT. It is my experience that SISCOM can improve confidence when interpreting subtle blood flow changes in extratemporal lobe epilepsy and can draw attention to areas overlooked on the initial visual inspection. However reliance on SISCOM images alone is not recommended, as imprecise co-registration of images will generate misleading subtraction results (51).

Statistical parametric mapping

Statistical parametric mapping is an image analysis tool that assesses the significance of cerebral blood flow changes on a voxel-by-voxel basis by automated statistical comparison to a group of normal subjects. SPM can be used to analyze *ictal* SPECT, either by comparison to a normal control group (78, 32) or comparison of a subtraction image to images of variation between repeated scans in normal subjects (76). While the feasibility has been demonstrated, there is as yet no evidence of improved accuracy for SPM analysis verses visual side-by-side or subtraction analysis.

REFERENCES

1. Casse R, Rowe CC, Newton MD, et al. Positron emission tomography and epilepsy. *Mol Imag Biol* 2002;4:338–351.
2. Engel J, Brown WJ, Kuhl DE, et al. Pathological findings underlying focal temporal lobe hypometabolism in partial epilepsy. *Ann Neurol* 1982;12:518–528.
3. Hudson LP, Munoz DG, Miller L, et al. Amygdaloid sclerosis in temporal lobe epilepsy. *Ann Neurol* 1993;33:622–631.
4. Hougaard K, Oikawa T, Sveinsdottir E, et al. Regional cerebral blood flow in focal cortical epilepsy. *Arch Neurol* 1979;33:527–535.
5. Engel J, Kuhl DE, Phelps ME, et al. Local cerebral metabolism during partial seizures. *Neurology* 1983;133:400–413.
6. Horsley V. An address on the origin and seat of epileptic disturbance. *Br Med J* 1892;1:693–696.
7. Ingvar DH. Regional cerebral blood flow in focal cortical epilepsy. *Stroke* 1973;4:359–360.
8. Rowe CC, Berkovic SF, Austin MC, et al. Patterns of postictal cerebral blood flow in temporal lobe epilepsy: qualitative and quantitative analysis. *Neurology* 1991;41:1096–1103.
9. Rowe CC, Berkovic SF, Sia STB, et al. Localization of epileptic foci with postictal single photon emission computed tomography. *Ann Neurol* 1989;26:660–668.
10. Newton MR, Austin MC, Chan JG, et al. Ictal SPECT using Tc-99m HMPAO: methods for rapid preparation and optimal deployment of tracer during spontaneous seizures. *J Nucl Med* 1993; 34:666–670.
11. Duncan R, Patterson J, Roberts R, et al. Ictal/postictal SPECT in the pre-surgical localization of complex partial seizures. *J Neurol Neurosurg Psychiatr* 1993;56:141–148.
12. Rowe CC, Berkovic SF, Austin MC et al. Visual and quantitative analysis of interictal SPECT with technetium-99m-HMPAO in temporal lobe epilepsy. *J Nucl Med* 1991;32:1688–1694.
13. Magistretti PL, Uren RF. Cerebral blood flow patterns in epilepsy. In: Nistico G, ed. Epilepsy: an update on research and therapy. New York: Alan R Liss, 1983:241–247.
14. Uren RF, Magistretti PL, Royal HD, et al. Single photon emission computed tomography: preliminary results in patients with epilepsy and stroke. *Med J Austr* 1983;1:411–413.
15. Devous MD Sr, Thisted RA, Morgan GF, et al. SPECT Brain imaging in epilepsy: a meta-analysis. *J Nucl Med* 1998;39:285–293.
16. Stefan H, Pawlik G, Bocher-Schwarz et al. Functional and morphological abnormalities in temporal lobe epilepsy: a comparison of interictal and ictal EEG, CT, MRI, SPECT, and PET. *J Neurol* 1987;234:377–384.
17. Ryvlin PR, Philippon B, Cinotti L et al. Functional neuroimaging strategy in temporal lobe epilepsy: a comparative study of FDG-PET and Tc-99m HMPAO SPECT. *Ann Neurol* 1992;31:650–656.
18. Theodore WH, Jabbari B, Leiderman D, et al. Positron emission tomography and single photon emission tomography in epilepsy: comparison of cerebral blood flow and glucose metabolism. *Ann Neurol* 1990;28:262.
19. Kuhl DE, Engel J, Phelps ME, Selin C. Epileptic patterns of local cerebral metabolism and perfusion in humans determined by emission computed tomography of ^{18}FDG and ^{13}NH3. *Ann Neurol* 1980;8:47–60.
20. Leiderman DB, Balish M, Sato S et al. Comparison of PET measurements of cerebral blood flow and glucose metabolism for the localization of human epileptic foci. *Epilepsy Res* 1992;13:153–157.
21. Gaillard WD, Fazilat S, White S, et al. Interictal metabolism and blood flow are uncoupled in temporal lobe cortex of patients with complex partial epilepsy. *Neurology* 1995;45:1871–1847.
22. Homan RW, Devous MD, LeRoy RF, Bonte FJ. Interictal focal cerebral blood flow elevations in partial seizures. *Neurology* 1989; 39(Suppl 1):300.
23. Duncan R, Patterson J, Hadley DM, et al. Tc-99m HMPAO single photon emission computed tomography in temporal lobe epilepsy. *Acta Neurol Scand* 1990;81:287–293.
24. Lee BI, Markand ON, Wellman HN et al. Interictal HIPDM-SPECT in patients with complex partial seizures. *Neurology* 1988; 38(Suppl 1):406.
25. Shen W, Lee BI, Park HM et al. HIPDM SPECT brain imaging in the presurgical evaluation of patients with intractable seizures. *J Nucl Med* 1990;31:1280–1284.
26. Grunwald F, Durwen HF, Bockisch A et al. Technetium-99m-HMPAO brain SPECT in medically intractable temporal lobe epilepsy: a postoperative evaluation. *J Nucl Med* 1991;32:388–394.
27. Bauer J, Stefan H, Feistel H et al. Ictal and interictal SPECT measurements using Tc-99m HMPAO in patients suffering from temporal lobe epilepsies. *Nervarzt* 1991;62:745–749.
28. Markand ON, Salanova V, Worth RM, et al. Ictal brain imaging in presurgical evaluation of patients with medically intractable complex partial seizures. *Acta Neurol Scand* 1994;152(Suppl):137–144.
29. Newton MR, Berkovic SF, Austin MC, et al. Ictal, postictal and interictal single-photon emission tomography in the lateralization of temporal lobe epilepsy. *Eur J Nucl Med* 1994;21:1067–1071.
30. Markand ON, Salanova V, Worth R, et al. Comparative study of interictal PET and ictal SPECT in complex partial seizures. *Acta Neurol Scand* 1997;95:129–136.
31. Lee SK, Lee SH, Kim SK, et al. The clinical usefulness of ictal SPECT in temporal lobe epilepsy: the lateralization of seizure focus and correlation with EEG. *Epilepsia* 2000;41:955–962.
32. Lee JD, Kim HJ, Lee BI, et al. Evaluation of ictal brain SPECT using statistical parametric mapping in temporal lobe epilepsy. *Eur J Nucl Med* 2000;27:1658–1665.
33. Weil S, Noachtar S, Arnold S, et al. Ictal ECD SPECT differentiates between temporal and extratemporal epilepsy: confirmation by excellent postoperative seizure control. *Nucl Med Commun* 2001;22:233–237.
34. Velasco TR, Wichert-Ana L, Leite JP, et al. Accuracy of ictal SPECT in mesial temporal lobe epilepsy with bilateral spikes. *Neurology* 2002;59:266–271.
35. Newton MR, Berkovic SF, Austin MC, et al. Postictal switch in blood flow distribution and temporal lobe seizures. *J Neurol Neurosurg Psychiatr* 1992;55:891–894.

36. Newton MR, Berkovic SF, Austin MC, et al. Dystonia, clinical lateralization, and regional blood flow changes in temporal lobe seizures. *Neurology* 1992;42:371–377.

37. Shin WC, Hong SB, Tae WS, Kim SE. Ictal hyperperfusion patterns according to the progression of temporal lobe seizures. *Neurology* 2002;58:373–380.

38. Ho SS, Berkovic SF, McKay WJ, et al. Temporal lobe epilepsy subtypes: differential patterns of cerebral perfusion on ictal SPECT. *Epilepsia* 1996;37:788–795.

39. Duncan R, Rahi S, Bernard AM et al. Ictal cerebral blood flow in seizures originating in the posterolateral cortex. *J Nucl Med* 1996;37:1946–1951.

40. Stefan H, Bauer J, Feistel H et al. Regional cerebral blood flow during focal seizures of temporal and frontocentral onset. *Ann Neurol* 1990;27:162–166.

41. Marks DA, Katz A, Hoffer P, Spencer SS. Localization of extratemporal epileptic foci during ictal single photon emission computed tomography. *Ann Neurol* 1992;31:250–255.

42. Harvey AS, Cook DJ, Bowe JM, et al. Ictal Tc-99m HMPAO SPECT in frontal lobe epilepsy. *Neurology* 1993;43:1966–1980.

43. Newton MR, Berkovic SF, Austin MC, et al. SPECT in the localization of extratemporal and temporal seizure foci. *J Neurol Neurosurg Psychiatr* 1995;59:26–30.

44. Hong KS, Lee SK, Kim JY, et al. Pre-surgical evaluation and surgical outcome of 41 patients with non-lesional neocortical epilepsy. *Seizure* 2002;11:184–192.

45. Hwang SI, Kim JH, Park SW, et al. Comparative analysis of MR imaging, positron emission tomography, and ictal single-photon emission CT in patients with neocortical epilepsy. *Am J Neuroradiol* 2001;22:937–946.

46. Ho SS, Berkovic SF, Newton MR, et al. Parietal lobe epilepsy: clinical features and seizure localization by ictal SPECT. *Neurology* 1994;44:2277–2284.

47. Kim SK, Lee DS, Lee SK, et al. Diagnostic performance of FDG-PET and ictal HMPAO SPECT in occipital lobe epilepsy. *Epilepsia* 2001;42:1531–1540.

48. Ebner A, Buschsieweke U, Tuxhorn I, et al. Supplementary sensorimotor area seizure and ictal single photon emission tomography. *Adv Neurol* 1996;70:363–368.

49. O'Brien TJ, So EL, Mullan BP et al. Subtraction ictal SPECT co-registered to MRI improves clinical usefulness of SPECT in localizing the surgical focus. *Neurology* 1998;445–454.

50. Spanaki MV, Spencer SS, Corsi M, et al. Sensitivity and specificity of quantitative difference SPECT analysis in seizure localization. *J Nucl Med* 1999;40:730–736.

51. Lewis PJ, Siegel A, Siegel AM, et al. Does performing image registration and subtraction in ictal brain SPECT help localize neocortical seizures? *J Nucl Med* 2000;41:1619–1626.

52. Valenti MP, Froelich S, Armspach JP, et al. Contribution of SISCOM imaging in the presurgical evaluation of temporal lobe epilepsy related to dysembryoplastic neuroepithelial tumors. *Epilepsia* 2002;43:270–276.

53. Ho SS, Berkovic SF, Berlangieri SU et al. Comparison of ictal SPECT and interictal PET in the presurgical evaluation of temporal lobe epilepsy. *Ann Neurol* 1995;37:738–745.

54. O'Brien TJ, So EL, Mullan BP, et al. Subtraction peri-ictal SPECT is predictive of extratemporal epilepsy surgery outcome. *Neurology* 2000;55:1668–1677.

55. Haginoya K, Munakata M, Yokoyama H, et al. Mechanism of tonic seizures in West syndrome viewed from ictal SPECT findings. *Brain Dev* 2001;23:496–501.

56. Carmant L, O'Tuama LA, Roach PJ, et al. Technetium-99m HMPAO brain SPECT and outcome of hemispherectomy for intractable seizures. *Pediatr Neurol* 1994;11:203–207.

57. Chugani HT, Mazziotta JC, Engel J, Phelps ME. The Lennox–Gastaut syndrome: metabolic subtypes by 2-deoxy-2 F-18fluoro-D-glucose positron emission tomography. *Ann Neurol* 1987;21:4–13.

58. Theodore WH, Rose D, Patronas N, et al. Cerebral glucose metabolism in the Lennox–Gastaut syndrome. *Ann Neurol* 1987;21:14–21.

59. English R, Soper N, Shepstone BJ, et al. Five patients with Rasmussen's syndrome investigated by single photon emission computed tomography. *Nucl Med Commun* 1988;10:5–14.

60. DiFazio MP, Davis RG. Utility of SPECT in neonatal gelastic epilepsy associated with hypothalamic hamartoma. *J Child Neurol* 2000;15:414–417.

61. Grunwald F, Durwen H, Bulau P, et al. HMPAO-SPECT in cerebral seizures. *Nukl Med* 1988;27:248–251.

62. Spanaki MV, Spencer SS, Corsi M, et al. The role of quantitative ictal SPECT analysis in the evaluation of non-epileptic seizures. *J Neuroimag* 1999;9:210–216.

63. Hietala S, Silfvenius H, Aasly J, et al. Brain perfusion with intracarotid injection of 99mTc-HMPAO in partial epilepsy during amobarbital testing. *Eur J Nucl Med* 1990;16:683–687.

64. Ryding E, Sjoholm H, Skeidsvoll D, Elmqvist D. Delayed decrease in hemispheric cerebral blood flow during Wada test demonstrated by 99m Tc-HMPAO single photon emission computer tomography. *Acta Neurol Scand* 1989;80:248–254.

65. Biersack HJ, Linke D, Brassel F et al. Technetium-99m HMPAO brain SPECT in epileptic patients before and during unilateral hemispheric anesthesia (Wada test). *J Nucl Med* 1987;28:1763–1767.

66. Savic I, Persson A, Roland P et al. In vivo demonstration of reduced benzodiazepine receptor binding in human epileptic foci. *Lancet* 1988;2:863–866.

67. Koepp MJ, Hand KS, Labbe C, et al. In vivo [^{11}C] flumazenil-PET correlates with ex vivo [^{3}H] flumazenil autoradiography in hippocampal sclerosis. *Ann Neurol* 1998;43:618–626.

68. Juhasz C, Chugani DC, Muzik O, et al. Relationship of flumazenil and glucose PET abnormalities to neocortical epilepsy surgery outcome. *Neurology* 2001;56:1650–1658.

69. Ferstl FJ, Cordes M, Cordes I et al. ^{123}I-iomazenil SPECT in patients with focal epilepsies – a comparative study with ^{99m}Tc-HMPAO SPECT, CT and MR. In: Kito S, ed. Neuroreceptor mechanisms in brain. New York: Plenum, 1991:405–412.

70. Debets RM, Sadzot B, van Isselt JW, et al. Is ^{11}C-flumazenil PET superior to ^{18}FDG PET and ^{123}I-iomazenil? *J Neurol Neurosurg Psychiatr* 1997;62:141–150.

71. Tanaka F, Yonekura Y, Ikeda A, et al. Presurgical identification of epileptic foci with iodine-123 iomazenil SPET: comparison with brain perfusion SPET and FDG PET. *Eur J Nucl Med* 1997;24:27–34.

72. Mueller-Gaertner HW, Fisher RS, Wilson AA et al. Decreased binding of I-123 iododexetimide to muscarinic cholinergic receptors in hippocampus in temporal lobe epilepsy (abstract). *J Nucl Med* 1992;33:928.

73. Boundy KL, Rowe CC, Black AB et al. Localization of temporal lobe epileptic foci with iodine-123 iododexetimide cholinergic neuroreceptor single-photon emission computed tomography. *Neurology* 1996;47:1015–1020.

74. Brinkmann BH, O'Brien TJ, Aharon S, et al. Quantitative and clinical analysis of SPECT image registration for epilepsy studies. *J Nucl Med* 1999;40:1098–1105.

75. Brinkmann BH, O'Brien TJ, Webster DB, et al. Voxel significance mapping using local image variances in subtraction ictal SPET. *Nucl Med Commun* 2000;21:545–551.

76. Chang DJ, Zubal IG, Gottschalk C, et al. Comparison of statistical parametric mapping and SPECT difference imaging in patients with temporal lobe epilepsy. *Epilepsia* 2002;43:68–74.

77. Kaiboriboon K, Lowe VJ, Chantarujikapong SI, Hogan RE. The usefulness of subtraction ictal SPECT coregistered to MRI in single and dual headed SPECT cameras in partial epilepsy. *Epilepsia* 2002;43:408–414.

78. Lee JD, Kim HJ, Lee BI, et al. Evaluation of ictal brain SPET using statistical parametric mapping in temporal lobe epilepsy. *Eur J Nucl Med* 2000;27:1658–1665.

CHAPTER 15

Positron-emission Tomography in Epilepsy

Csaba Juhász, Diane C. Chugani, Otto Muzik and Harry T. Chugani

POSITRON-EMISSION TOMOGRAPHY OF BRAIN GLUCOSE METABOLISM

Basic Technique and Principles

Positron-emission tomography (PET) is a noninvasive functional imaging method of measuring local chemical functions in various body organs. In the brain, PET has been applied in the study of local glucose and oxygen utilization, blood flow, protein and DNA synthesis, as well as neurotransmitter synthesis, uptake and receptor binding. Unlike structural cerebral imaging studies, PET images are functional representations of various aspects of brain activity. PET can be used to measure baseline functional activity as well as physiologic or pathologic changes and responses (e.g. elicited by behavioral or pharmacologic manipulations) in cerebral activity.

The PET technique employs a camera consisting of multiple pairs of oppositely situated detectors, which are used to record the paired high energy (511 keV) photons traveling in opposite ($\approx$180°) directions as a result of positron decay (1, 2). The size and cross-sectional geometry of the detectors largely determine the spatial accuracy of the localization of the positron-emitting source. Tracer kinetic models that mathematically describe physiologic or biochemical reaction sequences of compounds labeled with positron-emitting isotopes permit a characterization of the kinetics and the mathematical expression for calculating actual rates of the biologic process being studied (3). The amount of activity measured in an organ depends on the kinetics of the metabolic process, the transport properties between the blood and the cellular site of the process, and the amount and time course of delivery of the activity to the organ by the blood (1).

The most widely available PET tracer is 2-deoxy-2[18F] fluoro-D-glucose (FDG) to measure glucose metabolism of various organs. FDG is also the most commonly used tracer for epilepsy studies, although several other tracers have been used or proposed to image the epileptic brain (Table 15.1). FDG is similar to 2-[14C]deoxyglucose, an analog of glucose and a tracer used in autoradiography studies of various animals used in laboratory experiments. In FDG, hydrogen on the number 2 carbon is substituted with the positron emitter 18F (half-life: 110 min).

FDG is transported in tissue and phosphorylated to FDG-6-phosphate in the same manner as glucose. However, FDG-6-phosphate is not a substrate for the next reaction step of glycolysis, and also not a significant substrate for glycogen synthesis or for the pentose shunt. Thus, since it cannot immediately leave the cell, phosphorylated FDG gets trapped without significant further metabolism, and its location and amount can be measured by PET as the 18F decays. FDG is similar to glucose in its plasma to tissue transport and phosphorylation; thus, under steady-state conditions, FDG uptake reflects the utilization rate of exogenous glucose. In the brain, this rate is highly related to the synaptic density and functional activity of the brain tissue.

In order to quantify the measured process, e.g. to determine absolute glucose metabolic rates in various brain regions using FDG PET, it is necessary to perform independent measurements of the activity as a function of time in the arterial blood. Unlike for PET measurements of many other functions, accurate estimation of local cerebral metabolic rates can be achieved by obtaining a single set of PET images, provided that the arterial input function (from either timed arterial blood samples or dynamic PET scanning of the left ventricular blood pool) has been acquired. When analyzing pediatric PET scans, however, one has to keep in

TABLE 15.1. *PET Tracers and Their Clinical Use in Epilepsy*

Isotope	Half-life	Tracer	Target Function	Change in Epileptic Focus	Clinical Use
[18]F	109 min	2-deoxy-2[^{18}F]fluoro-D-glucose (FDG)	Glucose metabolism	Interictal decrease* Ictal increase	TLE (nonlesional) ETLE Childhood epilepsy
		^{18}F-cyclofoxy	Mu and kappa opiate receptors	Increase	n.e.
[11]C	20 min	[^{11}C]-flumazenil	GABA$_A$ receptors	Decrease	TLE/dual pathology ETLE
		α[^{11}C]-methyl-L-tryptophan	Tryptophan metabolism to serotonin or quinolinic acid	Increase	Tuberous sclerosis ETLE
		[^{11}C]FCWAY	5-HT$_{1A}$ receptors	Decrease	n.e.
		(S)-[N-methyl-[^{11}C]ketamine	NMDA receptors	Decrease	n.e.
		[^{11}C]doxepin	Histamine H$_1$ receptors	Increase	n.e.
		[^{11}C]carfentanil	Mu opiate receptors	Increase	n.e.
		[^{11}C]methyl-naltrindole	Delta opiate receptors	Increase	n.e.

* Except if cortex is actively spiking during uptake period.
ETLE, extra-temporal-lobe epilepsy; n.e., not established in clinical practice; TLE, temporal lobe epilepsy.

mind that absolute metabolic rates undergo major physiologic changes during brain development, with a temporary increase of brain metabolism above normal adult levels followed by a gradual decline to reach adult levels by the end of adolescence (4, 5). Furthermore, in patients with epilepsy, absolute glucose metabolic rates can be affected (usually decreased) by antiepileptic drugs (such as barbiturates, phenytoin, carbamazepine, benzodiazepines, or valproate) (6–8). These effects can be diminished by calculating metabolic rates normalized to the whole brain metabolism.

In clinical practice, however, absolute quantification is not always necessary. Since the regional *pattern* of cerebral glucose metabolic is largely fixed after 1 year of age (5), focal decreases or increases in FDG uptake can be reliably identified using activity images without calculating absolute glucose metabolic rates. In patients with unilateral seizure foci (that are potential candidates for epilepsy surgery if the seizures are medically intractable), use of asymmetry indices created from activity measured in various portions of the presumed epileptic hemisphere and from the contralateral homologous brain regions is a simple and sensitive method of detecting focal functional abnormalities of cortical and subcortical structures of the epileptic brain.

Clinical Use of FDG Positron-emission Tomography Studies in Epilepsy

Temporal Lobe Epilepsy

Initial FDG PET studies were performed more than two decades ago in patients with intractable complex partial seizures of temporal lobe origin, and showed localized glucose metabolic changes (interictal hypometabolism) that apparently coincided with the general location of the electroencephalography (EEG)-defined epileptic focus (Fig. 15.1) (9–11).

The sensitivity of PET to identify the epileptogenic temporal lobe has significantly improved, and is estimated to be around 85–90% or even beyond (12–15), largely as a result of the application of high-resolution scanners and advanced analytic methods. FDG PET can show relative temporal hypometabolism in more than 50% of patients with nonlateralized surface ictal EEG findings (16). Thus, application of PET in the evaluation of patients with intractable epilepsy has had a significant impact on management (16–18). In many cases, use of FDG PET could replace invasive EEG monitoring (depth electrodes) that, before the widespread application of advanced MRI techniques, was often otherwise inevitable.

Recent advances in analysis techniques of MRI (including application of fluid attenuation recovery techniques, hippocampal volumetry, and proton magnetic resonance spectroscopy) have led to very reliable noninvasive detection of hippocampal sclerosis by MRI, eliminating the need for functional imaging or invasive EEG monitoring in the majority of patients with temporal lobe epilepsy (TLE). In fact, FDG PET rarely provides additional clinical information when hippocampal atrophy is obvious on MRI (13). Therefore, PET is now generally reserved for those cases in which MRI fails to provide the necessary lateralization information. A recent study has lent support to this by showing that FDG PET is indeed able to lateralize the epileptic focus in TLE patients with subtle or absent quantitative MRI abnormalities (19). This study also demonstrated that glucose metabolism in medial temporal structures is often reduced over and above the severity of histopathologic changes, although the pathomechanism of hypometabolism remains to be determined.

A recent study on children with new-onset seizures found lower incidence of focal hypometabolism than expected from previous data obtained from patients with long-term, intractable epilepsy (20), suggesting that at least some of the hypometabolic areas may be the consequence of repeated seizures rather than simply indicating an area that is the

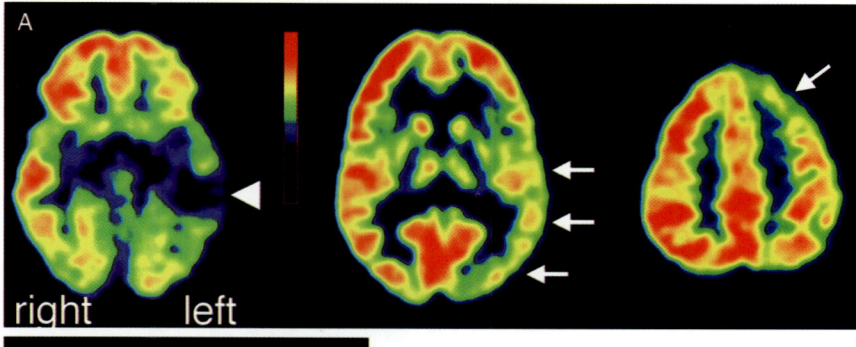

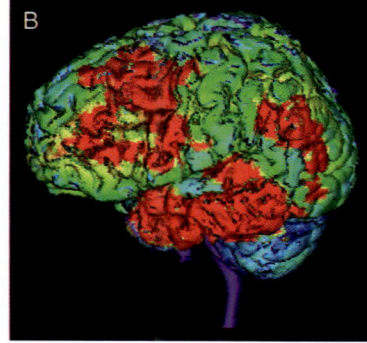

FIG. 15.1. FDG PET in left temporal lobe epilepsy. **A.** Severe hypometabolism in the left temporal region that corresponded to a developmental lesion (arrowhead) in a 10-year-old girl. Milder hypometabolism involving superior temporal, parietal and prefrontal cortex can be also seen (arrows). **B.** The three-dimensional surface reconstruction demonstrates the extent of hypometabolism (areas with more than 10% decrease of glucose metabolism as compared to contralateral homologous regions are indicated in *red*). Intracranial EEG monitoring with subdural grids demonstrated that the seizures originated from the inferior–medial temporal region, with occasional spread to the inferior frontal cortex. However, no independent epileptiform activity occurred in the frontal cortex and the large hypometabolic frontal area was 'silent' electrophysiologically.

primary site of seizures. Postoperative recovery of hypometabolism in remote areas in the frontal lobe after successful resection of the temporal focus (21, 22), also suggests that some of the hypometabolic areas are largely functional and potentially reversible if the primary epileptogenic region is excised.

It has been extensively demonstrated that interictal hypometabolic regions are not strictly confined to the presumed temporal epileptogenic zone or to the brain tissue showing pathologic changes, but commonly extend beyond temporal structures (12, 13, 23–25). Additional brain regions most commonly demonstrating interictal hypometabolism in TLE include ipsilateral parietal and frontal cortex as well as thalamus (Fig. 15.1B); these remote cortical regions, however, rarely show epileptiform activity on EEG and their resection is usually not necessary to alleviate seizures. Nevertheless, intracranial EEG studies should address extratemporal cortex with hypometabolism in cases where scalp ictal EEG abnormalities are not strictly confined to the temporal lobe but show a wider field potentially involving these extratemporal regions.

In addition to commonly extending beyond epileptogenic brain regions, the actual degree of glucose metabolic changes depends on the physiologic state of the tissue. For example, seizures during the tracer uptake and even frequent interictal spikes can significantly increase local glucose metabolism and can potentially mask or falsely lateralize hypometabolic epileptic foci (26–29). Therefore, continuous EEG monitoring during the FDG uptake period is essential to avoid false interpretation of focal abnormalities of glucose metabolism (30). Ictal FDG PET studies are often difficult

to interpret also because they often reveal complex patterns of increased and decreased glucose metabolism (reflecting a mixture of ictal and postictal metabolism). In these cases, FDG PET may have to be repeated in the interictal state or use of another PET tracer may become necessary.

Extratemporal Lobe Epilepsy

Early FDG PET studies in extratemporal epilepsy found focal, regional, or hemispheric hypometabolism in approximately two-thirds of adult patients with frontal lobe foci, and these abnormalities correlated well with electroclinical ictal localization (31). Using high-resolution PET scanning, da Silva et al. (32) reported unilateral frontal lobe hypometabolism in 85% of epileptic children with a frontal lobe focus and normal CT and MRI scan. The location of frontal lobe PET abnormality corresponded to the area of seizure onset in four-fifths of the patients. Recent studies have demonstrated consistently that computerized analysis of FDG PET scans may assist accurate and objective identification of extratemporal lobe epileptic foci (33–35).

When onset of frontal lobe seizures is in the neonatal period or in infancy, an underlying structural lesion is often present even when the MRI is normal (Fig. 15.2). Under these circumstances, FDG PET can be useful in defining an area of hypometabolism that both correlates with the extent of microdysgenesis (36) and delineates the general area of epileptogenicity. However, the extent of abnormal neocortical metabolism often exceeds the electrophysiologically defined epileptogenic region. Correlation studies between

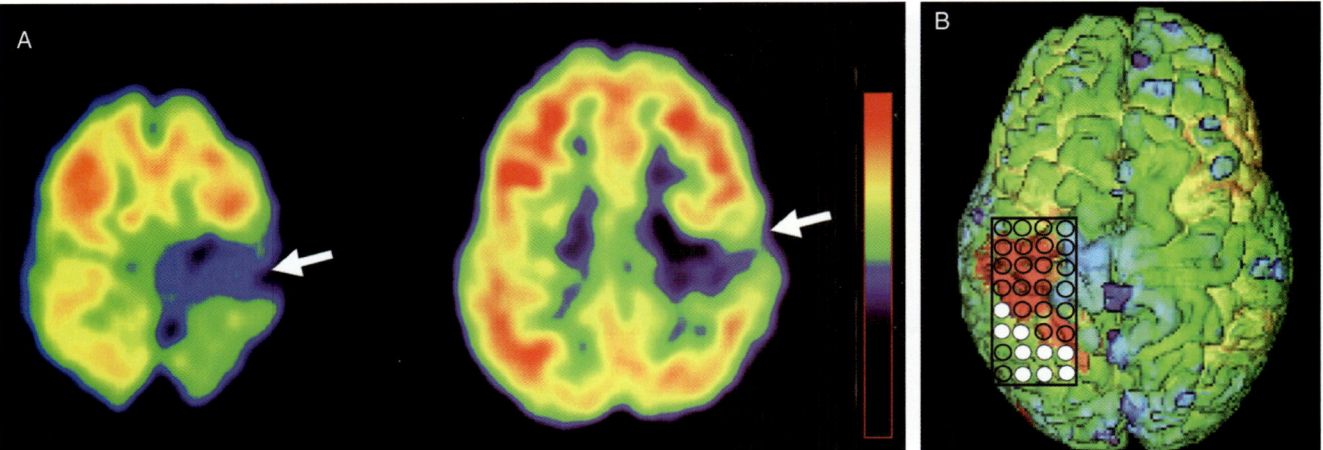

FIG. 15.2. A. FDG PET showing a well-defined area of hypometabolism in the superior parietal cortex of a 7.5-year-old girl with intractable seizures that started at 2 years of age. MRI was unremarkable but the abrupt decrease of cortical metabolism on PET suggested a lesion. **B.** Three-dimensional surface reconstruction from volumetric MRI (top view), superimposed with the FDG PET abnormality (>10% decrease of glucose metabolism; *red area*) as well as the subdural electrode array. The seizures originated from electrodes located behind the PET abnormality (white circles), while the hypometabolic cortex was 'silent' (these electrodes are represented by black open circles). Histology from the resected parietal tissue showed cortical dysplasia with balloon cells.

neocortical FDG PET abnormalities and ictal and interictal intracranial EEG data have demonstrated that, although FDG PET can detect abnormal cortical areas in patients with normal structural neuroimaging, and can correctly identify the general region of the epileptogenic cortex, it has limited specificity for the precise area of seizure onset (37, 38). Consistent with this, the extent of glucose hypometabolism ipsilateral to the seizure focus did not correlate with the epileptogenic tissue to be resected as determined by intracranial EEG (39). Nevertheless, findings from FDG PET can be useful to guide the placement of subdural electrodes, which otherwise must solely rely on seizure semiology and scalp electrode findings. Use of more specific tracers or application of other functional imaging modalities (e.g. ictal SPECT) can also help further, more precise, delineation of the epileptogenic tissue; this becomes particularly important when the epileptic focus potentially involves eloquent brain regions (primary motor, speech or visual areas).

Positron-emission Tomography Scanning of Epilepsy Syndromes in Childhood

Application of FDG PET has improved our understanding of the possible pathomechanism of epilepsy in various pediatric epilepsy syndromes and also has had an impact on their clinical management. For example, based on their electroclinical features, infantile spasms have been considered to be generalized seizures resulting from complex cortico-subcortical interactions. However, on PET scanning, most infants diagnosed with 'cryptogenic' spasms have focal or multifocal cortical regions of abnormal glucose utilization (Fig. 15.3). Histologic analysis of such regions (when a surgical resection

is undertaken) often reveals areas of cortical dysplasia that are commonly missed by MRI (40, 41).

When a single region of abnormal glucose utilization is apparent on PET, corresponding to the EEG focus, and the spasms are intractable, surgical removal of the focus with abnormal metabolism results not only in seizure control but also in reversal of the associated developmental delay.

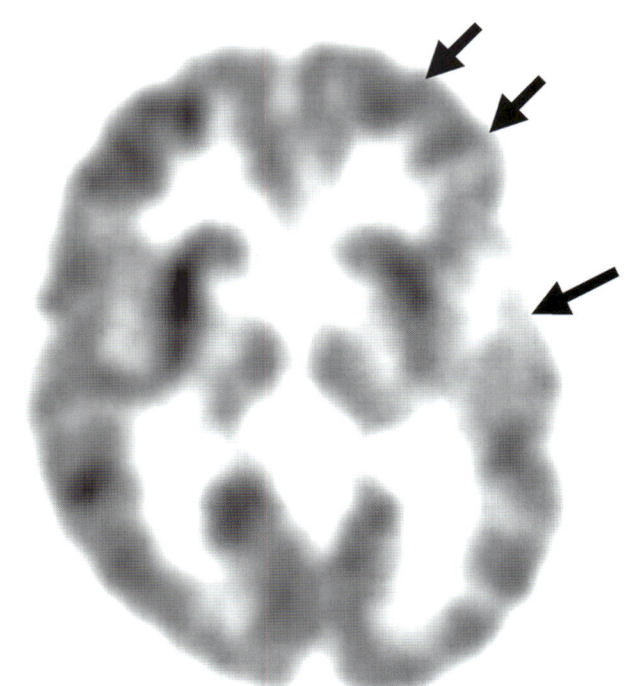

FIG. 15.3. Left frontal and temporal hypometabolism (arrows) in a 13-month-old boy with cryptogenic infantile spasms.

Most patients with bilateral multifocal areas of hypometabolism are not surgical candidates; however, if all seizures arise from one area, resective surgery may ameliorate the epilepsy but not improve cognitive status to the same extent as in those infants with a unifocal PET abnormality. When the pattern of glucose hypometabolism is generalized and symmetric, a lesional etiology is not likely and neurometabolic or neurogenetic disorders should be considered in further evaluating the child.

In children with *Lennox–Gastaut syndrome* (triad of multiple seizure types, developmental delay, and 1–2.5 Hz generalized 'slow' spike and wave EEG pattern), PET has provided a new classification based on metabolic anatomy. Four metabolic subtypes have been identified: unilateral focal, unilateral diffuse and bilateral diffuse hypometabolism, as well as normal patterns (42, 43). Patients with unilateral focal and unilateral diffuse patterns may be occasionally considered for cortical resection provided that there is concordance between PET and ictal EEG findings.

In patients at the advanced stage of *Sturge–Weber syndrome*, FDG PET typically reveals widespread unilateral hemispheric hypometabolism ipsilateral to the facial port wine stain in a distribution that commonly extends beyond the structural abnormalities depicted on CT or MRI scans (44, 45) (Fig. 15.4). The seizures often arise from the mildly hypometabolic cortex outside the region of the visible angioma or cortical atrophy.

The advantage of using PET in Sturge–Weber syndrome is to delineate the extent of functional involvement of cortical areas outside the region of the angioma, and MRI-detected atrophy, thus assisting in the assessment of candidacy for early hemispherectomy or focal cortical resection. FDG PET scans in these patients may also assess the rapidity of hemispheric demise and, indeed, those patients whose affected hemisphere becomes severely hypometabolic rapidly may not require surgical intervention

because, in a sense, they are undergoing 'autohemispherectomy' and forcing the contralateral hemisphere to undergo reorganization changes early and optimally. This is in contrast to those patients whose affected hemisphere shows mild hypometabolism associated with persistent seizures and cognitive delay; these are the subjects who require surgical intervention to enhance effective reorganization in the contralateral hemisphere while brain plasticity is at a maximum during development (45).

Hemimegalencephaly is a developmental brain malformation characterized by congenital hypertrophy of one cerebral hemisphere with ipsilateral ventriculomegaly. When the epilepsy is medically uncontrolled, cerebral hemispherectomy is recommended. Glucose metabolism PET studies suggest that children with hemimegalencephaly often show additional less pronounced abnormalities in the opposite hemisphere, thus accounting for the suboptimal cognitive outcome even with complete seizure control (46). FDG PET is, therefore, a useful diagnostic tool in such children to assess the functional integrity of the contralateral hemisphere prior to hemispherectomy and helps predict cognitive outcome, which, in children with hemimegalencephaly, is generally worse than in children who have undergone hemispherectomy for other conditions, such as congenital hemiplegic cerebral palsy, Sturge–Weber syndrome or Rasmussen's encephalitis.

Rasmussen's syndrome is an example where FDG PET can facilitate early diagnosis and management. In the early stage of this disease, CT and MRI are often unremarkable for several months after the clinical manifestation of the disease. In this stage of the disease, however, FDG PET scanning already shows areas of abnormal metabolism restricted mostly to the frontal and temporal regions, whereas the posterior cortex is usually preserved (47) (Fig. 15.5). Pathologic changes seen in the resected cortex are more pronounced in cortical areas of abnormal glucose metabolism than in

MRI **PET**

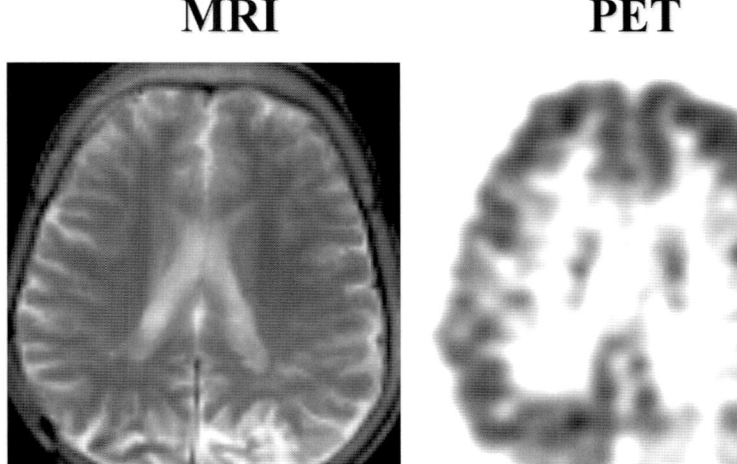

FIG. 15.4. MRI and FDG PET in Sturge–Weber syndrome. The child had a left occipital angioma with an underlying atrophy visualized on the MRI (arrowhead). This area showed minimal metabolism on PET, but a less severe hypometabolism extended far beyond the structural abnormality into the left parietal cortex (arrows). Seizures associated with Sturge–Weber syndrome often originate from moderately hypometabolic cortex.

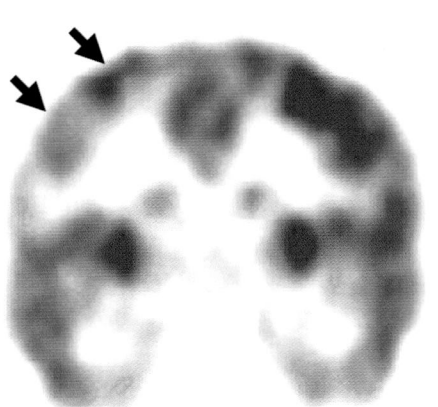

FIG. 15.5. Marked right frontal hypometabolism (arrows) in a child with Rasmussen's syndrome, 8 months after the onset of first seizure. MRI (including T2 and FLAIR sequences) was still unremarkable.

FDG PET

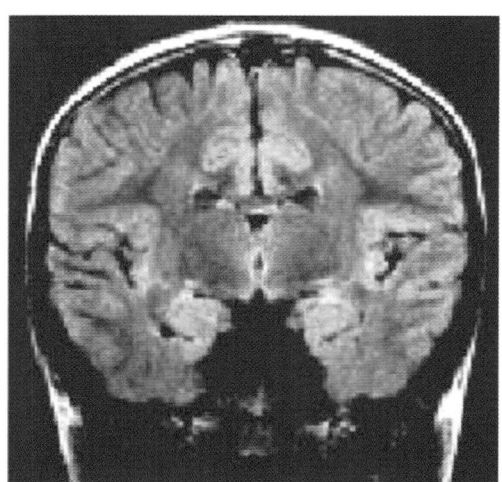

regions showing normal metabolism. Thus, FDG PET performed early during the course of Rasmussen's syndrome can facilitate the correct diagnosis and may also guide the site of brain biopsy when indicated.

Metabolic Correlates of Cognitive and Behavioral Abnormalities in Epilepsy

As discussed above, focal or regional glucose metabolic abnormalities on PET commonly extend beyond the presumed epileptogenic zone. These nonepileptogenic dysfunctional areas are of clinical interest because they often are associated with neuropsychological correlates. For example, in patients with unilateral TLE, presence of bitemporal glucose hypometabolism is associated with poor memory performance (48). In addition, TLE patients who perform poorly in tests of frontal lobe function often exhibit hypometabolism of the frontal lobe in addition to the temporal lobe epileptogenic zone, and impairment of verbal and performance intelligence measures in patients with TLE is associated with prefrontal involvement on the PET scan (49).

In infants with epileptic spasms, bilateral temporal hypometabolism (typically affecting both hippocampus and superior temporal gyri) is strongly associated with autistic features or pervasive developmental delay (50). A different pattern of bitemporal hypometabolism has been found in children with TLE and interictal aggressive behavior (51). In this latter group of patients, bitemporal hypometabolism was present in the temporal neocortex but the medial temporal (limbic) structures were relatively preserved in their glucose metabolism. Bilateral medial prefrontal hypometabolism was also a common finding in these patients, and the severity of temporal cortical hypometabolism in relation to the preserved medial temporal metabolism correlated well with the severity of aggression. These findings suggest that disinhibition of medial temporal lobe structures by temporal neocortex (and perhaps medial prefrontal cortex)

may be important in producing a phenotype of aggression. On the other hand, if the medial temporal lobe structures are also hypometabolic, an autistic phenotype is seen, as in monkeys that have been subjected to bilateral medial temporal lesions (52).

NEURO-RECEPTOR AND LIGAND POSITRON-EMISSION TOMOGRAPHY STUDIES

Positron-emission tomograph scanning of various neurotransmitter systems has been a rapidly evolving field of functional neuroimaging in neurology and psychiatry during the past decade. In epilepsy, the main emphasis of this effort is to find new PET tracers that are able to detect focal neurotransmitter and/or receptor abnormalities of the epileptic brain, thus providing a better, more specific noninvasive delineation of epileptic foci. Indeed, development of novel PET tracers targeting neurotransmitter systems has proved to be feasible, and a handful of these tracers are increasingly becoming clinically utilized in several epilepsy centers worldwide. In this section, we summarize the most important methodologic aspects and emerging clinical applications of these PET tracers in the study of human epilepsy, with special emphasis on patients with medically intractable seizures, and review the current role of these PET tracers during presurgical evaluation. We also demonstrate how correlation between structural MRI and ligand/neuroreceptor PET findings can facilitate more accurate detection of functional abnormalities in the epileptic brain, to provide new insights into the pathophysiology of human epilepsy.

Methodologic Aspects of Ligand/Neuroreceptor PET Scanning

One of the major targets of functional neuroimaging in epilepsy is the gamma-aminobutyric acid (GABA) system in the brain. GABA is the major inhibitory neurotransmitter in the human brain, and GABAergic mechanisms play a key role in regulating central nervous system excitability and susceptibility to seizures (53). The action of GABA is mediated in part by the GABA$_A$ receptor complex, the site of action of numerous therapeutic pharmacologic agents (such as benzodiazepines) and several drugs of abuse. Flumazenil is a benzodiazepine antagonist that binds to the alpha subunit of the GABA$_A$ receptor. The PET tracer [^{11}C]flumazenil (FMZ) can be used to obtain quantitative images of GABA$_A$ receptor binding.

Patients undergoing FMZ PET should not take drugs (such as benzodiazepines) that directly interact with the GABA$_A$ receptors. In clinical studies with FMZ PET, patients taking benzodiazepine drugs have generally been excluded, but the effects of drugs that result in allosteric interactions with GABA$_A$ receptors have not been well studied. Chronic vigabatrin treatment was associated with decreased regional GABA$_A$ receptor binding in young children with partial seizures or infantile spasms (106), but no similar effects were reported in adults (54). Age-related changes in FMZ binding have been reported in humans (55) and, in normal adult volunteers, baseline FMZ binding values are 25–50% lower (depending on the brain region) than those in children around 2 years of age (measured in the nonepileptic hemisphere of children with epilepsy).

During FMZ PET scanning in children, sedation is often unavoidable. Among commonly used sedatives, pentobarbital was reported to have no significant effect on in-vitro FMZ binding (56). Chloral hydrate (1000 mg taken orally) was found to cause a negligible increase of in-vivo FMZ binding of the whole brain in a small group of adults with partial epilepsy (55).

Quantification of FMZ PET images can be performed using a three-compartmental model (57) or a simpler two-compartmental model (58). This latter model yields parametric images of the volume of distribution (V_D) of the tracer in tissue and the ligand influx rate constant (K_1). V_D is a macroparameter incorporating both receptor density (B_{max}) and receptor affinity (K_D), and represents B_{max}/K_D. These two components can only be separated by applying more than one injection with different FMZ concentrations, i.e. to obtain multiple PET scans and produce a Scatchard plot. Such studies are feasible and may be useful to estimate receptor density and affinity in vivo (59) but are not practical. For example, even two PET studies in the same patient would allow for a suboptimal Scatchard analysis with only two points. On the other hand, V_D images allow visualization of a quantitative measure of GABA$_A$ receptor binding and are much easier to obtain.

Direct comparisons of in-vivo FMZ binding using PET with ex-vivo binding measured in resected epileptic tissues using [^{3}H]FMZ autoradiography showed that, after correction for partial volume effects, the degree of in-vivo FMZ binding correlated well with ex-vivo measurements of GABA$_A$ receptor binding in the epileptogenic hippocampi of patients with medial TLE (60). However, laminar analysis of resected spiking cortex from patients with TLE suggests that

decreased in-vivo FMZ binding is not necessarily due to decreased GABA$_A$ receptor density but may be due to complex changes that include both B_{max} and K_D in different cortical layers. In fact, [^{3}H]FMZ autoradiography studies showed increased B_{max} in cortical layers V–VI of spiking cortex but decreased receptor affinity that outweighed the increased binding such that the net effect was a decrease in V_D shown as an area of decreased FMZ uptake on the PET images (61).

The cortical-layer-specific increase of receptor number may be a compensatory mechanism for decreased GABAergic input. Limited spatial resolution of PET precludes laminar analysis of cortical FMZ binding in vivo, but the findings demonstrate that decreased FMZ binding on PET may be the result of spatial summation of multiple changes in GABA$_A$ receptor function. This may explain why, in some patients with focal epilepsy, no focal abnormalities of in-vivo FMZ binding can be detected in the EEG-determined epileptic focus, while others show focal increases of FMZ binding on PET.

A drawback of absolute quantification yielding FMZ V_D images is the requirement of arterial blood sampling to provide blood input function. Elimination of arterial blood sampling can facilitate more widespread clinical application of FMZ PET scanning and is particularly desirable in the pediatric patient population. In fact, visual as well as objective detection of focal cortical and subcortical abnormalities for clinical purposes can be reliably achieved using FMZ 'activity' images that do not require arterial blood sampling. Comparison of focal FMZ abnormalities in patients with neocortical epileptic foci showed that summed FMZ 'activity' images obtained between 10 and 20 minutes after tracer injection represented the best overall agreement between FMZ activity and V_D images, as compared to activity images obtained from an earlier (5–10 min) or later (15–30 min) time frame (62). Slight differences between the V_D and FMZ activity images can be caused by the tracer influx parameter K_1.

Another neurotransmitter system that has proved to be important in the functional neuroimaging of epilepsy is the serotonergic system and tryptophan metabolism. In-vitro observations showing increased serotonin (5-HT) content and immunoreactivity in human epileptic tissue (63, 64) have led to the application of the PET tracer α[^{11}C]methyl-L-tryptophan (AMT) in the study of epilepsy. AMT is an analog of tryptophan (the precursor of 5-HT), and is converted in the brain to α[^{11}C]methyl-serotonin, which is not a substrate for the degradative enzyme monoamine oxidase, and therefore accumulates in serotonergic terminals. This has been demonstrated in rats, where labeled AMT accumulated in high concentration in serotonergic cell bodies in the raphe nuclei (65). α[^{3}H]methyl-serotonin present in nerve terminals was released by K$^+$-induced depolarization, suggesting that this tracer is stored with the releasable pool of serotonin (66). Further, AMT, unlike tryptophan, is not incorporated into proteins in significant amounts (65, 67) and is therefore a suitable tracer for the measurement of serotonin synthesis in vivo in humans with PET, although it does not measure the absolute rate of serotonin synthesis.

Studies in animals (65, 68) and humans (69, 70) have suggested that the kinetic behavior of AMT can be described by a three-compartmental model using first-order rate constants. After transport of AMT across the blood–brain barrier, free AMT in the cytoplasm is either metabolized (to α[^{11}C]methyl-serotonin or via the kynurenine pathway; see below), or is irreversibly trapped, presumably in a serotonin synthesis precursor pool. The unidirectional uptake rate constant (K-complex) represents the combined unidirectional uptake into all three pools. The K-complex was found to be stable within an individual, and the rank order of regional brain values for this parameter is consistent with the rank order for serotonin content in the human brain (71).

An alternative route of tryptophan metabolism in the brain is via the enzymes 2,3-dioxygenase and indoleamine 2,3-dioxygenase, which are part of the kynurenine pathway. Under normal circumstances, levels of the metabolites of these pathways are 100–1000-fold lower than the concentration of tryptophan in the brain (72) and thus metabolites of the kynurenine pathway do not contribute significantly to the accumulation of AMT. Under pathologic conditions, however, induction of indoleamine 2,3-dioxygenase (e.g. by infections, viruses, or interferons) can lead to significant metabolism of tryptophan along the alternative kynurenine pathway. Among numerous metabolites of this pathway, quinolinic acid is neurotoxic, and a strong convulsant through its agonist action at the excitatory *N*-methyl-D-aspartate (NMDA) receptors. In fact, preliminary data from surgically resected brain tissue from children with tuberous sclerosis complex and intractable epilepsy have indicated that accumulation of quinolinic acid may contribute to the high in-vivo uptake of AMT in epileptogenic cortex (73).

In addition to using AMT for evaluating serotonin synthesis and tryptophan metabolism via the kynurenine pathway, an emerging approach is to image 5-HT$_{1A}$ receptors by PET. Using [^{11}C]-WAY, 5-HT$_{1A}$ receptor binding can be reliably measured in vivo (74). Preliminary PET studies in TLE showed decreased [^{18}F]FCWAY binding in the temporal lobe ipsilateral to the seizure focus as defined by EEG data (75).

Further PET tracers for in-vivo investigation of other neurotransmitter systems, such as [^{11}C]carfentanil (76), ^{11}C-diprenorphine (77), or 18F-cyclofoxy (78) for opiate receptors, [^{11}C]doxepin for histamine H$_1$ receptors (79), and (*S*)-[*N*-methyl-^{11}C]ketamine for NMDA-receptors (80) have not been adequately tested in epileptic patients but preliminary studies suggest that they may also be potentially useful in detecting epileptic cortex (see also Clinical applications, below).

Data Analysis

Qualitative visual analysis of ligand and neuroreceptor PET studies can be satisfactory for clinical purposes, with certain limitations. For example, since FMZ binding is relatively high in the medial temporal structures, unilateral decrease of FMZ binding in the hippocampus can be reliably identified, while bilateral symmetric decreases might be hard to interpret visually. Visual interpretation is also reliable to detect unilateral focal cortical decreases of FMZ binding but, again, is less reliable in detection of bilateral FMZ PET abnormalities and is not accurate in defining the extent of cortical areas with abnormal receptor binding.

Anatomical accuracy of ligand and neuroreceptor PET abnormalities can be enhanced by co-registering PET images with high-resolution MRI. This approach is especially useful when functional activity in very small brain structures, such as hippocampus, amygdala, or thalamic nuclei, is to be measured. High-resolution MRI-based partial volume correction enhances detection of FMZ binding in these structures (24, 81) and provides higher sensitivity to alterations than visual evaluation in patients with TLE, where focal decrease of FMZ binding in the medial temporal structures as well as in the thalamus ipsilateral to the seizure focus is common. One such study using PET/MRI co-registration found that the reduction in hippocampal FMZ binding is over and above what would be expected from loss of hippocampal volume, thus indicating that atrophy is not the sole determinant of GABA$_A$ receptor binding decrease in medial TLE and that other factors also contribute to decreased hippocampal FMZ binding (81).

Objective interpretation of PET images can be also performed using voxel-by-voxel analysis with statistical parametric mapping (SPM) (82). SPM is a robust, objective method of comparing patient groups with normal control groups, can detect common abnormalities of FMZ binding (83, 84), and is also applied to other types of PET measurement. This approach often reveals subtle abnormalities that are difficult to appreciate by visual or region-of-interest (ROI)-based image analysis. For example, using SPM and FMZ PET, involvement of the insular cortex was reported in 60% of patients with medial TLE (84). The presence or absence of such abnormalities did not predict surgical outcome but their regional distribution (anterior vs posterior insula) was related to ictal symptoms (emotional vs somesthetic symptoms, respectively).

The SPM analytic approach has been also useful to delineate focal abnormalities of cortical FMZ binding in patients with neocortical epileptic foci, including those with normal MRI and those with structural lesion (85, 86). Unlike previous ROI-based studies, these SPM studies consistently showed not only focal decreases but also increases of FMZ binding (85, 87), although the exact nature of these abnormalities is not entirely clear. Some of the areas showing increased FMZ binding coincide with focal cortical developmental malformations (88). Since no detailed EEG comparisons have been performed, the causative relationship between these focal abnormalities and epileptogenicity is not established.

In a recent study of 10 patients with malformations of cortical development, correction for partial volume effects for the area of MRI-defined malformation as well as for adjacent and overlying regions was applied (108). This study found decreased FMZ binding in some of the malformations but increased binding in some adjacent volumes of interest. Altogether, these studies demonstrate that objective analytic approaches are capable of identifying otherwise unappreciated abnormalities of abnormal FMZ binding that often extend beyond the structurally abnormal cortex representing functional abnormalities of GABA$_A$ receptors.

The SPM technique also allows objective analysis of FMZ binding in the white matter (which normally shows very low FMZ binding) by applying explicit white matter masking (90). These studies showed *increased* FMZ binding in the normal appearing temporal lobe white matter ipsilateral to the epileptic focus in patients with TLE and normal MRI. These white matter abnormalities were associated with microdysgenesis demonstrated by histopathology. In this case, FMZ V_D provided an in-vivo neuronal marker indicating increased number of white matter ectopic neurons in the epileptogenic temporal lobe. This is a potentially important finding, considering that ectopic neurons can contribute to epileptogenesis by providing an aberrant circuitry (91).

A drawback of voxel-based analytic approaches is that warping of native images to a predefined template requires smoothing, and results in a reduction of the original image resolution. An alternative objective method of delineating cortical PET abnormalities is based on analysis of asymmetries of small homologous cortical regions (33). The procedure uses native (unwarped) PET images and allows identification of abnormal cortical tracer content based on asymmetry indices derived from small bilateral homotopic cortical areas according to a predefined cutoff threshold (typically between 8% and 15%, depending on the PET tracer used), determined from PET scans of normal control subjects. The only major assumption made is that one of the hemispheres (contralateral to the presumed epileptic focus) is for the most part normal, and can serve as an internal control for the other hemisphere containing the epileptic focus. This, of course, is not always a valid assumption and is one of the pitfalls of the method.

The program marks all cortical segments in which the asymmetry of activity concentration exceeds the cutoff threshold. These marked PET images are then co-registered with the volumetric MRI image of the patient, and the PET abnormalities are surface-rendered, i.e. they are directly displayed on the cortical surface reconstructed from the patient's high-resolution MRI (Fig. 15.6). For patients undergoing subdural EEG recording, the locations of intracranial electrodes can be accurately identified and visualized on the three-dimensionally rendered brain surface by using digital X-ray images with fiducial markers (92, 93) or digital intraoperative photographs showing locations of electrode contacts on the cortex (94). These techniques allow direct comparison of objectively defined functional imaging abnormalities with ictal and interictal intracranial EEG datasets. Such comparisons provide a powerful way of exploring the functional relationship between ligand/neuroreceptor and electrophysiologic abnormalities of the epileptic cortex.

In patients with epilepsy and structural brain lesion(s), multimodal imaging of co-registered structural (MRI) and functional (PET or SPECT) abnormalities allows analysis of functional abnormalities in the lesions themselves as well as in the perilesional cortex (38, 95, 96). The benefit of simultaneous analysis of PET and MRI images has been well demonstrated in children with the tuberous sclerosis complex and intractable epilepsy (95). In these patients, MRI and FDG PET typically show multiple, typically bilateral lesions, but the seizures often originate from one of the lesions, as suggested by seizure semiology and ictal EEG.

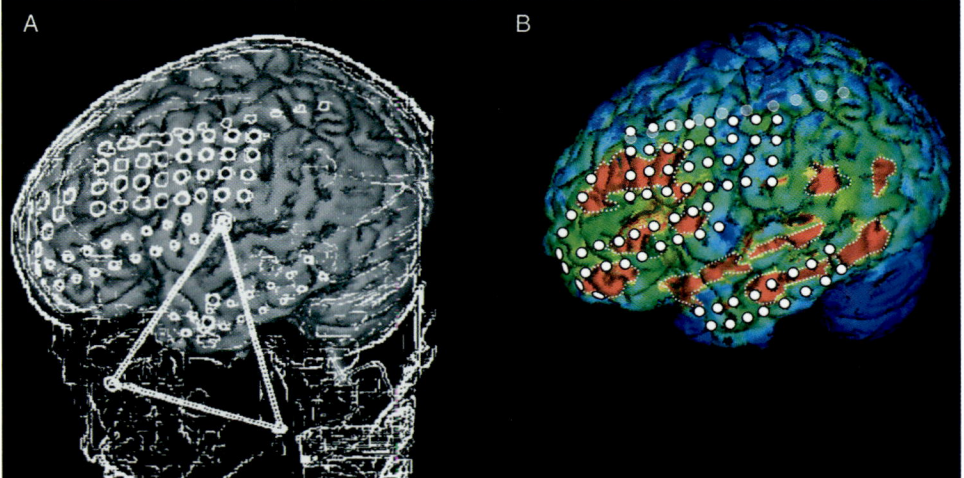

FIG. 15.6. X-ray-based identification of subdural grid electrodes for PET co-registration on the three-dimensional brain surface, reconstructed from volumetric MRI. **A.** The X-ray and MRI image datasets are co-registered using fiducial markers (two on the left and one on the right side), which form a triangle in the image space. **B.** Locations of the grid electrodes derived from the co-registered X-ray, superimposed to the brain surface, showing the objectively defined PET abnormalities in the left frontal and temporal cortex. A 1 × 10 electrode grid is located in the medial frontal–temporal area and cannot be directly visualized on the lateral surface.

However, neither MRI nor FDG PET can identify the epileptogenic lesion. In contrast, AMT PET often shows relatively increased uptake in the epileptogenic lesions and decreased uptake in the remaining ones (see Clinical applications, below). Thus, measurement of relative AMT uptake in the MRI-identified lesions can help differentiate epileptogenic from nonepileptogenic tubers.

Clinical Applications

Flumazenil Positron-emission Tomography Scanning of GABA_A Receptors

Among various neuroreceptor PET tracers used in epilepsy, FMZ is the one that has been most widely applied clinically. Initial studies using PET with FMZ showed significantly reduced binding in the epileptic focus of patients with partial epilepsy (97). Since then, several PET studies have demonstrated that areas of decreased FMZ binding commonly occur in patients with intractable partial epilepsy of both temporal and extratemporal origin, and that these abnormal regions tend to be spatially more restricted than corresponding regions of cortical glucose hypometabolism (15, 23, 59, 98).

Temporal Lobe Epilepsy

Flumazenil PET is highly sensitive in TLE and shows decreased FMZ binding in the sclerotic hippocampus in patients with medial TLE (23, 83). This high sensitivity of FMZ PET can be particularly useful in patients with a potentially epileptogenic cortical lesion when presence of dual pathology (co-existence of neocortical lesion and hippocampal sclerosis) is suspected (99) (Fig. 15.7). Undiagnosed dual pathology can be a source of surgical failure, since resection of both the cortical lesion and the affected hippocampus is necessary to optimize the surgical results. In some cases FMZ PET can detect multiple areas of decreased binding, including both the hippocampus and neocortical areas that do not show any obvious lesion on MRI. In such cases, intracranial EEG recordings are necessary to determine whether both the hippocampal and neocortical area is epileptogenic or, alternatively, one of them is the primary focus and the other may represent remote abnormality of GABA_A receptors; such areas are often targeted by rapid seizure spread (see also Extratemporal epilepsy, below).

Since decreased FMZ binding in pure medial TLE is largely (although not completely) confined to the affected temporal lobe, FMZ PET can be also helpful in patients where medial TLE is suspected (based on seizure semiology and/or ictal EEG recordings) but FDG PET shows additional extratemporal hypometabolism. Such regions of hypometabolism (most commonly in parietal or prefrontal cortex) may be seen with chronic epilepsy and do not necessarily indicate epileptogenicity, but may be associated with cognitive dysfunction. One comparative analysis of such cases suggested that decreased FMZ binding represents localized neuronal loss and/or receptor changes in the epileptogenic zone, whereas the more extensive glucose hypometabolism on FDG PET may reflect diaschisis (23). On the other hand, extratemporal cortical involvement on FMZ PET of patients with suspected TLE warrants caution, and may require consideration of intracranial EEG monitoring of the affected extratemporal areas, especially if the electroclinical findings cannot definitively exclude the extension of epileptogenic areas beyond the temporal lobe. Nevertheless, with clinical application of advanced MRI techniques, the overwhelming majority of patients with intractable TLE and hippocampal sclerosis do not require FMZ (or other types of) PET studies during their presurgical evaluation, and the use of FMZ PET is the subject of individual consideration.

The clinical significance of FMZ PET abnormalities in TLE and normal hippocampal volumes is less established.

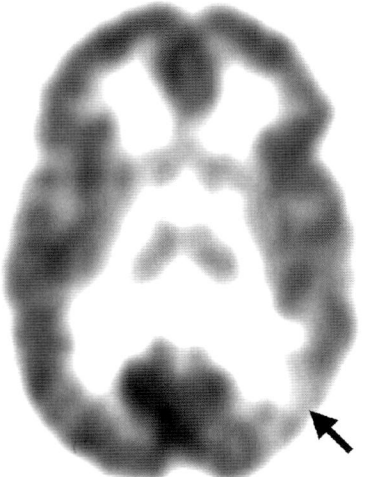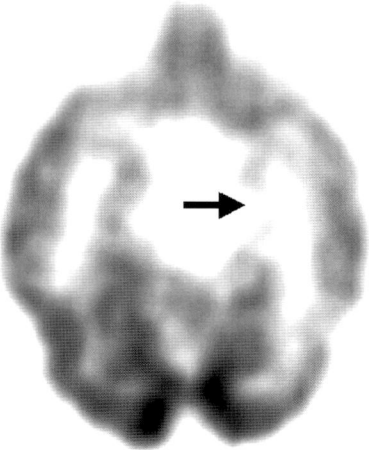

FIG. 15.7. [¹¹C]Flumazenil PET detecting dual pathology (arrows) consisting of a dysplastic area in the left posterior temporal region and decreased FMZ binding in the ipsilateral hippocampus indicating hippocampal sclerosis.

Transient and falsely lateralizing FMZ PET asymmetries have been reported in three patients with normal hippocampal MRI by Ryvlin et al. (100). In contrast, Lamusuo et al. (101) found decreased temporal FMZ binding ipsilateral to the EEG-defined seizure focus in 46% of medial TLE patients with normal hippocampal volumes. Histologic examination verified the presence of hippocampal damage in these cases, suggesting that FMZ PET can be useful to lateralize the epileptic temporal lobe in some TLE patients with normal volumetric MRI.

Using a more complex analytic method (by combining SPM and an MRI-based volume-of-interest approach with partial volume correction) in a similar group of MRI-negative TLE patients, Koepp et al. (102) found focal decreases and/or increases of FMZ binding ipsilateral to the presumed epileptic focus in 80% of the cases. However, these abnormalities did not consistently localize the epileptic focus. Altogether, these studies demonstrate a relatively high prevalence of focal FMZ binding abnormalities in TLE patients with normal MRI, but it remains unclear how these changes contribute to the presurgical evaluation of these patients and how they affect outcome after surgery.

Extratemporal Epilepsy

Since current surgical results remain suboptimal in extratemporal (neocortical) epilepsies, especially in the pediatric population, there has been a great deal of interest in applying neuroreceptor PET tracers in the presurgical evaluation of such patients, with special emphasis on those with normal MRI or cortical developmental malformations.

Studies to date indicate that FMZ PET is a promising imaging modality, which often shows decreased binding in the presumed epileptic focus shown on EEG even when the MRI appears normal (Fig. 15.8). Comparisons with intracranial ictal EEG findings have shown 57–100% sensitivity of FMZ PET in detecting neocortical epileptic foci, depending on the patient population and the applied analytic approach (15, 37, 103, 104). In a detailed comparison of objectively defined, surface-rendered FDG and FMZ PET abnormalities (using an asymmetry-based approach; see Analysis) and intracranial EEG data, Muzik et al. (37) found areas of decreased FMZ binding to be significantly more sensitive for detecting zones of seizure onset and frequent interictal spiking than areas of glucose hypometabolism. A close spatial relationship between seizure onset zone and the area showing reduced FMZ binding also has been reported in patients with cortical dysplasia (105).

Collectively, these findings suggest that FMZ PET is a useful clinical tool to further delineate potentially epileptogenic neocortex and to guide and enhance subdural electrode coverage for intracranial EEG monitoring. One of the few studies that have analyzed surgical outcome data in young patients who underwent cortical resection following FMZ PET scanning, found that complete resection of cortex with preoperative FMZ PET abnormalities was associated with excellent surgical outcome even in the absence of a structural lesion on MRI (39).

A subgroup of patients with neocortical epileptic foci shows area(s) of decreased FMZ binding remote from the seizure focus (Fig. 15.9). The exact nature of these abnormalities is not known. Comparisons with outcome data indicate that resection of such remote FMZ abnormalities is not

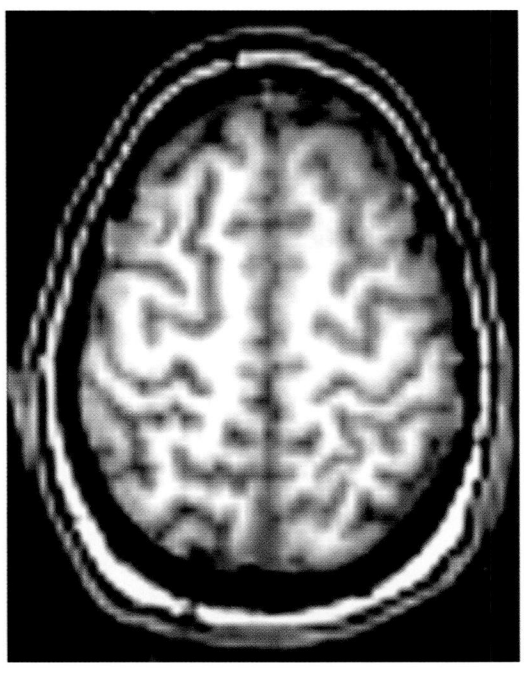

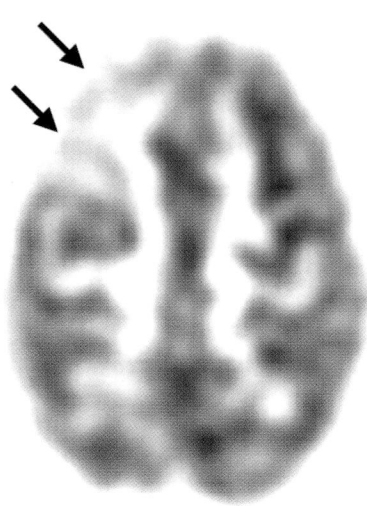

FIG. 15.8. Decreased [¹¹C]flumazenil binding in the right frontal cortex (arrows) in a patient with right frontal lobe epilepsy and normal MRI. The location of the seizure focus was verified by intracranial EEG monitoring.

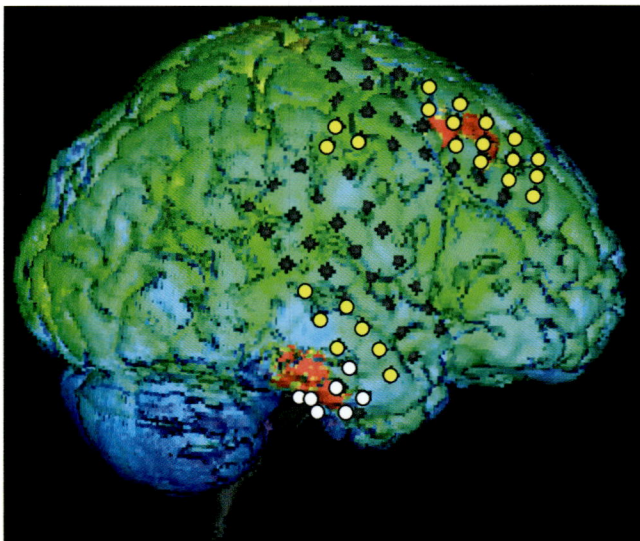

FIG. 15.9. Flumazenil (FMZ) PET abnormalities (red areas indicating areas with >10% decreases of FMZ binding on the three-dimensionally reconstructed surface) detecting the seizure focus (white electrodes in the right inferior temporal region) as well as a remote frontal cortical area that has shown frequent interictal spiking (yellow electrodes) on intracranial EEG.

connected regions, and were associated with seizure onset early in life and chronic intractable epilepsy (104).

Altogether, these data suggest that cortical areas with decreased FMZ binding, particularly if located in projection areas targeted by seizure propagation, may be related to repeated seizures over a relatively long period, and might represent potential areas of secondary epileptogenesis. This hypothesis, however, must be tested through further studies.

Occasionally, FMZ PET does not show any obvious focal abnormalities in patients with nonlesional extratemporal epilepsy. This is not common, but represents a limitation of FMZ PET. Further studies comparing FMZ with other PET tracers that have the capability of delineating epileptic brain regions will be useful. In fact, preliminary studies suggest that AMT PET may be helpful in some of these FMZ-negative cases (see below).

In patients with neocortical epilepsy and brain lesion, FMZ PET reliably detects most lesions, and the magnitude of decreased FMZ binding varies according to the type of lesion (98, 96, 99). Decreased FMZ binding, however, commonly extends to the perilesional cortex (Fig. 15.10), and the size of this perilesional abnormality is usually smaller than the corresponding perilesional hypometabolism shown with FDG PET (104, 96, 105). Perilesional FMZ PET abnormalities are often not concentric but eccentric, and show a good correspondence with epileptiform activity on intracranial EEG. Recently, Hammers et al (108). used a quantitative approach and found not only decreases but also increases of FMZ binding in cortex overlying or adjacent to focal cortical dysplasia. These studies support the notion that abnormal GABA$_A$ receptor binding is not confined to the cortical malformations visible on MRI, but extend beyond the structural lesion.

Objective, quantitative analysis of the FMZ PET images and their correlation with structural imaging and electrophysiologic findings are essential for optimal detection and interpretation of focal abnormalities. Further comparisons with new, emerging functional imaging modalities such as

always necessary to achieve long-term seizure freedom (provided that the seizure focus has been removed), although many of these remote areas appear to be targeted by rapid seizure spread as shown by intracranial ictal EEG recordings (104, 39). In fact, Savic et al. (107) reported postoperative recovery of such remote FMZ binding abnormalities (located in the primary projection areas of the seizure focus) in four patients with medial TLE following successful surgical resection of the primary epileptic focus. Furthermore, in patients with lesional epilepsy, remote cortical areas with decreased FMZ binding were located in ipsilateral synaptically

FIG. 15.10. [¹¹C]Flumazenil (FMZ) PET in a patient with a right frontal lesion (cyst) and intractable frontal lobe epilepsy. The lesion itself (delineated by dotted line) showed no FMZ binding, while the perilesional cortex showed decreased FMZ binding (arrows). The seizures originated from the right prefrontal cortex.

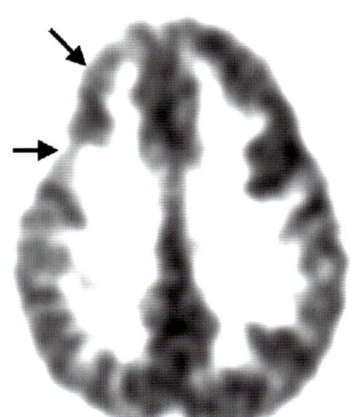

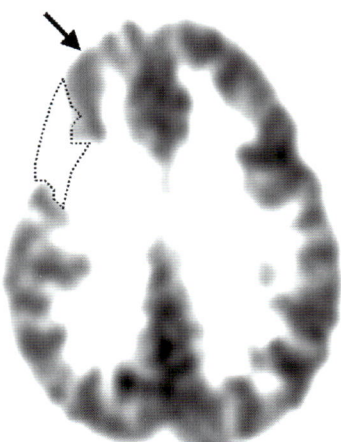

functional MRI, magnetic resonance spectroscopy, or magnetic source imaging may help further understand the significance of in-vivo GABA$_A$ receptor abnormalities in the pathogenesis of human partial epilepsy.

Idiopathic Generalized Epilepsy

Flumazenil PET studies in idiopathic generalized epilepsies have provided somewhat controversial findings. Savic et al. (109) first reported normal FMZ binding in cerebral cortex and decreased receptor density in the thalamus of adult patients with idiopathic generalized epilepsy. Prevett et al. (110, 111) found no differences in regional FMZ V_D values between at rest scans and images obtained during absence seizures, and also when compared to normal controls. In contrast, Koepp et al. (112) reported a significant global increase of FMZ V_D in the cortex, thalamus, and cerebellum in patients with idiopathic generalized epilepsy, with no effect from subsequent treatment with valproate. These findings are consistent with those from electrophysiologic studies in idiopathic generalized epilepsies and provide some support for the role of the thalamus in the pathogenesis of absence seizures. However, none of the studies have shown conclusively the initiation site of the seizures, and the role of ligand/receptor PET in the diagnosis of idiopathic generalized epilepsies remains limited.

Imaging Tryptophan Metabolism by Positron-emission Tomography

Although AMT PET is currently available in only a handful of epilepsy centers, it appears to have strong clinical applications in selected cases of epilepsy. The first successful clinical application of AMT PET in intractable epilepsy was demonstrated in children with the tuberous sclerosis complex who were being considered for resective epilepsy surgery (113). (Fig. 15.11). In fact, AMT PET was the first PET tracer capable of differentiating between epileptogenic and nonepileptogenic lesions in the interictal state in children with tuberous sclerosis. Subsequently, it was found to be useful also in patients with other types of neocortical epilepsy, by showing increased uptake of AMT in the epileptogenic regions.

While the specificity of focally increased AMT uptake for the epileptic focus appears to be very high, its sensitivity is suboptimal and seems to depend on the underlying etiology as well as the analytic approach applied. For example, in a cohort of 63 consecutive patients with tuberous sclerosis and intractable epilepsy, visual assessment identified increased AMT uptake in only 28 cases (44.4%) but when MRI-based quantitative assessment of the AMT images was applied, the sensitivity increased to 79% (114). This apparent discrepancy is due to the fact that nonepileptogenic tubers typically show decreased AMT uptake and that some epileptogenic

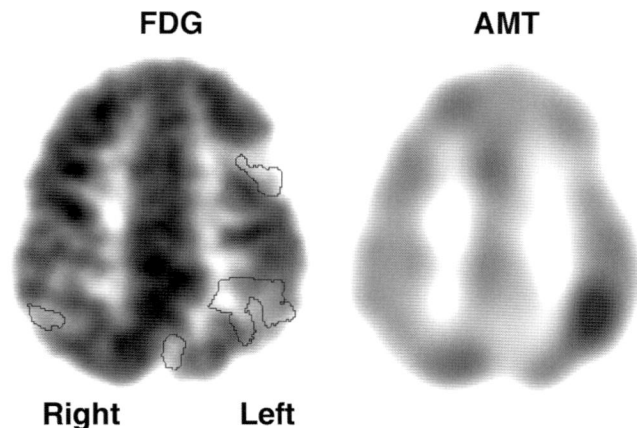

FDG **AMT**

Right **Left**

FIG. 15.11. FDG and α[^{11}C]methyl-L-tryptophan (AMT) PET scans in a patient with tuberous sclerosis and intractable seizures. FDG PET shows the typical finding of multiple areas with hypometabolism, consistent with multiple tubers. The outlined regions on the FDG PET represent individual tubers delineated on co-registered MRI images. AMT PET shows very high uptake (dark area) in the left parietal region, from where the seizures originated. The remaining tubers showed normal or decreased uptake.

tubers showing relatively increased AMT uptake cannot be easily differentiated from adjacent normal cortex without quantitative analysis following coregistration with MRI (95).

Recent studies in nontuberous sclerosis patients have shown that AMT PET can occasionally detect epileptic cortex in patients with normal MRI (115) and that histologically verified (macroscopic or microscopic) cortical dysplasia is associated with a higher occurrence of increased AMT uptake as compared to cases with nonspecific gliosis in the surgical specimen (116). This finding is consistent with previous human epileptic tissue studies showing serotonergic hyperinnervation in dysplastic tissues but not in cortex from patients with cryptogenic epilepsy (64). Comparisons with FDG PET also showed that the area of increased AMT uptake, if present, is significantly more restricted than the extent of corresponding glucose hypometabolism. Furthermore, in some instances, AMT PET can identify epileptogenic cortex even if FDG and/or FMZ PET do not show any obvious focal abnormality (Fig. 15.12).

Although clinical experience with AMT PET is limited in medial TLE, this method does not appear to be particularly useful in localizing medial temporal foci associated with hippocampal sclerosis. However, a recent study demonstrated that AMT PET can be useful to identify the epileptic focus in patients with TLE and normal hippocampal volumes (117). In addition, AMT PET scanning in patients with previously failed neocortical resection may disclose nonresected cortex with increased AMT uptake, especially if the histology had shown cortical developmental malformation. In these cases, AMT PET has the advantage of showing increased uptake in potentially epileptogenic areas and,

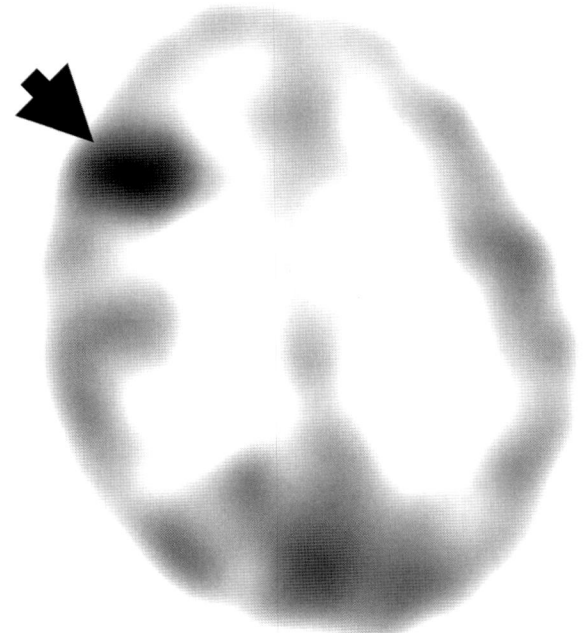

FIG. 15.12. α[¹¹C]Methyl-L-tryptophan (AMT) PET scan detecting epileptogenic cortex in a patient in whom neither FDG nor [¹¹C]flumazenil PET were localizing. Increased AMT uptake was seen in the epileptogenic right frontal lobe (arrow). The focus was verified by intracranial EEG. Histology showed cortical dysplasia in the surgical specimen following right frontal resection, which resulted in seizure freedom.

unlike MRI or interictal FDG or FMZ PET, can differentiate epileptogenic cortex from nonepileptic tissue damage caused by the initial surgery.

Opiate and Other Receptor Positron-emission Tomography Studies in Epilepsy

Clinical experience with opiate, histamine, and NMDA neuroreceptor PET tracers is limited, and their current role in presurgical evaluation is not well established. Endogenous opioid peptides modulate neural transmission in the hippocampus, and recurrent seizures induce changes in the expression of opioid peptides and receptors (118). Animal studies suggest that endogenous opioid release may play a role in termination of seizures (119). Consistent with this, serial absence seizures were found to be associated with an acute (15–41%) reduction of [¹¹C]diprenorphine (a nonspecific opiate receptor ligand) binding to association areas of neocortex (120), suggesting that occupation of opiate receptors by an endogenous opioid substance may contribute to seizure termination. Similarly, Koepp et al. (121) reported decreased [¹¹C]diprenorphine binding in the left parieto-temporo-occipital cortex of patients with reading induced epilepsy, scanned in the activated state. In addition, increased interictal binding of [¹¹C]carfentanil, a selective agonist for mu opiate

receptors, has been reported in the temporal neocortex ipsilateral to the seizure focus in patients with TLE (76, 77).

However, [¹¹C]diprenorphine binding was not significantly different between regions in the epileptic and contralateral temporal lobes. Similarly, there is a lack of overall asymmetry of [¹⁸F]cyclofoxy (which binds to both mu and kappa opiate receptors) binding, although some patients showed higher binding ipsilateral to the seizure focus (78). Finally, PET studies in TLE patients using the delta-receptor-selective antagonist [¹¹C]methylnaltrindole show a different regional pattern of increased binding as compared to [¹¹C]carfentanil (122). These studies suggest a differential regulation of opiate subtypes in TLE, with greater involvement of mu and delta receptors.

Kumlien et al. (80) reported a 9–34% decrease of (S)-[N-methyl-¹¹C]ketamine binding (a potential tracer for NMDA receptors) ipsilateral to the seizure focus in eight patients with medial TLE. It remains unclear whether these asymmetries are due to reduced NMDA-receptor density, reduced perfusion, focal atrophy (partial volume effects), or other factors. The same group of investigators have reported increased binding of [¹¹C]deuterium-deprenyl, an irreversible inhibitor of monoamine oxidase type B (MAO-B) with a very high affinity for the enzyme, in the epileptogenic temporal lobe, particularly in the medial temporal structures (124, 125). MAO-B is exclusively localized on astrocytes, and in-vitro studies had shown that its production is increased with gliosis in conjunction with neurodegenerative changes, mainly due to an increased number of reactive astrocytes. Interestingly, [¹¹C]deuterium-deprenyl binding was not increased in neocortical epileptic foci (124).

Thus, [¹¹C]deuterium-deprenyl PET seems to be more sensitive in TLE than in extratemporal epilepsy. This is in contrast to AMT PET, which may show increased uptake in neocortical foci but not in sclerotic hippocampus. These studies illustrate the specificity that PET is capable of providing in various types of epilepsy when appropriate tracers are selected. Finally, in patients with complex partial seizures, [¹¹C]doxepin PET demonstrated an increase of H₁ receptors in the seizure focus, which showed glucose hypometabolism on FDG PET (79) but these findings have not been replicated by other groups.

In summary, ligand/neuroreceptor PET studies provide new insights in the pathophysiology of human epilepsy and show differences in their sensitivity and specificity for temporal versus extratemporal lobe epilepsy. Unlike FDG, which characteristically shows decreased uptake in the region of the seizure focus interictally, some ligand and neuroreceptor tracers (such as AMT, [¹¹C]deuterium-deprenyl and [¹¹C]doxepin) show increased uptake in epileptogenic brain regions even in the interictal state. This represents a clear advantage over other imaging studies, especially when multiple structural lesions are present and potentially confound detection of the epileptogenic zone. The studies reviewed above also demonstrate that various tracers capture different aspects of the epileptic process and can provide complementary information regarding localization of epileptic foci. Multimodal registration of functional and structural images is a clinically useful tool to accurately delineate anatomical extent of functional abnormalities. Highly accurate software packages that allow detailed comparisons of ligand/neuroreceptor PET studies with scalp and intracranial EEG findings are now available, and their application will further establish the role of these new PET imaging modalities in the presurgical evaluation of intractable epilepsies.

REFERENCES

1. Hoffman EJ, Phelps ME. Positron emission tomography: principles and quantitation. In: Phelps ME, Mazziotta JC, Schelbert HR, eds. Positron emission tomography and autoradiography: principles and applications for the brain and heart. New York: Raven Press, 1986:237–286..

2. Ter Pogossian MM. Positron emission tomography. In: Wagner HN, Szabo Z, Buchanan JW, eds. Principles of nuclear medicine. London: WB Saunders, 1995:342–346.

3. Carson RE. Precision and accuracy considerations of physiological quantitation in PET. J Cereb Blood Flow Metab 1991;11:A45–A50.

4. Chugani HT, Phelps ME. Maturational changes in cerebral function in infants determined by 18FDG positron emission tomography. Science 1986;231:840–843.

5. Chugani HT, Phelps ME, Mazziotta JC. Positron emission tomography study of human brain functional development. Ann Neurol 1987;22:487–497.

6. Theodore WH. Antiepileptic drugs and cerebral glucose metabolism. Epilepsia 1988;29(Suppl 2):S48–S55.

7. Theodore WH, Bromfield E, Onorati L. The effect of carbamazepine on cerebral glucose metabolism. Ann Neurol 1989;25:516–520.

8. Leiderman DB, Balish M, Bromfield EB, Theodore WH. Effect of valproate on human cerebral glucose metabolism. Epilepsia 1991;32:417–422.

9. Kuhl DE, Engel J Jr, Phelps ME, Selin C. Epileptic patterns of local cerebral metabolism and perfusion in humans determined by emission computed tomography of 18FDG and 13NH3. Ann Neurol 1980;8:348–360.

10. Engel J Jr, Kuhl DE, Phelps ME. Patterns of human local cerebral glucose metabolism during epileptic seizures. Science 1982;218:64–66.

11. Engel J Jr, Kuhl DE, Phelps ME, Mazziotta JC. Interictal cerebral glucose metabolism in partial epilepsy and its relation to EEG changes. Ann Neurol 1982;12:510–517.

12. Swartz BE, Tomiyasu U, Delgado-Escueta AV, et al. Neuroimaging in temporal lobe epilepsy: test sensitivity and relationships to pathology and postoperative outcome. Epilepsia 1992;33:624–634.

13. Gaillard WD, Bhatia S, Bookheimer SY, et al. FDG-PET and volumetric MRI in the evaluation of patients with partial epilepsy. Neurology 1995;45:123–126.

14. Knowlton RC, Laxer KD, Ende G, et al. Presurgical multimodality neuroimaging in electroencephalographic lateralized temporal lobe epilepsy. Ann Neurol 1997;42:829–837.

15. Ryvlin P, Bouvard S, Le Bars D, et al. Clinical utility of flumazenil-PET versus [18F]fluorodeoxyglucose-PET and MRI in refractory partial epilepsy. A prospective study in 100 patients. Brain 1998;121:2067–2081.

16. Theodore WH, Sato S, Kufta CV, et al. FDG-positron emission tomography and invasive EEG: seizure focus detection and surgical outcome. Epilepsia 1997;38:81–86.

17. Engel J Jr, Henry TR, Risinger MW, et al. Presurgical evaluation for partial epilepsy: relative contributions of chronic depth-electrode recordings versus FDG-PET and scalp-sphenoidal ictal EEG. Neurology 1990;40:1670–1677.

18. Theodore WH, Sato S, Kufta C, et al. Temporal lobectomy for uncontrolled seizures: the role of positron emission tomography. Ann Neurol 1992;32:789–794.

19. Lamusuo S, Jutila L, Ylinen A, et al. [18F]FDG-PET reveals temporal hypometabolism in patients with temporal lobe epilepsy even when quantitative MRI and histopathological analysis show only mild hippocampal damage. Arch Neurol 2001;58:933–939.

20. Gaillard WD, Kopylev L, Weinstein S, et al. Low incidence of abnormal 18FDG-PET in children with new-onset partial epilepsy: a prospective study. Neurology 2002;58:717–724.

21. Akimura T, Yeh HS, Mantil JC, et al. Cerebral metabolism of the remote area after epilepsy surgery. Neurol Med Chir (Tokyo) 1999;39:16–25.

22. Spanaki MV, Kopylev L, DeCarli C, et al. Postoperative changes in cerebral metabolism in temporal lobe epilepsy. Arch Neurol 2000;57:1447–1452.

23. Henry TR, Frey KA, Sackellares JC, et al. In vivo cerebral metabolism and central benzodiazepine-receptor binding in temporal lobe epilepsy. Neurology 1993;43:1998–2006.

24. Juhász C, Nagy F, Watson C, et al. Glucose and [11C]flumazenil positron emission tomography abnormalities of thalamic nuclei in temporal lobe epilepsy. Neurology 1999;53:2037–2045.

25. Van Bogaert P, Massager N, Tugendhaft P, et al. Statistical parametric mapping of regional glucose metabolism in mesial temporal lobe epilepsy. Neuroimage 2000;12:129–138.

26. Chugani HT, Shewmon DA, Khanna S, et al. Interictal and postictal focal hypermetabolism on positron emission tomography. Pediatr Neurol 1993;9:10–15.

27. Chugani HT, Rintahaka PJ, Shewmon DA. Ictal patterns of cerebral glucose utilization in children with epilepsy. Epilepsia 1994;35:813–822.

28. Bittar RG, Andermann F, Olivier A, et al. Interictal spikes increase cerebral glucose metabolism and blood flow: a PET study. Epilepsia 1999;40:170–178.

29. Hong SB, Han HJ, Roh SY, et al. Hypometabolism and interictal spikes during positron emission tomography scanning in temporal lobe epilepsy. Eur Neurol 2002;48:65–70.

30. Sperling MR, Alavi A, Reivich M, et al. False lateralization of temporal lobe epilepsy with FDG positron emission tomography. Epilepsia 1995;36:722–727.

31. Swartz BE, Halgren E, Delgado-Escueta AV, et al. Neuroimaging in patients with seizures of probable frontal lobe origin. Epilepsia 1989;30:547–558.

32. Da Silva EA, Chugani DC, Muzik O, Chugani HT. Identification of frontal lobe epileptic foci in children using positron emission tomography. Epilepsia 1997;38:1198–1208.

33. Muzik O, Chugani DC, Shen C, et al. Objective method for localization of cortical asymmetries using positron emission tomography to aid surgical resection of epileptic foci. Comput Aided Surg 1998;3:74–82.

34. Drzezga A, Arnold S, Minoshima S, et al. 18F-FDG PET studies in patients with extratemporal and temporal epilepsy: evaluation of an observer-independent analysis. J Nucl Med 1999;40:737–746.

35. Kim YK, Lee DS, Lee SK, et al. 18F-FDG PET in localization of frontal lobe epilepsy: comparison of visual and SPM analysis. J Nucl Med 2002;43:1167–1174.

36. Chugani HT, Shewmon DA, Peacock WJ, et al. Surgical treatment of intractable neonatal-onset seizures: the role of positron emission tomography. Neurology 1988;38:1178–1188.

37. Muzik O, da Silva E, Juhász C, et al. Intracranial EEG vs flumazenil and glucose PET in children with extratemporal lobe epilepsy. Neurology 2000;54:171–179.

38. Juhász C, Chugani DC, Muzik O, et al. Is epileptogenic cortex truly hypometabolic on interictal positron emission tomography? Ann Neurol 2000;48:88–96.

39. Juhász C, Chugani DC, Muzik O, et al. Relationship of flumazenil and glucose PET abnormalities to neocortical epilepsy surgery outcome. Neurology 2001;56:1650–1658.

40. Chugani HT, Shields WD, Shewmon DA, et al. Infantile spasms: I. PET identifies focal cortical dysgenesis in cryptogenic cases for surgical treatment. *Ann Neurol* 1990;27:406–413.

41. Chugani HT, Shewmon DA, Shields WD, et al. Surgery for intractable infantile spasms: neuroimaging perspectives. *Epilepsia* 1993;34: 764–771.

42. Chugani HT, Mazziotta JC, Engel J Jr, Phelps ME. The Lennox-Gastaut syndrome: metabolic subtypes determined by 2-deoxy-2[^{18}F]fluoro-D-glucose positron emission tomography. *Ann Neurol* 1987;21:4–13.

43. Theodore WH, Rose D, Patronas N, et al. Cerebral glucose metabolism in the Lennox–Gastaut syndrome. *Ann Neurol* 1987;21:14–21.

44. Chugani HT, Mazziotta JC, Phelps ME. Sturge–Weber syndrome: a study of cerebral glucose utilization with positron emission tomography. *J Pediatr* 1989;114:244–253.

45. Lee JS, Asano E, Muzik O, et al. Sturge–Weber syndrome: correlation between clinical course and FDG PET findings. *Neurology* 2001;57:189–195.

46. Rintahaka PJ, Chugani HT, Messa C, Phelps ME. Hemimegalencephaly: evaluation with positron emission tomography. *Pediatr Neurol* 1993; 9; 21–28.

47. Lee JS, Juhász C, Kaddurah AK, Chugani HT. Patterns of cerebral glucose metabolism in early and late stages of Rasmussen's syndrome. *J Child Neurol* 2001;16:798–805.

48. Koutroumanidis M, Hennessy MJ, Seed PT, et al. Significance of interictal bilateral temporal hypometabolism in temporal lobe epilepsy. *Neurology* 2000;54:1811–1821.

49. Jokeit H, Seitz RJ, Markowitsch HJ, et al. Prefrontal asymmetric interictal glucose hypometabolism and cognitive impairment in patients with temporal lobe epilepsy. *Brain* 1997;120:2283–2294.

50. Chugani HT, Da Silva E, Chugani DC. Infantile spasms: III. Prognostic implications of bitemporal hypometabolism on positron emission tomography. *Ann Neurol* 1996;39:643–649.

51. Juhász C, Behen ME, Muzik O, et al. Bilateral medial prefrontal and temporal neocortical hypometabolism in children with epilepsy and aggression. *Epilepsia* 2001;42:991–1001.

52. Bachevalier J, Malkova L, Mishkin M. Effects of selective neonatal temporal lobe lesions on socioemotional behavior in infant rhesus monkeys (Macaca mulatta). *Behav Neurosci* 2001;115: 545–559.

53. Sivilotti L, Nistri A. GABA receptor mechanisms in the central nervous system. *Prog Neurobiol* 1991;36:35–92.

54. Verhoeff NP, Petroff OA, Hyder F, et al. Effects of vigabatrin on the GABAergic system as determined by [^{123}I]iomazenil SPECT and GABA MRS. *Epilepsia* 1999;40:1433–1438.

55. Chugani DC, Muzik O, Juhász C, et al. Postnatal maturation of human GABA$_A$ receptors measured with positron emission tomography. *Ann Neurol* 2001;49:618–626.

56. Bertz RJ, Reynolds IJ, Kroboth PD. Effect of neuroactive steroids on [^{3}H]flumazenil binding to the GABA$_A$ receptor complex in vitro. *Neuropharmacology* 1995;34:1169–1175.

57. Blomqvist G, Pauli S, Farde L, et al. Maps of receptor binding parameters in the human brain – a kinetic analysis of PET measurements. *Eur J Nucl Med* 1990;16:257–265.

58. Koeppe RA, Holthoff VA, Frey KA, et al. Compartmental analysis of [^{11}C]flumazenil kinetics for the estimation of ligand transport rate and receptor distribution using positron emission tomography. *J Cereb Blood Flow Metab* 1991;11:735–744.

59. Savic I, Ingvar M, Stone-Elander S. Comparison of [^{11}C]flumazenil and [^{18}F]FDG as PET markers of epileptic foci. *J Neurol Neurosurg Psychiatr* 1993;56:615–621.

60. Koepp MJ, Hand KS, Labbe C, et al. In vivo [^{11}C]flumazenil-PET correlates with ex vivo [^{3}H]flumazenil autoradiography in hippocampal sclerosis. *Ann Neurol* 1998;43:618–626.

61. Nagy F, Chugani DC, Juhász C, et al. Altered in vitro and in vivo flumazenil binding in human epileptogenic neocortex. *J Cereb Blood Flow Metab* 1999;19:939–947.

62. Niimura K, Muzik O, Chugani DC, et al. [^{11}C]flumazenil PET: activity images versus parametric images for the detection of neocortical epileptic foci. *J Nucl Med* 1999;40:1985–1991.

63. Pintor M, Mefford IN, Hutter I, et al. Levels of biogenic amines, their metabolites and tyrosine hydroxylase activity in the human epileptic temporal cortex. *Synapse* 1990;5:152–156.

64. Trottier S, Evrard B, Vignal JP, et al. The serotonergic innervation of the cerebral cortex in man and its changes in focal cortical dysplasia. *Epilepsy Res* 1996;25:79–106.

65. Diksic M, Nagahiro S, Sourkes TL, Yamamoto YL. A new method to measure brain serotonin synthesis in vivo. I. Theory and basic data for a biological model. *J Cereb Blood Flow Metab* 1990; 10:1–12.

66. Cohen Z, Tsuiki K, Takada A, et al. In vivo-synthesized radioactively labelled alpha-methyl serotonin as a selective tracer for visualization of brain serotonin neurons. *Synapse* 1995;21:21–28.

67. Madras BK, Sourkes,TL. Metabolism of α-methyl-tryptophan. *Biochem Pharmacol* 1965;14:1499–1506.

68. Diksic M, Nagahiro S, Chaly T, et al. Serotonin synthesis rate measured in living dog brain by positron emission tomography. *J Neurochem* 1991;56:153–162.

69. Muzik O, Chugani DC, Chakraborty P, et al. Analysis of [C-11]alpha-methyl-tryptophan kinetics for the estimation of serotonin synthesis rate in vivo. *J Cereb Blood Flow Metab* 1997;17:659–669.

70. Nishizawa S, Benkelfat C, Young SN, et al. Differences between males and females in rates of serotonin synthesis in human brain. *Proc Natl Acad Sci USA* 1997;94:5308–5313.

71. Chugani DC, Muzik O, Chakraborty P, et al. Human brain serotonin synthesis capacity measured in vivo with alpha-[C-11]methyl-L-tryptophan. *Synapse* 1998;28:33–43.

72. Saito K, Nowak TS Jr, Suyama K, et al. Kynurenine pathway enzymes in brain: responses to ischemic brain injury versus systemic immune activation. *J Neurochem* 1993;61:2061–2070.

73. Chugani DC, Muzik O. Alpha[C-11]methyl-L-tryptophan PET maps brain serotonin synthesis and kynurenine pathway metabolism. *J Cereb Blood Flow Metab* 2000;20:2–9.

74. Parsey RV, Oquendo MA, Simpson NR, et al. Effects of sex, age, and aggressive traits in man on brain serotonin 5-HT(1A) receptor binding potential measured by PET using [C-11]WAY-100635. *Brain Res* 2002;954:173–182.

75. Toczek MT, Carson RE, Lang L, et al. PET imaging of 5-HT1A receptor binding in patients with temporal lobe epilepsy. *Neurology* 2003;60:749–756.

76. Frost JJ, Mayberg HS, Fisher RS, et al. Mu-opiate receptors measured by positron emission tomography are increased in temporal lobe epilepsy. *Ann Neurol* 23:231–237.

77. Mayberg HS, Sadzot B, Meltzer CC, et al. 1991 Quantification of mu and non-mu opiate receptors in temporal lobe epilepsy using positron emission tomography. *Ann Neurol* 1988;30:3–11.

78. Theodore WH, Carson RE, Andreasen P, et al. PET imaging of opiate receptor binding in human epilepsy using [^{18}F]cyclofoxy. *Epilepsy Res* 1992;13:129–139.

79. Iinuma K, Yokoyama H, Otsuki T, et al. Histamine H$_1$ receptors in complex partial seizures. *Lancet* 1993;341:238.

80. Kumlien E, Hartvig P, Valind S, et al. NMDA-receptor activity visualized with (S)-[N-methyl-^{11}C]ketamine and positron emission tomography in patients with medial temporal lobe epilepsy. *Epilepsia* 1999;40:30–37.

81. Koepp MJ, Labbe C, Richardson MP, et al. Regional hippocampal [^{11}C]flumazenil PET in temporal lobe epilepsy with unilateral and bilateral hippocampal sclerosis. *Brain* 1997;120:1865–1876.

82. Friston KJ, Holmes AP, Worsley KJ, et al. Statistical parametric maps in functional imaging: a general linear approach. *Hum Brain Mapping* 1995;2:189–210.

83. Koepp MJ, Richardson MP, Brooks DJ, et al. Cerebral benzodiazepine receptors in hippocampal sclerosis. An objective in vivo analysis. *Brain* 1996;119:1677–1687.

84. Bouilleret V, Dupont S, Spelle L, et al. Insular cortex involvement in mesiotemporal lobe epilepsy: a positron emission tomography study. *Ann Neurol* 2002;51:202–208.

85. Richardson MP, Koepp MJ, Brooks DJ, et al. Benzodiazepine receptors in focal epilepsy with cortical dysgenesis: an ^{11}C-flumazenil PET study. *Ann Neurol* 1996;40:188–198.

86. Richardson MP, Koepp MJ, Brooks DJ, Duncan JS. ^{11}C-flumazenil PET in neocortical epilepsy. *Neurology* 1998;51:485–492.

87. Hammers A, Koepp MJ, Labbe C, et al. Neocortical abnormalities of ^{11}C]-flumazenil PET in mesial temporal lobe epilepsy. *Neurology* 2001;56:897–906.

88. Richardson MP, Friston KJ, Sisodiya SM, et al. Cortical grey matter and benzodiazepine receptors in malformations of cortical development. A voxel-based comparison of structural and functional imaging data. *Brain* 1997;120:1961–1973.

89. Richardson MP, Hammers A, Brooks DJ, Duncan JS. Benzodiazepine-GABA$_A$ receptor binding is very low in dysembryoplastic neuroepithelial tumor: a PET study. *Epilepsia* 2001;42:1327–1334.

90. Hammers A, Koepp MJ, Hurlemann R, et al. Abnormalities of grey and white matter ^{11}C]flumazenil binding in temporal lobe epilepsy with normal MRI. *Brain* 2002;125:2257–2271.

91. Chevassus-Au-Louis N, Congar P, Represa A, et al. Neuronal migration disorders: heterotopic neocortical neurons in CA1 provide a bridge between the hippocampus and the neocortex. *Proc Natl Acad Sci USA* 1998;95:10263–10268.

92. Von Stockhausen HM, Thiel A, Herholz K, Pietrzyk U. A convenient method for topographical localization of intracranial electrodes with MRI and a conventional radiograph. *Neuroimage* 1997;5:S514.

93. Muzik O, Chugani DC, Shen C, et al. Assessment of the performance of FDG and FMZ PET imaging against the gold standard of invasive EEG monitoring for the detection of extratemporal lobe epileptic foci in children. In: Gjedde A, Hansen SB, Knudsen GM, Paulson OB, eds. Physiological imaging of the brain with PET. San Diego, CA: Academic Press, 2001:381–387.

94. Wellmer J, von Oertzen J, Schaller C, et al. Digital photography and 3D MRI-based multimodal imaging for individualized planning of resective neocortical epilepsy surgery. *Epilepsia* 2002;43:1543–1550.

95. Asano E, Chugani DC, Muzik O, et al. Multimodality imaging for improved detection of epileptogenic lesions in children with tuberous sclerosis complex. *Neurology* 2000;54:1976–1984.

96. Szelies B, Sobesky J, Pawlik G, et al. Impaired benzodiazepine receptor binding in peri-lesional cortex of patients with symptomatic epilepsies studied by ^{11}C]-flumazenil PET. *Eur J Neurol* 2002;9:137–142.

97. Savic I, Persson A, Roland P, et al. In-vivo demonstration of reduced benzodiazepine receptor binding in human epileptic foci. *Lancet* 1988;2:863–866.

98. Szelies B, Weber-Luxenburger G, Pawlik G, et al. MRI-guided flumazenil- and FDG-PET in temporal lobe epilepsy. *Neuroimage* 1996;3:109–118.

99. Juhász C, Nagy F, Muzik O, et al. [11]C]flumazenil PET in patients with epilepsy with dual pathology. *Epilepsia* 1999;40:566–574.

100. Ryvlin P, Bouvard S, Le Bars D, Mauguiere F. Transient and falsely lateralizing flumazenil-PET asymmetries in temporal lobe epilepsy. *Neurology* 1999;53:1882–1885.

101. Lamusuo S, Pitkanen A, Jutila L, et al. [11]C]Flumazenil binding in the medial temporal lobe in patients with temporal lobe epilepsy: correlation with hippocampal MR volumetry, T2 relaxometry, and neuropathology. *Neurology* 2000;54:2252–2260.

102. Koepp MJ, Hammers A, Labbe C, et al. ^{11}C-flumazenil PET in patients with refractory temporal lobe epilepsy and normal MRI. *Neurology* 2000;54:332–339.

103. Savic I, Thorell JO, Roland P. [11]C]flumazenil positron emission tomography visualizes frontal epileptogenic regions. *Epilepsia* 1995;36:1225–1232.

104. Juhász C, Chugani DC, Muzik O, et al. Electroclinical correlates of flumazenil and fluorodeoxyglucose PET abnormalities in lesional epilepsy. *Neurology* 2000;55:825–834.

105. Arnold S, Berthele A, Drzezga A, et al. Reduction of benzodiazepine receptor binding is related to the seizure onset zone in extratemporal focal cortical dysplasia. *Epilepsia* 2000;41:818–824.

106. Juhász C, Muzik O, Chugani DC, et al. Chronic vigabatrin treatment modifies developmental changes of GABA$_A$ receptor binding in young children with epilepsy. *Epilepsia* 2001;42:1320–1326.

107. Savic I, Blomqvist G, Halldin C, Litton JE, Gulyas B. Regional increases in ^{11}C]flumazenil binding after epilepsy surgery. *Acta Neurol Scand* 1998;97:279–286.

108. Hammers A, Koepp MJ, Richardson MP, et al. Central benzodiazepine receptors in malformations of cortical development: a quantitative study. *Brain* 2001;124:1555–1565.

109. Savic I, Pauli S, Thorell JO, Blomqvist G. In vivo demonstration of altered benzodiazepine receptor density in patients with generalized epilepsy. *J Neurol Neurosurg Psychiatr* 1994;57:797–804.

110. Prevett MC, Lammertsma AA, Brooks DJ, et al. Benzodiazepine-GABA$_A$ receptors in idiopathic generalized epilepsy with ^{11}C]flumazenil and positron emission tomography. *Epilepsia* 1995;36:113–121.

111. Prevett MC, Lammertsma AA, Brooks DJ, et al. Benzodiazepine-GABA$_A$ receptor binding during absence seizures. *Epilepsia* 1995;36:592–599.

112. Koepp MJ, Richardson MP, Brooks DJ, et al. Central benzodiazepine/gamma-aminobutyric acid A receptors in idiopathic generalized epilepsy: an ^{11}C]flumazenil positron emission tomography study. *Epilepsia* 1997;38:1089–1097.

113. Chugani DC, Chugani HT, Muzik O, et al. Imaging epileptogenic tubers in children with tuberous sclerosis complex using alpha-^{11}C]methyl-L-tryptophan positron emission tomography. *Ann Neurol* 1998;44:858–866.

114. Juhász C, Chugani DC, Asano E, et al. Alpha[11]C]methyl-L-tryptophan positron emission tomography scanning in 176 patients with intractable epilepsy. *Ann Neurol* Suppl 2002;1:S118.

115. Fedi M, Reutens D, Okazawa H, et al. Localizing value of alpha-methyl-L-tryptophan PET in intractable epilepsy of neocortical origin. *Neurology* 2001;57:1629–1636.

116. Juhász C, Chugani DC, Muzik O, et al. Alpha-methyl-L-tryptophan PET detects epileptogenic cortex in children with intractable epilepsy. *Neurology* 2003;60:960–968.

117. Natsume J, Kumakura Y, Bernasconi N, et al. Alpha-^{11}C] methyl-L-tryptophan and glucose metabolism in patients with temporal lobe epilepsy. *Neurology* 2003;60:756–761.

118. Simmons ML, Chavkin C. Endogenous opioid regulation of hippocampal function. *Int Rev Neurobiol* 1996;39:145–196.

119. Tortella FC, Long JB, Holaday JW. Endogenous opioid systems: physiological role in the self-limitation of seizures. *Brain Res* 1985;332:174–178.

120. Bartenstein PA, Duncan JS, Prevett MC, et al. Investigation of the opioid system in absence seizures with positron emission tomography. *J Neurol Neurosurg Psychiatry* 1993;56:1295–1302.

121. Koepp MJ, Richardson MP, Brooks DJ, Duncan JS. Focal cortical release of endogenous opioids during reading-induced seizures. *Lancet* 1998;352:952–955.

122. Madar I, Lesser RP, Krauss G, et al. Imaging of delta- and mu-opioid receptors in temporal lobe epilepsy by positron emission tomography. *Ann Neurol* 1997;41:358–367.

123. Kumlien E, Bergstrom M, Lilja A, et al. Positron emission tomography with ^{11}C]deuterium-deprenyl in temporal lobe epilepsy. *Epilepsia* 1995;36:712–721.

124. Kumlien E, Nilsson A, Hagberg G, et al. PET with ^{11}C-deuterium-deprenyl and ^{18}F-FDG in focal epilepsy. *Acta Neurol Scand* 2001;103:360–366.

CHAPTER 16

Magnetoencephalography in Epilepsy

Robert C. Knowlton and William W. Sutherling

INTRODUCTION

Magnetoencephalography (MEG), also commonly referred to as magnetic source imaging (MSI), when combined with structural imaging, provides a new noninvasive tool for epilepsy localization (1). MEG is similar to electroencephalography (EEG); however, unlike electrical potentials measured with EEG, which are attenuated in strength and spatially blurred by tissues between brain and scalp surface, magnetic fields are minimally affected by intervening tissue layers (2). The potential advantage of MEG over EEG is based on greater accuracy of the observed signal at the scalp such that it allows cerebral sources to be modeled more simply; and this in turn allows for more clinically usable and reliable localization of brain activity (3).

Clinical applications of MEG center mostly on the ability of dipole source estimation to provide noninvasive information on cortical function and dysfunction localization. Because of the limitations of the most common model of source localization in clinical use, the single equivalent current dipole (ECD) model, present applications are restricted in attempts to localize truly focal sources that can be conveniently measured with high signal-to-noise ratio (SNR). Because of the typically high SNR of spikes and sharp waves, focal epileptiform paroxysms provide a unique opportunity for MEG source localization of clinically important spontaneous brain activity.

This chapter will focus on the clinical application of MEG epilepsy localization and brain mapping. The review will include those works in which the single ECD model has been demonstrated to be successful and times when it appears to be limited or inappropriate. Techniques that may allow a greater range of success for MEG source localization with more advanced spatiotemporal multidipole modeling will only be briefly covered. For more thorough reading on multiple source analysis see reviews by Scherg (4) and Ebersol (5).

Localization of the epileptogenic zone in patients with partial epilepsy is usually accomplished with video and EEG recording of seizures and a combination of structural and functional imaging (6). Magnetic resonance imaging (MRI), positron-emission tomography (PET), and *ictal* single-photon-emission tomography (SPECT) are established imaging modalities that can aid in identification of epileptogenic substrates. Neuroimaging findings, however, may be nonlocalizing when structural and functional disturbances are widely distributed, equivocal, or when no abnormality is revealed. Moreover, unlike EEG, which provides direct evidence of the origin of seizures, structural and metabolic imaging provides only indirect evidence of a potential epileptogenic substrate. Moreover, scalp-recorded EEG does not always yield clear localization of the epileptogenic zone either; and the relationship of EEG-detected abnormalities to structural lesions may be ambiguous.

Given these limitations of traditional techniques, the role of MEG in the evaluation of patients with medically refractory localization-related epilepsy can be defined. As demonstrated in numerous studies over the past 10 years, if MEG combined with source modeling can be used to accurately localize sources of epileptiform discharges (7–18), then it can play the role of delineating the functional epileptogenic significance of abnormalities depicted in imaging. Further, using image registration techniques, MEG can be combined with MRI, PET, and ictal SPECT to provide three dimensional (3D) mapping of the relationship of epileptiform activity to structural and metabolic anatomy, offering a novel noninvasive tool to obtain information about the location of the epileptogenic zone that often is not otherwise possible.

MAGNETOENCEPHALOGRAPHY BASICS

The Brain's Magnetic Field

The generation and localization of the magnetoencephalogram has been reviewed in several excellent papers and for further detail the reader is referred to Hamalainen et al. (19) The small electric currents in the neurons of the brain produce a small magnetic field according to the right hand rule of physics where, as in a small segment of wire, a current flowing in the direction of the thumb of the right hand produces a magnetic field that circulates in the direction of the curled fingers. Brain currents also produce the electroencephalogram. The current producing the MEG arises inside neurons. This is because volume currents outside neurons have a geometry that is symmetric and produces magnetic fields that are self-canceling, whereas the intracellular current has one direction at any instant and a high 'vorticity', which produces a detectable magnetic field outside the head. The volume currents outside the neurons travel through the extracellular space, cerebrospinal fluid, meninges, skull, and scalp to be recorded by EEG electrodes.

Whereas the EEG volume currents travel on paths determined by conductivity producing potentials on the surface of the scalp, the MEG produced by the intracellular currents is a field that is little affected by conductivities of the head compartments. Because of the geometry of the magnetic field, which is maximal perpendicular to the axis of current and zero along the axis of current, a current source that is radial to the surface of a spherical volume conductor (a good model of the head in the occipital region and convexity) does not produce an externally measured magnetic field. Thus, MEG measures that part of the current in a neuron that is tangential to the scalp and, therefore, measures a subset of currents in the brain. The EEG measures all currents. The minimal effect of conductivity on and the tangential field patterns of the MEG results in a simpler scalp topography. A small current source of any orientation produces a tangential dipole pattern with a maximum peak and a minimum valley and a null point between the two extremes, or sea level, in between. It is simpler to interpret patterns in MEG than in EEG.

Both the EEG and the MEG measured on the scalp result from the synchronous activity of a large ensemble of neurons by superimposition of the fields of many cells. The neurons, which have a parallel geometry allowing the fields to summate together, are the large pyramidal shaped neurons in layers 5 and 4 of the cerebral cortex. The currents producing the MEG probably arise in the apical dendrites of these neurons.

Detection and Measurement of the Magnetoencephalogram

There were two main problems that needed to be solved to measure the MEG: sensitivity and SNR.

Sensitivity

The brain's magnetic field is extremely small (a femtoTesla, about 10^{-15} T). This problem is solved by the use of the superconducting quantum interference device (SQUID) (20, 21). These detectors are sensitive enough to measure the gravitational potential change that occurs when a single electron moves 1 mm in the earth's gravitational field. Modern machines use dc-SQUIDs, which are more difficult to construct but more reliable, with less noise. The SQUIDs are immersed in liquid helium to give them their remarkable properties of such high sensitivity. When even a miniscule magnetic field threads through the central open space of the SQUID, it induces a change in the operation of the device from conducting to nonconducting – a dramatic electronic change that is easily amplified to a large signal and then viewed like a voltage versus time tracing similar to an EEG tracing. Figure 16.1 provides a schematic review of the process of recording human brain magnetic fields with a modern whole head magnetometer system.

Signal-to-Noise Ratio

Gradiometers, Magnetometers, and Shielded Rooms

The field is immersed in a hostile magnetic environment: The heart's magnetic field or MKG is 100 times larger. The earth's magnetic field is a billion times larger. MRI machines have magnets that are 10^{15} times larger. Such noise is eliminated in practice by specific pieces of equipment. First, a gradiometer coil is set up like two coaxial loops of metal wire, with a connecting wire between. When a magnetic field from far away threads the loops, it affects each in the same way and the loops are set up to cancel out the current induced in the loops if the currents are the same. When a magnetic field near one of the loops, but not the other, threads the loops, it produces a larger induced current in the nearby loop and a smaller current in the farther loop. This current, which is different in the two loops, is amplified. Thus, magnetic activity of the heart or environment is canceled and only the brain's magnetic field is amplified, since the head is placed near the coils.

Although a pick-up coil with only one loop (magnetometer) is more sensitive than a coil with two loops (gradiometer), the magnetometer is also sensitive to noise. Since the additional noise actually can decrease the SNR ratio and since the selective advantage of the MEG compared with EEG is dependent on a high SNR, gradiometers are usually used in a hospital environment. Even the resolving power of gradiometer coils is ineffective in canceling some of the ambient magnetic fields in a noisy hospital environment (fluorescent lights, MR magnet coils, pager systems). This problem has been solved by placing the MEG detector inside a large, magnetic-shielded room. The walls of the room are constructed of materials that are very magnetically permeable, so that most of the ambient magnetic fields are absorbed into the walls, do not enter the room, and do not reach the sensors.

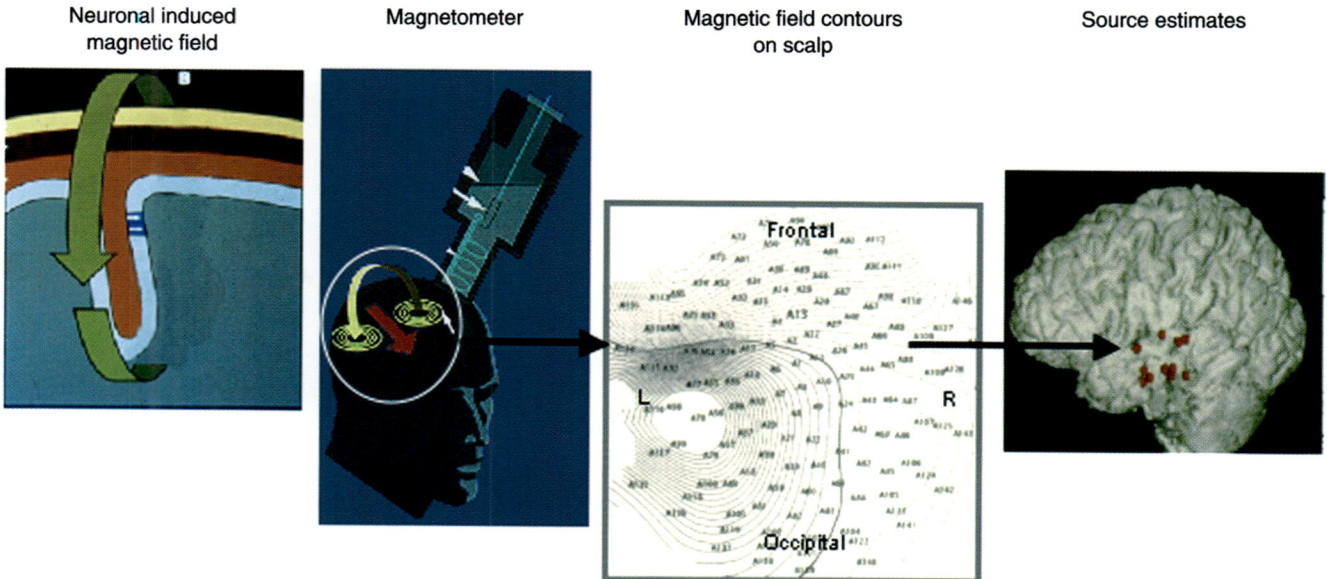

FIG. 16.1. Human magnetic field recordings of spontaneous paroxysmal brain activity and subsequent source localization.

Magnetoencephalography detects electrocorticographic (ECoG) spikes only during synchronous activation of an extended area of cortex when multiple ECoG electrodes are involved. Estimates from simultaneous EEG with ECoG strips have indicated that about 6 cm² is required for MEG detection (22). Synchronous cortical activity over about 2–3 cm² was required to produce a detectable extracranial spike in the MEG when MEG was compared to simultaneous recording from large ECoG grids where area could be quantified over the cortical surface (23). This is due to detection sensitivity and SNR. The MEG is better suited than EEG to extracranial–intracranial correlations because of the minimal effect of the volume conductor on MEG (13).

Source Localization

Localization is performed by comparing the measured field pattern to a computer-simulated field pattern (the forward solution) derived from equations for an equivalent point dipole source (like a small segment of wire) placed at multiple regions inside the skull at each region having varying orientations. In principle, superimposing the measured map on to the computer-generated forward solution map and mathematically determining the difference in the two patterns using the least-squared difference between them can solve the localization or inverse problem. Usually a searching algorithm, such as the downhill simplex, is used to optimize the least squares fit. The forward solution with the least-squares fit to the data is chosen as the correct inverse solution. Then the location and orientation of the equivalent dipole producing that forward solution is chosen as the location of the 'centroid' of the brain activity.

Realistic Models

The model of the source affects localization accuracy (24). SNR can be improved using such advanced models as the recursively applied multiple signal classification algorithm (RAP-MUSIC), which separates the signal from the noise subspace, increasing SNR. More realistic modeling therefore improves detection sensitivity of MEG. More realistic modeling has been used in excellent work by several investigators (25–31). Propagation is best assessed with the more realistic spatiotemporal dipole model (32).

The model of the volume conductor, or tissues of the head, also significantly affects localization accuracy of dipole and extended source models (19). Several mathematical and geometrical models of the human head as a volume conductor have been developed to correlate extracranially measured magnetic fields (MEG) and electric potentials (EEG) to their intracranial generators. Models such as single and multiple concentric spherical shells, boundary element model (BEM), and Finite element model (FEM) are among the most widely used (29). Skull effects dominate in volume conductor models. Recent detailed studies of conductivity have revealed the complexity of the skull's electrical properties (33–35). Inclusion of the results of such studies in the volume conductor model may improve the localizations from extracranial electric and magnetic measurements.

Electroencephalography

Although EEG is less accurate than MEG for spatial localization (19, 26, 36, 37) and the sensors more difficult to coregister with MRI, EEG has several complementary advantages. It is used routinely in all comprehensive epilepsy centers in the US. It is less expensive than MEG since it records only the voltage differences produced by scalp currents between two sites on the head, although recording of this easily obtainable quantity increases the complexity of the volume conductor necessary for analysis. Recording of epileptic activity is usually easier with EEG – availability of long-duration recordings allows a large spike sample across wake–sleep states to be captured. EEG measures the same current orientations as intracranial ECoG. EEG also measures more of the cerebral cortex than MEG, although, it concurrently increases the complexity for the source model required for analysis. The EEG combined with MEG gives more accurate localizations than MEG or EEG alone (27). More realistic volume conductor models are especially important to improve accuracy of the EEG and are essential to combine the MEG and EEG for localization (26–28, 31, 38).

Combined MEG and EEG modeling is the most sensitive noninvasive technique for radial and tangential sources. ECoG modeling is the most sensitive to gyri. Source models of combined MEG and EEG may allow more precise localization and separation of activity on postcentral versus precentral gyrus.

Magnetoencephalography Localization Accuracy

Phantom Studies – One Dipole and Two Dipoles Overlapping in Time

The localization error in MEG for a dry dipole phantom for one dipole and two dipoles. The MEG method analyzed with realistic modeling gives accurate localizations for one dipole and for two dipoles overlapping in time.

The dry phantom consisted of two plastic semicircles fitted together at a right angle to mimic a sphere (Neuromag, Helsinki; 4D Imaging, San Diego, CA). Small wire current dipoles were embedded in the plastic, tangential to the radii. This is used routinely as a calibration phantom. In this study a single dipole source and a two-dipole source at multiple locations were tested, using RAP-MUSIC. The phantom was attached mechanically to the bottom of the dewar inside the space for the head in a 100-SQUID 68 sensor channel whole cortex neuromagnetometer (CTF Systems, VSM Inc., Vancouver, Canada). The neuromagnetometer used 68 sensor first-derivative coaxial gradiometers and 19 reference channels to produce a synthetic third-derivative 68-sensor array which was flux-transformed to dc-SQUIDs. Coil parameters were baseline 5 cm and diameter 2 cm. Channel noise was 5–7 fT per root Hz.

Table 16.1 shows that, for one dipole activation, mean localization error was 1.0 mm (SE 0.4), with 95% confidence that the actual location was less than 2 mm from the estimated location. For two dipoles, overlapping in time but offset by 100 ms, mean error was 1.7 mm (SE 0.6) for each, with 95% confidence that each of the dipoles were within 3 mm of the estimate.

TABLE 16.1 *Magnetoencephalography Phantom Error One Dipole (mm)*

No	X	Y	Z	X′	Y′	Z′	Error
14	0.0	−27.0	47.6	−0.7	−27.5	47.8	0.88
25	0.0	32.5	56.3	0.2	32.5	56.1	0.28
26	0.0	27.5	47.6	0.0	27.6	47.5	0.14
14	0.0	−27.5	47.6	0.0	−27.5	46.3	1.30
15	0.0	−22.5	39.0	−0.2	−22.2	37.9	1.16
16	0.0	−17.5	30.3	−0.3	−17.7	29.5	0.88
1	56.3	0.0	32.5	56.3	−0.8	31.4	1.36
2	47.6	0.0	27.5	47.6	−0.8	26.7	1.13
4	30.3	0.0	17.5	30.5	−0.5	16.7	0.96
5	32.5	0.0	56.3	32.1	−0.6	55.0	1.49
6	27.5	0.0	47.6	27.5	−0.5	46.6	1.12
						Mean	0.97
						SEM	0.40

With perfectly synchronous activations of identical waveforms, errors were larger. Such synchrony may not be relevant to human cortex, because of delays from finite conduction speed of cortico-cortical association, U-fibers. Even in 3 Hz generalized spike-and-wave in primary generalized absence epilepsy (classic 'petit mal'), the prototype of generalized epileptic activity, interhemispheric conduction delays are 15 ms (39). In the case of source configurations with two dipoles within the same radius, for instance, in the auditory P300, which has components from superficial and deep structures in the temporal lobe, investigators have switched to study the visual P300, where the primary cortical response is in another lobe, occipital, and a later response is in the medial temporal lobe (40).

Additional studies with the 100-channel 68 sensor site MEG system have shown only slightly larger mean errors of localization when the experiments were repeated in a saline-filled sphere phantom with one dipole. In that case, the mean localization error was 1.4 mm and the SE was 0.9 mm (41).

Combined MEG and EEG methods may increase accuracy (36, 38, 42). In addition, comparison of the timing of an EEG component at the sphenoidal electrode versus the timing of a component at a lateral scalp electrode may help distinguish deep and superficial sources on MEG (43, 44).

Median Nerve Somatosensory Evoked Field From Central Fissure – Required Number of Channels and Reproducibility

Magnetoencephalography and EEG are accurate for localization of the central fissure for surgery and MEG is easier to integrate and reproduce with MRI for practical use of this information (7, 45, 46). The single moving dipole localizations of the median somatosensory evoked field N20m and P30m in the same subject were compared between a 100-channel 68-sensor site neuromagnetometer and a 200-channel 150-sensor site neuromagnetometer. The localization from each lab was co-registered onto the subject's MRI. The difference was 2.1 mm (SD 1.84), within 1 SD of the inherent error of MEG phantom dipole localization and co-registration in the saline-filled sphere (1.4 mm SD 0.9), similar to the 2–3 mm error in a phantom study on a 122-channel whole-head system (36).

Thus, within the error limits derived from phantom studies in two whole cortex neuromagnetometers, there was no detectable difference in localization of the early dipolar components of the median somatosensory evoked field between the 68-channel system and the 150-channel system (47). This confirms the results of a theoretical study, which predicts no significant difference between 64 channels and 128 channels for localization of one dipole and multiple dipole cortical sources (48). The accurate localization of the superficial, focal currents producing the early components of the SER is one of the most difficult tests of a localization method. A superficial source has the highest spatial frequency of topographical map isocontours (49).

MAGNETOENCEPHALOGRAPHY IN CLINICAL EPILEPSY AND BRAIN MAPPING

Magnetoencephalography Accuracy in Epilepsy Localization

Efforts at confirming accuracy of MEG in clinical localization of epilepsy have been addressed from numerous direct and indirect approaches. The direct methods mainly reflect work done with either implanted dipoles using special intracranial (IC) electrodes (8, 9) or simultaneous IC-EEG and MEG recordings (41, 50–52). Indirect confirmation mainly comes from studies demonstrating colocalization with known epileptogenic substrates either visible on functional or structural imaging or confirmed with subsequent IC-EEG and successful surgical outcomes with supportive histopathology (7, 10, 11, 13, 15, 16, 18, 53–60).

Recordings with implanted dipoles (created by a pair of special electrodes included with IC-EEG electrode implantation) provide the control of variables and parameters nearly equal to that in rigorous phantom studies but truly in vivo in human brain and skull. Results from dipoles placed in mesial, basal, and inferior lateral temporal regions showed that MEG predicted localizations were within 1, 2, and 4 mm respectively of the actual locations (8, 9). These findings provided fundamental support for validity of the entire system (from hardware to localization model to brain co-registration) to accurately localize sources in the human head. This type of testing, however, cannot account for the type of variable complex spontaneous paroxysmal discharges typical of most human partial epilepsies.

Although still few, simultaneous IC-EEG–MEG studies have increasingly been performed. The difficulties of these tests are not confined to logistical and safety issues of transporting patients with implanted IC electrodes for prolonged periods from a medical-surgical nursing hospital unit to the MEG laboratory (typically more of an outpatient setting); they also include frequent problems with artifact from electrical hardware and connections as well as cumbersome dressings that can negatively displace the MEG detectors from the closest possible position with scalp surface.

In spite of these issues, simultaneous IC-EEG–MEG studies elucidate details on the true capabilities and limitations of MEG to estimate various types and locations of spontaneous epileptiform paroxysms. With respect to depth of interictal spike sources in temporal lobe epilepsy it is clear that MEG detects few, if any, mesial or 'hippocampal-only' spikes recorded with subdural strip electrodes (50–52, 59). Basal temporal sources appear to require at least 6 cm² and lateral neocortical sources, 3–4 cm² of contiguous cortical activity. Similar to lateral temporal lobe sources, for MEG to detect the majority of spikes recorded from the dorsal lateral frontal lobe, activation of at least three subdural electrodes (1 cm apart) is required (51, 52). In the one reported case of mesial frontal-only spikes, MEG failed to record any epileptiform paroxysms.

Thus, it should be understood that MEG does not provide any clear advantage over EEG with respect to detection sensitivity of deep epileptiform sources. This does not mean that MEG cannot detect spikes that EEG does not (and vice versa) but rather that signal drop-off (inverse square of the distance) is generally similar, as should be expected. This parallel sensitivity excludes any patient specific skull or brain anatomy abnormalities that would affect electrical potentials and magnetic fields differentially, e.g. surgical skull defects, where MEG would be at an advantage. Furthermore, given the classical estimate of 6 cm² required for EEG to detect spikes, MEG may be more sensitive for convexity neocortical sources. Finally, MEG is intrinsically better at recording and detecting signals from sources that are primarily oriented tangentially to the convexity, such as intrasylvian cortex.

The most important difference between MEG and EEG is the accuracy of source localization. In one study that included both MEG and EEG dipole source localization, MEG was shown to be more accurate with the known source and tightness of dipole clustering (61). For clinical application this issue alone may support the use of MEG over EEG. However, new techniques using real head modeling with high resolution EEG (comparable to the resolution of sampling typically used in MEG) might provide similar accuracy or even better characterization of sources than MEG in certain circumstances. Ideally source localization should take advantage of the combination of MEG and EEG as complementary tools for optimally characterizing and localizing complex sources.

Although it is an indirect method of addressing accuracy of MEG, colocalization with focal epileptogenic substrates also may provide evidence for clinically relevant accuracy. Focal epileptogenic substrates may be represented by visible well delineated lesions on imaging or by electrophysiologically defining cryptogenic functional lesions, pathologies that when completely disrupted or removed surgically result in elimination of seizures. Because of the ability of highly accurate image co-registration, reliable in-vivo colocalization studies can be performed. With the greater ease and lower risk to validate localization, much of the reported work supporting MEG epilepsy source localization is indeed based on demonstrating concordance with imaging.

Well delineated lesion colocalization represents strong validation of MEG spike source localization, particularly with low-grade tumors or tumor-like lesions that clearly are the single focal cause of a given patient's epilepsy. Even in many cases when the lesion itself is not 'intrinsically' epileptogenic, immediately adjacent tissue is usually the source of spikes and seizure onset. This may not always be the case with developmental or tumor-like lesions (e.g. focal cortical dysplasias), where epileptiform discharges may extend up to several centimeters away from the MRI visible lesion. Still in nearly all cases a topographical relationship of spikes to the lesion can be delineated in a detailed fashion with IC-EEG and then compared with MEG localizations. Such studies have consistently shown MEG to be remarkably concordant with the IC-EEG findings, including various tumors and malformations of cortical development (15, 57, 60).

The best cases of confirmation with colocalization are seen in patients with intrinsically epileptogenic focal lesions (13, 15, 54, 57). Figure 16.2 shows a patient with a left peri-rolandic glial-neural complex. Trains of frequent spikes were recorded and nearly all clustered on the lesion itself. The MEG spike source estimates completely and tightly overlapped the lesion. Ultimate validation comes from colocalization with surgical removal of such lesions that render patients seizure free. The great confidence that this and other such lesions are the source of epileptiform discharges

shows without any doubt, that regardless of all issues involved with MEG methods, including the limits and assumptions associated with source modeling, that epilepsy MEG spike source localization can be remarkably accurate.

In contrast to the above example, other lesions are associated with peri-lesional epileptogenic tissue. One of the main challenges is to determine the eccentric location and extent of neighboring tissue that should be included in the resection that is in addition to the lesion removal. Otsubo et al. (60) addressed this issue specifically in their lesional MEG study in 12 children with neocortical epilepsy. The spatial relationship of spike sources with respect to the lesion correlated with ECoG findings in all cases. Thus, even with lesions that often suggest the obvious location of seizure sources, MEG spike source localization can not only confirm whether the lesion is epileptogenic but also delineate what neighboring tissue is epileptogenic and important to remove (Figure 16.3).

Cryptogenic lesions, those that are not visible on high-quality MRI, are true challenges in the sense of the 'needle-in-the-haystack' concept of epilepsy localization. Detection of these lesions is one of the main focuses of clinically applied functional epilepsy imaging – PET, SPECT, magnetic resonance spectroscopy (MRS), functional MRI (fMRI), and diffusion weighted imaging (DWI). MEG can play a similar, but even more important role by directly revealing the source of epileptiform disturbance in relation to the cryptic pathology, directly tying together the epileptogenic significance of focal functional abnormalities on imaging. This typically applies to cryptic cortical dysplasia that may or may not be associated with changes on PET or SPECT. Figure 16.4 demonstrates a typical example of this scenario both aiding detection of a cryptogenic substrate and confirming its functional epileptogenic significance. Only after MEG spike source localization was achieved was the lesion associated

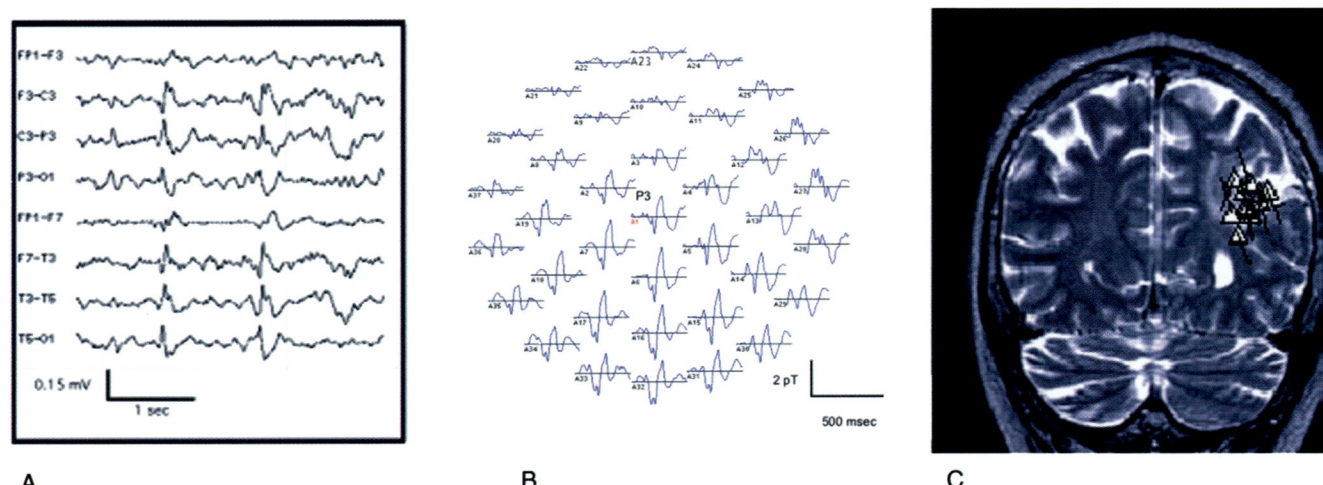

FIG. 16.2. MEG validation – epilepsy lesion colocalization. **A.** EEG spikes as recorded over the left central temporal and parietal regions; **B.** MEG recording of same spikes (37 channels centered over P3); **C.** Spike dipoles sources shown tightly overlapping left parietal glial neural complex as seen on T2-weighted MRI.

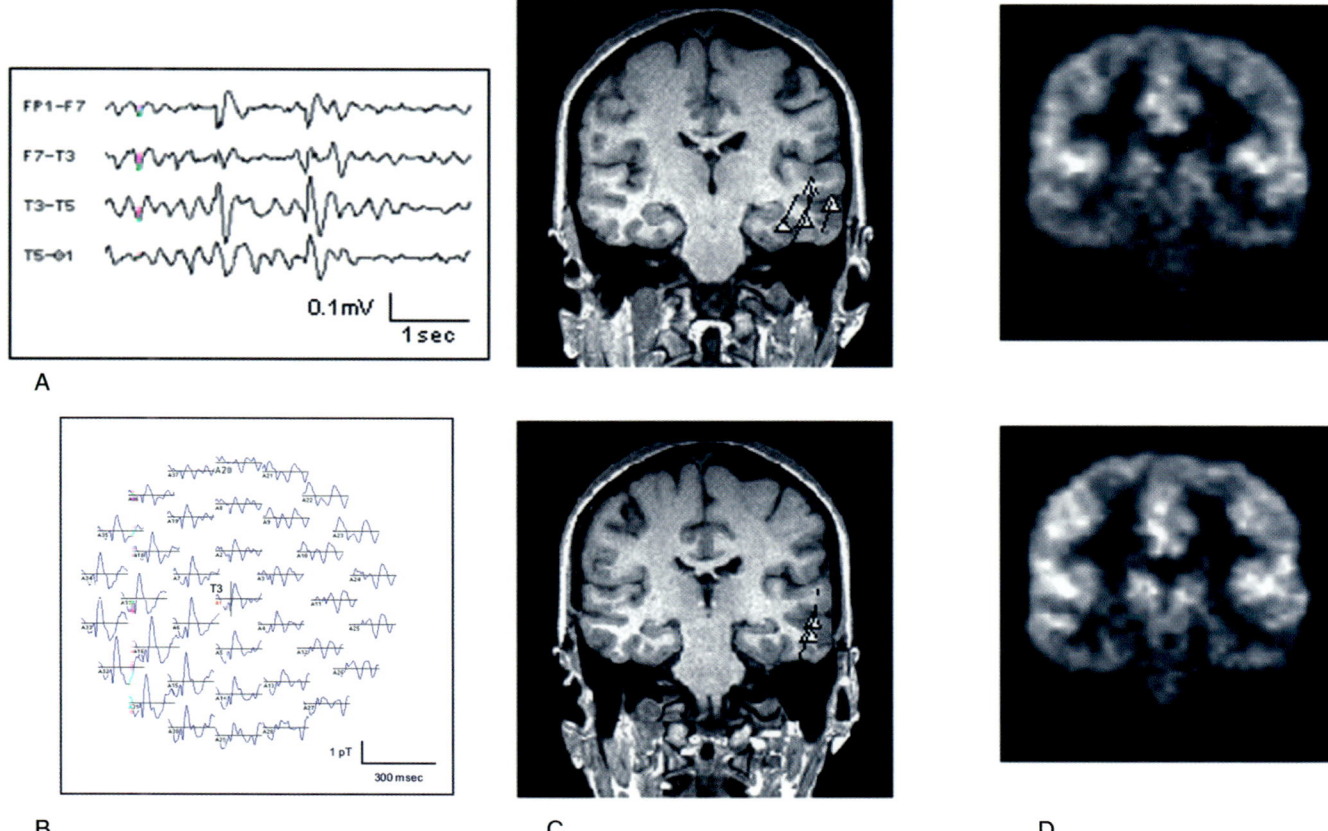

FIG. 16.3. MEG spike colocalization with MRI lesion of uncertain significance. **A.** Extracted epoch of spikes recorded with EEG over the left anterior temporal region. **B.** MEG sensor array tracing including a single spike as recorded with a 37-channel biomagnetometer centered over the mid left temporal region (T3). **C.** MRI images with MEG spike dipole sources (white triangles; attached tails represent dipole vector) overlying a questionable gray-matter lesion. **D.** Co-registered FDG-PET images revealing a focal functional defect that colocalizes with MEG spike sources. Histopathology after surgical resection showed findings of a ganglioglioma.

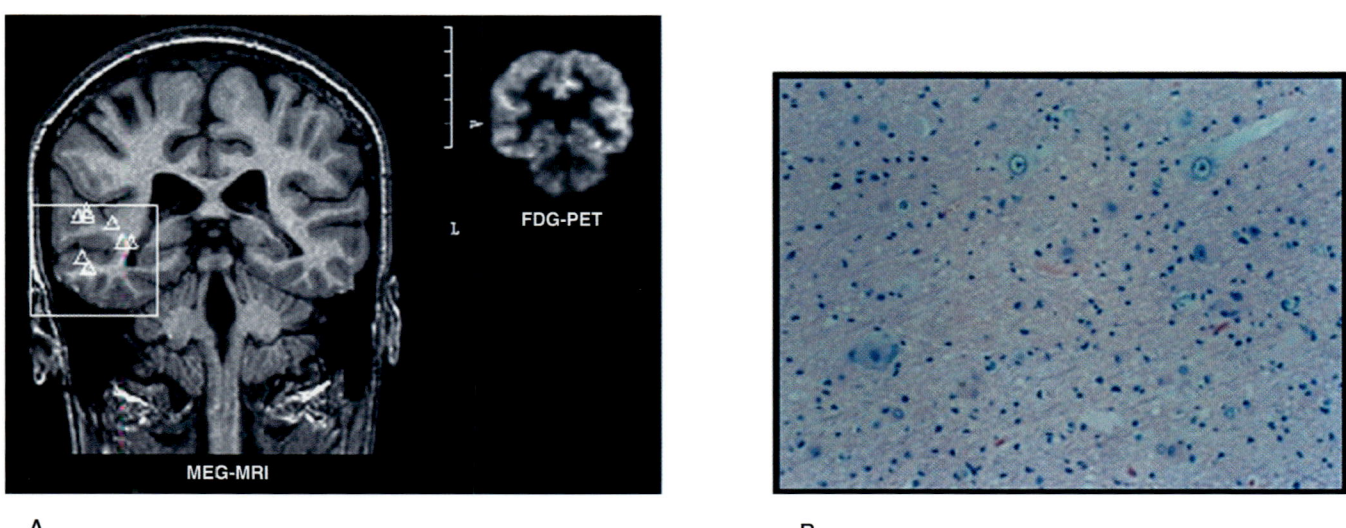

FIG. 16.4. MEG spike colocalization with a cryptic epileptogenic lesion. **A.** MRI with MEG spike dipole sources present in the right superior temporal gyrus and superior bank of the middle temporal gyrus (white triangles within boxed region). **Inset.** Co-registered FDG-PET image revealing a focal functional defect that colocalizes with MEG spike sources. **B.** Hematoxylin and eosin stain of surgical resection tissue from the location of spike sources showing a focal cortical dysplasia with Taylor type II balloon cells.

with focal relative hypometabolism appreciated on FDG-PET. Surgery guided by IC-EEG and intraoperative ECoG confirmed the focal neocortical temporal localization defined by MEG and histopathology revealed hamartomatous cortical dysplasia. Surgical resection yielded a seizure-free outcome.

Accepting that MEG spike localization may be accurate as a new noninvasive imaging tool, the first clinical application question is not necessarily whether it may replace IC-EEG but rather whether it can aid in the optimal placement of IC electrodes. Often hypotheses that influence IC electrode placement and distribution of coverage are based on relative low-resolution inference from scalp EEG with or without supplemental help from imaging. In fact, because it can only detect pathologic structural or functional disturbances that *indirectly* reflect the potential epileptogenic substrates, imaging can be misleading. Only neurophysiologic localization can provide confirmatory information directly reflecting epileptogenic tissue. Thus, it has been of great interest to determine whether MEG spike source localization correlates with IC-EEG recordings. Numerous reports

have shown that MEG can in most cases, especially in neocortical epilepsies, accurately predict localization of the most active epileptiform disturbances and seizures recorded with subdural grids (7, 11, 15, 16, 18, 56).

Still, an important issue will always remain, regardless of technical accuracy, is the fact that MEG conventionally only records and localizes interictal epileptiform activity. This limitation must always be acknowledged in ultimate clinical decision-making. As a result, in many cases, MEG should not be expected to replace IC-EEG ictal recordings. At the same time the value of localization of very active unifocal epileptiform paroxysms should not be underestimated, particularly in extratemporal lobe epilepsy. In such cases MEG should be able to at least optimally direct IC-EEG placement or even planning of craniotomy location and ECoG. With further ability to subgroup patients with the most robust unifocal active epileptiform disturbances, and concordant focal defects on advanced functional imaging, it should be possible to identify many patients who can skip IC-EEG all together. It is our experience that, although these

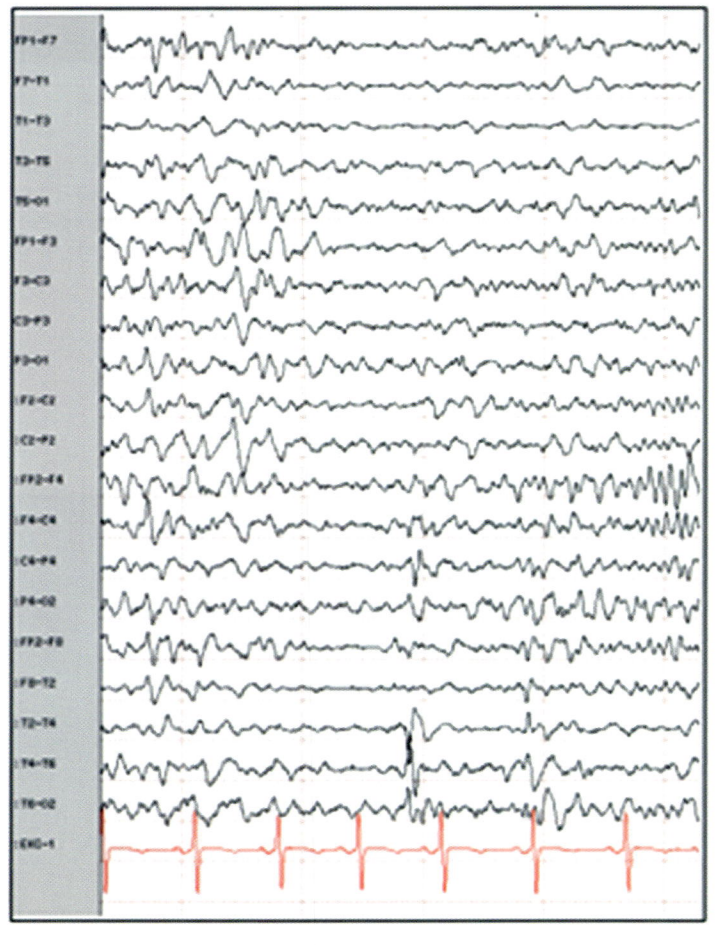

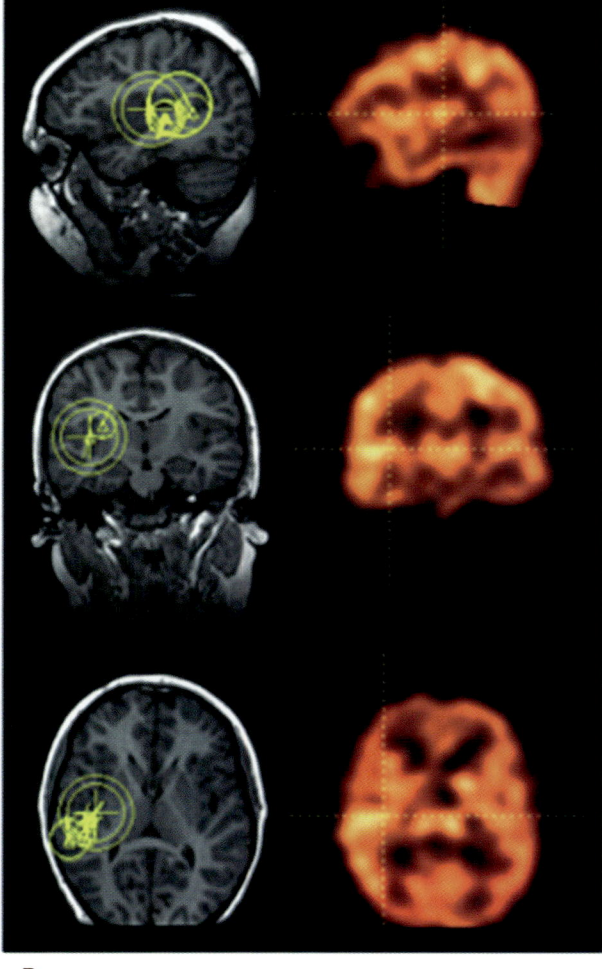

A   B

FIG. 16.5. MEG spike colocalization with ictal SPECT. **A.** EEG epoch with right mid-posterior temporal/inferior parietal spikes. **B.** MRI with MEG spike dipole sources present in the right superior temporal gyrus and deep intrasylvian cortex (yellow triangles; tails represent dipole vectors; circles represent 95% confidence volumes for source estimates). **C.** Co-registered ictal SPECT images of seizure related relative increase in blood flow colocalized to the area of clustered spike dipole sources.

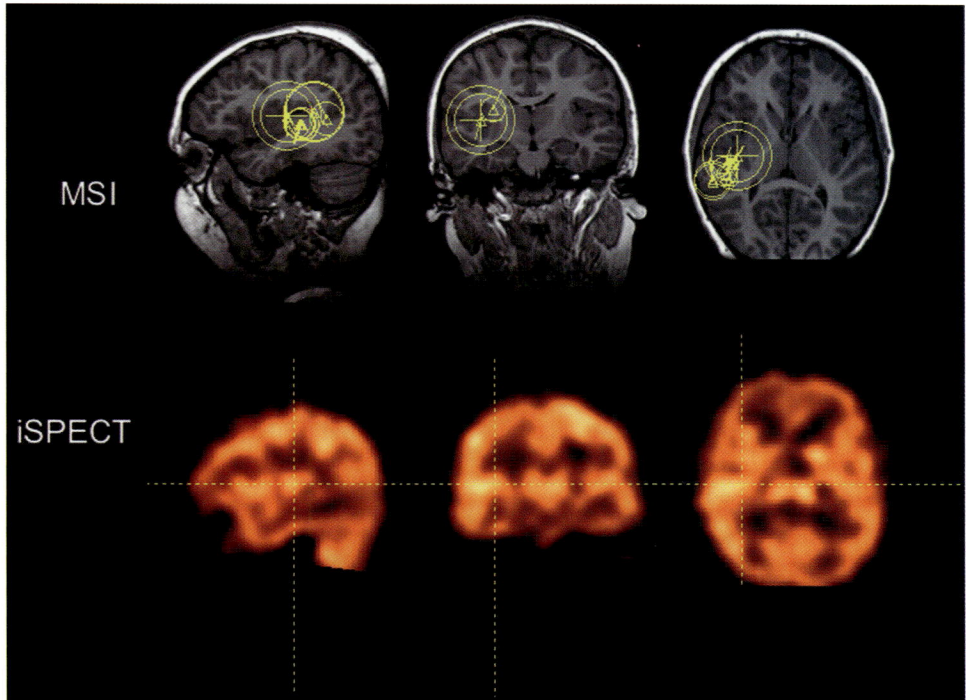

FIG. 16.6 Ictal MEG spike colocalization with ictal SPECT. **Top.** MRI with MEG spike dipole source localization estimates (yellow triangles; tails represent dipole vectors; circles represent 95% confidence volumes for source estimates) computed on rhythmic focal sharp waves seen on both EEG and MEG early in seizure evolution; same patient as in Figure 16.5). **B.** Co-registered ictal SPECT images of seizure related relative increase in blood flow colocalized to the area of initial seizure sharp-wave dipole sources.

cases are relatively rare, they are extremely important to recognize because they almost invariably have focal cryptogenic pathology and, most importantly, they comprise a subgroup of patients with extratemporal lobe epilepsy who have an excellent surgical prognosis.

Ictal MEG is not commonly performed but is feasible. The largest challenge in obtaining ictal MEG recordings is the logistics of capturing a seizure in the approximately 1–2 hour session of the typical examination. In a subset of the same patients for whom ictal SPECT can most readily be acquired, patients with frequent brief extratemporal seizures (mostly frontal lobe) can be recorded in the MEG suite. Movement related to the clinical onset can be a problem, but frequently at least a few seconds of *early* ictal cerebral activity can be recorded before clinical onset and can be analyzed by dipole source localization. Typically, individual spikes/sharp-waves of initial rhythmic ictal patterns are analyzed (Figure 16.6). Averaging of monomorphic spikes/sharp-waves is also possible (15).

As with interpretation of all ictal studies, one important issue is whether or not the sources reflect propagated seizure activity. This has to be of particular concern with mesial temporal seizures, where MEG is intrinsically limited to bias localization of propagated lateral temporal ictal activity. Still, in the few studies that have reported ictal MEG cases, results were promising, revealing consistent localization with IC-EEG and good surgical outcomes (41, 62–64). Notable also was the finding that ictal spikes agreed with interictal spike localization in most cases. Thus, if possible,

attempts should be made to perform ictal MEG in patients who have frequent seizures. This should especially be the case in the patients whose seizures are brief with rapid spread that would be difficult to localize with ictal SPECT, or when ictal SPECT may not be available.

SPECIAL LOCALIZATION ISSUES

Temporal Lobe Epilepsy

Magnetoencephalographic epilepsy localization in the temporal lobe depends greatly on whether the case of study is that of true mesial temporal lobe (MTLE) or lateral temporal lobe epilepsy (LTLE). For MTLE it is necessary to identify and characterize entorhinal, amygdala, and hippocampal spike sources as the predominant epileptiform disturbance of cerebral activity. However, the depth of mesial sources (3–4 cm) is such that their detection sensitivity is low. Moreover, spike propagation to basal and lateral cortex, as is required to generate a measurable MEG signal at the scalp, creates a complex net combination of biophysical magnetic field properties that can result in poor or inaccurate localization; the main issue is that MEG will be differentially more sensitive to the propagated activation in more superficial cortical regions.

Analysis of dipole orientations has provided a partial solution to this problem (5, 59, 61). Correlation with subsequent

IC-EEG recordings showed that anterior temporal dipole sources with a vertical orientation were associated with mesial onset seizures and imaging-defined hippocampal atrophy, whereas those anterior spike sources with predominantly horizontal orientation reflected basal and temporal polar sources more often. An even more important clinical distinction was that posterior vertical sources strongly correlated with lateral TLE. Thus, it has been proposed that dipole orientations are more important than absolute dipole localization in TLE (61).

Even with some of the localization limitations in MTLE, clinical value has been demonstrated with regard to distribution of spikes and seizure surgery outcome with anterior medial temporal lobectomy. Iwasaki and colleagues (65) classified spike localizations into two groups – anterior temporal (AT) and non AT localization – based on whether more than 70% of spike sources were anterior to a boundary line beginning at the point at which the central sulcus reaches the sylvian fissure and perpendicular to the chiasmatic commissural line (basically dividing the temporal lobe into anterior and posterior halves). Patients showing AT localization became seizure-free and spike-free following anterior temporal lobectomy. It is yet to be determined, but initial results suggest that patients with non-AT localizations (with or without evidence of MTS on MRI) should undergo IC-EEG evaluations to confirm localization and improve outcome.

Landau–Kleffner Syndrome

Landau–Kleffner syndrome (LKS) represents a unique and challenging epilepsy syndrome that may particularly benefit from MEG spike localization. LKS is an acquired epileptic aphasia or verbal agnosia occurring in a previously normal child, characterized by deterioration in language function in association with a seizure disorder and/or a paroxysmal EEG abnormality (66). The signature EEG abnormality is characterized by very frequent large-amplitude epileptiform discharges recorded with EEG in wide and varied distributions but mainly over the centrotemporal regions of either hemisphere. MEG studies in LKS patients have shown that the primary sources for the epileptiform disturbances lie predominantly in intra-sylvian cortex (67, 68).

Figure 16.7 is an example of MEG localization of very widespread typical epileptiform disturbances in a child with classic LKS. In spite of the large field, and even bilateral distribution (left-sided amplitude maximum), the source estimates based on MEG are remarkably unifocal and clustered tightly in the intrasylvian cortex. Extrasylvian sources appear to be secondary (from both cortico–cortical and transcallosal spread) when spatiotemporal analysis is performed (67). EEG detection and ability to localize deep fissural sources is limited compared to MEG because of overlapping secondary activation of radial sources in perisylvian convexity cortex. This activity in effect acts as noise, compromising the detection and optimal characterization of the intrasylvian

sources where over two-thirds of the regional cortical mantle lies.

One practical and important clinical consideration surrounding LKS source localization is the influence it may have on surgical treatment. Intra- and perisylvian multiple subpial transections can abolish the spikes (including secondary extrasylvian sources) and result in rapid reacquisition of language and speech function (67). The first challenge in LKS cases is to determine whether a predominant single source exists for what often appears on EEG to be widely distributed and bisynchronous. The second challenge (if a single unilateral source is strongly suspected) is to determine the location and extent of the critical sources. Both are crucial in surgical decision making – the former to determine who are best candidates for surgery and the latter to aid in minimizing risk (limiting as much as possible the opening of the sylvian tissue) and optimizing the likelihood that the correct location will be targeted.

Focal Slow-wave Localization

Slow-wave source localization is a potential application of MEG to aid presurgical evaluation. Persistent and intermittent (including postictal) relative focal slowing can be of localizing value because such nonepileptiform disturbances usually reflect pathology responsible for partial epilepsy, pathology that sometimes is cryptic on MRI. Source localization in general can be performed with EEG or MEG but, for the same reasons that spike source localization is advantageous with MEG, slow-wave sources can be more reliably estimated with MEG. Only a few studies have directly examined MEG slow-wave source localization in presurgical epilepsy evaluations. Although sensitivity, specificity, and validation have not been thoroughly demonstrated, results do confirm that the technique colocalizes slow-wave sources with confirmed lesions (69, 70). The need for further study is clear because of the implications for easily capturing these disturbances in the interictal state without the need to capture spikes that may be absent in routine MEG recordings.

Secondary Bilateral Synchrony

A relatively common epilepsy localization problem in extratemporal lobe epilepsy is that of secondary bilateral synchrony. This is variably defined depending on the strictness of the criteria chosen by electroencephalographers. Blume and Pillay's definition, 'sequential focal spikes or sharp waves leading directly to bilaterally synchronous epileptiform paroxysms,' might be the most reliably identified (71). Scalp EEG is poorly suited to address this problem in many cases.

The first problem, to determine if secondary bilateral synchrony actually applies in a given patient, can be the most difficult if a criterion requiring a single lateralized

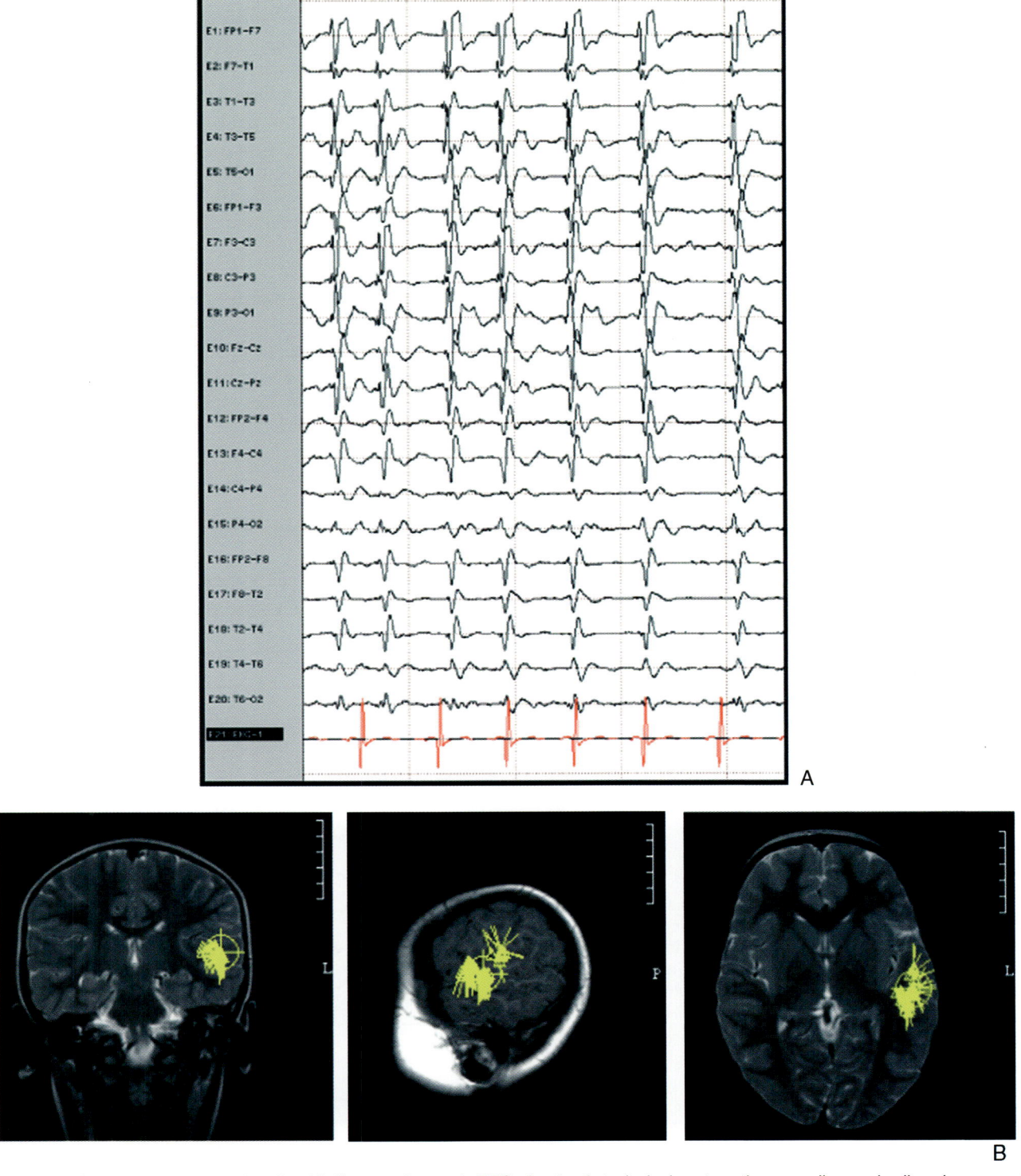

FIG. 16.7. MEG spike localization in Landau–Kleffner syndrome. **A.** EEG of patient's typical, almost continuous spikes and spike–slow-wave discharges recorded during sleep; discharges are widespread but consistently maximal over the left hemisphere. **B.** MEG spike dipole source estimates (yellow triangles; tails represent dipole vectors; circle represents a typical 95% confidence volume from a selected spike source) for those discharges seen on EEG are tightly localized to a relatively focal region in the deep left intrasylvian cortex.

predominant spike source in addition to bilateral synchronous paroxysms is not used. For cases with only bilaterally synchronous spike slow-wave discharges, MEG probably confers no particular advantage over EEG. For both methods, equally high temporal resolution requirements exist in order to separate sequential source activations within as little as 15 ms. Although this problem can be handled with very high recording sampling rates to address lateralization, localization remains difficult. Logically, the single ECD model should not be suited for valid localization. However, in the author's experience, the single ECD model may actually work in some instances, precisely because of its limitation of assuming one temporally isolated source.

Figure 16.8 provides an example of MEG lateralization of a patient with frontal lobe epilepsy and secondary bilateral synchrony. In this patient the single ECD model consistently lateralized the bisynchronous appearing discharges to the right. An explanation for this lateralization is put forward

based on the existence of sufficient temporal resolution at the onset of the discharges such that the model can be successful and will only be so for the primary source. Once activation of the secondary source has occurred the model will fail. Because of propagation latency variability, analysis of many discharges will not yield any localizable single dipole sources but, in those it does, the sources should be consistently lateralized to the primary side. This is one area of future MEG study that will most certainly be developed with more routine usage of multidipole spatiotemporal modeling.

Postsurgical Epilepsy Localization

Another unique application advantage of MEG over EEG is in patients who have had previous craniotomies and surgical resections. In these patients electrical potentials recorded at the scalp are distorted by cranial defects and the

FIG. 16.8. MEG spike localization in a patient with secondary bilateral synchrony. **A.** EEG showing widespread, bilateral epileptiform discharge with a left-sided amplitude emphasis (typical for this patient, although many discharges did not have any amplitude asymmetry). *Figure continued on facing page*

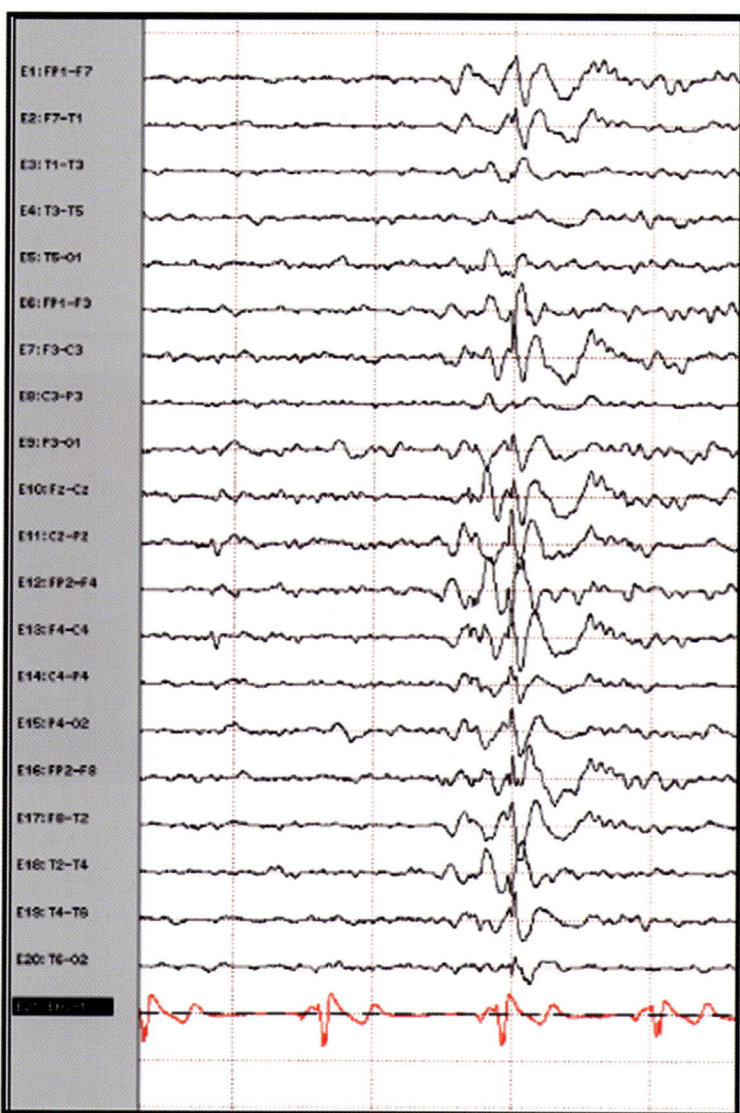

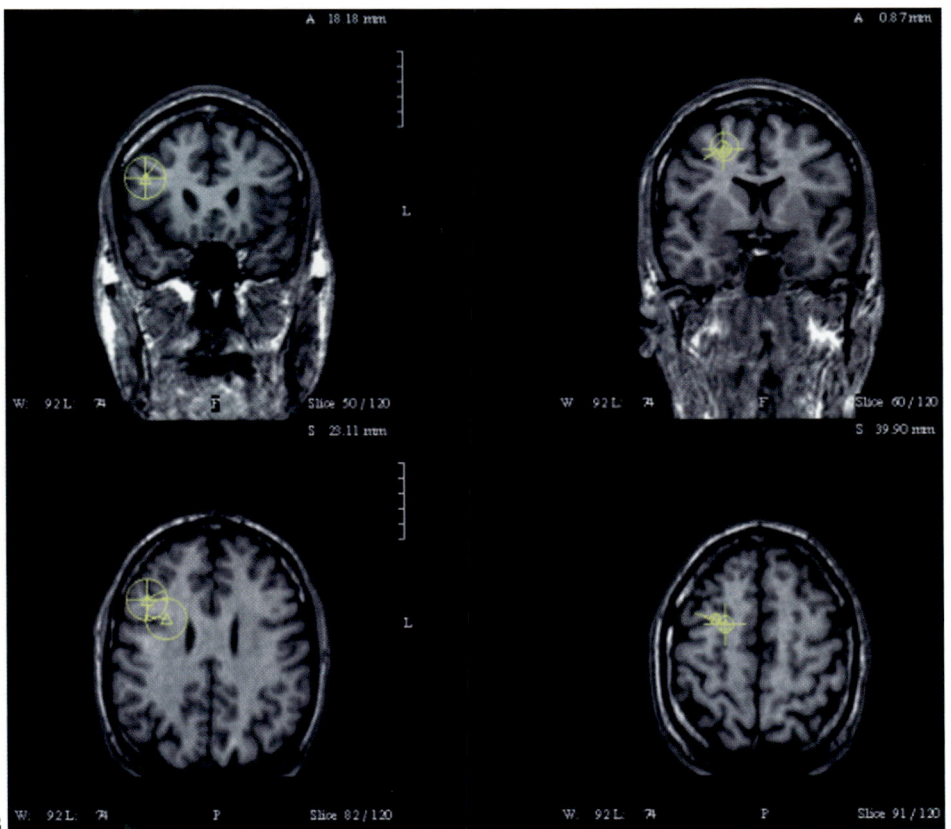

FIG. 16.8.—*Cont.* B. MEG spiked dipole source estimates (yellow triangles; tails represent dipole vectors; circle represents a typical 95% confidence volume from a selected spike source) were found consistently in the right frontal lobe. Following a large right frontal lobectomy, the patient became completely seizure-free, a result confirming secondary bilateral synchrony and localization.

biophysical disturbances of brain volume changes. This situation is particularly applicable in patients with recurrent seizures after epilepsy surgery for whom repeat surgery is contemplated. It has been confirmed with IC-EEG that MEG can be successful in localizing postsurgical epileptiform disturbances (72). Aiding or eliminating difficult repeat IC-EEG studies (because of dural adhesions) would be a true contribution for MEG. Further, prognostic studies are anticipated that evaluate more formally the extent of MEG spike sources included in the surgical resection cavities.

MAGNETOENCEPHALOGRAPHIC FUNCTIONAL LOCALIZATION

Localization of normal and abnormal task-specific function in the brain cannot rely on anatomic landmarks alone. Frameless stereotaxy systems have helped this situation greatly as they have become increasingly available. Certainly the capability of presurgical noninvasive structural imaging to guide intraoperative surgical approaches in real-time interactive fashion is valuable. However, this methodology remains limited if accurate mapping of function is not associated with structure.

Brain mapping (function localization mapped on structural anatomy) is now an established clinical tool of MEG with FDA approval and CPT codes in the United States. The basis

for this approval comes from numerous basic and clinical validation studies showing a high degree of accuracy for mapping of primary cortical functions, especially somatosensory and motor cortex. Conventional mapping with intraoperative ECoG with and without direct electrical cortical stimulation does not allow for preoperative planning and decision-making. The next section of this chapter reviews the most common methodologies of clinical MEG brain mapping, validation studies, and specific applications with case examples.

The goals of clinical imaging-based brain mapping are the same whether MEG or other functional imaging techniques are employed. Namely, it is expected that noninvasive preoperative mapping can provide aid in surgical decision-making (even whether to proceed with surgery), surgical planning strategy, and intraoperative guidance – all to optimize effectiveness of surgery with the least morbidity for significant neurologic deficits. Effectiveness of surgery typically includes maximal extent of resection (or disconnection) for tumors and other lesions, as well as epileptogenic tissue. Compromise in extent of resection due to inability to accurately define functional tissue can have consequences that are arguably as problematic as the deficits one is trying to avoid.

The basis of conventional MEG brain mapping is that of stimulus-induced magnetic field responses that can be recorded in a fashion analogous to electrical evoked potentials. By synchronizing recordings to task timing and averaging hundreds of stimulus epochs, strong SNRs can be obtained for multiple functional modalities to be adequately recorded and mapped. The advantage of MEG spatial resolution over EEG, as with spike source localization, rests on the near absence of attenuation and distortion of induced magnetic field as compared to evoked potentials. And if evoked cortical activation sources are focal and temporally isolated, MEG source localization can have a resolution on the order of millimeters (73, 74).

Moreover, when spatially separate predominant sources are sequentially activated, MEG allows temporal resolution (milliseconds) that is not possible with other functional imaging modalities. This type of resolution can be critical in mapping of complex cognitive functions such as language, where clinically important task-specific function may not be discerned among numerous scattered areas of increased rCBF as depicted with fMRI or [^{15}O]PET exams. Solving questions surrounding this problem is why MEG stands as a crucial component of future research in both basic and clinical brain mapping in spite of rapid advances in fMRI.

Primary somatosensory cortical localization is the most established clinical mapping method of MEG. It is noninvasive, can be rapidly performed, and is completely passive (allowing patients who are unable to cooperate or perform motor tasks to be studied). Numerous studies have examined MEG somatosensory mapping with respect to validity and effects on surgical decision-making (46, 74–79). The validation studies have mostly been performed with comparison to direct cortical stimulation (with both intraoperative maps and chronically implanted subdural grids). From these studies it is clear that the MEG somatosensory mapping is robust and accurate.

One difficulty with measuring comparisons of MEG to direct electrical stimulation to cortical surface must be emphasized. Even with the accuracy of image-based mapping comparison afforded by MEG data that is integrated with frameless stereotaxy systems (77, 79–81), direct measures of differences in localization cannot be performed because the intrinsic tendency of sulcal localizations with MEG versus surface maps with electrical stimulation.

Magnetoencephalographic somatosensory mapping employs various stimuli. The most common techniques use either airpuffs applied to skin surface or electrical stimulation of median and tibial nerves. Examinations typically require 256–512 repetitions for maximal SNRs with averaging. In contrast to electrical stimulation, the latency for the initial largest dipolar magnetic fields with airpuffs has a large variance across subjects and stimulus conditions – values for hand digit stimulation typically range from 35 to 70 ms. Major peaks at later latencies are also identified; these later peaks are believed to reflect processing in association cortices.

Detailed homuncular maps have been reported in normal subjects (73). Remarkably, most localizations of the main initial source mappings are found in the posterior bank of the central sulcus, generally following the Penfield homunculus (82), including some variation into the precentral gyrus.

In presurgical studies, mapping is usually confined to a few digits, toes, and lip for practical purposes. These examinations can be completed within 1–2 hours with results integrated into frameless stereotaxy systems for intraoperative use. However, one of the greatest values of MEG mapping studies is aiding the preoperative planning of surgery, especially surgical approaches in patients with distorted anatomy from lesions, abnormalities that can preclude accurate predictions of sensory-motor function localization based on anatomy (74, 79). Figure 16.9 shows the mapping of digit somatosensory function in a patient with a left central/rolandic tumor. In this case an initial biopsy was performed, taking an anterior approach in the belief that primary sensory-motor cortex was located at the posterior margin of the lesion. After the biopsy the patient had a transient right hemiparesis. When mapping was performed for planning surgical resection, the anterior margin of the tumor was shown to be the location of primary somatosensory cortex.

Motor mapping can be performed by synchronizing movement initiation to electromyographic (EMG) input. As with evoked electrical potentials a premovement 'readiness potential' or 'Bereitschaftspotential' can be recorded as an MEG readiness field (RF), lasting approximately 500 ms and occurring 1–2 seconds before EMG onset (83). Motor evoked fields begin with peaks 20–50 ms after EMG onset, followed by variable but typically identified larger-amplitude components occurring at approximately 100, 200, and 300 ms after movement onset. A postmotor field may be detected at latencies between 400 and 500 ms (83). The problem with mapping motor activated neural activity for clinical purposes is the complexity as compared to primary somatomotor sensory mapping. In fact, even with simple spontaneous repetitive finger movement, proprioceptive activation of sensory cortex may predominate, for a significant proportion of neural activation with motor mapping is localized to the postcentral gyrus.

Cortical Reorganization

In a further extension of the concept of mapping function location altered by pathology, is that of cortical reorganization (plasticity) resulting from early acquired or developmental lesions. Even more than with late acquired mass lesions such as tumors, congenital or early childhood alterations of normal anatomic development can result in anomalous, unpredictable localization of function. The implications of this issue arise not infrequently in the surgical treatment of epilepsy where epileptogenic substrates are commonly malformations of cortical development or early-acquired brain injuries such as perinatal strokes. In such cases, knowledge of alterations in function localization may play a critical role in surgical decision-making. This includes the decision to proceed with surgery or not as well as decisions about the extent of resection; all that can effect seizure outcome.

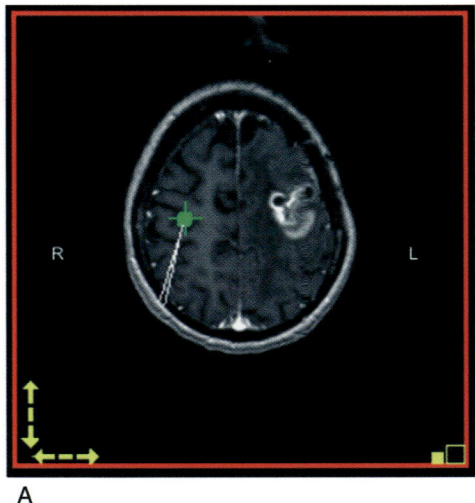 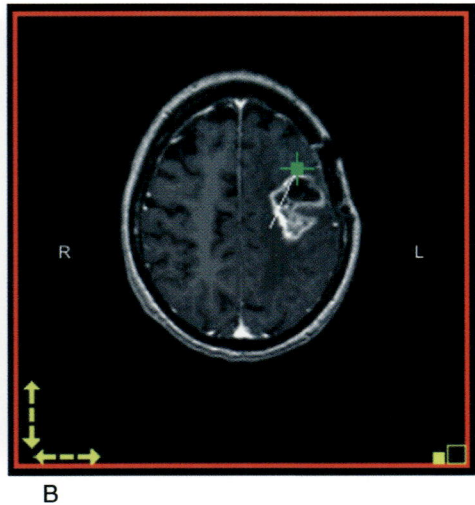

A   B

FIG. 16.9. MEG somatosensory mapping (SOM) in a central/rolandic tumor case. **A.** MEG SOM of left second finger activation (green squares; tails represent dipole vectors) localizes to the central sulcus in the unaffected right hemisphere. **B.** MEG SOM of right second finger activation localizes to the anterior margin of the left hemisphere tumor, an unexpected finding, as the primary motor and sensory cortex was suspected to be at the posterior margin of the tumor based on anatomic landmarks alone.

One example regarding the decision to proceed with surgery is that of hemispherectomy in patients with static lesions who have diminished but important residual motor-sensory function in affected limbs. Figure 16.10 shows the somatosensory mapping in a patient with large perinatal infarct involving the entire middle cerebral artery. Left side digit stimulation activated left hemisphere intrasylvian inferior parietal cortex. Following complete right anatomic hemispherectomy the patient became seizure-free and incurred no neurologic sensory-motor deficits.

Malformations of cortical development create particular challenges. First, the extent of epileptogenic pathology necessary to resect with resulting seizure-free outcome is usually greater than the lesion seen on MRI. This leads to the need for aggressive resections that often may encroach into functionally important tissue, cortex requiring careful delineation in order to obtain optimal resection. Second, the location of eloquent function may be anomalous, depending on the nature of the malformation. Figure 16.11 shows the somatosensory mapping of patients with complex malformations of cortical development, including extensive perirolandic polymicrogyria. Localizations of cortical activity from sensory stimulations of the digits and lip are within the malformation in what would be the best anatomic estimate

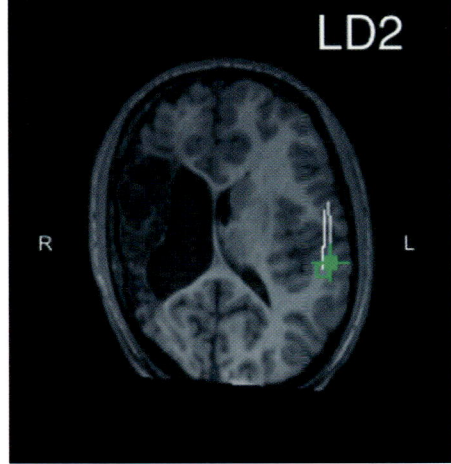 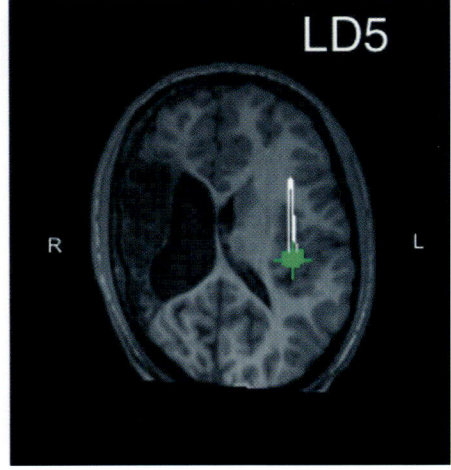

FIG. 16.10. MEG somatosensory mapping (SOM) in a patient with intractable epilepsy symptomatic of an early (perinatal) right middle cerebral artery stroke. SOM of left second and fifth finger (LD2 and LD5) activations – both in the left hemisphere. These localizations demonstrate complete reorganization of hemisphere lateralization. Additionally, the inferior parietal cortical localization represents aberrant intrahemispheric localization – centimeters inferior to typical rolandic homuncular localization for hand digits.

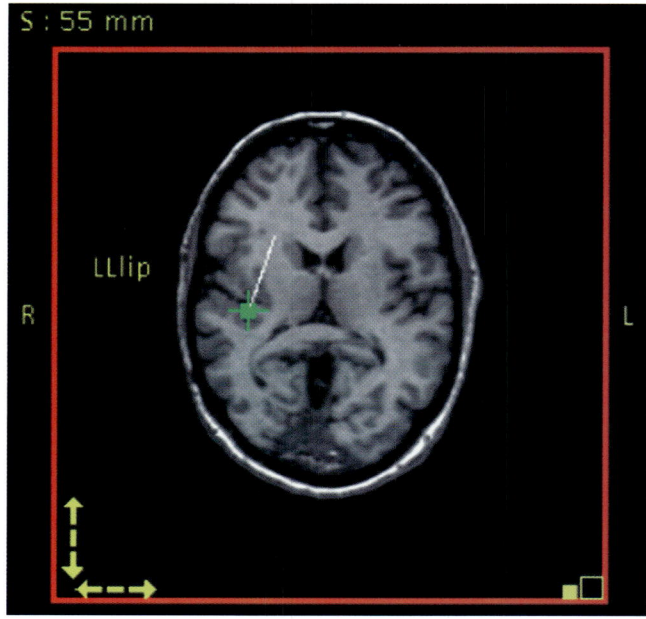

A

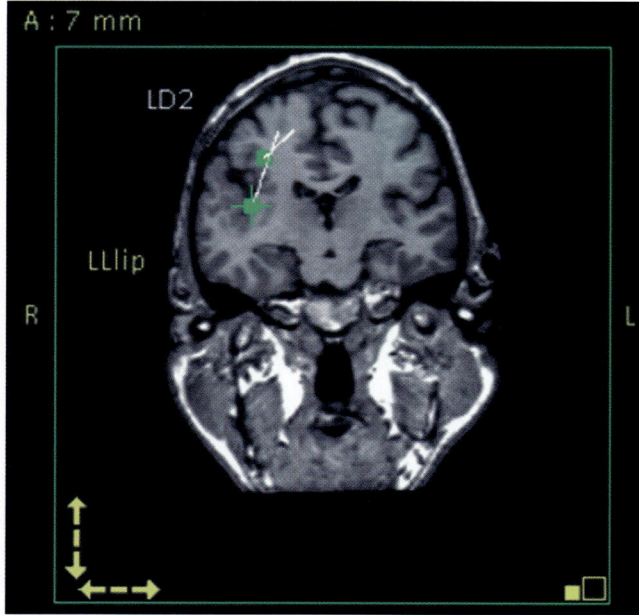

B

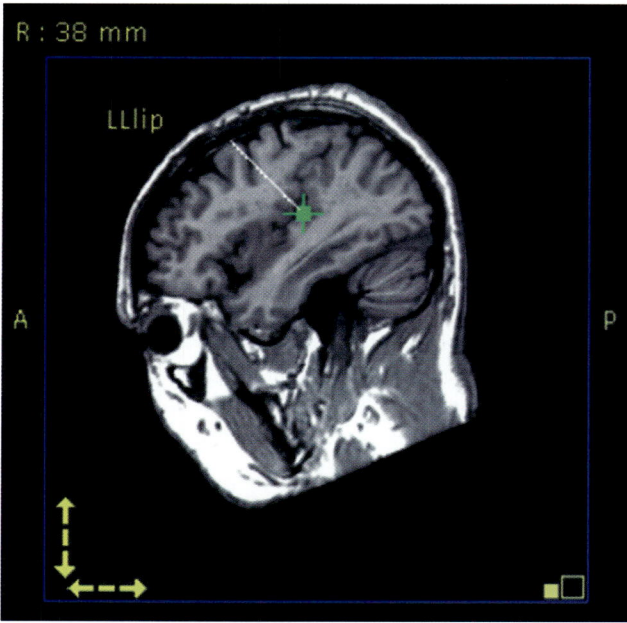

C

FIG. 16.11. MEG somatosensory mapping (SOM) in a patient with intractable epilepsy symptomatic of a malformation of cortical development. SOM localizations are overlaid on the patient's MRI (**A.** Transverse, **B.** Coronal, and **C.** Sagittal). In spite of the distorted anatomy, SOM of the left lower lip (Lllip) and the second digit of the left hand (LD2) activations are within the malformation – polymicrogyria – in what would be the best anatomic estimate for such activations based on typical homuncular organization.

for such activations based on typical homuncular organization. In contrast, localization of function in patients with absence of developed brain or when severe true dysplasias are present in anatomic areas expected to serve primary function is expected to be reorganized in a fashion that cannot be predicted without functional mapping.

Other sensory modality localizations with MEG, including visual and auditory mapping, show similar behavior to somatosensory mapping in the presence of various developmental or early-acquired lesions (84). Primary auditory cortex can be exquisitely mapped with MEG in response to tones, vowels, synthesized words, and other types of acoustic or phonetic stimulation (85). Very reproducible, tightly organized, tonotopic maps are demonstrated in the posterior planum of the superior temporal gyrus (86). The most prominent peak upon which auditory mapping is based is located at approximately 100 ms (m100), and is typically larger in amplitude and slightly earlier in cortex contralateral to the stimulation. The high degree of accuracy and reproducibility of m100 organization allows for sensitive detection of mapping derangements related to clinical disorders, including schizophrenia and epilepsy (87, 88).

A good example is the case of a patient with focal cryptogenic (normal MRI) neocortical TLE in whom auditory cortex mapping was shifted downward into the middle temporal gyrus. The patient's seizures and spikes were localized predominantly in the superior temporal gyrus, where focal cortical dysplasia with Taylor type II balloon cells was present as revealed under histopathologic exam following surgical resection. All such cases simply emphasize the complexity and unpredictable mapping of a common group of epilepsy patients who frequently undergo surgical evaluation and treatment for intractable seizures. MEG in such cases allows a combined approach to solving the difficult localization questions for both the epilepsy and functional mapping in a noninvasive fashion and like no other imaging modality.

CONCLUSIONS

The application of MEG to epilepsy localization is no longer a technological tool in development. Over the past several years the evolution to whole-head systems capable of routine clinical examination has been realized. Reports validating accurate estimation of focal epileptiform spike sources have come from multiple levels of concordance with other methods of epilepsy localization ranging from colocalization with visible epileptogenic lesions to confirmation by both subsequent and simultaneous implanted IC-EEG recordings.

The greatest value of epilepsy MEG source localization is in patients with neocortical seizure disorders. It is increasingly clear that if the epileptogenic zone is neocortical (especially in the dorsal lateral convexity or lateral temporal lobe) and characterized by tightly clustered unifocal spikes on MEG, then it is likely that IC-EEG recordings will add little to the evaluation. In such patients, even if no lesion is visible on MRI, focal deficits are frequently seen on functional imaging that are concordant with MEG. As more formal experience is gained with this subgroup of patients, it is expected that IC-EEG can be avoided in more patients.

Some specific epilepsy localization issues can be addressed by intrinsic attributes of MEG. LKS is one issue in particular in which MEG appears to be clearly at an advantage to evaluate for presurgical localization. MEG is uniquely capable of resolving localization of the complex primary intrasylvian epileptiform disturbances associated with LKS. In similar fashion, secondary bilateral synchrony can be addressed with MEG, although more routine investigation with multidipole spatiotemporal analysis should be performed. Advances in MEG localization of nonepileptiform disturbances (focal slowing) may offer additional sensitivity and delineation of epileptogenic pathology that can be gained without the necessity of capturing sometimes infrequent epileptiform discharges. Finally, because there is less distortion from cranial defects, MEG allows better evaluation of patients with prior craniotomies and surgical resections, in particular patients with unsuccessful prior epilepsy surgery for whom repeat surgery is contemplated.

The limitations of MEG need to be recognized. Deep sources of epileptiform activity still cannot be detected without extensive propagation of neuronal activation; for example, spikes originating from the hippocampus have to propagate over several square centimeters of basal or lateral temporal cortex to be detected in spontaneous recordings. Also, since typical recordings are of interictal epileptiform activity, even if MEG source localization attempts are successful and accurate, findings may not necessarily reflect where seizures begin. Fortunately, in the vast majority of cases in which MEG reveals well localized, mostly unifocal epileptiform disturbances, ictal IC-EEG has shown concordant ictal onset zones. Furthermore, ictal MEG can be performed in a substantial number of patients who have frequent seizures, which is often the case of those with extratemporal lobe epilepsy. Additionally, an exciting opportunity arises that specific characterization of interictal MEG spike localization can be discovered that predicts reliability of epilepsy localization and surgical prognosis.

The ultimate goal of completely noninvasive presurgical epilepsy evaluations can be met with the combination of epilepsy localization with brain mapping (of eloquent cortical function). MEG is particularly well suited to contribute greatly to this goal, as it is a tool capable of accomplishing both tasks.

ACKNOWLEDGMENTS

Robert Knowlton's work was supported by an NIH/NINDS sponsored Mentored Clinical Scientist Development Award. K-23 NS02218–01

William Sutherling's work was supported by Public Health Service research grants RO1 NS20806 from the Epilepsy Branch, National Institute of Neurological Diseases and Stroke; shared instrumentation grant S10 RR13276 from the National Center for Research Resources, research grant RO1 MH53213 from the National Institutes of Mental Health.

REFERENCES

1. Gallen C, Hirschkoff E, Buchanan D. Magnetoencephalography and magnetic source imaging. *Neuroimag Clin North Am* 1995;5:227–249.
2. Ricci GB, Romani GL, Salustri C, et al. Study of focal epilepsy by multichannel neuromagnetic measurements. *Electroencephalogr Clin Neurophysiol* 1987;66:358–368.
3. Ebersole JS. Magnetoencephalography/magnetic source imaging in the assessment of patients with epilepsy. *Epilepsia* 1997;38(Suppl 4):S1–S5.
4. Scherg M. Functional imaging and localization of electromagnetic brain activity. *Brain Topogr* 1992;5:103–112.
5. Ebersole JS. Non-invasive pre-surgical evaluation with EEG/MEG source analysis. *Electroencephalogr Clin Neurophysiol Suppl* 1999;50:167–174.
6. Laxer KD, Garcia PA. Magnetic resonance imaging, magnetic resonance spectroscopy, positron emission tomography scanning, and single photon emission tomography. *Neurosurg Clin North Am* 1993;4:199–209.

7. Sutherling WW, Crandall PH, Cahan LD, Barth DS. The magnetic field of epileptic spikes agrees with intracranial localizations in complex partial epilepsy. *Neurology* 1988;38:778–786.

8. Balish M, Sato S, Connaughton P, Kufta C. Localization of implanted dipoles by magnetoencephalography. *Neurology* 1991;41:1072–1076.

9. Rose DF, Sato S, Ducla-Soares E, Kufta CV. Magnetoencephalographic localization of subdural dipoles in a patient with temporal lobe epilepsy. *Epilepsia* 1991;32:635–641.

10. Paetau R, Kajola M, Karhu J, et al. Magnetoencephalographic localization of epileptic cortex – impact on surgical treatment. *Ann Neurol* 1992;32:106–109.

11. Stefan H, Schneider S, Feistel H, et al. Ictal and interictal activity in partial epilepsy recorded with multichannel magneto-electroencephalography: correlation of electroencephalography/ electrocorticography, magnetic resonance imaging, single photon emission computed tomography, and positron emission tomography findings. *Epilepsia* 1992;33:874–887.

12. Ioannides AA, Muratore R, Balish M, Sato S. In vivo validation of distributed source solutions for the biomagnetic inverse problem. *Brain Topogr* 1993;5:263–273.

13. Nakasato N, Levesque MF, Barth DS, et al. Comparisons of MEG, EEG, and ECoG source localization in neocortical partial epilepsy in humans. *Electroencephalogr Clin Neurophysiol* 1994;91:171–178.

14. Smith JR, Gallen C, Orrison W, et al. Role of multichannel magnetoencephalography in the evaluation of ablative seizure surgery candidates. *Stereotact Funct Neurosurg* 1994;62:238–244.

15. Knowlton RC, Laxer KD, Aminoff MJ, et al. Magnetoencephalography in partial epilepsy: clinical yield and localization accuracy. *Ann Neurol* 1997;42:622–631.

16. Minassian BA, Otsubo H, Weiss S, et al. Magnetoencephalographic localization in pediatric epilepsy surgery: comparison with invasive intracranial electroencephalography. *Ann Neurol* 1999;46:627–633.

17. Wheless JW, Willmore LJ, Breier JI, et al. A comparison of magnetoencephalography, MRI, and V-EEG in patients evaluated for epilepsy surgery. *Epilepsia* 1999;40:931–941.

18. Mamelak AN, Lopez N, Akhtari M, Sutherling WW. Magneto-encephalography-directed surgery in patients with neocortical epilepsy. *J Neurosurg* 2002;97:865–873.

19. Hamalainen M, Hari R, Ilmoniemi R, et al. Magnetoencephalography – theory, instrumentation, and applications to noninvasive studies of the working human brain. *Rev Mod Physics* 1993;65:413–497.

20. Feynman RP, Leighton RB, Sands M. The Feynman lectures on physics. Vol. III. Quantum mechanics. New York: Addison-Wesley, 1965.

21. Rose-Innes AC, Rhoderick EH. Introduction to superconductivity, 2nd ed. New York: Pergamon Press, 1978.

22. Cooper A, Winter A, Crow H, Walter W. Comparison of subcortical, cortical, and scalp activity using chronically indwelling electrodes in man. *Electroenceph Clin Neurophysiol* 1965:217–228.

23. Baumgartner C, Barth D, Levesque M, et al. Detection sensitivity of spontaneous magnetoencephalography spike recordings in frontal lobe epilepsy. *Epilepsia* 1989;30:665.

24. Stok C. The influence of model parameters on EEG/MEG single dipole source estimation. *IEEE Trans Biomed Eng* 1987;34:289–296.

25. Buchner H, Knoll G, Fuchs M, et al. Inverse localization of electric dipole current sources in finite element models of the human head. *Electroenceph Clin Neurophysiol* 1997;102:276–278.

26. Van den Broek SP, Reinder F, Donderwinkel M, Peters MJ. Volume conduction effects in EEG and MEG. *Electroenceph Clin Neurophysiol* 1998;106:522–534.

27. Fuchs M, Wagner M, Wischmann HA, et al. Improving source reconstructions by combining bioelectric and biomagnetic data. *Electroenceph Clin Neurophysiol* 1998;107:93–111.

28. Yan Y, Nunez P, Hart R. Finite-element model of the human head: scalp potentials due to dipole sources. *Med Biol Eng Comput* 1991:475–481.

29. Hamalainen M, Sarvas J. Realistic conductivity geometry model of the human head for interpretation of neuromagnetic data. *IEEE Tran Biomed Eng* 1989;36:165–171.

30. Sarvas J. Basic mathematical and electromagnetic concepts of the biomagnetic inverse problem. *Phys Med Biol* 1987;32:11–22.

31. Megis J, Peters MJ, Oosterom V. Computation of MEGs and EEGs using a realistically shaped multicompartment model of the head. *Med Biol Eng Comput* 1985;23:36–37.

32. Barth DS, Baugartner C, Sutherling W. Neuromagnetic field modeling of multiple brain regions producing interictal spikes in human epilepsy. *Electroenceph Clin Neurophysiol* 1989;73:389–402.

33. Sinstra JG, Peters MJ. The volume conductor may act as a temporal filter on the ECG and EEG. *Med Biol Eng Comput* 1998;36:711–716.

34. Akhtari M, Bryant H, Mamelak A, et al. Conductivities of three-layer human skull. *Brain Topogr* 2000;13:1–4.

35. Akhtari M, Bryant HC, Mamelak AN, et al. Conductivities of three-layer live human skull. *Brain Topogr* 2002;14:151–167.

36. Leahy RM, Mosher JC, Spencer ME, et al. A study of dipole localization accuracy for MEG and EEG using a human skull phantom. *Electroenceph Clin Neurophysiol* 1998;107:159–173.

37. Mosher J, Spencer M, Leahy R, Lewis P. Error bounds for EEG and MEG dipole source localization. *Electroenceph Clin Neurophysiol* 1993;86:303–320.

38. Fuchs M, Drenckhahn R, Wischmann HA, Wagner M. An improved boundary element method for realistic volume-conductor modeling. *Trans Biomed Eng* 1998;45:980–997.

39. Lueders H, Daube J, Johnson J, Klass D. Computer analysis of generalized spike-and-wave complexes. *Epilepsia* 1980;21:183.

40. Rogers R, Basile L, Taylor S, et al. Laterality of hippocampal responses to infrequent and unpredictable omissions of visual stimuli. *Brain Topogr* 1996;9:15–20.

41. Sutherling WW, Akhtari M, Mamelak AN, et al. Dipole localization of human induced focal afterdischarge seizure in simultaneous magnetoencephalography and electrocorticography. *Brain Topogr* 2001;14:101–116.

42. Wood C, Cohen D, Cuffin B, et al. Electrical sources in the human somatosensory cortex: Identification by combined magnetic and electric potential recordings. *Science* 1985:1051–1053.

43. Sutherling W, Barth D. Selective EEG electrode triggering of averaged magnetic data reduces the constraints of the inverse problem of neuromagnetic localization: a principle of relativity in the nervous system due to finite conduction delays. *Phys Med Biol* 1987;32:143–144.

44. Sutherling WW, Barth DS. Neocortical propagation in temporal lobe spike foci on magnetoencephalography and electroencephalography. *Ann Neurol* 1989;25:373–381.

45. Gallen C, Sobel D, Lewine J, et al. Neuromagnetic mapping of brain function. *Radiology* 1993;187:863–867.

46. Sobel D, Gallen C, Schwartz B, et al. Locating the central sulcus: comparison of MR anatomic and magneto encephalographic functional methods. *Am J Neuroradiol* 1993;14:915–925.

47. Sutherling W. Localization precision of whole cortex neuro-magnetometer system for human epilepsy studies. *Epilepsia* 2001; 42 (supp 7).

48. Mosher J, Spencer M, Leahy R, Lewis P. Source localization using recursively applied and projected (RAP) MUSIC. *IEEE Trans Signal Process* 1999;47:332–340.

49. Cuffin B, Cohen D. Comparison of the magnetoencephalogram and electroencephalogram. *Electroenceph Clin Neurophysiol* 1979: 132–146.

50. Mikuni N, Nagamine T, Ikeda A, et al. Simultaneous recording of epileptiform discharges by MEG and subdural electrodes in temporal lobe epilepsy. *Neuroimage* 1997;5:298–306.

51. Oishi M, Otsubo H, Kameyama S, et al. Epileptic spikes: magnetoencephalography versus simultaneous electrocorticography. *Epilepsia* 2002;43:1390–1395.

52. Shigeto H, Morioka T, Hisada K, et al. Feasibility and limitations of magnetoencephalographic detection of epileptic discharges: simultaneous recording of magnetic fields and electrocorticography. *Neurol Res* 2002;24:531–536.

53. Stefan H, Schneider S, Abraham-Fuchs K, et al. Magnetic source localization in focal epilepsy. Multichannel magnetoencephalography correlated with magnetic resonance brain imaging. *Brain* 1990; 113:1347–1359.

54. Minami T, Tasaki K, Yamamoto T, et al. Magneto-encephalographical analysis of focal cortical heterotopia. *Dev Med Child Neurol* 1996;38:945–949.

55. Taniguchi M, Yoshimine T, Kato A, et al. Dysembryoplastic neuroepithelial tumor in the insular cortex. Three dimensional magnetoencephalographic localization of epileptic discharges. *Neurol Res* 1998;20:433–438.

56. Lamusuo S, Forss N, Ruottinen HM, et al. [¹⁸F]FDG-PET and whole-scalp MEG localization of epileptogenic cortex. *Epilepsia* 1999;40: 921–930.

57. Morioka T, Nishio S, Ishibashi H, et al. Intrinsic epileptogenicity of focal cortical dysplasia as revealed by magnetoencephalography and electrocorticography. *Epilepsy Res* 1999;33:177–187.

58. Otsubo H, Sharma R, Elliott I, et al. Confirmation of two magnetoencephalographic epileptic foci by invasive monitoring from subdural electrodes in an adolescent with right frontocentral epilepsy. *Epilepsia* 1999;40:608–613.

59. Baumgartner C, Pataraia E, Lindinger G, Deecke L. Neuromagnetic recordings in temporal lobe epilepsy. *J Clin Neurophysiol* 2000; 17:177–189.

60. Otsubo H, Ochi A, Elliott I, et al. MEG predicts epileptic zone in lesional extrahippocampal epilepsy: 12 pediatric surgery cases. *Epilepsia* 2001;42:1523–1530.

61. Ebersole JS, Squires K, Gamelin J, et al. Dipole models of temporal lobe spikes from simultaneous MEG and EEG. In: Bea C, ed. Biomagnetism: fundamental research and clinical applications. Amsterdam: Elsevier Science, 1995: 20–22.

62. Ishibashi H, Morioka T, Shigeto H, et al. Three-dimensional localization of subclinical ictal activity by magnetoencephalography: correlation with invasive monitoring. *Surg Neurol* 1998; 50:157–163.

63. Oishi M, Kameyama S, Morota N, et al. Fusiform gyrus epilepsy: the use of ictal magnetoencephalography. Case report. *J Neurosurg* 2002;97:200–204.

64. Eliashiv DS, Elsas SM, Squires K, et al. Ictal magnetic source imaging as a localizing tool in partial epilepsy. *Neurology* 2002;59:1600–1610.

65. Iwasaki M, Nakasato N, Shamoto H, et al. Surgical implications of neuromagnetic spike localization in temporal lobe epilepsy. *Epilepsia* 2002;43:415–424.

66. Landau WM, Kleffner F. Syndrome of acquired aphasia with convulsive disorder in children. *Neurology* 1957;7:523–530.

67. Paetau R, Granstrom ML, Blomstedt G, et al. Magnetoencephalography in presurgical evaluation of children with the Landau–Kleffner syndrome. *Epilepsia* 1999;40:326–335.

68. Sobel DF, Aung M, Otsubo H, Smith MC. Magnetoencephalography in children with Landau–Kleffner syndrome and acquired epileptic aphasia. *Am J Neuroradiol* 2000;21:301–307.

69. Gallen CC, Tecoma E, Iragui V, et al. Magnetic source imaging of abnormal low-frequency magnetic activity in presurgical evaluations of epilepsy. *Epilepsia* 1997;38:452–460.

70. Ishibashi H, Simos PG, Castillo EM, et al. Detection and significance of focal, interictal, slow-wave activity visualized by magnetoencephalography for localization of a primary epileptogenic region. *J Neurosurg* 2002;96:724–730.

71. Blume WT, Pillay N. Electrographic and clinical correlates of secondary bilateral synchrony. *Epilepsia* 1985;26:636–641.

72. Kirchberger K, Hummel C, Stefan H. Postoperative multichannel magnetoencephalography in patients with recurrent seizures after epilepsy surgery. *Acta Neurol Scand* 1998;98:1–7.

73. Yang TT, Gallen CC, Schwartz BJ, Bloom FE. Noninvasive somatosensory homunculus mapping in humans by using a large-array biomagnetometer. *Proc Natl Acad Sci USA* 1993;90:3098–3102.

74. Gallen C, Sobel D, Waltz T, et al. Noninvasive presurgical neuromagnetic mapping of somatosensory cortex. *Neurosurgery* 1993; 33:260–268.

75. Sutherling WW, Crandall PH, Darcey TM, et al. The magnetic and electric fields agree with intracranial localizations of somatosensory cortex. *Neurology* 1988;38:1705–1714.

76. Orrison WW, Rose DF, Hart BL, et al. Noninvasive preoperative cortical localization by magnetic source imaging. *Am J Neuroradiol* 1992;13:1124–1128.

77. Gallen CC, Bucholz R, Sobel DF. Intracranial neurosurgery guided by functional imaging. *Surg Neurol* 1994;42:523–530.

78. Gallen CC, Schwartz BJ, Bucholz RD, et al. Presurgical localization of functional cortex using magnetic source imaging. *J Neurosurg* 1995;82:988–994.

79. Roberts TPL, Zusman E, McDermott M, et al. Correlation of functional magnetic source imaging with intraoperative cortical stimulation in neurosurgical patients. *J Image Guided Surg* 1995;1:339–347.

80. Rezai AR, Hund M, Kronberg E, et al. The interactive use of magnetoencephalography in stereotactic image-guided neurosurgery. *Neurosurgery* 1996;39:92–102.

81. Rezai AR, Mogilner AY, Cappell J, et al. Integration of functional brain mapping in image-guided neurosurgery. *Acta Neurochir* 1997;68(Suppl):85–89.

82. Penfield W, Bouldrey E. Somatic motor and sensory representation in the cerebral cortex of man as studied by electrical stimulation. *Brain* 1937;60:389–443.

83. Kristeva R, Cheyne D, Deecke L. Neuromagnetic fields accompanying unilateral and bilateral voluntary movements: topography and analysis of cortical sources. *Electroencephalogr Clin Neurophysiol* 1991;81: 284–298.

84. Nakasato N, Seki K, Kawamura T, et al. Functional brain mapping using an MRI-linked whole head magnetoencephalography (MEG) system. *Funct Neurosci* 1996;(EEG Suppl. 46):32–39.

85. Starr A, Kristeva R, Cheyne D, et al. Localization of brain activity during auditory verbal short-term memory derived from magnetic recordings. *Brain Res* 1991;558:181–190.

86. Pantev C, Bertrand O, Eulitz C, et al. Specific tonotopic organizations of different areas of the human auditory cortex revealed by simultaneous magnetic and electric recordings. *Electroencephalogr Clin Neurophysiol* 1995;94:26–40.

87. Rowley HA, Knowlton RC, Roberts TP, Laxer KD. Value of MEG and image coregistration in an unusual case of neocortical epilepsy. *Neurology* 1995;45:314.

88. Rojas DC, Bawn SD, Carlson JP, et al. Alterations in tonotopy and auditory cerebral asymmetry in schizophrenia. *Biol Psychiatry* 2002; 52:32–39.

Index

Agyria–Pachygyria complex 230–2

Ambiguous genitalia 232

Ammon's horn sclerosis 104

AMT PET, tryptophan metabolism 407

Amygdala sclerosis 108, 135

Anaplastic oligodendroglioma 185

Animal models, fMRI/EEG 311

Anisotropic diffusion 316

Anterior temporal lobe (AT)
    abnormalities, magnetic resonance imaging (MRI) 141–6
    changes in 143–5
    histopathologic findings 143
    signal change 144, 145

Antiepileptic drugs 356–7, 362–3

Apparent diffusion coefficient (ADC) 27, 316–17, 319, 323

Arbitrary associative learning 273, 276–7

Arterial spin-labeling (ASL) 28, 282–3, 285, 319, 321
    long transit times 322

Arteriovenous malformation (AVM) 158

Astrocytic neoplasms, magnetic resonance imaging (MRI) 153

Astrocytic tumors 151–2

Astrocytoma 154

Asymmetric field of view 23

Atomic nuclei, magnetic properties of 18–19

Atrophic sclerosis 200

Aura 100

Autosomal dominant nocturnal frontal lobe epilepsy 9

Bacterial abscess 213

Bacterial infections 212–13

Balloon cells
    focal cortical dysplasia (FCD) with 186–7, 224–6
    focal cortical dysplasia (FCD) without 243

Band heterotopia 238–9

Behavioral abnormalities 400

Benzodiazepine receptor studies 392

Beta-hydroxybutyrate, measurement of 342–3

Bilateral frontoparietal polymicrogyria 242

Bilateral open lip schizencephaly 243

Bilateral temporal lobe epilepsy 278

Blood-oxygenation-level-dependent contrast see BOLD
    BOLD contrast 282, 299, 312
    BOLD fMRI 283, 292
    BOLD functional magnetic resonance imaging 282
    BOLD images 284
    BOLD response 306
    BOLD signals 284–5, 301, 310–11

Bolus tracking magnetic resonance imaging 320–2, 329
    deconvolution analysis 320
    summary parameters 320–1

Brain, magnetic field 414

Brain anatomy 29–96
    inferior aspect 37
    overview 29–30

Brain damage, seizure-induced 10–11

Brain development 100

Brain mapping 417–21
    MEG 425

Brain metabolites, signal strength 20–1

^{13}C spectroscopy 348–50, 377
    information content 348
    polarization transfer methods 349

Calcification involving frontal lobe 135

Callosal agenesis 233

Callosal hypogenesis 234

Carbamazepine 357

Cavernous angiomas 159–60, 186

Cell proliferation 221

Cellular glutamate 356–7
    in hippocampus 357

Central nervous system (CNS)
    infections 209–14
    NAA in 367–8

Cerebral artery infarction 199

Cerebral blood flow (CBF) 27, 281, 283, 285, 319–20, 327, 329
    in partial seizures 385

Cerebral blood volume (CBV) 320, 327, 329

Cerebral cortex, development of see Cortical development

Cerebrospinal fluid (CSF) 112, 125, 252

Chemical shift 19–20
Chemical shift imaging (CSI) 19
Childhood, FDG PET in 398–400
Choline, measurement of 339–40
Cholinergic receptor studies 392
Cingulate gyrus seizures 179
Classical sclerosis 107
Cobblestone cortex 233
Cognitive abnormalities 400
Complex partial seizures (CPS) 100, 139
Congenital hemiplegia 241
Congenital muscular dystrophies 233
Congenital right body hemiplegia 142
Continuous ASL (CASL) 321
    perfusion studies 328–9
Cortex, abnormality 147
Cortical development
    categories of malformations 224
    cellular stages 222
    imaging of malformations 222–4
    imaging techniques 223–4
    major processes 221–2
    principles of 221–2
Cortical dysplasia, occipital lobe 194
Cortical excitability and GABA content 361
Cortical lobar displasia 187
Cortical malformations 3, 184–8, 221–48
    classification 223
    secondary to abnormal cortical organization 239–43
    secondary to abnormal neuronal migration 230–9
    secondary to abnormal stem cell formation 224–30
Cortical mantle, shape analysis 254–6
Cortical reorganization, MEG 426–9
Cortical stimulation mapping 290
Cortical thickness measurements 256–7
Cortical tube 228–9
Cranial injuries 160
Creatine, measurement of 339–40
Curvilinear multiplanar reformatting (CMPR) 250–1
Cystic cavity secondary to neonatal intraparenchymal
    bleed 199
Cysticercosis 215–16

Declarative memory, functional neuroanatomy of 273
2-Deoxy-2[S18sF]fluoro-D-glucose (FDG) 395
Diffuse prenatal anoxia 201
Diffusion, use of term 315
Diffusion imaging, applications 322–7
Diffusion tensor imaging (DTI) 27, 316
    biologic applications 316–19
    fiber-tracking 317–19
    orientation-independent parameters 316–17
Diffusion-weighted imaging (DWI) 315–16
    mechanisms of signal changes 319
Double cortex 238–9

Dual pathology 137–40
Dynamic susceptibility contrast (DSC) MRI 319
Dysembryoplastic neuroepithelial tumors (DNT) 153–8

Echinococcosis 217
Echo planar imaging (EPI) 26
EEG 5, 7, 205, 249, 351
    and MEG 415–16
    combined with functional MRI (fMRI) see fMRI/EEG
    Rasmussen's encephalitis 208
    temporal lobe epilepsy (TLE) 101–2
    see also fMRI/EEG
EEG–MEG, intracranial studies 417
Electrocorticographic (ECoG) spikes 415
Electroecephalography see EEG
Electroencephalogram 2–3
Electrophysiological data 13
Encephalomalacia 183
End-folium sclerosis 107
Engel JJ 6
Epidemiology of epilepsy 7
Epilepsy
    basic mechanisms 8
    classification 1–7
    definitions 1–7
    epidemiology 7
    important concepts 4
    international classification 6
    introduction to 1–16
    mechanisms 7
    MR-negative 132
    origin of modern view 1
    prevalence 7
    terminology 1–7
    unified model 10
Epilepsy syndromes 5–7
Epileptic focus and hippocampal sclerosis (HS) 108
Epileptic seizures see Seizures
Epileptic seizures, temporal lobe epilepsy (TLE) 100
Epileptogenesis
    after initial precipitating event 149
    mechanisms 7
    modern view 8
    secondary 10
Epileptogenic lesion 11
Epileptogenic region 11
Extrahippocampal lesion 140
Extrahippocampal pathology associated with hippocampal
    sclerosis 137–40
Extratemporal lobe epilepsy 422
    FDG PET 397–8
    FMZ PET 406–8
    magnetic resonance imaging (MRI) 177–96
    proton magnetic resonance spectroscopy 375
Extratemporal lobe seizures, surface coil study 189

FAIR-HASTE 329
Fast spin echo (FSE) 26
FDG PET 355, 390, 395–411
　clinical use 396–400
　extratemporal lobe epilepsy 397–8
　in childhood 398–400
　temporal lobe epilepsy (TLE) 396–7
Febrile seizures 9
Ferrier, David 1–2
Fibrillary astrocytoma 152
Fibromeningeal cortical scarring 181
Field-of-view (FOV) 23
Fluid-attenuated inversion recovery (FLAIR) 112–14,
　223, 229
Flumazenil positron-emission tomography scanning of
　GABAUAL receptors 404–7
fMRI 2–3, 5, 7, 18, 26–7, 281–98
　biophysical basis 282–5
　combined with EEG see fMRI/EEG
　cortical activity 309
　data acquisition 284
　data analysis 285–6
　episodic memory in temporal lobe epilepsy (TLE) 293
　experimental design 285–6
　group average activation patterns 288
　image distortion 284
　language activation maps, tailoring resections 291
　language activation protocols 291
　language maps 290
　memory lateralization 292–3
　motor activation 286
　somatosensory activation 286–7
　spatial resolution 284
fMRI/EEG 299–314
　acquisition of EEG within MRI scanner 302
　activation/deactivation 308
　animal models 311
　application to epilepsy 306–13
　areas identified 301
　benign epilepsy with centrotemporal spikes 308
　clinical use 308
　focal epilepsy 311
　functional connectivity 312–13
　gradient-induced artifacts 303–4
　image analysis 305–6
　interleaved techniques 303–4
　magnetic field attractive force 301
　movement-induced artifacts 304
　MRI artifacts 302
　novel approaches to epilepsy imaging 312
　patient safety 301
　practical issues 301–4
　radiofrequency burning 301–2
　role in epilepsy investigations 300–1
　scale of movement induced artifacts 304–5
　simultaneous and continuous data 304–6

spike-triggered acquisition 303
technical considerations 300–1
FMZ binding 402
FMZ PET
　extratemporal lobe epilepsy 406–8
　idiopathic generalized epilepsy 407
　temporal lobe epilepsy (TLE) 404–5
Focal cortical dysplasia (FCD) 260, 262–5
　conditions associated with 243
　with balloon cells 186–7, 224–6
Focal cortical dysplasia (TCD), without balloon cells 243
Focal epilepsy
　fMRI/EEG 311
　model for 272–3
Focal seizures 12
Focal subcortical heterotopia 237–8
Focal transmantle dysplasia 187–8, 224
Foreign tissue legions 151–60
Fractional anisotropy (FA) 27
Frontal lobe epilepsy 177–88
　clinical and anatomic features 185–6
　clinical aspects 177–8
　pathology and magnetic resonance imaging (MRI) 180
　post-traumatic pathology 180–1
　topographic distribution 180
Frontal lobe malignant astrocytoma 184
Frontal lobe syndromes 178–9
Frontal meningioma 1
Frontal pole, anterior aspect 39
Frontopolar seizures 179
Fukuyama congenital muscular dystrophy (FCMD) 233–5
Functional abnormality 3–4
Functional connectivity, fMRI/EEG 312–13
Functional MRI see fMRI
Functional neuroanatomy, of declarative memory 273
Functional neuroimaging
　future directions 279
　goal of 281
　left temporal specialization 276
　physiology 281
Fungal infections 214–15

GABA 9, 224, 334
　and cortical excitability 361
　and epileptogenesis 360–1
　measurement of 342–3
GABA metabolism 357–63
　homocarnosine in 363–5
GABA-ergic inhibition 9
GABA–glutamate cycle 360
GABA–glutamine cycle 359
GABA receptor 392
GABA-trasaminase (GABA-T) 353
GABAUAu receptors, flumazenil PET tomography scanning 404–7
Gabapentin 357, 362–3, 366

Gamma-amino butyric acid *see* GABA

Ganglioglioma 157

Gelastic epilepsy 391

Gelastic seizures 204–6

Generalized spike and slow wave discharges (S&W) 310–11

Giant cell tumors 228

Glial lesions 153

Glucose, brain metabolism 395–400

Glutamate 334
    concentrations in epilepsy 355–7
    measurement of 340–2
    metabolism 351–2

Glutamate–glutamine cycle 352–7
    measurement of 353–5
        epileptic human hippocampus 355
        steady-state using 2-S13sC glucose 353–4
        using 2-S13sC acetate 354–5

Glutamate–glutamine cycle/TCA cycle ratio 352, 355

Glutamine, measurement of 340–2

Glutamine synthetase (GS) 351

GM–CSF surface 256

GM–WM boundary 260–1

Gowers, William 1, 7

Gradient-echo images 27

Gradient-echo sequences 26

Gradiometers 414–15

Grand mal 4

Gray matter (GM) 252
    density 260
    reduction 259
    segmentation 253–4

S1sH spectroscopy 334–43, 370–1
    high-concentration multiplets 335
    high-concentration singlets 334–5
    information content 334
    lipid suppression 337
    localization 337–9
    low-concentration multiplets 335–6
    spectroscopic imaging 339
    water suppression 336–7

Hamartoma 163–4, 204–6, 227, 391

Helminthic infections 215

Hemimegalencephaly 229–30, 399

Hemispheres 29
    see also Left hemisphere; Right hemisphere

Herpes simplex virus (HSV) 210

Heterotopia 235–9

Hippocampal anatomy 30

Hippocampal atrophy 103, 117

Hippocampal axis 51

Hippocampal body 30
    coronal section 66–7

Hippocampal boundaries 125

Hippocampal cell loss, anterior versus posterior 106

Hippocampal damage 147

Hippocampal dysplasia 135
    with collection of abnormal cells 137

Hippocampal head 30
    coronal section 58–65

Hippocampal internal structure 122

Hippocampal malformation 136

Hippocampal sclerosis (HS) 100, 103–4, 160
    absence of epilepsy 134
    acquired etiology 149
    and epileptic focus 108
    and memory function 134
    anterior temporal lobe signal and volume changes associated with 140–6
    as acquired, subsequently epileptogenic lesion 148–9
    as combination of several factors 149–50
    as developmental lesion 149
    bilateral 108–9
    classic features 121
    classical 116
    coronal image 117
    development 129–30
    dual pathology 140
    examples 114
    extrahippocampal pathology associated with 137–40
    genesis of 148
    in addition to another clearly identified lesion 147
    in normal population 107–8
    initial precipitating insults 148
    left-sided 120
    loss of normal internal structure 118
    magnetic resonance features 112, 124
    magnetic resonance imaging (MRI) 146–7
    magnetic resonance visualization 275
    mesial temporal lobe epilepsy with 150
    origins of 146
    outcome after temporal lobe resection 150
    pathologic correlates 133–4
    pathophysiology 129–35
    progression 130–1
    quantitative cell counts 107
    quantitative measurements 123–9
    severity grading 131–3
    subtypes 105–7
    T2-weighted image 123
    types 104, 146–7
    unilateral 139
    use of term 104
    variants 104
    visual diagnosis 112
    with incomplete MR features 134

Hippocampal shape analysis 255

Hippocampal signal hypointensity on T1-weighted images 115

Hippocampal signal increase without hippocampal atrophy 133

Hippocampal T2-signal increase
    and clinical findings 134
    with hippocampal volume deficit 133
Hippocampal T2-weighted signal 112–15
Hippocampal tail 30–1
    coronal section 68–73
Hippocampal volumetry 130
Hippocampus 29
    abnormal 135
    anterior–posterior borders 126
    axial section 74–85
    cellular glutamate in 357
    chronic changes in 130–1
    general relations with adjacent nervous
        structures 49
    glutamate–glutamine cycle measurement 355
    internal structure 120, 122
    intracellular glutamate in 356
    left 136
    loss of definition of internal architecture 117–21
    medial aspect 52–3
    morphology 135
    normal 110, 115–16, 121
    optimized imaging 123
    orientation 111
    parasagittal image 112
    pyramidal neurons 120
    relations with surrounding nervous structures 31
    relative anisotropy 124
    right 137
    sagittal section 86–97
    sectional anatomy 57
    segmentation 253
    shape analysis 254
    signal characteristics 135
    structure 30
    T1-weighted sequence 118–19
    transverse section 54
    volume distribution 126
    volumetrics 124–6
Homocarnosine 361
    in GABA metabolism 363–5
Horsley, Victor 1–2
Hydrocephalus 234
Hypomyelination 234
Hypoperfusion patterns 387
Hypothalamic hamartoma 204–6, 391

Ictal blood flow and metabolism 385
Ictal cerebral blood flow 387–8
Ictal diffusion imaging 323
Ictal fMRI 306–8
Ictal imaging technologies 2
Ictal MEG 421
Ictal perfusion magnetic resonance imaging 327–8

Ictal SPECT 139, 387, 389–90
    and surgical outcome 390
Idiopathic generalized epilepsy (IGE) 310–11
    FMZ PET 407
Image acquisition 249–51
Image pre-processing 252
Image processing
    future directions 263–5
    overview 251–2
Image selected in vivo spectroscopy (ISIS) 19
Incongruous memory 278–9
Infectious and postinfectious disorders 207–17
Inferior frontal gyrus seizures 178
Inflammatory conditions 207–17
In-plane spatial resolution 23
Interictal blood flow and metabolism 385
Interictal diffusion imaging 323–6
    extrahippocampal 324–6
    hippocampal 323–4
Interictal perfusion magnetic resonance imaging 328
Interictal SPECT 386
    clinical role 387
Intermediate dorsal lateral frontal seizures 179
Intermediate medial frontal region seizures 179
International Classification of Epilepsies, Epileptic Syndromes, and
    related Seizure Disorders 100
International League Against Epilepsy (ILAE) 5–6, 109
Intracellular GABA 361
Intracellular glutamate in hippocampus 356
Intracranial (IC) EEG–MEG studies 417
Intractable epilepsy 7, 200
Intractable neonatal and early infantile seizures 390
Intractable partial epilepsy 151
Intractable partial seizures 155
Intractable temporal lobe epilepsy (TLE) 142–3, 278
Intralimbic gyrus 29
Inversion recovery 26
Ischemic injury 197–201
Ischemic stroke 202
Isotropic diffusion 316

Jackson, John Hughlings 1–2, 8
Jacksonian seizures 1

Lactate, measurement of 342–3
Laminar heterotopia 239
Landau–Kleffner syndrome (LKS), MEG 422
Language activation protocols 287–8
Language lateralization 288
Language mapping, normative studies 288–9
Language outcome prediction 290–1
Language systems, preoperative mapping 287
LASER sequence 339
Lateral-memory patterns in left temporal lobe epilepsy 277–8

Lateral temporal lobe epilepsy (LTLE) 421
Left frontal lobe seizure focus 389
Left hemisphere
    lateral aspect 33
    medial aspect 45
    occipital pole 42
    superior aspect 34
Left hippocampal sclerosis 275–6
Left lateral temporal lobe epilepsy 277
Left mesial temporal lobe epilepsy 277
    neuropsychological features of 278
Left superior temporal gyrus, superior aspect 43
Left temporal lobe epilepsy
    lateral-memory patterns in 277–8
    mesial-memory patterns in 277–8
Left temporal specialization, functional neuroimaging in 276
Left-sided foci 279
Lennox–Gastaut syndrome 390, 399
Leptomeningeal vessels
    right hemisphere
        inferior view 48
        lateral view 46
        medial view 47
Levetiracetam 366
Ligand-gated channel genes 9
Ligand/neuroreceptor PET scanning 400–2
Limbic lobe 29
Lissencephaly 230–3
    classical 231–2
    incomplete 232
    secondary to *RELN* mutation 232–3
Lower mesencephalon, horizontal section 56

Macewen, William 1
Magnetic field, brain 414
Magnetic field gradients 21
Magnetic fields used in MR studies 21
Magnetic properties of atomic nuclei 18–19
Magnetic resonance diffusion imaging 315–19
Magnetic resonance imaging (MRI) 2, 249
    anterior temporal lobe (AT) abnormalities 141–3
    biological effects 19
    changes in morphology 117–22
    changes in tissue signal 112–17
    compared to X-rays 19
    contrast 24
    coronal 120
    detection of pathology 112
    development 3
    diffusion contrast 27
    energy used 19
    evolving and expanding role 299–300
    extra-temporal lobe epilepsy 177–96
    hippocampal sclerosis (HS) 146–9
    ideal imaging sequence 22, 250

imaging time 24
    mesial temporal sclerosis 110
    optimization 22
    parallel imaging 28
    physics of 18–19
    principles of 17–28
    problems of movement 24
    recommended use 109
    sequences 109
    special conditions 197–219
    techniques 22
    temporal lobe epilepsy (TLE) 99–176
    terminology 18
    types of examination 17–18
Magnetic resonance perfusion imaging 27, 319–22, 327–31
Magnetic resonance signal 19
Magnetic resonance spectroscopy (MRS) 3, 19, 333–83
    biochemistry 351–69
    clinical applications 370–8
    contralateral abnormalities 373
    future direction 377–8
    high-field 377–8
    nuclei for 377
    overview 333
    principles and techniques 334–50
    see also S13sC spectroscopy; S1sH spectroscopy; S31sP spectroscopy;
        Proton magnetic resonance spectroscopy
Magnetic resonance techniques 11–14
Magnetic source imaging (MSI) 413
Magnetoencephalogram, detection and measurement 414–15
Magnetoencephalography (MEG) 413–31
    accuracy in localization 417
    basics 414
    brain mapping 425
    clinical applications 413
    cortical reorganization 426–9
    focal slow-wave localization 422
    functional localization 425–9
    Landau–Kleffner syndrome (LKS) 422
    localization accuracy 416–17
    phantom studies 416
    postsurgical epilepsy localization 424–5
    realistic models 415
    secondary bilateral synchrony 422–4
    somatosensory mapping (SOM) 427–8
    source localization 415
    special localization issues 421–5
    spike colocalization 419–21
    temporal lobe epilepsy (TLE) 421–2
    use in clinical epilepsy 417–21
    validation 418
Magnetometers 414–15
Malignant paraganglioma 191
Mean transit time (MTT) 320
Medial temporal lobe memory systems, preoperative mapping 292–4
Median nerve somatosensory evoked field from central fissure 416–17

Memory, cognitive architecture 272–3
Memory function 272–3
  and hippocampal sclerosis (HS) 134
Memory patterns in right and bilateral temporal
    lobe epilepsy 277–8
Meningioangiomatosis 165
Mesencephalon 31
Mesial memory patterns in left temporal lobe epilepsy 277–8
Mesial temporal abnormality and nonepileptogenic
    secondary damage 135
Mesial temporal cyst 165
Mesial temporal lobe epilepsy (MTLE) 421
  with hippocampal sclerosis (HS) 150–1
Mesial temporal pathology 276–7
Mesial temporal sclerosis 103–9
  magnetic resonance imaging (MRI) 110
Metastatic disease 158
Microcephaly with simplified gyral pattern (MSG) 224–5
Miller–Dieker syndrome 231
Mixed glial lesions 153
Molecular genetics 8–9
Motor phenomena 101
Muscle–eye–brain disease 233, 235

N-acetyl aspartate (NAA)
  measurement of 339–40
  metabolism 366–9
N-methyl D-aspartate (NMDA) 9
NAA
  in central nervous system 367–8
  in temporal lobe epilepsy (TLE) 372–3
  ipsilateral to seizure focus 368–9
Neocortical glutamate 356
Neonatal intraparenchymal bleed, cystic cavity
    secondary to 199
Neoplasms 151–7, 181–4
Neurocysticercosis 215
Neuroimaging 2, 271
Neuronal circuits 9–10
Neuronal migration 221
Neuropsychological assessment 278
Neuropsychological features of left mesial temporal
    lobe epilepsy 278
Neuropsychological model building 271
Neuropsychology 271–80
  future directions 279
  overview 271–2
Neuroreceptors
  clinical role 392
  imaging 392
  PET 400
Neuro-transmitter systems, PET 400
Nonepileptogenic secondary damage, and mesial temporal
    abnormality 135
Nuclear magnetic resonance (NMR) 18

Occipital GABA 362
Occipital horn dilation 192
Occipital lobe 29
  cortical dysplasia 194
Occipital lobe epilepsy 189–90
Occipital pole
  left hemisphere 42
  right hemisphere 41
Occipitoparietal epilepsy 188–94
  clinical aspects 188–90
  congenital acquired and developmental lesions 192–3
  imaging findings 190–1
  pathology 190
  tumors 191–2
Occipitoparietal oligodendroglioma 191
Oligoastrocytoma, intractable partial complex seizures 157
Oligodendroglioma 153, 156
Orbital lobe 38
Orbitofrontal seizures 179

S31sP spectroscopy 343–8, 376
  and temporal lobe epilepsy (TLE) 376
  information content 343–4
  localization 344
  metabolite heterogeneity 346–7
  single-voxel localization: ISIS 344
  spectroscopic imaging 344–6
  voxel positioning 347–8
Pacemaker zone 11
Pachygyria 232
Parahippocampal epilepsy 138
Parahippocampal gyrus 29, 137
  abnormalities 135–7
Parasitic infections 215
Parenchymal cysts 229
Parietal lobe epilepsy 190
Partial epilepsy 151
  seizure focus in 109–10
Partial seizures 5, 156, 198, 201
  cerebral blood flow in 385
  incidence 7
  metabolism in 385
Penfield, Wilder 2, 4
Perfusion functional magnetic resonance imaging 282–4
Perfusion magnetic resonance imaging 27, 319–22, 327–31
Perinatal diseases 200
Perinatal injury 193
Perinatal ischemic stroke 199
Periventricular infarcts 200
Periventricular polymicrogyria 140
PET 5, 224, 271, 281, 300, 307, 319, 385, 395–411
  basic technique and principles 395–6
  brain glucose metabolism 395–400
  clinical applications 404–9
  data analysis 402–4

PET (*Continued*)

  neuro-receptors 400

  neuro-transmitter systems 400

  opiate and other receptor studies 408–9

  tracers and their clinical use in epilepsy 396

Petit mal 4

Phenytoin 357

Pilocystic astrocytoma 152, 155–6

Pleomorphic xanthoastrocytoma 152

Point-resolved spectroscopy (PRESS) 19, 338–9

Polymerase-chain-reaction (PCR) analysis 210

Polymicrogyria 232, 239–42

  imaging of 240–2

  syndromes associated with 240

Porencephalic cyst formation 192

Porencephaly 198–200

  following intraparenchymal hemorrhage 193

Positron-emission tomography *see* PET

Post-traumatic epilepsy 161

Post-traumatic lesions 160

Postictal cerebral blood flow 388

Postictal SPECT 387

Postnatal occlusive diseases 200

Posttraumatic epilepsy 182–3

Prenatal infarction 198

Prenatal injuries 197–8

Primary memory and its intersection with
    language 273–4

Proton density contrast 24

Proton magnetic resonance imaging 19

Proton magnetic resonance spectroscopy 20, 370–1

  abnormalities 375

  extratemporal lobe epilepsy 375

  temporal lobe epilepsy (TLE) 371–5

Proton observe carbon edit (POCE) 350

Pseudoseizures 391

Pulse sequences 21–2, 25–8

Pulsed arterial spin labeling (PASL) 321–2, 329

Quantitative extrahippocampal abnormality 134

Radiofrequency (RF) pulse 19, 21–2

Rapid acquisition with relaxation enhancement (RARE) 26

Rasmussen's encephalitis 166, 207–9

  clinical features 207–8

  EEG 208

  end-stage disease 212

  imaging studies 208–9

  neuropathologic aspects 208

Rasmussen's syndrome 391, 399–400

Reading epilepsy 308–10

Recursively applied multiple signal classification
    algorithm (RAP-MUSIC) 415

Regional cerebral blood flow (rCBF) 385

Relaxation times 24

RELN mutation 232–3

Ribbon heterotopia 239

Right frontal lobe, lateral aspect 40

Right hemisphere

  inferomedial aspect 36

  leptomeningeal vessels

    inferior view 48

    lateral view 46

    medial view 47

  medial aspect 35

  occipital pole 41

  superior aspect 34

Right hippocampal sclerosis 275

Right hippocampus, intraventricular aspect 50

Right insula, lateral aspect 44

Right-sided foci 279

Right temporal lobe epilepsy 277

Right temporal lobe seizure focus 388

Rolandic area, seizures from 178

Schizencephaly 242–3

Secondary damage from seizures 160–5

Secondary memory 274

  disorders in temporal lobe epilepsy 274–8

Seizure-associated damage, histopathologic
    evidence 160–2

Seizure-associated injury, magnetic resonance
    evidence 162–5

Seizure focus 2

  in partial epilepsy 109–10

Seizure-induced brain damage 10–11

Seizure surgery, origins of 1–2

Seizures 4–5

  incidence 7

  international classification 5

  mechanisms of spread 10

  secondary damage from 160–5

SENSE 28

Sensorimotor cortex, preoperative mapping 286–7

Shape analysis 254

Shielded rooms 414–15

Signal-to-noise ratio (SNR) 22–3, 321–2, 414–15

Simple partial seizures (SPS) 100

Single equivalent current dipole (ECD) model 413

Single-photon-emission computed tomography *see* SPECT

SISCOM 392–3

Slice thickness 24

SMASH 28

Smoldering encephalitis 391

Spatial localization 19

SPECT 2, 5, 205, 224, 300, 307, 319, 330, 385–94

  extratemporal lobe epilepsy 388–90

  image analysis 392–3

  interictal variability 386–7

optimal image presentation 386
preoperative localization 385–6
sensitivity 387
temporal lobe epilepsy (TLE) 386–7
Spin-echo sequence 25
Statistical parametric mapping (SPM) 392–3
Stimulated echo acquisition mode (STEAM) 338
Stroke
after seizures study (SASS) 202
incidence 202
location and seizures 202
Structural abnormality 3–4
Structural analysis 249–69
Sturge–Weber syndrome 202–4, 399
clinical features 202–3
forme fruste of 204
imaging findings 203
Subependymal hamartomas 227
Subependymal heterotopia 236–7
Subependymal linear heterotopia 239
Sudden unexpected death (SUDEP) 7
Sulci, shape analysis 254–6
Superconducting quantum interference device (SQUID) 414
Supernumerary lobe 29
Supplementary motor seizures 179

T1-relaxation time 24–5
T1-weighted images 240
hippocampal signal hypointensity on 115
T1-weighted inversion recovery sequence 123
T2-relaxation time 25, 127–9
T2-relaxometry 126–9, 130–5
Taenia solium 215
Temporal clustering analysis 312
Temporal horn 31
Temporal lobe 29, 31
development and functions 99–100
Temporal lobe epilepsy (TLE) 249, 252
classification 100
clinical features 99–103
clinical problem 100
definitions 100
disorders of secondary memory 274–8
EEG 101–2
epileptic seizures 100
epileptogenic processes 146–51
FDG PET 396–7
FMZ PET 404–5
intractable 142–3, 278
magnetic resonance imaging (MRI) 99–176
MEG 421–2
NAA in 372–3
other than hippocampus 135–7
pathologic abnormalities 160
pathologic findings 103–9

pathology correlations 143–6
phosphorus magnetic resonance spectroscopy 376
proton magnetic resonance spectroscopy 371–5
seizure semiology 100–1
SPECT 386–7
temporal origin or spread to temporal structures 102–3
visual analysis of images 123
visual assessment of contralateral and bilateral
abnormality 123
Temporal lobe fibrodysplasia 164
Temporal lobe hyperperfusion 387
Temporal lobe resection 150
Temporal lobe trauma 162
Temporal lobectomy, actuarial analysis 151
Texture analysis 260–3
Tissue classification 252–4
Tissue segmentation 252–4
Topiramate 362–3, 366
Toxoplasmosis 215
Transmantle dysplasia 225–6
Transmitter systems 9
Tricarboxylic acid (TCA) cycle 351–2
Tryptophan metabolism, AMT PET 407
Tuberculoma 215
Tuberculosis 213–14
Tuberous sclerosis 226–9
diagnostic criteria 227
forme fruste 225
neuroimaging 227–9
Tumors, occipitoparietal epilepsy 191–2
Turbo spin echo (TSE) 26

Ulegyria 192, 200–1
Unilateral amytal hemispheric anesthesia 391
Unilateral megalencephaly 229–30
Unilateral open-lip schizencephaly 243
Upper mesencephalon, horizontal section 55

Valproate 357
Vascular injury 197–201
Vascular lesions 184
Vascular malformations 158–60, 193
Verbal-specific memory impairments and left hippocampal
sclerosis 275–6
Vigabatrin 357, 362–4, 366
Viral infections 209–11
Visuospatial-specific impairments and right hippocampal
sclerosis 275
Volumetric data acquisition 249–51
Voxel-based morphometry (VBM) 258–60

Wada–fMRI language lateralization comparisons 289–90
Wada test 287, 391

Walker–Warburg syndrome 233–4
White matter (WM) 252
  density 260
  reduction 259
  segmentation 253–4
WM–GM surface 256

X-linked lissencephaly 231
  with agenesis of the corpus callosum and ambiguous
    genitalia 233
Xanthoastrocytomas 152
X-rays, compared to magnetic resonance 19

Z-shimming techniques 284
Zero filling 23
Zonisamide 362